ANESTHESIA AND PERIOPERATIVE COMPLICATIONS

ANESTHESIA AND PERIOPERATIVE COMPLICATIONS

Edited by

JONATHAN L. BENUMOF, M.D.
Professor of Anesthesiology
University of California, San Diego
School of Medicine
La Jolla, California

LAWRENCE J. SAIDMAN, M.D.
Professor of Anesthesiology
University of California, San Diego
School of Medicine
La Jolla, California

with **49** *contributors*
with **188** *illustrations*

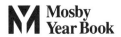
Mosby
Year Book

St. Louis Baltimore Boston Chicago London Philadelphia Sydney Toronto

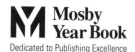

Mosby Year Book
Dedicated to Publishing Excellence

Editor: *Susan Gay*
Senior Developmental Editor: *Kathryn H. Falk*
Project Manager: *Mark Spann*
Production Editor: *Carl Masthay*
Book design: *Jeanne Wolfgeher*

q
RD82.5
.A54
1991

Printed in the United States of America

Mosby–Year Book, Inc.
11830 Westline Industrial Drive
St. Louis, Missouri 63146

Library of Congress Cataloging-in-Publication Data

Anesthesia and perioperative complications / edited by Jonathan L.
  Benumof, Lawrence J. Saidman ; with 49 contributors.—1st ed.
      p.   cm.
    Includes index.
    ISBN 0-8016-0586-5
    1. Anesthesia—Complications and sequelae. 2. Anesthetics—Side
effects. I. Benumof, Jonathan,   . II. Saidman, Lawrence
J.,   .
    [DNLM: 1. Anesthesia—adverse effects. 2. Intraoperative Care—
-adverse effects. 3. Intraoperative Complications—etiology.
4. Intraoperative Complications—prevention & control. WO 245
A5783]
    RD82.5.A54 1991
    617.9′6041—dc20
    DNLM/DLC
    for Library of Congress   91-18509
                                                                  CIP

C/MY 9 8 7 6 5 4 3

Contributors

Stephen E. Abram, M.D.
Professor and Vice-Chairman
Department of Anesthesiology
Medical College of Wisconsin
Milwaukee, Wisconsin

Jonathan M. Anagnostou, M.D.
Assistant Professor of Anesthesia
Department of Anesthesia
Indiana University School of Medicine
Indianapolis, Indiana

Cedric R. Bainton, M.D.
Professor of Anesthesia
Unviersity of California, San Francisco
School of Medicine;
Chief of Anesthesia
San Francisco General Hospital
San Francisco, California

Frederic A. Berry, M.D.
Professor of Anesthesiology and Pediatrics
University of Virginia Health Sciences Center,
Charlottesville, Virginia

Janice M. Bitetti, M.D.
formerly Assistant Professor of Anesthesiology
and Medicine
George Washington University Hospital
Washington, D.C.

Jay B. Brodsky, M.D.
Professor (Clinical) of Anesthesiology
Stanford University School of Medicine
Stanford, California

Robert A. Caplan, M.D.
Associate Clinical Professor of Anesthesiology
University of Washington School of Medicine;
Staff Anesthesiologist
Virginia Mason Medical Center
Seattle, Washington

H.S. Chadwick, M.D.
Associate Professor of Anesthesiology
Director of Obstetric Anesthesiology
University of Washington School of Medicine
Seattle, Washington

Frederick W. Cheney, M.D.
Professor of Anesthesiology

University of Washington School of Medicine
Seattle, Washington

Bart Chernow, M.D., F.A.C.P., F.C.C.P.
Physician-in-Chief, Sinai Hospital of Baltimore;
Professor of Medicine, Anesthesia, and Critical Care
Johns Hopkins University School of Medicine
Baltimore, Maryland

Albert T. Cheung, M.D.
Lecturer in Anesthesia, Department of Anesthesia
University of Pennsylvania
Philadelphia, Pennsylvania

Gregory Crosby, M.D.
Assistant Professor of Anesthesia
Harvard Medical School;
Assistant Anesthetist and Director of Neuroanesthesia
Department of Anesthesia
Massachusetts General Hospital
Boston, Massachusetts

John H. Eichhorn, M.D.
Professor and Chairman
Department of Anesthesiology
The University of Mississippi Medical Center
Jackson, Mississippi

James B. Eisenkraft, M.D.
Professor of Anesthesiology
Mount Sinai School of Medicine of the City University
of New York
New York, New York

Norig Ellison, M.D.
Professor of Anesthesia
University of Pennsylvania School of Medicine
Philadelphia, Pennsylvania

John Peder Erickson, M.D.
Assistant Professor of Anesthesia and Critical Care
and Pediatrics
University of Chicago
Division of Biological Sciences
Pritzker School of Medicine
Chicago, Illinois

Ronald J. Faust, M.D.
Associate Professor of Anesthesiology
Mayo Medical School
Rochester, Minnesota

v

Thomas J. Gal, M.D.
Professor of Anesthesiology
University of Virginia Health Sciences Center
Charlottesville, Virginia

Simon Gelman, M.D., Ph.D
Professor and Chairman,
Department of Anesthesiology
Professor of Physiology and Biophysics
University of Alabama Hospitals
Birmingham, Alabama

William W. Hesson, J.D.
Senior Assistant Director and Legal Council
University of Iowa Hospitals and Clinics
Iowa City, Iowa

Quinn H. Hogan, M.D.
Assistant Professor
Department of Anesthesiology
Medical College of Wisconsin
Milwaukee, Wisconsin

Jan Charles Horrow, M.D.
Associate Professor
Department of Anesthesiology
Director, Cardiac Anesthesia
Hahnemann University
Philadelphia, Pennsylvania

Joel A. Kaplan, M.D.
Horace W. Goldsmith Professor and Chairman
Department of Anesthesiology
Mount Sinai School of Medicine
New York, New York

Charles J. Kopriva, M.D.
Professor of Anesthesiology
Director of Cardiac Anesthesia
Yale University School of Medicine
Yale–New Haven Hospital
New Haven, Connecticut

Philip K. Kraker, D.O.
Assistant Professor of Anesthesiology
Yale University School of Medicine
Yale–New Haven Hospital
New Haven, Connecticut

Jerrold H. Levy, M.D.
Associate Professor of Anesthesiology
Emory University School of Medicine;
Division of Cardiothoracic Anesthesia
and Critical Care
Emory Clinic
Atlanta, Georgia

Anne C.P. Lui, M.D., F.R.C.P.C.
Active Attending Staff Anaesthetist
and Clinical Lecturer
University of Ottawa
Ottawa, Ontario, Canada

Mervyn Maze, M.D., Ch.B.
Associate Professor
Stanford University School of Medicine
Stanford, California

Anthony M. Mills, M.D.
Assistant Professor
Department of Anesthesiology
Columbia University College of Physicians and Surgeons
New York, New York

Terence M. Murphy, M.B., Ch.B., F.F.A.R.C.S.
Professor of Anesthesiology
University of Washington School of Medicine
Seattle, Washington

Nancy A. Nussmeier, M.D.
Assistant Professor
Department of Anesthesiology
University of Washington School of Medicine
Seattle, Washington

Declan O'Keeffe, M.B., Ch.B., F.F.A.R.C.S
Assistant Professor
Department of Anesthesiology
University of Washington School of Medicine
Seattle, Washington

Nathan Leon Pace, M.D.
Professor of Anesthesiology
Adjunct Professor of Bioengineering
University of Utah
Salt Lake City, Utah

James D. Pearson, M.D.
Assistant Professor of Anesthesiology
University of Alabama Hospitals
Birmingham, Alabama

Donald S. Prough, M.D.
Professor of Anesthesia and Neurology
Head, Section on Critical Care
Bowman Gray School of Medicine
Wake Forest University
Winston-Salem, North Carolina

David L. Reich, M.D.
Assistant Professor of Anesthesiology and Director
of Cardiothoracic Anesthesiology
Mount Sinai Medical Center
New York, New York

Michael F. Roizen, M.D.
Professor and Chairman
Department of Anesthesia and Critical Care
Professor of Medicine
University of Chicago
Division of Biological Sciences
Pritzker School of Medicine
Chicago, Illinois

Henry Rosenberg, M.D.
Professor and Chairman
Department of Anesthesiology
Hahnemann University
Philadelphia, Pennsylvania

Brian K. Ross, Ph.D., M.D.
Assistant Professor of Anesthesiology
University of Washington School of Medicine
Seattle, Washington

Roger L. Royster, M.D.
Associate Professor of Anesthesia
Associate in Cardiology
The Bowman Gray School of Medicine
Wake Forest University
Winston-Salem, North Carolina

Richard M. Sommer, M.D.
Assistant Professor of Anesthesiology
New York University School of Medicine;
Chief of Anesthesiology
Department of Veterans Affairs Medical Center
New York, New York

Robert K. Stoelting, M.D.
Professor and Chairman
Department of Anesthesia
Indiana University School of Medicine
Indianapolis, Indiana

Gale E. Thompson, M.D.
Chief of Anesthesiology
The Mason Clinic
Seattle, Washington

John H. Tinker, M.D.
Professor and Head
Department of Anesthesia
University of Iowa College of Medicine
Iowa City, Iowa

Terry S. Vitez, M.D.
Medical Group Resident
Premier Anesthesia
Atlanta, Georgia

John D. Wasnick, M.D.
Assistant Professor of Anesthesiology
Cornell University Medical College;
Director, Post-Anesthesia Care Unit
The New York Hospital
New York, New York

Herbert D. Weintraub, M.A., B.M., B.Ch.
(Oxon)
Professor of Anesthesiology
George Washington University Hospital
Washington, D.C.

Michael E. Weiss, M.D.
Clinical Assistant Professor of Medicine
Division of Allergy
University of Washington School of Medicine
Seattle, Washington

Gary Zaloga, M.D.
Professor of Anesthesia (Critical Care) and Medicine
Bowman Gray School of Medicine
Wake Forest University
Winston-Salem, North Carolina

To our colleagues whose professional lives have been
or will be touched by an anesthetic-related complication.

JONATHAN L. BENUMOF

LAWRENCE J. SAIDMAN

Preface

Anesthesia care providers expend much effort in preventing complications caused by anesthesia. When a complication or an unexpected outcome does occur, the anesthesia care provider will immediately want to know as much about the complication as possible: How often does it occur? Did I cause it? What are other possible causes? How should the complication be managed? What are the medicolegal and socioeconomic consequences of the complication?

During the past decade the anesthesia community has expressed a great interest in and concern about standards of anesthesia care and perioperative complications. This interest is reflected by the creation of the Anesthesia Patient Safety Foundation, the publication by the American Society of Anesthesiologists of standards related to anesthesia care and by the Food and Drug Administration of standards related to use of anesthesia machines, the advent of quality assurance programs, and the continued and perhaps just beginning to be successful battle against the inexorable increase in malpractice insurance rates. For all the above reasons, we felt that a textbook that covers the complete breadth and depth of anesthesia and perioperative complications is very much needed.

The book is organized according to the way we believe anesthesia care providers approach complications caused by anesthesia. The first approach (Part One) addresses the question, Did I cause the complication? by discussing complications attributable to specific anesthetic events (such as attempted internal jugular vein catheterization causing tension pneumothorax). However, many important complications cannot be characterized or understood by such a simple cause-and-effect relationship. Therefore the second approach (Part Two) examines all causes of a complication to or failure in an important system (most commonly a major organ). Of course, some overlap is an inherent byproduct of this organization, but we have, where possible, tried to minimize redundancy and maximize the transmitted information. Part Three of the book discusses the important medicolegal and socioeconomic ramifications of complications such as risk, epidemiology, costs, quality assurance, and malpractice suits; it is essential that complications be properly set in the larger context of these contemporary societal issues.

Our thanks to an outstanding group of authors both for sharing their expertise and for their attention to our timetable, to Susan M. Gay and Kathryn H. Falk, our editors from Mosby who supported our proposal, and to Pamela Smiley, who provided us with expert secretarial assistance.

JONATHAN L. BENUMOF

LAWRENCE J. SAIDMAN

Contents

PART THREE

Medicolegal Considerations

PART ONE

Complications From Specific Anesthetic Events

Management of the Airway

Cedric R. Bainton

Closed claims analysis[1] reveals that adverse outcomes associated with respiratory events constitute the single largest injury to patients. Three mechanisms—failure to ventilate (38%), failure to recognize esophageal intubation (18%), and difficult or failed intubation (17%)—accounted for 75% of the adverse events. Death or brain damage occurred in 85% of these cases. In most cases these were errors of omission, that is, failure to recognize the magnitude of a problem, failure to make appropriate observations, or failure to act in a timely manner.

Other injuries are those of commission with a spectrum from trivial to life threatening. Injury to the lips and to the nasal, oral, pharyngeal, laryngeal, and tracheal passages is an unavoidable fact of anesthetic practice. As we force entry into the pharynx for a view of the glottis or blindly probe to find this structure, we introduce sharply pointed metal and hard plastic objects to achieve our goal. For the most part we are successful and do not violate the delicate mucosal surfaces of these structures as long as we obey the rules to be gentle; never force; lift, do not pry; be conservative; opt if possible for a direct view; and avoid forceful, blind probing.

To minimize injury we must examine the airway carefully, identify the hurdles that must be overcome, devise a plan with minimal risk for injury, have practiced our skills ahead of time, and have sufficient time to follow out our plan. If time is short, some of these cautions may be pushed aside. For example, in the "no-ventilate, difficult-to-intubate" situation, to lose a tooth in the process of intubation is insignificant when survival is in the balance. In all situations, common sense should prevail. Quality assurance bodies assume that when injury occurs a mistake has been made. The suggestion of guilt for each injury implies that full knowledge is possible. Instead, medical knowledge is incomplete and continues to evolve. Complications are to be evaluated for the new insights and revelations they bring and not simply the rules we may have trespassed. Mistakes can be both logical and technical and can happen at any point in our management, knowledge base, problem evaluation, conception of a plan, execution of the plan, thinking on our feet, and evaluation of what went wrong. Problems also come in the use of new devices and techniques. We must explore these new possibilities but accept the fact that as we gain experience we will discover defects and difficulties we could not possibly have anticipated. This chapter is a review of the long list of potential pitfalls we can fall into in management of the airway, with the hope that the collective experience of our colleagues can reduce the need for each of us, individually, to experience all problems before our education is complete.

I. USE OF THE MASK

As innocuous as it may seem the anesthetic mask itself can be the source of several complications as the act of mask ventilation can.

A. Chemical burns

If a reusable mask is employed, it should be checked for any pinhole defects in the air-filled bladder before it is applied to the patient. If air or fluid is expressed when pressure is applied to the air bladder, the mask must be discarded. Durkan and Fleming[2] report how sterilizing solutions found access to the air bladder of such a mask in the process of cleaning. During anesthetic induction the solution leaked onto the patient's face causing burning and irritation of the patient's eye. Parenthetically, cold sterilizing solutions must be thoroughly washed from all surfaces of any reusable item. For example Grigsby et al.[3] incriminate residual gluteraldehyde on an improperly rinsed laryngoscope blade as the cause of life-threatening allergic glossitis. As a more subtle example, it is easy to forget that the suction channel of a fiberoptic laryngobronchoscope (fiberscope) may be a source of caustic gluteraldehyde. The channel must be thoroughly rinsed through with water after the cold sterilizing process or gluteraldehyde will drip on the larynx and trachea during laryngoscopy, and burns will result. Similarly the strict rules for ethylene oxide shelf time must be adhered to so that ethylene oxide does not have contact with mucosal surfaces of the patient.

B. Difficulties with mask fit and maintenance of airway

During anesthetic induction the mask is gently placed on the face for preoxygenation. It is important to notice whether the complaint air-filled portion of the mask is properly inflated such that the rigid parts of the mask do not make contact with the bridge of the nose or mandible. Otherwise bruising will occur at these contact points as pressure is more firmly applied. As induction proceeds, firmer mask pressure will be necessary to provide positive airway pressure to distend pharyngeal structures, maintain pharyngeal air space, and provide ventilation. It will be necessary to apply pressure with fingers to the angle of the mandible to maintain a tight mask fit. It is important not to depress the soft submandibular tissues, particularly in the child, or airway obstruction can occur. As greater pressure is applied to the mandible, it may be hard to avoid the mandibular branch of the facial nerve as it crosses over the mandible. Glauber[4] describes how he managed to injure this nerve in a physician colleague who he hoped to avoid intubating for risk of a sore throat. Instead the physician had facial nerve paresis for 3 weeks. Azar and Lear[5] report numbness of the lower lip in two patients. They attribute the injury to excessive pressure exerted by the rim of the mask on the mental nerves where they emerge from the mental foramina in the mandible. Positive airway pressure does not always distend and lift pharyngeal structures. Andersen et al.[6] describe how a large lax epiglottis was pushed caudally to impinge in the glottic opening and cause airway obstruction with continuous positive pressure breathing. As induction proceeds, the tongue may fall to the back of the pharynx and obstruct the airway. Oral airways need to be inserted gently to avoid scratching the mucosal surfaces, breaking teeth, or forcing the epiglottis into the glottic opening. Equal care should be given to insertion of a nasal airway to avoid a troublesome nosebleed. At some point it may be necessary to apply firm lifting pressure on the angle of the mandible and even subluxate the temporomandibular joint. Patients may later complain of bruising and pain over these points, and some may have persistent dislocation of the jaw. With airway obstruction, positive pressure may force air quite easily into the stomach instead of the trachea. The stomach may distend making the patient more prone to regurgitation with increased risk for aspiration. Cricoid pressure can help reduce the possibility of gastric ventilation during this difficult time. Edentulous patients are difficult to mask ventilate. Other patients who are difficult to ventilate by mask are those with full beards, large tongues, heavy jaw muscles (which resist subluxation of the mandible), poor atlanto-occipital extension, uncertain pharyngeal pathosis, and burns to the face or facial deformities. In such cases it may be best to avoid mask ventilation and opt instead for direct laryngoscopy, if judged to be easy, or awake fiberoptic laryngoscopy.

C. Prolonged mask use

When a mask is used for a prolonged period, it is important to examine pressure points frequently to make sure the blood supply is not being compromised. The bridge of the nose and skin over the mandible are most vulnerable. These areas can be massaged and the mask replaced, or it may be necessary to abandon mask ventilation if there is concern. Mask ventilation does not isolate the trachea; thus the patient is at risk for aspiration from silent regurgitation. The anesthetist must be alert to any sign of unexpected coughing or airway noise. Transparent masks are superior to opaque in that they permit a good view of the lips while the mask is in place and permit more prompt recognition of vomitus. Corneal abrasion is a real possibility. It is important to keep the eyelids closed and avoid undo mask pressure, particularly where there is an open globe injury. Patients with basilar skull fractures are at risk for pneumocephalus[7,8] with continuous-pressure mask ventilation. Rarely otorrhagia can occur.[9]

II. NASOTRACHEAL INTUBATION
A. Cranial intubations

Nasotracheal intubation can be hazardous. The classic picture of a nasogastric tube sitting inside the cranium passing through a basilar skull fracture[10] is now accompanied by the even more frightening picture of an endotracheal tube sitting in that same location.[11] Patients with major facial trauma and basilar skull fractures are not candidates for this approach.

B. Nasal injury and foreign bodies

All too common and particularly troublesome are nosebleeds. It is so much easier to prevent than to treat one. Thus every consideration must be made for prevention. One can minimize nosebleeds by using a small endotracheal (ET) tube, constricting the nasal mucosa, inserting a soft stint over which the tube can slide, and never using extreme force. An adult male can actually breathe adequately through a 5.0 mm tube; thus *think small!* A vasoconstrictor must be applied to the nasal mucosa. A dose of 0.5% neosynephrine in 4% lidocaine works well, just as 4% cocaine does. One approach is to dilate the nasal passage with nasal airways of progressively increasing size before ET tube insertion. I prefer to gently pass a well-lubricated pediatric esophageal stethoscope through the nose to establish that a channel exists and to gain entrance to the pharynx. The ET tube can then be passed over this stethoscope as a stint. This method prevents the sharp tip of the ET tube from cutting into the nasal and pharyngeal mucosa to cause bleeding or even a false submucosal passage. Such rents can progress to a retropharyngeal abscess.[12] It also protects the turbinates,[13,14] adenoids, and tonsils from partial excision and minimizes the chance to penetrate a pointing abscess. The esophageal stethoscope can then be removed and the tube suctioned for any blood, saliva, or debris. A similar technique can be used to insert a "split" tube when nasogastric (NG) tube placement is troublesome and a rigid split channel is necessary to guide the NG tube into the esophagus. If a nose bleed does occur, it is important to leave the ET tube in place in an attempt to tampon the bleed. The cuff of the ET tube can be inflated and the ET tube retracted to impact into the nasopharynx until bleeding stops. Foreign bodies in the nares are legion. Smith et al.[15] describe a rhinolith formed around a rubber tire of a toy car that was dislodged during nasal intubation 30 years later. The rhinolith had caused no symptoms. Once the trachea is intubated it is important to position the ET tube centrally as it enters the naris. Distortion of the naris can lead to ischemia and necrosis and nasal adhesion. Postintubation sequelae can occur. Sherry and Murday[16] describe an obstructing adhesion extending from the septum to the inferior turbinate occurring 4 months after nasal intubation. Although paranasal sinusitis tends to occur some days after nasal intubation,[17,18] nasal septal abscess and retropharyngeal abscess can occur after short-term intubation.[12].

III. OROTRACHEAL INTUBATION
A. Anatomic requirements

There are four anatomic requirements for successful oral laryngoscopy. If any of these is lacking, oral laryngoscopy will be difficult to impossible. Unless these requirements are thought through carefully the anesthetist may choose an approach that will increase the chance for injury and complications or leave the anesthetist in the difficult position of "failed intubation." These requirements are adequate oral entry, sufficient pharyngeal space, compliant submandibular tissue, and adequate atlanto-occipital extension.

Oral entry may be limited by facial scars, temporomandibular joint disease, a large tongue, and, most important, dental disease. Blind nasal or fiberoptic techniques can obviate these problems.

The pharyngeal space can be restricted by tumors, infection, and edema or disrupted by trauma or surgery. Whenever the anatomy is distorted, it is important to create the best possible view. There is great merit in intubation while the patient is awake, since wakefulness imparts greater pharyngeal space. A tubular blade[19] may be necessary. It is imperative to identify structures properly. If an ET tube is unwittingly passed through rents in the mucosa of the pharynx, the results can be disastrous.

Compliance of submandibular tissue is essential in direct laryngoscopy if the tongue is to be displaced from the pharynx to view the glottis. Compliance is decreased by scarring, after radiation, and with submandibular infection. Direct laryngoscopy will be very difficult in such circumstances, increasing the risk for injury if one persists. It is prudent to start with blind nasal or fiberoptic techniques since they are safer, quicker, and less injury prone in this circumstance.

Atlanto-occipital (AO) extension is essential to lift the epiglottis off the posterior wall of the pharynx during direct laryngoscopy. If the epiglottis cannot be elevated, glottic structures will not be seen. The fused, fixed, or unstable spine will thus be a problem. Blind nasal or fiberoptic techniques should be utilized to minimize injury.

B. Dental injury

Dental injury from the administration of general anesthesia is one of the most common anesthesia-related malpractice claims.[20] Injury is variously reported to range from 1:150 to 1:1000.[21] In New Zealand damage to teeth is viewed as an accepted risk of general anesthesia and not therefore compensatable.[22] Thus anesthesiologists may be liable for these expensive repairs. Teeth are dislodged because of poor bony support structure. Children's primary dentition is poorly supported. Children should be asked to identify teeth that are mobile and be notified that it would be to their advantage to have these removed before or at the time of general anesthesia. When orthodontic braces are removed, the teeth are quite mobile with poor structural support for many months. Periodontal disease destroys structural support for teeth. Minimal pressures applied to these teeth can extract them. If extraction occurs, the tooth should be retrieved and saved in moist gauze

without cleansing. The oral surgeon or dentist should be notified. Some teeth, reimplanted and braced, will survive. Carious teeth, capped teeth, and bridges are fragile and easily broken if not removed. Thus teeth can be injured easily in what might otherwise be considered easy intubation circumstances. If other anatomic difficulties for intubation are present, the risk for dental injury greatly increases. The prudent choice, where risk is high and time permits, is to do an awake blind nasal or fiberoptic intubation to avoid this hazard.

It is extremely important to make a careful dental examination before intubation. All diseased, loose, chipped, and capped teeth are identified, a note is made on the chart, and the patient is advised as to the risk of damage. Teeth protectors can be used but may be awkward and can obstruct vision.[23]

C. Cervical problems

If the neck is fused because of ankylosing spondylitis, attempts at direct laryngoscopy have limited chance for success and may create cervical fractures and quadriplegia.[24] The head fixed in a halo brace attached to a rigid jacket does not permit atlanto-occipital extension and has limited chance to succeed at direct laryngoscopy. These problems lend themselves to blind nasal or fiberoptic intubation as the greatest chance for success. The unstable neck because of acute cervical fracture can be supported by axial traction if intubation must proceed promptly. Special concern should be noted for C1 and C2 injuries where any degree of extension might be disastrous for spinal cord survival. If time permits, blind nasal and fiberoptic techniques are preferable. Down's syndrome and other congenital anomalies are associated with atlantoaxial subluxation.[25] Williams et al.[26] describe a child with Down's syndrome who complained of severe neck pain on attempted motion 1 month after anesthesia. The child had rotary subluxation of the atlantoaxial joint but no other neurologic symptoms. The child was successfully treated with C1-C2 fusion. In these patients a test of full range of motion and degree of atlanto-occipital extension should be established while the patient is awake. If any question exists, neurosurgeons should be consulted. Again, blind nasal fiberoptic techniques should be utilized to minimize potential injury.

Dong[27] points up the hazard of intubation in undiagnosed Arnold-Chiari malformations. Cerebellar tonsil herniation occurred during intubation for tonsillectomy. One week after intubation the child presented with acquired torticollis, clonus, and hyperactive deep tendon reflexes.

Surgical correction was successful, and symptoms resolved.

D. Intubation in the presence of preexisting laryngotracheal trauma

If injury is suspected in larynx or trachea, it is imperative that the lesion be visualized directly or with a fiberscope. The fiber can be passed distal to the lesion, and the ET tube can be passed over the fiber as a stint without further injury. If this approach is not used, the results can be disastrous (for example, passing the ET tube through a disruption into the mediastinum). If time does not permit fiber use, the smallest possible tube must be passed gently through the glottic opening. If the tube meets any resistance, the tube must be removed and a tracheostomy performed.

E. Corneal abrasion

Corneal abrasion is possible during the act of intubation. Loosely fitting watch bands, identification tags, and jewelry can scrape the cornea.[28] The ubiquitous stethoscope slung around the neck can fall forward to strike the forehead and come very close to the eyes.

F. Vocal cord paralysis

Several authors[29-32] report vocal cord paralysis after intubation with no other obvious cause for paralysis. Cavo[30] and Brandwein et al.[29] believe that the likely site of injury is pressure of the cuff on the recurrent laryngeal nerve close to or slightly caudad to the vocal process of the arytenoid. Inflating the cuff below this area would seem an obvious solution. The paralysis is usually temporary.

Mayhew et al.[33] remind us that vocal cord paralysis can have a central origin as well and report paralysis of the left vocal cord in an infant with a Dandy-Walker cyst after insertion of a cyst-to-peritoneum shunt.

G. Other nerve injuries

Teichner[34] reports a compression injury to the lingual nerve during a difficult intubation with loss of tongue sensation for 1 month. Aucott et al.[35] identify two patients who presented with signs of aspiration attributable to supraglottic anesthesia. The authors postulate that the internal branch of the superior laryngeal nerve was damaged during difficult intubation.

H. Macroglossia

Macroglossia developed 20 minutes after extubation in a 16-month-old child after craniotomy in the sitting position.[36] The case was long, 5 hours, and the head was in an extreme flexed position. There was no oral airway or bite block present. The cause is not clear. Teeple et al.[37] describe a similar problem in a 56-year-old woman, despite following the suggestions to avoid oral airway, bite block, soft-tissue compression of the chin, and extreme flexion of the head. They suggest that the endotracheal tube may have severely compressed circulation to the right side of the tongue. They recommend hourly checks of tongue intraoperatively to identify the problem. Macroglossia was accompanied by pronounced swelling of the head and neck in a procedure with the head in severe flexion. The authors[38] suggest that major venous compression was the cause. These three cases point to the hazards of severe neck flexion over a long period of surgery. Pressure from the ET tube on the tongue may play a role though a cause is not clear at this time.

Patane and White[39] point to the insidious development of macroglossia after prolonged cleft-palate repair. They caution careful postoperative observation where the tongue is severely retracted and the procedure lasts more than 3 hours. Although anesthetic maneuvers may have played no role in producing these cases of macroglossia, the postoperative sequelae of life-threatening airway obstruction are very much our concern.

I. Aspiration

Aspiration of gastric contents is a constant concern when one is intubating the trachea of a patient with a full stomach. The use of cricoid pressure has taken a great deal of worry out of the "crash induction." Cricoid pressure is effective even in the presence of a nasogastric tube.[40] It is imperative to make a careful assessment of "ease of intubation" when considering a crash intubation because it is very troublesome to be caught unable to intubate after giving paralyzing drugs. Clearly any patient with limited oral entry, restricted pharyngeal space, diminished submandibular tissue compliance, and limited AO extension will be poor candidates for a "crash" induction. If ease of intubation is uncertain, it is advisable to secure additional information while the patient is awake. Using oral analgesia, one can perform limited pharyngoscopy to determine if there will be adequate pharyngeal space. If uncertainty persists, awake blind or fiberoptic techniques should be used.

Harris et al.[41] report an unusual case with the potential for aspiration. The patient had percutaneous lithotripsy for intrahepatic cholelithiasis. At the conclusion of the procedure, 7 liters of 0.9% saline solution were infused into the common duct for irrigation. Saline refluxed through an "incompetent" pyloric sphincter. During emergence, the patient vomited 1 liter of thin watery gastric contents to the surprise of anesthetists. Vomiting was repeated in the recovery room.

J. Esophageal intubation

Esophageal intubation must be recognized promptly. A direct view of the endotracheal tube passing through the glottic opening is very reassuring but not always achieved. It is important to see that the arytenoids are inferior to the endotracheal tube. Ford[42] describes how posterior displacement of the tube toward the palate assists in providing this view. End-tidal P_{CO_2} values confirm proper intratracheal tube placement. The sharp upslope and downslope of a breath-by-breath P_{CO_2} tracing marching across the oscilloscope ends all doubt. All other signs, such as good breath sounds, axillary breath sounds, and absence of gastric breath sounds, can be misleading. Esophageal intubation can briefly produce an end-tidal P_{CO_2}[43] tracing, but the concentration decreases rapidly and disappears within 5 breaths. However, tracheal intubation is not invariably confirmed by capnography if there is profound bronchospasm[44] or no P_{CO_2} delivery to the lung because of absent cardiac output.

K. Lesions of the larynx

Kambic and Radsel[45] examined 1000 patients for laryngeal lesions after intubation; 6.2% had severe lesions, and 4.5% had hematoma of the vocal cord. Hematoma of the supraglottic region and laceration of the vocal cord mucosa were approximately 1% each. They suggest that since intubation almost always has some degree of trauma the anesthetists should examine the larynx before and after intubation so that lesions can be recognized and proper therapy implemented.

Peppard and Dickens[46] found a small but significant number of patients with laryngeal injury after short-term intubation. Recovery was generally prompt.

Arytenoid displacement is a rare event. Frink and Pattison[47] report a case that followed a traumatic endotracheal intubation. They suggest the natural curve of the ET tube from mouth to larynx places a force against the arytenoid sufficient to cause dislocation. In other cases it is likely that the forceful technique necessary in a difficult intubation is the cause.[48] Debo et al. report arytenoid subluxation after blind intubation with a lighted wand.[49]

Repeated intubations may result in laryngeal

trauma. Wackym et al.[50] report recrudescence of herpes zoster of the larynx under such circumstances.

The vocal process of the arytenoid is the most likely site of damage from the ET tube as it sits between the cords. Bishop et al.[51] show clearly that the degree of injury increases with increasing size of ET tube. It is this point that is the most common site for later granulation formation. Granulations are usually a late complication after long-term intubation but can occur after short intubation as well.[52] Longer term intubation results in varying degrees of laryngeal edema[53] and vocal fold ulceration.[53,54]

L. Bronchial intubation

Bronchial intubation occurs frequently and is sometimes hard to identify. Undetected, it leads to atelectasis and hypoxemia. Kramer et al.[55] describe three cases of pulmonary edema after intubation of the right mainstem bronchus. Measurement of tube length can be estimated by placement of the tube alongside the face and neck with bifurcation of the trachea taken at the angle of Louis. Palpation of the sharply inflated cuff in the neck above the sternal notch is also very useful. Transmitted light from a light wand can allow identification of the tip of the ET tube in the neck[56] just as a fiberoptic bronchoscope can. The tube can be deliberately passed into a mainstem bronchus and then removed until bilateral breath sounds are equal. If there is any question, a fiberscope can give the definitive answer. The tube can advance into a mainstem bronchus with flexion of the head or a steep Trendelenburg position. Thus the tube position should be checked after repositioning of the patient.

M. Tracheal trauma

Tracheal trauma can occur from the use of oversized ET tubes, overzealous inflation of ET tube cuffs, and sharp stylets that protrude from the ET tube. These injuries can produce mucosal tears, hemorrhage, and rupture of the trachea progressing to mediastinal emphysema and pneumothorax. Seitz and Gravenstein[57] report endobronchial rupture from use of an endotracheal tube guide or tube changer. They recommend special caution in the use of these guides.

ET tube cuffs inflated to a pressure greater than 30 torr (capillary perfusion pressure) run the risk of devitalizing the mucosa, which progresses to ulceration, necrosis, and loss of structural integrity of the trachea. If the patient is hypotensive, this problem will occur at progressively lower pressures. The need for larger cuff volumes to sustain a positive tracheal seal is an ominous sign that may herald tracheomalacia. The patient with Mounier-Kuhn syndrome (tracheobronchomegaly) is particularly vulnerable to this problem even at very low pressures.[58] It may be necessary to manage these patients with an uncuffed ET tube and pack the throat with gauze to maintain an airway seal. Massive gastric distension in the intubated patient may herald the presence of a tracheoesophageal fistula as the cuff continues to erode into the esophagus.[59] Patients bleeding more than 10 ml from the ET tube without cause are suspect for tracheo–carotid artery fistula.[60]

N. Double-lumen tubes

Benumof et al.[61] have defined the limits for safe placement of modern double-lumen endotracheal tubes. In large part fiberoptic bronchoscopes have taken the mystery out of proper tube placement. The tube can be placed blindly with fiber confirmation and readjustment. Alternatively the fiber can be passed through the right or left channel into the appropriate mainstem bronchus and the double lumen tube inserted over the fiber as a stint. Problems intraoperatively are again best confirmed and resolved by direct fiber observation. Injuries can occur. Bronchial rupture is a serious complication that must be attended to immediately. Precautions are listed: remove the stylet after the tip of the tube is passed through the cords, deflate the cuffs when repositioning the patient, and never overinflate the cuffs. Wagner et al.[62] were unable to explain the cause of the rupture of the membranous trachea in their patient. Hannallah and Gomes[63] believed the endotracheal tube was too large for their small patient resulting in rupture of the left mainstem bronchus.

Benumof[64] provides a technique to prevent overinflation of the left bronchial cuff. With the tracheal cuff inflated and the tracheal lumen open to the air the lung served by the bronchial lumen is inflated. The bronchial cuff is then inflated until the leak disappears.

O. Barotrauma

Barotrauma occurs with high-pressure distension of normal pulmonary structures or at much lower intrapulmonary pressures where disease has weakened tissue. Most notable are high-flow insufflation techniques with a small catheter distal to the larynx. If laryngospasm or some other form of expiratory obstruction develops, there is suddenly no egress for oxygen, and before the anesthesiologist recognizes the problem the lungs may become overdistended

and rupture. These problems are not uncommon in microlaryngeal surgery where jet ventilation is used.[65-69] Egol et al.[67] suggest that direct impingement of the catheter tip on the mucosal surface is a possible cause. They report the problem using the suction part of a fiberoptic laryngoscope for jet delivery of oxygen. Safety mechanisms must be in place to stop oxygen flow if intrapulmonary pressure increases to a dangerous level. For diseased pulmonary tissue as seen in pneumocystic pneumonia it is important to devise ways to ventilate at minimal intrapulmonary pressure to avoid disruption of pulmonary tissue. This holds true for the trauma victim with blunt trauma to the chest and subcutaneous emphysema. The patient has an intrapulmonary bronchial leak until proved otherwise, and low-pressure ventilation must be sustained if possible until the lesion is located. Chest tubes obviously help relieve the problem until definitive surgery can be done.

P. Esophageal perforation and retropharyngeal abscess

Perforation of the esophagus can occur with nasogastric and endotracheal intubation.[70-77] Perforation occurs most often over the cricopharyngeal muscle on the posterior wall of the esophagus. The esophagus is very thin and narrowed in this location. Bacterial contamination leads to diffuse cellulitis. Early diagnosis and treatment is extremely important. If mediastinitis results, mortality is over 50%. Life-threatening airway emergency, subcutaneous emphysema, and pneumothorax can result. Esophageal perforation can also occur in the delivery suite during aggressive airway management of meconium aspiration.[78] Esophageal perforation should be suspected in a patient with subcutaneous emphysema, fever, dysphagia, and a history of difficult intubation.

Q. Nasogastric tubes and esophageal stethoscopes

Placement of nasogastric tubes can cause many of the same problems of placement caused by endotracheal tubes: nosebleed, retropharyngeal dissection, perforation of the esophagus, and intracranial intubation.[10] The not-uncommon occurrence of finding that the nasogastric tube has passed into the trachea is repeated by Wood et al.[79] In this case the peculiar circumstance of changing head position unkinked the nasogastric tube that was coiled up in the mouth. The nasogastric tube, not functioning up to that time, suddenly began to evacuate the lung and activated the low-pressure airway alarm.

The esophageal stethoscope can also find its

way into the trachea. Pickard and Reid[80] report that a stethoscope found its way into the right lower lobe bronchus causing collapse of that lobe and significant hypoxemia until it was recognized.

R. Laryngospasm

Reflex responses to intubation can be troublesome. Laryngospasm as described by Fink[81] is more than spastic closure of vocal cords. Rather it constitutes an infolding of arytenoids and aryepiglottic folds, which are then covered by the epiglottis. This explains why vigorous anteriorly directed pressure on the angle of the jaw helps to break the spasm; the pressure elevates the hyoid, which puts a stretch on the hyoepiglottic ligament, the epiglottis, and aryepiglottic folds and thereby opens the forced closure of the glottis. Positive mask airway pressure may be helpful but not necessarily sufficient to break laryngospasm. Thus succinylcholine may be necessary if hypoxia is to be avoided. Prevention of laryngospasm is the real objective. It is extremely important that no saliva, blood, or gastric contents touch the glottic structures to incite spasm. In situations where every measure must be taken to assure a laryngospasm-free awakening from anesthesia it is wise to perform direct laryngoscopy while the patient is deeply anesthetized and to suction any suspicious material away from the glottis. Traditional wisdom indicates that the patient should then be extubated while a "deep" level of anesthesia exists or oppositely when the patient is responding appropriately to verbal commands. The danger period between these two states should be avoided for extubation. The patient with a full stomach must have intact pharyngolaryngeal reflexes if aspiration and laryngospasm are to be avoided. These patients fall into the group that must be responding to verbal commands before extubation is contemplated.

S. Bronchospasm

Bronchospasm occurs in response to tracheal irritation of the endotracheal tube and can be quite intense. It can be broken with inhalation of a beta-receptor agonist,[2] deepening inhalant anesthetic, or epinephrine. The best plan is to avoid the problem entirely. In patients with reactive airways, ketamine and inhalant drugs are ideal. A "deep" level of anesthesia should be achieved before the trachea is instrumented. Tracheal lidocaine can be administered as a spray before actual intubation. Sometimes the bronchospasm from this alone is alarming but usually short lived. Intravenously administered lidocaine can also be given before instrumentation.

T. Coughing and bucking

Coughing and bucking are responses to tracheal intubation and are to be avoided when there is increased intracranial pressure, when blood pressure must not be elevated, or when increased abdominal pressure could rupture an abdominal incision. While the patient is well anesthetized, the trachea can be sprayed with lidocaine particularly at the level of the irritating ET cuff. Lidocaine can be given intravenously just before extubation, and again the tube can be removed while a "deep" level of anesthesia persists. It is extremely important to clean the pharynx of any irritating material before extubation as described.

U. Apnea

Apnea is occasionally seen as a reflex tracheal response to irritation of the endotracheal tube. If the patient is not narcotized and has a light level of anesthesia and no other central explanation for apnea exists, consideration should be given to removing the ET tube to see if breathing will begin. Of course reintubation may be necessary.

V. Vomiting

Vomiting as a response to tracheal irritation is not unexpected with a full stomach. However, it need not be a problem. If the airway is secure, the ET tube must simply be kept in place until the patient clearly responds to verbal commands in a comprehensible fashion. At that point it is safe to remove the ET tube, but only then.

IV. PROBLEMS WHILE THE TRACHEA IS INTUBATED
A. Airway obstruction

Airway obstruction can occur in every imaginable form. Tubes can kink, be bitten to closure, and be obstructed with blood, mucus casts, foreign bodies, and lubricant. The plastic coating having been sheared from a stylet has been described.[82,83] Obstruction of an ET tube by a prominent aortic knuckle is reported.[84] Gas bubbles trapped in the walls of an ET tube expanded in the presence of nitrous oxide (N_2O) to obstruct the ET tube.[85] The anode wire tube is not immune to problems. It can kink at a point between the end of the ET tube adapter and before the support wire begins. The soft distal tip can fold into the tube and obstruct. Despite the added strength of an anode wire tube, a patient can bite through it.[86] If an anode tube is placed through a tracheostomy no farther than the proximal edge of the cuff, the inflated cuff can alter the tube position and abut the tube bevel against the tracheal wall and obstruct.[87] The inflated cuff may compress the ET tube inward.[88] The cuff may herniate over the tip.[89] The practical solution when confronted by these problems is to pass a suction catheter or fiberoptic bronchoscope down the lumen if time permits. If time does not permit, the tube should be removed and the patient re-intubated.

B. Laser fires

The risk of tracheal tube contact with a laser beam is 1:2.[90] Laser fires are commonplace. The laser penetrates the plastic ET tube. If high concentrations of oxygen are present, the laser creates a fire that propagates in both directions. A "blow torch" is created, fed by the combustible fuel of pyrolysis and intensified by high oxygen flow rates. To quench the fire, oxygen and all anesthetics should be turned off and the tube removed. The fire should be extinguished with saline solution. The airway should be examined for damage and the need for reintubation assessed. Pashayan et al.[91] offer a "helium protocol" to reduce fires. It consists of helium in a concentration of 60% to 80%, the use of unmarked polyvinylchloride tubes, a limit to laser power, and surgical technique characterized by short repeated bursts of power. Nitrogen works equally well to retard combustion at 80% concentration but obviously prevents an enriched oxygen environment. N_2O must not be used[92] because N_2O supports combustion. Barium sulfate strip and markings make polyvinylchloride more flammable.[93-95] Sosis and Dillon[96] have identified the best protective tapes. The new Xomed Laser Shield is not effective.[97] Intermittent apneic techniques and metal Laser Flex tubes work well.[98] A rigid bronchoscope can also be used effectively.

V. PROBLEMS OF EXTUBATION

Sometimes the endotracheal tube cannot be removed. Surgeons may inadvertently include the ET tube in their suturing process. Care must be taken to observe the proximity of surgical sutures. Lang et al.[99] advise the frequent inward-outward movement of the tube to identify fixation if the possibility is suspect as well as routine fiberoptic bronchoscopy through the tube to check for surgical proximity to the ET tube. When ET tube cuffs cannot be deflated, piercing the cuff with a transtracheal needle is recommended.

VI. EARLY POSTEXTUBATION PROBLEMS
A. Hoarseness

Lesser and Williams[100] believe that hoarseness, though transient, is attributable to laryngeal damage, since subjective change correlates well with objective changes in the voice-frequency histogram. Beckford et al.[101] on the other hand, found little evidence of intrinsic vocal fold trauma. They postulate that extralaryngeal factors may be equally important. Several investigators suggest that acoustical measures may be very useful in the identification and monitoring of minor intubation-related trauma.[102,103]

B. Postobstructive pulmonary edema

Postobstructive pulmonary edema has been described in a variety of circumstances.[104-108] The cause is not clear. A common denominator is hypoxia even for brief periods of time. Other theories indicate a possible role for negative intrathoracic pressure that develops against a closed glottis and catecholamine activation.[106] The onset can be delayed for some time after the episode of obstruction.[109] It is uncertain how to avoid the problem other than preventing hypoxia. Any period of airway obstruction with hypoxia is suspect. The condition should be recognized promptly. Reintubation, oxygen, and positive end-expiratory pressure are curative. The condition is usually self-limited when promptly treated.

C. Sore throats

Sore throat is a common symptom of patients after intubation. Monroe et al.[110] could find no difference in incidence if plastic oropharyngeal airways or gauze bite blocks were used. The incidence was in the range of 40% for both. The incidence was increased to 65% when blood was found on airway instruments. They incriminate aggressive oral suctioning as the likely cause. Klemola et al.[111] suggest that lidocaine jelly not be used. The incidence of sore throat was greatest when it was used in combination with lidocaine spray.

VII. PROBLEMS WITH SPECIAL TECHNIQUES
A. Lighted stylet

The lighted stylet is a recent innovation that uses a light at the tip of a flexible stylet to blindly probe for the glottis. It can be effective[112] but again has the disadvantage of any blind procedure. Recently arytenoid dislocation[98] was reported with its use.

B. Retrograde wire intubation

Retrograde wire intubation is an ingenious way to secure a difficult airway. It has the disadvantage that it is done blindly without view of the glottis and takes some time to accomplish. It is probably important to spray the larynx with lidocaine so that the retrograde wire, blood, or saliva do not irritate the vocal cords and act to initiate laryngospasm. Faithful[113] describes injury to multiple terminal branches of the maxillary and mandibular branches of the trigeminal nerve in its use.

C. Fiberoptic naso-orotracheal intubations

The fiberscope has made its place in anesthetic practice. It combines direct vision with the flexibility to probe the pharynx where oral laryngoscopy is difficult or impossible. It takes time to perform and requires practice and patience, but the rewards are worth it. Nosebleeds associated with nasal intubation have been discussed. The only other potential hazard to the patient is the practice of oxygen insufflation down the suction channel. This has the advantage of helping to keep the fiber tip clean as well as being a means to insufflate oxygen. However, I have experienced the sharp fiber tip cutting the mucosa. Insufflated oxygen then dissected the tissue to create significant emphysema of the pharynx, face, and perioptic areas. The same can happen intratracheally if the fiber tip goes submucosally.[67] Ovassapian[114] describes a technical problem with the fiber that failed to withdraw because it passed through the Murphy eye of the ET tube.

D. Transtracheal ventilation

Transtracheal ventilation is an elegant method to promptly salvage a "can't ventilate–can't intubate" situation.[115-117] Yealy et al.[118] demonstrate that the technique can effectively prevent aspiration in a canine model at specific frequencies and head elevation. It can be an aid to fiberoptic intubation.[119] The most serious problems are subcutaneous emphysema and barotrauma.[120] Massive subcutaneous emphysema can progress to mediastinal emphysema, pneumothorax, and death. This occurs when the catheter tip through which oxygen is being delivered migrates subcutaneously. The natural movement of compliant skin can be 3 to 4 inches. A catheter of this length sutured to the skin can migrate to the subcutaneous position if tension is inadvertently placed on the skin suture site, for example, if someone stumbles over the oxygen source hose. The answer to this problem is to use an 8-inch catheter. Barotrauma occurs when there is no egress of oxygen from the partially obstructed glottis and the anesthetist is not attentive to overinflation of the chest. Slow intratracheal bleeding has been a problem to internists who use the technique for tracheal sputum samples, but to anesthesiologists who will use this technique acutely and then secure the airway by some other method, this is less of a hazard.

VIII. SUMMARY

This chapter presents a discussion of the complications anesthesiologists may encounter in the management of the airway. Errors can be both in technique and in judgment. We need to study these events for the lessons we can learn (see Chapter 28). To minimize problems, it is important to think out problems ahead of time, devise safe plans, instrument under direct vision, be gentle, avoid sharp objects, be conservative, and use common sense.

REFERENCES

1. Caplan RA et al, Adverse respiratory events in anesthesia: a closed claims analysis, Anesthesiology 72:828-833, 1990.
2. Durkan W and Fleming N: Potential eye damage from reusable masks, Anesthesiology 67:444, 1987.
3. Grigsby EJ et al: Massive tongue swelling after uncomplicated general anaesthesia, Can J Anaesth 37(7):825-826, 1990.
4. Glauber DT: Facial paralysis after general anesthesia, Anesthesiology 65:516-517, 1986.
5. Azar I and Lear E: Lower lip numbness following general anesthesia, Anesthesiology 65:450-451, 1986.
6. Andersen APD et al: Obstructive sleep apnea initiated by lax epiglottis: a contraindication for continuous positive airway pressure, Chest 91(4):621-623, 1987.
7. Jarjour NN and Wilson P: Pneumocephalus associated with nasal continuous positive airway pressure in a patient with sleep apnea syndrome, Chest 96(6):1425-1426, 1989.
8. Klopfenstein CE, Forster A, and Suter PM: Pneumocephalus: a complication of continuous positive airway pressure after trauma, Chest 78(4):656-657, 1980.
9. Weaver LK, Fairfax WR, and Greenway L: Bilateral otorrhagia associated with continuous positive airway pressure, Chest 93(4):878-879, 1988.
10. Seebacher J, Nozik D, and Mathieu A: Inadvertent intracranial introduction of a nasogastric tube: a complication of severe maxillofacial trauma, Anesthesiology 42(1):100-101, 1975.
11. Horellou MF, Mathe D, and Feiss P: A hazard of naso-tracheal intubation, Anaesthesia 33:73-74, 1978.
12. Hariri MA and Duncan PW: Infective complications of brief nasotracheal intubation, J Laryngol Otol 103:1217-1218, 1989.
13. Cooper R: Bloodless turbinectomy following blind nasal intubation, Anesthesiology 71:469, 1989.
14. Wilkinson JA, Mathis RD, and Dire DJ: Turbinate destruction: a rare complication of nasotracheal intubation, J Emerg Med 4(3):209-212, 1986.
15. Smith WD, Timms MS, and Sutcliffe H: Unusual complication of nasopharyngeal intubation, Anaesthesia 44(7):615-616, 1989.
16. Sherry KM and Murday A: A nasal adhesion following prolonged nasotracheal intubation, Anaesthesia 42(6):651-653, 1987.
17. Arens JF, LeJeune FE Jr, and Webre DR: Maxillary sinusitis, a complication of nasotracheal intubation, Anesthesiology 40(4):415-416, 1974.
18. Fassoulaki A and Pamouktsoglou P: Prolonged na-

sotracheal intubation and its association with inflammation of paranasal sinuses, Anesth Analg 69:50-52, 1989.

19. Bainton CR: A new laryngoscope blade to overcome pharyngeal obstruction, Anesthesiology 67:767-770, 1987.
20. Rosenberg MB: Anesthesia-induced dental injury, Int Anesthesiol Clin 27(2):120-125, 1989.
21. Lockhart PB et al: Dental complications during and after tracheal intubation, J Am Dent Assoc 112(4):480-483, 1986.
22. Burton JF and Baker AB: Dental damage during anaesthesia and surgery, Anaesth Intensive Care 15:262-268, 1987.
23. Aromaa U et al: Difficulties with tooth protectors in endotracheal intubation, Acta Anaesthesiol Scand 32:304-307, 1988.
24. Salathé M and Jöhr M: Unsuspected cervical fractures: a common problem in ankylosing spondylitis, Anesthesiology 70:869-870, 1989.
25. Crosby ET and Lui A: The adult cervical spine: implications for airway management, Can J Anaesth 37:77-93, 1990.
26. Williams JP et al: Atlanto-axial subluxation and trisomy-21: another perioperative complication, Anesthesiology 67:253-254, 1987.
27. Dong ML: Arnold-Chiari malformation type I appearing after tonsillectomy, Anesthesiology 67:120-122, 1987.
28. Watson WJ and Moran RL: Corneal abrasion during induction, Anesthesiology 66:440, 1987.
29. Brandwein M, Abramson AL, and Shikowitz MJ: Bilateral vocal cord paralysis following endotracheal intubation, Arch Otolaryngol Head Neck Surg 112(8):877-882, 1986.
30. Cavo JW Jr: True vocal cord paralysis following intubation, Laryngoscope 95(11):1352-1359, 1985.
31. Lim EK, Chia KS, and NG BK: Recurrent laryngeal nerve palsy following endotracheal intubation, Anaesth Intensive Care 15(3):342-345, 1987.
32. Nuutinen J and Kärjä J: Bilateral vocal cord paralysis following general anesthesia, Laryngoscope 91(1):83-86, 1981.
33. Mayhew JF, Miner ME, and Denneny J: Upper airway obstruction following cyst-to-peritoneal shunt in a child with a Dandy-Walker cyst, Anesthesiology 62:183-184, 1985.
34. Teichner RL: Lingual nerve injury: a complication of orotracheal intubation, Br J Anaesth 43:413, 1971.
35. Aucott W, Prinsley P, and Madden G: Laryngeal anaesthesia with aspiration following intubation, Anaesthesia 44:230-231, 1989.
36. Mayhew JF, Miner M, and Katz J: Macroglossia in a 16-month-old child after a craniotomy, Anesthesiology 62:683-684, 1985.
37. Teeple E, Maroon J, and Rueger R: Hemimacroglossia and unilateral ischemic necrosis of the tongue in a long-duration neurosurgical procedure, Anesthesiology 64:845-846, 1986.
38. Ellis SC, Bryan-Brown CW, and Hyderally H: Massive swelling of the head and neck, Anesthesiology 42:102-103, 1975.
39. Patane PS and White SE: Macroglossia causing airway obstruction following cleft palate repair, Anesthesiology 71:995-996, 1989.
40. Salem MR et al: Cricoid compression is effective in obliterating the esophageal lumen in the presence of a nasogastric tube, Anesthesiology 63:443-446, 1985.
41. Harris M et al: Gastroduodenal reflux of irrigating solution during percutaneous lithotripsy for intrahepatic cholelithiasis, Anesthesiology 62:182-183, 1985.
42. Ford RWJ: Confirming tracheal intubation: a simple manoeuvre, Can Anaesth Soc J 30:191-193, 1983.
43. Sum Ping ST: Esophageal intubation, Anesth Analg 66:483, 1987.
44. Dunn SM et al: Tracheal intubation is not invariably confirmed by capnography, Anesthesiology 73:1285-1287, 1990.
45. Kambic V and Radsel Z: Intubation lesions of the larynx, Br J Anaesth 50:587-590, 1978.
46. Peppard SB and Dickens JH: Laryngeal injury following short-term intubation, Ann Otol Rhinol Laryngol 92(4 pt 1):327-330, 1983.
47. Frink EJ and Pattison BD: Posterior arytenoid dislocation following uneventful endotracheal intubation and anesthesia, Anesthesiology 70:358-360, 1989.
48. Gray B, Huggins NJ, and Hirsch N: An unusual complication of tracheal intubation, Anaesthesia 45:558-560, 1990.
49. Debo RF et al: Cricoarytenoid subluxation: complication of blind intubation with a lighted stylet, Ear Nose Throat J 68(7):517-520, 1989.
50. Wackym PA, Gray GF Jr, and Avant GR: Herpes zoster of the larynx after intubational trauma, J Laryngol Otol 100(7):839-841, 1986.
51. Bishop MJ, Weymuller EA Jr, and Fink BR: Laryngeal effects of prolonged intubation, Anesth Analg 63:335-342, 1984.
52. Drosnes DL and Zwillenberg DA: Laryngeal granulomatous polyp after short-term intubation of a child, Ann Otol Rhinol Laryngol 99:183-186, 1990.
53. Alessi DM, Hanson DG, and Berci G: Bedside videolaryngoscopic assessment of intubation trauma, Ann Otol Rhinol Laryngol 98:586-590, 1989.
54. Colice GL, Stukel TA, and Dain B: Laryngeal complications of prolonged intubation, Chest 96(4):877-884, 1989.
55. Kramer MR, Melzer E, and Sprung CL: Unilateral pulmonary edema after intubation of the right mainstem bronchus, Crit Care Med 17(5):472-474, 1989.
56. Mehta S: Guided orotracheal intubation in the operating room using a lighted stylet, Anesthesiology 66:105, 1987.
57. Seitz PA and Gravenstein N: Endobronchial rupture from endotracheal reintubation with an endotracheal tube guide, J Clin Anesth 1(3):214-217, 1989.
58. Messahel FM: Tracheal dilatation followed by stenosis in Mounier-Kuhn syndrome, Anaesthesia 44:227-229, 1989.
59. Tessler S et al: Massive gastric distention in the intubated patient, Arch Intern Med 150:318-320, 1990.
60. LoCicero J III: Tracheo-carotid artery erosion following endotracheal intubation, J Trauma 24(10):907-909, 1984.
61. Benumof JL et al: Margin of safety in positioning modern double-lumen endotracheal tubes, Anesthesiology 67:729-738, 1987.
62. Wagner DL, Gammage GW, and Wong ML: Tracheal rupture following the insertion of a disposable double-lumen endotracheal tube, Anesthesiology 63:698-700, 1985.
63. Hannallah M and Gomes M: Bronchial rupture associated with the use of double-lumen tube in a small adult, Anesthesiology 71:457-459, 1989.
64. Benumof JL: Physiology of the open chest and one lung ventilation. In Kaplan J, editor: Thoracic anesthesia, New York, 1983, Churchill Livingstone.
65. Badran I and Jamal M: Pneumomediastinum due to venturi system during microlaryngoscopy, Middle East J Anesthesiol 9(6):561-564, 1988.
66. Chang JL, Bleyaert A, and Bedger R: Unilateral pneumothorax following jet ventilation during gen-

eral anesthesia, Anesthesiology 53(3):244-246, 1980.

67. Egol A, Culpepper JA, and Snyder JV: Barotrauma and hypotension resulting from jet ventilation in critically ill patients, Chest 88(1):98-102, 1985.

68. O'Sullivan TJ and Healy GB: Complications of venturi jet ventilation during microlaryngeal surgery, Arch Otolaryngol 111(2):127-131, 1985.

69. Wetmore SJ, Key JM, and Suen JY: Complications of laser surgery for laryngeal papillomatosis, Laryngoscope 95(7 pt 1):798-801, 1985.

70. Eldor J, Ofek B, and Abramowitz HB: Perforation of oesophagus by tracheal tube during resuscitation, Anaesthesia 45:70-71, 1990.

71. Johnson KG and Hood DD: Esophageal perforation associated with endotracheal intubation, Anesthesiology 64:281-283, 1986.

72. Kras JF and Marchmont-Robinson H: Pharyngeal perforation during intubation in a patient with Crohn's disease, J Oral Maxillofac Surg 47:405-407, 1989.

73. Levine PA: Hypopharyngeal perforation: an untoward complication of endotracheal intubation, Arch Otolaryngol 106(9):578-580, 1980.

74. Majumdar B, Stevens RW, and Obara LG: Retropharyngeal abscess following tracheal intubation, Anaesthesia 37:67-70, 1982.

75. Norman EA and Sosis M: Iatrogenic oesophageal perforation due to tracheal or nasogastric intubation, Can Anaesth Soc J 33(2):222-226, 1986.

76. à Wengen DF: Piriform fossa perforation during attempted tracheal intubation, Anaesthesia 42(5):519-521, 1987.

77. Young PN and Robinson JM: Cellulitis as a complication of difficult tracheal intubation Anesthesia 42(5):569, 1987 [letter].

78. Topsis J, Kinas HY, and Kandall SR: Esophageal perforation: a complication of neonatal resuscitation, Anesth Analg 69:532-534, 1989.

79. Wood G et al: Ventilatory failure due to an improperly placed nasogastric tube, Can J Anaesth 37(5):587-588, 1990.

80. Pickard WA and Reid L: Hypoxia caused by an esophageal stethoscope, Anesthesiology 65:534-536, 1986.

81. Fink BR: Laryngeal complications of general anesthesia. In Orkin FK and Cooperman LH, editors: Complications in anesthesiology, Philadelphia, 1983, JB Lippincott.

82. Cook WP and Schultetus RR: Obstruction of an endotracheal tube by the plastic coating sheared from a stylet, Anesthesiology 62:803-804, 1985.

83. Zmyslowski WP, Kam D, and Simpson GT: An unusual cause of endotracheal tube obstruction, Anesthesiology 70:883, 1989 [letter].

84. Sapsford DJ and Snowdon SL: If in doubt, take it out: obstruction of tracheal tube by prominent aortic knuckle, Anaesthesia 40(6):552-554, 1985.

85. Populaire C, Robard S, and Souron R: An armoured endotracheal tube obstruction in a child, Can J Anaesth 36(3 pt 1):331-332, 1989.

86. Gemma M and Ferrazza C: "Dental trauma" to oral airways, Can J Anaesth 37:951, 1990.

87. Riley RH, Mason SA, and Barber CD: Obstruction of a preformed armoured tracheostomy tube, Can J Anaesth 37:824, 1990.

88. Wright PJ, Mundy JVB, and Mansfield CJ: Obstruction of armoured tracheal tubes: case report and discussion, Can J Anaesth 35(2):195-197, 1988.

89. Treffers R and de Lange JJ: An unusual case of cuff herniation, Acta Anaesthesiol Belg 40(1):87-90, 1989.

90. Pashayan AG and Gravenstein N: High incidence of CO_2 laser beam contact with the tracheal tube during operations on the upper airway, J Clin Anesth 1(5):354-357, 1989.

91. Pashayan AG et al: The helium protocol for laryngotracheal operations with CO_2 laser: a retrospective review of 523 cases, Anesthesiology 68:801-804, 1988.

92. Wolf GL and Simpson JI: Flammability of endotracheal tubes in oxygen and nitrous oxide enriched atmosphere, Anesthesiology 67:236-239, 1987.

93. Geffin B et al: Flammability of endotracheal tubes during Nd-YAG laser application in the airway, Anesthesiology 65:511-515, 1986.

94. Pashayan AG and Gravenstein JS: Helium retards endotracheal tube fires from carbon dioxide lasers, Anesthesiology 62:274-277, 1985.

95. Pashayan AG and Gravenstein JS: On reducing the flammability of PVC, Anesthesiology 68:173, 1988.

96. Sosis MB and Dillon F: What is the safest foil tape for endotracheal tube protection during Nd-YAG laser surgery? A comparative study, Anesthesiology 72:553-555, 1990.

97. Sosis MB: Airway fire during CO_2 laser surgery using a Xomed® laser endotracheal tube, Anesthesiology 72:747-749, 1990.

98. Hawkins DB and Joseph MM: Avoiding a wrapped endotracheal tube in laser laryngeal surgery: experiences with apneic anesthesia and metal Laser-Flex® endotracheal tubes, Laryngoscope 100:1283-1287, 1990.

99. Lang S et al: Difficult tracheal extubation, Can J Anaesth 36(3 pt 1): 340-342, 1989.

100. Lesser T and Williams G: Laryngographic investigation of postoperative hoarseness, Clin Otolaryngol 13:37-42, 1988.

101. Beckford NS et al: Effects of short-term endotracheal intubation on vocal function, Laryngoscope 100:331-336, 1990.

102. Priebe H-J, Henke W, and Hedley-Whyte J: Effects of tracheal intubation on laryngeal acoustic waveforms, Anesth Analg 67:219-227, 1988.

103. Yonick TA et al: Acoustical effects of endotracheal intubation, Speech Hearing Disord 55:427-433, 1990.

104. Frank LP and Schreiber GC: Pulmonary edema following acute upper airway obstruction, Anesthesiology 65:106, 1986.

105. Herrick IA, Mahendran B, and Penny FJ: Postobstructive pulmonary edema following anesthesia, J Clin Anesth 2(2):116-120, 1990.

106. Lang SA et al: Pulmonary oedema associated with airway obstruction, Can J Anaesth 37(2):210-218, 1990.

107. Warner LO, Beach TP, and Martino JD: Negative pressure pulmonary oedema secondary to airway obstruction in an intubated infant, Can J Anaesth 35(5):507-510, 1988.

108. Wilder RT and Belani KG: Fiberoptic intubation complicated by pulmonary edema in a 12-year-old child with Hurler syndrome, Anesthesiology 72:205-207, 1990.

109. Glasser SA and Siler JN: Delayed onset of laryngospasm-induced pulmonary edema in an adult outpatient, Anesthesiology 62:370-371, 1985.

110. Monroe MC, Gravenstein N, and Saga-Rumley S: Postoperative sore throat: effect of oropharyngeal airway in orotracheally intubated patients, Anesth Analg 70:512-516, 1990.

111. Klemola U-M, Saarnivaara L, and Yrjölä H: Post-operative sore throat: effect of lignocaine jelly and spray with endotracheal intubation, Eur J Anesthesiol 5:391-399, 1988.

112. Ellis DG et al: Guided orotracheal intubation in the operating room using a lighted stylet: a comparison with direct laryngoscopic technique, Anesthesiology 64:823-826, 1986.

113. Faithfull NS: Injury to terminal branches of the trigeminal nerve following tracheal intubation, Br J Anaesth 57(5):535-537, 1985.

114. Ovassapian A: Failure to withdraw flexible fiberoptic laryngoscope after nasotracheal intubation, Anesthesiology 63:124-125, 1985.

115. Benumof JL and Scheller MS: The importance of transtracheal jet ventilation in the management of the difficult airway, Anesthesiology 71:769-778, 1989.

116. Weymuller EA Jr et al: Management of difficult airway problems with percutaneous transtracheal ventilation, Ann Otol Rhinol Laryngol 96(1 pt 1):34-37, 1987.

117. Yealy DM and Stewart RD: Translaryngeal cannula ventilation: continuing misconceptions, Anesthesiology 67:445-446, 1987.

118. Yealy DM et al: Manual translaryngeal jet ventilation and the risk of aspiration in a canine model, Ann Emerg Med 19(11):1238-1241, 1990.

119. Todesco JM and Williams RT: Percutaneous transtracheal high-frequency jet ventilation as an aid to fiberoptic intubation, Anesthesiology 68:298, 1988 [letter].

120. Craft TM et al: Two cases of barotrauma associated with transtracheal jet ventilation, Br J Anaesth 64(4):524-527, 1990.

Chapter 2

Complications of Cardiovascular Access

David L. Reich

Joel A. Kaplan

I. **Electrocardiographic Monitoring**
   A. Electrical Hazards
   B. Burn Hazard
II. **Peripheral Intravenous Catheters**
   A. Infection
   B. Phlebitis
   C. Hematoma
   D. Extravasation
III. **Noninvasive Blood Pressure Monitoring**
IV. **Invasive Arterial Pressure Monitoring**
   A. Sites
      1. Radial and ulnar arteries
      2. Brachial or axillary arteries
      3. Femoral artery
      4. Dorsalis pedis artery
      5. Superficial temporal artery
   B. Contraindications to Arterial Cannulation
      1. Local infection
      2. Coagulopathy
      3. Proximal obstruction
      4. Raynaud's syndrome
   C. Surgical Considerations
   D. Infectious Risk
   E. Hemorrhage
   F. Thrombosis and Distal Ischemia
   G. Embolization
   H. Skin Necrosis
   I. Hematoma and Neurologic Injury
   J. Late Vascular Complications
   K. Inaccurate Pressure Readings
V. **Central Venous Pressure Monitoring**
   A. Measurement System Problems
   B. Sites
      1. Internal jugular vein
      2. External jugular vein
      3. Subclavian vein
      4. Antecubital veins
      5. Femoral vein
   C. Contraindications
      1. Absolute
      2. Relative
   D. Complications
      1. Arterial puncture

2. Pneumothorax
3. Hydrothorax
4. Chylothorax
5. Pericardial effusion and tamponade
6. Venous air embolism
7. Particulate embolism
8. Nerve injury
9. Dysrhythmias

VI. **Pulmonary Artery Monitoring**
   A. Measurement System Problems
   B. Sites
   C. Flotation of the Catheter
   D. Contraindications
      1. Absolute
      2. Relative
   E. Complications
      1. Dysrhythmias
      2. Complete heart block
      3. Endobronchial hemorrhage
      4. Pulmonary infarction
      5. Catheter knotting
      6. Valvular damage
      7. Thrombocytopenia
      8. Incorrect placement
      9. Catheter electrode detachment
      10. Ventricular perforation risk (Paceport pacing wires)
VII. **Determination of Cardiac Output**
   A. Fick Method
   B. Mixed Venous Oxygen Saturation
   C. Thermodilution
   D. Pulmonary Artery Doppler Probe
   E. Transtracheal Doppler Probe
   F. Thoracic Bioimpedance
   G. Transesophageal Echocardiography and Doppler Probes
      1. Incorrect interpretation
VIII. **Complications of Cardioversion**
   A. Dysrhythmias
   B. Airway Complications
   C. Burns
   D. Electrical Hazards to Health Care Personnel

16

Anesthesiologists are more frequently confronted with patients with cardiovascular disease as a consequence of the aging of the population and advances in surgical therapy. It is generally accepted that cardiovascular monitoring improves patient care and probably improves outcome. Noninvasive monitoring would be ideal because of the low incidence of complications. Unfortunately, noninvasive monitoring provides limited information. Thus invasive monitoring is becoming more prevalent during the intraoperative period. The aim of this chapter is to review the complications associated with various forms of cardiovascular monitoring. This should enable you to make educated decisions regarding cardiovascular monitoring based on the known benefits and risks.

I. ELECTROCARDIOGRAPHIC MONITORING
A. Electrical hazards

The application of large voltages or currents to skin or tissue represents a *macroshock*. All modern operating room monitoring equipment has electrically isolated patient connections. However, faulty equipment could result in leakage of electrical current that could reach the patient through ECG electrodes or other conductive materials in contact with the patient's body. Death from electrocution has resulted when ECG electrodes inadvertently came into contact with a power cord.[1]

According to National Fire Protection Association (NFPA) standards, the upper threshold for electrical safety for *external* application is 50 microamperes (μA).[2] All patient monitoring equipment must be regularly inspected by biomedical engineering personnel for leakage current.

The application of small amounts of electrical power to the heart represents a *microshock* (Fig. 2-1). The current may reach the heart by way of internal ECG leads, fluid-filled catheters, or internal equipment (List 2-1). The NFPA standard for electrical contract with the *heart* is a maximal leakage current of 10 μA. Thus pacing wires and intracardiac electrodes should always be covered with an insulating material and should never be touched with bare hands.

B. Burn hazard

Unipolar electrocautery is based on the principle that a high current density at the tip of the instrument burns the tissue. This current traverses the body and leaves via a grounding pad with a large surface area. The large surface area ensures a low current density at the exit

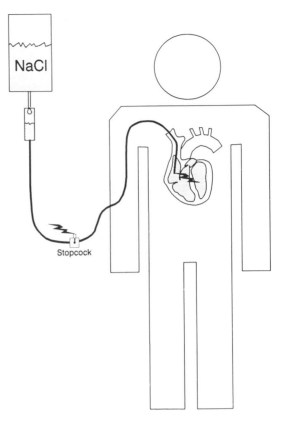

Fig. 2-1. Microshock is a potential hazard whenever a direct electrical connection to the heart exists. In the diagram, a saline-filled central venous catheter serves as an electrical conductor from the stopcock to the heart. Microshock currents as low as 100μAmp could result in ventricular fibrillation.

List 2-1. Sources of Microshock Hazard

ECG leads
Esophageal electrodes
Pacing wires
Pulmonary artery catheter electrodes

Intravascular catheters filled with electrolyte solution (saline)
Peripheral intravenous catheters
Central venous catheters
Pulmonary artery catheters
Arterial catheters

Internal equipment
Endoscopic probes
Transesophageal echocardiography probes
Esophageal temperature probes

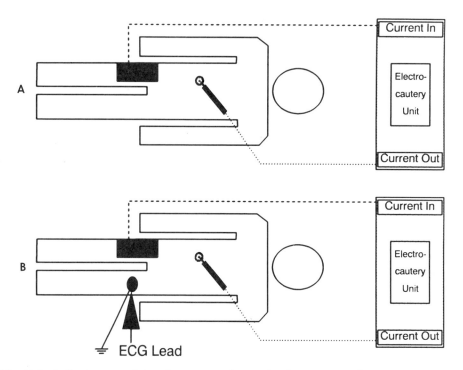

Fig. 2-2. A, In the normal situation, current leaves the electrocautery device and enters the patient through a small tip. The high current density at the instrument tip cauterizes the tissue. The current leaves the patient through the return pad (incorrectly termed a "grounding pad"). The pad has a large surface area, which results in a low current density and minimal heat generation. **B,** An ECG lead on the patient's thigh has inadvertently become grounded, short-circuiting the normal route through the return ("grounding") pad. As electrocautery current leaves through the small surface area of the ECG lead, a burn results from the high current density.

site, with little heat production. If an ECG lead inadvertently becomes the grounding site for unipolar electrocautery, a burn will result because of the relatively small surface area of the lead (Fig. 2-2). This problem can be prevented by use of electrically isolated monitoring equipment and preventing contact between ECG leads and wires with potentially grounded conductors, such as the metallic components of operating room tables.

II. PERIPHERAL INTRAVENOUS CATHETERS
A. Infection

The reasons intravenous catheters become infected include insertion through an infected skin site, poor aseptic technique during insertion or maintenance, sepsis with seeding of the catheter, and prolonged duration of cannulation with colonization by skin flora. Whenever infection at the cannulation site is identified, the catheter must be removed. The catheter is a foreign body that will never be sterilized with antibiotic therapy.

Lymphangitic streaks or cellulitis may occur as a result of intravenous catheter infection. These problems require systemic antibiotic therapy.

B. Phlebitis

The injection of irritating drugs, such as diazepam (propylene glycol vehicle), or hypertonic fluids will sometimes result in phlebitis because of a direct intimal injury. The vein is tender with surrounding edema and erythema. The intravenous catheter must be discontinued, and anti-inflammatory drugs administered. Antibiotic therapy will be required if suppurative phlebitis is present.

C. Hematoma

Elderly patients with fragile veins and lax subcutaneous tissues are prone to developing hematomas during peripheral venous cannulation attempts. These not only are painful but may also become infected. Pressure should be applied to prevent hematomas after unsuccessful cannulation. The treatment is warm soaks or heating pads to accelerate the breakdown of extravasated blood.

Massive hematomas may occur if blood extravasates during transfusions. This is especially dangerous when blood is administered under pressure to patients with precarious intravenous lines. The hematoma exerts pressure on the surrounding tissues, producing limb ischemia, or serves as a nidus for infection.

D. Extravasation

The extravasation of caustic substances (vasopressors, thiopental) may result in tissue necrosis and skin sloughing. It is preferable to administer irritating drugs in large-bore intravenous tubing along with rapid flow of a concurrent intravenous fluid. An alternative is to administer these substances in a central venous line if that is an option.

III. NONINVASIVE BLOOD PRESSURE MONITORING

The proliferation of noninvasive blood pressure monitoring devices has introduced the potential for a new set of complications. These devices inflate a cuff to a suprasystolic pressure and then slowly deflate to determine blood pressure by the oscillometric method. The rate of cuff deflation is directly proportional to the heart rate.

The innervation of the extremity is ischemic during the period of cuff inflation. Neurologic injury has resulted from too frequent or prolonged cuff inflation.[3] Ecchymoses and petechial hemorrhages also occur with high cuff pressures.

Prolonged cycling time may occur with irregular heart rhythms or impaired perfusion. The risk is that therapeutic interventions may be delayed while one is waiting for the results of repeat measurements.

IV. INVASIVE ARTERIAL PRESSURE MONITORING
A. Sites

1. Radial and ulnar arteries. The ulnar artery provides the majority of blood flow to the hand in about 90% of humans.[4] The radial and ulnar arteries are connected by a palmar arch, which provides collateral flow to the hand in the event of radial artery occlusion. Many clinicians routinely perform an Allen test before radial artery cannulation.

One performs an Allen test by occluding both the radial and ulnar arteries by compression and exercising the hand until it is pale. The ulnar artery is then released (with the hand open loosely), and the time until the hand regains its normal color is noted.[5] With a normal collateral circulation, the color returns to the hand in about 5 seconds. If, however, the hand takes longer than 15 seconds to return to its normal color, cannulation of the radial artery on that side is somewhat controversial. The hand may remain pale if the fingers are hyperextended or widely spread apart, even in the presence of a normal collateral circulation.[6] Variations on the Allen's test include using a Doppler probe or pulse oximeter to document collateral flow.[7,8]

Recently the value of the Allen test has been challenged. Slogoff et al. cannulated the radial artery in 16 patients with poor ulnar collateral circulation (assessed using the Allen test) without any complications.[9] An incidence of zero in a study sample of only 16 patients, however, does not guarantee that the true incidence of the complication is negligible. In contrast, Mangano and Hickey reported a case of hand ischemia requiring amputation in a patient with a normal preoperative Allen's test.[10] Thus the predictive value of Allen's test is questionable.

Allen's test remains, however, the best standard for assessment of the adequacy of collateral flow in the palmar circulation. If the Allen's test demonstrates that the hand is dependent on the radial artery for adequate perfusion, the other hand may be selected. If other cannulation sites are not available and Allen's test is abnormal, the ulnar artery may be used.

2. Brachial or axillary arteries. The brachial artery lies medially to the bicipital tendon in the antecubital fossa, in proximity to the median nerve. The complications from percutaneous brachial artery catheter monitoring are lower than those after brachial artery cutdown for cardiac catheterization.[11] Brachial artery pressure tracings resemble those in the femoral artery, with less systolic augmentation than radial artery tracings.[12]

In a recent study of 170 patients, brachial arterial pressures were found to more accurately reflect central aortic pressures than radial arterial pressures both before and after cardiopulmonary bypass.[13] Two large series of perioperative brachial arterial monitoring have documented the safety of this technique.[14,15]

The axillary artery may be cannulated by the Seldinger technique near the junction of the deltoid and pectoral muscles. This has been recommended for long-term catheterization in the intensive care unit[16] and in patients with peripheral vascular disease.[17] Since the tip of the 15 to 20 cm catheter may lie in the aortic arch, the use of the left axillary artery is recommended to minimize the chance of cerebral embolization during flushing.

3. Femoral artery. The femoral artery may be cannulated using any of the above techniques. It is usually cannulated for monitoring purposes when other sites are not accessible, or other pulses are not palpable. The use of this site remains controversial because of the high rate of ischemic complications and pseudonaneurysm formation after diagnostic angiographic and cardiac catheterization procedures.[18] However, the size of monitoring catheters is considerably smaller than that of diagnostic catheters, and the incidence of these complications should be much less. Older literature stated that the femoral area was intrinsically dirty and that catheter sepsis and mortality were significantly increased compared to other monitoring sites. More recent evidence indicates that femoral artery cannulation may be safe but that long-term cannulation (>4 days) is associated with an 8% to 17% incidence of catheter-related infections.[19]

The femoral artery is a less desirable choice as an arterial monitoring site in patients with peripheral vascular disease. Aortic inflow obstruction may decrease the arterial pressure in the femoral artery, or the femoral artery may have atheromatous plaques that could embolize and cause distal ischemia. However, the patient undergoing thoracic or upper abdominal aortic reconstruction may require femoral arterial monitoring in addition to monitoring in one of the upper extremities. In these operations, distal aortic perfusion (using partial cardiopulmonary or left-sided heart bypass) may be performed during aortic cross-clamping to preserve spinal cord and visceral organ blood flow. It is important to measure the distal aortic pressure at the femoral (or dorsalis pedis) artery to optimize the distal perfusion pressure.

4. Dorsalis pedis artery. The dorsalis pedis is a relatively small artery that may be cannulated when other sites are not available. Because of its small size, the incidence of failed cannulation is up to 20%, and the incidence of thrombotic occlusion is around 8%.[20] The dorsalis pedis arterial wave form tends to have higher systolic and lower diastolic pressures than simultaneously measured radial or brachial pressures.[21] The mean arterial pressure is the most consistent measurement obtained from different cannulation sites. Dorsalis pedis arterial monitoring is contraindicated in surgery for lower extremity revascularization.

5. Superficial temporal artery. The superficial artery is a branch of the external carotid that passes anteriorly to the ear. It has a variable course, and this may be determined with a Doppler probe.[22] The artery may be quite tortuous and difficult to cannulate. The tip of the catheter must be positioned carefully so that embolization via the internal carotid to the cerebral circulation will not occur. This approach is not recommended in patients with carotid occlusive or cerebrovascular disease.

B. Contraindications to arterial cannulation

1. Local infection. Placement of an arterial cannula through cellulitic or purulent tissue is likely to result in catheter sepsis. If signs of infection develop at an existing arterial cannulation site, the catheter must be removed. A separate cannulation site free of infection should be found. Strict aseptic technique is necessary during the insertion and maintenance of arterial cannulas.

2. Coagulopathy. Coagulopathy may result in hematoma formation during arterial cannulation at peripheral sites, such as the radial and dorsalis pedis arteries. However, there is a more significant risk of massive hematoma formation causing vascular or neurologic compromise during axillary and femoral cannulation attempts. Thus, in anticoagulated patients, it is recommended that more peripheral arterial cannulation sites be used when this form of monitoring is required.

3. Proximal obstruction. Anatomic factors may lead to intra-arterial pressure readings that greatly underestimate the central aortic pressure. The thoracic outlet syndrome and congenital anomalies of the aortic arch vessels will obstruct flow to the upper extremities. Aortic coarctation or atheromatous disease of the aorta and iliac vessels will diminish flow to the lower extremities. Arterial pressure distal to a previous arterial cutdown site may be lower than the central aortic pressure because of stenosis at the cutdown site.

4. Raynaud's syndrome. Radial and brachial arterial cannulation are contraindicated in patients with a history of Raynaud's syndrome or Buerger's disease (thromboangiitis obliterans). This is especially important in the perioperative setting because hypothermia of the hand is the main trigger for vasospastic attacks in Raynaud's syndrome.[23] It is recommended that large arteries, such as the femoral or axillary, be used for intra-arterial monitoring if indicated in patients with either of these diseases.

C. Surgical considerations

Several surgical maneuvers may interfere with intra-arterial monitoring. During mediastinoscopy, the scope intermittently obstructs the innominate artery by compressing it against the manubrium. Extreme retraction of the thoracic cage during internal mammary artery dissection results in damping of the arterial wave form on the ipsilateral side. The lateral decubitus position may compromise flow to the downward arm if an axillary roll is not properly positioned.

In situations where the arterial wave form damping is intermittent, such as mediastinoscopy procedures, it is advantageous to monitor radial artery pressure on the affected side. Thus the surgeon can be informed whenever compression of the innominate artery occurs. However, in situations where the damping is prolonged, such as internal mammary artery dissections, it is best to monitor arterial pressure at a different site.

D. Infectious risk

One complication that is common to all forms of invasive monitoring is the risk of infection. Infectious organisms may contaminate the catheter before insertion (poor manufacturing standards), during insertion (poor aseptic technique), or after final placement (bacteremia, poor aseptic technique, or infection at the insertion site). Other factors that are associated with catheter infection include nondisposable transducer domes, dextrose flush solutions, and duration of insertion.[24-26]

E. Hemorrhage

The use of an intra-arterial catheter carries the potential risk of exsanguination if the catheter or tubing assembly becomes disconnected. The use of Luer-Lok (instead of tapered) connections and monitors with low-pressure alarms should decrease the risk of this complication.[27]

F. Thrombosis and distal ischemia

The incidence of radial artery thrombosis after cannulation has been extensively studied. Thrombosis has been found to correlate with the following factors: prolonged duration of cannulation,[28] larger catheters,[29] and smaller radial artery size (that is, a greater proportion of the artery is occupied by the catheter).[30] Other factors associated with thrombosis in adults (but not in children) include polypropylene catheters[31] and tapered catheters[32] (List 2-2).

The incidence of thrombosis is not affected by the technique of cannulation[33] but is lowered with aspirin before treatment.[34] Bedford recommended removing arterial catheters with continuous aspiration of the catheter by syringe, during proximal and distal occlusion of the vessel, in order to remove accumulated thrombus.[35]

The relationship between radial artery thrombosis and ischemia of the hand is less certain. As discussed earlier, the ability of the Allen test

---

List 2-2. Causes of Arterial Thrombosis After Cannulation

Increased duration of cannulation

Increased proportion of lumen occupied by catheter
Larger catheter size
Smaller wrist size
Smaller arterial lumen

Catheter type
Tapered catheters
Polypropylene catheters?

---

to predict hand complications after radial artery cannulation has been challenged.[9] And, despite the widespread use of radial artery cannulation, hand complications are rarely reported.

Generalized atherosclerosis should predispose to distal ischemia. The hand should be closely examined at regular intervals in patients with atherosclerosis who have undergone axillary, brachial, radial, or ulnar arterial catheterization. Since thrombosis may appear several days after the catheter has been removed,[36] the examinations should be continued through the postoperative period. Although recanalization of a thrombosed artery can be expected in an average of 13 days,[37] the collateral blood flow may be inadequate during this period. Any evidence of hand ischemia should be aggressively investigated and promptly treated to prevent morbidity.[38]

The treatment plan should involve consultation with a vascular, hand, or plastic surgeon. Treatment has traditionally been conservative. However, fibrinolytic agents, such as streptokinase, stellate ganglion blockade, and surgical intervention are modalities that should be considered.

G. Embolization

Flushing of an arterial catheter forces any particulate matter or air to move distally or proximally within the artery. Distal embolization could potentially result in hand ischemia with tissue necrosis or loss of function. Forceful or prolonged flushing causes proximal embolization and could even result in cerebral embolization. Axillary or temporal catheters are the most likely sources for cerebral embolization, but brachial and radial catheters are also potential sources.[39] Emboli from the right arm are more likely to reach the cerebral circulation than the left arm because of the anatomy and direction of blood flow in the aortic arch. Other factors that influence the likelihood of cerebral embolization include the volume of flush solution and the rapidity of injection.[40]

H. Skin necrosis

Skin necrosis over the volar aspect of the forearm has been reported in eight patients after radial arterial cannulation.[41,42] In all of these patients the area of necrosis was proximal to the arterial puncture site. This has lead to full-thickness skin loss. The skin necrosis is presumably attributable to thrombosis of the radial artery with proximal propagation of the thrombosis to involve the cutaneous branches of the radial artery.

I. Hematoma and neurologic injury

Hematoma formation may complicate any arterial puncture or cannulation attempt and is particularly common in anticoagulated patients or those with coagulopathies. If a large hematoma develops, the resultant pressure may compress adjacent arteries or veins and cause distal ischemia. Compression of an adjacent nerve may result in a neuropathy. Nerve damage is especially likely if the nerve and artery lie in a limited tissue compartment, such as the fibrous sheath surrounding the brachial plexus. Hematoma formation should be prevented by the application of direct pressure after arterial punctures and the correction of any underlying coagulopathy. Surgical consultation should be obtained if massive hematoma formation or neurologic dysfunction develop, and surgical exploration and drainage may be necessary if conservative measures are ineffective.

Direct nerve injuries may also occur from needle trauma during attempts at arterial cannulation. Many arteries are in close anatomic relation to nerves. For example, the median nerve is in proximity to the brachial artery, and the axillary artery lies within the brachial plexus sheath.

J. Late vascular complications

Traumatic arterial cannulation may result in partial disruption of the wall of an artery. This could eventually result in pseudoaneurysm formation. The wall of a pseudoaneurysm is composed of fibrous tissue that continues to expand. If a pseudoaneurysm ruptures into a vein, or if a vein and an artery are injured simultaneously, an arteriovenous fistula results. The treatment for these lesions is surgical repair.[43]

K. Inaccurate pressure readings

Despite the great advantages of intra-arterial monitoring, it does not always yield accurate pressure values. The monitoring system may be incorrectly zeroed in and calibrated, or the transducers may not be at the appropriate level. The wave form will be damped if the catheter is kinked, or partially thrombosed. This would lead to underestimation of the systolic pressure and overestimation of the diastolic pressure. The wave form will be amplified (underdamped) if the pressure tubing is too long or the natural frequency of the transducer system is too low. This would lead to overestimation of the systolic pressure and underestimation of the diastolic pressure.

In extremely vasoconstricted patients, the brachial and radial artery pressures may be significantly lower than the central aortic pressure. Another possible cause for inaccurate measurements is unsuspected arterial stenosis proximal to the arterial cannula, as occurs with thoracic outlet syndrome and subclavian stenosis. Raynaud's syndrome will also yield unreliable pressure readings from peripheral arteries.

Concomitant use of a noninvasive pressure measurement system will often aid in the recognition of incorrect invasive measurements. A cuff placed on the same arm as a brachial or radial artery catheter can be slowly deflated until the first systole is detected on the arterial waveform tracing. This gives a good indication of the systolic pressure and is a useful method for checking the accuracy of invasively measured pressure.

V. CENTRAL VENOUS PRESSURE MONITORING

A. Measurement system problems

Central venous pressure (CVP) catheters are used to measure the filling pressure of the right ventricle and to give an assessment of the intravascular volume and right ventricular function. The distal end of the catheter must lie within one of the large intrathoracic veins or the right atrium. Although water manometers have been used, an electronic system is preferred. It allows the observation of the right atrial wave form, which provides additional information. In any pressure-monitoring system, it is necessary to have a reproducible landmark (such as the midaxillary line) as a zero reference. This is especially important in venous monitoring because small changes in transducer height produce proportionately larger errors than in arterial monitoring.

B. Sites

Percutaneous central venous cannulation may be accomplished by catheter-through-the-needle, catheter-over-the-needle, or catheter-over-a-wire (Seldinger) techniques.[44] A modification of the Seldinger technique that is designed to minimize the risk of complications is described here.

The vein is located using a syringe attached to a small (22- to 25-gauge) "finder" needle. This reduces the risk of inadvertent arterial puncture and tissue trauma if localization of the vein is difficult. When venous blood is aspirated through the "finder" needle, the syringe and needle are withdrawn, leaving a small trail of blood on the drape to indicate the direction of the vein. An 18-gauge intravenous catheter (attached to a syringe) is then inserted in an identical fashion. When venous blood is aspirated freely into the syringe, the whole assembly is advanced an additional 1 to 2 mm until the tip of the catheter is within the lumen of the vein. The catheter is then threaded into the vein, and the syringe and needle are removed.

An empty syringe is attached to the cannula and a sample of blood is withdrawn. To confirm that an artery has not been inadvertently cannulated, it is essential to compare the color of the blood sample to an arterial sample drawn simultaneously. If this is inconclusive or there is no arterial catheter in place, the cannula may be attached to a transducer by sterile tubing for observation of the pressure wave form. Another option is to attach the cannula to sterile tubing and allow blood to flow retrogradely into the tubing. The tubing is then held upright as a venous manometer, and the height of the blood column is observed. If the catheter is in a vein, it will stop rising at a level consistent with the central venous pressure and demonstrate respiratory variation. A guide wire is then passed through the 18-gauge cannula, and the cannula is exchanged over the wire for a central venous pressure catheter.

The considerations for selecting the site of cannulation include the experience of the operator, ease of access, anatomic anomalies, and the ability of the patient to tolerate the position required for catheter insertion.

1. Internal jugular vein. The internal jugular vein is preferred by many anesthesiologists. It is a clean area that is easily accessible during most surgical procedures. The likelihood of cannulating the superior vena cava is very high with right internal jugular approach, because of the straight path that the catheter follows.[45] The technique is contraindicated in patients with previous neck surgery, neck tumors, and superior vena cava obstruction. If severe carotid occlusive disease is present, caution must be exercised when one is palpating for landmarks, so as not to dislodge an atheromatous plaque and cause a stroke.

2. External jugular vein. Although the external jugular vein is another, often tempting, means of reaching the central circulation, the success rate with this approach is lower because of the tortuous path followed by the vein. In addition, a valve is usually present at the point where the external jugular vein perforates the fascia to empty into the subclavian vein. However, a success rate of 90% was reported using a J-wire to slide past obstructions to the central circulation.[46] The main advantage of this technique is that there is no need to advance a needle into the deeper structures of the neck. Thus the risk of carotid puncture is negligible. There remains, however, the risk of external jugular or subclavian vein perforation if the wire is forced past obstructions, or a straight-tipped guide wire is utilized.

3. Subclavian vein. The subclavian vein is readily accessible from supraclavicular or infraclavicular approaches and is often used for central venous access.[47] The success rate is higher than the external jugular approach but lower than the right internal jugular approach. Cannulation of the subclavian vein is associated with a higher incidence of pneumothorax and hemothorax than the internal jugular approach. However, this may be the cannulation site of choice in head and neck surgery when central venous access is required. It is also useful for parenteral nutrition or for prolonged central venous pressure access because the site is easily dressed and well tolerated by patients.

The *infraclavicular approach* is performed with the patient in the Trendelenburg position with a folded sheet between the scapulas to increase the distance between the clavicle and the first rib. The needle should not be advanced too far posteriorly in order to avoid the pleura and the subclavian artery. The *supraclavicular approach* is performed with the patient in the Trendelenburg position with the head turned away from the side of the insertion. The vessel is very superficial (about 1 to 2 cm) and lies very close to the innominate artery and the pleura. These approaches are usually not performed on the left side because of the risk of a thoracic duct injury.

4. Antecubital veins. The basilic and cephalic veins provide another route for central venous cannulation. The advantages of this approach are the low likelihood of complications and the ease of access intraoperatively, if the arm is exposed. The major disadvantage is that it is often difficult to assure placement of the catheter in a central vein. Studies have indicated that blind advancement will result in central venous cannulation in 59% to 75% of attempts.[48,49] Unsuccessful attempts result most frequently from failure to pass the catheter past the shoulder, or cannulation of the ipsilateral internal jugular vein. Turning the head to the ipsilateral side may help prevent internal jugular placement of the catheter.[50]

Artru et al. have reported a high success rate (92%) for the placement of multiorificed catheters from the antecubital veins using intravascular electrocardiography.[51] These catheters are positioned at the superior vena cava–right atrium junction and are used for the aspiration of air emboli in neurosurgical patients.

5. Femoral vein. The femoral vein is rarely cannulated in the adult patient for monitoring purposes. However, cannulation of this vein is technically simple, and the success rate is high. Although older literature reported a high rate of catheter sepsis and thrombophlebitis with this approach,[52,53] this may no longer be valid with disposable catheter kits and improved catheter technology.

In patients with superior vena cava obstruction who require central venous monitoring, the femoral approach will be needed to obtain true central pressures. The catheter should be long so that the distal tip lies in the mediastinal segment of the inferior vena cava.

C. Contraindications

1. Absolute. Superior vena cava syndrome is a contraindication to the placement of a central venous pressure catheter in the neck, subclavian area, or the upper extremities. Venous pressures in the head and upper extremities are elevated by the superior vena cava obstruction and do not reflect right atrial pressure. In addition, the risk of hematoma formation is extremely high.

2. Relative. Whenever there is infection at the site of insertion, there is a high risk that the catheter will also become infected and become a source for sepsis.

Coagulopathy predisposes to hemorrhagic complications of central venous catheterization. Massive neck hematomas may cause tracheal obstruction, and resolving hematomas are prone to infection. An otherwise insignificant hemothorax caused by laceration of a vessel may become life threatening in the presence of a coagulopathy.

Newly inserted pacemaker wires may be dislodged or entangled during the insertion of central venous pressure catheters. This could result in a severe bradydysrhythmia (if the patient is pacemaker dependent) or right ventricular perforation and pericardial tamponade.

D. Complications

1. Arterial puncture. Inadvertent arterial puncture during central venous cannulation is reported to occur with an incidence of 1.9 to 3.6%.[54-56] The two reasons why this occurs are (1) that all the veins commonly used for cannulation lie in proximity to arteries (except the external jugular and cephalic) and (2) venous anatomy is quite variable. Localized hematoma formation is the usual consequence. This may be minimized if a small-gauge needle (such as 22 gauge) is used to localize the vein before cannulation with a larger needle or cannula.[57]

If the arterial puncture is large or direct pressure is not applied, or the patient has a coagulopathy, a massive hematoma may form. In the neck, this may lead to upper airway obstruction requiring tracheal intubation. In the arm or leg, venous obstruction may occur. Arteriovenous fistula is also a reported complication of central venous cannulation.[58] Pseudoaneurysm formation is also a possibility.

A particularly difficult clinical problem arises when large catheter introducers (such as 8.5 French) are inadvertently placed in the carotid or subclavian arteries. The large hole in the artery usually but not always closes with direct pressure when the introducer is simply removed. Consultation with a vascular surgeon is recommended, since there is the potential for massive hematoma formation with airway obstruction, hemothorax, or mediastinal hematoma. In some institutions, the introducer is removed by surgical cutdown, and the arterial puncture site is repaired.

Hemothorax is a potential complication if the subclavian artery is lacerated during cannulation attempts. The symptoms of hypovolemia will predominate because of the large volume necessary to fill the hemithorax. Hemothorax may also occur if an indwelling catheter erodes through a venous structure into the pleural cavity. Obviously, hypoxemia may accompany any hemothorax.

2. Pneumothorax. If the pleural cavity is entered and lung tissue is punctured during a cannulation attempt, a pneumothorax may result. Tension pneumothorax is possible if air continues to accumulate because of a "ball-valve" effect. Pneumothorax is most common with subclavian punctures and occurs only rarely with internal jugular cannulation.[59]

The treatment of pneumothorax depends on the hemodynamic status of the patient. If the patient is in shock with distended neck veins and a hyperresonant hemithorax, immediate therapy is indicated to relieve tension pneumothorax. A large-bore intravenous cannula may be placed through the second intercostal space in the midclavicular line into the thoracic cav-

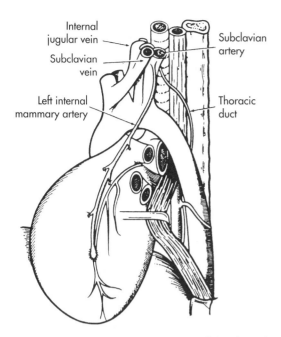

Internal
jugular vein

Subclavian
vein

Left internal
mammary artery

Subclavian
artery

Thoracic
duct

Fig. 2-3. The anatomic relationship of the thoracic duct to the left internal jugular and subclavian veins is diagramed. (From Di Lello F, Werner PH, Kleinman LH, et al: Ann Thorac Surg 44:660-661, 1987.)

ity. A rush of air will be detected, and the patient's clinical status will rapidly improve as the pressure within the hemithorax is relieved. Surgical consultation may then be obtained for placement of a chest (thoracostomy) tube.

3. Hydrothorax. If the catheter tip is placed extravascularly in the pleural cavity or erodes into this position, the fluid that is infused into the catheter will accumulate in the pleural cavity. The diagnosis is made by auscultation, percussion, and radiography of the chest. The treatment is discontinuation of the catheter and percutaneous pleurocentesis.

4. Chylothorax. Injury to the thoracic duct has been reported after left internal jugular and left subclavian venous cannulation.[60] This injury generally occurs near the insertion of the thoracic duct at the confluence of the left internal jugular and left subclavian veins (Fig. 2-3). Chylothorax then results from the accumulation of lymphatic drainage in the left hemithorax. The chylous leak often persists despite conservative management (chest tube drainage and low-fat diet). The consequences of a chronic chylothorax are nutritional depletion and possibly immunosuppression. This is a serious complication that may require surgical ligation of the thoracic duct for definitive treatment.[61] Fear of this complication is one of the major reasons for selecting the right side for internal

and subclavian cannulations whenever possible.[62]

5. Pericardial effusion and tamponade. If the right atrium or ventricle is perforated during central venous cannulation, pericardial effusion or tamponade may result. The likelihood of this complication is increased when inflexible guide wires or catheters are used. This complication has also been reported with the use of an indwelling polyethylene catheter.[63] Modern flexible catheters and J-tipped guide wires have made this a rarely reported complication.

The physiologic nature of fluid accumulation in the pericardial sac is such that sudden cardiovascular collapse occurs once a critical volume has been reached. This is explained by the compliance of the normal pericardium. The pressure is stable until the critical volume is reached and then rises steeply with any further increment in volume.

If pericardial tamponade is imminent, immediate pericardiocentesis is indicated. A long needle attached to a syringe is directed through the skin at the junction of the xyphoid process and the sternum on the left side and is directed toward the left shoulder. The needle is advanced while suction is maintained with the syringe until free-flowing blood is obtained. An ECG electrode will show injury current (ST-segment elevation) when the needle is within the pericardial sac. The withdrawal of small volumes of blood will result in considerable marked hemodynamic improvement because of the nature of the pericardial compliance.

6. Venous air embolism. Venous air embolism is a potentially fatal complication that can occur whenever there is negative pressure in the venous system that is open to the atmosphere. These conditions are met when patients are in the semiupright or sitting position, or generate a strong inspiratory effort. Patients with inspiratory airway obstruction (snoring) generate significant negative intrathoracic pressure and are at risk for air embolism during central venous cannulation. Paradoxical embolization is a risk if there is a patent foramen ovale or an atrial or ventricular septal defect.

During central venous cannulation, air embolism can usually be prevented with positional maneuvers, such as the Trendelenburg position, which increases the venous pressure in the vessel. Once the central venous catheter is placed, it is important to assure that the catheter is firmly attached to its connecting tubing. The complication may even occur after the catheter has been removed if the subcutaneous tract has failed to close.[64]

The diagnosis of venous air embolism is

likely when there is a sudden onset of tachycardia associated with pulmonary hypertension and systemic hypotension. A new murmur caused by turbulent flow in the right ventricular outflow tract may be heard. Two-dimensional echocardiography (transesophageal or transthoracic) and precordial Doppler probe monitoring are highly sensitive methods of detecting air embolism.

Venous air embolism is most effectively treated by aspiration of the air through a right atrial catheter. An older (and probably less effective) method involves turning the patient to the left lateral decubitus position to move the embolus out of the right ventricular outflow tract.

7. Particulate embolism. Catheter fragments may be sheared off and embolize to the right side of the heart and pulmonary circulation. This is especially likely when attempts are made to withdraw catheters through large-bore inserting needles but may also occur when needles are reinserted through intravenous cannulas, or guide wires are forced through kinked cannulas. Defective catheter manufacturing could also result in breakage and embolization. Paradoxical embolization is possible if systemic-pulmonary connections exist.

This problem can almost always be avoided using proper technique. A catheter must never be withdrawn through the inserting needle. During unsuccessful cannulation attempts, the needle and catheter must be withdrawn simultaneously. Reinsertion of needles into standard (catheter-over-the-needle) intravenous cannulas cannot be recommended but should certainly never be performed if the cannula is kinked or resistance is encountered. Similarly, guide wires should not be inserted through cannulas if blood return is not present, or forcefully inserted if resistance is encountered. The catheter-fragment position within the circulation will determine whether surgery or percutaneous techniques are necessary for its removal.[65]

8. Nerve injury. The brachial plexus, stellate ganglion, and phrenic nerve all lie in proximity to the internal jugular vein. These nerves may be injured during cannulation attempts. Paresthesias of the brachial plexus are not uncommonly obtained during attempts to localize the internal jugular vein. Horner's syndrome has been reported after internal jugular cannulation.[66]

Direct needle trauma is the most likely cause of paresthesias or motor deficits, and this risk is somewhat increased by the long-beveled needles used for vascular access.[67] Transient deficits may result from the deposition of local anesthetic in the brachial plexus, stellate ganglion, cervical plexus, and so forth. A large hematoma might also cause nerve injury if an inadvertent arterial puncture occurred, or if a coagulopathy were present.

9. Dysrhythmias. Transient atrial or ventricular dysrhythmias occur commonly as the guide wire is passed into the right atrium or ventricle during central venous cannulation using the Seldinger technique. This most likely results from the relatively inflexible guide wire causing extrasystoles as it contacts the endocardium. A case of ventricular fibrillation during guide-wire insertion has been reported.[68] The same authors reported a 70% reduction in the incidence of dysrhythmias when guide-wire insertion was limited to 22 cm.

There is a recent report of complete heart block caused by guide-wire insertion during central venous cannulation.[69] This case was successfully managed using a temporary transvenous pacemaker. This complication has previously been reported with right-sided heart and pulmonary artery catheterization (see p. 27). The problem most likely resulted from excessive insertion of the guide wire, with impingement of the wire in the region of the right bundle branch. It is recommended that the length of guide-wire insertion be limited to the length necessary to reach the superior vena cava–right atrial junction to avoid these complications.

VI. PULMONARY ARTERY MONITORING

A. Measurement system problems

Flow-directed pulmonary artery catheters (PAC) have been a major advance in the monitoring of patients during the perioperative period. Unfortunately a new set of complications related to this form of monitoring has become prevalent since the introduction of PACs in the 1970s.[70] Although the present older, more diseased population is likely to benefit from this "quantum leap" in monitoring, an effort must be made to reduce the morbidity and potential mortality from complications related to the technique.

Specific information that can be gathered with the PAC includes pulmonary artery systolic pressure (PASP), pulmonary artery diastolic pressure (PADP), mean pulmonary arterial pressure (MPAP), pulmonary capillary wedge pressure (PCWP), mixed venous blood gases, and cardiac output by thermodilution. Special purpose PACs for continuous mixed venous oximetry, pacing, and thermodilution right ventricular ejection fraction are also available.

The reason for measuring PCWP and PADP

is that they are estimates of left atrial pressure, which, in turn, is an estimate of left ventricular end-diastolic pressure (LVEDP). However, the PCW and PAD pressures will not accurately measure LVEDP in the presence of pulmonary vascular disease, positive end-expiratory pressure,[71] or mitral valvular disease.[72]

Left ventricular end-diastolic pressure is an index of left ventricular end-diastolic volume, or left ventricular preload.[73] The relationship between left ventricular end-diastolic pressure and end-diastolic volume is described by the left ventricular compliance curve. This curve is nonlinear and is affected by many factors, such as ventricular hypertrophy and myocardial ischemia.[74,75]

The patency of vascular channels between the distal port of the PAC and the left atrium is necessary to ensure a close relationship between the PCWP and left atrial pressure. This condition is met only in the dependent portions of the lung (West's zone III), where the pulmonary venous pressure exceeds the alveolar pressure.[76] Otherwise the PCWP will reflect the alveolar pressure, not the left atrial pressure. Since positive end-expiratory pressure decreases the size of West's zone III, it has been shown to adversely affect the correlation between PCWP and left atrial pressures.[77] Interestingly, ARDS seems to prevent the transmission of increased alveolar pressure to the pulmonary interstitium. This preserves the relationship between PCWP and left ventricular end-diastolic pressure during the application of positive end-expiratory pressure.[78]

B. Sites

The considerations for avoiding complications during the insertion PACs are the same as for CVP catheters (discussed on pp. 23 and 24). The right internal jugular approach remains the easiest because of the direct path between this vessel and the right atrium.

C. Flotation of the catheter

Passage of the PAC from the vessel introducer to the pulmonary artery can be accomplished by monitoring of the pressure wave form from the distal port of the catheter, or under fluoroscopic guidance. Wave-form monitoring is the more common technique for perioperative insertions. After the catheter tip has been advanced 15 to 20 cm through the vessel introducer, the balloon is inflated to facilitate the catheter's progress in the bloodstream.

The right atrial (RA) wave form is seen until the catheter tip crosses the tricuspid valve and enters the right ventricle. In the right ventricle, there is a sudden increase in systolic pressure but little change in diastolic pressure compared to the RA tracing. Dysrhythmias, particularly premature ventricle complexes, usually occur at this point but almost always resolve without treatment once the catheter tip has crossed the pulmonic valve. The catheter is advanced rapidly through the right ventricle toward the pulmonary artery. Slight reverse Trendelenburg position and right lateral tilt facilitate passage of the catheter through the right ventricular cavity (see below).

As the catheter crosses the pulmonic valve, a dicrotic notch appears in the pressure wave form, and there is a sudden increase in diastolic pressure. One obtains the pulmonary capillary wedge tracing by passing the catheter (approximately 3 to 5 cm) farther until there is a change in the wave form associated with a drop in the measured mean pressure. Deflation of the balloon results in reappearance of the pulmonary arterial wave form and an increase in the mean pressure value.

D. Contraindications

One unresolved issue is whether PAC monitoring improves outcome in critically ill patients. Several studies support the concept that PAC monitoring improves patient outcome because of improved management of alterations in cardiovascular status.[79,80] However, a large prospective study of patients undergoing elective coronary artery surgery did not identify differences in outcome between the CVP and the PAC monitoring groups.[81]

The indications for pulmonary artery catheterization in the perioperative period remain controversial and vary in different institutions. Contraindications to the use of a PAC include the following.

1. Absolute. In the presence of significant tricuspid or pulmonic valvular stenosis it is unlikely that a PAC would be able to cross the valve, and it would worsen the obstruction to flow if it did. Right atrial or right ventricular masses (that is, tumor, thrombus) or a part thereof can be dislodged by a PAC, causing pulmonary or paradoxical embolization. In patients with tetralogy of Fallot the right ventricular outflow tract is hypersensitive to pressure or touch and a PAC might induce a hypercyanotic episode because of "infundibular spasm."

2. Relative. Transient atrial and ventricular dysrhythmias are common during PAC placement in normal patients. The risk of inducing a dysrhythmia in a patient prone to malignant dysrhythmias must be weighed against the potential benefits of the information gained from PAC monitoring.

Coagulopathy is a relative contraindication to PAC insertion for the same reason it is to central venous access (see p. 24).

Finally, newly inserted pacemaker wires may be displaced by the catheter during insertion or withdrawal.

E. Complications

The complications associated with PAC placement include almost all those detailed in the section on CVP placement (see above). The only exception is atrial or ventricular perforation, which has never been reported with balloon-tipped catheters. Additional complications that are unique to the PAC are detailed here.

1. Dysrhythmias. The most common complication associated with PAC insertion is transient dysrhythmias, especially premature ventricular contractions (PVCs).[54] However, fatal dysrhythmias have also been rarely reported.[82] Intravenous lidocaine has been used in attempts to suppress these dysrhythmias with mixed results.[83,84] However, a positional maneuver entailing 5-degree head up and right lateral tilt was associated with a statistically significant decrease in malignant dysrhythmias (compared to the Trendelenburg position) during PAC insertion.[85]

2. Complete heart block. Complete heart block may develop during pulmonary artery catheterization in patients with preexisting left bundle-branch block.[86,87] This potentially fatal complication is most likely attributable to pressure from the catheter tip causing transient right bundle-branch block as it passes through the right ventricular outflow tract. The incidence of developing right bundle-branch block was 3% in a prospective series of patients undergoing pulmonary artery catheterization.[88] However, none of the patients with preexisting left bundle-branch block developed complete heart block in that series. In another study of 47 patients with left bundle-branch block, there were two cases of complete heart block but only in patients with recent onset of left bundle-branch block.[89] It is imperative to have an external pacemaker immediately available or to use a pacing catheter when placing a PAC in patients with left bundle-branch block.

3. Endobronchial hemorrhage. Iatrogenic rupture of the pulmonary artery (PA) with endobronchial hemorrhage has become more common, since the advent of PAC monitoring in the intensive care unit and the operating room. Over thirty cases have been recorded in the medical literature.[90] The incidence of PA-induced endobronchial hemorrhage is 0.064% to 0.20%.[91,92] Hannan et al. reported a 46% mortality in a review of 28 cases of PA-induced endobronchial hemorrhage, but the mortality was 75% in the anticoagulated patients.[93] Out of these reports, several risk factors have emerged: advanced age, female sex, pulmonary hypertension, mitral stenosis, coagulopathy, distal placement of the catheter, and balloon hyperinflation.

It is important to consider the cause of the hemorrhage when one is forming a therapeutic plan. If the hemorrhage is minimal and a coagulopathy coexists, correction of the coagulopathy may be the only necessary therapy. Protection of the uninvolved lung is of prime importance. Tilting the patient toward the affected side and performing an endobronchial intubation are maneuvers for protecting the contralateral lung.[94] Strategies proposed to stop the hemorrhage include the application of positive end-expiratory pressure, placement of bronchial blockers, rigid or flexible bronchoscopy, injection of clotted blood through the PAC, hyperinflation of the PAC balloon, and pulmonary resection.[95]

The clinician is obviously at a disadvantage unless the site of hemorrhage is known. A chest roentgenogram will usually indicate the general location of the lesion (Fig. 2-4). A small amount of radiographic contrast dye may help to pinpoint the lesion if active hemorrhage is present. Although the cause of endobronchial hemorrhage may be unclear, the bleeding site must be unequivocally located before surgical treatment is attempted.

4. Pulmonary infarction. This is currently a rare complication of PAC monitoring. An early report suggested that there was a 7.2% incidence of pulmonary infarction with PAC use.[96] However, continuously monitoring the pulmonary arterial wave form and keeping the balloon deflated when not determining the PCWP (to prevent inadvertent wedging of the catheter) were not standard practice at that time. Distal migration of PACs may also occur intraoperatively because of the action of the right ventricle. Inadvertent catheter wedging occurs during cardiopulmonary bypass because of the diminished right ventricular chamber size. Embolization of thrombus formed on a PAC could also result in pulmonary infarction.

5. Catheter knotting. Knotting of a PAC usually occurs as a result of coiling of the catheter within the right ventricle. Insertion of an appropriately sized guide wire under fluoroscopic guidance may aid in unknotting the catheter.[97] Alternatively the knot may be tight-

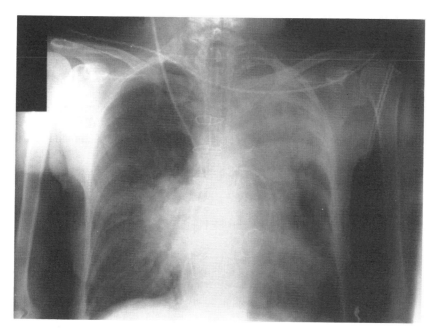

Fig. 2-4. A case of endobronchial hemorrhage caused by catheter-induced pulmonary artery rupture. A left-sided double-lumen endotracheal tube has been placed to protect the uninvolved lung.

ened and withdrawn percutaneously along with the introducer if no intracardiac structures are entangled.[98] If cardiac structures, such as the papillary muscles, are entangled in the knotted catheter, surgical intervention may be required.

6. Valvular damage. Withdrawal of the catheter with the balloon inflated may result in injury to the tricuspid[99] or pulmonic valves.[100] Septic endocarditis has also resulted from an indwelling PAC.[101]

7. Thrombocytopenia. Mild thrombocytopenia has been reported in dogs and humans with indwelling PACs.[102] This probably results from increased platelet consumption. Heparin-coated PACs might trigger the rare disease of heparin-induced thrombocytopenia, though this has not yet been reported. This disease has a high morbidity and mortality and is probably attributable to an autoimmune response to heparin that results in thrombotic events and thrombocytopenia caused by increased platelet consumption.[103]

8. Incorrect placement. The catheter may pass through an interatrial or interventricular communication into the left side of the heart. It is then possible for the catheter to enter the aorta through the left ventricular outflow tract. A similar complication has been reported where the catheter crossed a surgically repaired tear in the superior vena cava into the left side of the heart.[104] This complication should be recognized by the similarity between the "pulmonary artery" and systemic arterial wave forms.

9. Catheter electrode detachment. The multipurpose PAC (Pacing TD Catheter, American Edwards Laboratories, Santa Ana, California) contains five electrodes for bipolar atrial, ventricular, or AV sequential pacing. With appropriate filtering, the catheter may also be used for the recording of an intracardiac ECG. The intraoperative success rate for atrial, ventricular, and AV sequential capture have been reported as 80%, 93%, and 73% respectively.[105] Electrode detachment has been reported twice with the multipurpose catheter: with prolonged placement (60 hours)[106] and during catheter withdrawal.[107]

10. Ventricular perforation risk (Paceport pacing wires). The thin wires using for endocardial atrial and ventricular pacing in the Paceport PAC are relatively rigid. If the PAC were to move distally, as occurs during balloon inflation, the wire could perforate the right atrium or ventricle. Although this has not yet been reported, it is recommended not to insert the PAC further or inflate the balloon once the pacing wire or wires have been passed into the atrium or ventricle.

VII. DETERMINATION OF CARDIAC OUTPUT

A. Fick method

The major limitations of the direct Fick technique are related to errors in sampling and analysis or to the inability to maintain steady-state hemodynamic and respiratory conditions.[108,109] To minimize errors in sampling, one must ascertain that the venous blood is truly mixed venous blood and that the samples represent average rather than instantaneous samples.

The most serious errors in the measurement of cardiac output by the direct Fick technique result from changes in pulmonary volumes. Indeed, the methods used to measure oxygen consumption, measure the uptake of oxygen by the lungs $(F_IO_2 - F_EO_2)\dot{V}_E$, rather than by the blood. Since lung volumes can change, the tissues' oxygen consumption is not necessarily being measured. The use of calculated values for oxygen consumption is also fraught with errors, as recently demonstrated by Kendrick et al.[110] They noted that differences between measured and assumed oxygen values were often greater than 25% in either direction.

With the widespread availability of mass spectrometry, several investigators have attempted to continuously measure cardiac output by means of the Fick principle.[111-116] In comparisons with the thermodilution technique, good correlations have usually been obtained. In some studies, the reproducibility of the measurements was found to be better for Fick than for thermodilution.

B. Mixed venous oxygen saturation

The addition of fiberoptic bundles to pulmonary artery catheters has enabled the continuous monitoring of mixed venous oxygen saturation using reflectance spectrophotometry. The catheter is connected to a device that includes a light-emitting diode and a sensor to detect the light returning from the pulmonary artery. Mixed venous oxygen saturation is calculated from the differential absorption of various wavelengths of light by the saturated and desaturated hemoglobin.[117]

In vivo, continuous monitoring of mixed oxygen saturation has been complicated by artifacts attributable to the vessel wall, clot formation on the catheter with loss of light intensity, and varying hematocrit. Getting et al.[118] demonstrated that a three-wavelength system (Opticath, Oximetrix Inc., Mountain View, California) is more accurate than a two-wavelength system (Swan-Ganz, American Edwards Laboratories, Santa Ana, California). Reinhart et al. investigated the accuracy and mechanical dependability of both systems during long-term use in critically ill patients.[119] They noted that values obtained with either system showed similar correlations with in vitro mixed venous oxygen saturation measurements.

C. Thermodilution

The use of thermal indicator has eliminated some but not all of the limitations associated with dye cardiac outputs. Handling of the indicator is undoubtedly easier with thermal than with dye indicator. The computer calibration procedures are greatly simplified and blood withdrawal is not necessary. Some common problems, however, remain. Extrapolation of the tail end of the time-concentration curve remains essential. Various manufacturers have handled this problem differently and inconsistencies can sometimes be observed when substituting one cardiac output computer for another.[120]

Pulmonary artery catheterization is not without problems, and, as seen above, the list of reported complications is long. Additionally the determination of cardiac output remains intermittent, and frequent measurements could lead to fluid overload. Complications have also been attributed to the rapid injection of cold indicator into the right atrium. Slowing of the heart rate was described by Nishikawa.[121] In a prospective study, Harris et al. observed that with the use of iced injectate a decrease in heart rate of more than 10% occurred in 22% of the determinations.[122] Recently, Nishikawa et al. have reported that heart-rate slowing was more likely in patients with low cardiac index, low mean pulmonary artery pressure, and high systemic vascular resistance.[123]

Thermodilution cardiac output determination requires the frequent injection of boluses of room temperature or iced solution. As injectate syringes are refilled and reconnected to the injectate port, small bubbles are introduced, especially at stopcocks. Echocardiography and precordial Doppler probe scanning usually reveal a shower of air emboli during injections. Although the majority of patients tolerate these emboli with no sequelae, approximately 1 in 20 patients has a patent foramen ovale. Thus there is a risk of paradoxical air embolism with systemic infarction in this subset of patients.

D. Pulmonary artery Doppler probe

A newly developed pulmonary artery catheter that incorporates an ultrasonic transducer has been developed. The catheter is curved in such a way as to maintain contact with the wall of the pulmonary artery. Using the Doppler principle, instantaneous stroke volume is calculated from the mean velocity of blood flow in the main pulmonary artery.[124] The accuracy of this technique was favorable compared to an electromagnetic flow probe when tested in a bench model and an in vivo animal model.

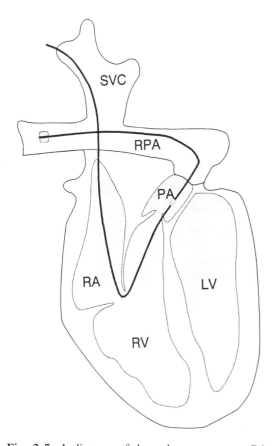

Fig. 2-5. A diagram of the pulmonary artery, *PA,* catheter modified for continuous Doppler cardiac output determination. Notice the sharp curvature of the catheter necessary to maintain the Doppler transducers laterally within the main pulmonary artery. The catheter is straightened and stiffened for insertion using a wire (not shown). The text describes potential complications that could occur with this catheter design. *LV,* left ventricle; *RA,* right atrium; *RPA,* right pulmonary artery; *RV,* right ventricle; *SVC,* superior vena cava.

The practicality of this device in clinical management remains to be proved. The higher degree of accuracy (if it holds up in clinical studies) is unlikely to result in changes in clinical management, and the additional cost may be prohibitive. However, the potential for research applications, such as investigations of right ventricular function and pulmonary vascular impedance, is promising.[125]

The potential complications of this device are related to its design. The relatively sharp curve of the catheter holds it laterally within the main pulmonary artery (Fig. 2-5). If the catheter is present for prolonged periods, contact with the wall of the pulmonary artery might erode through the vessel. The insertion of the catheter is facilitated using a straightening wire that presumably gives the catheter additional stiffness. The added stiffness could increase the risk of atrial, ventricular, or pulmonary artery perforation. In addition, the piezoelectric crystals could potentially become loose and be dislodged from the catheter.

E. Transtracheal Doppler probe

Preliminary work in a canine model has shown that Doppler cardiac output may be determined transtracheally. The equipment consists of a 5 mm ultrasonic transducer bonded to the distal end of an endotracheal tube. The shape of the cuff is ellipsoidal to ensure contact between the transducer and the anterolateral wall of the trachea (Fig. 2-6). The technique correlated well ($r^2 = 0.82$) with thermodilution cardiac output determinations.[126]

The technique is similar to transesophageal Doppler techniques in that the calculation of cardiac output is based on approximations of

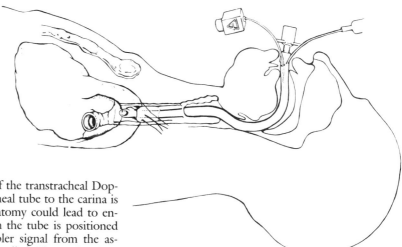

Fig. 2-6. The relationship of the transtracheal Doppler cardiac output endotracheal tube to the carina is diagramed. Variations in anatomy could lead to endobronchial intubation when the tube is positioned to obtain the optimal Doppler signal from the ascending aorta. (Courtesy Applied Biometrics, Inc, Minnetonka, Minn, 1990.)

the aortic area and the angle of incidence between the ultrasound beam and the transverse plane of the aorta. Theoretical advantages of this method over the transesophageal approach include measurement of blood flow in the ascending aorta (proximal to the arch vessels) and a more constant anatomic relationship between the trachea and the ascending aorta.

Potential complications include the potential for compromising ventilation (by endobronchial intubation) during positioning of the ultrasonic probe. It is also possible that the probe (which protrudes slightly) might damage airway structures, such as the larynx or carina.

F. Thoracic bioimpedance

It is questionable whether the accuracy of thoracic bioimpedance is adequate to justify its use as a clinical monitor of cardiac output. The potential problems with this monitor are similar to ECG monitoring. A macroshock hazard is created by the multiple electrical connections. These connections could also potentially result in a burn if grounding of unipolar electrocautery occurred.

G. Transesophageal echocardiography and Doppler probes

Although transesophageal echocardiography (TEE) and Doppler probe insertions have been performed in many thousands of patients, there are remarkably few reports of complications. The risks of intraoperative transesophageal echo and Doppler probing should theoretically be higher than that for awake transesophageal echo or upper gastrointestinal endoscopy because (1) the patient cannot indicate discomfort, (2) the duration of monitoring is lengthy, and (3) the probe is not guided endoscopically.

Potential complications include damage to pharyngeal, laryngeal, esophageal, and gastric structures, resulting in perforation, laceration, abrasion, or hemorrhage. Additional risks include internal burns and microshock. O'Shea et al. evaluated the effects of transesophageal echo in animals by excising the entire esophagus after variable durations of continuous TEE use.[127] They observed no significant mucosal or thermal injuries. In a human study, 5 of 6 patients had low contact pressure between the transducer and the esophagus, but 1 patient had a greatly elevated (>60 mm Hg) contact pressure.[128]

Vocal cord paresis has been attributed to intraoperative transesophageal echocardiography in 2 patients who were undergoing craniotomies in the sitting position with considerable cervical flexion.[129] A recent case report described a Mallory-Weiss tear caused by transesophageal echo in an elderly female undergoing elective aortic valve replacement.[130] The resultant bleeding resolved spontaneously with correction of a coagulopathy, and the diagnosis was confirmed by endoscopy. Humphrey[131] described a patient in whom manipulations of the transesophageal transducer led to the undetected displacement of an esophageal stethoscope into the stomach. The missing stethoscope was discovered several weeks later and was removed endoscopically.

Certain principles should be followed to decrease the already low rate of complications from transesophageal echo. The probe should be well-lubricated before introduction and positioning. The tip of the probe should not be flexed or extended (retroflexed) for prolonged periods of time or forcefully manipulated at any time. The probe should remain in the neutral position during cardiopulmonary bypass because high-pressure contact in the presence of a low tissue-perfusion pressure may result in tissue necrosis and ulceration. This form of monitoring should be avoided in patients with esophageal pathosis, such as achalasia, strictures, and varices.

The short-axis view of the left ventricle is actually a transgastric view. Thus it is reasonable to weigh the potential risks versus the benefits of transesophageal echo in patients with a gastric pathosis. Transesophageal echo is usually avoided in patients with severe hiatal hernia because the image quality is often poor.

The rate of complications associated with transesophageal continuous-wave Doppler cardiac output probes should be somewhat less than that associated with echo probes. The continuous-wave Doppler probes do not flex or extend, and this probably prevents the probe from exerting excessive pressure on the esophageal mucosa.

1. Incorrect interpretation. The complications related to the mechanical aspects of transesophageal echocardiography have fortunately been very minimal. However, the complications related to incorrect interpretation have not yet been evaluated. These could be of much greater magnitude as echocardiography assumes a greater role in guiding anesthetic and surgical management. A series of recent reports have highlighted some of the difficulties and technical limitations that may be encountered when using Doppler color flow technology to assess valvular function.

Stevenson has demonstrated that gain setting, pulse-repetition frequency, and carrier frequency significantly affected the size of regurgitant valve lesions.[132] Findings by Yoshida et al. have suggested that with the introduction of highly sensitive techniques like Doppler color flow mapping, the limits of normality may need to be redefined.[133] These investigators examined valvular function with transthoracic Doppler color flow mapping in 211 apparently healthy volunteers. In their normal subjects the prevalence of mitral regurgitation was 38% to 45%, of tricuspid regurgitation was 15% to 77%, and of pulmonary regurgitation 28% to 88%. Regurgitant flow signals were never detected at the aortic valve. In an accompanying editorial, Sahn and Maciel discussed the clinical implications of these observations.[134] They also indicated that the esophageal echo window significantly increases the sensitivity of Doppler color flow mapping for intracardiac flow events. If transesophageal echocardiography is used as a gold standard, the incidence of detectable valve regurgitation in healthy subjects will become substantially higher.

Although wall-motion abnormalities are sensitive indicators of myocardial ischemia,[135] their specificity and predictive value are less certain.[136] In a study of 156 high-risk patients, 20% developed new or worsened segmental wall-motion abnormalities.[137] However, these episodes correlated poorly with electrocardiographic changes and postoperative cardiac events. There are also difficulties with on-line echo image interpretation and interobserver variability. Thus there is the potential for altering anesthetic or surgical management inappropriately based on erroneous echo interpretation.

VIII. COMPLICATIONS OF CARDIOVERSION
A. Dysrhythmias

Cardioversion is undertaken to convert supraventricular or ventricular tachydysrhythmias or atrial fibrillation to normal sinus rhythm. The key differences between cardioversion and defibrillation are that the energy delivered is usually lower and the shock is synchronized to the QRS complex (in cardioversion). The synchronization is performed so that depolarization does not occur during the vulnerable period of repolarization, the "R-on-T" phenomenon.

The most common complications of cardioversion are dysrhythmias, such as ventricular ectopic beats, ventricular tachycardia, and ventricular fibrillation. Predisposing factors include digitalis toxicity and electrolyte abnormalities (potassium depletion). The treatment of choice is repeat cardioversion or defibrillation. Artifact or low quality of the ECG signal used for cardioversion might cause the shock to be initiated during the vulnerable period.

B. Airway complications

Cardioversion is usually performed as an emergent or semiemergent procedure in critically ill patients. A full stomach is often present, and the cardioversion is usually not performed in a location with ideal airway management equipment.

Thus it is critical to assess the potential for airway obstruction, regurgitation, and aspiration of gastric contents in any cardioversion patient. In the presence of a full stomach, benzodiazepine sedation is acceptable, but general anesthesia should not be induced. Despite this precaution, unsuccessful cardioversion may result in severe hypotension and loss of consciousness. Thus suction and appropriate airway management equipment must be prepared.

C. Burns

Large amounts of conductive gel or saline-soaked gauze are utilized to deliver the shock to the chest wall. Inadequate electrical contact results in arcing and skin burns. If multiple high-energy (>200 joules) shocks are required, skeletal and myocardial cell injury will also occur.

D. Electrical hazards to health care personnel

Health care personnel attending the cardioversion or defibrillation patient are at risk of macroshock. No physical contact with the patient or the patient's bed or stretcher should occur during the shock. The person delivering the shock should give a verbal warning before the discharge to prevent injury to others.

REFERENCES

1. Katcher ML and Shapiro MM: Severe burns and death associated with electronic monitors, N Engl J Med 317:56, 1987 [letter].
2. NFPA no 76C. High frequency electricity in health care facilities, Quincy, Mass, 1975, National Fire Protection Association.
3. Sy WP: Ulnar nerve palsy related to use of automatically cycled blood pressure cuff, Anesth Analg 60:687, 1981.
4. Mozersky DJ, Buckley CJ, Hagood C, et al: Ultrasonic evaluation of the palmar circulation, Am J Surg 126:810-812, 1973.
5. Allen EV: Thromboangiitis obliterans: methods of diagnosis of chronic occlusive arterial lesions distal to the wrist with illustrated cases, Am J Med Sci 178:237-244, 1929.
6. Greenhow DE: Incorrect performance of Allen's test: ulnar artery flow erroneously presumed inadequate, Anesthesiology 37:356-357, 1972.
7. Brodsky JB: A simple method to determine patency of the ulnar artery intraoperatively prior to radial artery cannulation, Anesthesiology 42:626-627, 1975.

8. Nowak GS, Moorthy SS, and McNiece WL: Use of pulse oximetry for assessment of collateral arterial flow, Anesthesiology 64:527, 1986 [letter].

9. Slogoff S, Keats AS, and Arlund C: On the safety of radial artery cannulation, Anesthesiology 59:42-47, 1983.

10. Mangano DT and Hickey RF: Ischemic injury following uncomplicated radial artery catheterization, Anesth Analg 58:55-57, 1979.

11. Barnes RW, Foster E, Jansen GA, et al: Safety of brachial artery catheters as monitors in the intensive care unit: prospective evaluation with the Doppler ultrasonic velocity detector, Anesthesiology 44:260-264, 1976.

12. Pascarelli EF and Bertrand CA: Comparison of blood pressures in the arms and legs, N Engl J Med 270:693-698, 1964.

13. Bazaral MG, Welch M, Golding LAR, and Badhwar K: Comparison of brachial and radial arterial pressure monitoring in patients undergoing coronary artery bypass surgery, Anesthesiology 73:38-45, 1990.

14. Barnes RW, Foster EJ, Janssen GA, and Boutros AR: Safety of brachial arterial catheters as monitors in the intensive care unit: prospective evaluation with the Doppler ultrasonic velocity detector, Anesthesiology 44:260-264, 1976.

15. Gravlee GP, Wong AB, Adkins TG, et al: Comparison of radial, brachial, and aortic pressures after cardiopulmonary bypass, J Cardiothoracic Anesth 3:20-26, 1989.

16. Gurman GM and Kriemerman S: Cannulation of big arteries in critically ill patients, Crit Care Med 13:217-220, 1985.

17. Yacoub OF, Bacaling JH, and Kelly M: Monitoring of axillary arterial pressure in a patient with Buerger's disease requiring clipping of an intracranial aneurysm, Br J Anaesth 59:1056-1058, 1987.

18. Eriksson I and Jorulf H: Surgical complications associated with arterial catheterization, Scand J Thorac Cardiovasc Surg 4:69, 1970.

19. Bedford RF: Invasive blood pressure monitoring. In Blitt CD, editor: Monitoring in anesthesia and critical care medicine, New York, 1989, Churchill Livingstone.

20. Youngberg JA and Miller ED: Evaluation of percutaneous cannulations of the dorsalis pedis artery, Anesthesiology 44:80, 1976.

21. Husum B, Palm T and Eriksen J: Percutaneous cannulation of the dorsalis pedis artery, Br J Anaesth 51:1055, 1979.

22. Prian GW: New proximal approach works well in temporal artery catheterization, JAMA 235:2693-2694, 1976.

23. Porter JM: Raynaud's syndrome. In Sabiston DC, editor: Textbook of surgery, Philadelphia, 1985, WB Saunders.

24. Band JD and Maki DG: Infection caused by arterial catheters used for hemodynamic monitoring, Am J Med 67:735-741, 1979.

25. Shinozaki T, Deane R, Mazuzan JE, et al: Bacterial contamination of arterial lines: a prospective study, JAMA 249:223-225, 1983.

26. Weinstein RA, Stamm WE, and Kramer L: Pressure monitoring devices: overlooked sources of nosocomial infection, JAMA 236:936-938, 1976.

27. Pierson DJ and Hudson LD: Monitoring hemodynamics in the critically ill, Med Clin North Am 67:1343-1360, 1983.

28. Bedford RF and Wollman H: Complications of percutaneous radial-artery cannulation: an objective prospective study in man, Anesthesiology 38:228-236, 1973.

29. Bedford RF: Radial arterial function following percutaneous cannulation with 18- and 20-gauge catheters, Anesthesiology 47:37-39, 1977.

30. Bedford RF: Wrist circumference predicts the risk of radial-arterial occlusion after cannulation, Anesthesiology 48:377-378, 1978.

31. Davis FM and Steward JM: Radial artery cannulation, BR J Anaesth 52:674-684, 1980.

32. Downs JB, Rackstein AD, Klein EF, and Hawkins IF: Hazards of radial-artery catheterization, Anesthesiology 38:283-286, 1973.

33. Jones RM, Hill AB, Nahrwold ML, and Bolles RE: The effect of method of radial artery cannulation on postcannulation blood flow and thrombus formation, Anesthesiology 55:76-78, 1981.

34. Bedford RF and Ashford TP: Aspirin pretreatment prevents post-cannulation radial-artery thrombosis, Anesthesiology 51:176-178, 1979.

35. Bedford RF: Removal of radial-artery thrombi following percutaneous cannulation for monitoring, Anesthesiology 46:430-432, 1977.

36. Bedford RF and Wollman H: Complications of percutaneous radial-artery cannulation: an objective prospective study in man, Anesthesiology 38:228-236, 1973.

37. Kim JM, Arakawa K, and Bliss J: Arterial cannulation: factors in the development of occlusion, Anesth Analg 54:836-841, 1975.

38. Vender JS and Watts RD: Differential diagnosis of hand ischemia in the presence of an arterial cannula, Anesth Analg 61:465-468, 1982.

39. Chang C, Dughi J, Shitabata P, et al: Air embolism and the radial arterial line, Crit Care Med 16:141-143, 1988.

40. Lowenstein E, Little JW, and Lo HH: Prevention of cerebral embolization from flushing radial artery cannulae, N Engl J Med 285:1414-1415, 1971.

41. Goldstein RD and Gordon MJV: Volar proximal skin necrosis after radial artery cannulation, NY State J Med 90:375-376, 1990.

42. Wyatt R, Glaves I, and Cooper DJ: Proximal skin necrosis after radial-artery cannulation, Lancet 1:1135-1138, 1974.

43. Freeark RJ and Baker WH: Arterial Injuries. In Sabiston DC, editor: Textbook of surgery, Philadelphia, 1986, WB Saunders.

44. Kaplan JA: Hemodynamic monitoring. In Kaplan JA, editor: Cardiac anesthesia, ed 2, Philadelphia, 1987, Grune & Stratton.

45. English IC, Frew RM, Pigott JF, et al: Percutaneous catheterization of the internal jugular vein, Anaesthesia 24:521-531, 1969.

46. Blitt CD, Wright WA, Petty WC, et al: Cardiovascular catheterization via the external jugular vein: a technique employing the J-wire, JAMA 229:817-818, 1974.

47. Defalque RJ: Subclavian venipuncture: a review, Anesth Analg 47:677-682, 1968.

48. Kellner GA and Smart JF: Percutaneous placement of catheters to monitor "central venous pressure," Anesthesiology 36:515-516, 1972.

49. Webre DR and Arens JF: Use of cephalic and basilic veins for introduction of cardiovascular catheters, Anesthesiology 38:389-392, 1973.

50. Burgess GE, Marino RJ, and Peuler MJ: Effect of head position on the location of venous catheters inserted via the basilic vein, Anesthesiology 46:212-213, 1977.

51. Artru AA and Colley PS: Placement of multiorificed CVP catheters via antecubital veins using intravascular electrocardiography, Anesthesiology 69:132, 1988.

52. Burri C and Ahnefeld FW: The caval catheter, Berlin, 1978, Springer-Verlag.
53. Bansmer G, Keith D, and Tesluk H: Complications following the use of indwelling catheters of the inferior vena cava, JAMA 167:1606-1611, 1958.
54. Shah KB, Rao TLK, Laughlin S, and El-Etr AA: A review of pulmonary artery catheterization in 6245 patients, Anesthesiology 61:271-275, 1984.
55. Davies MJ, Cronin KD, and Domaingue CM: Pulmonary artery catheterization: an assessment of risks and benefits in 220 surgical patients, Anaesth Intensive Care 10:9, 1982.
56. Sise MJ, Hollingworth P, Brimm JE, et al: Complications of the flow-directed pulmonary-artery catheter: a prospective analysis in 219 patients, Crit Care Med 9:315, 1981.
57. Jobes DR, Schwartz AJ, Greenhow DE, et al: Safer jugular vein cannulation: recognition of arterial puncture, Anesthesiology 59:353-355, 1983.
58. Ortiz J, Dean WF, Zumbro GL, et al: Arteriovenous fistula as a complication of percutaneous internal jugular vein catheterization, Milit Med 141:171, 1976.
59. Cook TL and Deuker CW: Tension pneumothorax following internal jugular cannulation and general anesthesia, Anesthesiology 45:554-555, 1976.
60. Khalil DG, Parker FB, Mukherjee N, and Webb WR: Thoracic duct injury: a complication of jugular vein catheterization, JAMA 221:908-909, 1972.
61. Teba L, Dedhia HV, Bowen R, and Alexander JC: Chylothorax review, Crit Care Med 13:49-52, 1985.
62. Arditis J, Giala M, and Anagnostidou A: Accidental puncture of the right lymphatic duct during pulmonary artery catheterization, Acta Anaesthiol Scand 32:67-68, 1988.
63. Friedman BA and Jergeleit HC: Perforation of atrium by polyethylene central venous catheter, JAMA 203:1141-1142, 1968.
64. Green HL and Nemir P Jr: Air embolism as a complication during parenteral alimentation, Am J Surg 121:614-616, 1971.
65. Smyth NPD and Rogers JB: Transvenous removal of catheter emboli from the heart and great veins by endoscopic forceps, Ann Thorac Surg 11:403-408, 1971.
66. Parikh RD: Horner's syndrome: a complication of percutaneous catheterization of the internal jugular vein, Anaesthesia 27:327-329, 1972.
67. Selander D, Dhuner K-G, and Lundborg G: Peripheral nerve injury due to injection needles used for regional anesthesia: an experimental study of the acute effects of needle point trauma, Acta Anaesthesiol Scand 21:182, 1977.
68. Royster RL, Johnston WE, Gravlee GP, et al: Arrhythmias during venous cannulation prior to pulmonary artery catheter insertion, Anesth Analg 64:1214-1216, 1985.
69. Eissa NT and Kvetan V: Guide wire as a cause of complete heart block in patients with preexisting left bundle branch block, Anesthesiology 73:772-774, 1990.
70. Swan HJC, Ganz W, Forrester JS, et al: Catheterization of the heart in man with the use of a flow-directed balloon-tipped catheter, N Engl J Med 283:447-451, 1970.
71. Lorzman J, Powers SR, Older T, et al: Correlation of pulmonary wedge and left atrial pressure: a study in the patient receiving positive end-expiratory pressure ventilation, Arch Surg 109:270-277, 1974.
72. Manjuran RS et al: Relationship of pulmonary artery diastolic and pulmonary artery wedge pressures in mitral stenosis, Am Heart J 89:207-211, 1975.
73. Lappas D, Lell WA, Gabel JC, et al: Indirect measurement of left-atrial pressure in surgical patients: pulmonary capillary wedge and pulmonary artery diastolic pressures compared with left atrial pressure, Anesthesiology 38:394-397, 1973.
74. Raper R and Sibbald WJ: Misled by the wedge? Chest 89:427-434, 1986.
75. Nadeau S and Noble WH: Misinterpretation of pressure measurements from the pulmonary artery catheter, Can Anaesth Soc J 33:352-363, 1986.
76. West JB: Ventilation/blood flow and gas exchange, ed, Oxford, 1970, Blackwell Scientific Publications.
77. Shasby DM, Dauber IM, Pfister S, et al: Swan-Ganz catheter location and left atrial pressure determine the accuracy of the wedge pressure when positive end-expiratory pressure is used, Chest 80:666-670, 1980.
78. Teboul J-L, Zapol WM, Brun-Buisson C, et al: A comparison of pulmonary artery occlusion pressure and left ventricular end-diastolic pressure during mechanical ventilation with PEEP in patients with severe ARDS, Anesthesiology 70:261-266, 1989.
79. Rao TLK, Jacobs KH, and El-Etr AA: Reinfarction following anesthesia in patients with myocardial infarction, Anesthesiology 59:499-505, 1983.
80. Moore CH, Lombardo TR, Allums JA, and Gordon FT: Left main coronary artery stenosis: hemodynamic monitoring to reduce mortality, Ann Thorac Surg 26:445-451, 1978.
81. Tuman KJ, McCarthy RJ, Spiess BD, et al: Effect of pulmonary artery catheterization on outcome in patients undergoing coronary artery surgery, Anesthesiology 70:199-206, 1989.
82. Spring CL, Pozen RG, Rozanski JJ, et al: Advanced ventricular arrhythmias during bedside pulmonary artery catheterization, Am J Med 72:203-208, 1982.
83. Salmenperä M, Peltola K, and Rosenberg P: Does prophylactic lidocaine control cardiac arrhythmias associated with pulmonary artery catheterization? Anesthesiology 56:210-212, 1982.
84. Shaw TJI: The Swan-Ganz pulmonary artery catheter: incidence of complications with particular reference to ventricular dysrhythmias and their prevention, Anesthesia 34:651-656, 1979.
85. Keusch DJ, Winters S, and Thys DM: The patient's position influences the incidence of dysrhythmias during pulmonary artery catheterization, Anesthesiology 70:582-584, 1989.
86. Abernathy WS: Complete heart block caused by a Swan-Ganz catheter, Chest 65:349, 1974.
87. Thomson IR, Dalton BC, Lappas DG, et al: Right bundle branch block and complete heart block caused by the Swan-Ganz catheter, Anesthesiology 51:359-362, 1979.
88. Sprung CL, Elser B, Schein RMH, et al: Risk of right bundle-branch block and complete heart block during pulmonary artery catheterization, Crit Care Med 17:1-3, 1989.
89. Morris D, Mulvihill D, and Lew WYW: Risk of developing complete heart block during bedside pulmonary artery catheterization in patients with left bundle-branch block, Arch Intern Med 147:2005-2010, 1987.
90. McDaniel DD, Stone JG, Faltas AN, et al: Catheter-induced pulmonary artery hemorrhage, J Thorac Cardiovasc Surg 82:1-4, 1981.
91. Shah KB, Rao TLK, Laughlin S, and El-Etr AA: A review of pulmonary artery catheterization in 6,245 patients, Anesthesiology 61:271-275, 1984.
92. Dhamee MS and Pattison CZ: Pulmonary artery rupture during cardiopulmonary bypass, J Cardiothoracic Anesthesia 1:51-56, 1987.

93. Hannan AT, Brown M, and Bigman O: Pulmonary artery catheter-induced hemorrhage, Chest 85:128-131, 1984.

94. Stein JM and Lisbon A: Pulmonary hemorrhage from pulmonary artery catheterization treated with endo-bronchial intubation, Anesthesiology 55:698-699, 1981.

95. Gourin A and Garzon AA: Operative treatment of massive hemoptysis, Ann Thorac Surg 18:52, 1974.

96. Foote GA, Schabel SI, and Hodges M: Pulmonary complications of the flow-directed balloon-tipped catheter, N Engl J Med 290:927-931, 1974.

97. Mond HG, Clark DW, Nesbitt SJ, and Schlant RC: A technique for unknotting an intracardiac flow-directed balloon catheter, Chest 67:731-733, 1975.

98. Lipp H, O'Donoghue K, and Resnekov L: Intracardiac knotting of a flow-directed balloon catheter, N Eng J Med 284:220, 1971.

99. Boscoe MJ and deLange S: Damage to the tricuspid valve with a Swan-Ganz catheter, Br Med J 283:346-347, 1981.

100. O'Toole JD, Wurtzbacher JJ, Wearner NE, and Jain AC: Pulmonary-valve injury and insufficiency during pulmonary-artery catheterization, N Eng J Med 301:1167-1168, 1979.

101. Greene JF Jr, Fitzwater JE, and Clemmer TP: Septic endocarditis and indwelling pulmonary artery catheters, JAMA 233:891-892, 1975.

102. Kim YL, Richman KA, and Marshall BE: Thrombo-cytopenia associated with Swan-Ganz catheterization in patients, Anesthesiology 53:261-262, 1980.

103. King DJ and Kelton JG: Heparin-associated throm-bocytopenia, Ann Intern Med 100:535-540, 1984.

104. Allyn J, Lichtenstein A, Koski G, et al: Inadvertent passage of a pulmonary artery catheter from the superior vena cava through the left atrium and left ventricle into the aorta, Anesthesiology 70:1019-1021, 1989.

105. Zaidan J and Freniere S: Use of a pacing pulmonary artery catheter during cardiac surgery, Ann Thorac Surg 35:633-636, 1983.

106. Macander PJ, Kuhnlein JL, Buiteweg J, et al: Electrode detachment: a complication of the indwelling pacing Swan-Ganz catheter, N Engl J Med 314:1711, 1986.

107. Heiselman DE, Maxwell JS, and Petro V: Electrode displacement from a multipurpose Swan-Ganz catheter, PACE 9:134-135, 1986.

108. Grossman W: Fick oxygen method. In Cardiac catheterization and angiography, ed 3, Philadelphia, 1986, Lea & Febiger.

109. Guyton AC: The Fick principle. In Guyton AC, Jones CE, and Coleman TG, editors: Circulatory physiology: cardiac output and its regulation, ed 2, WB Saunders, Philadelphia 1973.

110. Kendrick AH, West J, Papouchado M, et al: Direct Fick cardiac output: Are assumed values of oxygen consumption acceptable? Eur Heart J 9:337-342, 1988.

111. Heneghan CPH, Gillbe CE, and Brantwaithe MA: Measurement of metabolic gas exchange during anesthesia, Br J Anaesth 53:73, 1981.

112. Heneghan CPH and Brantwaithe MA: Non-invasive measurement of cardiac output during anaesthesia, Br J Anaesth 53:351, 1981.

113. Davies G, Hess D, and Jebson P: Continuous Fick cardiac output compared to continuous pulmonary artery electromagnetic flow measurements in pigs, Anesthesiology 66:805, 1987.

114. Davies GG, Jebson PJR, Glasgow BM, and Hess DR: Continuous Fick cardiac output compared to ther-

115. Rieke H, Weyland A, Hoeft A, et al: Continuous measurement of cardiac output based on the Fick principle in cardiac anesthesia, Anaesthetist 39:13-21, 1990.

116. Carpenter JP, Nair S, and Staw I: Cardiac output determination: thermodilution versus a new computerized Fick method, Crit Care Med 13:576, 1985.

117. Krouskop RW, Cabatu EE, Chelliah BP, et al: Accuracy and clinical utility of an oxygen saturation catheter, Crit Care Med 11:744-749, 1983.

118. Getting A, DeTraglia MC, and Glass DD: In vivo comparison of two mixed venous saturation catheters, Anesthesiology 66:373-375, 1987.

119. Reinhart K, Moser N, Rudolph T, et al: Accuracy of two mixed venous saturation catheters during long-term use in critically ill patients, Anesthesiology 69:769-773, 1988.

120. Matthew EB and Vender JS. Comparison of cardiac output measured by different computers, Crit Care Med 15:989, 1987.

121. Nishikawa T and Dohi S: Slowing of heart rate during cardiac output measurement by thermodilution, Anesthesiology 57:538, 1982.

122. Harris AP, Miller CF, Beattie C, et al: The slowing of sinus rhythm during thermodilution cardiac output determination and the effect of altering injectate temperature, Anesthesiology 63:540, 1985.

123. Nishikawa T and Dohi S: Hemodynamic status susceptible to slowing of heart rate during thermodilution cardiac output determination in anesthetized patients, Crit Care Med 18:841-844, 1990.

124. Segal J, Pearl RG, Ford AJ, et al: Instantaneous and continuous cardiac output obtained with a Doppler pulmonary artery catheter, J Am Coll Cardiol 13:1382-1392, 1989.

125. Nishimura RA: Another measurement of cardiac output: Is it truly needed? J Am Coll Cardiol 13:1393-1394, 1989.

126. Abrams JH, Weber RE, and Holmen KD: Transtracheal Doppler: a new procedure for continuous cardiac output measurement Anesthesiology 70:134-138, 1989.

127. O'Shea J, D'Ambra M, Magro C, et al: Transesophageal echocardiography: Is it safe to the esophagus? An in vivo study, Circulation 78(II):1756, 1988.

128. Urbanowicz JH, Kernoff RS, Oppenheim G, et al: Transesophageal echocardiography and its potential for esophageal damage, Anesthesiology 72:40-43, 1990.

129. Cucchiara RF, Nugent M, Seward JB, et al: Air embolism in upright neurosurgical patients: detection and localization by two-dimensional transesophageal echocardiography, Anesthesiology 60:353, 1984.

130. Dewhirst WE, Stragand JJ, and Fleming BM: Mallory-Weiss tear complicating intraoperative transesophageal echocardiography in a patient undergoing aortic valve replacement, Anesthesiology 73:777-778, 1990.

131. Humphrey LS: Esophageal stethoscope loss complicating transesophageal echo-cardiography, J Cardiothoracic Anesthesia 2:356, 1988.

132. Stevenson JG. Two-dimensional color Doppler estimation of the severity of atrioventricular valve regurgitation: important effects of instrument gain setting, pulse repetition frequency, and carrier frequency, J Am Soc Echocardiography 2:1-10, 1989.

133. Yoshida K, Yoshikawa J, Shakudo M, et al: Color Doppler evaluation of valvular regurgitation in normal subjects, Circulation 78:840-847, 1988.

134. Sahn DJ and Maciel BC: Physiological valvular regurgitation: Doppler echocardiography and the potential for iatrogenic heart disease, Circulation 78:1075-1077, 1988.

135. Smith JS, Cahalan MK, Benefiel DJ, et al: Intraoperative detection of myocardial ischemia in high-risk patients: electrocardiography versus two-dimensional transesophageal echocardiography, Circulation 72:1015-1021, 1985.

136. Thys DM: The intraoperative assessment of regional myocardial performance: Is the cart before the horse? J Cardiothoracic Anesthesia 1:273-275, 1987.

137. London MJ, Tubau JF, Wong MG, et al: The "natural history" of segmental wall motion abnormalities in patients undergoing non-cardiac surgery, Anesthesiology 73:644-655, 1990.

Chapter 3

Complications of Spinal, Epidural, and Caudal Anesthesia

Terence M. Murphy
Declan O'Keeffe

Stimulated by the development of dural puncture by Quincke,[1] August Bier proceeded to undergo spinal anesthesia at the hands of his assistant Hilderbrandt.[2] It was a less than complete block and so the procedure was repeated on his assistant. Within the next 24 hours they developed the first and second reported instances of post–spinal anesthesia headache! Upon recovery from the block, Hilderbrandt also complained of postoperative pain from bruising to his pretibial area while anesthetized—the first report of complications from too vigorous assessment of block effectiveness—apparently Bier kicked him in the shin to see if the block was effective![3] Although widely embraced by the medical profession as a most useful procedure in patients undergoing elective surgery, the profound sympathetic blockade produced by spinal anesthesia proved disastrous to the hypovolemic patient, and just as in a later global conflict when the newly introduced

drug thiopental proved deadly when given to traumatized soldiers at Pearl Harbor,[4] so too at the Battle of Jutland in 1906[5] Admiral Sir Gordon Taylor of His Majesty's Royal Navy declared that "spinal anesthesia was a most effective form of euthanasia for the 'war injured' "! Since these earlier times, delivering local anesthetics to the neuraxis has become much better understood but is still associated with problems, and an integral part of anesthesia practice is recognizing and treating the complications associated with delivering this type of anesthesia care to patients.

The use of local anesthetics around the neuraxis in spinal and epidural (both lumbar and caudal) techniques is associated with a variety of complications ranging from the common and usually easily treated, such as the milder forms of hypotension; which are an accompaniment rather than a complication of spinal and epidural anesthesia, through to the rare but sometimes disastrous neurodestructive complications that might occur because of erroneous administration of chemical or infectious noxious substances through the administering needle. Examples of this latter disaster occurred in the United Kingdom, in the now infamous *Woolley and Roe* case, which unfortunately caused the virtual abandonment of spinal and epidural anesthesia in Britain for almost three decades.[6] As a fledgling house surgeon in Liverpool in 1961, I (T.M.M.) asked a senior urologic surgeon why spinal anesthesia wasn't used anymore. I was told, "We keep our spinal anesthetics with the leeches!"

As in many anesthesia endeavors, prevention is better than cure, and knowledge of the sound anatomic, physiologic, and pharmacologic basic principles involved in administering local anesthetics around the neuraxis will reduce to a minimum the complication rate and, one would hope, prevent the more serious side effects, the occurrence of which is rare and is often unexplainable in individual cases.

I. COMPLICATIONS OF NEURAXIAL REGIONAL ANESTHETIC TECHNIQUES
A. Failure

Although not often considered a conventional complication, failure is perhaps one of the most frustrating aspects of the use of regional anesthesia. Unlike general anesthesia, which for the most part can be delivered successfully (albeit not always safely) all the time, it is not yet possible to achieve this degree of success with regional anesthesia. Because of the difficulty of positioning a needle at a deep anatomic site with less than perfect control over the distal end of the needle, some degree of failure is common to all percutaneous needle techniques. There will always, even with experienced practitioners, be a small percentage of failures, until some more perfect feedback is obtained for correct placement at the intended target site.

There may well be anatomic impediments to epidural spread. Midline septa and other abnormal anatomic barriers have been invoked as being important factors in preventing satisfactory spread of anesthetic agent. Although it is tempting to often invoke the existence of such impediments when faced with a unilateral or imperfect epidural block, one series of 200 patients had an incidence of 6% unilateral anesthesia and the authors Asato et al.[7] were not of the opinion that epidural septa could be blamed. Other factors such as epidural catheters passing through paravertebral foramina into the paravertebral gutter could be invoked and indi-

cate that one might withdraw the catheter a few centimeters when such complications occur.

Because subarachnoid placement has the very positive identification of cerebrospinal fluid, this is perhaps the most successful of all the percutaneous needling techniques, though every anesthesiologist can remember those instances where cerebrospinal fluid appears to have been adequately sampled at the beginning and end of a spinal needle placement and yet failure or inadequate anesthesia has resulted. We just do not yet understand all the factors involved in the satisfactory production of such anesthesia to explain some of these failures, and it is vitally important that all anesthesiologists have a backup plan to cope with incomplete blocks. With experience and increasing expertise, these failures will become less frequent, and with the improving expertise and understanding of regional anesthesia these days it is now possible to provide quite efficient spinal and epidural anesthesia in most cases.

B. Backache

Backache is ubiquitous in society and occurs in about 50%[8] to 80%[9] of the population, irrespective of their receiving spinal or epidural anesthesia! The physical trespass of introducing a needle into and around the vertebral column may leave painful sequelae. In most cases this is borne with appropriate fortitude by most patients and is controlled usually with the simplest of analgesic regimens. It is brief and time limited.

Backache is a pain complaint that seems to come with the bipedal gait. Backache after and associated specifically with spinal anesthesia is relatively uncommon. It can be caused by any traumatic sequelae to the needling process, that is, hematoma, ligament injury, or associated reflex muscle spasms. Because of the many other symptomatic diversions in the postoperative period, the relatively minor sequelae of spinal and epidural needle puncture may well be underreported. Other factors can, of course, contribute to back pain. The length of time on the operating table or the surgical position as with lithotomy may well lead to lumbar ligamentous strain, particularly when muscle relaxants reduce the muscular support of the spinal column. Flatten[10] reported a 55% incidence of back pain in outpatients, and Perz[11] noted a 32% incidence with almost a fourth of these patients reporting their back pain as severe. Most complaints of backache, however, are usually of a mild nature. Males reported significantly less (50%) than females in this study.

There is a subgroup of patients in society

whose lives are blighted with significant and severe back pain. Many of these patients undergo trespass with spinal and epidural needles as part of their back pain treatment (myelograms, epidural anesthetics, and so on) or from unrelated surgeries, and backache can be a frequent postanesthetic complaint of such patients. Such persons may well need more extensive therapy in the postoperative period, using stronger analgesics, stimulation-produced analgesia (TNS, or transcutaneous neural stimulation, units), and so on, but unless there is some obvious signs of neurologic trespass or deficit, restoration of function must be built into the treatment recommended, and active physical therapy is entirely appropriate if one assumes that the postsurgical condition permits it.

It is interesting to notice recent reports of the appearances of backache associated with the newer epidural preparation of 2-chloroprocaine. Significant localized paralumbar muscle pain has been reported in as high as 40% of patients receiving this drug in 2% and 3% concentrations epidurally.[12] This does not seem to be associated with any neurologic deficit. It appears to be time limited, and the addition of the disodium EDTA preservative to replace the bisulfite contained in earlier preparations of this local anesthetic has been implicated. Until clarification of this particular complication is forthcoming, it needs to be acknowledged as a possible sequel to the administration of 2-chloroprocaine epidural solutions. The pain could be reduced by further treatment with alternative local anesthetic solutions in the epidural space, which should provide analgesia that would outlast the dissipation of the precipitating ingredients (? EDTA) in the 2-chloroprocaine.

Dirks[13] speculates that disodium EDTA could bind calcium and create a state of hypocalcemia leading to spasm of the paravertebral muscles. He treated a patient with this problem by slow intravenous infusion of 300 mg of calcium chloride with dramatic improvement in 15 minutes.

C. Infection

Infection associated with spinal and epidural techniques is very rare indeed, though there are intermittent reports of same. Local anesthetic agents may well be bacteriostatic if not bactericidal,[14] and unless there is some gross breakdown of sterile technique, these procedures seem to be remarkably free of infectious sequelae. Instances of epidural abscesses[15] and bacterial meningitis do occur from time to time, and current standards of asepsis need to be rigidly maintained with the administering equipment (needles, catheters, drugs, trays, and anesthesiologists hands).[16] Local infection at the site of insertion of the needle or indwelling epidural catheter is not uncommon, but epidural or subarachnoid space infections are rare, though of course, more serious.[17]

Because the outcome of epidural or subarachnoid infections seems to depend on the severity and duration of the process before instituting treatment, early diagnosis is paramount. If diagnosed early and treated promptly and vigorously, recovery is quite feasible.[18]

Perhaps of more current concern is the possibility of the utilization of epidural and spinal anesthesia in what appears to be an increasing population of patients suffering from acquired immunodeficiency syndrome (AIDS). Apparently, 20% of such patients can develop degenerative process in the spinal cord, and although there is not as yet any significant incidence of such complications associated with regional anesthesia techniques in patients with AIDS, warnings have been issued.[19]

D. Headache

Headache, like backache, is very common in society, and a diagnostic evaluation is necessary, after complaints of headache in the postoperative period, in those patients who have received spinal or epidural anesthesia. The classic post–dural puncture headache is often confused with the much more common tension-migraine headache spectrum. This latter is usually associated with a fairly lengthy history of such symptoms, and in those at the migraine end of the spectrum the presentation is often unilateral. Perhaps most significantly, these forms of chronic headache are not associated with any specific relationship to posture, whereas usually the most significant differential characteristic of the post–dural puncture headaches is that they are classically exacerbated when the upright posture is assumed.

Serious causes of spinal headache would be much more rare and include bacterial or perhaps more common aseptic meningitis, where the symptoms are those of meningeal irritation, usually a constant headache unrelated to position. In the case of bacterial meningitis, cerebrospinal fluid sampling and appropriate antibiotic therapy is indicated. Persistence of symptoms unrelated to posture and associated with hyperpyrexia should arouse an index of suspicion and a neurologic consultation.

Although rare, cortical vein thrombosis is another condition that can create a severe headache often in the postpartum period that can be confused with dural puncture headache.[20,21]

Another very rare cause of headache would be a cerebral or epidural hematoma that could possibly arise as a result of previous head trauma, or anticoagulant therapy associated with epidural or spinal anesthesia. This would be differentiated from the traditional post–dural puncture headache by the lack of postural character and may well involve more localizing focal, neurologic signs requiring expeditious neurologic assessment.

The classic post–dural puncture headache is believed to result from decreased pressure in the neuraxis, caused by leakage of cerebrospinal fluid through the dural puncture site. The headache is classically posture related, that is, made worse by upright posture and relieved by lying down. In probably 90% or more of such headaches, it commences within 3 days after the dural tap. It usually resolves spontaneously in a further 2 to 3 days and rarely lasts longer than a week.

Traction on the trigeminal, glossopharyngeal, or vagal innervation of the meninges is believed to be the mechanism involved in such pain.[22,23] Most of the patients have pain referred classically to the frontal and occipital area, though some patients will complain of diffuse neck pain believed to be mediated by the upper cervical nerves. Probably 1% of patients or more have auditory (see later) and visual disturbances that can accompany the headache, and certainly dizziness, tinnitus, and photophobia are classic associated symptoms.

In an evaluation of this problem, Jones[24] reported that the symptoms of the post–dural puncture headache are usually slight in about 50% of such patients and often do not interfere with normal activity. Approximately 35% of people with post–spinal anesthesia headache will need to assume the recumbent position for varying periods of time to obtain relief, and only about 15% of patients have headaches so severe that they cannot sit up long enough to attend to important functions such as eating or bathroom trips. These are the patients that we, as anesthesiologists, often see in consultation for consideration for epidural blood patches.

It is critically important to carefully evaluate the history and physical signs as outlined above so that dural puncture headache may not be confused with more "mundane" causes of headache such as muscle tension and migraine, as opposed to the more serious but fortunately much more rare meningitis, cortical vein thrombosis, and cerebral hematoma.

1. Causes of post–dural puncture headache

a. Size of dural puncture needle. Much has been and continues to be written about prevention of the problem of post–dural puncture headache. Virtually all studies looked at up to now show that the incidence of post–dural puncture headache decreases with the use of smaller needles and that this incidence of headache can be minimized by use of the tiny 29- or 30-gauge needles where an incidence of less than 1% has been reported. The problem, however, in using such delicate filiform needles is an increased failure rate than that experienced with the more "robust" 25- or 22-gauge needles. The varying incidence of spinal headache with use of similar-gauged needles in comparable patients may depend on several factors, which probably include the configuration of the needle point, the effect of its bevel, and its orientation to dural fibers, as well as the subsequent trauma and nature of the defect produced in the dura. Needles such as the Greene, Whitaker, and Sprotte needles have been produced in an attempt to separate rather than sever dural fibers, theoretically resulting in a less traumatic defect in the dura that will close more effectively once the needle is removed. In a group of obstetric patients Snyder[25] demonstrated that a 26-gauge Quincke needle resulted in a 25% incidence of headache compared to a 4% incidence with a 22-gauge Whitaker needle in obstetric patients. Neal[26] recently reported a 5.5% and 3.8% incidence of spinal headache when he compared the 26-gauge Quincke needle and the 22-gauge Greene needle in a nonobstetric population. Another very important factor also mentioned in this report was the influence of age, with headache being more frequent in the younger age groups. In patients under 40 years of age the incidence of headache with the 26-gauge Quincke needle was 10.5% and with the 22-gauge Greene needle was 5.3%. Over 40 years of age there was a similar incidence of approximately 3% in both groups.

b. Orientation of the tip of dural puncture needle. Mihic [27] has reported that the incidence of spinal headache can be reduced dramatically depending on the orientation of the needle puncture. With a 22-gauge needle he reduced the incidence of spinal headache from 17% to 0.24% and with a 25-gauge needle from 15% to 0% by inserting the spinal needle bevel parallel to the dural fibers. Morris[28] has noted a similar reduction in post–dural puncture headache after accidental dural puncture with a large Touhy needle. The headache incidence was 30% when the bevel direction was parallel to the dural fibers as compared to 73% when perpendicular to it.

In a large series of over 1000 spinal anesthetics, Lybecker[29] has demonstrated that it is even

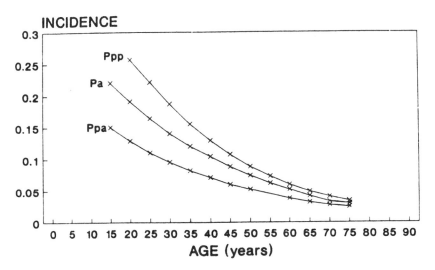

Fig. 3-1. Logistic regression of post – dural puncture headache as a function of age. Average punctures, *Pa*, and parallel, *Ppa*, or perpendicular, *Ppp*, insertion of the bevel of the needle in relation to the longitudinal dural fibers. (From Lybecker H et al: Anesth Analg 70:389, 1990.)

possible to predict outcome with respect to the risks of post–dural puncture headache, which can be estimated from the age of the patient and the bevel direction of the spinal needle (Fig. 3-1).

Hatfalvi suggests that the incidence of spinal headache may be decreased by using paramedian as opposed to midline approaches to spinal puncture.[30] This thesis has recently been tested by use of samples of dura, and the fluid that leaked could be reduced by a more acute angle of puncture (30 degrees) as opposed to 60- or 90-degree needle punctures.[31]

c. Skin-preparation fluids. Skin-preparation fluids have recently been incriminated in the genesis of post–dural puncture headache by Gurmarnik.[32] He has recently reported that one can reduce the incidence of spinal headache by meticulous removal of the povidone-iodine (Betadine) skin preparation used to clean the puncture site before inserting the needle. Six-percent incidence of spinal headache was reported if the Betadine was not removed, and no incidence of spinal headache was reported if the Betadine was carefully removed.

d. Age. Virtually all authors who have evaluated post–dural puncture headache attest to the fact that there is a decreasing incidence with age, invoking explanations of decreased pain sensibility with age, or loss of sensibility of pain-sensitive structures within the cranium. There is also narrowing of the paravertebral foramina with age, and therefore perhaps it reduces the cerebrospinal fluid loss from the neuraxis and perhaps maintains a higher epi-

dural-space pressure and so reducing cerebrospinal fluid leak. The use of a standard 22-gauge spinal needle has an incidence of spinal headache of approximately 5% in patients over 50 years of age. It can be two to four times this incidence in patients younger than 50. The incidence of post–dural puncture headache increases after accidental dural puncture with larger 18-gauge epidural needles. As noted above it is also much reduced in patients beyond the sixth decade of life for unknown reasons. Perhaps, as Stone has recently suggested, the relatively more "closed" epidural space of the elderly prevents paravertebral leakage of the cerebrospinal fluid, which remains in the spinal canal and equilibrates pressures across the dura mater and so reducing cerebrospinal fluid flowout through the dural defect,[33] and in fact continuous spinal anesthesia with conventional-sized epidural catheters passed through an 18-gauge needle are used in my own practice in septuagenarians and older persons and carries an acceptably low incidence of post–dural puncture headache.

e. Sex. There appears to be a difference between the sexes in the incidence of post–dural puncture headache, being almost universally reported to be higher in women than in men, and the reason is unclear. Even if one ignores the possible complicating factors associated with obstetrical practice, there is still a higher incidence of post–dural puncture headache of approximately double, or more in outpatients,[11] in females as opposed to males below 50 years of age. The local anesthetic agent does not seem to influence the incidence or occurrence of post–dural puncture headache, and of course such headaches occur in diagnostic dural puncture with or without the use of the local anesthetic agents.

f. Concentration of local anesthetic. It is of interest, however, that Naulty[34] has recently suggested the influence of local anesthetic solutions on post–dural puncture headache, speculating that low concentrations of the local anesthetic in the cerebrospinal fluid can cause vasoconstriction followed by a reactive hyperemia of intracranial blood vessels with resulting headache.

The same authors in follow-up correspondence[35] suggest that headache complicates otherwise normal epidural anesthesia in from 10% to 30% of parturients, such that patients who received 2% lidocaine may have had a higher incidence of headache (34%) compared with those receiving weaker bupivacaine solutions (16%).

The true contribution of the anesthetic agent to post–dural puncture headaches remains to be adequately clarified and, in consideration of the ubiquitous nature of headache in society, will need rigorously controlled studies to determine what, if any, influence local anesthetic drugs have on this symptom.

2. Treatment of post–dural puncture headache. In most cases, probably 75% or more, post–dural puncture headache is mild or moderate and self-limiting and resolves within a week. Conservative therapy using analgesics, bedrest, and increased fluid intake will be associated with a successful resolution in a matter of days. Although the supine position is certainly advised and comfortable, if postural headache occurs, it probably is not necessary as a preventive measure against the occurrence of such headache, and, in fact, ambulation should not be discouraged after spinal punctures though patients probably should be advised to maintain a good state of hydration.

If and when post–dural puncture headache occurs, as with all pain problems, an appropriate explanation of the mechanisms of the pain should be given to the patient in terms he or she can understand. This often brings with it a reduction of the anxiety and suffering components and may well then permit such headaches to be treated by conservative bed rest, hydration, and the prescribing of appropriate analgesics, either nonopioid for milder headaches, or more powerful opioids if one has to resort to them for the short duration they are likely to be needed. If the headache persists despite these conservative measures, an epidural blood patch should be considered if the patient or the atten-

dants are reluctant to persist with the conservative measures mentioned above. One performs this by placing an epidural needle in the vicinity of the dural puncture and aseptically drawing 10 to 15 ml of the patient's own blood from a previously sited large-bore intravenous catheter in an antecubital vein. This blood is immediately (and observing aseptic principles) injected into the epidural space. This method is usually 90% successful, and if relief does not follow, it can be repeated. If the headache symptoms fail to respond to epidural blood patches, it is appropriate to reevaluate the diagnosis of the headache symptoms. This innovative therapy has been remarkably effective and safe and should be available to that small percentage of patients who cannot or will not persist in the conservative therapy outlined above.[36]

Because epidural blood injections spread cephalad more effectively than caudad, the needle to inject the blood patch should be inserted at a spinal level below the original dural puncture site and 10 to 15 ml of autologous blood injected.[37]

Of patients who have experienced postdural puncture headache, only 43% declared they would be willing to undergo spinal anesthesia again and then only if they could be assured of getting an epidural blood patch in the event of a post–dural puncture headache.[38]

More recently, caffeine has been evaluated by either oral or systemic intravenous administration as a therapy for post–dural puncture headache. Jarvis and colleagues demonstrated an 80% improvement in patients with post–dural puncture headache after an infusion of 50 mg of caffeine–sodium benzoate administered intravenously in a liter of lactated Ringer's solution followed by ongoing hydration.[39] Orally taken caffeine also appears to be effective.[40]

E. Unplanned dural puncture

Accidental dural punctures can occur during attempted epidural anesthesia and, in addition to complicating the anesthetic administration at the time, can compromise subsequent epidural anesthetic attempts. In reviewing the records of 200 patients who had accidental dural punctures during insertion of epidural catheters, Ong[41] reported on the subsequent administration of epidural anesthesia in those who were treated with and without epidural blood patches. He showed that a previous dural puncture significantly reduced success of a subsequent epidural anesthetic. If a blood patch had been administered, only 59% of the patients had an uncomplicated successful second epidural anesthetic. In the event of a dural puncture but with no blood patch, the success rate was 65%. This compared unfavorably with the 90% success rate in parturients who had previous epidural anesthesia without dural puncture.

F. Problems after use of microcatheters

In an attempt to utilize continuous techniques and at the same time minimize the severity of "spinal" headaches, microcatheters have recently been introduced for continuous spinal anesthesia.[42] The early experience with these tiny catheters is still being assessed. They pose some very practical problems in being able to be safely and effectively negotiated through the needle and into position. Kinking and blockage occur, and if any blood enters the needle during insertion, it can be difficult if not impossible to retract the needle over the catheter.[43]

It appears, furthermore, that there have been anecdotal adverse neural deficits reported[44] that have recently resulted in the temporary cessation of the use of these catheters in some institutions until this problem and these reports are more clearly understood.

G. Cardiovascular and respiratory complications

1. Test doses. To prevent the profound cardiorespiratory complications that can follow an accidental injection of a large dose of local anesthetic agent into an epidural vein, or subarachnoid space, test doses are used. These have traditionally contained enough local anesthetic agent to produce a spinal anesthetic effect if introduced into the subarachnoid space (such as 60 mg of lidocaine), and sufficient epinephrine to produce a tachycardia if injected intravenously (such as 15 µg).[45] Although controversy exists in this regard, this is still the standard practice. Recently suggested was a novel method of detecting intravascular catheter placement by use of a Doppler ultrasound probe placed over the precordium and noting heart tone changes after air injection.[46] One cubic centimeter of air was injected through an epidural catheter while heart tones were continually monitored in patients in labor. Injections of such a small quantity of air appear to be safe and correlated well with conventional test doses, though false-positive results did occur in 2% of patients.

2. Development of high spinal anesthesia. Most spinal anesthetics are performed for surgeries on the lower part of the body, and in such circumstances there is rarely need to provide anesthesia to a level higher than lower thoracic levels, and then cardiovascular and respiratory stability is usually well maintained. In the event that spinal anesthesia, either intentionally or accidentally, involves increasingly more cephalad spread, such that sympathetic control of the cardiovascular system is interrupted, significant hypotension can occur. Anesthesia of the cardiac accelerator fibers from the high thoracic outflow can produce bradycardia, and with continuing ascendancy of the block, paralysis of the phrenic nerve supply to the diaphragm and hence respiration can be compromised. Even higher cortical functions can be affected in the case of "total spinal" block.

In young healthy subjects even total spinal blocks are often surprisingly well tolerated if respiration and blood pressure are maintained and, in fact, have been used as a form of elective global anesthesia.[47] However, the same healthy person, if hypotensive, tolerates such high sympathetic blockade poorly.[48] Similarly, in the older debilitated patient, especially those with cardiovascular compromise, high spinal (or high epidural) anesthetics can and sometimes do require lifesaving treatment.

It should be noted that total spinal blocks are difficult to produce electively—requiring 30 to 40 ml of 1% lidocaine to achieve a 95% success rate, and because the duration is variable (1 to 2 hours), it has not proved practical yet to be adopted for routine surgical use.[47]

The cranial spread of anesthetic from the initial spinal or epidural administration in the lumbar area usually occurs in the first few minutes after such an administration. It is, however, very important to realize that it can occur at any time. This unexpected event has been emphasized with the recent closed-claim analysis where Caplan et al.[49] reported this rare but significant complication concerning 14 cases of unexpected sudden cardiac arrest associated with apparently stable hemodynamics. Six of these patients died and seven sustained permanent neurologic injury. Speculation concerning the genesis of same included possible myocardial ischemia secondary to decreased blood pressure, associated coronary artery disease or intrinsic atrioventricular nodal disease, and maybe unopposed vagal tone attributable to what may well have been a complete chemical sympathectomy. It is critically important to acknowledge the possible contribution of opioids and sedative hypnotic agents that are frequently used in combination with spinal epidural anesthesia for "sedation." This may have been responsible for approximately half the cases reported in this closed-claim study, and Knill[50] issued caveats along these lines, but such problems continue to occur.[51] Obviously meticulous monitoring throughout the duration of the case is always as necessary in regional as it is in general anesthesia.

With the onset of spinal or epidural anesthesia to high thoracic levels, anxious and unprepared patients may well experience significant apprehension and agitation that comes with the deafferentation, particularly if complicated by the nausea that often accompanies the hypotension associated with the sympathetic block. It is thus often tempting and appropriate to treat the anxiety with appropriate sedatives and hypnotics. Because of the duration of long cases, patients are also often administered analgesic opioids to minimize the discomfort of unblocked areas of the body during what can often be long periods of a potentially uncomfortable position on the operating table.

3. Resuscitation from cardiac arrest associated with either spinal or epidural anesthesia. Controversy exists over the optimal resuscitation of patients who have experienced delayed cardiac arrest associated with either spinal or epidural anesthesia. The basic principles of administration of oxygen and supporting of the circulation with both volume and vasoactive drugs are appropriate. Caplan,[49] however, speculates that the appropriate use of a more potent alpha-adrenergic agonist (such as epinephrine) by promoting peripheral vasoconstriction could increase venous return to the heart and improve cardiac output during the resuscitation efforts. Associated peripheral vasoconstriction may increase diastolic blood pressure as well as cardiac perfusion to speed the recovery of cardiac function. Conventional efforts to improve venous return (by the Trendelenburg position, elevating or wrapping legs, and so on) should also be used.

With the progression of spinal anesthesia to high thoracic or cervical levels, unconsciousness may well occur secondary to a decreasing blood pressure causing cerebral ischemia. Treatment for this is administration of fluids, enhancing venous return, and the administration of a vasopressor. If the high spinal or epidural spread of local anesthetics anesthetizes the cervical origins of the phrenic nerves, that is, C3 to C5, respiratory support will be necessary, with tracheal intubation and positive-pressure ventilation. Even in a high spinal or epidural block that does not produce respiratory paralysis but does anesthetize the abdominal and thoracic wall, it may well be necessary to intubate the trachea both to protect the airway (they cannot cough) and to facilitate ventilation, especially in patients with preexisting respiratory compromise (the obese, pregnant, and others). Usually, when a high spinal block with conventional doses of local anesthetic drug has progressed to a "total spinal" block producing phrenic nerve paralysis, it is relatively short lived. The amount of spinal anesthetic reaching cervical levels is small, and restoration of respiratory function usually occurs in 30 to 60 minutes. If one assumes that blood pressure and heart rate can be maintained, it is eminently feasible to proceed with the planned surgery. It is usually appropriate to administer general anesthesia either by inhalational or intravenous routes until the operation is completed and the trachea is extubated.[52]

4. Patients with preexisting coronary artery disease. In patients with preexisting coronary artery disease the use of a lumbar epidural anesthesia has recently been shown to produce abnormalities in myocardial segmental wall motion.[53] This moderate to severe worsening of the wall motion seems to occur simultaneously with the decreased blood pressure that is associated with lumbar epidural anesthesia. A group of healthy control patients also demonstrated transiently decreased blood pressure and an increase in segmental wall motion abnormalities indicating that changes in the diastolic arterial pressure subsequent to the onset of lumbar epidural anesthesia may impair myocardial profusion, which could conceivably aggravate the potential for ischemia in patients with coronary arterial disease who may already may have compromised coronary profusion.

5. Reversal of regional anesthesia. Unlike general anesthesia, regional anesthesia, once established, has not as yet proved amenable to reversal techniques. However, in a recent publication, Johnson[54] has reduced the duration of motor block from epidural anesthesia by diluting the epidural anesthetic with additional 15 ml aliquots of crystalloid solutions on three occasions in the immediate recovery period. Lactated Ringer's solution or normal saline was shown to decrease the duration of motor block by 50%. The sensory blockade, however, was not influenced significantly (Fig. 3-2).

H. Nausea and vomiting

Nausea and vomiting is a frequent accompaniment of hypotension during high spinal or epidural anesthesia and may be a symptom of cerebral hypoxia. It usually responds dramatically to restoration of the blood pressure with intravenous fluid therapy, head-down position, the administration of a vasopressor (such as ephedrine 5 to 25 mg), the administration of oxygen therapy, or all four.[52] If the initial arterial pressure decrease is treated immediately, usually nausea and vomiting can be avoided.

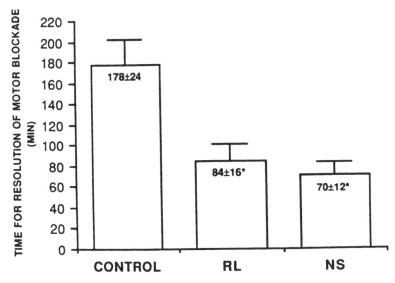

Fig. 3-2. Epidural reversal with crystalloid infusion. Effect of epidural crystalloid (*RL*, lactated Ringer's solution; *NS*, normal saline solution) versus control on the time between conclusion of operation and complete resolution of motor blockade. Bar heights represent mean times, and error bars show standard error of the mean. *P <0.05. (From Johnson MD et al: Anesth Analg 70:395, 1990.)

Another potential cause for nausea during neuraxial anesthesia is traction on abdominal viscera in the upper abdomen. This occurs typically in an otherwise satisfactory lower abdominal procedure with a low thoracic level of epidural or spinal anesthesia (T8 or so). Before completing the operation, the surgeon may elect to examine the upper abdomen by manually palpating retrohepatic areas and producing traction on the upper abdominal viscera, which often still have intact neural connections via the splanchnic nerves to spinal cord levels above the blocked segments. In such circumstances, the patient may suddenly become nauseated and may even retch and vomit. The administration of atropine (0.4 to 1.0 mg IV) and having the surgeon desist from such manipulation will usually resolve this problem. If the upper abdominal manipulation is essential for completion of the operation, one may need in such circumstances to raise the level of the block by administering more local anesthetic through the epidural or subarachnoid catheter if one is in place and, if it is not in place, proceeding to tracheal intubation with general anesthesia, which may even be necessary to resolve the discomfort and protect the airway in the face of nausea that cannot be controlled by other means.[55]

I. Major neurologic complications

These are the *bêtes noires* of the regional anesthesiologist, that is, concerns of producing paralysis, weakness, or incontinence after spinal and epidural anesthesia. Needle trespass on the spinal nerves or spinal cord itself is exceedingly rare (or is not reported!). Although hypotension and bradycardia are to be expected and have been reported to occur 10% and 2% respectively in a large series,[56] the incidence of dural puncture is low, even in epidural procedures in the cervical region.[56,57] Fortunately nerve damage from such techniques seems to be exceedingly rare.

Kane[58] revealed only a single permanent lesion possibly related to the spinal anesthetic in a large series. Other reviewers, Vandam and Dripps[59] and Moore,[60] have found only rare neurologic lesions. Although they can and do occur with often tragic results, it must be appreciated that such disasters also occur with general anesthesia.[61]

Overall the risks of major neurologic deficits after any form of anesthesia are exceedingly rare. In a recent review of nerve injury in 227 patients associated with anesthesia,[61] the mechanism of injury was unclear despite extensive analysis in most of the cases. It is interesting that although nerve damage seems to be a significant source of anesthesia-related claims the median payment for such nerve damage involving disabling injuries was $56,000, significantly lower than the $225,000 median payment for other disabling injury claims that did not involve nerve damage. The reviewers concluded that for the most part the standard of anesthesia care had been met more often in claims involving nerve damage than in claims not involving nerve damage. The other salient feature was that the relatively common ulnar nerve injuries often seem to occur without any identifiable mechanism. With the advent of automatically cycled blood pressure cuffs, Sy[62] a decade ago suggested that this could contribute to ulnar nerve palsy. Alexander[63] has recently reminded us of the same possibility, though such an explanation is still only speculative without adequate documentation of the site of the blood pressure cuff on a large series of patients.

It should be noted that most of the nerve-damage claims, in fact, were associated with general anesthesia, and it was only the lumbosacral nerve injuries having an identifiable anesthetic cause that seemed to be associated with regional anesthesia where paresthesia or pain occurred during the placement of spinal or epidural needles, or where pain occurred after the injection of the local anesthetic that a claim was made. Of the 82 regional anesthetics involved, the most frequent technique used was subarachnoid block 35%, lumbar epidural block 20%, and caudal epidural block 6%.

The neural deficits noted some years ago in association with chloroprocaine were shown to be attributable to the neurotoxic effects of the contained preservative sodium bisulfite.[64] With the removal of this preservative, chloroprocaine is now used, and no further episodes of neural deficit have been described though, as mentioned above, there is now a recent association with significant severe back pain during the recovery period after epidural use of this agent.[12,13]

Alas, the precise mechanism of nerve injuries associated with both regional and general anesthesia is all too often usually unknown.[65] Unfortunately, prospective studies of such infrequent injuries are very difficult to do but may be necessary to improve our understanding of such mechanisms and to more predictably prevent such unfortunate anesthetic sequelae.

In the event that neurologic complications occur after spinal or epidural anesthesia, a comprehensive neurologic assessment and evaluation should be undertaken with appropriate prompt neurologic consultation, to obtain early documentation of the clinical condition. It is obviously important to ascertain neurologic status before embarking upon anesthesia so that any preexisting neurologic disease will be documented before anesthesia, rather than subsequently being attributed to the anesthetic or surgical experience.

1. Risk of anticoagulation. Another complication associated with spinal or epidural anes-

thesia is that of spinal or epidural hematoma. These are quite rare but, as with some of the events listed above, can result in permanent and catastrophic paralysis. A major concern about epidural or subarachnoid hematomas centers largely around the concomitant use of these anesthetic techniques when patients are undergoing anticoagulation.[66]

In the face of frank and efficient anticoagulant therapy, needle trespass into the spinal canal is contraindicated in all but the most extenuating circumstances. It has, however, proved eminently feasible to combine regional anesthesia and the use of anticoagulants. Rao and El-Etr[67] successfully introduced epidural placement of catheters before and removed them after anticoagulation in association with major vascular surgery without any incidents of epidural hematomas complicating their large series. Machers and Abrams[68] also performed intrathecal puncture, administering morphine, before the induction of general anesthesia and high-dose heparin to patients undergoing cardiopulmonary bypass without any symptoms of spinal hematoma resulting.

The increasing use of minidose heparin is a controversial issue, and epidural or spinal anesthesia is unsafe and should not be used if such minidose heparin results in abnormal coagulation studies (partial thromboplastin time or activated clotting time). However, if results of these studies are within the limits of normal, it may be possible to use spinal or epidural anesthesia as long as frequent checks are made to verify the function of the nervous system. This is quite feasible with the advent of the use of neuraxial opioids for postoperative pain control, and it is often feasible to utilize epidural or spinal local anesthetics for the duration of surgery and epidural or spinal opioids for postoperative pain control, which permits ongoing monitoring of the integrity of the neuraxis.

Should neurologic compromise be suspected in association with spinal or epidural anesthesia, prompt neurosurgical consultation should be sought. Left unattended, epidural hematoma, which causes spinal cord compression, rapidly leads to irreversible paralysis within hours. If these forms of regional anesthesia are to be used in association with anticoagulation, probably shorter acting local anesthetic agents (such as lidocaine) would be a more appropriate choice than the long-acting bupivacaine or etidocaine so that neurologic function can be evaluated rapidly after the termination of surgery.

2. Chemical meningitis. Intermittently there have been reports of epidemics of chemical meningitis.[69,70] It is usually characterized by fever, headache, cervical rigidity, nausea, vomiting, and occasionally transient neurologic signs, even prostration, and can progress to coma. Despite these symptoms, the cerebrospinal fluid is often sterile though it can contain increased white cells. Treatment is for the most part symptomatic, and fortunately this complication of meningitis is now much less frequent with the advent of improved techniques and the widespread adoption of disposable equipment. However, it still continues to occur from time to time.[71]

3. Cauda equina syndrome. Cauda equina syndrome is so called because the neurologic defects are localized to that area innervated by the lumbar and sacral nerves. It can be produced by chemical or other injury to the area associated with either the needle or the injection of caustic substances.

In the infamous *Woolley and Roe* case in Great Britain 50 years ago, the anesthetic ampules were stored in phenol solution that apparently seeped into the spinal anesthetic through cracks in the glass ampules resulting in two cases of severe neurologic complications. This unfortunate happening received wide medicolegal publicity and, except for a few isolated practitioners such as J.A. Lee,[72] led to the virtual abandonment of spinal and epidural anesthesia for three decades in the United Kingdom.

4. Adhesive arachnoiditis. The central nervous system condition called "adhesive arachnoiditis" usually is associated with infection, chemical insult, or trauma, to the neuraxis. The epidural and subarachnoid spaces can be obliterated by adhesions with dense attachments to the arachnoid or dura. The resulting inflammatory process can lead to a wide variety of neurologic deficits. In the more advanced progressive adhesive arachnoiditis, the condition can lead to hydrocephalus, syringomyelia, the whole spectrum of paraplegia and quadriplegia, or all three.

Such disasters fortunately have not been recorded in recent times in association with anesthesia, but continued vigilance needs to be maintained in the practice of regional anesthesia techniques. It is all too easy to accidentally introduce unintended solutions into the neuraxis.[73,74] Fortunately, the improved pharmaceutical standards and sterility associated with modern operating room practice has minimized this clinical catastrophe.

In the event that neurotoxic substances are accidentally injected into the subarachnoid space, it is feasible to "wash them out." Such a technique was recently described by Tartiere,[75]

who introduced a second subarachnoid conduit to treat an accidental intrathecal injection of hypertonic solution of Angiografin (meglumine amidotrizoate). Ten milliliter aliquots of saline were injected through a preexisting thoracic intrathecal catheter in this patient and withdrawn through a second catheter inserted in the lumbar subarachnoid space. A total of 180 ml of saline were used, and despite the onset of neurotoxic signs of spastic paresis, bilateral lower extremity pain, tachycardia, and ST-segment depression, no permanent cardiovascular or neurologic complications persisted.

J. Miscellaneous complications

1. Hearing loss after spinal anesthesia. Recent reports have described hearing loss after spinal anesthesia. It would seem that this, like post–dural puncture headache, seems to parallel the size of the dural defect.

Fog[76] using postoperative audiograms found a threefold increase in hearing loss at 10 decibels or more in those patients who underwent a spinal puncture with a 22-gauge needle as opposed to a 26-gauge needle (Fig. 3-3).

Apparently none of these patients had a post–spinal anesthesia headache, a finding indicating in fact that audiometry may be a more sensitive indication of cerebrospinal leak than post–spinal anesthesia headache! For the most part, this appears to be an eminently reversible phenomena.

2. Particulate contamination. Although particulate contamination of solutions from glass ampules occurs,[77] and small particles have been implicated in instances of phlebitis and pulmonary emboli, there is as yet no information available on such contaminants during subarachnoid or epidural injections. Although filtering of agents for injections into the subarachnoid space is practiced by some anesthesiologists, it is not as yet a universal practice.

II. COMPLICATIONS OF PEDIATRIC EPIDURAL AND SPINAL ANESTHESIA

Since the recent increase in the use of regional anesthesia and analgesia in children, there is as yet relatively limited information of the complications associated with these techniques. Broadman[78] has reported experiences with 1154 cases of caudal anesthesia, none of whom had any complications in the immediate postanesthetic period and no complications were detected later in a random sample interviewed by telephone!

More recently, this ongoing experience has now been performed in excess of 3500 children and the safe record continues.[79] Broadman

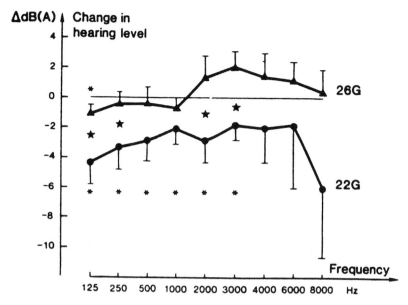

Fig. 3-3. Hearing loss after spinal anesthesia. Mean changes in hearing level ± standard error of the mean on "worse side" is shown at each frequency. Negative values indicate decreased hearing. *Asterisk,* statistically significant change in hearing level compared with preoperative values; *star,* statistically significant intergroup differences. (From Fog J et al: Anesth Analg 70:517, 1990.)

does, however, report three serious events involving respiratory compromise, a total spinal block, and a tonic clonic seizure. All these three infants were less than 6 months of age, and all recovered without any further problems. Thus an overall incidence of significant perioperative complications was only 3 out of 3500 (0.09%)!

Dalens[80] reporting on 750 caudal blocks reported a failure rate of 3.5%, with most of the failures occurring in children over 7 years of age. This is probably related to the fact that the sacral hiatus is so much more easily identified in infants and small children and becomes progressively more difficult to identify with increasing age.

It should be mentioned that in both of the above studies by Broadman and Dalens regional anesthesia was instituted in patients already under general anesthesia. This would not only facilitate patient acceptance but because of the improved respiratory and cardiovascular maintenance and monitoring associated with modern general anesthesia would also have, perhaps, added a protective factor.

Subarachnoid blocks in infants and children have also been enjoying renewed popularity.[81] "Bloody taps" would appear to be encountered 25% of the time in infants less than 30 weeks of gestational age.[79] Another interesting observation is that of a "dry tap" where cerebrospinal fluid cannot be obtained after apparent correct

placement in the subarachnoid space. This has been reported in infants and neonates who have been fasting for more than 6 hours. Broadman who has recently reported this[79] suggests gentle aspiration with a 1 ml syringe and abandoning the procedure if one is unable to aspirate clear fluid.

Valley[82] has reviewed the use of caudal morphine in a large series of pediatric patients including 54 patients who were under 1 year of age. Like others, they have demonstrated beneficial analgesic effect with 75% of the patients not requiring supplemental analgesics for the first 10 hours after a single caudal epidural dose. In contrast to earlier studies, the incidence of clinically important respiratory depression was as high as 8% (almost double that reported in adults), and 10 of the 11 cases of respiratory depression in this study occurred in patients less than 1 year of age and weighing less than 9 kg. All the patients who developed respiratory depression had been administered supplementary intravenous opioids. This study also demonstrated the other complications of the neuraxial narcotics with a 51% incidence of urinary tract retention, 7% vomiting, and 3% pruritus.

In former preterm infants undergoing inguinal hernia repair Welborn[83] noted that spinal anesthesia with tetracaine alone was well tolerated but if the spinal anesthesia was supplemented with ketamine 89% of infants developed prolonged apnea. This was more than twice the effect observed when ketamine was used to supplement general anesthesia.

A recent review by Lloyd-Thomas attests to the popularity and surprising cardiovascular stability in the use of spinal and epidural anesthesia in younger children, even with blocks as high as T3 to T5 and the gratifying lack of complications except to point out that nausea and vomiting are common after caudal block for unknown reasons.[84]

III. CONCLUSIONS

Spinal, lumbar, and caudal epidural anesthetics are most useful techniques, and their safe use requires the ability to recognize and treat the complications associated with their use. It is very important to understand the applied anatomy of these blocks, to detect the degree of blockade, to monitor the patient at all times, and to prevent accidental intravascular injections by always aspirating before all injections of local anesthetic agents. It is critically important to always have a functioning intravenous catheter in place for administration of emergency drugs. It is advisable to perform these procedures when the patient is awake and can give meaningful feedback, though it seems that pediatric anesthesiologists are successfully using these techniques in patients receiving general anesthetics.

REFERENCES

1. Quinke H: Die Lumbalpunction des Hydrocephalus, Ber Klin Wochenschr 28:929, 1891.
2. Bier A: Versuche über Cocainisirung des Rückenmarkes, Dtsch Z Chir 51:361, 1899.
3. Fink BR: History of neural blockade. In Cousins MJ and Bridenbaugh PO, editors: Neural blockade, Philadelphia, 1988, JB Lippincott.
4. Halford FJ: A critique of intravenous anesthesia in war surgery, Anesthesiology 4:67, 1943.
5. Davis DA: Historical vignettes of modern anesthesia, Clinical Anesthesia series, Philadelphia, 1968, FA Davis.
6. Cope RW. The *Woolley and Roe* case: *Woolley and Roe vs. The Ministry of Health and Others,* Anaesthesia 9:249-270, 1954.
7. Asato F, Kirakawa N, Oda M, et al: A midline epidural septum is not a common cause of unilateral epidural blockade, Anesth Analg 71:427-429, 1990.
8. Taylor H and Curran NM: The Nuprin pain report, New York, Lewis, Harris & Assoc 1985.
9. Von Korf M, Dworkin SF, Resche L, and Kruger A: An epidemiological comparison of pain complaints, Pain 32:173-183, 1988.
10. Flatten H and Araeder J: Spinal anesthesia for outpatient surgery, Anaesthesia 40:1108-1111, 1985.
11. Perz RR, Johnson DL, and Shinozaki T: Spinal anesthesia for outpatient surgery, Anesth Analg 67:S168, 1988.
12. Fibuch EE and Opper SE: Back pain following epidurally administered Nesacaine, Anesth Analg 69:113-115, 1989.
13. Dirks WE: Treatment of Nesacaine-NPF induced back pain with calcium chloride, Anesth Analg 70:461-462, 1990.
14. Schmidt RN and Rosenkranz HS: Antimicrobial activity of local anesthetics, J Infect Dis 121:597-607, 1970.
15. Goucke CR and Graziotti P: Extradural abscess following local anesthestic and steroid injection for chronic low back pain, Br J Anesth 65:427-429, 1990.
16. James FM, George RH, Halen H, and White GJ: Bacteriological aspects of epidural analgesia, Anesth Analg 55:187-190, 1976.
17. Baker AS, Ojemann RG, Swartz MN, and Richardson EP: Spinal epidural abscess, N Engl J Med 293:463-468, 1975.
18. Ready LB and Helfer Đ: Bacterial meningitis in patients after epidural anesthesia, Anesthesiology 71:988-990, 1989.
19. Greene ER: Spinal and epidural anesthesia in patients with the acquired immunodeficiency syndrome, Anesth Analg 65:1089-1093, 1986.
20. Hubbert CH: Dural puncture headache suspected: cortical vein thrombosis diagnosed, Anesth Analg 66:285, 1986.
21. Swirtz EC, Costen N, and Marks GF: Cortical vein thrombosis may mimic post dural puncture headache, Reg Anaesth 12:188-190, 1987.
22. Bonica JJ: The management of pain, Philadelphia, 1953, Lea & Febiger, pp 493-494.
23. Atkinson RS and Lee JA: Spinal anesthesia in day care surgery, Anaesthesia 40:1059-1060, 1985 [editorial].
24. Jones RJ: The role of recumbency in the prevention and treatment of post-spinal headache, Anesth Analg 53:788-796, 1974.
25. Snyder GE, Person DL, and Flor CE: Headache in obstetrical patients: comparison of Whitaker needle vs. Quincke needle, Anesthesiology 71:A860, 1989.
26. Neal JN, Bridenbaugh LD, Mulroy MF, and Palmen BD: Instance of postdural puncture headache is similar between 22 g, Greene and 26 g. Quincke spinal needles, Anesthesiology 71:A678, 1989.
27. Mihic DN: Postspinal headache and relationship with needle bevel, Reg Anaesth 10:76-81, 1985.
28. Morris MC, Leighton BL, and Desimone CA: Needle bevel direction in headache after inadvertent dural puncture, Anesthesiology 70:729-731, 1989.
29. Lybecker H, Møller JT, May O, and Nielsen HK: Incidence and prediction of postdural puncture headache: a prospective study of 1021 spinal anesthesias, Anesth Analg 70:389-394, 1990.
30. Hatfalvi BI: The dynamics of postspinal headache, Headache 17:64-67, 1977.
31. Ready LB, Caplan S, Haschke RH, and Nessley M: Spinal needle determines the rate of transdural fluid leak, Anesth Analg 69:457-460, 1989.
32. Gurmarnik S: Skin preparation and spinal headache, Anesthesiology 43:1037, 1989.
33. Stone DJ and DiFazio CA: Postspinal headache in older patients, Anesth Analg 70:222, 1990 [letter].
34. Naulty JS, Hertwig L, Hurt CL, et al: Influence of local anesthetic solutions on postdural puncture headache, Anesthesiology 72:450-454, 1990.
35. Naulty JS: Local anesthetics and postdural puncture headaches, Anesthesiology 73:587-588, 1990.
36. DiGiovanni AJ and Dunbar BS: Epidural injections for autologous blood for postlumbar-puncture headache, Anesth Analg 49:268-271, 1970.
37. Szeinfeld M, Ihneidan IH, Moser MN, et al: Epidural blood patch: the evaluation of the volume and spread of blood injected into the epidural space, Anesthesiology 64:820-822, 1986.

38. Tarkkila PJ, Miralles JA, and Palomakie A: Subjective complications and efficacy of the epidural blood patch with the treatment of postdural puncture headache, Reg Anaesth 14:247-250, 1989.

39. Jarvis AP, Greenwald W, and Fagraus L: Intravenous caffeine for postdural puncture headache, Anesth Analg 65:316-317, 1986.

40. Cammann WR, Murray RS, Mushlind PS, and Lambert DH: Effects of caffeine on postdural puncture headache: a double blind placebo controlled trial, Anesth Analg 70:181-184, 1989.

41. Ong BY, Graham CR, Ringalert KRA, et al: Impaired epidural analgesia after dural puncture with and without subsequent blood patch, Anesth Analg 70:76-79, 1990.

42. Hurley RJ, and Lambert DH: Continuous spinal anesthesia with a microcatheter technique: preliminary experience, Anesth Analg 70:97-102, 1990.

43. Nagle GJ, McQuay HJ, and Glynn CJ: 32-gauge spinal catheters through 26-gauge needles, Anaesthesia 45:1052-1054, 1990.

44. Kendall Healthcare Products Company, 15 Hampshire St, Mansfield, MA 02048; 1-(800)-346-7197, Ext. 8074.

45. Moore DC and Batra MS: The components of an effective test dose prior to epidural block, Anesthesiology 55:693, 1974.

46. Leighton BL, Norris MC, DeSimone CA, et al: The air test as a clinically useful indicator of intravenously placed epidural catheters, Anesthesiology 73:610-613, 1990.

47. Evans TI: Total spinal anesthesia, Anesth Intensive Care 2:158-163, 1974.

48. Bonica J, Kennedy WF, Akamatsu TJ, and Gerbershagen HU: Circulatory effects of epidural block. 111. Effects of acute blood loss, Anesthesiology 36:219, 1972.

49. Caplan RA, Ward RJ, Posner K, and Chaney FW: Unexpected cardiac arrest during spinal anesthesia: a closed claim analysis of predisposing factors, Anesthesiology 68:5-11, 1988.

50. Knill RL: Arrest during spinal anesthesia. Unexpected? Anesthesiology 69:6-9, 1988.

51. Gild W and Crilley P: Sudden cardiac arrest during epidural anesthesia, Anesthesiology 73:1296, 1990.

52. Lambert DH: Complications of spinal anesthesia, Int Anesth Clin 27:320, 1989.

53. Saada M, Duval AN, Bonnet F, et al: Abnormalities in myocardial segmental wall motion during lumbar epidural anesthesia, Anesthesiology 71:26-32, 1989.

54. Johnson MD, Burger GA, Mushlin PS, et al: Reversal of bupivacaine epidural anesthesia by intermittent epidural injections of crystalloid solutions, Anesth Analg 70:395-399, 1990.

55. Crocker JS and Vandam LD: Concerning nausea and vomiting during spinal anesthesia, Anaesthesia 20:587, 1959.

56. Bonnet F, Derosier JP, Pluskwa F, et al: Cervical epidural anaesthesia for carotid artery surgery, Can J Anaesth 37:353-358, 1990.

57. Waldman SD: Complications of cervical epidural nerve blocks with steroids: a prospective study of 790 consecutive blocks, Reg Anaesth 14:149-151, 1989.

58. Kane RE: Neurological deficits following epidural or spinal anesthesia, Anesth Analg 60:150, 1981.

59. Vandam LD and Dripps RD: A long-term follow-up of patients who received 10,098 spinal anesthetics. II: Incidence and analysis: minor sensory neurological defects, Surgery 38:463, 1955.

60. Moore DC and Bridenbaugh LD: Spinal (subarachnoid) block: a review of 11,574 cases, JAMA 195:907, 1966.

61. Kroll DA, Caplan RA, Posner K, et al: Nerve injuries

associated with anesthesia, Anesthesiology 73:202-207, 1990.

62. Sy WP: Ulnar nerve damage possibly related to the use of automatically cycled blood pressure cuff, Anesth Analg 66:687-688, 1981.

63. Alexander GD: Mechanism of ulnar nerve injury, Anesthesiology 73:1294-1295, 1990.

64. Wang BC, Hillman DE, Spielholz NI, and Turndorf H: Chronic neurological deficits and Nesacaine-CE— an effect of the anesthetic, 2-chloroprocaine or the antioxidant, sodium bisulfite Anesth Analg 63:445-447, 1984.

65. Dawson DM, and Crarup C: Perioperative nerve lesions, Arch Neurol 46:1355-1360, 1989.

66. Owen EL, Casten GW, and Hessel EA: Spinal subarachnoid hematomas after lumbar puncture and heparinization: a case report, review of the literature, and discussion of anesthetic implications, Anesth Analg 65:1201-1207, 1986.

67. Rao TL and El-Etr AA: Anticoagulation following placement of epidural and subarachnoid catheters: an evaluation of neurologic sequelae, Anesthesiology 55:618-620, 1981.

68. Machers ET and Abrams LD: Intrathecal morphine in open heart surgery, Lancet 2:543, 1980.

69. Goldman WW and Sanford JP: An "epidemic" of chemical meningitis, Am J Med 29:94, 1960.

70. DiGiovanni AJ: Chemical meningitis associated with cleaning fluid, JAMA 214:129, 1970.

71. Ready LB and Helfer D: Bacterial meningitis in parturients after epidural anesthesia, Anesthesiology 71:988-990, 1978.

72. Lee JA: A synopsis of anaesthesia, Bristol, 1947, John Wright & Sons.

73. Tessler MJ, White I, Naugler Colville EN, and Biehl DR: Inadvertent epidural administration of potassium chloride: a case report, Can J Anaesth 35:631-633, 1988.

74. McGuinness JP and Cantees KK: Epidural injection of phenol containing ranitidine preparation, Anesthesiology 73:553-555, 1990.

75. Tartiere J, Gerard JL, Peny J, et al: Acute treatment after accidental intrathecal injection of hypertonic contrast media, Anesthesiology 71:169, 1989 [letter].

76. Fog J, Wang LP, Sundberg A, and Mucchiano C: Hearing loss after spinal anesthesia is related to needle size, Anesth Analg 70:517-522, 1990.

77. Finkelstein A, Lochandwala BS, and Pandey NS: Particulate contamination of an intact glass ampule, Anesthesiology 73:362-363, 1990.

78. Broadman LM, Hannallah RS, Norden JN, and McGill WA: "Kiddie caudals": experience with 1,154 consecutive cases without complications, Anesth Analg 66:S18, 1987.

79. Broadman LM: Regional anesthesia in pediatric patients, ASA Annual Refresher Course Lectures, no. 264, Park Ridge, Ill, 1990, American Society of Anesthesiologists.

80. Dalens D and Hasnaoui A: Caudal anesthesia in pediatric surgery success rate and adverse effects in 750 consecutive patients, Anesth Analg 68:83-89, 1989.

81. Abajian JC, Mellish PWP, et al: Spinal anesthesia for surgery in the high risk infant, Anesth Analg 63:359-362, 1984.

82. Valley RD and Bailey AG: Caudal morphine for postoperative analgesia in infants and children: a report of 138 cases, Anesth Analg 72:120-124, 1991.

83. Welborn LG, Rice LJ, Hannallah RS, et al: Postoperative apnea in former pre-term infants: prospective comparison of spinal and general anesthesia, Anesthesiology 72:838-842, 1990.

84. Lloyd-Thomas AR: Pain management in pediatric patients, Br J Anaesth 64:85-104, 1990.

Chapter 4

Complications of Nerve Blocks

Stephen E. Abram
Quinn H. Hogan

The consideration of risks and complications carries special importance when one is performing nerve blocks for surgical anesthesia, obstetrics, or pain control. There is a qualitative difference between general and regional anesthesia in the nature of the adverse outcomes that may occur. Many of the complications during or after a general anesthetic are the consequence of the patient's coexisting disease, such as intraoperative myocardial ischemia or postoperative pulmonary dysfunction. Although the anesthetic may have failed to prevent these developments, they are often viewed as, at least in part, the patient's fault. With nerve blocks, however, the complications are in most cases solely the direct consequence of the actions of the anesthesiologist, requiring a heightened awareness of the complications and the means of avoiding them. A further burden for those performing a nerve block is the still common notion held by many physicians and patients that since general anesthesia is risk free, except when bungled, why subject the patient to the clear risk of a needle-induced injury to nerves, vessels, and organs? This relative risk can be put into perspective by the information in the other chapters in this book.

The most obvious and common complication of nerve block anesthesia is its failure, which often results in the patient being exposed to additional risks. Additional blocks may be attempted, causing higher systemic concentrations of local anesthetic. Increasing sedation might be produced by supplementation with intravenous and inhaled drugs in an attempt to salvage a block, putting the patient at risk of hemodynamic and ventilatory complications,[1,2] especially if the patient has already been positioned in such a way that monitoring or airway management are impeded. Ultimately the risks of a general anesthetic might be added to those to which the patient was exposed during the failed block, increasing the total risk. In these ways, a failed block can initiate a sequence of events leading to further complications.

Although this chapter does not cover in detail the reported failure rates for various blocks, it is important to bear in mind that nerve blocks are in part a technical exercise, with success dependent not only on knowledge, but also on skill and experience. Series reported from training centers give the worst case, and a practitioner can expect improved results with repetition. With regard to the complication of failure, regional anesthesia again suffers comparison to general anesthesia, which gives the appearance of always working. However, in important ways, general anesthesia rarely succeeds completely: humoral and neural manifestations of nociception are nearly universal,[3] and degrees of awareness (though without spontaneous recall) are frequent.[4,5] When the surgeon asks the question, "Is he or she feeling this?" only during successful regional anesthesia can the anesthetist truly answer, "No."

In this chapter we first discuss the pathogenic mechanisms of complications during nerve blocks, after which each type of block considered. Complications following spinal and epidural block are considered in Chapter 10.

I. PATHOLOGIC PROCESSES INVOLVED IN COMPLICATIONS OF NERVE BLOCK
A. Toxicity of injected solution

A local anesthetic, by definition, has a reversible effect on nerve function. The rarity of neuropathy after nerve block procedures demonstrates the safety of applying local anesthetics to nerves. It has become clear, however, that local anesthetics deviate from the defined ideal and may cause prolonged functional and structural

changes in nerves and surrounding tissue. A discussion of these matters requires a digression into the details of peripheral nerve anatomy (Fig. 4-1).

The outermost layer of a peripheral nerve, the epineurium, is made of loose connective tissue in continuity at the intervertebral foramen with the dura of the nerve root. Within this inert supporting tissue, the individual axons are organized into fascicles by a surrounding sheath, the perineurium. The endoneurium within the fascicles provides the connective tissue between the axons. Far from being merely a structural element, the perineurium includes multiple layers of metabolically active epithelium.[6] Since the perineurium and pia-arachnoid membranes are in continuity anatomically and since the cells of both membranes share common histologic features and enzyme histochemistry, it is highly probable that the perineurium controls the endoneural milieu in the same fashion as the pia-arachnoid does for the central nervous system. By providing a diffusion barrier, the endothelium of the endoneural vessels and the perineurium act as a "blood-nerve barrier" for the fascicles.[6]

Local anesthetics produce a variety of cytotoxic effects in cell cultures, including inhibi-

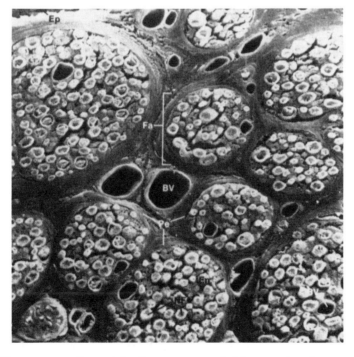

Fig. 4-1. The anatomy of a peripheral nerve as revealed by scanning electron microscopy. The nerve fibers, *NF*, are grouped into fascicles, *Fa*, by a perineural sheath, *Pe*. Between and around the fascicles is the epineural connective tissue, *Ep*. Blood vessels, *BV*, are found in the epineural tissue as well as in the endoneural space, *En*, the area enclosed by perineurium. (From Kessel RG and Kardon RH: Tissue and organs, New York, 1979, WH Freeman & Co.)

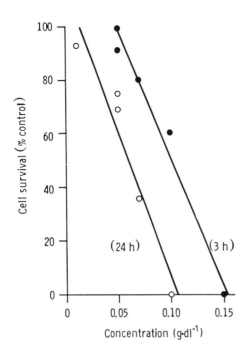

Fig. 4-2. The survival of cells grown in culture, as a percentage of control. Survival diminishes with increasing bupivacaine concentration and with duration of exposure (in hours). (From Sturrock JE and Nunn JF: Br J Anaesth 51:273, 1979.)

tion of cell growth, motility, and survival, as well as morphologic changes.[7] The extent of these effects are proportionate to the duration the cells are exposed to the local anesthetic solution (Fig. 4-2) and occur using local anesthetic concentrations in the range used clinically. Within this range, the cytotoxic changes are greater as concentrations increase (Fig. 4-2). It is not clear how to extrapolate the pattern of these findings from cell cultures to that of nerves in vivo. The inhibition of cell growth and division in fibroblast cultures, however, may have direct relevance as the mechanism by which local anesthetics impede healing when injected into a wound.[8,9] Local anesthetics have been shown to damage skeletal muscle as well, with customary concentrations producing degeneration of muscle fibers after a single injection.[10] Regeneration takes place over the subsequent 2 weeks, and no clinical consequences of this phenomenon have been observed.

Cytotoxic changes have also been found to follow the in vivo exposure of nerves to clinically used concentrations of local anesthetics. The exact site of the local anesthetic deposition, whether inside or outside the perineural membrane that surrounds the fascicle, plays an important role in determining the pathogenic potential. After the extrafascicular application of local anesthetics, the regulatory function of the perineurial and endothelial "blood-nerve barrier" is subtly compromised. The normally hypertonic endoneural fluid becomes hypotonic, with the accumulation of edema, increased perineural permeability, and increased fluid pressures within the fascicles.[11] Inflammatory changes as well as myelin and Schwann cell injury have been identified.[11,22] Ester local anesthetics in comparison to amides are especially prone to producing these changes.[22] Local anesthetic-induced alterations in nerve blood flow may potentiate these direct cytotoxic effects because lidocaine progressively diminishes nerve blood flow with increasing concentrations.[13]

Animal models using intrathecal injection of local anesthetics have failed to show consistent changes in nerve structure, though extensive functional impairment may occur while the nerves retain a normal histologic appearance.[14,15] As with the effects of local anesthetics in cell cultures, the duration of exposure[14] and concentration of local anesthetic [15] is important in determining the incidence of local anesthetic-induced residual paralysis. The clinical importance of these changes after extra-fascicular injections has not been determined, but it is prudent to use only the minimum necessary local anesthetic concentrations. Since small fiber neurons are more sensitive to chemical damage, the manifestations of local anesthetic nerve damage would include spontaneous paresthesias and deficits in pain and temperature perception but not loss of motor, touch, or proprioceptive function.[16]

There is less doubt about the clinical importance of local anesthetic neurotoxicity when the drug is injected intrafascicularly (Fig. 4-3). Although axonal degeneration and a damaged blood-nerve barrier are inconsistent[17] or absent[12] after the intrafascicular injection of saline alone, lidocaine 1% and bupivacaine 0.5% injection results in evidence of axonal degeneration and barrier changes. Findings are progressively worse with increasing concentrations of both agents, especially in concentrations above the clinically used range.[12,17] Ester local anesthetics and carbonated lidocaine produce widespread and severe damage of the nerve fibers and the blood-nerve barriers when injected within the fascicles.[17] This evidence leads to the conclusion that the surrounding perineurium plays an important role in protecting the fascicular contents from the cytotoxic effects of local anesthetics.

In humans, nerve conduction evidence may show neuropathy after intraneural injection of local anesthetics even in the absence of symp-

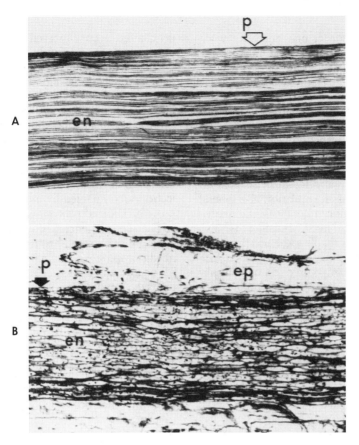

Fig. 4-3. A, The normal appearance of a peripheral nerve. *p,* Perineurium; *en,* endoneural space; longitudinal section. **B,** Twelve days after the intraperineural injection of 0.5% bupivacaine with epinephrine, 5 μg/ml, the axons are fragmented and partially digested by Schwann cells. *ep,* Epineural connective tissue. (**A** and **B** from Selander D, Brattsand R, Lundborg G, et al: Acta Anaesthesiol Scand 23:127, 1979.)

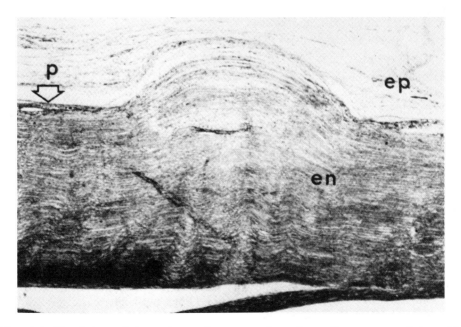

Fig. 4-4. Herniation of the endoneural contents through needle puncture of the perineurium. *en,* Endoneural space; *ep,* epineural connective tissue; *p,* perineurium. (From Selander D, Brattsand R, Lundborg G, et al: Acta Anaesthesiol Scand 23:127, 1979.)

toms.[18] Since this disorder may emerge a week or more after the injection, it may not present until well past the anesthesiologist's postoperative visit.

Additives to the local anesthetic solutions may cause neuropathologic changes. Most notable is the injury caused by sodium bisulfite, an antioxidant added to preparations of chloroprocaine. When combined with low pH solutions, sodium bisulfite has a pronounced neurotoxic effect intrathecally[19,20] and for this reason is no longer available in this formulation. Peripheral nerves appear to be more tolerant of the neurotoxic effects of bisulfite.[21] Bisulfite is also present in currently available local anesthetic solutions containing epinephrine added before packaging. Even though no reports have implicated this mixture in a neurotoxic complication, it is probably best to avoid bisulfite by adding fresh epinephrine to the local anesthetic at the time of the block.

The addition of epinephrine has been shown to increase the neurotoxicity of bisulfite-containing chloroprocaine solutions [22] and to increase the axonal degeneration that follows intrafascicular bupivacaine injection.[12,17] Nerve blood flow, especially in the large epineural feeding arteries, is sensitive to the vasoconstrictive effect of injected epinephrine at usual concentrations.[13] Because of these issues, epinephrine should be added to local anesthetic solutions only if prolongation of the block cannot be achieved by use of a different local anesthetic, or if maximal doses are used and systemic toxicity is possible. Chlorocresol, an antimicrobial preservative added to multiuse vials, is neurotoxic and should not be used in nerve block solutions.

B. Mechanical nerve damage

Injury to the nerve during needle insertion for nerve block anesthesia is an unavoidable risk. The interruption of the perineural tissue around the nerve fascicles breaches the blood-nerve barrier and produces edema of the nerve and herniation of the endoneural contents through the rent (Fig. 4-4). With sharp-beveled needles, a fascicular injury is more likely to result from needle-point contact with the nerve than with a blunt-beveled needle,[23] and it can similarly be expected that a fine needle (such as 25-gauge) will penetrate the nerve more frequently than a larger (22-gauge) needle will. Needle-tip penetration of the nerve may not itself be the cause of clinical complications.[18,24] No functional change is evident in humans after the passage of a needle into the ulnar nerve if local anesthetic is not injected intraneurally.[18] In a rat model,

no changes were observed in microscopic anatomy or in the adequacy of diffusion barriers within the nerve after the penetration of the fascicle with a needle and the injection of saline solution,[12] despite the creation of intrafascicular pressures that transiently exceed the nerve capillary perfusion pressure.[25] Nonetheless, the placement of a needle within the nerve is a source of concern, since injection of local anesthetic subperineurally is likely to result in axonal degeneration[17] as discussed above. Any injection accompanied by intense lancinating pain must be aborted promptly.

The consequences of eliciting paresthesias during block procedures is unknown. When the needle impinges upon the nerve, some degree of nerve injury might occur, but this is unproved. A clinical study by Selander is the most pertinent regarding paresthesias during nerve blocks.[26] Symptomatic nerve lesions were apparent postoperatively in 2.8% of patients after axillary blocks in whom paresthesias were sought and in 0.8% of patients in whom the injection was made on either side of the artery (of whom 40% had unintentional paresthesias). The difference between the groups was not significant, though only patients who experienced paresthesias developed postblock neuropathy. It needs to be noted, however, that epinephrine was used uniformly in the paresthesia group but only in half of the artery group, and sharp pointed needles were used. In a contrasting study in a nontraining situation,[27] 3 patients (0.36%) developed postblock neuropathy from a group of 835 brachial plexus blocks done with the intentional production of paresthesias. All three patients had multiple paresthesias during the block. A prudent approach would include the use of blunt needles and gentle technique. If a paresthesia is provoked, injection at this site should be done with no further needle advancement, or a slight withdrawal of the needle. Injection should halt immediately if it initiates or intensifies a paresthesia. Seeking multiple paresthesias may be accompanied by an increased incidence of neuropathy because the initial local anesthetic deposit may conceal needle contact with nerves. It is usually unwise to attempt a major nerve block in a patient who is unable to report a paresthesia, such as a deeply sedated or generally anesthetized patient.

Many authors have advised against nerve blocks at confined fascial spaces, such as the ulnar nerve at the elbow or the peroneal nerve at the fibular head. There is a concern that neuropathy is more likely after these blocks, either because of the pressure that develops in the enclosed space on the injection of the anesthetic

Changes in nerves compressed by tourniquet

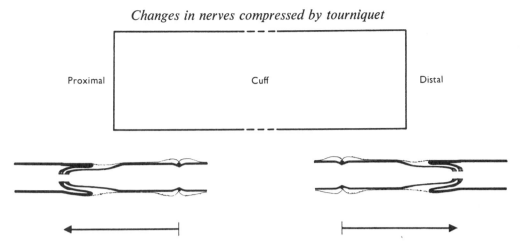

Fig. 4-5. Nerve injury from tourniquets represented diagramatically, showing maximal deformation at the margins of a tourniquet. A pressure gradient is created, *arrows,* causing intussusception of the node of Ranvier into the adjacent perinodal myelin sheath. (From Ochoa J, Fouler TJ, and Gilliat RW: J Anat 113:433, 1972.)

solution or because the nerve is fixed in position and unable to recede from the encroaching needle. However, evidence is generally lacking to prove this increased risk.

Other sources of neuropathy must be considered when one is evaluating a nerve injury after a nerve block. Tourniquets may cause nerve damage either by ischemia or mechanical deformation, though distortion of the nerve under the tourniquet (Fig. 4-5) is the more likely mechanism of prolonged nerve dysfunction. Even when ischemic periods last 6 hours, ischemia alone fails to produce lasting structural changes in nerves,[28] and nerve function returns within 6 hours if ischemic times are less than 2 hours.[29] However, the portion of the nerve under the proximal edge of the pneumatic cuff, where the mechanical distortion of the nerve is maximal, may suffer irreversible damage after 2 to 4 hours of tourniquet inflation.[30] One may minimize nerve damage by using wide cuffs and inflation pressures just adequate for arterial occlusion[31] and by keeping inflation times as brief as possible. Alternating between the two cuffs of a double-cuff tourniquet may allow prolonged ischemia with diminished mechanical damage to the nerves, since neither site is compressed for more than an hour.[32] With this arrangement, ischemic changes such as tissue edema and sensory deficits occurred but resolved within 3 weeks, and permanent changes were rare. Large fibers are the neural components most susceptible to both ischemic and mechanical damage. The main findings of tourniquet-induced neuropathy are motor loss and diminished touch, vibration, and position

sense, with preserved senses of heat, cold, and pain and the absence of spontaneous paresthesias.[33]

Special care must be used to avoid positioning injuries after nerve blocks, since an anesthetized limb may be malpositioned without resulting pain. The most common upper extremity injuries that result from malpositioning are ulnar damage, caused by direct pressure on the nerve at the elbow, and brachial plexus injury, caused by prolonged stretching of the plexus. Tension on the brachial plexus occurs when the arm is abducted excessively (over 90 degrees) and is further increased by extension of the shoulder.[34] The most frequent lower extremity malposition injury is common peroneal nerve damage, which results from direct pressure over the fibular head. Other causes of postoperative neuropathy include deficits that predate the operation, surgical injuries, and compression from compartment syndromes or casts. These considerations make a careful preblock neurologic examination of the limb imperative. Should a deficit develop, early consultation should be considered with specialists for detailed neurologic and electrophysiologic diagnosis.

II. MISCELLANEOUS COMPLICATIONS RELATED TO THE PERFORMANCE OF A NERVE BLOCK
A. Systemic complications from local anesthetics

The prevention of adverse systemic responses to the local anesthetic injected during nerve blocks must be a matter of close attention by the physician. These blocks may be chosen to avoid the perceived greater risk of a general anesthetic or major neuraxial block or may be performed away from the operating room for therapeutic or diagnostic purposes. The result may be a lessened expectation of systemic sequelae and a diminished preparedness to treat an adverse response. However, when large doses of local anesthetic are administered for nerve blocks, patient monitoring must be as intense as for a general, spinal, or epidural anesthetic, and resuscitation equipment and drugs must be immediately available.

In the setting of nerve blocks, toxic reactions may be early, because of intravascular injection of the drug, or delayed until an extravascular bolus is absorbed. Many of the major nerves are in the vicinity of large vessels. Since the failure to aspirate blood from the block needle does not ensure that the injectate will not enter a vessel, the injection should proceed slowly and incrementally to allow the identification of intravascular injection before the full dose is administered. If 30 ml of 1.5% lidocaine is to be injected, for example, 7 ml might be injected at a time, with a wait of perhaps a minute between injections.

The peak serum concentration of local anesthetic and the likelihood of a resulting toxic response vary when a given dose is injected at different sites.[35] The concentrations after intercostal blocks are the highest, probably because the drug is distributed throughout a large area by multiple small injections at different intercostal spaces and the tissue is highly vascular. The deposition of the same dose in a single mass, as with a lumbar sympathetic or celiac block, diminishes the exposure of the drug to absorption compared to a dispersed injection. Placement of the anesthetic solution into a sheathed enclosure or a fatty and minimally vascular tissue plane, as with brachial plexus blocks or sciatic-femoral blocks, results in the lowest blood concentration of anesthetic, provided that the injection is outside the vessels.

The addition of epinephrine to local anesthetic solutions diminishes the peak blood concentration after nerve block procedures.[36] This effect is greatest with mepivacaine, prilocaine, and lidocaine, especially when they are used for intercostal and paracervical administration. Whereas etidocaine and bupivacaine blood concentrations after epidural block are not much affected by the addition of epinephrine, a significant diminution is seen in most studies of plexus and peripheral nerve blocks with these drugs, though not so pronounced an effect as with the shorter acting amides. The benefit of

epinephrine for reducing blood concentrations of anesthetic must be weighed against the potential of increased neurotoxicity as described above.

Although peak blood concentrations of local anesthetic are reached in most cases by 20 minutes after the injection, it is important to realize that peak concentrations may occur up to 60 minutes after the injection.[36]

The performance of a nerve block may be stressful to patients,[16] and sedation is commonly used. Benzodiazapines have been shown to increase the local anesthetic blood concentration required to cause central nervous system toxicity[37,38] and would thus appear to protect the patient. Preventing central nervous system manifestations may, however, delay the discovery of blood concentrations high enough to cause cardiovascular toxicity, the threshold for which is not raised by benzodiazapines.[37,38] More importantly, the early signs of toxicity require communication with the patient to elicit perceptions such as circumoral numbness, dizziness, and tinnitus, as well as changes in speech and mental status. Identification of paresthesias likewise requires a responsive patient. For these reasons, aggressive sedation should be avoided in most nerve block procedures, with the goal being a comfortable but responsive patient.

If local anesthetic is introduced into the arterial circulation of the brain, central nervous system toxicity can be prompt and profound. As little as 0.5 ml of 0.5% bupivacaine can cause seizures when injected into the vertebral artery.[39,40] Other presentations may include loss of consciousness, transient blindness, aphasia, or hemiparesis.[40-42] The greatest risk of direct cerebrovascular administration of local anesthetics is via the vertebral or carotid arteries during blocks of the stellate ganglion, brachial plexus, and cervical plexus. However, it has been demonstrated in baboons that retrograde arterial flow can deliver local anesthetic to the brain arterial supply from forcible injections into the lingual, brachial, and even femoral arteries.[43]

B. Vascular complications during nerve blocks

Since major vessels are often in proximity to the desired target of the nerve block needle, vascular punctures are impossible to avoid with certainty. In most cases, such punctures are innocuous. Indeed, some techniques use the penetration of a major artery as the landmark to ensure effective needle placement, as in the transarterial technique of axillary brachial plexus blockade[44] and the transaortic technique of celiac plexus blockade.[45] Nonetheless, complications may result in a variety of ways from vascular punctures. Of greatest importance is the deposition of a portion of the injectate intravascularly, causing high blood concentrations of local anesthetic and systemic toxicity (see p. 58). There is rarely any direct toxicity to the vessels from a properly chosen injectate, though the intra-arterial injection of solutions with epinephrine may produce a transient vasospasm of the large arteries of the limb[46,47] and the microvasculature of the nerves, producing a sharp decrease in nerve blood flow.[48] Compartment syndromes have been reported, however, when directly toxic solutions have been mistakenly injected during nerve block in the place of the desired local anesthetic solution.[49] Even when epinephrine is placed extravascularly, its action on distal terminal arteries may cause ischemia and tissue loss[50] and should be avoided at such sites as the digits, penis, ears, and perhaps the nose and ankle, depending on the adequacy of the patient's circulation.

The injection of solution into closed fascial spaces such as the axillary sheath may transiently produce intrasheath pressures greater than the mean arterial pressure.[51] In a similar way, the development of a carotid bruit may signal the compression of the vessel after an interscalene bolus injection.[52] There is no evidence that this mechanism can produce vascular compromise. Circulatory disturbance may result, however, from vessel damage by the block needle. Case reports have documented the development of artery occlusion from subintimal administration of the local anesthetic[53] and venous narrowing and aneurysm formation after axillary block.[54] The absence of vascular occlusive complications from large series of regional anesthetics would indicate that these are rare complications. This optimistic view must be tempered by the knowledge that these problems may appear weeks after the block, making their incidence difficult to ascertain. The formation of hematomas after nerve blocks is well recognized.[16,55] Vascular punctures are common during nerve blockade, but hematomas are infrequent and are usually harmless, though they may rarely contribute to nerve damage.[16]

The avoidance of vessel injury requires the use of needles no larger than 22 gauge and an orderly and gentle use of the needle so as to penetrate vessels the fewest possible times. A technique should be adopted so that the needle is advanced only in the axis of its shaft and never moved laterally within the body, a movement that may cause lacerations by the needle tip. Redirection of the needle should take place only after the needle is withdrawn to the skin. When possible, firm pressure should be placed on the puncture site after blockade to minimize bleeding, especially if blood has been aspirated during the procedure. By comparing vital signs and vascular status after the block to those noted before the block, one can identify problems and treat promptly. Therapy usually requires only pressure to the area, but early surgical consultation may avoid tissue loss.

Anticoagulation presents a difficult decision for the physician considering nerve block injections. In the presence of full heparinization, nerve blocks may lead to problematic bleeding,[56] and other options should be chosen if possible. Heparinization after nerve blockade is frequently done without ill effects. However, a case report[57] has implicated heparin administered after a subclavian perivascular brachial plexus block as a causative factor in the development of a hemothorax. Many patients coming for nerve blocks have compromised platelet function from nonsteroidal anti-inflammatory drugs, including aspirin. Although this is probably not a contraindication to nerve blocks in general, a rational approach would include careful consideration of the expected benefits from the nerve block, the relative desirability of alternative techniques, and other associated risk factors such as anemia, vascular disease, and frail tissues that might potentiate problems from vascular punctures. Blocks at sites where extravasation can be monitored directly and compression applied create less of a risk than blocks in which bleeding may not be apparent, such as celiac or intercostal blocks. A bleeding time may be useful in deciding to proceed or not. An even more uncertain relative contraindication is the use of small doses of subcutaneous heparin for pulmonary embolism prophylaxis. No simple rule can be applied as a substitute for a balanced judgment based on the nature of the block, the patient, and the disease.

C. Pulmonary complications

Any needle insertion into the chest or neck may transgress the boundaries of the chest wall and lead to damage of the visceral pleura, initiating a slow leakage of air from the pulmonary parenchyma. Fear of causing a pneumothorax discourages many anesthetists from using these blocks. This may be an overreaction, however. The incidence in most studies is quite low, as is enumerated in the discussions of the individual blocks later. The risk of pneumothorax accompanying the placement of an interpleural catheter is uncertain because studies differ greatly in their results. Obtaining a chest roentgenogram after procedures such as intercostal, supraclavicular, and stellate blocks is not necessary in most situations. Since the small needles used for nerve blocks cause slow leaks, a developing pneumothorax is likely to be missed by a chest roentgenogram obtained soon after the block. Six to 12 hours may elapse before intrapleural air accumulates and symptoms arise. Also, since it is not necessary to treat small, asymptomatic pneumothoraces,[58] their discovery may be irrelevant. But when a needle procedure about the chest is followed by chest pain, coughing, or shortness of breath, a chest roentgenogram should be obtained. With a pneumothorax, the physical exam may show hyperresonance or loss of breath sounds on the side of the procedure. The presence of subcutaneous emphysema is strong evidence of the development of a pneumothorax. Even less commonly, the chest may fill with blood from needle damage to an intercostal[56] or subclavian[57] artery or with chyle from damage to the thoracic duct.[59]

To minimize the frequency of pneumothoraces after nerve blocks, large needles and repeated deep probing should be avoided, and care should be used in patient selection. Agitated or coughing patients or those with emphysema have an increased risk of developing a pneumothorax. General anesthesia may occasionally be administered after a block employing needles near the pleura, perhaps after a failed block. In these cases, it is best to avoid the use of positive-pressure ventilation and nitrous oxide, both of which may expand any pneumothorax present. The bilateral use of blocks having a pneumothorax risk is usually unwise. If patients are to be discharged home within 12 hours of a nerve block, procedures with a minimal risk of pneumothorax are desirable. For example, an epidural block may be a better choice than intercostal blocks, or an axillary block may be preferred to a supraclavicular block.

When a pneumothorax is identified, the treatment will depend on the extent of the lung collapse and the patient's condition. In the most common situation in which the collapse is less than 25% of the lung volume, reinflation is likely to be spontaneous. If the patient is not in distress, care should be conservative, with repeat chest roentgenograms to confirm the lack of progression and with attentive monitoring of the patient's condition. Larger accumulations are less likely to resolve,[60] especially when over 50% of the lung has collapsed, and consultation with a surgeon regarding the insertion of a chest tube should take place. Discussion with the surgeon should include the fact that, unlike

most other pulmonary air leaks, the ones caused by block needles are slow, and aggressive therapy with large thoracostomy tubes should be tempered by this fact. If hemodynamic collapse follows a nerve block procedure near the lungs, especially if the neck veins are distended and the trachea is deviated to the side opposite the side blocked, a tension pneumothorax must be suspected. There may be occasions in which the rapid onset of a cardiopulmonary crisis precludes the performance of a chest roentgenogram. In this setting, decompression of the pneumothorax by the passage of a large intravenous catheter in the second intercostal space at the midclavicular line may be lifesaving.

The proper expansion of the lungs depends on a complex interaction of diaphragm, intercostal, abdominal, and accessory muscle mechanics.[61] Interference with the motor nerves driving these muscles produces subtle deficits in mechanics that are well tolerated in healthy persons. Bilateral intercostal blocks from T6 to T12 results only in the minor loss in peak expiratory flows and endurance, with no deficit in resting lung volumes or vital capacity.[62] The loss of a single phrenic nerve also produces changes in respiratory performance that are tolerable to most otherwise fit persons, as demonstrated in studies of phrenic paralysis after brachial plexus blocks above the clavicle in which the diaphragm is shown to be immobile but the patients are asymptomatic.[63-66] It is fortunate that these changes are well tolerated because a degree of intercostal motor block is likely to follow all intercostal blocks, and diaphragmatic weakness is common after brachial plexus blocks in the neck, either because of misplacement of the local anesthetic anterior to the scalenus anticus, which separates the phrenic from the plexus, or more commonly because of the spread of anesthetic cephalad to the roots of C3 to C5. Bilateral phrenic block is less innocuous. Even though minimal change in tidal volume occurs after bilateral phrenic blocks in healthy volunteers, there is a 25% decrease in vital capacity.[67] In patients with compromised pulmonary function, this could result in ventilatory insufficiency.

Even the unilateral loss of respiratory muscle activity is not always harmless, as demonstrated by the various case reports of respiratory distress after intercostal blocks[68,69] and brachial plexus blocks in the neck.[70,71] Advanced emphysema is accompanied by flattening of the diaphragm and expansion of the anteroposterior dimensions of the chest, diminishing the ability of the diaphragm to expand the chest.[72] Since ventilation in these patients is especially dependent on intercostal activity, they may be more prone to the adverse effects of intercostal paralysis. However, complications resulting from either intercostal or phrenic paralysis may also develop in patients without any preexisting pulmonary disease.

Ventilatory motor interference should be considered a possibility whenever dyspnea follows a nerve block in the neck or an intercostal block. Unlike a pneumothorax, the onset is usually within 1 or 2 hours of the procedure. Confirmation of phrenic paresis requires x-ray or ultrasound examination. The frequency with which asymptomatic phrenic paresis is identified after brachial plexus blocks in the neck depends on the thoroughness of the radiologic study. A routine roentgenogram showed phrenic involvement in 10% to 36% of patients,[64,73] whereas other studies showed a 67% incidence when fluoroscopy was used[65] and 80% when inspiratory and expiratory chest roentgenograms were compared.[63] Using ultrasound imaging to detect paradoxical diaphragm motion revealed phrenic paralysis in all of 12 subjects.[74] Since diaphragmatic weakness is such a common finding after these blocks, the real value in obtaining a chest roentgenogram is elimination of the alternative diagnosis of pneumothorax.

The risk of ventilatory motor block can be minimized by careful patient selection, cautious technique, use of solutions of anesthetic no more concentrated than necessary for an adequate result, and avoidance of the bilateral use of such blocks, especially ones carrying the risk of phrenic block. The therapy for this complication is supplemental oxygen administration and ventilatory support until the motor block has resolved.

D. Undesired extension of blockade

Minute amounts of local anesthetic are needed to achieve a thorough block when the drug is placed in the immediate vicinity of the targeted axons. As an example, 1 ml of 1% lidocaine produces a block when placed within the ulnar nerve of human subjects.[15] The requirement for doses of 5 to 60 ml for the various nerve blocks is attributable to the need to deliver the drug to the target nerve without requiring the perfection of needle placement that minimal doses would demand. For single nerves such as the lateral femoral cutaneous, an injection of 5 or 10 ml allows delivery from a pool of anesthetic by diffusion and bulk flow. For many blocks, large volumes are needed to reach nerves at a distance from the needle. The paratracheal stellate block anesthetizes the ganglion that resides at the T1 level by a needle placed at C6. A brachial plexus block at any level requires an adequate volume of injectate to reach the multiple components of the plexus, and a celiac block likewise uses the bulk flow of a large injected volume to reach the entirety of the ganglion. The problems arise because the drug also travels to undesired destinations, causing blockade of neural components with pathologic as well as therapeutic consequences.

The list of case reports in which local anesthetic gets to unintended nerves is a catalog that proves the axiom, "If it can go wrong, it will," as in the following.

Subarachnoid injection, often with a resulting total spinal anesthetic, may follow retrobulbar block,[75-77] brachial plexus block,[78,79] facet joint injection,[80] or intercostal block, especially when administered by the intrathoracic route during surgery.[81-85] In many of these cases, the presentation was cardiac arrest. Also reported is postural headaches in 3 of 24 patients receiving one or more thoracic paravertebral somatic nerve blocks, probably caused by dural puncture.[86]

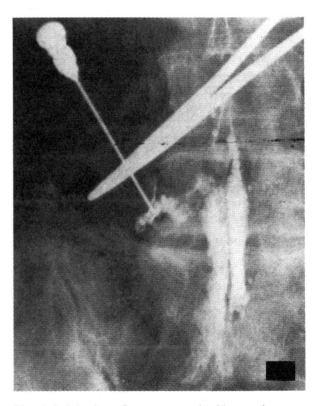

Fig. 4-6. Injection of a nerve root, in this case the fifth lumbar, may not be selective unless small volumes are used. Spread to the epidural space is demonstrated in this roentgenogram. (From Krempen JS, Smith B, and DeFreest LJ: Orthop Clin North Am 6:311, 1975.)

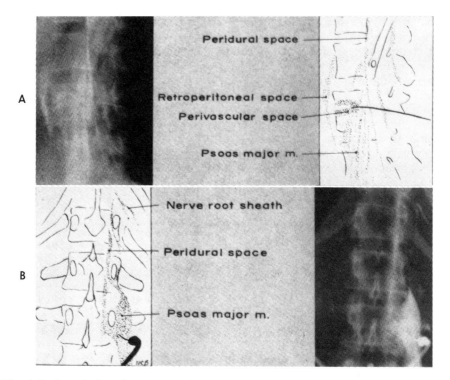

Fig. 4-7. Lateral, **A,** and posteroanterior, **B,** views of epidural spread of injectate after a lumbar paravertebral sympathetic block. Interpretation of injections designed to produce differential blockade of the sympathetic nerves must be cautious in light of the possibility of spillover into somatic nerves. (From Evans JA, Dobben GD, and Gay GR: JAMA 200:93, 1967.)

Epidural spread of anesthetic can result from brachial plexus block,[87-90] intercostal block,[91] segmental somatic blocks[92] (Fig. 4-6), and facet injections.[93-94]

Spread to the paravertebral sympathetic chain may follow brachial plexus block[95] or intercostal block.[96-98] Spread to the contralateral sympathetic chain may occur during stellate ganglion block.[99] Contrariwise, somatic blockade can develop with injections of the lumbar sympathetic chain[100] (Fig. 4-7) or the cervicothoracic sympathetic chain.[100,101]

Finally, undesired peripheral nerve blocks may develop from the injection at other sites.[102-104]

The misplacement of needles certainly may contribute to these undesired outcomes, as when an improperly angled needle enters a cervical neural foramen during interscalene block. However, accurate needle placement may still result in undesired blocks. Several pathways are possible. As proved by MacIntosh in 1947,[105] the paravertebral spaces communicate with the epidural space (Fig. 4-6) and with each other. Also, the intercostal space allows passage of drugs into the paravertebral space.[106] By such communicating tissue planes, in other parts of the body as well, bulk flow of anesthetic may lead to blockade of undesired neural elements.

Passage of local anesthetic into the cerebro-spinal fluid produces an extensive response. The common explanation is the injection of drug into an extension of the subarachnoid space continuing out the neural foramen around the segmental nerve as a dural sleeve or cuff. There is no doubt that these extensions exist because they can be seen on myelography.[107] But the usual termination of the subarachnoid space is at the dorsal root ganglion in or medial to the intervertebral foramen.[108] A more likely pathway leading to spinal anesthesia during peripheral nerve blocks is intraneural injection.[109,110] When injectate is introduced into the epineurium of peripheral nerves, only a localized bleb forms.[25] In contrast, when a solution is injected into a fascicle within a nerve, there is extensive subperineural spread, with the injectate eventually reaching the subpial and then the subarachnoid spaces (Fig. 4-8). The nerve fascicle is thus topographically an extension of the central nervous system, and it is fortuitous that nerve fascicles are entered with difficulty.[18] When spinal anesthesia results from a nerve block, the onset is typically within minutes of the injection. It is important to realize, however, that the transit of local anesthetic to the cerebrospinal fluid may require 15 to 30 minutes, allowing the delayed development of total

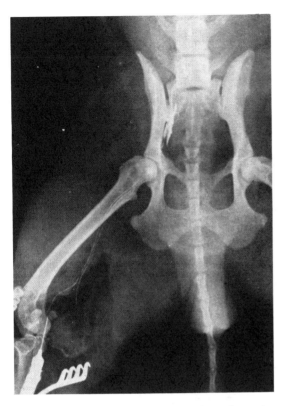

Fig. 4-8. Contrast medium injected into the endoneural space of a peripheral nerve in a dog flowing proximally to the plexus and appearing in the subarachnoid space, as well as passing distally in another fascicle after rupture in the plexus. (From French JD, Strain WH, and Jones GE: J Neuropathol Exp Neurol 7:47, 1948.)

spinal anesthesia.[110] The proper treatment of this event requires prompt ventilatory and hemodynamic support.

Because of the impossibility of limiting the spread of local anesthetics entirely to the desired nerves, diagnostic nerve block procedures should be interpreted with caution. For example, the epidural spread of anesthetic injected into facet joints and near segmental nerves is common (Fig. 4-7), as is the spread from sympathetic blocks to somatic nerves and the reverse. If a diagnosis of a pain mechanism is made on the basis of a block that is in fact more extensive than believed, inappropriate therapeutic procedures might be performed, including surgical ablations. This concern should encourage the use of small volumes when blocks are done for diagnosis.

E. Infections

It is rare for the site of needle insertion for nerve blocks to become infected, though cases have been reported occurring after pudendal and paracervical blocks for obstetrics.[111,112]

The low incidence of this complication may be in part attributable to the broad antimicrobial activity of local anesthetics.[113] As with many of the other complications of nerve blocks, because infections are rare and unexpected, the possibility might not be considered and early signs may be missed. Puncture sites should always be examined on the following days for signs of inflammation.

F. Fetal complications

Pudendal and paracervical blocks have been used by obstetricians to provide analgesia for labor and delivery. The advantage to the obstetrician is that specialized anesthesia training is not required for the administration of these procedures. Paracervical block provides analgesia for uterine contractions and cervical dilatation, whereas pudendal block provides analgesia for perineal and vaginal distension.

Pudendal block is considered a safe and effective method for providing analgesia for vaginal delivery. The tissues injected are more vascular than the epidural space, and peak local anesthetic blood concentrations may be somewhat higher than for epidural analgesia. In addition, injection is generally performed within a short interval of delivery, at a time that maternal blood concentrations are near peak. Despite this potential for fetal local anesthetic toxicity, reports of adverse reactions, either fetal or maternal, are rare, and fetal local anesthetic blood concentrations are considerably lower than maternal.[114] Merkow et al.[114] were unable to demonstrate significant neurobehavioral depression among infants delivered after pudendal blocks with meplvacaine, chloroprocaine, or bupivacaine.

On the other hand, paracervical block is associated with a high incidence of fetal bradycardia, ranging from 2% to 70%.[115] The incidence is related to local anesthetic dose. Although it has been postulated that the phenomenon may be caused by changes in uterine tone or blood flow, the majority of evidence points to high fetal blood concentration as the cause.[116] Fetal concentrations of local anesthetic in excess of those in maternal blood have been documented,[116] leading to postulates that direct diffusion of drug into the uterine artery may occur. Direct uterine arterial injection and injection directly into the fetal presenting part may also occur with this block, leading to profound fetal toxicity or death.

III. COMPLICATIONS OF NEUROLYTIC BLOCKS

Ethanol and phenol are the agents used most extensively to produce neurolytic neural blockade. Alcohol causes extraction of phospholipids, cholesterol, and cerebrosides and precipitation of lipoproteins and mucoproteins.[117] The neurolytic effect of phenol is mainly the result of protein denaturation. When these drugs are administered in proximity to peripheral nerves, they cause axonal damage that results in wallerian degeneration. Less severe damage can result in local demyelination, producing a temporary neural deficit that recovers in a period of days to weeks. Injury to the cell body of a neuron produces cell death and permanent loss of function. Damage to the optic nerve by neurolytic agents generally results in permanent blindness.

Alcohol and phenol both have effects on other tissues and are capable of producing sclerosis of small blood vessels and local tissue irritation. Both drugs also have systemic effects. Those of alcohol are well known. High blood concentrations of phenol produce toxicity similar to that of local anesthetics.

The complications of neurolytic blocks will be divided into four categories: damage to peripheral neural structures, spread to neuraxial structures, local tissue effects, and systemic effects.

A. Damage to peripheral nerves

Peripheral neurolytic blocks may produce unwanted effects by spread of drug to adjacent peripheral nerves. The most devastating consequences involve damage to motor nerves. Spread of drug to the facial nerve during trigeminal neurolytic blocks is an example. Other examples include overflow of drug to the brachial plexus during stellate ganglion block, spread of drug to somatic nerve roots during celiac, splanchnic, or lumbar sympathetic blocks, and overflow to the glossopharyngeal nerve during gasserian ganglion block.[118] Meticulous needle placement, use of a small local anesthetic test dose, and use of small volumes of neurolytic agents should minimize such complications. A thorough knowledge of the anatomy of the peripheral nervous system is a prerequisite to performance of neurolytic blocks, and neurolytic agents should be avoided around important motor nerves, such as the common peroneal nerve, damage to which may produce footdrop.

Another consequence of peripheral neurolytic block is neuropathic pain, a phenomenon commonly termed "neuritis"[118,119] that is seen more commonly with alcohol than with phenol.[119] It occurs sufficiently often to discourage many practitioners from using neurolytic agents on peripheral nerves. It may occur soon after the block or may come on weeks to months later, as function in the blocked nerve returns. Denervation dysesthesia, also termed "anesthesia dolorosa" is another potential consequence of neurolytic blockade. It is the result of loss of neural input from the affected area and may cause disruption of normal gating mechanisms in the dorsal horn or may lead to sensitization or spontaneous activity in dorsal horn neurons that are involved with nociceptive transmission. Unfortunately, prognostic local anesthetic blocks do not predict the occurrence of this problem. Denervation dysesthesia responds poorly to opioids but may be ameliorated by centrally acting drugs such as tricyclic antidepressants or anticonvulsants.

Even when peripheral blocks are performed without apparent complications, untoward effects can result from the loss of function of the nerve blocked. For instance, mandibular block may produce weakness of mastication. Block of the maxillary division of the trigeminal nerve can result in loss of corneal reflexes and keratitis.[120] Loss of sensation may result in repeated burns or injury to insensible areas, and some patients find the loss of sensation as distressing as their original pain.

B. Spread to neuraxial structures

The use of neurolytic agents in the epidural or subarachnoid space is recognized as a useful analgesic technique. However, the unintentional spread of neurolytic agents to these areas during attempted peripheral blocks may be devastating, especially since the volumes of drug used are generally higher than those used neuraxially. The resulting damage to the spinal cord and nerve roots may produce permanent or long-lasting sensory and motor block, bowel and bladder dysfunction, vasomotor instability, and, when blockade is extensive, paraplegia, quadriplegia, or death.

Neuraxial spread may occur whenever blocks are performed relatively near the midline posteriorly. Splanchnic, celiac, and lumbar sympathetic blocks have been associated with epidural and subarachnoid spread of drug, which results when the needle is placed too superficially and enters the neural foramen. Biplane fluoroscopy or computerized tomography should be used whenever these blocks are performed with neurolytic agents. Other blocks that are associated with neuraxial spread are stellate ganglion block, paravertebral somatic root block, intercostal blocks, and facet rhizolysis. Subarachnoid spread of neurolytic agents can result from injection directly into the subarachnoid space, into the dural root sleeve, or from intraneural spread associated with intrafascicular injection.[25]

Subarachnoid injection is also a potential complication of certain cranial nerve blocks, such as gasserian ganglion block, and may result in permanent damage to other cranial nerves and vasomotor fibers (see next column for the discussion of trigeminal nerve block complications).

Surgical distortion of anatomy may lead to unexpected complications. I (S.E.A.) have seen the subarachnoid spread of local anesthetic during a lesser occipital nerve block in a patient who had undergone craniotomy for acoustic neuroma. The needle apparently entered the dura through the craniotomy defect. Injection of lidocaine produced transient hypotension and loss of consciousness. Such an injection with a neurolytic agent would be devastating.

C. Local tissue effects

Gangrene and slough of tissues has been reported occurring after neurolytic block, particularly after block of the infraorbital nerve.[118,121] The mechanism of slough after infraorbital block is unclear. Whenever alcohol or phenol is injected superficially, skin necrosis may occur, probably as a result of sclerosis of cutaneous blood vessels.

Pain, swelling, cellulitis, and abscess formation in the area of injection of neurolytic agents have been reported.[118] Histologic studies of lytic drug injection into muscles have shown the development of pallor and coagulation followed by necrosis, degeneration, and lymphocyte and macrophage infiltration.[122] New capillaries and fibroblasts appear in 7 to 10 days, and regeneration is complete in 2 to 3 weeks. Given the degree of tissue damage caused by neurolytic agents, one would anticipate significant damage to organs injected with these drugs. Renal and ureteral damage can occur during neurolytic lumbar sympathetic block. One can reduce damage to these organs and spread of drug to other neural structures along a needle track by clearing the needle of neurolytic agent with local anesthetic or saline before needle withdrawal.

D. Systemic effects

Ethanol has relatively little systemic effect, even in relatively large doses. Fifty milliliters of 50% ethanol, a dose commonly used for celiac plexus block, is roughly equivalent to 2 ounces of whiskey in its alcohol content. However, when alcohol metabolism is abnormal, as in patients taking disulfiram (Antabuse), even small quantities of alcohol can produce dramatic reactions, related to accumulation of acetaldehyde. Symptoms include flushing, palpitations, headache, nausea, vomiting, and vertigo. Blood pressure may decrease precipitously. As little as 7 ml of alcohol may cause such reactions in patients taking disulfiram.[123] Acetaldehyde syndrome may also occur after alcohol blocks in patients deficient in aldehyde dehydrogenase[124] (ALDH) or in patients taking drugs that, like disulfiram, suppress ALDH activity. Carmofur, used as an antitumor agent, has been associated with acetaldehyde syndrome in patients who have undergone alcohol celiac plexus blocks.[125]

Use of large volumes of phenol or the intravascular injection of phenol produces systemic effects similar to those of local anesthetics. Increasing blood levels produce tinnitus and flushing,[126] with high levels causing seizures, loss of consciousness, and hypotension.[119]

IV. COMPLICATIONS OF SPECIFIC BLOCKS

Following is a discussion of the more common complications associated with specific types of blocks. Discussion is confined to those blocks that are used in practice with some frequency.

Essentially all local anesthetic blocks may be associated with local anesthetic toxicity either through relative overdose or through intravascular injection. Discussion of the management of local anesthetic toxicity can be found elsewhere in this text, and systemic reactions to local anesthetics is mentioned only for those blocks that carry a particularly high risk of toxic reactions. Likewise, damage to a nerve by a block needle and local infection can result from any type of block. Again, discussion of such complications is confined to blocks for which such complications are particularly likely.

A. Trigeminal nerve and its branches

Block of the gasserian ganglion is now done infrequently. Alcohol injection of the gasserian ganglion was at one time a common treatment for tic douloureux. In recent years it has been found that many cases respond dramatically to anticonvulsants, particularly carbamazapine. For those cases for which neural ablation is elected, radiofrequency coagulation is more commonly used, since it is more accurate and controllable.

Spread of drug in the cerebrospinal fluid surrounding the gasserian ganglion can result in more widespread involvement affecting other cranial nerves. Small quantities of local anesthetic injected into the adjacent subarachnoid space can produce widespread cranial nerve block and loss of consciousness.[127] Advancing

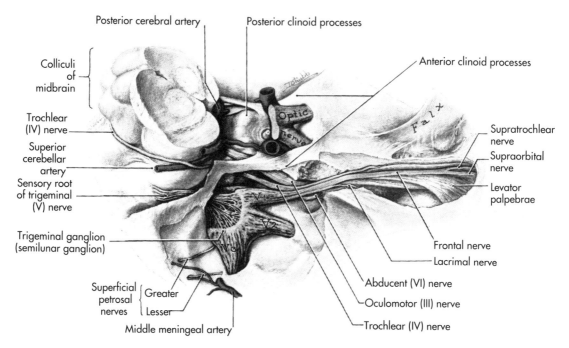

Fig. 4-9. Relationship of the trigeminal ganglion to major intracranial neural and vascular structures. (From Grant JCB: An atlas of anatomy, ed 5, Baltimore, 1962, The Williams & Wilkins Co.)

the needle too far may produce damage to cranial nerves III and VI or to the substance of the brain itself (Fig. 4-9).

Alcohol injection of the trigeminal ganglion is associated with a variety of potentially serious problems. Anesthesia of the second division can result in keratitis and corneal ulceration through loss of corneal sensation and interference with corneal reflexes. An ophthalmologist should be consulted to help manage this potential complication. Blockade of paratrigeminal sympathetic fibers may cause ipsilateral Horner's syndrome, whereas blockade of motor fibers to the masseter muscle can result in weakness of mastication.[128] Block of the oculomotor or abducens nerves will produce diplopia, which usually improves after a few days.[119] Other complications resulting from spread of the alcohol beyond the area of the ganglion include damage to the facial nerve with resulting paresis, involvement of the vestibular and auditory portions of nerve VIII with dizziness, nausea, and nystagmus, hearing loss, and damage to the optic nerve. Injury to the glossopharyngeal nerve can result in dysphagia.

Denervation dysesthesia is a fairly common sequela to correctly performed gasserian ganglion alcohol block, producing a constant burning sensation in the affected area. It has been reported in about 10% of patients.[119] Herpes simplex of the lip, mucous membrane erosion

of the mouth, and nasal ulceration are trophic disturbances that can occur subsequently to gasserian ganglion ablation.

Glycerol injection of the gasserian ganglion produces analgesia in many tic patients without the potential complications of alcohol.[129] Anesthesia is less profound, but recurrence of the original symptoms weeks to months later can occur.

Hemorrhage into the temporal fossa and cheek may result from puncture of vessels in the subtemporal region. Intra-arterial injection of even small quantities of local anesthesic into the middle meningeal or carotid artery can produce central nervous system toxicity.

Supraorbital block with local anesthetic is likely to produce considerable swelling of the upper eyelid, but it is easily controlled with direct pressure. Injection of alcohol or phenol can produce slough of skin over the injection site. Neurolytic agents can spread into the orbit, and so volume should be kept low (less than 0.5 ml).

Block of the infraorbital area can be done at the level of the foramen rotundum or at the infraorbital foramen. Gangrene and slough of areas supplied by the nerve have been reported.[130] The cause of this complication is not known. One case of ocular muscle palsy after infraorbital alcohol block has been reported.[131] In that case, the nerve was injected under direct vision during a Caldwell-Luc procedure.

Intra-arterial injection is a likely possibility when one is blocking the mandibular nerve because of the proximity to the maxillary and middle meningeal arteries. Again, central nervous system toxicity can occur after injection of very small doses.

Neurolytic block of the mandibular nerve can produce weakness of mastication, since it contains motor branches to the masseter muscle. Facial nerve injury is a possible complication. A death related to carotid artery injury during the performance of this block has been reported.[132]

B. Retrobulbar block

Puncture of a vessel, particularly an artery, within the orbit may lead to serious problems because of increasing pressure within a relatively closed space.[130] Hematoma formation initially produces palpebral edema and exophthalmus. As pressure increases, diplopia may occur. Eventually, vision may be compromised or even lost because of pressure on the optic nerve or ophthalmic artery.

Injection of even minute amounts of local anesthetic into the ophthalmic artery may produce convulsions because of retrograde spread of anesthetic within the ophthalmic artery to the internal carotid artery with subsequent rapid flow to the brain.[133] If large doses are injected rapidly, the phase of central nervous system irritability may be bypassed with rapid development of apnea, hypotension, and loss of consciousness.[134]

Life-threatening reactions can also result from spread of drug to the intracranial subarachnoid space. Spread of local anesthetic to the cerebrospinal fluid after retrobulbar block is well documented[75] and probably occurs through injection within the dural sheath of the optic nerve. Onset time of central nervous system symptoms is generally several minutes as opposed to the instantaneous onset seen with intra-arterial injection. Signs and symptoms of intracranial subarachnoid local anesthetic spread include drowsiness, blindness (including the contralateral eye), apnea, hemiplegia, aphasia, loss of consciousness, seizures, shivering, and cardiac arrest.[75] The practice of instructing the patient to look upward and medially during the block pulls the optic nerve forward, perhaps increasing the likelihood of subarachnoid spread.[76]

C. Occipital nerve block

In general, there is little risk associated with occipital nerve block. Volumes used are small, and, despite the high vascularity of the region, risk of toxic reaction is low. Neuralgia of the greater or lesser occipital nerves is occasionally encountered in patients who have had posterior fossa craniotomy or removal of cerebellopontine angle tumors. If a bony defect exists at the site of the occipital block, it is possible for local anesthetic to spread to the intracranial subarachnoid space. Symptoms would depend on the structures anesthetized, but hypotension, apnea, and loss of consciousness would be likely. If the craniectomy defect is large, dura and even brain could be herniated into the soft tissues of the occipital region, and so injection into brain substance may be possible.

D. Cervical plexus block

The most likely serious complications of cervical plexus block are vertebral artery injection and subarachnoid injection. These complications can be minimized by cessation of injection if pain on injection occurs or if blood or cerebrospinal fluid is aspirated. Epidural spread may occur, even with correct needle placement, and generally would not cause serious consequences unless high local anesthetic volumes and concentrations were used. Epidural and subarachnoid block are more likely to occur if the needle angle is somewhat cephalad, allowing the needle to advance through the neural foramen.

Since the phrenic nerve arises from the cervical plexus, respiratory embarrassment related to phrenic blockade is a concern, particularly if bilateral cervical plexus block is contemplated.[127] However, the occurrence of even bilateral phrenic block is unlikely to produce serious respiratory embarrassment in the absence of preexisting pulmonary compromise.

E. Stellate ganglion block

The proximity of the carotid and vertebral arteries to the cervicothoracic sympathetic chain creates a significant risk of central nervous system toxicity, which, as previously stated, can occur with very small doses. Seizures have been reported after injection of 15 mg of lidocaine.[135] Other central nervous system effects, without convulsions, have been reported occurring after intra-arterial injection. Szeinfeld et al.[136] reported a case of transient aphasia and blindness without seizure after injection of 2.5 mg of bupivacaine. Scott et al.[137] reported a case of loss of consciousness followed by transient aphasia and hemiparesis, again without convulsions, after injection of 20 mg of lidocaine. Hematoma formation can occur after puncture of a vessel in the neck with potential compromise of the airway. This complication is rare in the absence of coagulopathy.

The carotid artery lies superficial to the sympathetic chain but is retracted laterally during the performance of cervicothoracic sympathetic block. One should feel the carotid pulsation on the pads of the retracting fingers before needle insertion. The vertebral artery traverses the C7 transverse process and then enters a foramen to ascend behind the anterior tubercle of C6. Although there is moderate risk of intra-arterial injection with a C7 approach, the risk is considerably less if the needle is positioned on the C6 anterior tubercle. There is still some risk with the C6 approach, since the needle may slip off the anterior tubercle during injection, and in a small percent of cases the vertebral artery may pass anterior to the C6 anterior tubercle[138] (Fig. 4-10).

Injection at the C7 level or deep to the C6 anterior tubercle may cause blockade of the adjacent nerve roots. Local anesthetic can spread from these locations to the brachial plexus and epidural space. Positioning the needle within the dural sheath of a nerve root may lead to subarachnoid spread. Such an injection of neurolytic agents will lead to devastating consequences (Fig. 4-11).

Pneumothorax is occasionally encountered after a C7 approach to the sympathetic chain. It is very unlikely when the C6 approach is used. Hoarseness is often seen after stellate ganglion block. It has generally been attributed to recurrent laryngeal nerve block, and it would seem prudent to advise patients not to eat or drink until the hoarseness resolves because of the risk of aspiration. When contemplating performance of bilateral stellate block, one should wait a sufficient length of time to ensure that no hoarseness has occurred after the first side is done before attempting the second side. Bilateral tension pneumothorax can result from bilateral blocks and is an added reason that some physicians are unwilling to block both sides in 1 day.

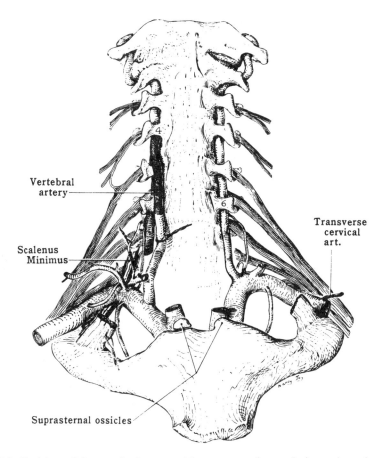

Fig. 4-10. Position of the vertebral artery with respect to the cervical anterior tubercles. The artery passes anterior to the C6 anterior tubercle in 6.4% of cases. (From Grant JCB: An atlas of anatomy, ed 5, Baltimore, 1962, The Williams & Wilkins Co.)

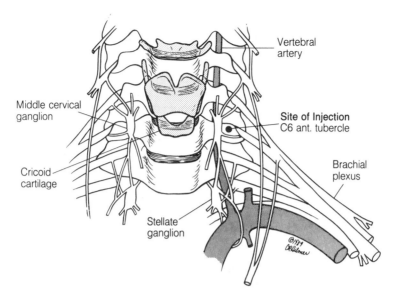

Fig. 4-11. Relationship of the C6 anterior tubercle, the usual site of injection for cervicothoracic sympathetic block, to adjacent neural and vascular structures. Notice that there is no anterior tubercle at C7 and that the chain lies even closer to the vertebral artery and roots of the brachial plexus at that level. (From Abram SE and Boas RA: Sympathetic and visceral nerve blocks. In Benumof JL, editor: Clinical procedures in anesthesia and intensive care, Philadelphia, 1991, JB Lippincott Co.)

Trauma to the thoracic duct has been reported after left stellate ganglion block.[139] The problem resolved after 5 days of pleural drainage. Patients should be followed carefully for several weeks because chyle may reaccumulate after initial resolution. Esophageal puncture can occur if the needle is angled medially. A bitter taste occurs without other symptoms. Leak of esophageal contents after needle puncture is unlikely.

The risks of performing a neurolytic stellate ganglion block are considerable. The complications that occurred in a case reported by Superville-Sovak et al.[140] illustrate the dangers of this procedure. After injection of 3 ml of 6% phenol in glycerin their patient experienced hemiplegia, paralysis of one hemidiaphragm, considerable reduction in vital capacity, and eventually death. Autopsy revealed a spinal cord infarct in the distribution of the anterior spinal artery involving one half of the spinal cord from C3 to C5, thrombosis of the vertebral artery, and direct neurolytic damage to the cervical cord and nerve roots. It would seem that few if any indications warrant exposing a patient to such devastating potential consequences.

F. Upper and lower extremity blocks

Neurologic dysfunction after extremity blocks can result from a variety of causes. These include preexisting, often unrecognized, neurologic deficits, nerve damage from surgical trauma, tourniquets, or malpositioning, as well as damage to a nerve during performance of a block. Preexisting neurologic problems should be documented by a careful preoperative neurologic assessment. It is particularly important to assess preexisting nerve damage in trauma patients. The most common upper extremity injuries that result from malpositioning are ulnar damage, caused by direct pressure on the nerve at the elbow, and brachial plexus injury, caused by stretching of the plexus. The most frequent lower extremity malposition injury is common peroneal nerve damage, which results from direct pressure over the fibular head. Even when intraoperative positioning is managed properly, compression or malpositioning injuries may occur postoperatively while the block persists.

As previously discussed in this chapter, injury to the brachial plexus can result from needle trauma. Most cases are probably associated with intraneural injection. Studies examining the consequences of eliciting paresthesias[26,141] have not clearly implicated this practice as a cause of neurologic damage. The overall incidence of nerve injury after axillary block is between 0.4% and 5.5%.[16,26,27,141] The incidence of neurologic sequelae occurring after continuous blocks was reported to be less than 1%.[142] We have found no studies that assess the incidence of nerve lesions occurring after interscalene or supraclavicular approaches. Persistent radiculopathy[143] and phrenic nerve damage[144] have been reported after interscalene block, and plexus injury has been reported after supraclavicular block.[145] There are few reports of neurologic damage after femoral plexus or sciatic blocks. Perhaps the preponderance of reports of injury after upper extremity blocks is a reflection of their much higher frequency of use.

There are few reports of nerve injury after block of the peripheral branches of the brachial or femoral plexus. Born[146] reported neurologic deficits in 7 of 49 patients who underwent wrist or metacarpal blocks. Although the authors attributed the complications to injection of bupivacaine into a confined space, it seems much more likely that their high complication rate was related to the use of 27-gauge needles, which probably predispose to intraneural injection. The safety of bupivacaine for wrist block is documented in a study by Nyström et al,[147] who compared the incidence of neurologic complications from wrist block for 0.5% bupivacaine versus 2% lidocaine in a double-blind, randomized trial. They reported only one patient among 71 who developed nerve damage unrelated to surgical manipulation, and that patient received lidocaine. Block of the ulnar nerve within the ulnar groove at the elbow and the common peroneal nerve behind the fibular head are believed to be associated with a high frequency of neurologic damage, though little data on the subject are available.

Both arterial[148] and venous[149] insufficiency requiring vascular reconstruction have been reported after axillary block. These complications were believed to be related to needle trauma to the vessel wall.

Interscalene brachial plexus block is associated with essentially the same potential complications as stellate ganglion block, including vertebral artery injection, phrenic nerve block, recurrent laryngeal block, and subarachnoid and epidural block. Pneumothorax is the most common serious complication associated with supraclavicular block. The incidence varies between 0.6% and 6%.[34] Winnie[34] suggests that the subclavian perivascular approach is associated with a much lower incidence than that associated with more classical approaches. Risk is theoretically greater on the right because of the higher dome of the lung on that side. It is also more likely in tall, thin patients and in patients with emphysema. Mani et al.[57] reported a case of hemopneumothorax after subclavian perivascular block in a heparin-anticoagulated patient.

There are relatively few reports of hemorrhagic complications occurring after extremity blocks. Those that have been reported are usually associated with the use of anticoagulants.

In addition to the case of hemopneumothorax mentioned above,[57] Parziale et al.[149] reported a case of compartment syndrome that followed a median nerve block at the elbow in a patient receiving sodium warfarin (Coumadin). Hematoma formation without neurologic consequences has been reported in several series[1] but was associated with neuropathic changes in two patients in Woolley and Vandam's series.[16] Johr[150] reported a case of femoral nerve compression by a hematoma after continuous femoral nerve block. The patient had been treated with dextran 70.

Gangrene of the digits after digital nerve block with epinephrine-containing solutions has been reported,[19] and warnings against the use of epinephrine for digital and penile blocks are common in regional anesthesia texts. It is not clear how common such injuries are or what concentrations of epinephrine are associated with them, but it would seem prudent to avoid all vasoconstrictors in anesthetic solutions when performing digital blocks.

G. Intravenous regional anesthesia

The complications of intravenous regional anesthesia are related to the hazards of tourniquet inflation and those of local anesthetic toxicity. Since the duration of intravenous regional anesthesia is generally limited to 1½ hours or less, the incidence of tourniquet-related nerve damage is very low. However, a case of permanent motor nerve damage was reported occurring after an intravenous regional anesthetic in a previously healthy young patient.[151] The surgical procedure in that case lasted only 50 minutes. If intravenous regional anesthesia is used for a surgical procedure for which a tourniquet is unnecessary, the risk of the tourniquet is added to the risk of anesthesia. Again, because of the relatively short period of tourniquet inflation, the release of accumulated metabolic products such as lactic acid and potassium at the time of cuff deflation is unlikely to cause problems. On the other hand, the reactive hyperemia that ensues can produce some hemodynamic changes. Under most circumstances, such changes are insignificant. However, a sudden decrease in vascular resistance in the limb can cause a drop in the subclavian artery pressure if there is proximal stenosis, resulting in reduced vertebral artery flow, a phenomenon termed "subclavian steal." Two cases of tourniquet-induced subclavian steal were reported by Carney.[152] One case occurred in a previously healthy 9 year old who suffered permanent neurologic dysfunction. Although neither of these cases occurred after intravenous regional anesthesia, I (Q.H.H.) have witnessed such cases and are aware of others in which severe bradycardia and transient cortical blindness occurred after deflation of tourniquets that were used for intravenous regional anesthesia. Venous thrombosis is another reported complication of the use of an intraoperative tourniquet.[153]

Local anesthetic toxicity during intravenous regional block can occur at the time of tourniquet deflation or as a result of leaking of anesthetic beneath the cuff. Premature accidental cuff deflation is likely to cause acute local anesthetic toxicity if it occurs during the first 10 to 15 minutes, before the anesthetic has had time to diffuse out of the venous system into the tissues. There are very few reports of serious local anesthetic toxic reactions associated with the use of 0.5% lidocaine or prilocaine. On the other hand, Heath[154] reported that there were seven recorded deaths in the United Kingdom between 1979 and 1983 as a result of bupivacaine Bier blocks. In at least some of the recorded cases, 0.2% bupivacaine in a dose of 1.5 ml/kg was used, and early tourniquet inflation did not occur. The usual bupivacaine concentration for intravenous regional anesthesia is 0.25%, which is comparable in potency and toxity to 1% lidocaine or prilocaine. In light of the documented deaths associated with intravenous regional bupivacaine and the need for higher relative concentrations with the drug, it would seem prudent to avoid its use altogether for this technique.

Toxic reactions related to leak of anesthetic under the cuff can occur when injection pressure exceeds cuff occlusion pressure. Davies et al.[155] reported that local anesthetic gained access to the general circulation in 13 of 52 cases. This is more likely to occur if arterial flow is not completely occluded and venous congestion occurs.[156] Systolic blood pressure appears to be an unreliable guide to determining tourniquet pressure, and it has been suggested that tourniquet pressure should be set at 100 mm Hg above occlusion pressure, the tourniquet pressure that abolishes arterial pulsation in the limb. Since exsanguination of the limb with an Esmarch bandage reduces the peak injection pressure,[157] it would be likely to reduce the risk of anesthetic leaking past the cuff. Even when exsanguination is carried out, toxic reactions can occur if large anesthetic volumes are used. Rosenberg et al.[158] reported a local anesthetic convulsion that occurred in a 120 kg patient after injection of 80 ml of 0.25% bupivacaine. The tourniquet was set at 300 mm Hg, and the patient's blood pressure at the time of injection was 160/80. This report also illustrates the potential for local anesthetic toxicity with the use of bupivacaine.

H. Intercostal nerve blocks

Despite the fact that the intercostal spaces are fairly vascular, the reported incidence of systemic toxic reactions is low. Moore[159] reported only five cases of local anesthetic convulsions among 17,000 patients. All five convulsions occurred among surgical patients who had bilateral blocks of the lower seven intercostal nerves. In a study of 10 patients who underwent bilateral intercostal blocks with 400 mg of bupivacaine (0.5% with epinephrine 1:320,000), Moore et al.[160] found that mean peak arterial levels ranged from 1.7 to 4.0 μg/ml (mean 3.3). Peak levels occurred 10 to 30 minutes after injection.

Pneumothorax is a recognized complication of intercostal block. The incidence depends on the skill of the anesthesiologist and the diligence with which one looks for subclinical cases. Reported incidence ranges from less than 0.1% in a series of 17,000 cases reported by Moore[159] to 19%.[161] Clinically significant pneumothorax is probably caused either by rupture of an emphysematous bleb or by laceration of the visceral pleura by the needle. One may reduce needle trauma by asking the patient to hold the breath as the needle is walked off the lower border of the rib and injected.

Intraneural injection may result in spread of drug proximally to the subarachnoid space or spinal cord. Since the volumes of local anesthetic injected at any one intercostal space are generally low, the chances of developing a very high or total spinal are relatively low. However, if such intraneural spread occurs with neurolytic agents, the resulting effect on the cord may be devastating. It is essential therefore that great care be exercised and that small volumes be used in the performance of neurolytic intercostal block. As with other blocks, local bleeding can occur in anticoagulated patients[56] and can lead to significant accumulation of blood in the pleural space.

I. Paravertebral somatic and sympathetic blocks

Because of the proximity of the somatic nerve roots and the sympathetic chain in the lumbar and thoracic areas, the complications of both types of blocks will be considered together. The complications of cervical somatic root block are the same as those described for cervical plexus block.

The principal risk of these procedures is spread of drug to the epidural or subarachnoid space, which is generally the result of placement of the needle into the dural cuff, which extends over the nerve root. If small local anesthetic volumes appropriate to diagnostic or prognostic nerve root blocks are used, the consequences of subarachnoid spread are minimal. If lumbar sympathetic block is performed by use of an approach that begins 8 to 10 cm lateral to the midline, the needle may enter the neural foramen, leading to epidural or subarachnoid spread. If large volumes are used, total spinal anesthesia can ensue.[162] Neurolytic lumbar sympathetic blocks can result in damage to somatic neural structures when needle position is faulty. In addition, it is possible for drug to spread posteriorly along the rami communicantes to the somatic roots even when the needle position is satisfactory.[162]

We have encountered one patient who developed a post–lumbar puncture headache after an L3 paravertebral root block that resulted in subarachnoid spread of local anesthetic. Sharrock[86] reported three cases of postural headache among 24 patients who underwent a total of 39 thoracic paravertebral somatic nerve blocks.

Pneumothorax is a potential complication of high lumbar and thoracic paravertebral blocks. There is little or no space between the thoracic sympathetic chain and the pleura. We have treated a patient with an L1 nerve block who developed a 20% pneumothorax that resolved without intervention. A fatal pneumothorax in a patient with severe pulmonary dysfunction was reported by de Krey.[163]

Hematuria resulting from needle puncture of a kidney or ureter is occasionally encountered after lumbar sympathetic block. It is generally without serious consequences. However, injection of neurolytic agents into a kidney or ureter can produce significant damage. Kuzmarov et al.[164] reported a case of ureteral damage requiring surgical repair that resulted from alcohol injected into the ureter during attempted sympathetic block.

Postsympathectomy limb pain, also referred to as "sympathalgia," is commonly seen after surgical or neurolytic sympathectomy. In some series, it has occurred in nearly every case.[165] There is generally a 2-week period after the sympathectomy followed by the onset of deep, boring pain, usually in the anterior thigh and often worse at night. Soft tissues of the thigh are very tender. The pain usually subsides spontaneously in several days to several weeks. The cause of this condition is unclear.

J. Celiac plexus and splanchnic nerve block

Celiac plexus block is associated with a low complication rate. Even when neurolytic agents are used, the incidence of neurologic damage is low.[166] Brown et al.[167] had no neurologic complications in a series of 136 patients. However, paraplegia has been reported with both alcohol and phenol,[168,169] and biplanar fluoroscopy or CT scan should be used when this block is performed with neurolytic agents.

Pnuemothorax is an occasional complication. It is somewhat more likely with splanchnic block because needle position is farther cephalad, at the anterolateral border of T12. Brown[167] reported two cases of pneumothorax in his series of 136 celiac plexus blocks. Both resolved without need for thoracostomy.

Orthostatic hypotension occurs occasionally after celiac plexus block. It is more likely to occur if the needle position is retrocrural, close to the vertebral body, allowing drug spread to the lumbar sympathetic chain. It is generally short lived, even when neurolytic agents are used. All the cases we have encountered resolved within 48 hours.

Retroperitoneal fibrosis has been reported after repeated celiac plexus alcohol injections for chronic pancreatitis.[170] No apparent sequelae were noted except for the inability to continue treatment with these injections. Chest pain is common after celiac alcohol block. It usually resolves within an hour. Pleural effusion is occasionally seen in the postblock period.[171]

K. Blocks of the perineum

The fetal complications of paracervical blocks were discussed earlier in this chapter. Both pudendal and paracervical blocks are associated with occasional retropsoas abscesses.[112,172] As with epidural blocks, there is some evidence that pudendal blocks diminish the bearing-down reflex during labor and may prolong the second stage.[173]

As with digital nerve blocks, penile block with epinephrine-containing solutions may lead to ischemia and gangrene of tissues distal to the block. This complication probably results from a combination of pressure on vessels by the injected solution and vasoconstriction of the small arteries by the epinephrine. Unlike other areas of the body, no collateral flow is possible beyond the block.

REFERENCES

1. Caplan RA, Ward RJ, Posner K, and Cheney FW: Unexpected cardiac arrest during spinal anesthesia: a closed claims analysis of predisposing factors, Anesthesiology 68(1):5-11, 1988.
2. Smith DC and Crul JF: Oxygen desaturation following sedation for regional analgesia, Br J. Anaesth 62:206-209, 1989.
3. Kehlet H: Modification of responses to surgery by neural blockade: clinical publications. In Cousins M and Bridenbaugh P, editors: Neural blockade, ed 2, Philadelphia, 1988, JB Lippincott Co.

4. Levinson BW: States of awareness during general anaesthesia: preliminary communication, Br J Anaesth 37:544-546, 1965.

5. Rosen M and Lunn J, editors: Consciousness, awareness and pain in general anesthesia, London, 1987, Butterworth & Co.

6. Shanthaveerappa TR and Bourne GH: Perineural epithelium: a new concept of its role in the integrity of the peripheral nervous system, Science 154:1464-1467, 1966.

7. Sturrock JE and Nunn JF: Cytotoxic effects of procaine, lignocaine and bupivacaine, Br J Anaesth 51:273-280, 1979.

8. Morris T and Tracey J: Lignocaine: its effects on wound healing, Br J Surg 64:902, 1977.

9. Bodvall B and Rais O: Effects of infiltration anaesthesia on the healing of incisions in traumatized and non-traumatized tissues, Acta Chir Scand 123:83-91, 1962.

10. Benoit PW and Belt WD: Destruction and regeneration of skeletal muscle after treatment with a local anaesthetic, bupivacaine (Marcaine), J Anat 107(3):547-556, 1970.

11. Myers RR, Kalichman MW, Reisner LS, and Powell HC: Neurotoxicity of local anesthetics: altered perineurial permeability, edema, and nerve fiber injury, Anesthesiology 64(1):29-35, 1986.

12. Gentill F, Hudson AR, Hunter D, and Kline DG: Nerve injection injury with local anesthetic agents: a light and electron microscopic, fluorescent microscopic, and horseradish peroxidase study, Neurosurgery 6(3):263-272, 1980.

13. Myers RR and Heckman HM: Effects of local anesthesia on nerve blood flow: studies using lidocaine with and without epinephrine, Anesthesiology 71:757-762, 1989.

14. Li DF, Bahar M, Cole G, and Rosen M: Neurological toxicity of the subarachnoid infusion of bupivacaine, lignocaine or 2-chloroprocaine in the rat, Br J Anaesth 57:424-429, 1985.

15. Ready LB, Plumer MH, Haschke RH, et al: Neurotoxicity of intrathecal local anesthetics in rabbits, Anesthesiology 63(4):364-370, 1985.

16. Woolley EJ and Vandam LD: Neurological sequelae of brachial plexus nerve block, Ann Surg 149(1):53-60, 1959.

17. Selander D, Brattsand R, Lundborg G, et al: Local anesthetics: Importance of mode of application, concentration and adrenaline for the appearance of nerve lesions, Acta Anaesth Scand 23:127-136, 1979.

18. Löfström B, Wennberg A, and Wién L: Late disturbances in nerve function after block with local anaesthetic agents, Acta Anaesth Scand 10:111-122, 1966.

19. Gissen AJ, Datta S, and Lambert D: The chloroprocaine controversy II. Is chloroprocaine neurotoxic? Reg Anaesth 9:135, 1984.

20. Wang BC, Hillman DE, Spielholz NI, and Turndorf H: Chronic neurological deficits and Nesacaine-CE: an effect of the anesthetic, 2-chloroprocaine, or the antioxidant, sodium bisulfite? Anesth Analg 63:445-447, 1984.

21. Covino B: Clinical pharmacology of local anesthetic agents. In Cousins MJ and Bridenbaugh PO, editors: Neural blockade, Philadelphia, 1988, JB Lippincott, p. 130.

22. Barsa J, Batra M, Fink BR, and Sumi SM: A comparative in vivo study of local neurotoxicity of lidocaine, bupivacaine, 2-chloroprocaine, and a mixture of 2-chloroprocaine and bupivacaine, Anesth Analg 61(12):961-967, 1982.

23. Selander D, Dhuner KG, and Lundborg G: Peripheral nerve injury due to injection needles used for regional anesthesia, Acta Anaesth Scand 21:182-188, 1977.

24. Moore DC: Complications of regional anesthesia, Springfield, Ill, 1955, Charles C Thomas, Publisher, p. 114.

25. Selander D and Sjöstrand J: Longitudinal spread of intraneurally injected local anesthetics, Acta Anaesth Scand 22:622-634, 1978.

26. Selander D, Edshage S, and Wolff T: Paresthesiae or no paresthesiae? Acta Anaesthesiol Scand 23:27-33, 1979.

27. Winchell SW and Wolfe R: The incidence of neuropathy following upper extremity nerve blocks, Reg Anaesth 10(1):12-15, 1985.

28. Tountas CP and Bergman RA: Tourniquet ischemia: ultrastructural and histochemical observations of ischemic human muscle and of monkey muscle and nerve, J Hand Surg 2(1):31-37, 1977.

29. Lundborg G: Structure and function of the intraneural microvessels as related to trauma, edema, formation and nerve function, J Bone Joint Surg 57A:938-948, 1975.

30. Ochoa J, Fouler TJ, and Gilliatt RW: Anatomical changes in peripheral nerve compressed by a pneumatic tourniquet, J Anat 113:433-455, 1972.

31. Moore MR, Garfin SR, and Hargens AR: Wide tourniquets eliminate blood flow at low inflation pressures, J Hand Surg 12A(6):1006-1011, 1987.

32. Dreyfuss UY and Smith RJ: Sensory changes with prolonged double-cuff tourniquet time in hand surgery, J Hand Surg 13A(5):736-740, 1988.

33. Mullick S: The tourniquet in operations upon the extremities, Surg Gynecol Obstet 146:821-826, 1978.

34. Winnie AP (Håakasson L, editor): Plexus anesthesia, vol 1: Perivascular techniques of brachial plexus block, Philadelphia, 1983, WB Saunders Co, pp. 221-265.

35. Coveno B and Vassalo H: Local anesthetics, New York, 1976, Grune & Stratton, pp. 95-96.

36. Tucker GT and Mather LE: Properties, absorption, and disposition of local anesthetic agents. In Cousins M and Bridenbaugh PO, editors: Neural blockade, ed 2, Philadelphia, 1990, JB Lippincott Co, pp. 47-110.

37. Bernards CM, Carpenter RL, Rupp SM, et al: Effect of midazolam and diazepam premedication on central nervous system and cardiovascular toxicity of bupivacaine in pigs, Anesthesiology 70(2):318-823, 1989.

38. Torbiner ML, Yagiela JA, and Mito RS: Effect of midazolam pretreatment on the intravenous toxicity of lidocaine with and without epinephrine in rats, Anesth Analg 68(6):744-749, 1989.

39. Korevaar WC, Burney RG, and Moore PA: Convulsions during stellate ganglion block: a case report, Anesth Analg 58(2):329-330, 1979.

40. Kozody R, Ready LB, Barsa JE, and Murphy TM: Dose requirement of local anaesthetic to produce grand mal seizure during stellate ganglion block, Can Anaesth Soc J 29(5):489-491, 1982.

41. Szienfeld M, Laurencio M, and Pallares V: Total reversible blindness following attempted stellate ganglion block, Anesth Analg 60(9):689-690, 1981.

42. Scott DL, Ghia JN, and Teeple E: Aphasia and hemiparesis following stellate ganglion block, Anesth Analg 62:1038-1040, 1983.

43. Aldrete JA, Romo-Salas F, Arora S, et al: Reverse arterial blood flow as a pathway for central nervous system toxic responses following injection of local anesthetics, Anesth Analg 57:428-433, 1978.

44. Cockings E, Moore PL, and Lewis RC: Transarterial brachial plexus blockade using high doses of 1.5% mepivacaine, Reg Anaesth 12(4):159-164, 1987.

45. Ischia S, Luzzani A, Ischia A, and Faggion S: A new approach to the neurolytic block of the coeliac plexus: the transaortic technique, Pain 16:333-341, 1983.

46. Merrill DG, Brodsky JB, and Hentz RV: Vascular insufficiency following axillary block of the brachial plexus, Anesth Analg 60(3):162-164, 1981.

47. Nishimura N, Morioka T, Sato S, and Kuba T: Effects of local anesthetic agents on the peripheral vascular system, Anesth Analg 44(1):135-139, 1965.

48. Selander D, Mansson L, Karlsson L, and Svanvik J: Adrenergic vasoconstriction in peripheral nerves of the rabbit, Anesthesiology 62:6-10, 1985.

49. Hastings H II and Misamore G: Compartment syndrome resulting from intravenous regional anesthesia, J Hand Surg 12A(4):559-562, 1987.

50. Moore DC: Complications of regional anesthesia, Springfield, Ill, 1955, Charles C Thomas, Publisher, pp. 97-99.

51. Lennon RL and Linstromberg JW: Brachial plexus anesthesia and axillary sheath elastance, Anesth Analg 62:215-217, 1983.

52. Siler JN, Lief PL, and Davis JF: A new complication of interscalene brachial-plexus block, Anesthesiology 38(6):590-591, 1973.

53. Ott B, Neuberger L, and Frey HP: Obliteration of the axillary artery after axillary block, Anaesthesia 44:773-774, 1989.

54. Restelli L, Pinciroli D, Conoscente F, and Cammelli F: Insufficient venous drainage following axillary approach to brachial plexus blockade, Br J Anaesth 56:1051-1053, 1984.

55. Moore, DC: Complications of regional anesthesia, Springfield, Ill, 1955, Charles C Thomas, Publisher, pp. 87-92.

56. Nielsen CH: Bleeding after intercostal nerve block in a patient anticoagulated with heparin, Anesthesiology 71(1):162-164, 1989.

57. Mani M, Ramamurthy N, Rao TLK, et al: An unusual complication of brachial plexus block and heparin therapy, Anesthesiology 48(3):213-214, 1978.

58. Moore, DC: Complications of regional anesthesia, Springfield, Ill, 1955, Charles C Thomas, Publisher, pp. 55-68.

59. Thompson KJ, Melding P, and Hatangdi VS: Pneumochylothorax: a rare complication of stellate ganglion block, Anesthesiology 55(5):589-591, 1981.

60. Winnie AP (Håkansson L, editor): Plexus anesthesia, vol 1: Perivascular techniques of brachial plexus block, Philadelphia, 1983, WB Saunders Co, p. 229.

61. Derenne J-P, Macklem PT, and Roussos C: The respiratory muscles: mechanics, control, and pathophysiology, part I, Am Rev Respir Dis 118:119-133, 1978.

62. Hecker BR, Bjurstrom R, and Schoene RB: Effect of intercostal nerve blockade on respiratory mechanics and CO_2 raise chemosensitivity at rest and exercise, Anesthesiology 70:13-18, 1989.

63. Shaw, WM: Paralysis of the phrenic nerve during brachial plexus anesthesia, Anesthesiology 10:627-628, 1949.

64. Harley N and Gjessing J: A critical assessment of supraclavicular brachial plexus block, Anaesthesia 24(4):564-570, 1969.

65. Knoblanche GE: The incidence and aetiology of phrenic nerve blockade associated with supraclavicular brachial plexus block, Anaesth Intensive Care 7:346-349, 1979.

66. Hickey R and Ramamurthy S: The diagnosis of phrenic nerve block on chest xray by a double-exposure technique, Anesthesiology 70(4):704-707, 1989.

67. Eisele JH, Noble MIM, Katz J, et al: Bilateral phrenic-nerve block in man: technical problems and respiratory effects, Anesthesiology 37(1):64-69, 1972.

68. Cory PC and Mulroy MF: Postoperative respiratory failure following intercostal block, Anesthesiology 54:418-419, 1981.

69. Casey WF: Respiratory failure following intercostal nerve blockade, Anaesthesia 39:351-354, 1984.

70. Hood J and Knoblanche G: Respiratory failure following brachial plexus block, Anaesth Intensive Care 7(3):285-286, 1979.

71. Kayerker UM and Dick MM: Phrenic nerve paralysis following interscalene brachial plexus block, Anesth Analg 62:536-537, 1983.

72. Sharp JT, Goldberg NB, Druz WS, et al: Thoracoabdominal motion in chronic obstructive pulmonary disease, Am Rev Respir Dis 115:47-56, 1977.

73. Farrar MD, Scheybani M, and Nolte H: Upper extremity block effectiveness and complications, Reg Anaesth 6:133-134, 1981.

74. Urmey WF, Talts KH, Schraft S, and Sharrock NE: Ipsilateral hemidiaphragm paresis associated with interscalene brachial plexus anesthesia, Anesthesiology 71(3A):A728, 1989.

75. Nicoll JMV, Acharya PA, Ahlen K, et al: Central nervous system complications after 6000 retrobulbar blocks, 66:1298-1302, Anesth Analg 1987.

76. Rigg JD and James RH: Apnoea after retrobulbar block, Anaesthesia 44:26-27, 1989.

77. Wang BC, Bogart B, Hillman DE, and Turndorf H: Subarachnoid injection: a potential complication of retrobulbar block, Anesthesiology 71:845-847, 1989.

78. Ross S and Scarborough D: Total spinal anesthesia following brachial-plexus block, Anesthesiology 39(4):458, 1973.

79. Edde RR and Deutsch S: Cardiac arrest after interscalene brachial-plexus block, Anesth Analg 56(3):446-447, 1977.

80. Goldstone JC and Pennant JH: Spinal anaesthesia following facet joint injection, Anaesthesia 42:754-756, 1987.

81. Benumof JL and Semenza J: Total spinal anesthesia following intrathoracic intercostal nerve blocks, Anesthesiology 43(1):124-125, 1975.

82. Otto CW and Wall CL: Total spinal anesthesia: a rare complication of intrathoracic intercostal nerve block, Ann Thorac Surg 22(3):289-292, 1976.

83. Chester SC and Gutteridge GA: Subtotal spinal anaesthesia as a complication of intrathoracic intercostal nerve blocks, Anaesth Intensive Care 9:387-389, 1981.

84. Gallo JA Jr, Lebowitz PW, Battit GE, and Bruner JMR: Complications of intercostal nerve blocks performed under direct vision during thoracotomy: a repeat of two cases, J Thorac Cardiovasc Surg 86(4):628-630, 1983.

85. Sury MRJ and Bingham RM: Accidental spinal anaesthesia following intrathoracic intercostal nerve blockade, Anaesthesia 41:401-403, 1986.

86. Sharrock NE: Postural headache following thoracic somatic paravertebral nerve block, Anesthesiology 52:360-362, 1980.

87. Kumar A, Battit GE, Froese AB, and Long MC: Bilateral cervical and thoracic epidural blockade complicating interscalene brachial plexus block: report of two cases, Anesthesiology 35(6):650-652, 1971.

88. Muravchick S and Owens WD: An unusual complication of lumbosacral plexus block: a case report, Anesth Analg 55(3):350-352, 1976.

89. Scammell SJ: Inadvertent epidural anaesthesia as a complication of interscalene brachial plexus block, Anaesth Intensive Care 7(1):56-57, 1979.

90. Lombard TP and Couper JL: Bilateral spread of analgesia following interscalene brachial plexus block, Anesthesiology 58:472-473, 1983.

91. Middaugh RE, Menk EJ, Reynolds WJ, et al: Epidural block using large volumes of local anesthetic solution for intercostal nerve block, Anesthesiology 63:214-216, 1985.

92. Krempen JS, Smith B, and DeFreest LJ: Selective nerve root infiltration for the evaluation of sciatica, Orthop Clin North Am 6(1):311-315, 1975.

93. Moran R, O'Connell D, and Walsh MG: The diagnostic value of facet joint injections, Spine 13(12):1407-1410, 1988.

94. Raymond J and Dumas JM: Intraarticular facet block: diagnostic test or therapeutic procedure? Radiology 151(2):334-336, 1984.

95. Seltzer JL: Hoarseness and Horner's syndrome after interscalene brachial plexus block, Anesth Analg 56(4):585-586, 1977.

96. Skretting P: Hypotension after intercostal nerve block during thoracotomy under general anaesthesia, Br J Anaesth 53:527-529, 1981.

97. Purcell-Jones G, Speedy HM, and Justins DM: Upper limb sympathetic blockade following intercostal nerve blocks, Anaesthesia 42:984-986, 1987.

98. Brown RH and Tewes PA: Cervical sympathetic blockade after thoracic intercostal injection of local anesthetic, Anesthesiology 70:1011-1012, 1989.

99. Allen G and Samson B: Contralateral Horner's syndrome following stellate ganglion block, Can Anaesth Soc J 33:112-113, 1986 [letter].

100. Evans JA, Dobben GD, and Gay GR: Peridural effusion of drugs following sympathetic blockade, JAMA 200(7):93-98, 1967.

101. Moore DC: Complications of regional anesthesia, Springfield, Ill, 1955, Charles C Thomas, Publisher, pp. 53-54.

102. Sharrock NE: Inadvertent "3-in-1 block" following injection of the lateral cutaneous nerve of the thigh, Anesth Analg 59:887-888, 1980.

103. Huang KC, Fitzgerald MR, and Tsueda K: Bilateral block of cervical and brachial plexuses following interscalene block, Anaesth Intensive Care 14(1):87-88, 1986.

104. Manara AR: Brachial plexus block: unilateral thoraco-abdominal blockade following the supraclavicular approach, Anaesthesia 42:757-759, 1987.

105. Macintosh RR and Mushin WM: Observations on the epidural space, Anaesthesia 2:100-104, 1947.

106. Nunn JF and Slavin G: Posterior intercostal nerve block for pain relief after cholecystectomy, Br J Anaesth 52:253-259, 1980.

107. Taveras JM and Wood EH: Diagnostic neuroradiology, vol 2, Baltimore, 1976, Williams & Wilkins, pp. 1144-1150.

108. Shantha TR and Evans JA: The relationship of epidural anesthesia to neural membranes and arachnoid villi, Anesthesiology 37(5):543-557, 1972.

109. French JD, Strain WH, and Jones GE: Mode of extension of contrast substances injected into peripheral nerves, J Neuropathol Exp Neurol 7:47-58, 1948.

110. Moore DC, Hain RF, Ward A, and Bridenbaugh LD Jr: Importance of the perineural spaces in nerve blocking, JAMA 13:1050-1053, 1954.

111. Wenger DR and Gitchell RG: Severe infections following pudendal block anesthesia: need for orthopaedic awareness, J Bone Joint Surg 55A(1):202-207, 1973.

112. Svancarek W, Chirino O, Schaefer G, and Blythe JG: Retropsoas and subgluteal abscesses following paracervical and pudendal anesthesia, JAMA 237(9):892-894, 1977.

113. Schmidt RM and Rosenkranz HS: Antimicrobial activity of local anesthetics: lidocaine and procaine, J Infect Dis 121(6):597-607, 1970.

114. Merkow AJ, McGuinness GA, Erenberg A, et al: The neonatal neurobehavioral effects of bupivacaine, mepivacaine and 2-chloroprocaine used for pudendal block, Anesthesiology 52:309-312, 1980.

115. Hamilton LA and Gottschalk W: Paracervical block: advantages and disadvantages, Clin Obstet Gynecol 17:199-210, 1974.

116. Ralston DH and Schnider SM: The fetal and neonatal effects of regional anesthesia in obstetrics, Anesthesiology 48:34-64, 1978.

117. Katy J and Joseph JW: Neuropathology of neurolytic and semidestructive agents. In Cousins MJ and Bridenbaugh PO, editors: Neural blockade, Philadelphia, 1982, JB Lippincott, pp. 122-132.

118. Moore DC: Complications of regional anesthesia, Springfield, Ill, 1955, Charles C Thomas, Publisher.

119. Swerdlow M: Complications of neurolytic neural blockade. In Cousins MJ and Bridenbaugh PO, editors: Neural blockade, Philadelphia, 1982, JB Lippincott, pp. 543-553.

120. Murphy TM: Complications of neurolytic blocks. In Orkin FK and Cooperman LH, editors: Complications in anesthesiology, Philadelphia, 1983, JB Lippincott, pp. 117-122.

121. Macomber DW: Necrosis of nose and cheek secondary to treatment of trigeminal neuralgia, Plast Reconstruct Surg 11:337-340, 1953.

122. Mannheimer W, Pizzolato P, and Adriani J: Mode of action and effects on tissues of long-acting local anesthetics, JAMA 154:29-32, 1953.

123. Ritchie JM: The aliphatic alcohols. In Gilman AG et al, editors: The pharmacological basis of therapeutics, ed 7, New York, 1985, MacMillan Co, pp. 372-386.

124. Noda J, Umeda S, Mori K, et al: Acetaldehyde syndrome after celiac plexus alcohol block, Anesth Analg 65:1300-1302, 1986.

125. Noda J, Umeda S, Mori K, et al: Disulfiram-like reaction associated with carmofur after celiac plexus alcohol block, Anesthesiology 67:809-810, 1987.

126. 126. Reid W, Watt JK, and Gray TG: Phenol injection of sympathetic chain, Br J Surg 47:45-48, 1970.

127. Murphy TM: Complications of diagnostic and therapeutic nerve blocks. In Orkin FK and Cooperman LH, editors: Complications in anesthesiology, Philadelphia, 1983, JB Lippincott, pp. 106-122.

128. Crimeni R: Clinical experience with mepivacaine and alcohol in neuralgia of the trigeminal nerve, Acta Anaesthesiol Scand 24(suppl):173, 1966.

129. Håkanson S: Trigeminal neuralgia treated by the injection of glycerol into the trigeminal cistern, Neurosurgery 9:638-646, 1967.

130. Moore DC: Complications of regional anesthesia, Springfield, Ill, 1955, Charles C Thomas, Publisher, pp. 121-122.

131. Morrison WV and Kalina RE: Ocular muscle palsy: results following alcohol injection of infraorbital nerve, Arch Otolaryngol 94:571-573, 1971.

132. Horowitz NH and Rizzoli HV: Postoperative complications in neurosurgical practice, Baltimore, 1967, Williams & Wilkins, pp. 666.

133. Meyers EF, Ramirez RC, and Boniuk I: Grand mal seizures after retrobulbar block, Arch Ophthalmol 96:847, 1978.

134. Rosenblatt RM, May DR, and Barsoumian K: Cardiopulmonary arrest after retrobulbar block, Am J Ophthalmol 90:425-427, 1980.

135. Korevaar WC, Burney RG, and Moore PA: Convulsions during stellate ganglion block: a case report, Anesth Analg 58:329-330, 1979.

136. Szeinfeld M, Laurencio M, and Pallares VS: Total reversible blindness following attempted stellate ganglion block, Anesth Analg 60:689-690, 1981.

137. Scott DL, Ghia JN, and Teeple E: Aphasia and hemiparesis following stellate ganglion block, Anesth Analg 62:1038-1040, 1983.

138. Grant JCB: An atlas of anatomy, ed 5, Baltimore, 1962, Williams & Wilkins, p. 567.

139. Thompson KJ, Melding P, and Hatangdi VS: Pneumochylothorax: a rare complication of stellate ganglion block, Anesthesiology 55:589-591, 1981.

140. Superville-Sovak B, Raminsky M, and Finlayson MH: Complications of phenol neurolysis, Arch Neurol 32:226-228, 1975.

141. Plevak DJ, Linstromberg JW, and Danielson DR: Paresthesia vs nonparesthesia: the axillary block, Anesthesiology 59:A216, 1983.

142. Sada T, Kobayashi T, and Murakami S: Continuous axillary brachial plexus block, Can Anaesth Soc J 30:201-205, 1983.

143. Barutell C, Vidal F, Raich M, et al: A neurological complication following interscalene brachial plexus block, Anaesthesia 35:365-367, 1980.

144. Bashein G, Robertson HT, and Kennedy WF: Persistent phrenic nerve paresis following interscalene brachial plexus block, Anesthesiology 63:102-104, 1985.

145. Lim EK and Pareira R: Brachial plexus injury following brachial plexus block, Anaesthesia 39:691-694, 1984.

146. Born G: Neuropathy after bupivacaine (Marcaine) wrist and metacarpal blocks, J Hand Surg 9A:109-112, 1984.

147. Nyström A, Lindström G, Reiz S, and Hanel DP: Bupivacaine: a safe local anesthetic for wrist blocks, J Hand Surg 14:495-498, 1989.

148. Ott B, Neuberger L, and Frey HP: Obliteration of the axillary artery after axillary block, Anaesthesia 44:773-774, 1989.

149. Parziale JR, Marino AR, and Herndon JH: Diagnostic peripheral nerve block resulting in compartment syndrome: case report, Am J Phys Med Rehabil 67:82-84, 1988.

150. Johr M: Späte Komplikation der kontinuierlichen Blockade des N. femoralis, Reg Anaesth 37:37-38, 1987.

151. Larsen UT and Hommelgaard P: Pneumatic tourniquet paralysis following intravenous regional analgesia, Anaesthesia 42(5):526-528, 1987.

152. Carney AL and Anderson EM: Tourniquet subclavian steal: brainstem ischemia and cortical blindness—clinical significance and testing. Adv Neurol 30:283-290, New York, 1981, Raven Press.

153. Krose AJ and Stiris G: The risk of deep vein thrombosis after operations on a bloodless lower limb: a venographic study, Injury 7:271-273, 1976.

154. Heath ML: Bupivacaine toxicity and Bier blocks, Anesthesiology 59:481, 1983.

155. Davies JAH, Wilkey AD, and Hall ID: Bupivacaine leak past inflated tourniquets during intravenous regional analgesia, Anaesthesia 39:996-999, 1984.

156. Davies JAH, Hall ID, Wilkey AD, et al: Intravenous regional anesthesia, Anaesthesia 39:416-421, 1983.

157. Haasio J, Hiippala S, and Rosenberg PH: Intravenous regional anesthesia of the arm, Anaesthesia 44:19-21, 1989.

158. Rosenberg PH, Kalso EA, Tuominen MK, et al: Acute bupivacaine toxicity as a result of venous leakage under the tourniquet cuff during a Bier block, Anesthesiology 58:95-98, 1983.

159. Moore DC: Intercostal nerve block and celiac plexus block for pain therapy. In Benedetti C et al, editors: Advances in Pain Research and Therapy 7:309-329, New York, 1984, Raven Press.

160. Moore DC, Mather LE, Bridenbaugh PO, et al: Arterial and venous plasma levels of bupivacaine following epidural and intercostal nerve blocks, Anesthesiology 45:39-45, 1976.

161. Chivers EM: Pulmonary complications following regional anesthesia for abdominal operations, Br J Anaesth 20:55-59, 1946.

162. Gay GR and Evans JA: Total spinal anesthesia following lumbar paravertebral block: a potentially lethal complication, Anesth Analg 50:344-347, 1971.

163. de Krey JA, Schroeder CF, and Buechel DR: Selective chemical sympathectomy, Anesth Analg 47:633-637, 1968.

164. Kuzmarov IW, MacIsaac SG, Sioufi, J, et al: Iatrogenic ureteral injury secondary to lumbar sympathetic ganglion blockade, Urology 16:617-619, 1980.

165. Litwin MS: Postsympathectomy neuralgia, Acta Surg 84:121-125, 1962.

166. Moore DC, Bush WH, and Burnett LL: Celiac plexus block: a roentgenographic, anatomic study of technique and spread of solution in patients and corpses, Anesth Analg 60:369-379, 1981.

167. Brown DL, Bulley K, and Quiel EL: Neurolytic celiac plexus block for pancreatic cancer pain, Anesth Analg 66:869-873, 1987.

168. Cherry DA and Lamberty J: Paraplegia following celiac plexus block, Anaesth Intensive Care 12:59-72, 1984.

169. Galizia EJ and Lahira SK: Paraplegia following celiac plexus block with phenol: case report, Br J Anaesth 46:539-540, 1974.

170. Pateman J, Williams MP, and Filshie J: Retroperitoneal fibrosis after multiple celiac plexus blocks, Anaesthesia 45:309-310, 1990.

171. Fujita Y and Takaori M: Pleural effusion after CT-guided alcohol celiac plexus block, Anesth Analg 66:911-912, 1987.

172. Mercado AO, Naz JF, and Ataya KM: Postabortal paracervical abscess as a complication of paracervical block anesthesia, J Reproduct Med 34:247-249, 1989.

173. Langhoff-Roos J and Lindmark G: Analgesia and maternal side effects of pudendal block at delivery: a comparison of three local anesthetics, Acta Obstet Gynecol Scand 64:269-272, 1985.

Chapter 5

Equipment Failure: Anesthesia Delivery Systems

James B. Eisenkraft
Richard M. Sommer

Failure of the anesthesia delivery system, though uncommon, may result in patient injury or even death. More common than total failure of a delivery system component is operator error and misuse of the system. A sound understanding of the anesthesia delivery system is therefore essential for the safe practice of anesthesia.

Cooper et al.[1] collected 1089 descriptions of "critical incidents" during anesthesia of which approximately 30% were related to equipment failure, including breathing circuit disconnection, gas flow-control errors, loss of gas supply, leaks, misconnections, and ventilator malfunctions. Seventy of the 1089 incidents resulted in a "substantive negative outcome" for the patient, and of these only three were attributable to equipment failure. This confirmed a previous impression that human error is the dominant problem in anesthesia mishaps.[2] Although equipment failure is rarely the cause of death during anesthesia, critical incidents related to equipment are not infrequent and have prompted improvements in machine design and construction.[3]

Buffington et al.[4] intentionally created five faults in a standard anesthesia machine and then invited 190 attendees at a postgraduate assembly of the New York State Society of Anesthesiologists to identify them within 10 minutes. The average number of discovered faults was 2.2, and 7.3% of participants found no faults and only 3.4% found all five. The authors concluded that greater emphasis was needed in educational programs on the fundamentals of anesthesia machine design and detection of hazards.[4]

Kumar et al.[5] conducted a random survey of 169 anesthesia machines and ancillary monitors in 45 hospitals in the State of Iowa. The machines ranged in age between 1 and 28 years (the oldest being of 1958 vintage). Five machines had no backup source of oxygen, 60 had no functioning oxygen analyzer, 15 had gas leaks of greater than 500 ml/min (2 proximal to and 13 distal to the common gas outlet, that is, the patient circuit). Fourteen of the 383 vaporizers tested did not meet the manufacturer's calibration standards, and 20 had been added downstream of the machine common gas outlet. Of the 123 machines with ventilators, 16 had no alarm for low airway pressure and only 31 had a high-pressure alarm. Of the ventilators surveyed, 59% were of the hanging bellows design and 41% of the standing design. Of the machines surveyed, 95.5% had a scavenging system but in 24.3% the scavenging circuit connectors were indistinguishable from the breathing circuit connectors, a potentially hazardous design.[5] From the foregoing it is apparent that the potential for development of delivery system–related problems is great and that equipment users may not be as educated as they should be to detect such problems.

With patient safety as the primary concern, over the past several years the basic "gas machine" has evolved into the present more sophisticated anesthesia delivery systems. Safety of the delivery system has been enhanced in two basic ways: (1) pneumatic and mechanical design features (such as proportioning systems, vaporizer interlocks) have been incorporated into the systems, and (2) system monitors with alarms (such as volume, pressure, O_2 concentration) to alert to system malfunctions have been added.

The most current voluntary consensus standard describing the features of a modern machine is that published by the American Society for Testing and Materials (ASTM) in March 1989, which describes the minimum performance and safety requirements to be used in the design of anesthesia machines for human use.[6] This standard supersedes the Z79.8-1979 document published by the American National Standards Institute in 1979 (ANSI).[7] It is anticipated that use of a state-of-the-art delivery system, which includes certain basic system monitors, together with adoption of the Standards for Basic Intraoperative Monitoring, as published by the American Society of Anesthesiologists (ASA) in 1986 and periodically updated,[8] will enhance patient safety, though (as in the case of monitoring standards)absolute confirmation by demonstration of a statistically significant difference may be difficult.[9]

Complications of the anesthesia delivery system may be operator induced (misuse) or attributable to failure of a component. The approach taken in this chapter is to first trace the normal flow of gases and vapors from their sources of storage through the various components of the delivery system and to consider the function of each. In this way the effects of individual component failure will be more readily appreciated. The structure and function of the anesthesia delivery system are discussed in greater detail elsewhere.[10-12] Delivery-system failure and operator error are then discussed from the patient aspect under the general categories of oxygenation, carbon dioxide, circuit pressures and volumes, anesthetic agent delivery, humidification of inhaled gases, and electrical failure. Finally, since prevention of failures or errors is preferable to their occurrence, delivery system checkouts and standards are discussed.

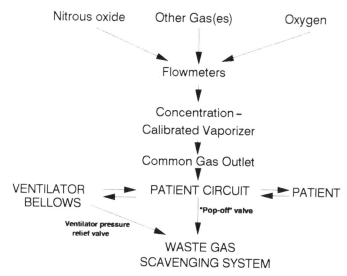

Fig. 5-1. Schema of generic anesthesia delivery system. (From Eisenkraft JB: The anesthesia delivery system. In Rogers MC, Tinker JH, and Covino BG, editors: Principles and practice of anesthesiology, St. Louis, 1992, Mosby−Year Book, Inc.

I. THE ANESTHESIA DELIVERY SYSTEM: STRUCTURE AND FUNCTION
A. Overview

The components of a modern basic anesthesia delivery system are depicted in Fig. 5-1. These include the anesthesia machine itself, which receives the gases O_2, N_2O, and perhaps a third and fourth gas (such as helium, air, CO_2) delivered under pressure. A controlled gas mixture in terms of concentration of O_2 and other gas or gases, as well as total gas flow rates, is delivered to a concentration-calibrated vaporizer where a measured amount of a potent inhaled agent may be added. The resulting fresh gas mixture of known composition and metered production rate leaves the anesthesia machine by the common gas outlet and flows to the patient circuit. The patient circuit represents a minienvironment with which the patient makes respiratory exchange and with whose contained gas tensions the patient's arterial blood and brain will equilibrate to produce the desired depth of anesthesia, as well as controlled tensions of CO_2, O_2, and other gases. Connected to the circuit may be an anesthesia ventilator bellows whereby the patient may be mechanically ventilated. Excess gases are vented from the anesthesia circuit through either the adjustable pressure-limiting (APL, or "pop-off") valve or the ventilator pressure−relief valve. The vented gases enter the waste gas scavenging system and are removed from the operating room, usually through the hospital suction.

Presently, in the United States, the two largest manufacturers of anesthesia delivery systems (machines, ventilators, vaporizers, scavenging systems) are North American Dräger (Telford, Pennsylvania)and Ohmeda (a division of BOC Health Care, Madison, Wisconsin). The features of a basic anesthesia delivery system are reviewed with reference to the Dräger and Ohmeda products where there are important differences. We emphasize at the outset that the machine manufacturer's operator's and service manuals represent the most comprehensive source of reference for any individual model of machine, and you are strongly encouraged to review the manual or manuals relevant to your equipment.

B. Basic anesthesia machine

The flow arrangements of a basic two-gas anesthesia machine are shown in Fig. 5-2. The machine receives each of the two basic gases, oxygen and nitrous oxide, from two supply sources: a tank or cylinder source and a pipeline source.

1. Oxygen. Oxygen tanks form a backup supply to the machine in case of pipeline failure. Machines are usually equipped with one or two E cylinders, which hang on gas-specific O_2 yokes. The pin-index safety system (PISS) ensures that the correct medical gas tank is hung in the correct gas yoke. The system consists of two pins in the yoke that fit into two holes in the tank valve. The two pins are in a unique configuration for O_2 and should never be removed from the hanger yoke. Specific pin con-

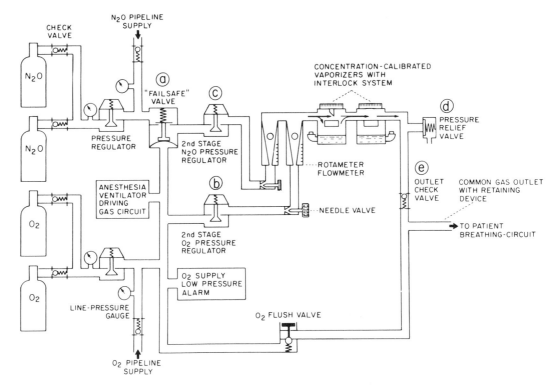

Fig. 5-2. Schema of flow arrangements of a contemporary anesthesia machine. (Adapted from "Check-Out": a guide for preoperative inspection of an anesthesia machine, Park Ridge, Ill, 1987, American Society of Anesthesiologists.)

a. Fail-safe valve in Ohmeda machines is termed a "pressure sensor shutoff valve"; in Dräger machines it is referred to as the "oxygen-failure protection device."

b. Second stage O_2 pressure regulator is used in Ohmeda (but not in Dräger Narkomed) machines.

c. Second stage N_2O pressure regulator is used in Ohmeda Modulus machines having the Link-25 proportion limiting system but not used in Dräger machines.

d. Pressure relief valve used in Ohmeda machines. In Dräger machines excesses of pressure are relieved by a pressure-relief mechanism, as in the Dräger Vapor 19.1 Vaporizer.

e. Outlet check valve used in Ohmeda Machines except Modulus II Plus and Modulus CD Models but not used in Dräger machines.

figurations exist for each of the medical gases supplied in small cylinders to prevent misconnections of gas supplies. A tank should therefore never be force fitted to a yoke. In this way only oxygen should enter the O_2 piping system of the machine.

Before a new O_2 tank is hung in the yoke, the plastic wrapper surrounding the tank valve should be removed and the tank valve opened briefly so that the emerging O_2 will blow out any debris from the valve. If the wrapper is not removed before one hangs the tank, a small disk of plastic will lodge in the yoke O_2 inlet and may totally obstruct O_2 flow from the tank.

Oxygen tanks are filled at the factory to a pressure of 1900 to 2200 PSIG at room temperature.[11] A full E cylinder of O_2 (internal volume approximately 5 liters) at a pressure of 1900 PSIG will evolve 660 liters of gaseous O_2

at atmospheric pressure (14.7 PSIA, or 760 mm Hg).* If the O_2 tank pressure is 1000 PSIG, the tank is 52% full (1000/1900) and will generate only or 340 liters (660 × 52%) of O_2. It is important to understand these principles when O_2 cylinders are in use to supply the machine or to transport a ventilated patient. If the anesthesia machine is equipped with two E cylinders of O_2, only one should be open at any one time so that both are not emptied simultaneously.

In the hanger yoke for O_2 (and other medical gases) is a check valve to prevent leakage of gas out through the yoke if no cylinder is hanging in place and the machine is being supplied by

---

*PSIG, Pounds per square inch for gauge pressure; PSIA, pounds per square inch for absolute pressure. Thus 0 PSIG = 14.7 PSIA = 760 mm Hg pressure at sea level.

the pipeline or from a second O_2 tank (Fig. 5-2). If two O_2 tanks are hanging, the check valve in the yoke prevents transfilling of gas from one tank to the other. These check valves may leak, and so if a hanger yoke does not have a tank hanging in it, a yoke plug should be inserted. This is to prevent leakage of gas in the event of an incompetent check valve, which might otherwise cause depletion of O_2.

In many medical facilities the O_2 pipeline is supplied from a bulk liquid source. Alarms and safety devices, including relief valves and shut-off valves, ensure the safe functioning of the bulk O_2 storage and pipeline systems. Pipeline O_2 is available in the operating rooms through manufacturer- and gas-specific outlets or gas-specific "quick couplers."[11]

Although the wall connectors are noninterchangeable among medical gases so that a N_2O hose connector cannot be connected to an O_2 outlet, these connectors are also manufacturer specific (such as Schraeder, Ohmeda, Chemetron). At the machine end of the pipeline hose is a connector that is gas specific by a national standard.[13] The Diameter Index Safety System (DISS) specifies that on the machine the medical gas inlet connectors for different medical gases be of different diameter. The DISS and PISS are designed to ensure that the correct medical gas enters the correct part of the anesthesia machine.[13,14] It is possible, however, for tanks (E cylinders or bulk storage) to be erroneously filled, in which case a hypoxic gas would enter the O_2 designated parts of the machine. In one hospital the O_2 pipeline was connected to a bulk supply of N_2 causing at least one catastrophe.[15] Pipeline crossovers during hospital construction or maintenance may also result in failure of O_2 delivery.[16-18] Such crossovers may also occur in the tubing connecting the machine to the wall piped-gas supply. It is also possible for the correct gas to be supplied to the correct inlet but for the supply to be contaminated by other chemicals. This occurred recently when the solution used to clean the O_2 supply tubing between the tanker and the hospital pipeline had not been flushed out. In this case all the hospital outlets had to be shut down and patients switched to tank supplies while the pipeline system was flushed out with fresh oxygen.[19]

Whereas O_2 from the pipeline supply enters the machine at a pressure of 50 PSIG, O_2 from a full tank supply enters the yoke at pressures of around 1900 PSIG. The O_2 tank source is therefore regulated (oxygen passes through a regulator valve) and enters the machine at a nominal pressure of 45 PSIG (Fig. 5-2). Pres-

sure regulators are devices that reduce a variable high input pressure (in this case 1900 PSIG) to a constant low output pressure (in this case 45 PSIG) for the gas whose pressure is being regulated. Regulators can malfunction and may deteriorate with age. If excessively high pressure builds up, a pressure relief valve in the regulator opens to vent the gas to atmosphere and protect the machine low-pressure system from exposure to extremely high pressures.[11,20] If the regulator's diaphragm should rupture, oxygen at high pressure and velocity will flow to atmosphere around the adjustment screw, causing a hissing noise. In this case a new machine is needed, since a large leak is created and even oxygen supplied through the pipeline will be leaked (Fig. 5-2). If the pressure loss is excessive, the low O_2 supply pressure alarm may be annunciated.

Once it has been checked, the tank supply should be turned *off* if the pipeline source is being used. If the O_2 tank or tanks remain turned *on* while the machine is being supplied from the pipeline, O_2 is drawn preferentially from the pipeline (50 PSIG) because the regulator that controls flow from the oxygen tanks will permit flow only when the pressure in the machine falls below about 45 PSIG (Fig. 5-2). However the pipeline pressure may at times fluctuate to below 45 PSIG, in which case O_2 would be drawn from an open tank and the backup tank supply would be inadvertently depleted.

At the pipeline inlet for all gases supplied to the machine is a check valve to prevent leakage of gas if the pipeline is disconnected and the tanks are in use.[21] Malfunction of this valve during supply of the machine from the O_2 pipeline may result in interference with the O_2 supply.[22]

O_2 entering the machine at a pressure of 45 PSIG (from tank or pipeline) may flow or pressurize in at least five directions (Fig. 5-2):

1. When the O_2 flush valve is opened, O_2 flows to the common gas outlet of the machine at a steady rate of 35 to 75 L/min.[6] The O_2 flush bypasses the vaporizers, and the pressure in the patient circuit can be high (pipeline pressure up to 50 PSIG) when the flush is operated. Furthermore the valve may stick in the open position.[23] Caution is therefore necessary when one is using the O_2 flush so as to prevent barotrauma.[24]

2. Oxygen pressurizes an O_2 supply failure alarm system such that if the O_2 supply pressure falls (usually below 30 PSIG) an alarm is annunciated. In the Ohmeda Modulus I, Modulus II, Modules and Excel machines a pressurized canister is used. This emits an audible

alarm for at least 7 seconds when the pressure falls below threshold. In Dräger Narkomed[25] and in Ohmeda Modulus II Plus and Modulus CD machines[25] a pressure-operated electrical switch ensures a continuous audible alarm whenever the O_2 supply pressure falls below the threshold setting. Failure of O_2 supply may be attributable to a pipeline interruption or malfunction, or the O_2 pipeline control valve outside the operating room may have been inadvertently turned off.[16-18]

If the alarm sounds during use of the O_2 pipeline, one of the O_2 backup supply tanks on the machine is opened and supply pressure should be restored to the machine, satisfying the alarm. When one is using a backup tank, the lowest possible flow of O_2 (and other gases) should be used to conserve O_2, and if an O_2-powered anesthesia ventilator is being used, it should be turned off and manual (bag) ventilation instituted. Failure of the O_2 pipeline supply pressure will also actuate alarms in the hospital so that the engineering or other departments responsible for supply and pipeline maintenance are alerted.[16]

3. Oxygen provides a power source for a pneumatically driven anesthesia ventilator.[25,26]

4. In fail-safe valves, oxygen pressurizes and holds open a pressure-sensor shutoff valve that reduces or interrupts the supply of N_2O and other gases (such as CO_2 He, air) to their flowmeters if the O_2 supply pressure falls below the threshold setting. This, in relation to N_2O supply control, is the so-called *fail-safe system* designed to prevent the unintentional delivery of a hypoxic mixture to the flowmeters. The fail-safe system differs between Dräger and Ohmeda machines.

In Ohmeda machines, when the O_2 supply pressure falls below 20 PSIG, the flows of N_2O and other gases to other flowmeters are interrupted. The pressure-sensor shutoff valve used by Ohmeda is an all-or-nothing, or threshold, arrangement, open at O_2 pressures greater than 20 PSIG, closed at pressures below that.[26]

The fail-safe valve in Dräger Narkomed machines is called an *oxygen failure protection device* (OFPD), and there is one for each of the gases supplied to the machine.[25,27] As the O_2 supply pressure falls, OFPDs proportionately reduce the supply pressure of other gases to their flowmeters. The supply of N_2O and other gases is completely interrupted when the O_2 supply pressure falls to below 12 ± 4 PSIG.[25] The "fail-safe system" ensures that at low or zero O_2 supply pressures only O_2 may be delivered to the common gas outlet of the machine. However, as long as there is adequate O_2 supply

pressure, other gases may flow to their flowmeters. The fail-safe system does not require a *flow* O_2 from its flowmeter, only a supply pressure. Thus a normally functioning fail-safe valve will permit *flow* of 100% N_2O provided that the machine has an adequate O_2 supply *pressure*. The term "fail-safe system" may therefore represent something of a misnomer, since it does not ensure O_2 *flow* (see below).

5. Oxygen flows to the O_2 flow control valve (flowmeter, rotameter). Gas supply to the O_2 flowmeters differs between Ohmeda and Dräger machines.

In modern Ohmeda machines the O_2 supply pressure to the flowmeter is regulated to 14 PSIG by a second-stage regulator.[26] This regulator (Fig. 5-2) ensures a constant supply pressure to the Ohmeda O_2 flowmeter. Thus, even if the O_2 supply pressure to the machine decreases below 45 to 50 PSIG, as long as it exceeds 14 PSIG the flow set on the O_2 flowmeter will be maintained. Without this second-stage O_2 regulator, if the O_2 supply pressure were to fall, the O_2 flow would decrease at the flowmeter and if another gas (such as N_2O) were being used simultaneously a hypoxic gas mixture could result at the flowmeter level.

Dräger Narkomed anesthesia machine design does not require a second-stage O_2 pressure regulator valve (Fig. 5-2).[25] Narkomed machines have OFPDs that interface the supply pressure of O_2 with that of N_2O and any other gas supplied to the machine.[25,27] A decrease in O_2 supply pressure causes a proportionate decrease in the supply pressure of each of the other gases to their flowmeters. As the O_2 supply pressure and flow decrease, all other gas flows are decreased in proportion to prevent creation of a hypoxic gas mixture at the flowmeter level (see also the discussion of the fail-safe system above).

The use (in Ohmeda machines) or nonuse (in Dräger machines) of a second-stage O_2 regulator will affect the total gas flow emerging from the common gas outlet of the machine if the O_2 supply pressure were to decrease. In an Ohmeda machine, as long as the O_2 supply pressure exceeds 20 PSIG all gas flows are maintained as set on the flowmeters. In a Dräger machine, if the O_2 supply pressure falls from normal (45 to 50 PSIG), all gas flows decrease in proportion. A decrease in total gas flow from the machine common gas outlet may cause rebreathing, depending on the patient circuit in use, with a Mapleson (rebreathing) system being affected more than a system with CO_2 absorption (circle system).

2. Nitrous oxide. Like oxygen, nitrous oxide

(N_2O) may be supplied from the pipeline system at a pressure of 50 PSIG or from a backup E cylinder supply on the machine. Because it has a critical temperature* of 36.5° C (critical pressure 1054 PSIG), N_2O can exist as a liquid at room temperature (20° C).[28,29] E cylinders of N_2O are factory filled to 90% to 95% capacity with liquid N_2O.[11] Above the liquid in the tank is N_2O vapor, and because the liquid agent is in equilibrium with its gas phase, the pressure exerted by the gaseous N_2O is its saturated vapor pressure (SVP) at the ambient temperature. At 20° C the SVP of N_2O is 750 PSIG.[28,29]

A full E tank of N_2O will generate approximately 1600 liters of gas at 1 atmosphere pressure at sea level (14.7 PSIA). As long as some liquid N_2O is present in the tank and the ambient temperature remains at 20° C, the pressure in the N_2O tank will remain at 750 PSIG, which is the SVP of N_2O at 20° C.[20,28,29]

Nitrous oxide from the tank supply enters the yoke at pressures of up to 750 PSIG (at 20° C) and then passes through a regulator that reduces this pressure to a nominal 45 PSIG (Fig. 5-2). The pin-index safety system is designed to ensure that only a N_2O tank may hang in a N_2O hanger yoke. As with O_2, a check valve in each yoke prevents the backleakage of N_2O if no tank is hung in the yoke.

The N_2O pipeline is supplied from banks of large tanks of N_2O, usually H cylinders, each of which evolves 16,000 liters of gas at atmospheric pressure.[11] The pressure in the N_2O pipeline is regulated to 50 PSIG to supply the outlets in the operating room. Having entered the anesthesia machine, N_2O has to flow past the "fail-safe" valve in order to reach its flow-control valve and rotameter.

In Ohmeda Modulus anesthesia machines that have the Link-25 Proportion Limiting System a second-stage N_2O regulator further reduces gas pressure so that N_2O is supplied to its flowmeter at a nominal pressure of 26 PSIG (Figs. 5-1 and 5-3). The actual downstream pressure of this regulator is adjusted at the factory or by a field service representative to ensure correct functioning of the proportioning system.

3. Flowmeters. The proportions of O_2 and N_2O and other medical gases controlled by the machine, as well as total gas flows delivered to the patient circuit, are adjusted by means of flow-control valves and flowmeters (rotameters).[20,27,29] There may be one rotameter, or two rotameters (Fig. 5-3) in series for each gas.[6,27] Two flowmeters in parallel for the same gas (that is, low flow and high flow O_2 and N_2O) are not a modern arrangement and may be hazardous if a low flow of O_2 is set inadvertently together with a high flow of N_2O. The ASTM standard requires that modern machines have only *one* flow-control knob for each gas emerging at the common gas outlet.[6] If two flow tubes are present for a gas, the first permits accurate measurement of low flows (usually up to 1 L/min) and the other of flows of up to 10 to 12 L/min. In North America the oxygen flowmeter is positioned on the right side of the rotameter bank, downstream of the other flowmeters and closest to the common gas outlet. In the event of a leak in one of the other flowmeter tubes, this position is the one least likely to result in a hypoxic mixture.[30,31]

Rotameters are precision instruments.[11,29,32] Flow tubes are manufactured for specific gases, calibrated with a unique float, and for use within a certain range of temperatures and pressures. Flowmeters are not interchangeable among medical gases, and if a gas is passed through a rotameter for which it was not calibrated, the flow shown would likely be incorrect. Theoretical exceptions to this would be that at *low* flows, flow rates of gases with *similar viscosities* would be read identically (such as O_2 and He, 202 and 194 micropoises respectively) and at *high flows* gases of *similar density* (such as N_2O and CO_2, both having molecular weights of 44) would be read identically.[10,32] Again, it is emphasized that flowmeters are *not* interchangeable among medical gases and for the Ohmeda machines they are now manufactured key indexed so that they cannot be interchanged.[26]

The gas flow to the rotameter tube is controlled by a touch- and color-coded knob that is linked to a needle valve.[20] In the United States the O_2 flow–control knob is color-coded green, is fluted, and is larger in diameter than the other gas flow–control knobs. The N_2O flow–control knob is smaller, color-coded blue, and not fluted. The flow-control knobs are now commonly also protected by a bar or some other protective device so that their settings are not inadvertently changed when items are being arranged on the machine's table surface.

Anesthesia machine manufacturers offer, as an option, an O_2 flow that cannot be discontinued completely because either a stop is provided to ensure a minimum oxygen flow of 200 to 300 ml/min past the needle valve (Oh-

---

*Critical temperature is the highest temperature at which a gas may exist in liquid form. The pressure that must be applied to permit liquefaction of the gas at this temperature is the critical pressure.

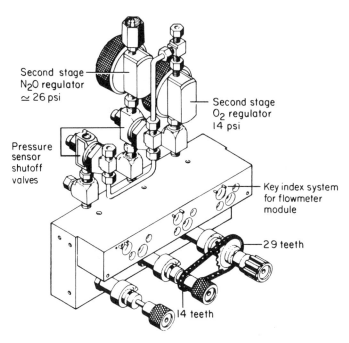

Fig. 5-3. Ohmeda Link-25 proportion-limiting system, which ensures at least a 25% oxygen mixture at the level of the flowmeters when O_2 and N_2O are being used[26,36]. When the supply pressure to the second-stage oxygen regulator falls below a nominal 26 PSIG, the pressure sensors cause the supply of N_2O and other gases to be shut off. (Adapted from Modulus II Plus® Anesthesia Machine: Preoperative checklists: Operation and maintenance manual, Madison, Wisc, 1988, permission granted by Ohmeda, a division of B.O.C. Healthcare Inc.)

meda),[20,26] or a gas-flow resistor, which permits a flow of 200 to 300 ml/min O_2 to bypass a totally closed oxygen flow-control needle valve, is provided (Dräger Narkomed).[25] In modern Dräger Narkomed machines, the minimum oxygen flow feature functions only in the O_2/N_2O mode but not in the "all gases" mode.[25]

Flowmeters are also subject to failure. Thus a needle valve may break[33,34] or a stop mechanism for the flow-control knob may malfunction,[35] in either case preventing the delivery of oxygen (or other gases). The flow tubes are also subject to breakage and leakage.[11,27]

4. Oxygen-ratio monitoring and proportioning systems. A major consideration in the design of modern anesthesia machines is the prevention of the delivery of a hypoxic gas mixture.[6] The "fail-safe" system described above serves only to interrupt (Ohmeda) or proportionately reduce and ultimately interrupt (Dräger OFPD) the supplies of N_2O and other gases (such as air or helium) to their flowmeters if the O_2 supply pressure to the machine is reduced. It does not prevent the delivery of a hypoxic mixture to the common gas outlet and the term "fail-safe" is therefore somewhat of a misnomer.

In modern machines, O_2 and N_2O flow controls are physically interlinked either mechanically (Ohmeda),[26] or mechanically and pneumatically (Dräger),[25,27] so that a fresh gas mixture containing at least 25% O_2 is created at the level of the flowmeters when N_2O and O_2 are being used.

Ohmeda anesthesia machines use the Link-25 Proportion Limiting Control System to ensure an adequate percentage of O_2 in the gas mixture created.[26] In Modulus machines having this system a gear with 14 teeth is mounted on and integral with the N_2O flow–control spindle while a gear with 29 teeth is mounted and "floats" on a threaded O_2 flow–control valve spindle (Fig. 5-3).[36] The two gears are connected together by a precision stainless steel link chain. For every 2.07 revolutions of the N_2O flow–control spindle, an O_2 flow control, set to the lowest oxygen flow, will rotate once because of the 29:14 ratio of gear teeth. Because the gear on the O_2 flow–control spindle is thread mounted so that it can ride ("float") on the control valve spindle (rather than being integral with the spindle), O_2 flow can be increased independently of N_2O. However, regardless of the O_2 flow set, if the flow of N_2O

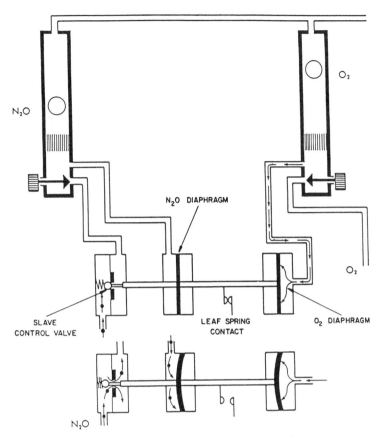

Fig. 5-4. Oxygen ratio monitor controller (ORMC). See text for details of operation. (From Schreiber P: Safety guidelines for anesthesia systems, Telford, Penn, 1985, North American Dräger, Inc.)

is increased sufficiently, the gear on the O spindle will engage with the O_2 flow–control knob, causing it to rotate and thereby cause O_2 flow to increase.[36] If N_2O flow is now reduced, the O_2 flow will remain high unless it is deliberately reduced by the user. The 75% N_2O : 25% O_2 proportioning is completed because the N_2O flow–control valve is supplied from a second-stage gas regulator that reduces N_2O pressure to a nominal 26 PSIG before it reaches the flow–control valve, whereas the O_2 flow–control valve is supplied at a pressure of 14 PSIG from a second-stage O_2 regulator (Figs. 5-2 and 5-3). The Link-25 system permits the N_2O and O_2 flow–control valves to be set independently of one another, but whenever what would be a N_2O concentration of more than 75% is inadvertently set, the O_2 flow is automatically increased to maintain at least 25% O_2 in the resulting gas mixture. This system thus *increases the minimum flow of O_2 according to the N_2O flow set*. Ohmeda Excel machines have a system similar in principle but with a 24:48 ratio of gear teeth.

It should be noted that the Link-25 system interconnects only the N_2O and O_2 flow–control valves. If the anesthesia machine has flow controls for other gases, such as helium or air, a gas mixture containing less than 25% O_2 could potentially be set at the level of the flowmeters.

In Dräger Narkomed machines, the *Oxygen Ratio Monitor Controller (ORMC)* (Fig. 5-4) serves to limit the flow of N_2O *according to the O_2 flow* and create a mixture of at least 25% O_2 at the flowmeter level when these two gases are being used.[25,27] At O_2 flow rates of less than 1 L/min, even higher concentrations of O_2 are delivered. In addition, an alarm is activated when the ORMC is functioning to prevent a hypoxic mixture when the Narkomed machine is used in the "N_2O/O_2" mode but not in the "all gases" mode (that is, when air, helium, and so on might be switched into the system).[25]

The ORMC works as follows (Fig. 5-4). As O_2 flows past its flow-control valve and up the rotameter tube, it encounters a resistor, which creates a backpressure that is applied to the O_2 diaphragm. As N_2O flows past its flow-control valve and up its rotameter tube, it also encounters a resistor, which causes a backpressure on the N_2O diaphragm. The two diaphragms are linked by a connecting shaft, the ultimate position of which depends on the relative backpressures and therefore flows of N_2O and O_2. The left-hand end of the connecting shaft controls the orifice of a slave valve, which in turn controls the supply pressure of N_2O to its flow-control valve. When the oxygen flow is high, the shaft moves to the left and opens the slave control valve. Conversely, if the flow of N_2O is increased excessively, the shaft moves to the right, closing the slave valve orifice and limiting the supply pressure and thereby the flow of N_2O to its flow-control valve. When the ORMC is acting to prevent a hypoxic mixture, the leaf spring contacts (Fig. 5-4) are closed, annunciating an alarm. This alarm is disabled if the machine is in the "all gases" mode.[25]

Like the Link-25 system, the ORMC functions only between N_2O and O_2, and there is no interlinking of O_2 with other gases such as air or helium, which might also be deliverable by the machine. Thus, whenever a third or fourth gas is in use, the proportioning systems afford no protection against creation of a hypoxic mixture. Although of elegant design, both the ORMC and Link-25 systems are potentially subject to mechanical or pneumatic failure. In the case of the Link-25 system, breakage of the link chain[37] and incorrect mounting of the O_2 flow–control knob on its spindle causing late engagement of the floating gear and hence late increase in O_2 flow,[36] both potentially resulting in hypoxic mixtures, have been reported. Because of these limitations, total reliance should never be placed on a proportioning system. When one is setting gas flows, O_2 should always be increased first or decreased last and adequacy should always be confirmed by checking the flows on the gas rotameters. Furthermore, even if the systems are functioning correctly, they ensure adequacy of only greater than 25% oxygen at the flowmeter level. An O_2 leak downstream of the flowmeters could result in a hypoxic mixture emerging from the machine common gas outlet.[27] A functional and enabled oxygen analyzer in the patient circuit is therefore essential if a potentially hypoxic mixture is to be detected and thereby prevented. The controlled flows of O_2, N_2O, and other gases are then mixed in the manifold at the top of the flowmeter bank and flow to a calibrated anesthesia vaporizer (see Fig. 5-2).

C. Anesthesia vaporizers

A vapor is the gas phase of an agent that is normally a liquid at room temperature and atmospheric pressure. Modern vaporizers are devices that facilitate the change of a liquid anesthetic into its vapor phase and add a controlled amount of this vapor to the flow of gases passing to the patient circuit.[10]

1. Regulating vaporizer output: variable bypass versus measured flow. The saturated vapor

Table 5-1. Physical properties of volatile agents

Agent or parameter	Halothane	Enflurane	Isoflurane	Methoxyflurane
Structure	$CHBrClCF_3$	$CHFClCF_2OCHF_2$	$CF_2HOCHClCF_3$	$CHCl_2CF_2OCH_3$
Molecular Weight	197.4	184.5	184.5	165.0
Boiling point at 760 mm Hg (°C)	50.2	56.5	48.5	104.7
Saturated vapor pressure at 20° C (mm Hg)	243	175	238	20.3
Saturated vapor concentration at 20° C and 1 ATA (vol %)	32	23	31	2.7
MAC at 1 ATA (vol %)	0.75	1.68	1.15	0.16
P_{MAC1} (mm Hg)	5.7	12.8	8.7	1.22
Specific gravity of liquid at 20° C	1.86	1.52	1.50	1.41
1 g of liquid produces... L of vapor at 20° C	0.123	0.130	0.130	0.145
1 ml of liquid produces... L of vapor at 20° C	0.226	0.196	0.195	0.204

From Eisenkraft JB: Vaporizers and vaporization of volatile anesthetics, Progress in Anesthesiology, vol 2, no 24, San Antonio, Texas, 1988, Dannemiller Memorial Educational Foundation.
1 ATA, 1 atmosphere, absolute; *MAC,* minimum alveolar concentration.

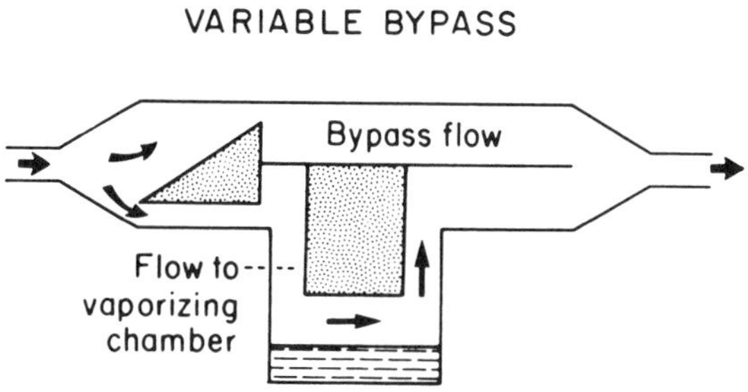

VARIABLE BYPASS

Bypass flow

Flow to vaporizing chamber

Fig. 5-5. Variable bypass vaporizer. (From Eisenkraft JB: Vaporizers and vaporization of volatile anesthetics, Progress in Anesthesiology, vol 2, no 24, San Antonio, Texas, 1988, Dannemiller Memorial Educational Foundation.)

MEASURED FLOW VAPORIZER
(Copper Kettle, Verni-Trol)

Main flow meters

To patient

Measured flow to vaporizer (bubble-through)

Vaporizing chamber
Liquid anesthetic

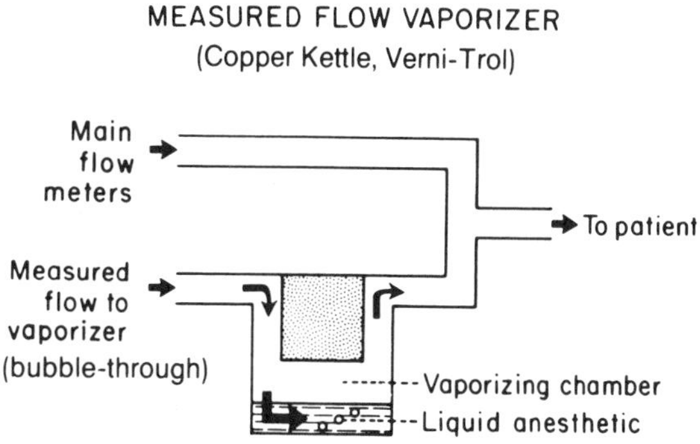

Fig. 5-6. Measured flow vaporizer (Copper Kettle, Verni-Trol). (From Eisenkraft JB: Vaporizers and vaporization of volatile anesthetics, Progress in Anesthesiology, vol 2, no 24, San Antonio, Texas, 1988, Dannemiller Memorial Educational Foundation.)

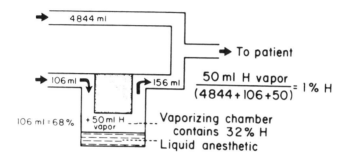

4844 ml

To patient

$$\frac{50 \text{ ml H vapor}}{(4844+106+50)} = 1\% \text{ H}$$

106 ml   156 ml

106 ml ≈ 68%   +50 ml H vapor

Vaporizing chamber contains 32% H
Liquid anesthetic

In practice main flow is set to 5 L/min, vaporizer flow is set to 100 ml/min and H output is 0.913%,

i.e., 47 ml H vapor diluted in (5000 + 100 + 47) ml

Fig. 5-7. Preparation of 1% (vol/vol) halothane by a measured flow vaporizer. (From Eisenkraft JB: Vaporizers and vaporization of volatile anesthetics, Progress in Anesthesiology, vol 2, no 24, San Antonio, Texas, 1988, Dannemiller Memorial Educational Foundation.)

pressures of the three most commonly used potent inhaled agents halothane, enflurane, and isoflurane at room temperature are 243, 175, and 238 mm Hg respectively and far in excess of those required clinically (Table 5-1). The vaporizer therefore first creates a saturated vapor that must then be diluted by the bypass gas flow to result in clinically useful concentrations. If this were not done, a lethal concentration of agent could be delivered to the anesthesia circuit.

Modern anesthesia vaporizers are concentration calibrated and of the variable bypass design.[6] In a variable bypass vaporizer (such as Tec series from Ohmeda; Dräger Vapor 19.1) the total fresh gas flow from the anesthesia machine flowmeters passes to the vaporizer.

The vaporizer (Fig. 5-5) splits the incoming gas into a smaller flow, which enters the vaporizing chamber of the vaporizer to emerge with saturated vapor concentrations of the agent, and a larger bypass flow, which, when mixed with the vaporizing chamber output, results in the desired or "dialed-in" concentration.[10,38]

In the virtually now obsolete measured flow (non–concentration calibrated) vaporizers, such as Copper Kettle (Foregger/Puritan-Bennett) or Verni-Trol (Ohmeda), a measured flow of O_2 is set on a separate flowmeter to pass to the vaporizer, from which vapor at its saturated vapor pressure emerges (Fig. 5-6). This flow is then diluted by an additional measured flow of gases from other flowmeters on the anesthesia machine. With this type of arrangement, several calculations are necessary to determine the anesthetic vapor concentration in the emerging gas mixture.

2. Measured-flow vaporizers (Copper Kettle, Verni-Trol). Although measured-flow vaporizers are no longer considered desirable[6] and are not mentioned in the ASTM F 1161-88 standard, it is helpful to first review the function of a measured-flow vaporizer (such as Copper Kettle). Suppose 1% (vol/vol) halothane is required at a total fresh gas flow rate to the patient circuit of 5 L/min (Fig. 5-7). This requires 50 ml of halothane vapor to be evolved per minute by the vaporizer (1% × 5000 ml).

In the vaporizing chamber, halothane represents 32% (243/760) of the atmosphere, if one assumes that the temperature is kept constant at 20° C, and therefore saturated vapor pressure is maintained at 243 mm Hg (Table 5-1). Now, if 50 ml of halothane vapor represent 32%, the carrier gas (O_2) must represent the other 68%, or 106 ml ([50/32] × 68); alternatively:

$$\frac{243}{760} = \frac{50}{Y + 50}$$

where Y = carrier gas (O_2) flow = 106 ml.

Thus, if 106 ml/min of O_2 flow into a Copper Kettle vaporizer, 156 ml/min of gas will emerge, of which 50 ml will be halothane vapor and 106 ml the O_2 that was supplied to the vaporizer. This vaporizer output of 156 ml/min must be diluted by an additional fresh gas flow of 4844 ml/min (5000 − 156) to create a precise 1% halothane mixture (since 50 ml of halothane diluted in a total volume of 5000 ml = 1% halothane by volume).

In clinical practice, however, the anesthetist would likely set flows of 100 ml/min to the Copper Kettle vaporizer and 5 L/min of fresh gas on the main flowmeters, which results in a little less than 1% halothane (actually [47/5147] = 0.91%). Multiples of these numbers are used to create other concentrations of halothane from a Copper Kettle vaporizer. Thus a 100 ml/min gas flow to the vaporizer and a 2500 ml/min flow on the main flowmeters would give about 2% halothane (actually 1.78%).[38] It is important to realize that if there is O_2 flow only to the vaporizer and no diluent fresh gas flow is set on the main flowmeters, lethal concentrations (approaching 32%) of halothane would be delivered to the anesthesia circuit, albeit at low flow rates.[10,38]

3. Variable bypass (concentration-calibrated) vaporizers. In the foregoing examples it was necessary to calculate both the O_2 flow to the measured flow vaporizer and the total diluent gas flow needed to produce the desired output concentration of vapor. This is inconvenient and may give rise to errors, but it is important to understand the principles underlying the calculations involved because such vaporizing systems may still be in use.

In the concentration-calibrated variable bypass design the vaporizer splits the total flow of gas arriving from the machine flowmeters between a variable bypass and the vaporizer chamber containing the liquid anesthetic agent (Fig. 5-5). The ratio of these flows, the *splitting ratio*, depends on the anesthetic agent, the temperature, and the desired vapor concentration set to be delivered to the patient circuit. The splitting ratios for variable bypass vaporizers used at 20° C are shown in Table 5-2.[38]

Concentration-calibrated vaporizers are agent specific and should be used only with the agent for which the unit is designed and calibrated. In order to produce a 1% vapor concentration, a halothane vaporizer makes a flow split of 46:1, whereas an enflurane vaporizer makes a flow split of 28.7:1 (Table 5-2). If an empty enflurane vaporizer set to deliver 1% were filled with halothane, the halothane vapor emerging would be in excess of 1% (actually [46/28.7] = 1.6%). An understanding of splitting ratios enables fairly accurate prediction of the concentration output of an empty agent-specific variable bypass vaporizer that has been erroneously filled with an agent for which it was not designed (see below).

4. Temperature compensation. Agent-specific concentration-calibrated vaporizers are located in the fresh gas pathway between the flowmeters on the anesthesia machine and the

Table 5-2. Gas-flow splitting ratios at 20° C

	Halothane	Enflurane	Isoflurane	Methoxyflurane
1%	46:1	29:1	44:1	1.7:1
2%	22:1	14:1	21:1	0.36:1
3%	14:1	9:1	14:1	Maximum possible is 2.7% at 20° C

From Eisenkraft JB: Vaporizers and vaporization of volatile anesthetics, Progress in Anesthesiology, vol 2, no 24, San Antonio, Texas, 1988, Dannemiller Memorial Educational Foundation.

common gas outlet. The vaporizers must be efficient and produce steady concentrations of agent over a fairly wide range of incoming gas-flow rates. However, as the agent is vaporized and the liquid temperature falls, saturated vapor pressure (SVP) decreases and vaporizing chamber output would tend to decrease. In the case of a measured-flow situation (as with Copper Kettle) or an uncompensated variable bypass vaporizer, this would result in delivery of less anesthetic vapor to the patient circuit. For this reason, all vaporizing systems must be temperature compensated. This compensation may be manually or automatically achieved.[10,38]

Measured-flow vaporizers (Copper Kettle, Verni-Trol) incorporate a thermometer that measures the temperature of the liquid agent in the vaporizing chamber. A lower temperature translates to a lower saturated vapor pressure in this chamber, and reference to the vapor pressure curves enables a resetting of either the vaporizer or diluent main gas flows or both to ensure correct output at the prevailing temperature. Such an arrangement can be tedious, but it does ensure the most accurate and rapid temperature compensation. Modern variable bypass vaporizers (such as Ohmeda Tec series, Dräger Vapor 19.1) have automatic temperature compensation achieved by a temperature-sensitive valve in the bypass gas flow. When temperature rises, the valve in the bypass opens wider to create a higher splitting ratio. More gas flows through the bypass, and less gas enters the vaporizing chamber. A smaller volume of a higher concentration of vapor emerges from the vaporizing chamber that, when mixed with an increased bypass gas flow, maintains the vaporizer output reasonably constant when temperature changes are gradual and not extreme. Dräger Vapor 19.1 vaporizers are specified as accurate to ±15% of the concentration set when used within the temperature range of +15° to +35° C at normal atmospheric pressure.* At temperatures outside of this range the resulting concentration increases beyond the upper tolerance limit despite continuing compensation. The boiling point of the volatile agent must never be reached in the current variable bypass vaporizers designed for halothane, enflurane, and isoflurane because otherwise the vapor output concentration would be totally uncontrolled and lethal.

It is also important to recognize that there is a certain amount of inertia in any temperature-compensating mechanism. An increase in temperature would result in increased evaporation of liquid agent and therefore increased cooling (because of heat loss) of the remaining liquid. This would tend to lower the saturated vapor pressure of the agent. Changes in ambient temperature, unless drastic, therefore usually do not result in major changes in vaporizer output. In the Dräger Vapor 19.1 series vaporizers a sudden change in temperature requires a compensation time of 6 min/° C to maintain output concentration within the limits stated previously.* In the case of an increase in temperature, vaporizer output would be in excess of that shown on the dial until compensation had occurred.

In some older design vaporizers (such as Fluotec Mark II), the temperature-compensation valve was in the vaporizing chamber itself. The thymol preservatives added to halothane could cause sticking of this valve, so that in the later models and other modern vaporizers the temperature-compensating valve is in the bypass gas flow.[11]

5. *Arrangement of vaporizers.* Older anesthesia machines had up to three variable bypass vaporizers arranged in series such that fresh gas passed through each vaporizer (albeit all through the bypass flow) to reach the common gas outlet of the anesthesia machine. Without an interlock system, which permits only one vaporizer to be in use at any one time, it was possible to have all three vaporizers on simultaneously. Apart from potentially overdosing the patient, the agent from the upstream vaporizer could contaminate the agent or agents in those downstream. During subsequent use, the output of the downstream vaporizer would be contaminated. The resulting concentrations in the emerging gas and vapor mixture would be indeterminate and might even be lethal.[10,38]

With modern arrangements, only one vaporizer can be on at any time. The ASTM F1161-88 standard requires that to prevent cross-contamination of the contents of one vaporizer with agent from another, a system shall be provided that isolates the vaporizers from each other and prevents gas from passing through the vaporizing chamber of one vaporizer and then through that of another.[6] This specification is met by use of an interlock system. Contemporary Dräger and Ohmeda anesthesia machines incorporate manufacturer-specific interlock systems.[25,26]

6. *Calibration and checking of vaporizer outputs.* Vaporizers should be regularly serviced and their outputs checked to ensure that a malfunction does not exist. Thus the vaporizer is set to deliver a certain vapor concentration,

---

*Operating Manual, Vapor 19.1, Lübeck, FDR, March 1986, Drägerwerk AG.

and the actual output concentration is measured by an anesthetic-agent analyzer sampling gas via a connector placed at the common gas outlet of the anesthesia machine.

Currently available practical vapor-analysis methods include mass spectrometry, multiwavelength infrared (IR) spectroscopy, and laser-Raman spectroscopy. These three methods enable *multiple* agents to be identified and quantified in the presence of one another. Other technologies, such as single-wavelength IR spectroscopy, photoacoustic spectroscopy, vibrating crystal, and refractometry, are accurate and reliable if only one agent is present and has been qualitatively identified to the analyzer. They are inaccurate in the presence of multiple agents. Refer elsewhere for a more detailed discussion of these technologies.[39]

7. Desflurane (Suprane). Desflurane (Suprane; Anaquest, Liberty Corner, New Jersey) is a new potent inhaled volatile anesthetic currently undergoing clinical investigation in the United States. The physical properties are shown in List 5-1. With a saturated vapor pressure of 664 mm Hg at 20° C and a boiling point of 23.5° C at 760 mm Hg atmosphere pressure this agent is extremely volatile, which presents certain problems when it comes to vaporization and production of controlled concentrations of vapor. There are at least four possible methods for controlling the vapor output concentration.

1. *Heated, pressurized vaporizer.* The technique is employed in the Ohio DM (Direct Metering) 5000 machine which has a heated, pressurized, measured flow vaporizer.[11] The DM 5000 machine is currently being used for clinical trials only.

2. *Heated, pressurized variable bypass vaporizer.* Desflurane could be heated to more than 24° C to form a gas under pressure that is then metered into the main gas flow using a separate flow-control system. A heated, pressurized variable bypass vaporizing system (as distinct from the measured-flow system above) would address these considerations.

3. *Liquid injection.* Desflurane liquid in small metered or pulsed doses could be vaporized into known fresh gas flows to produce clinically useful concentrations.

4. *Cooled variable bypass vaporizer.* If cooled to 5° C, desflurane has a saturated vapor pressure of about 250 mm Hg and could thus be administered using a conventional variable bypass (Tec type) vaporizer. Cooling a vaporizer presents many technical problems and is energy inefficient.

If and when desflurane becomes available for general clinical use, the vaporizing system will clearly be different from those in use for the presently available potent inhaled agents and will require a source of energy (electricity). General requirements of the desflurane vaporizer will be that it will deliver accurate concentrations over a wide range of gas flows and that it be easily retrofitted to modern anesthesia machines, replacing one of the existing machine-mounted and interlocked vaporizers. An agent-specific filling device will be essential with this agent. The reason is that with its high vapor pressure at room temperature, erroneous filling of another vaporizer with this agent would likely lead to severe overdosage.

D. Common gas outlet, outlet check valves, and pressure-relief valves

The fresh gas mixture produced by the settings of the flowmeters for O_2, N_2O with or without other gases, and vapor from one concentration-calibrated vaporizer leave the machine through the common gas outlet. Situated between the vaporizer and the common gas outlet, Ohmeda Modulus I, Modulus II, and Excel machines have (1) an outlet check valve and (2) a pressure-relief valve (Fig. 5-2).[10] The pressure-relief valve, as its name indicates, prevents the buildup of excessive pressures upstream of the outlet check valve. These components are located upstream from where the oxygen flush flow would join to pass to the common gas outlet. The pressure-relief valve also prevents buildup of pressure in the anesthesia machine if the common gas outlet should become obstructed. This may occur if the tubing connecting the common gas outlet to the anesthesia circuit becomes obstructed or kinked.

The purpose of the outlet check valve, where present (Ohmeda Modulus I, Modulus II, Excel but not Modulus II Plus or Modulus CD machines), is to prevent reverse gas flow, which

---

List 5-1. Desflurane (Suprane) physical properties

Formula: $CF_2H—O—CFH—CF_3$
Molecular weight: 168
Specific gravity: 1.45
Boiling point: 23.5° C at 760 mm Hg
Saturated vapor pressure: at 20° C = 664 mm Hg
Odor: ethereal
Preservative free
Minimum alveolar concentration (MAC): 6.0% to 7.25% (age-related)* at 760 mm Hg

---

Data Courtesy of Anaquest, Research and Development, Liberty Corner, NJ.
*Datum from Rampil IJ, Lockhart SH, Zwass MS, et al: Anesthesiology 74:429-433, 1991.

could cause gas to go back into the vaporizer ("pumping effect") if the latter did not have its own outlet check valve or specialized design. This effect, if not prevented, would cause increased vaporizer output concentrations.

Dräger Narkomed machines are designed so as not to require an outlet check valve, with any pumping effect being eliminated by special design of the Vapor 19.1 vaporizer. The Ohmeda Modulus II Plus and Modulus CD machines are equipped with Ohmeda TEC 4 or TEC 5 vaporizers, which incorporate a baffle system and specially designed manifold to prevent the pumping effect, making an outlet check valve unnecessary on these machines. Nevertheless, the Ohmeda Modulus II Plus and Modulus CD Machines do have a pressure-relief valve, which opens at 135 ± 15 mm Hg (2.2 PSIG)[26] (Fig. 5-2). Dräger Narkomed machines do not require a separate pressure-relief valve. In these machines pressure relief, if required, takes place through the specially designed Vapor 19.1 vaporizers when the pressure exceeds about 18 PSIG. The presence or absence of an outlet check valve and pressure-relief valve is of some significance when it comes to leak testing the low-pressure system of the anesthesia machine (see below). Also, if a transtracheal jet ventilation system has been configured to be connected to the machine common gas outlet and ventiliation achieved by intermittent depression of the oxygen flush button,[39a,39b] the driving pressure of such a system would be limited by the opening pressure of the pressure-relief valve. In the case of the Modulus II Plus and Modulus CD machines this would be approximately 2.2 PSIG; in the case of Dräger Narkomed machines equipped with Vapor 19.1 vaporizers it would be 18 PSIG, and in the case of Modulus II and Excel machines (outlet check valve present) or Dräger Norkomed machines without vaporizers (no pressure-relief system) it would be 45 to 55 PSIG, depending on whether the tank or pipeline oxygen supply to the machine was in use (Fig. 5-2).

The ASTM F1161-88 standard requires that machines should have only one common gas outlet and that when the common gas outlet is connected to the breathing system by a fresh gas supply hose (the usual arrangement in most operating rooms) the common gas outlet shall be provided with a manufacturer-specific retaining device.[6] The purpose of the retaining device is to help prevent disconnection or misconnections between the machine common gas outlet and the patient circuit, which could result in patient injury.[26] Thus a disconnection here could result in entrainment of room air, which might result in a hypoxic mixture in the circuit,

as well as failure of delivery of inhaled anesthetic.[40,41] Dräger Narkomed machines have a bar type of retaining device, whereas Ohmeda machines use a spring-loaded bayonet-fitting retaining device.[25-27]

E. Anesthesia circuits

The anesthesia circuit represents a minienvironment with which the patient makes respiratory exchange. The fresh gas flow from the anesthesia machine delivers metered concentrations of O_2, N_2O, and potent inhaled anesthetic to the circuit and gases are vented from the circuit to the scavenging system. In some arrangements high fresh gas flows are used, in which case the patient's inspired gas concentrations will approximate those in the fresh gas supply. Other circuits, such as the adult circle system, use lower fresh gas flows and rely upon an absorption system for CO_2. In the circle system using low gas flows, the composition of the inspired gas may be quite different from that of the fresh gas inflow.

Patient breathing circuits are generally composed of corrugated 22 mm diameter tubing, a reservoir bag, and connecting piece or elbow to the patient's airway. They may or may not also include a valve or valves. The way in which these items are arranged gives the resulting circuit its functional characteristics.[42] Incorrect arrangement of components may give rise to circuit malfunction. Breathing systems are generally classified as rebreathing, having no CO_2 absorption system (that is, Mapleson classification circuits A-F), or nonrebreathing, having a carbon dioxide absorber (such as a circle system).[10]

1. Rebreathing systems (Fig. 5-8). The rebreathing circuits, assigned letters according to Mapleson's classification, are discussed in more detail elsewhere.[10,11,27,42-46] Since there is no CO_2 absorber in any of these systems, the potential exists for the patient to inhale alveolar gas that has been previously exhaled and contains CO_2. The extent of rebreathing will depend on the circuit anatomy, the patient's minute ventilation, pattern of ventilation, fresh gas flow rate, and whether ventilation is spontaneous or controlled. An understanding of the functional characteristics is therefore essential to their appropriate use. Only the more commonly used coaxial Mapleson D (Bain) and F (the Jackson-Rees modification of Ayre's system) are briefly described here.

a. Coaxial Mapleson D (Bain system). The Coaxial Mapleson D system is shown in Fig. 5-9. Fresh gas from the anesthesia machine enters the inner (smaller-bore) tubing and is delivered to the patient end. Exhaled gas is carried

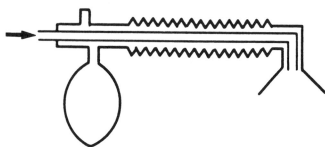

Fig. 5-9. Bain circuit. Coaxial Mapleson D.

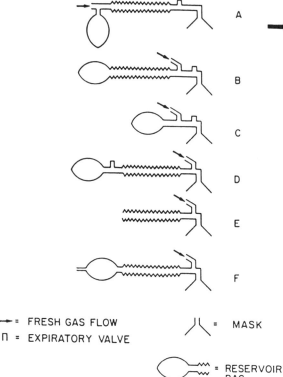

= FRESH GAS FLOW

Π **= EXPIRATORY VALVE**

= MASK

= RESERVOIR BAG

Fig. 5-8. Mapleson classification of rebreathing systems. The Mapleson A circuit is also known as the Magill attachment. (From Conway CM: Br J Anaesth 57:649, 1985.)

through the outer tubing to the reservoir bag and pop-off valve. Both reusable and disposable versions are available. The outer tubing is now made from transparent material so that the inner tubing may be inspected for kinking or disconnection. Clearly if the latter were to occur at the machine end, the whole system would become apparatus dead space and result in excessive rebreathing.

A ventilation nomogram shows that during controlled ventilation, the $P_{A}CO_2$ can be estimated from a combination of fresh gas flow (FGF) and minute ventilation (V_E).[47] At high FGF, $P_{A}CO_2$ becomes independent of FGF and dependent on V_E. At high V_E, $P_{A}CO_2$ is independent of V_E and becomes dependent on FGF. The Bain circuit can thus be used to provide controlled rebreathing with hyperventilation, resulting in normal $P_{A}CO_2$. The pop-off valve in the Bain circuit is located close to the anesthesia machine, therefore scavenging from the Bain circuit is not generally a problem.

A pre-use check of the Bain circuit is essential to ensure that the inner gas delivery tube has not become disconnected. If this occurred, it could lead to rebreathing. Two checkout methods have been described. In one,[48] the patient end of the whole system is occluded, the pop-off valve is closed, and the system is filled with

oxygen until the reservoir bag is distended. The patient end is then unoccluded, and oxygen is flushed into the circuit through the inner tube. The high flow of oxygen produces a Venturi effect at the patient end of the circuit, with the low pressure created at the end of the outer tubing causing oxygen to be drawn along the outer tubing from the reservoir bag, causing the bag to deflate. If there is a disconnection or a leak in the inner tubing, flushing the circuit with oxygen would allow the high pressure to be transmitted from the inner to the outer tubing and the reservoir bag would remain inflated or distend further.[48] A second method[49] is to set a 50 ml/min flow on the oxygen flowmeter and then occlude the distal (patient) end of the inner tube using the plunger of a small syringe. If the inner tube is intact, this sequence should cause the gas flow to cease and the oxygen flowmeter bobbin to fall. The second test is preferred because if the inner tube has been omitted the first test may give no indication that anything is wrong.[11]

b. Mapleson F. The Mapleson F circuit is the Jackson-Rees modification of Ayre's T-piece (Mapleson E) system.[10] In this system (Fig. 5-8), to the end of the expiratory limb tubing is added a reservoir bag and a means for venting waste gases. The latter is usually a valve with an adjustable orifice that is connected to a waste gas–scavenging system.

The system functions similarly to the Mapleson E except that during exhalation a mixture of exhaled and fresh gas collects in the bag and on the next inspiration the patient inhales fresh gas both from the machine common gas outlet and that stored in the expiratory limb and bag. Addition of the reservoir bag to the E system provides a means to qualitatively monitor ventilation during spontaneous breathing, as well as a means to control ventilation by manually squeezing the reservoir bag. Prevention of rebreathing is achieved by use of fresh gas flows of two to three times minute ventilation.[43]

2. Circle system

a. Structure. In this system the components form a circle into which fresh gas can enter and from which excess gas can leave. Although sev-

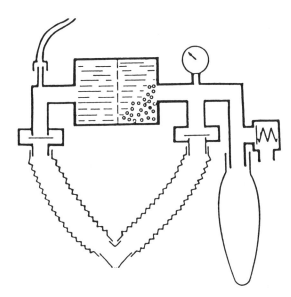

Fig. 5-10. Contemporary anesthesia circle system arrangement. *P,* Patient. (From Schreiber P: Safety guidelines for anesthesia systems, Telford, Penn, 1985, North American Dräger, Inc.)

eral configurations are possible,[45] the arrangements of the components of a modern circle system are shown in Fig. 5-10. Fresh gas enters just upstream of the inspiratory unidirectional valve and, during inspiration, passes down the inspiratory limb of the circle to the Y-piece connector. During expiration, gas passes along the expiratory limb to the expiratory unidirectional valve. Just beyond the expiratory valve are the adjustable pressure-limiting (APL, or "pop-off") valve and a reservoir bag. Gas then passes through a canister containing a CO_2 absorbent (such as soda lime) and emerges to rejoin fresh gas entering the circuit from the anesthesia machine just upstream of the inspiratory valve.

In the system described, rebreathing of CO_2 is prevented by the absorption of CO_2 from exhaled gas before it is reinspired. At high fresh gas flows, however, CO_2 absorption becomes unnecessary and some older circle systems even permitted bypass of the absorber canister.[11] At lower fresh gas flows CO_2 absorption is necessary, and Eger[45] has suggested three basic rules for preventing CO_2 rebreathing in a circle system. These are as follows:

1. There must be a unidirectional valve between the reservoir bag and the patient on both the inspiratory and expiratory sides.
2. Fresh gas must not enter the system between the expiratory unidirectional valve and the patient.
3. The overflow valve must not be placed between the patient and the inspiratory unidirectional valve.

Incompetence of either of the unidirectional valves permits bidirectional gas flow in the corrugated patient tubing, leading to rebreathing of previously exhaled CO_2.

The circle system is currently the most popular patient circuit in use in the United States. It has the advantages of permitting low fresh gas flows, reduction of operating room pollution, and conservation of heat and humidity. Disadvantages of the circle system include a somewhat complex design with multiple components that could malfunction or be arranged incorrectly.[27] In addition is the difficulty of predicting inspired gas composition within the circle, particularly if low fresh gas flows are being used. The latter may cease to be a problem, however, as monitoring of anesthetic and respiratory gas concentrations becomes more common.

b. Absorption of carbon dioxide. The CO_2 absorber is the central component in a circle system. Modern canisters are large with a minimum gas space equal to the largest expected patient tidal volume. This design permits low gas flow rates, long dwell times, and thereby more complete removal ("scrubbing") of CO_2.[50] The two CO_2 absorbents in most common use are soda lime (Sodasorb, Dewey and Alny Chemical Division, Lexington, Massachusetts)[50] and barium hydroxide lime (Baralyme, Chemetron Medical Division, Allied Health Care Products, Inc., St. Louis, Missouri).[11]

Absorptive surface area and flow of gas through the absorbent are a function of granule size. The smaller the size, the larger is the area for absorption but the greater the resistance to gas flow. Conversely, large granules decrease absorptive surface area, offer less resistance to flow, and may encourage channeling of gases through the absorbent, thereby decreasing CO_2 absorption.[50]

Indicators are added to the absorbent granules to show when they are becoming exhausted. These indicators are pH-sensitive and are colorless when the absorbent is fresh but become colored when pH decreases. The most commonly used indicator is ethyl violet, which changes from colorless to purple as absorption proceeds.[11,50]

Recently it has been reported that ethyl violet, the indicator added to Sodasorb, may be deactivated by fluorescent lighting and even undergo temporal deactivation after a container of Sodasorb is opened, even if it is stored in the dark.[51] Such deactivation increases the hazard of using CO_2 absorption, but such a hazard would be offset by the use of continuous intraoperative capnography. It has been recommended that the deactivation problem be minimized by use of ultraviolet filters and incorporating additional ethyl violet in Sodasorb.[51]

When one is using CO_2 absorption, the absorbent must be compatible with the anesthetic gases in use. In this regard trichloroethylene may react with soda lime to produce dichloroacetylene, phosgene, and carbon monoxide, which are potentially neurotoxic gases. Trichloroethylene is not used in the United States but was commonly used in the United Kingdom.[10] Sevoflurane, a new potent inhaled anesthetic, is unstable in the presence of soda lime, but the effects are nontoxic.[52] Sevoflurane is, however, widely used in Japan, where nonrebreathing systems are popular.

F. Anesthesia ventilators

1. General considerations. Contemporary anesthesia ventilators, such as the Dräger AV-E and the Ohmeda 7000 and 7800 series, are examples of "bag-in-a-bottle" respirators.[53,54] The basic principle of operation is that the reservoir bag of an anesthesia circle system is replaced by a bellows in a bellows housing, and the adjustable pressure-limiting (APL, or pop-off) valve is replaced by a ventilator pressure-relief valve (PRV). Inspiration occurs when compressed (driving) gas enters the bellows housing. The bellows is compressed, and the PRV is held closed (Fig. 5-11). Gas contained within the bellows and fresh gas entering the patient circuit from the anesthesia machine are forced into the patient's lungs. At end-inspiration the bellows housing ceases to be pressurized, the bellows refills (by gravity in the case of a hanging

bellows as in Fig. 5-11), and the PRV is able to open, venting excess patient circuit gas to the waste gas–scavenging system.

Anesthesia ventilators are also described as double-circuit ventilators, one circuit being the driving gas circuit and the other the patient circuit. The interface between these two circuits is the ventilator bellows itself. Although both the Dräger AV-E and the Ohmeda models are double-circuit design ventilators, their mechanisms of operation differ in certain details.

2. Ohmeda 7000 ventilator. In the Ohmeda 7000 model (Fig. 5-12) the driving gas supply, oxygen at a nominal pressure of 50 PSIG, passes to a pressure regulator whose output is set to 38 PSIG at a 24 L/min flow. From here the pressure-regulated oxygen flow passes to a block containing five solenoid flow-control valves connected in parallel. These flow-control valves are electronically opened during the inspiratory phase to direct oxygen flow through calibrated tuned orifices. By controlling the duration of opening of each of the five solenoid valves, the control module determines the volume of oxygen that passes through into the collection chamber and then enters the bellows housing where it exerts pressure on the bellows and displaces an equal volume of anesthesia gas mixture from the bellows into the patient circuit. This displaced volume is the tidal volume.

The Ohmeda 7000 ventilator uses a standing bellows that empties until the predetermined tidal volume has been delivered. During inspiration the exhaust valve in the collection chamber is closed so that the driving gas does not es-

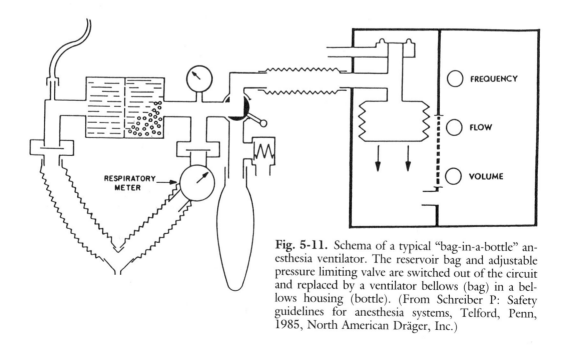

Fig. 5-11. Schema of a typical "bag-in-a-bottle" anesthesia ventilator. The reservoir bag and adjustable pressure limiting valve are switched out of the circuit and replaced by a ventilator bellows (bag) in a bellows housing (bottle). (From Schreiber P: Safety guidelines for anesthesia systems, Telford, Penn, 1985, North American Dräger, Inc.)

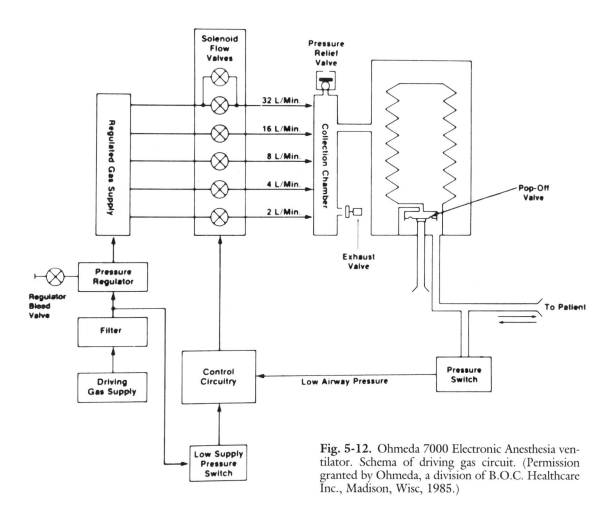

Fig. 5-12. Ohmeda 7000 Electronic Anesthesia ventilator. Schema of driving gas circuit. (Permission granted by Ohmeda, a division of B.O.C. Healthcare Inc., Madison, Wisc, 1985.)

cape. A ventilator pressure relief valve (pop-off valve) located in the base of the bellows is held closed by the driving gas pressure during inspiration so that gas passes from within the bellows to the patient circuit (Fig. 5-12). Exhalation begins when the driving gas exhaust valve, located in the control module, opens permitting driving gas to be vented from the bellows housing, as it is displaced by the bellows refilling with anesthesia gases from the patient's lungs and the fresh gas flow from the anesthesia machine. For the bellows to refill during exhalation, a slight positive pressure must be maintained in the patient circuit. The ventilator pressure relief (pop-off) valve is therefore a positive end-expiratory pressure (PEEP) valve exerting a pressure of about 2.5 cm H$_2$O on the gas contained within the patient circuit. At end expiration, when the bellows has reached its limit of expansion and the circuit pressure has risen to above 2.5 cm H$_2$O, the ventilator pressure–relief (pop-off) valve opens and excess gas from the patient circuit is vented to the waste gas–scavenging system.

3. Ohmeda 7800 Series ventilators. The Ohmeda 7800 Series ventilators are very similar to the model 7000 but differ in certain features.[54] The driving gas, oxygen at 50 PSIG, passes to a primary regulator whose output is controlled to 26 PSIG. From here the oxygen passes to a pneumatic manifold where its flowthrough into the bellows housing is controlled by a flow-control valve. This sophisticated valve varies the opening of a flow orifice according to the current supplied to the valve's coil, thereby controlling oxygen flow and therefore volume to the bellows housing.[10,54] The ventilator controls also differ between the two series.

4. Dräger Anesthesia Ventilator AV-E. This model ventilator is also of double-circuit pneumatically powered design.[10,25] A schema of this ventilator is shown in Fig. 5-13, to which reference should be made for the following description of operation. The ventilator is powered by oxygen at a nominal driving pressure of 50 PSIG *(2)*. When the ventilator on/off switch *(3)* is turned on, oxygen pressure is sup-

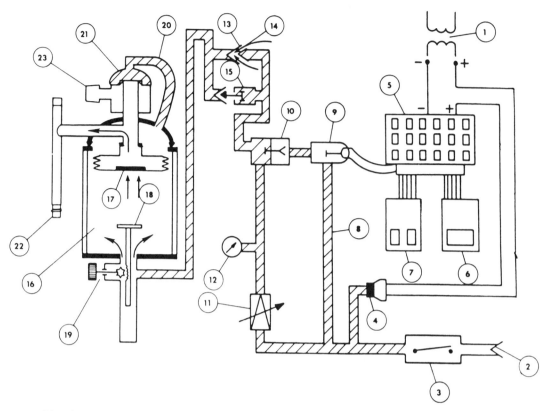

Fig. 5-13. Dräger AV-E ventilator. Schema of ventilator function during *inspiration*. See text for details of operation. (From North American Dräger, Inc., Telford, Penn, 1986.) *1*, Electric power supply (117 volts AC); *2*, gas supply—oxygen (50 PSIG); *3*, ventilator on-off switch; *4*, electrical supply on-off switch (1 PSIG pressure switch); *5*, AV-E—printed circuit board; *6*, inspiration:expiration (I:E) ratio control; *7*, frequency control; *8*, solenoid pilot pressure line; *9*, solenoid valve; *10*, control valve; *11*, flow regulator; *12*, flow indicator gauge; *13*, venturi; *14*, venturi entrainment port; *15*, pilot actuator; *16*, bellows chamber; *17*, bellows; *18*, tidal-volume adjustment plate; *19*, tidal-volume control; *20*, relief-valve pilot line; *21*, ventilator relief valve; *22*, patient breathing system connector; *23*, waste gas scavenging system connector.

plied to a 1 PSIG switch *(4)*, which is activated and energizes the electronic circuit. The respiratory rate *(7)* and I:E ratio *(6)* controls are set as desired. Inspiration (Fig. 5-13) occurs when the solenoid valve *(9)* receives an electrical signal from the control unit *(5)*. This signal remains throughout inspiration and activates the solenoid valve *(9)* to allow oxygen at 50 PSIG to pass through it to activate the control valve *(10)*. Opening of the control valve allows oxygen that has passed through the adjustable flow regulator *(11)* to pass through the control valve *(10)* to the venturi nozzle *(13)*. The inspiratory flow rate is adjusted by the flow regulator *(11)* (inspiratory flow–control knob), and the flow rate is monitored on a flow-indicator gauge *(12)*. This indicator is really a pressure gauge, measuring pressure downstream of the flow regulator. As the oxygen flows from venturi nozzle *(13)*, room air is entrained through the

muffler and entrainment port *(14)*. The mixture of oxygen and entrained air is directed into the bellows chamber *(16)*. As pressure rises in the bellows chamber, the bellows is compressed and anesthetic gases contained within the bellows are forced into the patient circuit through the breathing connector *(22)*. At the same time, driving gas pressure from the bellows housing *(16)* is transmitted through the relief-valve pilot line *(20)* to hold the ventilator pressure–relief valve *(21)* closed as long as the bellows housing is under pressure (that is, throughout inspiration). In this model ventilator the bellows is normally emptied completely with each inspiratory cycle so that the tidal volume is determined by the extent to which the bellows is allowed to expand during exhalation, which is in turn adjusted by the tidal-volume control knob *(19)* and bellows plate *(18)*. During the inspiratory pause the oxygen continues to flow from the

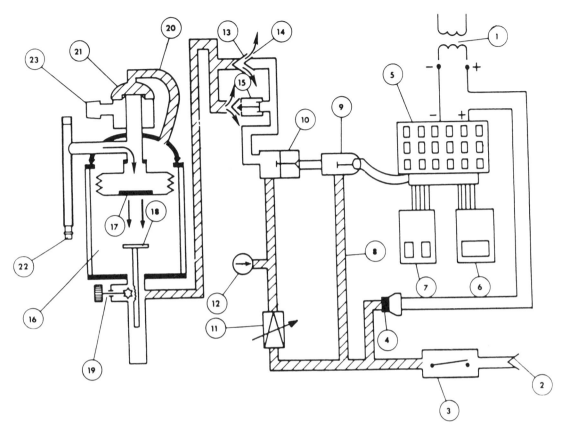

Fig. 5-14. Dräger AV-E ventilator. Schema of ventilator function during *expiration*. For numbers see Fig. 5-13. See text for details. (From North American Dräger, Inc., Telford, Penn.)

venturi nozzle *(13)*, but since the bellows is now fully compressed, no further air is entrained, with pressure being maintained in the bellows housing by the pressure of the oxygen jet from the venturi. Meanwhile the chamber *(16)* contains a mixture of air and oxygen.

Expiration (Fig. 5-14) begins when the electrical signal from the control unit *(5)* to the solenoid valve *(9)* stops. The latter valve is deactivated and closes, interrupting the supply of 50 PSIG oxygen to the control valve *(10)*, which therefore also closes. The preset oxygen flow from the flow regulator *(11)* is interrupted by control valve *(10)* causing a pressure drop at the venturi *(13)* and no back pressure is supplied to pilot actuator *(15)*. The latter opens to allow gas from the bellows chamber *(16)* to be vented through the pilot actuator *(15)* and the entrainment port *(14)* of the venturi *(13)*. As the pressure falls in the bellows chamber *(16)*, the bellows *(17)* begins to refill. As long as any pressure remains in the bellows chamber *(16)*, the ventilator pressure–relief valve *(2)* is also pressurized and held closed.

As with the standing bellows arrangement in the Ohmeda ventilators (7000 and 7800 series) and the standing-bellows version of the AV-E (Figs. 5-15 and 5-16), the ventilator pressure–relief valve applies about 2.5 cm of PEEP to the patient circuit. Once the standing bellows has reached its preset limit of expansion (the set tidal volume) and the patient circuit pressure exceeds 2.5 cm H_2O, the pressure-relief valve opens permitting excess circuit gas to enter the waste gas–scavenging system.

In the Dräger AV-E the ventilator pressure–relief valve is controlled by an external relief valve pilot line (Figs. 5-13 and 5-14, item *(20)*, which is essentially a short piece of plastic tubing. Kinking of this line can cause malfunction of the ventilator.[55] Incompetence of the pressure-relief valve itself may result in patient hypoventilation.[55-57]

5. Design differences

a. Standing versus hanging-bellows ventilators. Recent anesthesia ventilators are of the standing-bellows design; that is, they rise (fill by ascending) during exhalation and descend

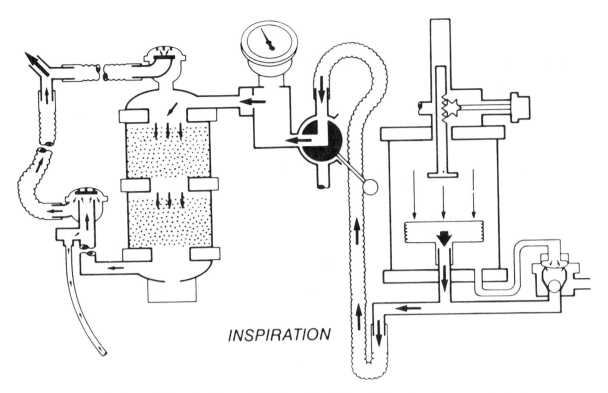

Fig. 5-15. North American Dräger AV-E standing bellows design showing events during inspiration. (From North American Dräger, Inc., Telford, Penn.)

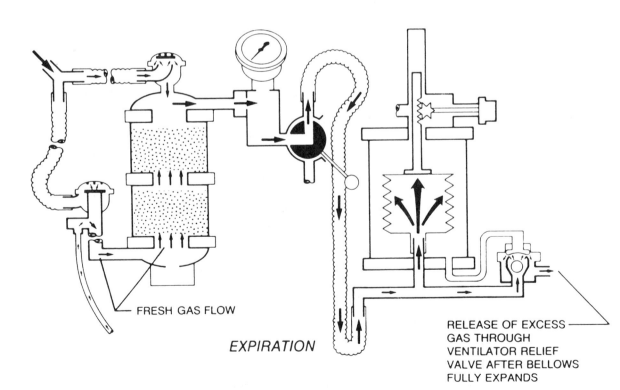

FRESH GAS FLOW

EXPIRATION

RELEASE OF EXCESS
GAS THROUGH
VENTILATOR RELIEF
VALVE AFTER BELLOWS
FULLY EXPANDS

Fig. 5-16. North American Dräger AV-E standing bellows design showing events during expiration. (From North American Dräger, Inc., Telford, Penn.)

(empty) during inspiration. In the event of a disconnection, where circuit pressure would become equal to atmospheric pressure, the bellows would not refill during exhalation.

In the hanging-bellows design (Figs. 5-11 and 5-13) the bellows fills by gravity during exhalation so that the ventilator pressure-relief valve does not require a PEEP design. In the event of a patient circuit disconnection room air would be entrained into the patient circuit through the leak and the bellows would refill, emptying through the leak on the next inspiration. For this reason the standing-bellows design is preferred, though it is not required by the most recent standard describing specifications for anesthesia ventilators.[58]

b. Dräger versus Ohmeda ventilators. The gas entering the bellows housing in an Ohmeda ventilator is 100% oxygen (Fig. 5-12), whereas in the Dräger AV-E it is an air/oxygen mixture (Figs. 5-13 and 5-14). In the event of a leak (hole) in the bellows, driving gas would enter the patient circuit and dilute the gases therein. This could cause oxygen enrichment with an Ohmeda ventilator but could cause a decrease in F_IO_2 with a Dräger AV-E.

In the Dräger AV-E one determines the tidal volume by setting the expansion limit of the bellows during expiration, since the bellows is emptied completely during inspiration. The Dräger AV-E standing bellows (Figs. 5-15 and 5-16) is graduated from 0 ml at the bottom to 2000 ml at the top of the housing. In the Ohmeda design, the bellows is graduated from 0 ml at the top to 1600 ml at the bottom of the bellows housing, since the tidal volume is displaced from the bellows by a metered volume of compressed oxygen from the ventilator control unit (Fig. 5-12).

The Dräger ventilator uses a venturi nozzle and an air/oxygen mixture to compress the bellows. This economizes on the use of compressed oxygen. In the Ohmeda ventilator, oxygen consumption is a little greater than the set minute ventilation.[59]

In the Ohmeda ventilator the circuit pressure–relief valve is flush-mounted inside the bellows itself (Fig. 5-12). The design does not use a relief-valve pilot line and is therefore not vulnerable to the effects of kinking of this line (Fig. 5-13, item *20*).[55] A potential advantage of the exposed ventilator pressure–relief valve, however, is that its function can be observed if there is any concern, whereas the Ohmeda valve is not normally visible.

Ohmeda ventilators incorporate a high pressure–relief valve in the driving gas circuit (Fig. 5-12). This may be preset to 65 cm H_2O (as in the 7000 model) or be adjustable (Ohmeda 7800 Series). In the 7800 series, when the pressure in the patient circuit exceeds the user-set limit, the ventilator is automatically cycled to the exhalation mode. Most of the originally supplied Dräger AV-E ventilators do not have a pressure-limiting valve in the driving gas circuit though a retrofittable Pressure Limit Control valve is available for certain Dräger AV-E ventilators (see the discussion of pressure and volume later).

Because the Dräger AV-E ventilator venturi nozzle requires entrainment of room air (Figs. 5-13 and 5-14), a clean muffler is essential. If the muffler becomes blocked for any reason, air is no longer entrained and inspiration cannot be completed. If blockage of the muffler occurs during exhalation, gas cannot leave the ventilator bellows housing, and the bellows remain compressed.[60]

6. Tidal volume considerations. Anesthesia ventilators are designed to work with an anesthesia circuit and continuous-flow anesthesia machine. During inspiration the ventilator pressure–relief valve is held closed so that gas contained in the bellows enters the patient circuit rather than the scavenging system (Fig. 5-11). Meanwhile fresh gas continues to enter the patient circuit from the anesthesia machine throughout the ventilatory cycle, according to the rotameter settings. This represents potential additional tidal volume for the patient.

When one is setting tidal volume on a ventilator to achieve a certain delivered patient tidal volume, it is important to consider the fresh gas flow rate from the anesthesia machine to the patient circuit.[61,62] Changing the fresh gas flow (FGF) respiratory rate (RR), or inspiration:expiration (I:E) ratio may have a profound effect on patient tidal volume (TV), alveolar ventilation, and Pa_{CO_2}.[62] The latter effect is illustrated in Fig. 5-17.

The additional minute ventilation to the circuit when one is using an anesthesia ventilator is approximated by the formula:

Additional minute ventilation = $(I/[I + E]) \times FGF$

This result is divided by the respiratory rate to determine the potential augmentation of each ventilator bellows tidal volume. In terms of tidal volume actually delivered to the patient this formula provides an approximation only. The actual augmentation of patient tidal volume also depends on the patient's total thoracic compliance compared with that of the anesthesia circuit components. If the patient's total thoracic compliance is low, additional fresh gas inflow from the machine may be accommo-

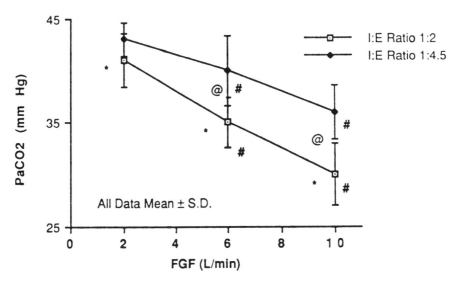

Fig. 5-17. Effect of fresh gas-flow (FGF) and inspiration:expiration (I:E) ratio on Pa_{CO_2} in patients ventilated with anesthesia ventilator set to a constant tidal volume (TV). Increasing FGF or the I:E ratio causes an increase in delivered TV, an increase in alveolar ventilation, and a decrease in Pa_{CO_2}. (From Scheller MS, Jones BL, and Benumof JL: J Cardiothorac Anesth 3:564, 1989.)

dated mainly by compression within the circuit. Thus patient minute volume (MV) is given by the following:

Set MV + (FGF × I/[I+E]) − Gas volume
    compressed in circuit at peak inspiratory pressure

The last term can be calculated as the product of circuit compliance and peak inspiratory pressure. These considerations do not apply to intensive care unit ventilators that are designed to be minute volume dividers.

7. Positive end-expiratory pressure. The deliberate application of positive end-expiratory pressure (PEEP) to the patient's airway is not uncommon during anesthesia. One may apply PEEP by adding a free-standing PEEP valve (such as Boehringer valve, Wynnewood, Pennsylvania) between the expiratory limb of the circle and the expiratory unidirectional valve. Free-standing PEEP valves function well, but there is always the possibility that they may be used erroneously and could totally occlude the circuit if incorrectly placed in the inspiratory limb of the circle.[9,27]

The machine manufacturers Dräger and Ohmeda provide, as an option, PEEP valves built into their recent anesthesia delivery systems. These valves are convenient and also avoid the risk of erroneous valve placement. The position of a PEEP valve in the anesthesia circuit deserves some consideration, however. At end exhalation, that part of the circuit between the PEEP valve and the inspiratory unidirectional valve will be at positive end-expira-

tory pressure as determined by the PEEP-valve setting. The remainder of the circuit is at 0 end-expiratory pressure (or +2.5 cm H_2O if a standing-bellows ventilator is in use) (Fig. 5-16). With the next inspiration, the emptying ventilator bellows must first compress gas in the patient circuit to the level set on the PEEP valve before any gas will flow past the inspiratory unidirectional valve to flow to the patient. If the ventilator bellows tidal volume is fixed, the additional compressible gas volume represents lost tidal volume for the patient. The closer the PEEP valve is to the ventilator bellows, the smaller is the ventilator-bellows tidal volume loss to compression of gas in the circuit up to the set level of the PEEP. Thus once ventilator settings have been made without PEEP the addition of a PEEP valve by the expiratory unidirectional valve will result in decreased minute ventilation for the patient.[63] This volume loss, attributable to compression of gas in the circuit, is greater with the Ohmeda ventilator design than with the Dräger AV-E because of the larger compressible gas volume remaining in an Ohmeda bellows at end inspiration (total bellows volume of 1600 ml minus tidal volume), compared with almost no compressible volume in the AV-E bellows, which empties completely with each inspiration.[64]

Advantages of placing the PEEP valve near the expiratory unidirectional valve, however, are that in these positions PEEP may be applied during spontaneous as a well as mechanical ventilation (Fig. 5-16).

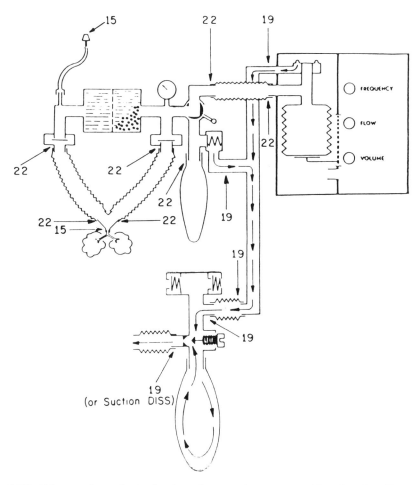

Fig. 5-18. Schema of anesthesia circuit and scavenging system tubing showing diameters in millimeters for hose connections. See text. (From Schreiber P: Safety guidelines for anesthesia systems, Telford, Penn, 1985, North American Dräger, Inc.)

G. Waste gas scavenging systems

Waste gases may leave the anesthesia circuit through the adjustable pressure-limiting (APL) valve or through the ventilator pressure–relief valve. In either case, 19 mm internal-diameter tubing is used, as distinct from the 22 mm internal-diameter anesthesia circuit and ventilator tubing and the 15 mm internal-diameter common gas outlet and endotracheal tube connector sizes (Fig. 5-18). The scavenging system acts to *interface* the gas flow out of the patient circuit with the hospital suction system.[11]

Scavenging systems may be open or closed. *Closed systems* use spring-loaded valves to ensure that excessively high or low pressures are not applied to the patient circuit (Fig. 5-19).[11,65] Thus, if the system is not connected to negative pressure (suction), excess pressure in the interface caused by gas entering it from the circuit would first cause distension of the interface reservoir bag, and then the excess would be vented via the positive pressure ("pop-off")–relief valve at about +5 cm H_2O. In the event that excessive suction might be applied to the circuit, the reservoir bag would first be sucked empty and then one (Ohmeda interface) or two (Dräger closed interface, Fig. 5-19) negative pressure–relief ("pop-in") valves (-0.25 to -1.80 cm H_2O), depending on the system would open to preferentially draw in room air and minimize the potential application of negative pressure to the patient circuit.[65]

Open-reservoir scavenging interfaces are valveless (Fig. 5-20) and use continually open relief ports to provide pressure relief.[66] Waste gas from the circuit is directed to the bottom of the canister, and hospital suction aspirates gas from the bottom of the canister. In this type of interface, the reservoir canister contains the excess waste gas and thereby accommodates a range of waste-gas flow rates from the patient circuit. Since this type of interface depends on relief

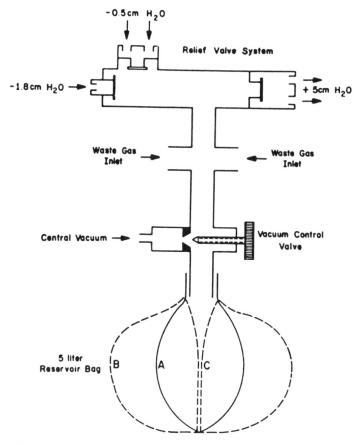

Fig. 5-19. Dräger closed scavenger interface. (From Schreiber P: Safety guidelines for anesthesia systems, Telford, Penn, 1985, North American Dräger, Inc.)

ports for pressure relief, care must be taken to ensure that these ports remain unoccluded at all times. Although the open reservoir system has the advantage of being valveless (and valves can become stuck or malfunction), there is no visual indication that the system is functioning, whereas with the closed interface the reservoir bag movement provides a constant indication of system function.

If the 19 mm diameter tubing (Fig. 5-18) connecting the APL valve or the ventilator pressure–relief valve with the interface becomes occluded, pressure will build up in the patient breathing system.

If the valves in a closed interface or the ports in an open interface were to become occluded, excesses of positive or negative pressure could develop in the circuit. Examples are discussed in a subsequent section.

H. Basic monitors and alarms

1. Oxygen analyzer and alarm. Anesthesia machines must be equipped with an oxygen analyzer that measures the O_2 concentration either within the inspiratory limb of the anesthesia breathing system or within the fresh gas mixture.[6] The analyzer must be enabled and functioning whenever the anesthesia machine is capable of delivering an anesthetic mixture. It must also annunciate a high-priority alarm when the measured O_2 concentration falls below the user-preset threshold.[6] Delivery system oxygen analyzers are usually located in the proximity of the inspiratory unidirectional valve. These analyzers (fuel cells) are specific for oxygen and are not fooled by other agents. Disasters associated with oxygen-delivery failure or delivery of a hypoxic mixture would likely have been avoided if a functioning oxygen analyzer with alarm had been in use.[15,18]

Schreiber[27] has stated that "the use of an oxygen analyzer with an anesthesia system is the single most important measure to prevent hypoxia." Furthermore, monitoring of oxygen in the patient breathing system during general anesthesia using an anesthesia machine is required by the ASA Standards for Basic Intraoperative Monitoring.[8]

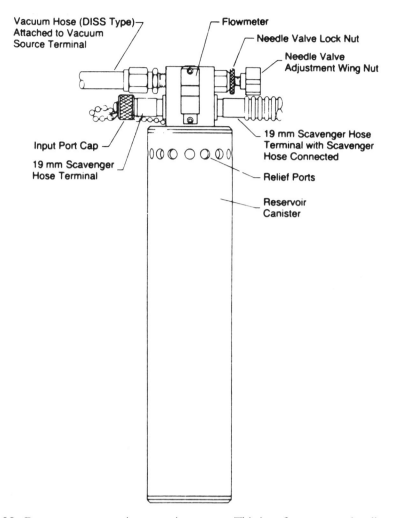

Fig. 5-20. Drager open reservoir scavenging system. This interface uses continually open relief ports to provide positive and negative pressure relief (compare with valves in Fig. 5-19). An adjustable needle valve regulates the waste-gas exhaust flow, which is indicated on an uncalibrated flowmeter. A flowmeter reading halfway between the two white lines corresponds to a suction flow rate of about 25 L/min. (From Open reservoir scavenger operator's instruction manual, Telford, Penn, Dec 1986, North American Dräger, Inc.)

An oxygen monitor and alarm system in the expiratory limb of a circle system with the alarm settings close to the expected expiratory O_2 concentration has been suggested as an effective backup system for detecting a disconnection.[67]

2. Monitoring of circuit pressures and volumes. The ASTM F1161-88 standard requires that the machine shall have breathing pressure monitoring as well as either exhaled volume or ventilatory CO_2 monitoring.[6] The machine must have a means to continually monitor pressure in the breathing system, and the pressure monitor must be designed to annunciate a visual and audible high-priority alarm when pressure in the system (1) exceeds a user-adjustable

limit for high pressure, (2) exceeds a user-adjustable limit for continuing positive airway pressure for more than 15 ±1 seconds. The latter alarm threshold should be adjustable between 10 and 30 cm H_2O. The pressure monitor and alarm must be enabled and functioning automatically whenever the anesthesia machine is in use.[6]

The ASA Standards for Basic Intraoperative Monitoring[8] requires that when ventilation is controlled by a mechanical ventilator there should be in continuous use a device that is capable of detecting disconnection of components of the breathing system. The device must emit an audible signal when its alarm threshold is exceeded. This is the circuit low-pressure alarm

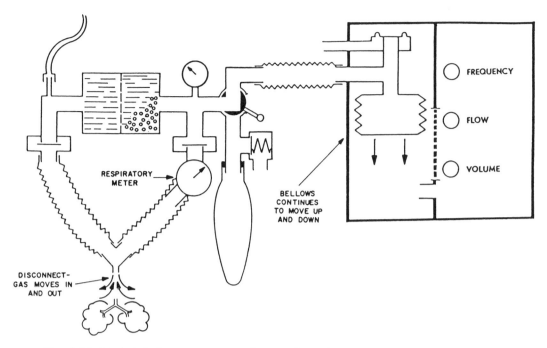

Fig. 5-21. Typical circle system connected to ventilator showing positions of pressure gauge (close to absorber) and spirometer (expiratory limb of circle). Notice that with use of the hanging bellows ventilator shown, a disconnect between the patient and the Y-piece allows room air to be entrained during exhalation. This air is "pulled" through the respiratory meter causing it to be "fooled." (From Schreiber P: Safety guidelines for anesthesia systems, Telford, Penn, 1985, North American Dräger, Inc.)

sometimes loosely termed the "disconnect alarm." If the pressure in the circuit does not exceed the user-set minimum within a set period (usually 15 seconds, but this may be set at 60 seconds to allow a slow respiratory rate to be deliberately set on the ventilator), the alarm is annunciated. Modern circuit pressure monitors also annunciate an alarm when the pressure in the breathing system falls below -10 cm H_2O at any time (subatmospheric pressure alarm).

Modern delivery systems incorporate a mechanical pressure gauge that is usually mounted on the absorber, and the circuit pressure may be measured at that point (Fig. 5-21). In addition, pressure may be sensed at almost any point in the circuit and be transmitted through pilot tubing to a remote electronic pressure monitor that incorporates audible and visual alarms. Ideally, pressure should be sensed at the patient connector, but water and sterilization problems make this site impractical.[27] Sensing pressure by the absorber may fail to detect abnormalities between the patient and the inspiratory and expiratory unidirectional valves. Thus, if a freestanding PEEP valve were inserted between the expiratory limb of the circuit and the exhalation unidirectional valve, the PEEP would not be detectable by a pressure monitor sensing pressure by the absorber (Fig. 5-21).

Although the circle system is the one most commonly used, other circuits such as the Bain or Mapleson F may be employed, and pressure-monitoring adapters are available for use in these situations.

The pressure monitoring and alarm connections in both the Dräger and Ohmeda absorber systems are self-sealing. If the pressure-monitoring sensor is disconnected from the absorber and the circle is then used, the low-pressure alarm will be activated (senses atmospheric pressure) yet the circuit pressure gauge will display normal pressures!

Monitoring of pressure at the absorber may also fail to detect a patient circuit disconnection during positive-pressure ventilation. Because the ventilator delivers its tidal volume in the proximity of the pressure alarm sensing point (Fig. 5-21), the low-pressure alarm limit may be satisfied if not set to be sensitive enough (that is, just below the usual peak inspiratory pressure). It therefore is important to recognize where in the circuit the pressure gauge senses pressure and where the pressure monitoring and alarm system is sensing pressure, if different. The ASTM F1161-88 standard also requires monitoring of exhaled volume or ventilatory CO_2.[6] An alarm is activated if the patient's exhaled volume falls below an operator-adjustable minimum. The monitor must be designed to be in an enabled condition and functioning automatically whenever the anesthesia machine is in use. When the volume monitor alarm is disabled, a low-priority alarm is to be annunciated.

Modern circle systems also incorporate a spirometer, which measures tidal and minute volumes, demonstrates reversal of gas flow if it should occur (because of incompetence of the exhalation unidirectional valve), and, if electronic, incorporates low and high alarm limits. Mechanical spirometers do not incorporate an alarm. In Dräger systems the spirometer is located on the absorber side (downstream) of the expiratory unidirectional valve. In Ohmeda systems it is usually placed just upstream of the expiratory valve so that in both systems it is the gas volume flowing through the expiratory limb of the circuit (exhaled volume) that is measured (Fig. 5-21).

Monitoring exhaled volumes is valuable when a low-volume alarm limit can be set to be sensitive, that is, just less than the set ventilation parameters (including tidal volume, rate, fresh gas flow, I:E ratio). A disconnection in the patient circuit should result in a decrease in displayed tidal volume and minute volume. Unlike the pressure gauge, which is sensing pressure at the absorber, the spirometer will usually give an indication of flow problems in the patient circuit.

In the event of a circuit disconnection, a spirometer in the expiratory limb may, however, be "fooled" if a hanging-bellows design of ventilator is being used. Thus during exhalation a weight in the hanging bellows causes it to descend, drawing room air in through the disconnection site, through the spirometer and into the descending bellows. Fig. 5-21 shows that fresh gas will also pass to the descending (hanging) bellows via the absorber, so that with such a scenario, the decrease in the tidal volume reading compared with the tidal volume before the disconnection occurred is that attributable to gas compressed in the patient circuit during exhalation. Unless the low-volume alarm limits have been set to be very sensitive, a disconnection of the patient circuit with a hanging-bellows ventilator will likely go undetected by a spirometer in the expiratory limb of the circle. A disconnection of the tubing between the ventilator and the breathing circuit would, however, be detectable by both the spirometer and the pressure monitor.

It has been mentioned previously that the standing-bellows design of ventilator is preferred because a disconnection is more obvious as the bellows fails to fill on exhalation and that an expiratory spirometer is less likely to be fooled. It is also possible for an expired spirometer to be fooled by a standing-bellows ventilator when there is a patient circuit disconnection. The mechanism is as follows. When the disconnection occurs, the standing bellows empties, falling to its bottom resting position as if the largest possible tidal volume had been delivered (Fig. 5-15). At end exhalation, the pressure in the driving gas circuit is zero, but the empty bellows contains a residual volume of patient circuit gas. On the next inspiration, driving gas pressure in the bellows housing rises and the bellows is actively compressed, discharging some of the contained residual gas volume. With the next exhalation cycle, the rubber bellows resumes its original unpressurized configuration and may aspirate gas from the patient circuit. Gas drawn into the bellows through the spirometer will cause the spirometer to record a volume of as much as 140 ml, depending on the size of the bellows and the fresh gas flow from the anesthesia machine.[68] An inappropriately set low-volume alarm thus might record an "adequate" tidal volume and be "fooled" in this circumstance.

Although monitoring of pressure and exhaled volume are now required in modern delivery systems, it is apparent from the above discussion that not all ventilation or pressure problems will be detectable when one is using these monitors as presently configured. Detection is improved by "bracketing" the user-adjustable alarm-limit thresholds close to the patient's normal high and low pressures and volumes. Some older monitors had fixed alarm limits and even some modern ones have default settings, which may not provide adequate warning of problems in the circuit. Problems associated with alarm limits being set too insensitive are discussed further in a subsequent section. A disposable pneumotachometer head placed by the patient's airway might represent an improvement over the current monitors, since it could (with corrections for gas composition and humidity) provide instantaneous measurements of flow, volume, and pressure at this important site. Such a system is currently being investigated for general clinical use.

II. COMPLICATIONS
A. Hypoxemia

Hypoxemia, defined as a Pao_2 of less than 60 mm Hg, may be caused by problems in the patient or problems with the anesthesia delivery system. In the setting of adequate ventilation and normal or expected alveolar oxygen, the patient pathosis will be the cause for hypoxemia. The pulmonary pathosis may be such that it causes shunting, venous admixture, or, significantly less likely, diffusion defects. Pneumonia, atelectasis, pulmonary edema, pneumothorax, hemothorax, pyothorax, pulmonary embolism, alveolar proteinosis, and bronchospasm are some of the pathologic conditions that may cause hypoxemia and are reviewed elsewhere in this volume.

The anesthesia-delivery system may cause hypoxemia by failing to deliver sufficient oxygen to the lungs and thereby cause low alveolar oxygen levels. Apnea and severe hypoventilation are well described causes of alveolar hypoxia. These problems can occur because of failure to initiate ventilation manually or mechanically or when a disconnect exists in the breathing system even though ventilation is attempted. The area that is particularly problematic with regard to insufficient alveolar oxygen is the delivery of a hypoxic mixture to the lungs.

The anesthesia machine may be the source of delivery of a hypoxic mixture to the breathing system and ultimately to the patient. The only way to know qualitatively and quantitatively the oxygen composition of the gas mixture in the breathing system is to measure the oxygen concentration with an analyzer in the breathing system. If a gas other than oxygen is flowing through the oxygen flowmeter, it may appear that 100% oxygen is being delivered to the breathing circuit when in fact the circuit is receiving no oxygen at all.[37]

Oxygen analyzers have certain limitations, however. First, the oxygen analyzer must be properly calibrated, the alarm limits set, and the alarm working. Second, it must actually be sampling the gases that the patient is breathing. An oxygen analyzer placed at the inspiratory unidirectional valve may show an adequate oxygen concentration, but the patient may not be receiving that gas if there is a circuit disconnection between the inspiratory valve and the patient. In those circumstances the patient may not receive adequate oxygen, but the analyzer may not indicate that to the anesthesiologist. In addition, vigilant observation of the integrity of the breathing circuit and machine is required for safe patient care.

The oxygen pipeline may have a gas other than oxygen flowing through it. The bulk liquid oxygen tank may be filled with liquid nitrogen.[15] The pipelines may be crossed so that nitrous oxide or some other gas may be flowing through the oxygen pipeline. Inside the operating room the hose from the wall nitrous oxide outlet may have an oxygen connector at the patient end. Connecting this to the anesthesia machine oxygen inlet would permit nitrous oxide to flow to the oxygen flowmeter.[11,17,69-71] If

such a situation is suspected, the oxygen pipeline connection to the machine should be disconnected and the oxygen tank turned on. Failure to disconnect the pipeline gas (at 50 to 55 PSIG) will prevent the flow of tank oxygen, which is regulated to enter the machine at 45 PSIG (see section I, B, 1).

The oxygen cylinder yokes can be a source of a gas other than oxygen; this gas would then flow through the oxygen flowmeter and eventually to the breathing system. An oxygen cylinder may be filled with a gas other than oxygen, and this cylinder may be attached to the oxygen yoke.[72] A nitrous oxide cylinder could be attached to an oxygen yoke if the pin-index system were defeated by removal of a pin or by placement of more than one washer between the yoke and the oxygen cylinder. Crossed pipes within the anesthesia machine could cause the gas delivered to the oxygen flowmeter to be some other gas.[73,74]

It is also possible for the oxygen flowmeter not to deliver any gas to the patient.[75] The liquid oxygen tank and backup central supply cylinders may be empty. The central system may be shut down for repairs or other purposes.[76] The pipeline system may not be connected from the wall to the anesthesia machine. The backup cylinders on the machine may be empty, absent, or turned off.[69] The oxygen flow–control valve or oxygen-piping system in the machine may be obstructed and thereby prevent the flow of oxygen to the flowmeter.[33,34] The flowmeter bobbin or rotameter may become stuck because of static electricity, grit, or dirt, and it may appear that gas is flowing from the oxygen flowmeter even when it is not.[27] Also a leak may exist in the flowmeter tubes, which results in loss of the oxygen before it reaches the common gas outlet of the machine.[77-80] On older anesthesia machines the nitrous oxide flowmeter may be turned on without the oxygen flowmeter being turned on. This type of problem should be prevented on anesthesia machines that have oxygen-ratio monitors and oxygen-flow controllers designed to prevent the delivery of a hypoxic mixture (see the next topic below). However, one should not rely upon these devices to prevent delivery of hypoxic mixtures.

The Ohmeda Link-25 system can be defeated if the needle valve is broken in the closed position, or if the linkage between the flowmeter controls fails.[33,36,81] This can result in a hypoxic mixture in the breathing circuit. In addition, a fundamental limitation of all oxygen-ratio monitor and controller systems is that they do not qualitatively analyze the gas that is flowing through the oxygen flowmeter. For this reason it is critical that the breathing circuit gas be continuously monitored with an oxygen analyzer.[27]

The anesthesia breathing system may contain a hypoxic mixture for many possible reasons. Valves in the circuit may be absent or incompetent. This would allow rebreathing of exhaled gas, which could become hypoxic if insufficient mixing with fresh gas occurred. This is a particular problem if both the inspiratory and expiratory valves were missing in a circle breathing system. In the Mapleson circuits interruption or loss of the fresh gas from the anesthesia machine could lead to severe rebreathing of a hypoxic mixture as the patient consumes the oxygen in the system and replaces it with CO_2. Failure of the fresh gas supply from the anesthesia machine to the breathing circle will also result in a circle system that becomes progressively hypoxic as the patient uses up the oxygen. Disconnections between the anesthesia machine or vaporizer and the breathing circuit will also cause the system to become hypoxic.[41,82-84]

Leaks in the breathing circuit will cause fresh gases to be lost (see below). If a hanging-bellows ventilator is being used, the fresh gases may be replaced with room air that is entrained into the breathing system as the bellows falls during the exhalation phase of the ventilatory cycle. This would cause room air to be substituted for the desired breathing mixture.[40] A standing bellows would merely collapse if a significant leak developed in the breathing system. Most importantly, leaks in the breathing system can also result in either severe hypoventilation or apnea. These leaks may occur in valve housings or inspiratory or expiratory hoses, at connection sites, ventilator hoses, or system, pressure-relief valves, or from subatmospheric pressure applied to the breathing system from a scavenger suction, or a nasogastric tube that is in the trachea and applied to suction.[11,27]

A leak in the ventilator bellows will result in driving gas or gases entering the breathing system. If air is the driving gas, the oxygen concentration in the breathing system will be reduced.[85]

During closed-system anesthesia the flow of fresh gases from the anesthesia machine is adjusted so that the total flow into the breathing system equals the total uptake and other gas loss from the circuit. The circuit may become hypoxic or hyperoxic if it is not carefully monitored for oxygen concentration throughout the anesthetic. This occurs because uptakes of oxygen and nitrous oxide change during the anesthetic. Initially nitrous oxide uptake is high, but

as the anesthetic progresses, nitrous oxide uptake declines. If a compensatory reduction in nitrous oxide flow is not undertaken, the system oxygen concentration will fall and the patient will become hypoxemic.

B. Hyperoxia

An oxygen concentration that is higher than anticipated is a problem that the anesthesiologist rarely confronts. It is always attributable to administration of a gas mixture that contains more oxygen than desired. In all circumstances an accurate and properly positioned oxygen analyzer will detect this problem. Insufficient nitrous oxide or air administered from the nitrous oxide and other gas flowmeters will cause the inspired oxygen to increase. Leaks from either of these flowmeters, inaccurate flowmeters, and flowmeters with stuck rotameters may cause these gases to be lost or not administered with a resultant rise in inspired oxygen. A leak in a hanging-bellows ventilator that causes entrainment or injection of driving gas from the bellows housing may cause the inspired oxygen to rise if the oxygen content of the entrained gas is higher than that delivered from the common gas outlet.[85,86]

C. Hypercarbia (hypercapnia)

Hypercarbia, defined as elevation of the arterial CO_2 tension ($Paco_2$) to levels greater than 45 mm Hg, occurs when CO_2 production exceeds elimination. During anesthesia and surgery, patient factors and anesthesia-delivery system conditions may combine or act individually to produce hypercarbia.

Patients who are breathing spontaneously and receiving inhaled anesthetics or intravenous agents may hypoventilate or become apneic because of the central respiratory depressant action of these agents. Airway obstruction caused by a central action of anesthetics, or by neuromuscular blocking drugs prevents adequate gas exchange and results in hypercarbia and hypoxia. Central nervous system, high spinal cord, or phrenic nerve pathosis may cause hypoventilation or apnea and result in hypercarbia. Muscle relaxants, by blocking the neuromuscular junction, and high spinal, epidural anesthesia, by interfering with the transmission of neural output at the spinal cord level, cause apnea and result in hypercarbia.

Pulmonary pathosis in patients who are breathing spontaneously and in those mechanically ventilated can cause hypercarbia. Patients with significant venous admixture will retain carbon dioxide if the minute ventilation is normal. However, hypercarbia is not a problem during one-lung anesthesia if the entire calculated minute ventilation is delivered to the ventilated lung and the pulmonary shunt is small.

Increased metabolic rate caused by fever, thyrotoxicosis, malignant hyperthermia, or hyperalimentation, will result in increased CO_2 production. If this condition is not compensated for by an increase in alveolar ventilation equal to the increase in metabolic rate above the calculated normal, the result will be CO_2 retention and hypercarbia.

The anesthesia delivery system, through misuse, malfunction, or a combination of both, can cause hypercarbia. Apnea from failure to turn on a ventilator, or failure to manually ventilate the patient, will cause hypercarbia. Turning on the ventilator but failing to provide an adequate tidal volume and ventilatory rate to a patient with normal CO_2 production will result in increased Pa_{CO_2}. Leaks in the anesthesia machine, breathing circuit, or ventilator or failure to initially fill the ventilator bellows because of insufficient fresh gas flow from the anesthesia machine may lead to inadequate ventilation and hypercarbia.[27]

Insufficient fresh gas supply to the breathing circuit can be caused by failure of the piped gas system centrally, valves that are closed to a particular operating room, leaks in the pipes, failure to connect the anesthesia machine to the piped gas supply system, or leaks in the hoses.[11,40,75] However, these problems are external to the anesthesia machine and can easily be overcome by utilization of the reserve gas cylinders on the anesthesia machine.

Within the machine leaks may develop at the oxygen cylinder–yoke interface and through a cylinder mount if the check valve is absent and there is no other cylinder present. An absent check valve on the pipeline system can create a large oxygen leak.[5] It is also possible for gas to leak from the pipes, flowmeters, vaporizers, vaporizer selector switches, and vaporizer mounts on the anesthesia machine.[11,27,87-92]

The interface between the anesthesia machine and the breathing circuit may be a source for leakage.[40,41,82-84] Disconnection of the gas hose from the common gas outlet or the anesthesia circuit will cause a leak. A leak in that hose or from the other hoses in the breathing circuit may cause sufficient gas volume loss as to result in hypoventilation and hypercarbia. Disconnections and leaks of anesthesia circuit hoses, valve housings, endotracheal tubes, ventilator hose, reservoir bag, ventilator bellows, and system-relief valves either in the ventilator or in the manual breathing system can reduce the breathing system volume and cause hypercarbia.[11,27,56,57,93-105] In addition, subatmospheric pressure in the breathing system, which may be caused by malfunction of the scavenger interface, sampling of gas for analysis of the breathing system contents, or suction on a nasogastric tube that was placed in the trachea, will cause gas to be lost from the breathing system and will result in a reduction in minute ventilation (see discussion of pressure and volume excesses, p. 110). Gas flow from the machine to the circuit may also be prevented by obstruction of the piping system in the machine or in the hose to the circuit.[106-109]

The anesthesia ventilator can be the source of hypoventilation if it is set in such a way that it fails to deliver an adequate alveolar minute ventilation. This can develop when the preset tidal volume is so small that only dead-space ventilation takes place. It may also occur with ventilators where the tidal volume, respiratory rate, inspiration-to-expiration ratio, and flow of compressing gases into the bellows chamber can be independently set. With such ventilators (such as Dräger AV-E) it is possible to set an adequate tidal volume and respiratory rate, but if the inspiratory time or driving gas flow is not sufficient, the preset tidal volume may not be completely delivered, resulting in significant hypoventilation. This problem can be prevented if one observes the ventilator bellows and ensures that they are adequately compressed and delivering the preset tidal volume before exhalation begins.

In patients with poor pulmonary compliance, despite the fact that adequate tidal volume and frequency are set on the ventilator, the lungs may not be adequately ventilated. The bellows may fail to deliver the desired volume because the lungs are too stiff. In addition, a significant volume may be lost to expansion of the compliant tubing of the breathing circuit when the lung compliance is poor (see the considerations of tidal volume, p. 99). When ventilators that are pressure cycled or have a high pressure limit are used for patients with poor compliance, it is very likely that the ventilator will cycle before delivering an adequate tidal volume. Each of these circumstances may result in hypercarbia because of hypoventilation.

The fresh gas flows from the anesthesia machine to the breathing circuit contribute to the tidal volume and minute ventilation. If the patient is normocarbic and these flows are significantly decreased, the result will be a decreased tidal volume, increased dead space–to–tidal volume ratio, and increased Pa_{CO_2}.[61,62,110]

The CO_2 absorber is frequently a source of problems with regard to hypoventilation or hypercarbia. Leaks from the absorber occur frequently when it is incorrectly closed. Absorbent granules may prevent the rubber gaskets from seating properly, or incorrectly applied gaskets may result in a leak. Simply failing to return the absorber handle to the closed and locked position will cause a huge gas leak.[111] Within the absorber, exhausted absorbent granules or channeling of gas flow through spent absorbent will allow the recycling of exhaled gas and rebreathing of previously exhaled CO_2. In addition, some anesthesia circuits have a switch that allows the anesthetic gases to bypass the absorber and thereby permit rebreathing of CO_2. Leaving the switch in the bypass position sets the stage for development of hypercarbia.

The anesthesiologist relies upon the color of the CO_2 absorbent indicator to determine if the absorbent has been exhausted. However, photodeactivation of the ethyl violet by fluorescent lights can give the false impression that the absorbent is fresh when in fact it has been exhausted. This can result in hypercarbia.[51] Some anesthesia machines are equipped to deliver CO_2. Inadvertently delivering CO_2 to the breathing circuit can cause hypercarbia to develop.[112,113]

Problems within the breathing circuit may lead to rebreathing of exhaled gas before CO_2 has been removed. The result of these problems is an increase in apparatus dead space and dead-space ventilation. Inspiratory or expiratory unidirectional values that are absent, broken, or malfunctioning in the open position will cause rebreathing of exhaled CO_2. At normal total minute ventilation the patient will become hypercarbic. Any large connecting tube, filter, adapter, and "artificial noses" placed between the Y-piece of the breathing circuit and the patient will also increase dead-space ventilation.

The arrangement of the components of the circle system must be set in such a way that breathing of exhaled CO_2 is prevented.[45] This is described on p. 93.

Although the circle system is designed to permit rebreathing of exhaled gas after absorption of CO_2, valveless (Mapleson) breathing systems do not have CO_2 absorbers (see p. 92).[10] If these systems are used incorrectly, hypercarbia will result. The Mapleson A system (Magill attachment) is designed to be used in spontaneously breathing patients only. To prevent rebreathing it is critical that the fresh gas flow rate be greater than 0.7 times the minute ventilation and that the hose between the patient and the reservoir bag be long enough to prevent CO_2-laden exhaled gas from reaching the reservoir bag.[43,44]

The Mapleson B and C systems are designed in such a way that rebreathing of exhaled CO_2 will always occur unless the fresh gas flow rate is equal to or greater than the peak inspiratory flow rate. In both systems CO_2 accumulates in a blind pouch (see Fig. 5-8). Even if one uses reasonable fresh gas flow rates, such as 1.5 to 2.5 times the minute ventilation, the patient must still be hyperventilated in order to prevent hypercarbia. Therefore, when these systems are employed, the patient must be hyperventilated and fresh gas flow must exceed minute ventilation. If the patient breathes spontaneously, the work of breathing will be increased because of the increased minute ventilation caused by rebreathing of exhaled CO_2. Controlled ventilation does not impose any additional metabolic demands, since no ventilatory work is performed.[43,44]

The Mapleson D, E, and F systems are essentially T-piece systems and function in a similar way. Hypercarbia can be prevented by administration of fresh gas at 2.5 to 3 times the minute ventilation and provision of normal minute ventilation. Alternatively, smaller fresh gas flows can be used, but to prevent CO_2 accumulation the patient must be hyperventilated. With all the Mapleson systems rebreathing and hypercarbia will occur if the fresh gas supply connection is disrupted. This disruption can be a particularly difficult problem with the Bain circuit because it may not be easy to detect a disconnected or kinked inner hose.[87,114,115]

Although uncommon, some machines may be equipped with a circle breathing system that does not have a CO_2 absorber. To prevent hypercarbia with this system the fresh gas flows must be raised to 2 to 3 times the minute ventilation. Alternatively the fresh flows can be set to 1.5 times the normal minute ventilation, and the patient can be hyperventilated to compensate for the partial rebreathing that will occur.

D. Hypocarbia (hypocapnia)

Unlike hypercarbia, hypocarbia results from hyperventilation to the point that CO_2 removal exceeds CO_2 production. Physiologic circumstances that reduce metabolic rate include sleep, general anesthesia, and hypothermia under general anesthesia. Therefore the predicted minute ventilation for an awake patient may result in hypocarbia for an unconscious or anesthetized patient.

Certain anesthesia machine-related situations can lead to unintended hyperventilation and resultant hypocarbia. The ventilator may be set to deliver significantly more than the required minute ventilation. One may increase this by setting the ventilatory rate or tidal volume too high. Alternatively the ventilator may be set correctly but the contribution to ventilation of the fresh gas flow from the anesthesia machine may not have been considered.[62,110] Failure to recognize this may be very significant in the patient with very compliant lungs. Leaks into the breathing circuit from a ventilator bellows that has a hole in it will cause an augmentation of tidal volume delivered and act to hyperventilate the patient.[129b] The gas that will be added to the breathing circuit will be the driving gas from the ventilator, which may be air, oxygen, a mixture of air and oxygen, or some other gas. Therefore the exact gas mixture that the patient breathes and the minute ventilation may be altered by leaks in the bellows.[85,86,116]

E. Circuit pressure and volume excesses

Essential to delivery of anesthesia to and oxygenation and ventilation of the patient is adequate movement of gases between the delivery system and the patient's lungs. Schreiber has described four basic causes of failure of this function,[27] as follows:

1. Occlusion in the inspiratory or expiratory pathway
2. Insufficient amount of gas in the breathing system
3. Failure to initiate artificial ventilation when required
4. Disconnection in the breathing system during mechanical ventilation

1. Occlusions. The anesthesia system comprises numerous tubes that may become occluded (Fig. 5-18).[117] In general such problems may be categorized generally as outside the tube, within the wall, or within the lumen of the tube. Tubing misconnections are now less common since standard diameters have been introduced. Nevertheless even with adapters, misconnections are still possible. In general, circuit tubing connections are 22 mm in diameter, scavenging tubing (but not the scavenging reservoir bag mount!) is 19 mm, and the common gas outlet and endotracheal tube connectors are 15 mm in diameter.[27] Accessories added to the circuit may cause an obstruction. Filters placed in the circuit,[118] incorrectly connected humidifiers,[119] and manufacturing defects in tubing have all been reported as causes of total occlusion of the breathing circuit.[11,120] A freestanding PEEP valve may cause obstruction if it is incorrectly placed in the inspiratory limb of a circle system.[9,27] The PEEP valves that use a weighted ball (such as those by Boehringer Company, Wynnewood, Pennsylvania) are designed to be mounted vertically on the expiratory side of a circle system. In one case, the weighted-ball PEEP valve was erroneously placed horizontally in the expiratory limb between the circuit and the exhalation unidirectional valve. At first the circuit was unobstructed (but there was no PEEP!). When the O_2 flush was operated, the metal ball was driven downstream, totally obstructing the PEEP valve and circuit and rendering ventilation of the patient impossible. Because of such potential user errors, freestanding PEEP valves are considered by many to be undesirable.[121]

Although total occlusion of the breathing circuit should activate a pressure or volume alarm in most cases, depending on the system used, these alarms may be fooled when the endotracheal tube is totally occluded.[9] Consider a breathing circuit with a pressure-monitoring system (such as the Dräger Pressure Monitor DPMS) incorporating three possible threshold settings for the low-pressure alarm (8, 12, 25 cm H_2O) and a fixed setting of +65 cm H_2O for the high-pressure alarm limit threshold used with a Dräger Narkomed 2A anesthesia machine and Dräger AV-E ventilator. When the tracheal tube becomes totally obstructed (kinked), during inspiration pressure rises in the circuit, satisfying the low-pressure alarm but unless it reaches +65 cm H_2O the high-pressure alarm is not activated. The peak pressure achieved in the circuit during inspiration depends on the inspiratory flow control setting (which determines the driving pressure available to compress the bellows) and the fresh gas inflow rate from the anesthesia machine (see p. 95). At low ventilator inspiratory flow settings the driving pressure of the AV-E ventilator may be 50 cm H_2O or less, which, combined with normal rates of fresh gas inflow from the machine, may result in failure of peak inspiratory pressure to reach the high-pressure alarm threshold of +65 cm H_2O. During exhalation, excess gas is released normally from the patient circuit. The volume alarm may also be fooled in this situation, depending on its low-limit threshold setting. In the system described the low-volume alarm threshold was fixed at 80 ml. This situation involved total failure to ventilate the patient and would be immediately detectable by continuous capnometry, or pressure and volume alarms whose thresholds can be set close to the normal values for that particular patient, or continuous monitoring of breath sounds.

Misconnections and obstructions may usually be prevented or detected by testing of the breathing circuit before use with all accessories in place and in spontaneous, assisted, and controlled ventilation modes. Occasionally an obstruction can develop because of failure of a component during the case.[122]

2. *Inadequate amount of gas in the breathing system.* An insufficient volume of gas in the breathing system may be attributable to inadequate delivery or excessive loss. Inadequate delivery may be caused by failure of gas delivery to the machine or from the common gas outlet.[41,117] A decrease in oxygen supply pressure to the machine may cause a decrease in gas flows set at the flowmeters. This has been discussed previously (see p. 83). Flow setting errors may occur. A disconnection, misconnection, or obstruction between the machine common gas outlet and the patient circuit have a similar effect.

Inadequate volume of gas in the circuit may be caused by excessive removal. An active scavenging system utilizes wall suction to remove the waste gases from the scavenging interface. Excessive negative pressure may be applied to the circuit if the negative pressure relief ("pop-in") valve or valves on the interface should become occluded.[123] A similar situation could arise with an open-reservoir scavenging system if the relief ports become occluded while suction is applied to the interface. A high subatmospheric pressure in the scavenging system may open the circuit adjustable pressure-limiting (APL) valve transmitting the subatmospheric pressure to the patient circuit. If a ventilator were being used, unrelieved excess negative pressure in the scavenging system would in most cases tend to hold the ventilator pressure–relief valve to its seat, preventing its opening on exhalation and causing a high pressure to develop in the circuit.[124]

A sidestream gas analyzer (such as a multiplexed mass spectrometer) connected to a patient circuit has been reported as the cause of excessive negative pressure in a breathing circuit where the fresh gas flow of 50 ml/min during cardiopulmonary bypass was less than the mass spectrometer's gas sampling rate of 250 ml/min.[124] Sampling rates of commonly used gas analyzers vary between less than 50 ml/min to as high as 800 ml/min; therefore considerable potential exists for creating negative pressure in the circuit if low fresh gas flow rates are being used.[124]

Excess gas removal by a sampling device during spontaneous ventilation creates a subatmospheric pressure in the circuit that in turn causes the APL valve to close, thereby preventing the scavenging system negative pressure relief valve or valves from relieving the negative pressure in the circuit (see Fig. 5-18). Maximum circuit subatmospheric pressure achieved by sidestream sampling devices during testing ranged from −11 to −148 mm Hg. Such low pressures, if transmitted to the patient's airway,

could result in barotrauma and cardiovascular dysfunction.[124]

Excessive volume loss resulting in negative pressures in the breathing system may occur if hospital suction is applied through the working channel of a fiberoptic bronchoscope that has been inserted into the system through an airway diaphragm adapter or by a suction catheter that has been inadvertently advanced alongside the tracheal tube into the trachea.

Inadequate circuit volume and negative pressure may occur during spontaneous ventilation in the presence of a low fresh gas flow rate and inadequate size of reservoir bag (such as the pediatric size used with an adult patient). During inspiration, the reservoir bag would collapse and a negative pressure would arise in the circuit. Circuit APL valves usually have a minimum opening pressure that is slightly greater than that needed to distend the reservoir bag. If the bag were of correct size but noncompliant, or the APL valve had a low opening pressure, during exhalation most of the gas would exit through the APL valve rather than fill the bag. The net result would be an inadequate reservoir volume for the next inspiration.[27]

Modern circuit pressure monitors incorporate a subatmospheric-pressure alarm such that when pressure is less than −10 cm H_2O at any time, audible and visual alarms are annunciated.[25,26]

3. *Failure to initiate artificial ventilation.* Failure to initiate artificial ventilation is usually attributable to an operator error. The error may be forgetting to turn on the ventilator (as after cardiopulmonary bypass), inadvertently setting a respiratory rate of zero breaths per minute, failure to select the "automatic" (ventilator) setting at the "manual/automatic" selector switch in the circuit, or failure to connect the ventilator circuit hose to the patient circuit connector by the selector switch or at the bag mount.[27] Because some older circuit volume and pressure alarms must be deliberately enabled or are enabled only when the ventilator is on, forgetting to turn on the ventilator may not be detectable by these monitors. In this respect continuous capnography provides the most sensitive monitor of ventilation. If the delivery system incorporates a standing-bellows ventilator, failure to connect to the ventilator tubing to the circuit will result in collapse of the bellows. With either bellows design, when a ventilator is turned on but the "manual" (bag) mode is selected at the selector switch, then during inspiration the bellows will attempt to empty against a total obstruction and failure of the bellows to empty will be readily observed (Fig. 5-21). Failure to ventilate in this situation is annunciated by both low pressure and volume alarms. Some older designs of circle system lack a "manual/automatic" selector switch, and the APL valve must be closed to effect intermittent positive-pressure ventilation (IPPV) when the ventilator hose is connected to the bag mount. Failure to close the APL valve is yet another cause of failure to initiate IPPV.

Even if the breathing system incorporates a selector switch, there are occasions when the primary anesthesia ventilator fails and a freestanding ventilator is brought in to provide IPPV. The foregoing considerations then apply if the new ventilator is connected to the circuit via the bag mount connection, that is, selecting the "manual" mode and closing the APL valve.

4. Leaks and disconnections in the breathing system. Breathing circuit disconnections and leaks are among the most common of anesthesia mishaps.[1,2,93,125] Anesthesia-breathing systems contain numerous basic connections as well as additional ones as more monitors, humidifiers, filters, and so forth are added (Fig. 5-18). Disconnections cannot be totally prevented, and indeed the 15 mm connector between the patient and the circuit has been considered by some as a safety fuse to prevent unintentional extubation.[27] Circuit disconnections and their detection have been the subject of several reviews.[1,2,9,93,125] Cooper et al.[1,2] found that disconnections of the patient from the machine were responsible for 7.5% of critical incidents involving human error or equipment failure. Of these disconnections about 70% occurred at the Y-piece.[1,2]

The risks of disconnection are reduced by secure locking of connecting components, use of "disconnect" (pressure, volume, capnography) alarms, and user education. When a disconnection occurs, the anesthetist must systematically trace the flow of gases through the breathing system looking for the disconnection in the same way as would be done in the event of a no-gas-flow or obstruction situation.

Most disconnections are detectable by the basic breathing system monitors of pressure and volume. Pressure monitors will annunciate an alarm if the peak inspiratory pressure in the circuit fails to reach the threshold low setting. It is important that the alarm setting on the monitor be user adjustable and be capable of being set to a level just below the usual peak inspiratory pressure. Some monitors provide a continuous graphic display of the circuit pressure as well as of the alarm threshold or thresholds.[25] A response algorithm for the low-pressure alarm condition has been described.[126]

The circuit low-pressure alarm can be fooled if not set to be very sensitive. Thus a circuit disconnection at the Y-piece combined with sufficient resistance at the patient connector end may not trigger the low-pressure alarm if inspiratory gas flow from the ventilator bellows is high enough and the low-pressure alarm threshold is crossed. Examples include unintended extubation of a patient who has a small-diameter tracheal tube where the tube connector offers high resistance to gas flow, or occlusion of the open patient connector by drapes.[27] A circuit low-pressure alarm sensing pressure in the absorber may be fooled if there is a high resistance between the inspiratory tubing connector and the Y-piece such as may be attributable to a cascade humidifier in the inspiratory limb of the circle.[127] Humidifiers may also represent the source of a detectable leak in the anesthesia circuit.[103]

A circuit low-pressure alarm is less likely fooled when a standing-bellows ventilator is being used, since failure of the bellows to fill adequately during exhalation will result in lower peak pressures on the next inspiration. With the hanging-bellows design, the peak inspiratory pressure will tend to be higher, with the bellows having filled completely during exhalation. A pressure alarm set to an inappropriately low threshold is therefore more likely to be fooled by a hanging-bellows ventilator.

Before the use of retaining devices at the common gas outlet, disconnections could occur here.[41] The diameter of the tubing connecting the common gas outlet with the circuit is relatively narrow and offers relatively high resistance to gas flow compared with the 22 mm diameter circuit tubing. If a hanging-bellows ventilator were being used with a large tidal volume setting, the machine-top-circuit connector-tubing resistance may be such that during inspiration the low-pressure alarm limit would be exceeded despite the leak.[41] During exhalation, room air would be entrained via the fresh gas inflow tubing to refill the bellows. A disconnection of this tubing may also lead to a hypoxic gas mixture in the circuit as air is entrained and O_2 is consumed. This type of disconnection associated with air entrainment is detectable by an O_2 analyzer with an appropriately set alarm in the patient circuit (see p. 106).

If, as is recommended, the circuit low-pressure alarm has been set to just below the peak inspiratory pressure, it should be recognized that more false-positive alarms will be generated. Thus for a given ventilator setting of tidal volume, a decrease in fresh gas flow, I:E ratio, or inspiratory flow rate, or an increase in respiratory rate will decrease the peak inspiratory pressure thereby triggering the alarm (see p. 99). A false-positive alarm with appropriate response is preferable to a false-negative alarm (provided that it does not lead to permanent silencing of the alarm or monitor) however.

Leaks from the circuit, other than those attributable to component disconnection, may also result in inadequate exchange of gas between system and patient. Leaks may occur in any component because of cracking,[103] incorrect assembly,[100] or malfunction of a system component, particularly the ventilator pressure–relief valve.[55-57]

During inspiration, the ventilator pressure–relief valve is normally held closed by driving gas circuit pressure from the bellows housing. If the pressure-relief valve is not held closed during inspiration, gas in the patient circuit leaves to the scavenging system rather than being driven into the patient's lungs (Fig. 5-18). Ventilator pressure–relief valve incompetence has been reported in connection with pilot-line disconnection or occlusion[94,128] and valve damage.[56,57] In such a situation, the loss of volume from the circuit would be detected by appropriately set pressure and volume alarms, but the source of the leak might be less obvious. If a closed-reservoir scavenging system is in use, one makes the diagnosis by observing the scavenging system reservoir bag.[94] The bag normally fills during exhalation, as gas is released from the patient circuit, and empties during inspiration, when the pressure-relief valve is closed (Fig. 5-18). If the pressure-relief valve is incompetent, the scavenging system reservoir bag will be seen to fill during inspiration, as the ventilator bellows empties its contained gas into the scavenging system and the scavenging reservoir bag empties during exhalation.[94]

Leaks and malfunctions in the patient circuit are sometimes first detected by an airway gas monitor capable of measuring nitrogen.[129] Application of negative pressure to the circuit by a malfunctioning scavenging system, or intermittently by a hanging-bellows ventilator during exhalation, may cause entrainment of air into the breathing system through a small leak otherwise unrecognized by pressure, volume, or even CO_2 monitoring.[129] A leak of room air or other gases into the patient circuit may result in dilution of the anesthesia gas mixture and, potentially in an extreme case, awareness under anesthesia.[129a] Leaks into the patient circuit may occur if there is a hole in the ventilator bellows, when the high pressure in the driving gas circuit during inspiration forces driving gas into the patient circuit. With an Ohmeda ventilator the diluting gas would be 100% O_2, but with a Dräger AV-E it would be an air/O_2 mix-

ture.[129b,c] Such an event might be detected by a change in F_IO_2, peak inspiratory pressure, tidal or minute volume, end-tidal CO_2, or a multigas or agent analyzer.

5. High pressures in the breathing system. The anesthesia machine provides a continuous flow of gas to the patient circuit. Whenever circuit gas inflow exceeds outflow rate, excessive pressures may develop. If these pressures are transmitted to the patient's lungs, severe cardiovascular compromise, barotrauma, and even pneumothorax may result.[130,131]

During spontaneous ventilation high pressure may result from inadequate opening (or even complete closure) of the adjustable pressure-limiting (APL) valve, kinking or occlusion of the tubing between the APL valve and the scavenging interface, or malfunction of the interface, that is, no suction and obstruction of the interface positive-pressure relief valve. During spontaneous ventilation, since the patient circuit reservoir bag is "in circuit," the bag will distend to accommodate the excess gas. Reservoir bags are highly distensible and limit the maximum circuit pressure to approximately 45 cm H_2O. Nevertheless, such an airway pressure could produce hypotension by inhibiting venous return. Increases in circuit pressure will be more rapid when the fresh gas inflow rate is high, as during prolonged use of the oxygen flush.[24]

Excessive circuit pressures may occur during use of an anesthesia ventilator. Thus during inspiration the ventilator pressure–relief valve (PRV) is normally held closed, opening during expiration to vent excess gas to the scavenging system. The effects of fresh gas flow, I:E ratio, and respiratory rate on tidal volume, alveolar ventilation, and by inference circuit pressure have been discussed in detail (see p. 99). Selection of a high inspiratory gas flow rate on the ventilator will be associated with increased peak pressures in the circuit.

There are many reports of ventilator malfunctions causing excessive circuit pressures. Failure of the ventilator to cycle from inspiration to expiration results in driving gas continuing to enter (Dräger) or enter but not leave (Ohmeda) the bellows housing.[24] This causes the ventilator pressure–relief valve (PRV) to remain closed and excess gas to build up pressure within the circuit. The pressure increase is limited by the driving gas pressure prevailing in the bellows housing. In Dräger ventilators this pressure depends on the setting of the inspiratory flow–control knob.[27,55]

Other reported causes of the ventilator pressure–relief valve failing to open normally include mechanical obstruction of the driving gas exhaust system (Dräger AV-E muffler),[60] kinking of a ventilator pressure–relief valve pilot line during inspiration,[55] and diffusion of N_2O into the space between the two pieces of rubber constituting the relief valve diaphragm, causing insidious PEEP.[132] Even with normal ventilator function high pressures in the circuit may be caused by occlusion of the tubing between the ventilator pressure–relief valve and the scavenging system, or obstruction of the scavenging interface "pop-off" valve (see Fig. 5-18). In such cases, as the pressure in the patient circuit rises, the ventilator bellows empties less completely and may even become distorted.

High pressures arising in the circuit are detected by the circuit pressure monitor, which incorporates two types of alarms.[27] A continuing-pressure alarm is annunciated usually when the circuit pressure remains in excess of +15 cm H_2O for more than 10 seconds. A high-pressure alarm is annunciated when the circuit pressure exceeds the threshold limit, which, in modern monitors, is set by the user but has a default setting of 50 to 65 cm H_2O depending on the unit. When either of these alarms is annunciated during mechanical ventilation, a problem should be suspected with the ventilator circuit. Circuit pressure can be immediately relieved by disconnection of the patient from the circuit at the Y-piece, or by selecting the manual (bag) mode and relieving pressure by the adjustable pressure-limiting valve. The incorporation of safety relief valves into the circuit as a protection against high pressures has not been popular, since these devices would limit the ability to ventilate a patient with poor compliance.[27]

As a protection against development of excessive pressures in the patient circuit during mechanical ventilation, circuit pressure–limiting devices are available from both Ohmeda and Dräger. The Ohmeda 7800 Series ventilators incorporate an inspiratory high-pressure limit such that when the selected threshold (pressure measured in patient circuit downstream of inspiratory unidirectional valve) is exceeded, the ventilator cycles to expiration, driving gas circuit pressure falls to zero, and excess patient circuit gas is discharged to the scavenging system via the ventilator pressure–relief valve.[53] Basic Dräger AV-E ventilators are not pressure limited but a pressure-limit control is available and may be retrofitted to certain standing-bellows design AV-E units.[133] The Dräger pressure-limit control device senses the pressure in the patient circuit at the bellows, and whenever the threshold high-pressure limit is exceeded, a valve opens in the driving gas circuit (bellows

housing) to release excess driving gas to the atmosphere, thereby limiting driving gas pressure such that patient circuit pressure does not exceed the set limit for the remainder of the inspiration. The time cycling of the Dräger AV-E is thus maintained,[133] in contrast with the Ohmeda 7800 Series ventilators.[53] Both the Dräger and the Ohmeda approaches to limiting pressure in the patient circuit require a normally functioning ventilator pressure–relief valve, since it is through this valve (the opening pressure of which is controlled by the pressure in the driving gas circuit) that excess gas and pressure is relieved from the patient circuit. If the PRV or its outflow path should become obstructed, neither the Dräger nor the Ohmeda pressure-limiting mechanisms would be effective in relieving pressure in the patient circuit.

F. Anesthetic agent dosage and administration problems

Complications to the patient may arise as a result of an anesthetic agent overdosage or underdosage or administration of an incorrect agent. Hazards of vaporizer malfunction causing anesthetic overdosage or underdosage are perhaps greater with a rebreathing than with a circle system. The reason is that in the former system high flows of fresh gas are delivered directly to the patient's airway whereas in the circle system, unless high flows are being used, there is a greater discrepancy between delivered and inspired agent concentrations.

1. Liquid agent in the fresh gas piping. Lethal anesthetic agent overdosage may occur when excessive amounts of saturated vapor or even liquid agent enter the fresh gas delivery system.[134] The former situation is more likely with a measured flow type of vaporizer arrangement (Copper Kettle or Verni-Trol), since calculation or flow setting errors can easily arise. In addition, some older designs of vaporizer can be overfilled so that excess liquid could enter the fresh gas delivery system. Modern vaporizers are concentration calibrated and are designed so as to prevent overfilling.[6]

Tilting or tipping of a vaporizer may result in liquid agent entering the fresh gas or bypass lines. Such an occurrence could result in lethal concentrations of vapor being delivered to the common gas outlet of the machine and thence to the patient circuit. One milliliter of liquid potent volatile agent will produce approximately 200 ml of vapor at 20° C (Table 5-1).[38] If 1 ml of liquid halothane were to enter the common gas tubing, it would require 10 liters of fresh gas to dilute the resulting vapor to a concentration of 2%, or a minimum alveolar

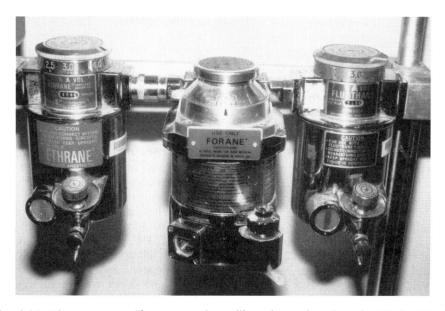

Fig. 5-22. Three agent-specific concentration calibrated vaporizers in series. Notice (1) absence of interlock system; (2) outer (Foregger) vaporizers produce increase in concentration when dial is rotated clockwise, whereas the center vaporizer is of the contemporary configuration such that counterclockwise dial rotation increases output concentration.

concentration of approximately 3 MAC. It is easy to appreciate how a relatively small volume of liquid agent in the wrong place could have a profound effect on a patient.

If a vaporizer has been tilted or tipped and there is concern that liquid agent may have leaked into the fresh gas delivery system, then with no patient connected to the system the vaporizer should be flushed with a high flow rate of oxygen from the flowmeter (*not* the O_2 flush, which bypasses the vaporizer) and with the vaporizer dial set to a high concentration. If any doubt still exists as to the safe function of the vaporizer, it should be withdrawn from clinical service until certified safe for use by an authorized service representative. Additional caution is needed with a halothane vaporizer that has been tipped. Liquid halothane contains thymol, a sticky preservative that does not evaporate. Thymol entering the flow control and temperature-compensating parts of a vaporizer could cause vaporizer malfunction even after the halothane has been flushed out of these parts.

Modern vaporizers are mounted on the back bar of the anesthesia machine. Ohmeda Tec 4 and Tec 5 vaporizers are designed to be easily mounted on or removed from Selectatec Series mounted manifolds.[135,136] Because they are designed to be removable, Tec vaporizers incorporate an antispill mechanism that prevents liquid agent from entering the bypass sections.[135,136] Dräger Vapor 19.1 vaporizers are not designed to be easily removable and are more permanently mounted on the Narkomed machine.[137] Removal of these vaporizers should be performed by authorized service personnel only. These vaporizers do not incorporate an antispill mechanism, with the risk of agent spillage being minimized by the "permanent" mounting. Nevertheless spillage of liquid agent could occur in such vaporizers if the whole Dräger Narkomed anesthesia machine were to be tilted or even laid on its side, as may occur if the machine is too close to an electrically powered operating table that is being raised!

2. Concentration dial design. Anesthetic agent overdosage may also occur if a vaporizer were to deliver unexpectedly high but not lethal concentrations. In modern vaporizers concentration is increased when one turns the dial counterclockwise.[6] In some older design vaporizers, turning the dial clockwise increased concentration. Some machines may still be equipped with the older design or even a combination of the two designs, which might therefore present a hazard if the dial is turned inappropriately. It is therefore important that the anesthetist deliberately observe the dial and calibration settings when changing a vaporizer dial concentration setting (Fig. 5-22).

3. Incorrect filling of vaporizers

a. Single agent. Anesthetic agent overdosage or underdosage can occur if an agent-specific vaporizer is filled wholly or partially with an incorrect agent.[10,38] If an empty concentration-calibrated vaporizer designed for one agent is filled with an agent for which it was not designed, the vaporizer concentration output may be erroneous.[138,139] Since at room temperature the vaporizing characteristics of halothane and isoflurane are almost identical, this problem currently really only applies to interchanging halothane or isoflurane with enflurane (see Table 5-1).

A more dangerous situation would obtain if a vaporizer designed for methoxyflurane (an agent with a saturated vapor pressure of 20.3 mm Hg at 20° C) were filled with halothane, enflurane, or isoflurane (see Table 5-1). A methoxyflurane vaporizer filled with halothane and set to deliver 1% methoxyflurane (6 MAC of methoxyflurane) would deliver 14.8% (approximately 20 MAC) halothane. Set to 1 MAC (0.16%) methoxyflurane, the vaporizer makes a flow split of 16:1, similar to that of a halothane or isoflurane variable bypass vaporizer set to deliver 2.7% (see Table 5-2). As the use of methoxyflurane has almost completely disappeared, such errors are now an unlikely occurrence.

The outputs of erroneously filled vaporizers are shown in Table 5-3. Erroneous filling affects the output concentration and consequently the MAC (minimum alveolar concentration) or potency output of the vaporizer.[138] Thus an enflurane vaporizer set to 2% (1.19 MAC) but filled with halothane will deliver 3.21% (4.01 MAC) of halothane, that is, 3.3 times the anticipated anesthetic potency output (Table 5-3).[138]

Erroneous filling of vaporizers may be prevented by careful attention to the specific agent and the vaporizer when filling is performed. Agent-specific keyed filling mechanisms, analogous to the pin-index system for medical gases, are available as options on modern vaporizers.[11,135-137] Liquid anesthetic agents are available packaged in bottles that have an agent-specific collar. An agent-specific filling device has one end that fits the collar on the agent bottle and the other end that fits only the vaporizer designed for that agent. These filling devices, though well intentioned, have up to now not gained much popularity in use. Thus agents are not always supplied in agent-specific "collared" bottles, and a problem with erroneous fitting of a collar to a bottle has even been reported.[140] The ASTM F1161-88 Standard states that the vaporizer filling mechanism *should* be fitted with a permanently attached standard, agent-specific keyed filling device to prevent accidental filling with the wrong agent.[6] Agent-specific filling devices will assume even greater importance if and when desflurane, an agent with a saturated vapor pressure of 664 mm Hg at 20° C (see List 5-1), is introduced into general clinical use. Filling a currently used and variable bypass vaporizer (such as Tec 4) with desflurane could result in very high concentration outputs of this agent. It can be calculated that an isoflurane variable bypass vaporizer set to deliver 1% isoflurane (0.87 MAC) but filled with desflurane will deliver approximately 13% desflurane (2.6 MAC) at 20° C. A small increase in temperature would result in a drastically increased output concentration and could become uncontrolled and potentially lethal if the desflurane were to boil. As discussed previously a special type of vaporizer will be required for this new agent (see p. 90).

b. Mixed agents. Perhaps a more likely scenario is that an agent-specific vaporizer that is partially filled with a correct agent is topped up with an incorrect agent.[138] The situation here is

Table 5-3. Output in O_2 in percent and MAC of erroneously filled vaporizers at 22° C

Vaporizers	Liquid	Setting%	Output%	Output MAC*
Halothane	Halothane	1.0	1.00	1.25
	Enflurane	1.0	0.62	0.37
	Isoflurane	1.0	0.96	0.84
Enflurane	Enflurane	2.0	2.00	1.19
	Isoflurane	2.0	3.09	2.69
	Halothane	2.0	3.21	4.01
Isoflurane	Isoflurane	1.5	1.50	1.30
	Halothane	1.5	1.56	1.95
	Enflurane	1.5	0.97	0.57

From Bruce DL and Linde HW: Anesthesiology 60:342-346, 1984.
*MAC, Minimum alveolar concentration in vol%.

Table 5-4. Vaporizer output after incorrect refilling from 25% full to 100% full

Vaporizer	Setting%	Refill liquid	Halothane		Enflurane		Isoflurane		Total MAC
			%	MAC*	%	MAC	%	MAC	
Halothane	1.0	Enflurane	0.33	0.41	0.64	0.38	—	—	0.79
	1.0	Isoflurane	0.41	0.51	—	—	0.90	0.78	1.29
Enflurane	2.0	Halothane	2.43	3.03	0.96	0.57	—	—	3.60
Isoflurane	1.5	Halothane	1.28	1.60	—	—	0.57	0.50	2.10

From Bruce DL and Linde HW: Anesthesiology 60:342-346, 1984.
* *MAC,* Minimum alveolar concentration in vol%.

more complex and less easily predicted in terms of vaporizer output, and large errors in delivered vapor administration can occur. Halothane, enflurane, and isoflurane, when mixed, do not react chemically but do influence the extent of each other's ease of vaporization.[141] Halothane facilitates the vaporization of both enflurane and isoflurane and in the process is itself more likely to vaporize.[141] The clinical consequences depend on the potencies of each of the mixed agents as well as the delivered vapor concentrations. If a halothane vaporizer 25% full is refilled to 100% with isoflurane and set to deliver 1%, the halothane output is 0.41% (0.51 MAC) and isoflurane output 0.9% (0.78 MAC) (see Table 5-4).[138] In this case, the output potency of 1.29 MAC is not far from the 1.25 MAC (1% halothane) expected.

On the other hand, an enflurane vaporizer 25% full and set to deliver 2% (1.19 MAC) enflurane, which is filled to 100% with halothane has an output of 2.43% (3.03 MAC) halothane and 0.96% (0.57 MAC) enflurane (see Table 5-4).[138] This represents a total MAC of 3.6, or more than twice that intended. In any event, it is important that erroneous filling of vaporizers be avoided and that, if suspected, the vaporizer should be emptied and, if necessary, serviced, flushed, and refilled with the correct agent.

4. Simultaneous use of more than one vaporizer. Modern anesthesia vaporizers incorporate an interlock system to prevent simultaneous use of more than one vaporizer and agent.[6] Older designs of anesthesia machine had up to three variable bypass vaporizers arranged in series such that fresh gas passed through each vaporizer (albeit the bypass flow) to reach the common gas outlet of the anesthesia machine. Without an interlock device, which would have permitted only one vaporizer to be in use at any time, it was possible to have all three vaporizers on simultaneously (Fig. 5-22). Apart from potentially overdosing the patient, the agent from

the upstream vaporizer could contaminate the agent or agents in those downstream.[14,2,143] During subsequent use, the output of the downstream vaporizer would be contaminated and the concentration and results of the emerging gas and vapor mixture would be indeterminant and might even be lethal. With such in-series arrangements care must be taken to ensure that only one vaporizer is on at any time and, to minimize risk in case cross-contamination should occur, the sequence of vaporizers from upstream to downstream should be such that the agent that has the lowest saturated vapor pressure is upstream (that is, farthest from the patient). The correct series sequence is therefore methoxyflurane, enflurane, isoflurane, halothane, with halothane being closest to the common gas outlet of the anesthesia machine. As the use of safety interlocking devices increases, the foregoing may be of historical interest only.

Although vaporizer interlock systems represent a desirable (and now standard) safety feature on modern machines,[6] failures of these systems have been reported.[108,144,145] Failure may result such that it is possible for more than one vaporizer to be on at one time.[144] Exclusion of the selected vaporizer has been described with a Selectatec system.[145] It is therefore important that the anesthetist check the interlock system periodically for correct function.

The good intentions for the vaporizer interlock system can also be defeated if a freestanding vaporizer is used in series with the fresh gas flow but downstream of the common gas outlet. Such arrangements configured by the user are potentially dangerous and should not be used.[146]

5. Pumping effect. Measured flow and some other older designs of concentration-calibrated vaporizers were subject to the so-called pumping effect, which could result in increased output concentrations during mechanical ventilation when low fresh gas flow rates were in use. The explanation for this effect is that, during positive-pressure ventilation, increases in pressure in the vaporizer caused bypass gas to enter the vaporizing chamber of the vaporizer, thereby increasing output.[11] Recent vaporizing systems are designed to be compensated for or protected against the pumping effect.[135-137] In older Ohmeda anesthesia machines vaporizer protection is afforded by an outlet check valve located just upstream of the common gas outlet (see Fig. 5-2), which prevents increases in pressure in the patient circuit from being transmitted back into the machine and thence to the vaporizer. Some older designs of vaporizer (such as Ohio Ethrane vaporizer) incorporated a check valve in the vaporizer outlet.[40]

The most modern vaporizers (Ohmeda Tec 4 and Tec 5 and Dräger Vapor 19.1) do not use check valves but use baffles or other design features to prevent the pumping effect.[135-137] If an anesthesia machine is to be used for a patient who is susceptible to malignant hyperthermia, it has been recommended that the vaporizers be removed and that the machine be flushed with O_2 at 10 L/min for 5 minutes, with replacement of the fresh gas outlet hose and use of a new disposable circle.[147] Others have disagreed with some of these recommendations.[148]

6. Anesthetic agent underdosage. Anesthetic agent underdosage may also occur, resulting in light anesthesia, patient movement, or even awareness. Perhaps the most common problem is forgetting to turn the vaporizer on. In some early vaporizer exclusion systems (Dräger Vapor, Ohio Selectatec), the vaporizer dial could be turned on while the vaporizer was excluded from the gas delivery system. In recent systems the exclusion mechanism is activated only when the vaporizer is turned on; thus this potential problem is avoided.[25,135-137]

7. Miscellaneous malfunctions. The unintentional delivery of high concentrations of anesthetic vapor may result from any kind of internal malfunction of the vaporizer, and so regular checking of function and output calibration are essential. Such checking should ideally be performed in the usual-use environment of the vaporizer. Thus the output of Ohmeda Tec 4 vaporizers has been found to be accurate in the proximity of a 1.5 Tesla magnet in a magnetic resonance imaging suite.[149,150]

Although numerous design features have helped to make contemporary vaporizing systems safer for the patient, ideally an agent-specific analyzer should be used in the patient circuit to monitor inhaled concentrations.[151] A variety of such units using various different technologies are available and all incorporate alarm features.

G. Humidification problems

Humidification of the inspired gases is desirable because it (1) prevents heat loss caused by evaporation of water from the tracheobronchial tree, (2) maintains moisture in the conducting airways and thereby facilitates ciliary function, and (3) prevents water loss from the patient by evaporation. Humidity can be provided by heat and moisture exchange devices that are attached to the endotracheal tube[152,153] and by moistening of the inside of the breathing tubes and reservoir bag with water before use. In addition, unheated water vaporizers can be employed to provide moisture to the patient. However, the disadvantage of any system that does not employ heat is that it will cool as evaporation takes place and the amount of humidity generated will therefore be reduced.[11]

Heated humidifiers (vaporizers) are devices through which the inspired gases are passed in order to saturate the gases with water at the temperature of the humidifier. The dry gases either bubble through the humidifier or pass over or blow by the surface of the water. The heat is usually provided by electricity.

The advantage of this type of system is that the inspired gases become saturated with water at an elevated temperature. However, as the gas cools on leaving the humidifier, condensation will occur in the tubing and the amount of humidity delivered to the patient will decrease. The condensation problem can be managed by heating the gases in the inspiratory hose either externally or internally with a heating wire. Keeping the distance from the humidifier to the patient as short as possible will also decrease the amount of condensation.

Another technique is to heat the humidifier to a temperature higher than body temperature so that as the inspired gases cool in the inspiratory tubing they enter the endotracheal tube at the desired temperature. One must be careful when using this technique in order to avoid burning the patient's tracheobronchial tree. It is therefore mandatory to monitor the temperature of the inspired gases at the endotracheal tube to ensure that the gases are not too hot. Since the gases that are delivered to the patient have at most 100% relative humidity, there is little chance that the patient will be fluid overloaded when a heated humidifier is employed.[11]

Hazards associated with the "artificial nose" (heat and moisture exchanger) include misconnection, obstruction, and disconnection.[154,155] A heated humidifier may cause bulk water delivery to the patient, thermal trauma to the airway, obstruction of the breathing circuit, and electrical and fire hazards. These devices are electrically powered; thermostat failure may result in superheating of the gases in the humidifier causing softening of the plastic inspiratory tubing.[11,156] Softening of the inspiratory hose may lead to complete occlusion of the inspiratory hose and thereby prevent the patient from being ventilated. One can avoid this problem by making sure that the gas flow through the humidifier is initiated before one turns the humidifier on.[157]

Other hazards, such as erroneously filling the humidifier with a liquid other than water, will create a hazard that is determined by the chemical used and the amount of exposure the patient receives.

Humidity can also be provided with a nebulizer technique. Nebulizers create droplets of water with either a jet of gas over the surface of the water or ultrasonically. Unlike the heated vaporizer, the nebulizer creates three hazards. It can act as a nidus for bacterial transmission, there may be increases in respiratory resistance, and the patient can become overhydrated. Therefore extreme care should be taken in cleaning the nebulizer, sterile water must be used, and the amount of water delivered must be carefully monitored. In addition, because of the risk of increased respiratory resistance, nebulizers should probably not be used in patients who are breathing spontaneously.

When using heated humidifiers or nebulizers, the anesthesiologist should guard against (1) fluid overload, (2) thermal injury, (3) additional sites for disconnection within the breathing circuit, (4) obstruction to gas flow, (5) burning of the equipment because of electrical malfunction, (6) shock hazards, and (7) the risk of infection transmission via the nebulizer.[11,156]

H. Electrical failures

Before the late 1970s most anesthesia machines were completely mechanical or pneumatic and had no electrical components. These machines consisted of the gas piping system, regulators, valves, flowmeters, vaporizers, and a ventilator that was completely pneumatic. Monitor and alarm systems were attached to the machine, and they were either pneumatic or battery powered.

During the 1980s the anesthesia machines were redesigned to include electrical systems that control the ventilator, alarm system, and integrated monitors. An example of this type of anesthesia machine is the North American Dräger Narkomed 2B.[158] The machine is equipped with a power cord and accepts an electrical input of 90 to 130 volts at 50 to 60 Hz. There are four electrical outlets (receptacles) on the anesthesia machine into which additional equipment can be plugged. There is a battery backup system that consists of a 12-volt rechargeable battery. The battery backup system is activated when the alternating-current (AC) power to the machine fails.

Before using the machine the operator should check the status of the AC power supply and the charge on the battery. No case should be started if the power has failed or the battery is not charged. A discharged battery takes 16 hours to recharge.[158]

The main on/off switch on the machine turns on the electrical supply and mechanically opens the flow of gases to the flowmeters. Even if the electrical system were to fail completely, the flow of gas to the flowmeter would continue uninterrupted. If the AC power were to fail, the battery backup system would take over. However, the backup battery provides only power to the ventilator control circuits, the monitors built into the machine, and the alarm system. Any peripheral device that is plugged into the AC receptacles that are built into the machine will lose power when the AC power to the machine fails. The battery backup does not energize those receptacles.

The backup battery system will provide power for at least 30 minutes. When the battery voltage drops to 10 volts, all electrical power to the anesthesia machine ceases in order to prevent the battery from deeply discharging. At that point the ventilator will stop, and the monitors and alarms in the machine will cease to function. The patient's ventilation must be performed manually until the power is restored.[158]

Some electrical problems occur commonly. The anesthesia machine may be left in the on position and the power cord disconnected from the wall. This will result in a discharge of the battery and a machine that will deliver gases when turned on but will have no electrical monitors or alarms functioning until the battery can be recharged. Alternatively the power cord from the machine may be plugged into a receptacle that is built into the machine. In this circumstance the machine is not powered by the external AC power supply and can run off only the battery system. In addition, any other device that is plugged into the other receptacles will not have any power delivered to them.

The Narkomed 2B anesthesia machine incorporates three circuit breakers. They are associated with the primary AC power supply, the battery, and the convenience receptacles. When the latter circuit breaker is in the open (tripped) position, the receptacles will not be energized. The source of the tripping of the circuit breaker should be sought, and then the breaker should be reset.[158]

When the AC power supply to the operating room fails completely, all electrical equipment that does not have a backup battery will cease to function. Therefore one should be aware that electrically powered monitors will cease to function unless AC power can be restored. In addition, important life-support devices such as the cardiopulmonary bypass machine will also stop, and they will require either manual or battery power in order to maintain the artificial circulation. Finally, the operating room lights may also fail during total loss of electricity, and this problem would have to be managed with flashlights.[159,160]

III. PREVENTION OF COMPLICATIONS
A. Preanesthetic check of the anesthesia delivery system

The purpose of the preanesthetic check is to determine that all the necessary equipment is present and functioning as expected before the induction of anesthesia. The usefulness of this is self-evident; moreover it is supported by an anesthesia literature that describes anesthesia machine malfunctions that could have been discovered before the case began if a thorough check of the equipment had been performed.[161] In August 1986 the Food and Drug Administration released its *Anesthesia Apparatus Checkout Recommendations*[162] and stated that "this checkout, or a reasonable equivalent, should be conducted before administering anesthesia. This is a guideline which users are encouraged to modify to accommodate differences in equipment design and variations in local clinical practice. Such local modifications should have appropriate peer review. *Users should refer to the operator's manual for special procedures or precautions.*" Many anesthesia departments have adopted these recommendations without modification, whereas others have modified them to suit their needs. Whichever approach is taken, it is absolutely critical that the machine be carefully inspected and checked before use.

When the delivery system is checked before the start of anesthesia, it is desirable to arrange it in the way it will be used during the case. Moving the machine after the case has begun, modifying the breathing circuit with a humidifier, or adding other components can affect the performance of the anesthesia delivery system. Inspecting the machine in the conditions in which it will be used during the operation will minimize this type of problem.[55] However, the preoperative equipment check does not guard against the problem of intraoperative equipment failure. The anesthesiologist must be vigilant in the monitoring of equipment performance and ready to intervene in any hazardous situation.

The generic FDA guidelines for machine inspection are self-explanatory (see Appendix, p. 123).[162] Steps 5, 7, 8, 10, 12, 13, 15, 16, 17, and 24 are set out in greater detail below.

STEP 5. CHECK THE OXYGEN CYLINDER SUPPLIES. You should first make sure that the oxygen-pressure gauge reads zero. The pipeline oxygen source should be disconnected, and one of the reserve oxygen cylinders should be opened. The pressure should be noted, the cylinder closed, and the system depressurized when the oxygen flush button is pressed. The second cylinder should be opened and its pressure noted. High-pressure gas leaks should be sought, the manifestation of which is a high-pitched hissing noise. When you are testing the pressure of each cylinder, it is critical that the pressure on the oxygen-pressure gauge be zero before you open the cylinder; otherwise the residual pressure in the oxygen piping system will be displayed, and the anesthesiologist may be misled in believing that the cylinder contains more oxygen than it does. At least one of the cylinders should be nearly full, and cylinders that are one quarter full or less should be replaced. At the conclusion of the cylinder checks the cylinder valves should be closed. This prevents the use of the cylinder supply without the anesthesiologist being aware of it.

STEP 7. CHECK THE NITROUS OXIDE AND OTHER CYLINDER GAS SUPPLIES. The nitrous oxide test is performed similar to the oxygen cylinder tests. However, the reading on the pressure gauge will remain at 745 PSIG until most of the liquid nitrous oxide has been used up. In order for you to know how much of this agent is in the cylinder it must be weighed.[10]

STEP 8. TEST THE FLOWMETERS. The floats should be at the bottom of the flow tubes. When the valves are opened, the floats should move smoothly and not stick. Make certain that the floats are not stuck at the top of the flow tubes.

STEP 10. TEST THE OXYGEN-PRESSURE FAILURE SYSTEM. Set the oxygen and other gas flows to midrange. Close the oxygen cylinder and release the pressure in the oxygen piping by pressing the oxygen flush valve. Verify that the flow of all gases falls to zero and that if an oxygen-pressure failure alarm is present it alarms when the oxygen pressure falls below the threshold. After the test is complete, reopen the oxygen cylinder and bleed all the gases from the piping system and close the flow-control valves.

STEP 12. ADD ANY ACCESSORY EQUIPMENT TO THE BREATHING SYSTEM. It is very important to have the entire breathing system fully assembled before testing it for leaks and proper function. This is because it is possible to modify the system with malfunctioning equipment after it has been checked. Under those circumstances the circuit check would fail to detect the system malfunction.

STEP 13. CALIBRATE THE OXYGEN MONITOR. The absolutely critical oxygen monitor should be calibrated to read 21% when exposed to room air. The alarm should be tested for proper function at low oxygen concentrations. The sensor should then be exposed to the breathing circuit, and 100% oxygen should be flowing through the system. The monitor should read close to 100%. Slight inaccuracy at the 100% end of the scale may be tolerated, but the monitor must be well calibrated at the 21% end.

STEP 15. CHECK UNIDIRECTIONAL VALVES. Each limb of the breathing circuit should be checked for valve function. You should not be able to exhale through the inspiratory hose or inhale through the expiratory hose of the circuit. After this test the circuit should be reassembled.

STEP 16. TEST THE LEAKS IN THE MACHINE AND BREATHING SYSTEM. The adjustable pressure limit (pop-off) valve should be closed, and the patient end of the breathing circuit should be occluded. The system should be pressurized to 20 cm H_2O by flowing oxygen from the flowmeter. With no gas entering the breathing circuit and without squeezing the reservoir bag you should maintain this pressure. If there is a decrease in pressure, the amount of leak can be quantitated by flowing oxygen until the pressure is held steady. On machines with a check valve proximal to the common gas outlet a negative-pressure leak test at the common gas outlet must be performed to rule out a leak upstream from that valve. See references 10 and 26 for more details.

STEP 17. EXHAUST VALVE AND SCAVENGER SYSTEM TEST. Open the adjustable pressure limit (APL) valve and observe that the pressure falls to zero. With the valve open observe that no positive or negative pressure exists in the circuit when there is no flow of gas and at high flow of gas from the oxygen flush. Positive pressure in the circuit would indicate that there is obstruction to flow at the APL valve or distal to it in the scavenging system. Negative pressure in the

circuit would probably be caused by a faulty negative-pressure–relief system or valve within the scavenger interface.

STEP 24. SET AIRWAY PRESSURE AND/OR VOLUME MONITOR ALARM LIMITS. If the alarm limits are adjustable, set the airway pressure limits several cm H_2O below the peak airway pressure for the minimum ventilation-pressure alarm, and approximately 10 cm H_2O above the peak airway pressure for the continuing-pressure and high-pressure alarms. Set the minimum volume alarm to a point close to but below the delivered minute volume. Setting the alarms in this way will make the system as sensitive as possible to changes in the patient or breathing system that may adversely effect the patient's ventilation.

It is again emphasized that the operator's manual should be consulted for specific delivery system check-out procedures.

B. Anesthesia machine standards and obsolescence

The American National Standards Institute (ANSI) Z-79.8 standard approved in 1979 did much to improve the design and safety features of the anesthesia machines produced in the subsequent decade.[7] In 1988 the American Society of Anesthesiologists (ASA) Committee on Equipment and Standards undertook the task of examining the issue of aging anesthesia gas machines. This began with a panel on anesthesia machine obsolescence at the 1988 annual ASA meeting in San Francisco.[163]

In March 1989 the ASA Board of Directors approved the following policy submitted by the Committee on Equipment and Standards.[164] "The age of an anesthesia gas machine has not been demonstrated to be a factor in anesthetic mishaps. An anesthesia gas machine, however, which no longer functions as designed and isn't modified to meet acceptable levels of performance and monitoring should not be used.

Each anesthesia department should establish a protocol to ensure that all anesthesia staff members are qualified in the operation of each type of gas machine, ventilator, and monitor before use."

The most recent anesthesia machine standard is the ASTM F1161-88.[6] Recent North American Dräger and Ohmeda machines far exceed this standard, and both companies offer an evaluation program with a view to upgrading or replacing older equipment that may no longer be considered acceptable.

Important aspects of the recent ASTM F1161-88 standard are listed below. Numbers in parentheses refer to sections in the standards document. You are encouraged to review the original document for further details.[6]

1. Flow control (Section 9.1). Only one flow-adjustment control for each gas delivered to the common gas outlet shall be provided. Thus banks of flowmeters in parallel with separate high and low flow controls for the same gas are now undesirable. Some new anesthesia machines include a separate flow control and delivery nipple for oxygen. This does not violate the Standard, since this oxygen is not being delivered to the common gas outlet.

2. Concentration-calibrated vaporizers (Section 12.1). All vaporizers located within the fresh gas circuit shall be concentration calibrated. Control of the vapor concentration shall be provided by means of calibrated knobs or dials (12.1.1). Measured flow vaporizers (Copper Kettle, Verni-Trol) are not mentioned and therefore are no longer to be considered up to date

3. Common gas outlet (Section 13.1.1). When the common gas outlet is connected to the breathing system by a fresh gas supply hose, the common gas outlet shall be provided with a retaining device. The outlet should have a manufacturer-specific fitting.

4. Alarms (Section 16). Alarm characteristics of monitors should be categorized as high, medium, or low priority. The alarms should be distinguishable audibly and visually, and the operator response should be immediate, prompt, or at least display an awareness, according to the clinical priority and appropriateness. Present machines should therefore incorporate an integrated and prioritized alarm system.

5. Oxygen supply precautions (Section 17). The machine shall be designed so that whenever the O_2 supply pressure is reduced from normal (manufacturer specified) and until flow ceases, the set O_2 *concentration* shall not de-

crease at the common gas outlet. The anesthesia circuit oxygen concentration shall be measured, and the analyzer will annunciate a high-priority alarm when the concentration falls below the preset threshold. The machine is designed so that the oxygen analyzer is enabled and functioning anytime the machine is capable of delivering an anesthetic mixture.

6. Ventilatory monitoring (Section 18). The anesthesia machine shall have breathing pressure monitoring as well as having either exhaled volume, or ventilatory CO_2 monitoring.

The alarms associated with these monitors are to be enabled and functioning automatically whenever the machine is in use.

Refer to the original document for further information and for the rationale for the stated requirements.[6]

IV. CONCLUSIONS

The anesthesia delivery system may cause complications to the patient because of misuse or component failure. The delivery system continues to evolve as more is learned about patient safety and as design and monitoring features are added. Clearly a basic understanding of the delivery-system structure and function will enhance patient safety by avoiding misuse and facilitating troubleshooting or alternative techniques if a component should fail. All anesthetizing locations should have immediately available a fresh tank supply of oxygen and a resuscitation bag for use in the event of a total machine failure.

Although some states (in particular New York and New Jersey) have implemented regulation with regard to the practice of anesthesiology, as of December 1990 only the State of New Jersey has published regulations concerning requirements for anesthesia equipment, safety, maintenance, and inspection.[165] Other states may well follow.

ANESTHESIA APPARATUS CHECKOUT RECOMMENDATIONS⊕

This checkout, or a reasonable equivalent, should be conducted before administering anesthesia. This is a guideline which users are encouraged to modify to accommodate differences in equipment design and variations in local clinical practice. Such local modifications should have appropriate peer review. Users should refer to the operator's manual for special procedures or precautions.

*1. **INSPECT ANESTHESIA MACHINE FOR:**
machine identification number
valid inspection sticker
undamaged flowmeters, vaporizers, gauges, supply hoses
complete, undamaged breathing system with adequate CO_2 absorbent
correct mounting of cylinders in yokes
presence of cylinder wrench

*2. **INSPECT AND TURN ON:**
electrical equipment requiring warm-up. (ECG/pressure monitor, oxygen monitor, etc.)

*3. **CONNECT WASTE GAS SCAVENGING SYSTEM:**
Adjust vacuum as required

*4. **CHECK THAT:**
flow-control valves are off
vaporizers are off
vaporizers are filled (not overfilled)
filler caps are sealed tightly
CO_2 absorber bypass (if any) is off

*5. **CHECK OXYGEN (O_2) CYLINDER SUPPLIES:**
a. Disconnect pipeline supply (if connected) and return cylinder and pipeline pressure gauges to zero with O_2 flush valve.
b. Open O_2 cylinder; check pressure; close cylinder and observe gauge for evidence of high pressure leak.
c. With the O_2 flush valve, flush to empty piping.
d. Repeat as in b. and c. above for second O_2 cylinder, if present.
e. Replace any cylinder less than about 600 psig. At least one should be nearly full.
f. Open less full cylinder.

*6. **TURN ON MASTER SWITCH (if present)**

*7. **CHECK NITROUS OXIDE (N_2O) AND OTHER GAS CYLINDER SUPPLIES:**
Use same procedure as described in 5a. & b. above, but open and *CLOSE* flow-control valve to empty piping.
Note: N_2O pressure below 745 psig. indicates that the cylinder is less than $1/4$ full.

*8. **TEST FLOWMETERS:**
a. Check that float is at bottom of tube with flow-control valves closed (or at min. O_2 flow if so equipped).
b. Adjust flow of all gases through their full range and check for erratic movements of floats.

*9. **TEST RATIO PROTECTION/WARNING SYSTEM (if present):**
Attempt to create hypoxic O_2/N_2O mixture, and verify correct change in gas flows and/or alarm.

*10. **TEST O_2 PRESSURE FAILURE SYSTEM:**
a. Set O_2 and other gas flows to midrange.
b. Close O_2 cylinder and flush to release O_2 pressure.
c. Verify that all flows fall to zero. Open O_2 cylinder.
d. Close all other cylinders and bleed piping pressures.
e. Close O_2 cylinder and bleed piping pressure.
f. CLOSE FLOW-CONTROL VALVES.

*If an anesthetist uses the same machine in successive cases, these steps need not be repeated or may be abbreviated after the initial checkout.

†A vaporizer leak can be detected only if the vaporizer is turned on during this test. Even then, a relatively small but clinically significant leak may still be obscured.

⊕As developed by the FDA, August 1986.

*11. **TEST CENTRAL PIPELINE GAS SUPPLIES:**
a. Inspect supply hoses (should not be cracked or worn).
b. Connect supply hoses, verifying correct color coding.
c. Adjust all flows to at least midrange.
d. Verify that supply pressures hold (45-55 psig.).
e. Shut off flow-control valves.

*12. **ADD ANY ACCESSORY EQUIPMENT TO THE BREATHING SYSTEM:**
Add PEEP valve, humidifier, etc., if they might be used (if necessary remove after step 18 until needed).

13. **CALIBRATE O_2 MONITOR:**
*a. Calibrate O_2 monitor to read 21% in room air.
*b. Test low alarm.
c. Occlude breathing system at patient end; fill and empty system several times with 100% O_2.
d. Check that monitor reading is nearly 100%.

14. **SNIFF INSPIRATORY GAS:**
There should be no odor.

*15. **CHECK UNDIRECTIONAL VALVES:**
a. Inhale and exhale through a surgical mask into the breathing system (each limb individually, if possible).
b. Verify unidirectional flow in each limb.
c. Reconnect tubing firmly.

†16. **TEST FOR LEAKS IN MACHINE AND BREATHING SYSTEM:**
a. Close APL (pop-off) valve and occlude system at patient end.
b. Fill system via O_2 flush until bag is just full, but with negligible pressure in system. Set O_2 flow to 5 L/min.
c. Slowly decrease O_2 flow until pressure *no longer rises* above about 20 cm H_2O. This approximates total leak rate, which should be no greater than a few hundred ml/min. (less for closed circuit techniques). CAUTION: Check valves in some machines make it imperative to measure flow in step c. above when pressure *just stops rising*.
d. Squeeze bag to pressure of about 50 cm H_2O and verify that system is tight.

17. **EXHAUST VALVE AND SCAVENGER SYSTEM:**
a. Open APL valve and observe release of pressure.
b. Occlude breathing system at patient end and verify that negligible positive or negative pressure appears with either zero or 5 L/min. flow and exhaust relief valve (if present) opens with flush flow.

18. **TEST VENTILATOR:**
a. If switching valve is present, test function in both bag and ventilator mode.
b. Close APL valve if necessary and occlude system at patient end.
c. Test for leaks and pressure relief by appropriate cycling (exact procedure will vary with type of ventilator).
d. Attach reservoir bag at mask fitting, fill system and cycle ventilator Assure filling/emptying of bag.

19. **CHECK FOR APPROPRIATE LEVEL OF PATIENT SUCTION.**

20. **CHECK, CONNECT, AND CALIBRATE OTHER ELECTRONIC MONITORS.**

21. **CHECK FINAL POSITION OF ALL CONTROLS.**

22. **TURN ON AND SET OTHER APPROPRIATE ALARMS FOR EQUIPMENT TO BE USED.**
(Perform next two steps as soon as is practical)

23. **SET O_2 MONITOR ALARM LIMITS.**

24 **SET AIRWAY PRESSURE AND/OR VOLUME MONITOR ALARM LIMITS (if adjustable).**

REFERENCES

1. Cooper JB, Newbower RS, and Kitz RJ: An analysis of major error and equipment failures in anesthesia management: consideration for prevention and detection, Anesthesiology 60:34-42, 1984.
2. Cooper JB, Newbower RS, Long CD, and McPeek BJ: Preventable anesthesia mishaps: a study of human factors, Anesthesiology 49:399-406, 1978.
3. Sykes MK: Incidence of mortality and morbidity due to anaesthetic equipment failure, Eur J Anaesthesiol 4:198-199, 1987.
4. Buffington CW, Ramanathan S, and Turndorf H: Detection of anesthesia machine faults, Anesth Analg 63:79-82, 1984.
5. Kumar V, Hintze MS, and Jacob AM: A random survey of anesthesia machines and ancillary monitors in 45 hospitals, Anesth Analg 67:644-649, 1988.
6. American Society for Testing and Materials: Minimum performance and safety requirements for components and systems of anesthesia gas machines F1161-88, Philadelphia, March 1989, ASTM.
7. American National Standards Institute: Minimum performance and safety requirements for components and systems of continuous flow anesthesia machines for human use, ANSI Z79.8-1979, New York, 1979, the Institute.
8. Standards for basic intraoperative monitoring (last amended October 1990; effective Jan 1, 1991), American Society of Anesthesiologists; Park Ridge, Il, 1986.
9. Eichhorn JH: Prevention of intraoperative anesthesia accidents and related severe injury through safety monitoring, Anesthesiology 70:572-577, 1989.
10. Eisenkraft JB: The anesthesia delivery system. In Rogers MC, Tinker JH, and Covino BG, editors: Principles and practice of anesthesiology, St Louis, 1992, Mosby–Year Book, Inc.
11. Dorsch JA and Dorsch SE: Understanding anesthesia equipment, ed 2, Baltimore, 1984, Williams & Wilkins.
12. Petty C: The anesthesia machine, New York, 1987, Churchill Livingstone.
13. Diameter-index safety system, CGA V-5, New York, 1978, Compressed Gas Association, Inc.
14. Compressed gas cylinder valve outlet and inlet connections, CGA V-1, New York, 1977, Compressed Gas Association, Inc.
15. Holland R: Wrong gas disaster in Hong Kong, Anesthesia Patient Safety Foundation Newsletter 4:26, Park Ridge, Ill, Sept 1989, American Society of Anesthesiologists.
16. Eichhorn JH: Medical gas delivery systems, Int Anesthesiol Clin 19:1-26, 1981.
17. Feeley TW, McClelland KJ, and Malhotra IV: The hazards of bulk oxygen delivery systems, Lancet 1:1416, 1975.
18. Sprague DH and Archer GW: Intraoperative hypoxia from an erroneously filled liquid oxygen reservoir, Anesthesiology 42:360, 1975.
19. Gilmour IJ, McComb C, and Palahniuk RJ: Contamination of a hospital oxygen supply, Anesth Analg 71:302-304, 1990.
20. Bowie E and Huffman LM: The anesthesia machine: essentials for understanding, Madison, Wisc, 1986, Ohmeda, The BOC Group, Inc.
21. Heine JF and Adams PM: Another potential failure in an oxygen delivery system, Anesthesiology 63:335-336, 1985.
22. Varga DA, Guttery JS, and Grundy BL: Intermittent oxygen delivery in an Ohmeda Unitrol Anesthesia Machine due to a faulty O-ring check valve assembly, Anesth Analg 66:1200-1201, 1987.
23. Bailey PL: Failed release of an oxygen flush valve, Anesthesiology 59:480, 1983.
24. Sprung J, Samaan F, Hensler T, et al: Excessive airway pressure due to ventilator control valve malfunction during anesthesia for open heart surgery, Anesthesiology 73:1035-1038, 1990.
25. Narkomed 3 anesthesia system, operator's instruction manual, Telford, Penn, 1986, North American Dräger Inc.
26. Modulus II Plus[R] Anesthesia Machine, preoperative checklists, operation and maintenance manual, Madison, Wisc, Oct 1988, Ohmeda, The BOC Group, Inc.
27. Schreiber P: Safety guidelines for anesthesia systems, Telford, Penn, 1985, North American Dräger, Inc.
28. Rau JL and Rau MY: Fundamental respiratory therapy equipment, Sarasota, Fla, 1977, Glenn Educational Medical Series Inc.
29. Parbrook GD, Davis PD, and Parbrook EO: Basic physics and measurement in anesthesia, ed 2, Norwalk, Conn, 1986, Appleton-Century-Crofts.
30. Eger EI II, Hylton RR, Irwin RH, et al: Anesthetic flow meter sequence: a cause for hypoxia, Anesthesiology 24:396, 1963.
31. Williams AR and Hilton PJ: Selective oxygen leak: a potential cause of patient hypoxia, Anaesthesia 41:1133-1134, 1986.
32. Sykes MK, Vickers MD, and Hull CJ: Principles of measurement for anesthetists, Philadelphia, 1981, FA Davis Co.
33. Khahil SN and Neuman J: Failure of an oxygen flow control valve, Anesthesiology, 73:355-356, 1990.
34. Beudoin MG: Oxygen needle valve obstruction, Anaesth Intensive Care 16:130-131, 1988.
35. Rung GW and Schneider AJL: Oxygen flowmeter failure on the North American Dräger Narkomed 2A Anesthesia Machine, Anesth Analg 65:209-213, 1986.
36. Richards C: Failure of a nitrous oxide–oxygen proportioning device, Anesthesiology 71:997-999, 1989.
37. Abraham ZA and Basagoitia J: A potentially lethal anesthesia machine failure, Anesthesiology 66:589-590, 1987.
38. Eisenkraft JB: Vaporizers and vaporization of volatile anesthetics, Prog Anesthesiol, vol 2, no 24, San Antonio, Texas, 1988, 39. Dannemiller Memorial Educational Foundation.
39. Eisenkraft JB: Gas analysis in the operating room, review course lecture manual, 38th annual review course, San Antonio, Texas, Dannemiller Memorial Educational Foundation, 1991.
39a. Benumof JL and Scheller MS: The importance of transtracheal jet ventilation in the management of the difficult airway, Anesthesiology 71:769-778, 1989.
39b. Delaney WA and Kaiser RE: Percutaneous transtracheal jet ventilation made easy, Anesthesiology 74:952, 1991.
40. Capan L. Ramanathan S, Chalon J, et al: A possible hazard with use of the Ohio Ethrane vaporizer, Anesth Analg 59:65, 1980.
41. Ghanooni S, Wilks DH, and Finestone SC: A case report of an unusual disconnection, Anesth Analg 62:696-697, 1983.
42. Magee PT: Anesthetic breathing systems, Prog Anesthesiol, vol 4, chapt 11, San Antonio, Texas, 1990, Dannemiller Memorial Educational Foundation.
43. Sykes MK: Rebreathing circuits, a review, Br J Anaesth 40:666, 1960.
44. Conway CM: Anesthetic breathing systems, Br J Anaesth 57:649, 1985.
45. Eger EI II: Anesthetic systems: construction and function. In Anesthetic uptake and action. Baltimore, 1974, Williams, and Wilkins, 206-227.

46. Bain JA and Spoerel WE: Flow requirements for a modified Mapleson D system during controlled ventilation, Can Anaesth Soc J 20:629, 1973.

47. Seeley HF, Barnes PK, and Conway CM: Controlled ventilation with the Mapleson D system, Br J Anaesth 49:107, 1977.

48. Pethick SL: Correspondence, Can Anaesth Soc J 22:115, 1975.

49. Seed RF: A test for coaxial circuits, Anaesthesia 32:676, 1977.

50. The Sodasorb® manual of carbon dioxide absorption, Lexington, Mass, 1962, Dewey and Almy Chemical Division, of WR Grace & Co).

51. Andrews JJ, Johnston RV, Bee DE, and Arens JF: Photodeactivation of ethyl violet: a potential hazard of Sodasorb,® Anesthesiology 72:59-64, 1990.

52. Tanifuji Y, Takagi MS, Kobayashi K, et al: The interaction between sevoflurane and soda lime or Baralime, Anesth Analg 68:S285, 1989.

53. Ohmeda 7000 Electronic Anesthesia ventilator, service manual, Madison, Wisc, 1985, Ohmeda, The BOC Group Inc.

54. Ohmeda 7810 Electronic Anesthesia ventilator, service manual, Madison, Wisc, 1989, Ohmeda, The BOC Group Inc.

55. Eisenkraft JB: Potential for barotrauma or hypoventilation with the Dräger AV-E ventilator, J Clin Anesth 1:452-456, 1989.

56. Khahil SN, Gholston TK, Binderman J, and Antosh S: Flapper valve malfunction in an Ohio closed scavenging system, Anesth Analg 66:1334-1336, 1987.

57. Sommer RM, Bhalla GS, Jackson JM, and Cohen MI: Hypoventilation caused by ventilator valve rupture, Anesth Analg 67:999-1001, 1988.

58. American Society for Testing and Materials: Standard specification for ventilators intended for use during anesthesia, F1101-90, Philadelphia, May 1990, the Society.

59. Raessler KL, Kretzman WE, and Gravenstein N: Oxygen consumption by anesthesia ventilators, Anesthesiology 69 (3A):A271, 1988.

60. Roth S, Tweedie E, and Sommer RM: Excessive airway pressure due to a malfunctioning anesthesia ventilator, Anesthesiology 65:532, 1986.

61. Gravenstein N, Banner MJ, and McLaughlin G: Tidal volume changes due to the interaction of anesthesia machine and anesthesia ventilator, J Clin Monit 3:187-190, 1987.

62. Scheller MS, Jones BL, and Benumof JL: The influence of fresh gas flow and I:E ratio on tidal volume and arterial PCO_2 in mechanically ventilated surgical patients, J Cardiothorac Anesth 3:564, 1989.

63. Elliott WR, Harris AE, and Philip JH: Positive end-expiratory pressure: implications for tidal volume changes in anesthesia machine ventilation, J Clin Monit 5:100-104, 1989.

64. Pan PH and van der Aa JJ: Anesthesia ventilator performance, delivered tidal volume, and PEEP, Anesthesiology 73(3A):A420, 1990 [abstract].

65. Narkomed 2A anesthesia machine, technical service manual, operating principles, Telford, Penn, 1985, 1989, North American Dräger.

66. Open Reservoir Scavenger operator's instruction manual, Telford, Penn, Telford, Penn, Dec 1986, North American Dräger.

67. Knaack-Steinegger R and Thomson DA: The measurement of expiratory oxygen as a disconnection alarm, Anesthesiology 68. 70:343-344, 1989.

68. Gravenstein JS and Nederstigt JA: Monitoring for disconnection: ventilators with bellows rising on expiration can deliver tidal volumes after disconnection, J Clin Monit 6:207-210, 1990.

69. Feeley TW and Hedley-White J: Bulk oxygen delivery systems: design and dangers, Anesthesiology 44:301-305, 1976.

70. O'Connor CJ and Hobin KF: Bypassing the diameter-indexed safety system, Anesthesiology 71:318-319, 1989.

71. Anderson B and Chamley D: Wall outlet oxygen failure, Anaesth Intensive Care 15:468-469, 1987 [letter].

72. Jawan B and Lee JH: Cardiac arrest caused by an incorrectly filled oxygen cylinder: a case report, Br J Anaesth 64:749-751, 1990.

73. Bonsu AK and Stead AL: Accidental cross-connexion of oxygen and nitrous oxide in an anaesthetic machine, Anaesthesia 38:767-769, 1983.

74. Heath ML: Accidents associated with equipment, Anaesthesia 39:57-60, 1984.

75. Lacoumenta S and Hall GM: A burst oxygen pipeline, Anaesthesia 38:596-597, 1983 [letter].

76. Carley RH, Houghton IT, and Park GR: A near disaster from piped gases, Anaesthesia 39:891-893, 1984.

77. Williams AR and Hilton PJ: Selective oxygen leak: a potential cause of patient hypoxia, Anaesthesia 41:1133-1134, 1986.

78. Hanning CD, Kruchek D, and Chunara A: Preferential oxygen leak: an unusual case, Anaesthesia 42:1329-1330, 1987 [letter].

79. Moore JK and Railton R: Hypoxia caused by a leaking rotameter: the value of an oxygen analyser, Anaesthesia 39:380-381, 1984, [letter].

80. Cole AG, Thompson JB, Fodor IM, et al: Anaesthetic machine hazard from the Selectatec block, Anaesthesia 38:175-177, 1983 [letter].

81. Goodyear CM: Failure of nitrous oxide–oxygen proportioning device, Anesthesiology 72:397-398, 1990.

82. Rossiter SK: An unexpected disconnection of the gas supply to a Cape Waine 3 ventilator, Anaesthesia 38:180-180, 1983 [letter].

83. Henshaw J: Circle system disconnection, Anaesth Intensive Care 16:240-240, 1988 [letter].

84. Horan BF: Unusual disconnection, Anaesth Intensive Care 15:466-467, 1987 [letter].

85. Ripp CH and Chapin JW: A bellow's leak in an Ohio anesthesia ventilator, Anesth Analg 64:942-942, 1985 [letter].

86. Spoor J: Ventilator malfunction, Anaesth Intensive Care 14:329-329, 1986 [letter].

87. Berner MS: Profound hypercapnia due to disconnection within an anaesthetic machine, Can J Anaesth 34:622-626, 1987.

88. McQuillan PJ and Jackson IJ: Potential leaks from anaesthetic machines: potential leaks through open rotameter valves and empty cylinder yokes, Anaesthesia 42:1308-1312, 1987.

89. Bamber PA: Safety hazard with cylinder yoke on a Boyle's machine, Anaesthesia 41:1260-1262, 1986 [letter].

90. Jablonski J and Reynolds AC: A potential cause (and cure) of a major gas leak, Anesthesiology 62:842-843, 1985 [letter].

91. Jove F and Milliken RA: Loss of anesthetic gases due to defective safety equipment, Anesth Analg 62:369-370, 1983 [letter].

92. Pyles ST, Kaplan RF, and Munson ES: Gas loss from Ohio Modulus Vaporizer Selector-Interlock Valve, Anesth Analg 62:1052-1052, 1983, [letter].

93. Sara CA and Wark HJ: Disconnection: an appraisal, Anaesth Intensive Care 14(4):448-452, 1986.

94. Eisenkraft JB and Sommer RM: Flapper valve malfunction, Anesth Analg 66:1131, 1988.

95. Poulton TJ: Unusual corrugated tubing leak, Anesth Analg 65:1365-1365, 1986 [letter].
96. Nelson RA and Snowdon SL: Failure of an adjustable pressure limiting valve, Anaesthesia 44:788-789, 1989 [letter].
97. Cooper MG, Vouden J, and Rigg D: Circuit leaks, Anaesth Intensive Care 15: 359-360, 1987 [letter].
98. Hutchinson BR: An unusual leak, Anaesth Intensive Care 15:355-355, 1987 [letter].
99. Ferderbar PJ, Kettler RE, Jablonski J, and Sportiello R: A cause of breathing system leak during closed circuit anesthesia, Anesthesiology 65:661-663, 1986.
100. Raja SN and Geller H: Another potential source of a major gas leak, Anesthesiology 64:297-298, 1986.
101. Brown MR, Burris WR, and Hilley MD: Breathing circuit mishap resulting from Y-piece disintegration, Anesthesiology 69:436-437, 1988 [letter].
102. Colavita RD and Apfelbaum JL: An unusual source of leak in the anesthesia circuit, Anesthesiology 62:208-209, 1985 [letter].
103. Lamarche Y: Anaesthetic breathing circuit leak from cracked oxygen analyzer sensor connector, Can Anaesth Soc J 32:682-683, 1985 [letter].
104. Miller DC, Collins JW, and Wallace L: Failure of the expiratory valve on a Bain system, Anaesthesia 43:992-992, 1988 [letter].
105. Robblee JA, Crosby E, and Keon WJ: Hypoxemia after intraluminal oxygen line obstruction during cardiopulmonary bypass, Ann Thorac Surg 48:575-576, 1989 [see comments therein].
106. Wan YL and Swan M: Exotic obstruction, Anaesth Intensive Care 18:274-274, 1990 [letter].
107. Boscoe MJ and Baxter RC: Failure of anaesthetic gas supply, Anaesthesia 38:997-998, 1983 [letter].
108. Hogan TS: Selectatec switch malfunction, Anaesthesia 40:66-69, 1985.
109. Milliken RA and Bizzarri DV: An unusual cause of failure of anesthetic gas delivery to a patient circuit, Anesth Analg 63:1047-1048, 1984 [letter].
110. Ghani GA: Fresh gas flow affects minute volume during mechanical ventilation, Aneth Analg 63:619-619, 1984.
111. Birch AA and Fisher NA: Leak of soda lime seal after anesthesia machine check, J Clin Anesth 1:474-476, 1989 [letter].
112. Nunn JF: Carbon dioxide cylinders on anaesthetic apparatus, Br J Anaesth 65:15-156, 1990 [editorial].
113. Razis PA: Carbon dioxide: a survey of its use in anaesthesia in the U.K., Anaesthesia 44:348-351, 1989.
114. Sims C and Cullingford DW: Kinking of the Mera-F-Circuit, Anaesth Intensive Care 16:243-243, 1988 [letter].
115. Hewitt AJ and Campbell W: Unusual damage to a Bain system, Anaesthesia 41:882-883, 1986 [letter].
116. Neufeld PD, Walker EA, and Johnson DL: Survey on breathing system disconnexions, Anaesthesia 41:438-439, 1986 [letter].
117. Goldman JM and Phelps RW: No flow anesthesia, Anesth Analg 66:1337-1347, 1987.
118. Koga Y, Iwatsuki N. Takahashi M, and Hashimoto Y: A hazardous defect in a humidifier, Anesth Analg 71:712, 1990.
119. Schroff PK and Skerman JH: Humidifier malfunction: a cause of anesthesia circuit occlusion, Anesth Analg 67:710-711, 1988.
120. Spurring PW and Small LFG: Breathing circuit disconnections and misconnections, Anaesthesia 38:683-688, 1983.
121. Arellano R, Ross D, and Lee K: Inappropriate attachment of PEEP valve causing total obstruction of ventilation bag, Anesth Analg 6:1050-1051, 1987.
122. Anagnostou JM, Hults S, and Moorthy SS: PEEP valve barotrauma, Anesth Analg 70:674-675, 1990.
123. Sharrock NE and Leith DE: Potential pulmonary barotrauma when venting anesthetic gases to suction, Anesthesiology 46:152-154, 1977.
124. Mushlin PS, Mark JB, Elliott WR, et al: Inadvertent development of subatmospheric airway pressure during cardiopulmonary by-pass, Anesthesiology 712: 459-462, 1989.
125. McEwen JA, Small CF, and Jenkins LC: Detection of interruptions in the breathing gas of ventilated anaesthetized patients, Can J Anaesth 35:549-561, 1988.
126. Raphael DT, Weller RS, and Doran DJ: A response algorithm for the low pressure alarm condition, Anesth Analg 67:876-883, 1988.
127. Slee TA and Pavlin EG: Failure of a low pressure alarm associated with use of a humidifier, Anesthesiology 69:791-793, 1988.
128. Choi JJ, Guida J, and Wu W-H: Hypoventilatory hazard of an anesthetic scavenging device, Anesthesiology 65:126-127, 1986.
129. Lanier WL: Intraoperative air entrainment with an Ohio Modulus Anesthesia Machine, Anesthesiology 64:266-268, 1986.
129a. Baraka A and Muallem M: Awareness during anaesthesia due to a ventilator malfunction, Anaesthesia 34:678-679, 1979.
129b. Waterman PM, Pautler S, and Smith RB: Accidental ventilator induced hyperventilation, Anesthesiology 48:141, 1978.
129c. Longmuir J and Craig DB: Inadvertent increase in inspired oxygen concentration due to defect in ventilator bellows, Can Anaesth Soc J 23:327-329, 1976.
130. Dean HN, Parsons DE, and Raphaely RC: Bilateral tension pneumothorax from mechanical failure of anesthesia machine due to misplaced expiratory valve, Anesth Analg 50:195-198, 1971.
131. Sears BE and Bocar ND: Pneumothorax resulting from a closed anesthesia ventilator port, Anesthesiology 47:311-313, 1977.
132. Henzig D: Insidious PEEP from a defective ventilator gas evacuation outlet valve, Anesthesiology 57:251-252, 1982.
133. Pressure Limit Control, Operator's instruction manual, Telford, Penn, 1988, North American Dräger.
134. Kopriva CJ and Lowenstein E: An anesthetic accident: cardiovascular collapse from liquid halothane delivery, Anesthesiology 30:246, 1969.
135. Tec 5 Continuous flow vaporizer, operation and maintenance manual, Steeton, UK, 1989, Ohmeda.
136. Tec 4 Continuous flow vaporizer, operation manual, V5, Steeton, UK, 1987, Ohmeda.
137. Operator's manual, Dräger 19.1 Vaporizer, Lübeck, FDR, 1986, Drägerwerk AG.
138. Bruce DL and Linde HW: Vaporization of mixed anesthetic liquids, Anesthesiology 60:342-346, 1984.
139. Chilcoat RT: Hazards of mis-filled vaporizers: summary tables, Anesthesiology 63:726-727, 1985.
140. Riegle EV and Desertspring D: Failure of the agent-specific filling device, Anesthesiology 73:353-354, 1990.
141. Korman B and Ritchie IM: Chemistry of halothane-enflurane mixtures applied to anesthesia, Anesthesiology 63:152-156, 1985.
142. Murray WJ, Zsigmond EK, and Fleming P: Contamination of in-series vaporizers with halothane-methoxyflurane, Anesthesiology 38:487, 1973.
143. Dorsch SE and Dorsch JA: Chemical cross-contamination between vaporizers in series, Anesth Analg 52:176-180, 1973.
144. Silvasi DL, Haynes A, and Brown ACD: Potentially

lethal failure of the vapor exclusion system, Anesthesiology 71:289-291, 1990.

145. Cudmore J and Keogh J: Another Selectatec switch malfunction, Anaesthesia 45:754-756, 1990.

146. Marks WE and Bullard JR: Another hazard of free-standing vaporizers: increased anesthetic concentration with reversed flow of vaporizing gas, Anesthesiology 45:445, 1976.

147. Beebe JJ and Sessler DI: Preparation of anesthesia machines for patients susceptible to malignant hyperthermia, Anesthesiology 69:395-400, 1988.

148. Cooper JB and Philip JH: More on anesthesia machines and malignant hyperthermia, Anesthesiology 70:561-562, 1989.

149. Rao CC, Brandl R, and Mashak JN: Modification of Ohmeda Excel 210 anesthesia machine for use during MRI, Anesthesiology 71(3A):A365, 1989 [abstract].

150. Rao CC, Krishna G, and Emhardt J: Anesthesia machine for use during MRI, Anesthesiology 73:1054-1055, 1990.

151. Munshi C, Dhamee S, Bardeen-Henschel A, and Dhuruva S: Recognition of mixed anesthetic agents by mass spectrometer during anesthesia, J Clin Monit 2:121-124, 1986.

152. Bickler PE and Sessler DI: Efficiency of airway heat and moisture exchangers in anesthetized humans, Anesth Analg 71:415-418, 1990 .

153. Turner DA and Wright EM: Efficiency of heat and moisture exchangers, Anaesthesia 42:1117-1119, 1987 [letter].

154. Bengtsson M and Johnson A: Failure of a heat and moisture exchanger as a cause of disconnection during anaesthesia, Acta Anaesthesiol Scand 33:522-523, 1989.

155. Prasad KK and Chen L: Complications related to the use of a heat and moisture exchanger, Anesthesiology 72:958-958, 1990.

156. Ward CF, Reisner LS, and Zlott LS: Murphy's law and humidification, Anesth Analg 62:460-461, 1983.

157. Shroff PK and Skerman JH: Humidifier malfunction: a cause of anesthesia circuit occlusion, Anesth Analg 67:710-711, 1988 [letter].

158. Operators manual, North American Dräger Narkomed 2B, Telford, Penn, 1988, North American Dräger.

159. Greenhalgh DL and Thomas WA: Blackout during cardiopulmonary bypass, Anaesthesia 45:175-175, 1990 [letter].

160. Welch RH and Feldman JM: Anesthesia during total electrical failure, or what would you do if the lights went out? J Clin Anesth 1:358-362, 1989.

161. Crosby WM: Checking the anesthetic machine, drugs, and monitoring devices, Anaesth Intensive Care 16:32-35, 1988.

162. Food and Drug Administration: Anesthesia apparatus checkout recommendations, Rockville, Md, 1986, FDA.

163. Lees DE: Old anesthesia equipment target of study, panel, Anesthesia Patient Safety Foundation Newsletter 4:13-51, Park Ridge, Ill, 1989, American Society of Anesthesiologists.

164. Annual report, ASA Committee on Equipment and Standards, Sept 1989.

165. New Jersey register: Subchapter 18: Anesthesia 21 N.J.R. 503-504, Feb 21, 1989.

Chapter 6

Complications of Drugs Used in Anesthesia

Jonathan M. Anagnostou
Robert K. Stoelting

This chapter is a compilation of side effects of drugs commonly encountered in anesthetic practice. The purpose is not to restate the pharmacology of these drugs but rather to concentrate on their properties, which could be detrimental to the patient. Clearly, a certain pharmacologic effect that might be quite acceptable in one clinical circumstance could be undesirable in another. For example, the increase in heart rate seen with pancuronium might be acceptable in an otherwise healthy young adult, whereas this same effect (that is, tachycardia) in an elderly patient with severe atherosclerotic coronary artery disease could lead to myocardial ischemia.

The layout of this chapter consists of complimentary parts. Tables 6-1 and 6-2 list adverse effects and drug interactions and serve as rapid reference tools, and the accompanying text provides additional detail and explanation of the material presented in the tables. For certain drugs, refer to the appropriate chapter for more detailed explanations, though many important adverse effects are listed in the tables for rapid reference (Tables 6-1 and 6-2).

I. INHALATIONAL ANESTHETICS
A. Volatile drugs

Although many of the side effects of the volatile drugs are quite similar, clinically significant differences between these drugs do exist. These differences are best illustrated by comparisons at equivalent minimum alveolar concentrations (MAC), and statements regarding qualitative differences between agents are made with this understanding. (For a discussion of the hepatotoxic complications of the volatile anesthetics see Chapter 18.)

1. Central nervous system complications. While isoflurane causes electrical silence on the EEG at concentrations over 2 MAC[1,2] enflurane causes high voltage and high frequency rates of activity on the EEG, which may progress to spike-and-wave activity, especially at concentrations greater than 2 MAC and during periods of hyperventilation to Paco$_2$ of less than 30 mm Hg.[3] This may accompany myoclonic patient movements indistinguishable from seizures. This enflurane "seizure activity" may be enhanced by amitriptyline.[4]

Cerebral blood flow (CBF) may be increased by all the volatile drugs, with halothane causing the greatest increase and isoflurane the least.[5] The administration of 1.1 MAC of halothane during controlled ventilation to a Paco$_2$ of 40 mm Hg causes a 200% increase in CBF. The same 1.1 MAC of enflurane causes a 50% to 60% increase, whereas CBF does not increase under isoflurane anesthesia until concentrations of greater than 1.1 MAC are administered. Increases in intracranial pressure parallel the rises in CBF. These effects may be blunted by hyper-

Text continued on p. 137.

Table 6-1. Drug complications

Pharmaceutical class	Drug	Complications and potentially adverse effects
Inhalational anesthetics	Halothane	Myocardial depression, hypotension, dysrhythmias respiratory depression, hepatotoxicity increased intracranial pressure, uterine relaxation
	Enflurane	Myocardial depression, hypotension, tachycardia, dysrhythmias, respiratory depression, "seizures" increased intracranial pressure, nephrotoxicity, hepatotoxicity, uterine relaxation
	Isoflurane	Vasodilatation, hypotension, myocardial depression, tachycardia, dysrhythmias, respiratory depression increased intracranial pressure, ?hepatotoxicity, uterine relaxation
	Nitrous oxide	Expansion of closed spaces in the body, increased intracranial pressure, decreased hypoxic respiratory drive, myocardial depression, increased pulmonary artery pressures, megaloblastic anemia, neurotoxicity (chronic exposure)
Intravenous anesthetics	Barbiturates	Hypotension, vasodilatation, tachycardia, respiratory depression, phlebitis, tissue damage with extravasation or arterial injection
	Benzodiazepines	Respiratory depression, vasodilatation, amnesia, phlebitis and pain on injection (diazepam)
	Propofol	Hypotension, heart block, pain on injection, myoclonus, hiccups
	Etomidate	Pain on injection, myoclonus, activation of seizure foci, adrenal suppression, nausea
	Ketamine	Tachycardia, dysrhythmias, increased secretions, increased intracranial pressure, emergence delirium, transient cortical blindness, flashbacks
Drugs used in psychiatric disorders	Phenothiazines and butyrophenones	Dry mouth, blurred vision, urinary retention, tachycardia, orthostatic hypotension, heart blocks, arrhythmias, disorientation, dysphoria, impaired thermoregulation, lowered seizure threshold, neuroleptic malignant syndrome
	Tricyclics	Dry mouth, nausea, tremor, seizures, dysrhythmias, orthostatic hypotension
	MAOIs	Orthostatic hypotension, hepatotoxicity, seizures, fever
Opioid agonist drugs	Morphine	Respiratory depression, nausea, vasodilatation, hypotension, bradycardia, biliary spasm, urinary retention, delayed gastric emptying
	Meperidine	Respiratory depression, cardiovascular depression, hypotension, tachycardia, biliary spasm, nausea
	Fentanyl	Respiratory depression, chest wall rigidity, bradycardia
	Sufentanil	Similar to fentanyl, hypotension
	Alfentanyl	Similar to fentanyl, hypotension
Opioid antagonist drug	Naloxone	Hypertension, tachycardia, dysrhythmias, pulmonary edema, nausea and vomiting
Opioid agonist-antagonists	Butorphenol	Respiratory depression, diaphoresis, nausea, dysphoria, increased pulmonary artery pressures
	Nalbuphine	Respiratory depression, dizziness, nausea
	Pentazocine	Respiratory depression, dysphoria, nausea, tachycardia, increased pulmonary artery pressures, hypertension
	Buprenorphine	Respiratory depression, nausea, cardiovascular effects similar to morphine

Table 6-1—cont'd. Drug complications

Pharmaceutical class	Drug	Complications and potentially adverse effects
Local anesthetics	All	Tinnitus, agitation, blurred vision, drowsiness, seizures, coma, cardiovascular collapse Ester local anesthetics—cross-sensitivity to PABA
	Lidocaine	Arteriolar vasodilatation, myocardial depression, heart blocks, respiratory depression
	Mepivicaine	Similar to lidocaine, fetal depression
	Bupivicaine	Cardiotoxicity, lesser margin between central nervous system and cardiac toxicity
	Prilocaine	Methemoglobinemia
	Etidocaine	Similar to bupivacaine
	Chloroprocaine	Neurotoxicity with subarachnoid use (? drug versus preservative)
	Cocaine	Tachycardia, hypertension, myocardial ischemia, dysrhythmias, agitation
	Tetracaine	? Relatively high intravenous toxicity for anesthetic potency
	Benzocaine	Methemoglobinemia
Depolarizing relaxant	Succinylcholine	Increased intracranial and intraocular pressures, myalgias, hyperkalemia, myoglobinuria, dysrhythmias, sustained muscle contractions, triggering of malignant hyperthermia
Nondepolarizing relaxants	All	Respiratory embarrassment (incomplete reversal)
	d-Tubocurarine	Vasodilatation, histamine release, hypotension
	Metocurine	Similar to *d*-tubocurarine but of lesser magnitude
	Pancuronium	Tachycardia, hypertension, dysrhythmias
	Gallamine	Pronounced tachycardia, dysrhythmias
	Atracurium	Histamine release, vasodilatation, hypotension
	Vecuronium	Potentiation of opoiod-induced bradycardia
Cholinesterase inhibitors	All	Bradycardia, heart blocks, vasodilatation, salivation, abdominal cramping, bronchoconstriction, skeletal muscle weakness (high doses)
	Physostigmine	Agitation
Anticholinergic drugs	Atropine	Bradycardia (low dose), tachycardia, dysrhythmias, photophobia, blurred vision, urinary retention, dry skin, fever, mental status changes, thickening of bronchial secretions, increased intraocular pressure (in narrow-angle glaucoma), central anticholinergic syndrome
	Scopolamine	Similar to atropine, except produces sedation and amnesia
	Glycopyrrolate	Similar to atropine, but less tachycardia and no central nervous system effects
	Ipratropium	Systemic effects rare (not absorbed with inhalation)
Catecholamines	Epinephrine	Tachycardia, dysrhythmias, myocardial ischemia, hyperglycemia, hypertension
	Norepinephrine	Hypertension, peripheral ischemia, dysrhythmias, tissue necrosis with extravasation
	Isoproterenol	Tachycardia, dysrhythmias, vasodilatation, hypotension, myocardial ischemia

Continued.

Table 6-1—cont'd. Drug complications

Pharmaceutical class	Drug	Complications and potentially adverse effects
	Dopamine	Hypotension (low dose), tachycardia, dysrhythmias, myocardial ischemia, peripheral ischemia (high dose), tissue necrosis with extravasation, hypertension, nausea and vomiting
	Dobutamine	Tachycardia, dysrhythmias, hypotension, nausea, headache, muscle tremors
Noncatecholamine inotropes	Amrinone	Vasodilatation, hypotension, gastrointestinal upset, thrombocytopenia
	Milrinone	Vasodilatation, hypotension
	Digitalis	Dysrhythmias, heart blocks, myocardial and bowel ischemia, nausea and vomiting, visual disturbances, mental status changes, tissue irritation on extravasation
	Ephedrine	Similar to epinephrine but less severe, also tremor, agitation
	Mephentermine	Similar to ephedrine, decreases uterine blood flow in the parturient
	Metaraminol	Hypertension, bradycardia, hypotension if prolonged infusion is abruptly stopped
Selective beta$_2$-adrenergic receptor agonists	All	Tachycardia, dysrhythmias, hypokalemia; when used in premature labor, may also cause hypertension, pulmonary edema, worsening of diabetic control
Vasopressors	Phenylephrine	Hypertension, bradycardia
	Methoxamine	Similar to phenylephrine, decreased renal perfusion
Vasodilators	Nitroprusside	Hypotension, tachycardia, myocardial ischemia, nausea, restlessness, intracranial hypertension, hypoxemia Cyanide toxicity—metabolic acidosis Thiocyanate toxicity—tinnitus, mental status changes, muscle spasms, convulsions
	Nitroglycerin	Hypotension, headache, methemoglobinemia, hypoxemia
	Hydralazine	Hypotension, tachycardia, headache, cutaneous flushing, lupuslike syndrome
	Minoxidil	Similar to hydralazine, pericardial effusion, no lupuslike syndrome
	Diazoxide	Hypotension, tachycardia, myocardial ischemia, hyperglycemia, pain on extravasation
	Adenosine	Hypotension, heart blocks
Beta-adrenergic receptor blockers	Nonselective (e.g., propranolol)	Bradycardia, hypotension, bronchospasm, congestive heart failure (susceptible patients), Raynaud's phenomenon; exacerbation of hypoglycemia in diabetics; lethargy, fatigue
	Nadolol	As above, except lesser central nervous system problems
	Pindolol	As above, except less bradycardia; hypertension (higher doses)
	Timolol	As above; eye drops may cause intraoperative bradycardia
	Selective beta$_1$ (e.g., metoprolol)	As for nonselective beta blockers, but bronchospasm, Raynaud's phenomenon, and exacerbation of hypoglycemia in diabetics less likely

Table 6-1—cont'd. Drug complications

Pharmaceutical class	Drug	Complications and potentially adverse effects
Alpha-adrenergic receptor blockers	Phentolamine	Vasodilatation, hypotension, tachycardia, dysrhythmias, myocardial ischemia, abdominal pain, diarrhea
	Phenoxybenzamine	As for phentolamine,
	Prazosin	As for phentolamine, but less tachycardia; also dry mouth, lethargy, vertigo, syncope (especially first dose)
Mixed adrenergic blocker	Labetalol	Bradycardia, hypotension, fatigue, nausea, bronchospasm
Ganglionic blocker	Trimethaphan	Vasodilatation, hypotension, tachycardia, urinary retention, ileus, histamine release (high doses)
Central sympatholytics	Clonidine	Sedation, dry mouth, skin rash, constipation, rebound hypertension on abrupt discontinuation
	Methyldopa	Sedation, hepatotoxicity, anemia, orthostatic hypotension, rebound hypertension
	Reserpine	Dry mouth, sedation, orthostatic hypotension, bradycardia
Calcium-channel blockers	Verapamil	Myocardial depression, hypotension, heart blocks, dizziness, nausea, headache, hepatotoxicity, accelerated heart rate (in preexcitation syndromes)
	Nifedepine	Vasodilatation, hypotension, tachycardia, myocardial depression, rebound hypertension and angina
	Diltiazem	Bradycardia, hypotension, myocardial depression
Histamine-1 (H_1) blockers	All	Sedation, dizziness, dry mouth, tachycardia, seizures, hypotension (rapid intravenous injection)
	Promethazine	As above, plus tissue necrosis on extravasation or arterial injection
Histamine-2 (H_2) blockers	Cimetidine	Sedation, confusion, coma, hypotension (intravenous injection), bradycardia, heart block (intravenous injection), nephritis, neutropenia, thrombocytopenia
	Ranitidine	As for cimetidine, except no heart blocks, central nervous system effects
	Famotidine	As for ranitidine
Antacids	Aluminum hydroxide	Constipation, hypophosphatemia, nephrolithiasis, hypomagnesemia, aluminum toxicity (in renal failure), granulumatous reaction if aspirated
	Calcium carbonate	Hypercalcemia, hyperphosphatemia, acid rebound, milk-alkali syndrome, granulomatous reaction if aspirated, metabolic alkalosis
	Sodium bicarbonate	Metabolic alkalosis, sodium overload (in congestive heart failure)
	Sodium citrate	Poor taste, damage if aspirated less than particulate antacids
Diuretics	Furosemide	Vasodilatation, hypotension, hypovolemia, hyponatremia, hypokalemia, ototoxicity, interstitial nephritis, hyperuricemia
	Ethacrinic acid	As for furosemide except increased ototoxicity
	Thiazides	Hypochloremia, hypokalemia, hyperuricemia, metabolic alkalosis, hyperglycemia, thrombocytopenia, rashes
	Spironolactone	Hyperkalemia, nausea

Continued.

Table 6-1—cont'd. Drug complications

Pharmaceutical class	Drug	Complications and potentially adverse effects
	Thiazides	Hypochloremia, hypokalemia, hyperuricemia, metabolic alkalosis, hyperglycemia, thrombocytopenia, rashes
	Spironolactone	Hyperkalemia, nausea
	Mannitol	Hyponatremia, transient intravascular fluid shift
	Urea	As for mannitol; venous thrombosis, tissue necrosis if extravasated
	Acetazolamide	Drowziness, metabolic acidosis, rashes, paresthesias
Anticoagulants	Heparin	Bleeding, thrombocytopenia, cutaneous necrosis, paradoxical hypercoagulability, neuropathy, alopecia
	Coumarin	Bleeding, teratogenicity, skin necrosis
	Protamine	Histamine release, vasodilatation, hypotension, bronchoconstriction, tachycardia, increased pulmonary artery pressure
Thrombolytics	Streptokinase	Bleeding, fever, allergic reactions
	Urokinase and tissue plasminogen activators	As for streptokinase except less allergic responses
Antiplatelet drugs	Aspirin	Prolonged elevated bleeding times, tinnitus, nausea, confusion, hyperventilation
	Dipyridamole	Dizziness, headache, abdominal distress, rashes, vasodilatation and hypotension (intravenous injection)
	Dextrans	Anaphylaxis, acute renal failure (dextran 40), bleeding diathesis (dextran 70)
Antidysrhythmic drugs	Lidocaine	See under Local Anesthetics
	Verapamil	See under Calcium Entry Blockers
	Adenosine	See under Vasodilators
	Procainamide	Vasodilatation, hypotension, heart block, myocardial depression, fever, agranulocytosis, lupus-like syndrome, muscle weakness (myasthenics)
	Quinidine	Gastrointestinal disturbances, ventricular dysrhythmias, hypotension, tinnitus, vertigo, fever, thrombocytopenia, hepatotoxicity
	Bretylium	Tachycardia, hypertension, bradycardia, hypotension, nausea and vomiting
	Phenytoin	Nystagmus, dizziness, hypotension, heart blocks, asystole, gingival hyperplasia, hepatitis, hyperglycemia, rashes, peripheral neuropathy, anemia
	Disopyramide	Myocardial depression, heart blocks, dry mouth, urinary retention
	Amiodarone	Bradycardia, heart blocks, vasodilatation, hypotension, thyroid dysfunction, hepatotoxicity, neuropathy
Antibiotics	Penicillins and cephalosporins	Skin rashes, angioedema, anaphylaxis, up to 10% incidence of cross-reactivity
	Aminoglycosides	Ototoxicity, nephrotoxicity, skeletal muscle weakness
	Vancomycin	Bronchospasm, hypotension, flushing, ototoxicity, nephrotoxicity, ?myocardial depression
	Amphotericin B	Fever, hypotension, nephrotoxicity, hypokalemia, thrombocytopenia, anemia, seizures

Table 6-1—cont'd. Drug complications

Pharmaceutical class	Drug	Complications and potentially adverse effects
Miscellaneous drugs	Metoclopromide	Abdominal cramps, restlessness, extrapyramidal reactions, sedation, dysphoria, rashes
	Theophylline	Nausea and vomiting, headache, agitation, tachycardia, dysrhythmias, seizures
	Pentoxifylline	Dysrhythmias, hypotension, angina
	Doxapram	Hypertension, tachycardia, vomiting, fever, convulsions
	Dantrolene	Dizziness, nausea, diarrhea, sedation, skeletal muscle weakness, hepatitis

Table 6-2. Selected drug interactions

Drug	Combination	Adverse interaction
Volatile anesthetic	Nitrous oxide Opioids (including agonist-antagonists) Benzodiazepines Lidocaine Clonidine Methyldopa Reserpine	Increased depth of anesthesia (i.e., decrease in minimum alveolar concentration, MAC)
	Epinephrine and other beta-adrenergic receptor agonists	Dysrhythmias greatest with halothane
	Beta-adrenergic receptor blockers Calcium-channel blockers	Myocardial depression
	Timolol ophthalmic	Intraoperative bradycardia
	Amiodarone	Bradycardia, heart blocks
Halothane	Theophylline Pancuronium plus a tricyclic antidepressant	Dysrhythmias
Nitrous oxide	Opioids	Myocardial depression
Barbiturates	Central nervous system depressants	Increased respiratory depression
Benzodiazepines	Central nervous system depressants	Increased respiratory depression
	Alcohol	Increased absorption
	Opioids (high dose)	Myocardial depression
Diazepam	Cimetidine	Decreased diazepam clearance
Ketamine	Tricyclic antidepressants	Hypertension dysrhythmias
	Halothane	Hypertension, dysrhythmias Hypotension (myocardial depression)
Antipsychotics	Opioids	Potentiation of opioid sedation
Tricyclic antidepressants	Opioids	Potentiation of opioid sedation
	Halothane plus pancuronium Ketamine	Hypertension, dysrhythmias

Continued.

Table 6-2. Selected drug interactions—cont'd

Drug	Combination	Adverse interaction
Monoamine oxidase inhibitors (MAOIs)	Succinylcholine	Prolonged muscle relaxation
	Barbituates Opioids Alcohol	Increased sedation
	Meperidine (?other opioids)	Hypertension, seizures, hyperpyrexia
	Sympathomimetics	Exaggerated sympathomimetic response
Naloxone	Opioids	Hypertension, dysrhythmias, pulmonary edema ("sudden arousal")
Opioid agonist-antagonists	Opioids	Blunting of opioid analgesia
	Opioids (in physical dependency)	Precipitation of opioid withdrawal
Local anesthetics	Neuromuscular blockers	Enhanced muscle relaxation
Succinylcholine	Halothane	Classical malignant hyperthermia triggering combination
	Cholinesterase inhibitors Echothiophate, isoflurophate (ophthalmic) Trimethaphan Cyclophosphamide	Prolonged neuromuscular block
Nondepolarizing neuromuscular blockers	Aminoglycoside antibiotics	Enhanced muscle relaxation
Pancuronium	Digoxin	Dysrhythmias
Vecuronium	Potent opioids (sufentanil, fentanyl)	?Enhanced opioid bradycardia
Beta-adrenergic receptor agonists	Digoxin	Dysrhythmias
Dopamine	Bretylium	Hypertension on initiating bretylium
	Phenytoin	Hypotension
Sympathomimetics—direct acting	Reserpine	Enhanced symathomimetic effect
Verapamil	Beta-adrenergic receptor blockers Digoxin	Heart blocks
	Carbamazepine Oral hypoglycemic agents	Enhanced toxicity
Calcium-channel blockers	Neuromuscular blockers	Enhanced muscle relaxation
Promethazine	Opioids	Enhanced sedation
Cimetidine	Lidocaine, propranolol, diazepam, other hepatically metabolized drugs	Decreased elimination of other drug
Furosemide	Lithium compounds	Elevated lithium levels
	Neuromuscular blockers	Enhanced muscle relaxation
	Sulfonamides	Allergic cross-sensitivity

Table 6-2. Selected drug interactions—cont'd

Drug	Combination	Adverse interaction
Heparin	Certain protein-bound drugs (e.g., diazepam, propranolol)	Elevated free plasma levels of other drug
Coumarin	Salicylates, phenylbutazone	Increased bleeding diathesis
Protamine	NPH-insulin, ?fish	Allergic cross-sensitivity
Procainamide	Neuromuscular blockers	Enhanced muscle relaxation
Quinidine	Neuromuscular blockers	Enhanced muscle relaxation
Amiodarone	Digoxin	Increased digoxin blood levels
	Volatile anesthetics	Bradycardia, sinus arrest
Aminoglycosides	Neuromuscular blockers	Enhanced muscle relaxation
Metoclopramide	Opioids Anticholinergics	Impairment of metoclopramide's gastric emptying effect

ventilation to a $Paco_2$ of 30 mm Hg; however, it appears that in the case of halothane the hyperventilation must precede the administration of the drug to be effective.[6] In patients with intracranial tumors, significant increases in intracranial pressure occurring with the administration of isoflurane despite hyperventilation have been reported.[7]

2. Cardiovascular complications. In the absence of surgical stimulation, blood pressure decreases with all the volatile drugs, albeit by different mechanisms.[5] Isoflurane causes a decrease in peripheral vascular resistance while (at less than 2 MAC) cardiac output is maintained with a decrease in stroke volume and an increase in heart rate. Halothane causes a decrease in blood pressure because of depression of cardiac output with little change in peripheral resistance. Enflurane produces a decrease in both cardiac output and peripheral resistance while causing a dose-dependent increase in heart rate. The volatile agents may "sensitize" the heart to the cardiac dysrhythmic effects of epinephrine, with halothane being the most "sensitizing" and isoflurane the least.[8] (See also Chapter 10 for a discussion of the arrhythmogenic properties of the volatile anesthetics.)

It has been suggested that isoflurane may produce a coronary steal syndrome in patients with coronary artery disease by dilating nondiseased coronary vessels and thereby diverting flow from ischemic areas of myocardium.[9] Although it seems possible for this to occur, isoflurane may actually improve tolerance to pacing-induced ischemia,[10] and if hemodynamic factors effecting myocardial oxygen balance are controlled (that is, heart rate and blood pressure), ischemia is not a problem for the majority of patients with coronary artery disease receiving isoflurane during anesthesia.[11,12]

3. Renal complications. Methoxyflurane and enflurane are metabolized in the body to produce fluoride ions. Free fluoride ions may be toxic to the kidney, with renal dysfunction manifesting as a decreased concentrating ability.[13] Prolonged enflurane anesthesia (9.6 hours at 1 MAC) may produce a renal concentrating defect,[14] but a shorter exposure (2.7 hours at 1 MAC) does not.[15] Methoxyflurane metabolism produces fluoride in potentially nephrotoxic concentrations after lesser dose exposure than enflurane does.[13] Halothane[14] and isoflurane[16] are not metabolized to fluoride in amounts great enough to be nephrotoxic.

4. Uterine complications. All the volatile inhalational agents produce uterine relaxation, which may increase intraoperative uterine bleeding in the pregnant patient.[17] This effect can be minimized when one limits the dose of volatile drug to 0.6 MAC or less.[18]

5. Drug interactions. Many drugs produce a decreased minimum alveolar concentration (MAC) for the volatile anesthetics, and volatile anesthetic dosage should be altered accordingly to avoid an anesthetic overdose. Among these MAC-lowering drugs are opioids and opioid agonist-antagonists,[19] benzodiazepines,[20] nitrous oxide,[21] lidocaine,[22] clonidine,[23] reserpine,[24] and methyldopa.[24] Epinephrine[8] and other beta-adrenergic receptor agonists[25] are associated with cardiac dysrhythmias in the presence of halothane and, to a lesser extent, enflurane and isoflurane. The myocardial depression of the volatile anesthetics may be more pronounced in combination with beta-adrenergic receptor blockers[26] or calcium-channel blockers.[27] Halothane has been associated with significant cardiac dysrhythmias when administered to patients receiving theophylline[28] or the combination of pancuronium and a tricyclic antidepressant.[29] In patients receiving amiodarone, volatile anesthetics may be associated with heart block and sinus arrest and also with bradycardia resistant to atropine.[30,31] Volatile anesthetics, especially when administered with succinylcholine, have been implicated as the drugs most frequently associated with the triggering of malignant hyperthermia in susceptible patients.[32]

B. Nitrous oxide

Respiratory drive in response to carbon dioxide is not depressed, and the $Paco_2$ does not increase while one is breathing nitrous oxide alone.[33] Hypoxic ventilatory drive is blunted however.[34] Nitrous oxide may cause an increase in cerebral blood flow and intracranial pressure,[35] probably to a lesser degree than the volatile anesthetics.

Although nitrous oxide produces a mild sympathetic stimulation when administered to a patient receiving one of the volatile anesthetics,[36-38] significant cardiovascular depression (decreased cardiac output and increased cardiac filling pressures) may occur when nitrous oxide is added to an opioid anesthetic technique.[39] Nitrous oxide alone, even in an analgesic dose of 40%, can cause myocardial depression in patients with occlusive coronary artery disease.[40] Pulmonary artery pressures may rise with nitrous oxide administration, especially in patients with preexisting pulmonary hypertension.[41]

Inhibition of methionine synthetase, an enzyme involved in DNA synthesis, has been demonstrated with exposure to nitrous oxide.[42,43] Nitrous oxide oxidizes the cobalt in vitamin B_{12} to an inactive state,[42] thus inhibiting the activity of methionine synthetase and preventing the conversion of methyltetrahydrofolate to tetrahydrofolate, a compound required for DNA synthesis. This effect is likely responsible for several complications of nitrous oxide. Megaloblastic anemia may follow prolonged (many hours) administration,[44] and megaloblastic changes may be seen in critically ill patients after as little as 5 hours of exposure.[45] These changes are reversible upon discontinuation of the nitrous oxide. Chronic nonmedical abuse of nitrous oxide is associated with an anemia and neurologic damage usually manifest as a polyneuropathy.[46] Nitrous oxide is teratogenic in animals if exposure is early in pregnancy.[47] The significance of this in humans is unknown, though studies have failed to demonstrate an increased incidence of birth defects in children born to women exposed to nitrous oxide anesthesia during the first or second trimesters of pregnancy.[48,49]

Complications can result from the accumulation of nitrous oxide in closed spaces in the body because nitrous oxide diffuses into and out of body cavities faster than nitrogen does. This results in expansion of distensible spaces or increases in pressure of nondistensible ones.[50] The bowel may become distended during abdominal surgery, and a preexisting pneumothorax may greatly increase in size to become a tension pneumothorax.[51] Similarly a venous air embolism may enlarge.[52] During middle ear surgery, middle ear pressure may rise,[53] and tympanic membrane rupture has occurred.[54] Dislodgment of the tympanic membrane graft may follow the development of negative middle ear pressure upon the discontinuation of nitrous oxide after the closure of the previously open middle ear, as the nitrous oxide diffuses out of the closed space faster than nitrogen diffuses in.

II. INTRAVENOUS ANESTHETICS
A. Barbiturates

Although almost all of the barbiturates can exhibit somewhat similar side effects, it is clearly the ultra–short acting agents that are of the most interest to anesthesiologists. Thiopental is probably the prototypical drug of this class, though thiamylal and methohexital are also commonly used and display very similar adverse effects.[55] The barbiturates should be avoided in patients with acute intermittent porphyria because acute exacerbations of the disorder may result.[56] The effects of barbiturates may be exaggerated in patients taking monoamine oxide inhibitors (MAOIs), and prolonged sedation may follow thiopental administration in patients taking tricyclic antidepressants.[57]

1. Cardiovascular effects. Doses of barbiturates used in induction of anesthesia cause a moderate (10% to 20%) decrease in blood pressure attributable mainly to a decrease in peripheral vascular tone with venous pooling. There is a baroreceptor-mediated compensatory increase in heart rate, and cardiac output may fall because of decreased preload.[58] Hypotension may be severe in hypovolemic patients.[59] Occasional phlebitis may follow the administration of thiopental; this is more of a problem with the 5% than with the 2.5% solution of the drug.[60] Extravascular injection may cause tissue sloughing, and intra-arterial injection of thiopental may result in thrombosis and permanent neurovascular damage.[61]

2. Respiratory effects. The ultra–short acting barbiturates are potent respiratory depressants, and apnea usually accompanies anesthetic induction doses of these drugs.[62] Respiratory depression with thiopental is potentiated by the presence of other central nervous system depressants, especially the opioids.[63] With a smaller dose, or before the peak effect of an induction dose, hypersensitivity to pain and airway stimulation may occur with the potential for laryngospasm.[64]

B. Benzodiazepines

Although the benzodiazepines produce only a mild decrease in respiratory drive when used for sedation in healthy patients,[65] apnea may be induced in patients with preexisting pulmonary disease or in the presence of other central nervous system depressants such as opioids.[66] Midazolam often induces apnea when used in higher doses, as for induction of anesthesia.[67] Cardiovascular side effects are usually mild and consist in small decreases in blood pressure, peripheral vascular tone, and cardiac output.[68,69] Infrequently, even a low dose of diazepam may induce hypotension however.[70] Induction doses of midazolam produce a greater decrease in blood pressure than diazepam because of greater decreases in peripheral vascular tone.[71] Hypovolemia accentuates this hypotensive effect.[72] Diazepam may cause pain on intravenous injection and phlebitis.[73] The benzodiazepines often produce anterograde amnesia, which may be more profound with midazolam.[74] This effect can be advantageous, as during cardiac anesthesia, or a complication, as for a mother during delivery of her child.[75] Maternal intake of diazepam during pregnancy has been associated with fetal anomalies.[76]

Interactions of the benzodiazepines with other drugs include potentiation of their sedative effects by other central nervous system depressants as well as modification of their elimination. Alcohol particularly accentuates the central nervous system–depressant effects of diazepam because it enhances the systemic absorption of the benzodiazepine.[77] Diazepam in doses up to 0.2 mg/kg decreases the minimum alveolar concentration of halothane.[20] Cimetidine delays the hepatic clearance of diazepam, but not midazolam or lorazepam.[55] When added to a large-dose opioid anesthetic in patients undergoing cardiac surgery, benzodiazepines may cause significant decreases in cardiac output and blood pressure.[78]

C. Propofol

Propofol may cause pain on injection, especially when administered via a small vein.[79] Other bothersome side effects have included cough-

ing, hiccups, and involuntary skeletal muscle movements. Nausea and vomiting occur somewhat less frequently than with thiopental.[79] Cardiovascular depression occurs, and the hypotensive effect of propofol can be pronounced in patients with coronary artery disease.[80] Heart block has been reported with propofol as well.[81] It should be emphasized that propofol is packaged in a solution that supports bacterial growth and that the drug should be used promptly once a vial is opened.

D. Etomidate

In contrast to propofol, etomidate is generally associated with cardiovascular stability.[82] Pain on injection and phlebitis occur more often with etomidate than with thiopental administration.[83] Etomidate causes cerebral vasoconstriction and decreases intracranial pressure.[84] Although anticonvulsant activity has been documented in animals,[85] etomidate may activate seizure foci in humans.[86] Myoclonic movements not associated with epileptiform activity on EEG occurs in up to one third of patients, an incidence that may be decreased by pretreatment with an opioid or a benzodiazepine.[55] Etomidate increases respiratory rate while decreasing tidal volume but may also cause apnea.[87] Significant adrenocortical suppression may occur, especially with prolonged administration as when using the drug for sedation in a critical care setting.[88] The incidence of postoperative nausea and vomiting is higher than that associated with thiopental.[89]

E. Ketamine

Ketamine is a direct myocardial depressant in vitro[90] but increases sympathetic tone in vivo causing an increase in heart rate and blood pressure.[91] In critically ill patients who may be depleted of endogenous catecholamines, ketamine can cause significant falls in blood pressure.[92] Ventilation is usually not depressed, though apnea can occur, especially in the presence of other CNS depressants.[93] Airway reflexes are normally well maintained under ketamine, but this is not a reliable phenomenon.[94] Oropharyngeal secretions are often increased by ketamine, an effect that may be blunted by pretreatment with an antisialagogue such as glycopyrrolate.[55] Ketamine is a potent cerebral vasodilator and can increase intracranial pressure significantly.[95] Transient cortical blindness has been associated with this drug, but the mechanism of this is not known. Emergence delirium occurs in 5% to 30% of patients. This phenomenon is more likely to occur with anticholinergic or droperidol premedication, in patients under 16 years of age, in females, and in patients with a psychiatric history. The incidence is decreased with benzodiazepine premedication.[93] In patients receiving tricyclic antidepressants, ketamine may induce hypertension and cardiac dysrhythmias.[57] Hypotension may result from the administration of ketamine to a patient under halothane anesthesia.[95]

III. DRUGS USED IN PSYCHIATRIC DISORDERS
A. Antipsychotic agents

Antipsychotic agents most commonly utilized by anesthesiologists include the phenothiazines and the butyrophenones. The most commonly occurring adverse effects of these drugs are related to their cholinergic effects and include dry mouth, blurred vision, urinary retention, and tachycardia.[96] Orthostatic hypotension is relatively frequent and blood pressure may decrease because of a peripheral alpha-adrenergic receptor blockade, especially during hypovolemia.[97] Cardiac side effects may include prolongation of the PR and QT intervals and the QRS complex on the electrocardiogram (ECG). Preexisting heart block may be exaggerated. Sudden death from a cardiac dysrhythmia has been reported with large phenothiazine doses.[98] CNS complications can include disorientation, hallucinations, and extrapyramidal effects such as dystonias, akathisia, and tardive dyskinesia (after prolonged therapy).[97] Droperidol may also be associated with dysphoric reactions, which may be strong enough to cause the patient to refuse surgery.[99] The antipsychotics interfere with hypothalamic thermoregulation, an effect that can lead to hypothermic complications[100] but may be useful in treating postoperative shivering. The seizure threshold is decreased by antipsychotic drugs.[101] These drugs should be used with extreme caution if at all in patients with parkinsonism because they may worsen symptoms of the disease. The antipsychotics have minimal respiratory effects but can potentiate the respiratory depression of opioids.[102]

Neuroleptic malignant syndrome has been associated with the antipsychotics, usually early in the course of therapy.[103] This syndrome is clinically similar to malignant hyperthermia but probably is mediated by a somewhat different mechanism. Symptoms include fever, diaphoresis, dyspnea, skeletal muscle rigidity, tremors, and altered consciousness. Associated feature may include tachycardia, cardiac dysrhythmias, blood pressure changes, leukocytosis, and elevated plasma creatine phosphokinase and hepatic transaminase levels. Risk factors appear to be high ambient temperature, malnutrition, dehydration, and physical exertion. The syndrome

has a high mortality (approximately 20%). Treatment is symptomatic and includes discontinuation of antipsychotic medication, intravenous fluids, and cooling of the patient.[104] Bromocriptine (2 to 20 mg IV every 8 hours) and dantrolene sodium have been reported to help abort the syndrome.

1. Tricyclic antidepressants. Tricyclic antidepressants have significant anticholinergic adverse effects including nausea and vomiting, drying of mucous membranes, and difficulty with urination.[97] Sedation, tremor, and seizures can occur. Cardiovascular complications include orthostatic hypotension and cardiac dysrhythmias.[105] Tricyclic antidepressant overdose is a potentially life-threatening condition causing delirium, respiratory depression, seizures, cardiac dysrhythmias, and cardiac arrest.[106] Serious ventricular dysrhythmias have occurred in patients on tricyclic antidepressants during halothane anesthesia and in the presence of pancuronium.[57] Tricyclic antidepressants potentiate the CNS depressant effects of opioids.[107]

2. Monoamine oxidase inhibitors. Complications of the monoamine oxidase inhibitors (MAOIs) include mainly orthostatic hypotension, hepatotoxicity, and serious drug interactions.[108] Overdose with these compounds produces a syndrome of sympathetic nervous system hyperactivity, including blood pressure liability, agitation, hyperpyrexia, and seizures.[109] MAOIs potentiate the depressant effects of ethanol, barbiturates, and opioids[110] and may prolong the action of succinylcholine.[111] Hypertension, convulsions, and fever may occur if meperidine is administered to a patient receiving an MAOI.[112] Administration of sympathomimetic compounds, especially indirect-acting agents, is exaggerated in the presence of MAOIs. Hypotension in this setting is best treated by reduced doses of a direct-acting sympathomimetic (such as phenylephrine).[113] It has been traditionally recommended that MAOIs be discontinued for 2 weeks before elective surgery to avoid intraoperative hemodynamic instability; however, reports of stable anesthetic courses in these patients has led to the questioning of this recommendation.[114]

IV. OPIOID AGONISTS
A. Morphine

Morphine is the prototypical opioid agonist drug to which all other opioids are compared. Central nervous system complications include respiratory depression, apnea, nausea, and vomiting.[115] Although opioids are sedating, amnesia is not reliable and the complication of intraoperative awareness may accompany the use of large doses of an opioid as a sole anesthetic agent.[116] Euphoria and a feeling of well-being accompany morphine administration, and the drug has a high potential for abuse.

Adverse cardiovascular effects of morphine may include decreases in peripheral vascular tone and blood pressure because of histamine release.[117] These effects are especially pronounced in hypovolemic patients. Sinus bradycardia secondary to central vagal stimulation may accompany large-dose morphine administration.[118] (See also Chapter 10.)

Morphine causes constipation and spasm of the sphincter of Oddi.[119] Gastric emptying is delayed, and in patients with gastroesophageal reflux the severity of reflex symptoms is increased. This may increase the risk of aspiration during anesthesia.[120]

B. Meperidine

Meperidine causes less biliary spasm than morphine does.[119] Whereas at smaller doses, it is hemodynamically well tolerated in the healthy patient, larger dose meperidine (2 to 10 mg/kg IV) causes significant cardiovascular depression including decreases in peripheral vascular resistance, cardiac output, and blood pressure.[121] In contrast to morphine, meperidine can cause tachycardia,[121] perhaps because of its structural similarity to atropine. Like morphine, meperidine causes histamine release.[122] When administered in the presence of MAOIs, meperidine's effects may be considerably potentiated. Additionally a severe reaction consisting in convulsions, high fever, and hypotension may occur.[112]

C. Fentanyl

Like the other opioids, fentanyl is a potent respiratory depressant. Fentanyl may cause delayed respiratory depression occurring 30 to 60 minutes after apparent initial recovery from the drug.[123] Large doses of fentanyl can produce chest wall rigidity, making ventilation of the lungs difficult. This rigidity may be prevented by pretreatment with a nondepolarizing neuromuscular blocker or administration of a volatile anesthetic.[124] In contrast to morphine, fentanyl is not likely to produce decreases in peripheral vascular tone or blood pressure; however, fentanyl is more likely to induce bradycardia.[125] Unlike morphine, fentanyl does not cause histamine release.[122]

D. Sufentanil

The complications of sufentanil are very similar to those seen with fentanyl. Sufentanil may cause hypotension and bradycardia when used for induction of anesthesia in large doses.[126] Chest wall rigidity and delayed respiratory depression have occurred with sufentanil.[127]

E. Alfentanil

Adverse effects of alfentanil are comparable to fentanyl. When used in large doses (125 to 150 µg/kg) for induction of anesthesia in patients undergoing coronary artery bypass procedures, alfentanil may cause a significant decrease in blood pressure, which may be greater than that observed with fentanyl or sufentanil.[128]

F. Neuraxial opioids

The epidural or intrathecal administration of an opioid can produce adverse effects somewhat different from those after intravenous injection of the same drug. Respiratory depression after epidural morphine administration occurs in a biphasic course, with an early incidence within the first hour after injection and a later incidence occurring about 6 to 12 hours thereafter. More lipid-soluble opioids may be associated with a lower incidence of delayed respiratory depression. Other complications of neuroaxial opioids include pruritus, nausea, and urinary retention. These complications are all reversible with naloxone.[129]

V. OPIOID ANTAGONIST: NALOXONE

Naloxone is the prototypical opioid antagonist drug. When used to reverse the depressant effects of opioids, naloxone administration may cause hypertension, tachycardia, cardiac dysrhythmias, and pulmonary edema.[130] These complications are believed to be caused by a centrally mediated catecholamine release accompanying the sudden "pharmacologic arousal." Careful titration of small intravenous doses of naloxone in an attempt to reverse respiratory depression while maintaining analgesia should minimize this problem.[131] Naloxone can produce nausea and vomiting, a complication that may also be attenuated by slow administration.[131]

VI. OPIOID AGONIST-ANTAGONISTS

As a rule, the opioid agonist-antagonist drugs exhibit side effects similar to those seen with the true opioids. The respiratory depression of these compounds reaches a ceiling effect, beyond which additional doses do not produce additional depression[120]; however, clinically significant hypoventilation can occur.[132] Dysphoria is relatively common with the agonist-antagonist drugs, limiting their abuse potential.

These compounds are less likely to cause biliary spasm than the pure agonist drugs can.[119] The antagonist properties of these agents may blunt the analgesic effects of subsequently administered true agonist drugs[132] and may precipitate opioid withdrawal symptoms in opioid-dependent patients.[133]

A. Butorphanol

Side effects of butorphanol include sedation, diaphoresis, nausea and vomiting, and dysphoric reactions including hallucinations.[133] Butorphanol may cause significant increases in pulmonary arterial pressure with increased myocardial oxygen demand.[134]

B. Nalbuphine

Dysphoric reactions with nalbuphine are uncommon, though dizziness, nausea, and vomiting may occur.[135] In contrast to butorphanol, it does not increase pulmonary arterial pressure and myocardial work.[136]

C. Pentazocine

Common adverse effects of pentazocine include dizziness, diaphoresis, and nausea and vomiting.[137] Pentazocine causes increases in heart rate, pulmonary arterial and systemic blood pressure, and left ventricular filling pressure.[138] Although dysphoric reactions occur, pentazocine does have some abuse potential.[137]

D. Buprenorphine

The respiratory depression observed with buprenorphine may be difficult to treat because it is not easily reversed by naloxone.[139] Doxapram has been suggested as an alternative pharmacologic treatment.[140] The cardiovascular effects of buprenorphine are similar to morphine. As with the other agents in this class, sedation and nausea are side effects, but dysphoria is uncommon.

VII. LOCAL ANESTHETICS

Complications of local anesthetics are attributable to high blood levels of drug secondary to inadvertent intravascular injection.[141] In general, as blood levels increase, the patient may experience circumoral numbness, restlessness, tinnitus, and blurred vision. Drowsiness may occur with the amide local anesthetics. With even higher blood levels, seizures followed by central nervous system depression, apnea, and cardiovascular collapse occur. If local anesthetic blood levels increase rapidly, overt seizures may be the initial symptom. Local anesthetics can interfere with neuromuscular transmission and may potentiate the effects of neuromuscular blocking drugs.[142] (Chapter 10 contains a dis-

cussion of the cardiac dysrhythmias associated with local anesthetics.)

True allergic reactions to local anesthetics are most uncommon, probably accounting for less than 1% of all adverse reactions.[143] Often a patient's reaction is termed an allergy when in fact it is a manifestation of a toxic blood level of the local anesthetic. Many allergic reactions occurring with the use of a local anesthetic are attributable to an allergic response to preservatives such as methylparaben and not the local anesthetic.[144] With the ester local anesthetics, *para*-aminobenzoic acid (PABA) is often the offending compound. PABA is a metabolite of the ester local anesthetics, and therefore cross-sensitivity between these agents is to be expected. Since PABA is a common ingredient in many commercial sunscreen preparations, it might also be wise to avoid ester local anesthetics in a patient who reports an allergy to sunscreens. Patients allergic to esters do not appear to be at increased risk of allergic responses to amide local anesthetics.[145]

A. Lidocaine

In addition to central nervous system toxicity outlined above, lidocaine in high concentrations can produce profound myocardial depression.[146] Atrioventricular conduction may be slowed, and heart block may be induced.[147] Lidocaine depresses the ventilatory response to hypoxia, even at clinically relevant plasma concentrations.[148] Systemic toxicity of lidocaine may be enhanced in the presence of hyperkalemia.[149]

B. Mepivacaine

Although quite similar to lidocaine in most respects, mepivacaine causes neonatal depression when used for epidural anesthesia because it produces higher and longer lasting fetal blood levels.[150]

C. Bupivacaine

Bupivacaine appears to be relatively more cardiotoxic than most other local anesthetics and more likely to produce cardiac dysrhythmias.[151] This cardiotoxicity may be even more pronounced in pregnancy.[152] (See Chapters 10 and 22.)

D. Prilocaine

Prilocaine has been associated with methemoglobinemia probably mediated through its metabolite *o*-toluidine[153]

E. Etidocaine

Like bupivacaine, etidocaine appears to be more cardiotoxic than other less potent local anesthetics.[151] Etidocaine used for peridural anesthesia can be associated with a more profound motor than sensory blockade, an effect that may be of significant psychic stress to the patient.[154]

F. Chloroprocaine

The rapid plasma hydrolysis of chloroprocaine accounts for its extremely low systemic toxicity.[155] Neurologic deficits have been reported occurring after the inadvertent subarachnoid injection of chloroprocaine, possibly because of sodium bisulfite used as a preservative rather than the drug itself.[156]

G. Cocaine

The toxic effects of cocaine mainly stem from its ability to block catecholamine reuptake, both in the central nervous system and systemically.[157] Cardiovascular complications may include tachycardia, peripheral vasoconstriction, hypertension, myocardial ischemia, cardiac dysrhythmias, and death. Adverse CNS effects may include restlessness, headache, nausea, convulsions, coma, and respiratory failure secondary to medullary depression. In small doses, cocaine produces feelings of well-being and euphoria and is a drug of very significant abuse potential.

H. Tetracaine

For its local anesthetic potency, tetracaine may have relatively high intravenous toxicity when compared to that of other local anesthetics.[154]

I. Benzocaine

Benzocaine is a local anesthetic principally used for topical anesthesia and causes methemoglobinemia that may be severe enough to require treatment.[158]

VIII. NEUROMUSCULAR BLOCKERS
A. Depolarizing neuromuscular relaxants

1. Succinylcholine. Adverse effects of succinylcholine may include increases in intraocular, intracranial, and intragastric pressure.[159] These effects may be blunted but not abolished by pretreatment with a small dose of a nondepolarizing relaxant such as *d*-tubocurarine or metocurine. Myalgias, especially of the neck, back, and abdomen, occur frequently after succinylcholine administration and may also be attenuated by similar pretreatment. The serum potassium concentration increases after succinylcholine is administered, but this is not blocked by pretreatment with a nondepolarizing relaxant.[160] This increase in serum potassium may be sufficient to cause cardiac dysrhythmias and even cardiac arrest in patients with severe burns, upper motor neuron lesions, skeletal

muscle atrophy caused by denervation, and severe intra-abdominal infections.[161] Sustained skeletal muscle contraction has also been described in patients with myotonic dystrophy and myotonia congenita.[162] Myoglobinuria can occur after the administration of succinylcholine to normal pediatric patients.[163] Succinylcholine administered with a volatile anesthetic is the classical triggering anesthetic for malignant hyperthermia in susceptible patients.[33] Cardiac dysrhythmias may be induced by succinylcholine. (See Chapter 10.)

Prolonged paralysis can occur in the presence of drugs that interfere with pseudocholinesterase, the plasma enzyme that degrades succinylcholine, and in patients with abnormal or deficient pseudocholinesterase.[159] Compounds that may prolong the action of succinylcholine by this mechanism include certain insecticides, echothiophate eye drops, trimethaphan, and certain chemotherapeutic agents such as cyclophosphamide. Prolonged neuromuscular blockade with features of depolarizing blockade (phase II block) can also occur with larger doses of succinylcholine or in patients with deficient pseudocholinesterase activity.[164]

B. Nondepolarizing neuromuscular relaxants

One of the most dangerous complications of the nondepolarizing blockers is inadequate antagonism reversal or recovery from their skeletal muscle-relaxant effects. The resultant inability to support the airway leads to hypoventilation, hypercarbia, and hypoxemia most often in the postanesthesia care unit.[165]

1. d-Tubocurarine. The neuromuscular blocker *d*-tubocurarine induces a decrease in peripheral vascular tone and blood pressure by histamine release and some blockade of autonomic ganglia.[166]

2. Metocurine. The side effects of this agent are similar to *d*-tubocurarine but of lesser magnitude.[167]

3. Pancuronium. In contrast to *d*-tubocurarine, pancuronium increases heart rate, cardiac output, and blood pressure by increasing plasma catecholamines and selective vagal blockade.[166] These cardiovascular effects may precipitate myocardial ischemia in patients with atherosclerotic coronary artery disease. Patients receiving digoxin may be at increased risk of cardiac dysrhythmias after pancuronium administration.[168]

4. Gallamine. The drug gallamine induces pronounced (30% to 40%) increases in heart rate along with a small increase in blood pressure. Cardiac dysrhythmias may accompany administration of gallamine.[169]

5. *Atracurium.* At higher doses and with rapid intravenous administration, atracurium causes histamine release with resultant cutaneous flushing and decreases in peripheral vascular tone and blood pressure.[170]

6. *Vecuronium.* Vecuronium is remarkably devoid of cardiovascular side effects even at higher doses, though some believe that vecuronium may magnify the bradycardia produced by opioids.[171]

IX. CHOLINESTERASE INHIBITORS

The cholinesterase inhibitors include neostigmine, pyridostigmine, edrophonium, and physostigmine. Their effects and complications are largely related to their anticholinesterase activity, which leads to accumulation of acetylcholine at various cholinergic sites throughout the body.[161] The adverse effects of the cholinesterase inhibitors can include bradydysrhythmias, atrioventricular nodal block, peripheral vasodilatation, excess salivation, sweating, increased gastrointestinal motility, increased bladder tone, and bronchoconstriction. The muscarinic side effects of the cholinesterase inhibitors are minimized by the concurrent administration of an anticholinergic agent. In higher doses, the cholinesterase inhibitors may produce skeletal muscle weakness.[172] Neostigmine and pyridostigmine cause pronounced inhibition of plasma cholinesterase and can significantly prolong the action of a subsequently administered dose of succinylcholine.[173] The ophthalmic anticholinesterase drugs used in the treatment of glaucoma (echothiophate, isoflurophate, and demecarium bromide) produce a similar effect. Physostigmine crosses the blood-brain barrier and produces CNS stimulation, an effect that has been utilized therapeutically.[174]

X. ANTICHOLINERGIC AGENTS

The anticholinergic drugs are competitive muscarinic receptor blockers, and their adverse effects are largely predictable on that basis. These may include bradycardia (at small doses), tachycardia, dry mouth, photophobia, blurred vision, urinary retention, dry skin, fever, and mental status changes.[175] Intravenous administration of atropine has been reported to induce ventricular tachycardia and fibrillation.[176] Bronchial secretions are reduced, and this drying effect can lead to mucus plugging.[177] In patients with narrow-angle glaucoma scopolamine may cause a deleterious rise in intraocular pressure, and its use in these patients has been discouraged.[178] Atropine may produce the central anticholinergic syndrome, consisting in restlessness, mental status changes, and hyperpyrexia.[179] Scopol-

amine may also produce this syndrome but more commonly causes sedation and amnesia. Glycopyrrolate does not cause CNS complications because it does not readily cross the blood-brain barrier. Ipratropium bromide is a newer anticholinergic drug used by the inhalational route in the treatment of bronchospastic disorders. Since it is poorly absorbed, it rarely produces systemic complications.[177]

XI. VASOACTIVE DRUGS
A. Catecholamines

The complications of catecholamines are largely an extension of their pharmacologic effects and are usually predictable on that basis. Significant hypertension may be induced with epinephrine, norepinephrine, and dopamine if the dose administered is not carefully titrated.[180] Catecholamines may exacerbate digitalis-associated cardiac dysrhythmias, perhaps by shifting potassium intracellularly.[181]

1. *Epinephrine.* Epinephrine can cause significant tachycardia and cardiac dysrhythmias,[57] especially in the presence of halothane.[8] The drug may induce myocardial ischemia, especially in patients with preexisting cardiac disorders.[57] Epinephrine should not be added to local anesthetics for "ring blocks" of digits because the intense localized vasoconstriction caused by this catecholamine produces ischemia and necrosis of the digit.[154]

2. *Norepinephrine.* The intense alpha-adrenergic receptor effects of norepinephrine may produce ischemia of the extremities, particularly when administered in larger doses and in patients with peripheral vascular disease.[182] A metabolic acidosis can be induced by this peripheral vasoconstriction. This vasoconstriction and increased afterload may exacerbate myocardial ischemia.[183] Extravasation of norepinephrine may cause local tissue necrosis and sloughing. Prompt infiltration of the area of extravasation with a solution of 0.5% to 1% phentolamine may minimize this local tissue loss.

3. *Isoproterenol.* The intense beta-adrenergic receptor effects of isoproterenol may produce tachycardia, cardiac dysrhythmias, and hypotension because of peripheral vasodilatation.[180] Myocardial oxygen demand is increased, and myocardial ischemia may be exacerbated.

4. *Dopamine.* At low doses (less than 3 mg/kg/min) this drug may cause a decrease in blood pressure in the presence of hypovolemia because of renal and mesenteric vasodilatation by stimulation of dopaminergic receptors. At higher doses, beta$_1$-adrenergic receptor stimulation may produce tachycardia, tachydysrhythmias, increased myocardial oxygen consumption, and myocardial ischemia.[184] At doses above 15 to 20 mg/kg/min, the alpha-adrenergic receptor effects of dopamine can lead to limb ischemia and gangrene if therapy is prolonged.[185] Inadvertent subcutaneous infiltration may produce local tissue necrosis and may be treated as described for norepinephrine. Nausea and vomiting often occur when dopamine is administered to the awake patient. Significant hypertension may result if dopamine is given to a patient with a pheochromocytoma.

Dopamine may adversely interact with certain drugs. MAOIs may significantly enhance the hypertensive response to dopamine,[97] as the initial effect of bretylium does.[186] Administration of dopamine to a patient receiving phenytoin may induce hypotension.[187]

5. Dobutamine. Because of its beta-adrenergic receptor–stimulating properties, dobutamine can produce tachycardia, cardiac dysrhythmias, and myocardial ischemia. Blood pressure may decrease somewhat if the cardiac output does not increase in proportion to the decrease in peripheral vascular resistance. Nausea, headache, and skeletal muscle tremors are other potentially adverse effects of dobutamine.[21]

B. Noncatecholamine inotropic agents

1. Amrinone. In addition to its positive inotropic effects, amrinone decreases systemic vascular resistance and cardiac filling pressures.[188] Hypotension may be a significant problem, especially in the presence of hypovolemia. Amrinone should be used only for short-term therapy because prolonged administration of the drug can cause thrombocytopenia and gastrointestinal disturbances. Milrinone is a compound with pharmacologic properties similar to amrinone; however it has not been associated with gastrointestinal or thrombocytopenic complications.[189]

2. Digitalis. Complications with digitalis therapy are very common, occurring in up to 20% of patients.[190] A wide variety of cardiac dysrhythmias have been described with digitalis toxicity, but the most common rhythm disturbances include paroxysmal atrial tachycardia with atrioventricular block, accelerated junctional rhythms, premature atrial and ventricular contractions, and ventricular tachycardia. High degrees of AV block may also occur.[191] Digitalis causes constriction of the coronary and mesenteric vasculature and may produce myocardial and gastrointestinal ischemia. Other problems that may complicate therapy with digitalis include gastrointestinal disturbances

(anorexia, nausea, vomiting), visual disturbances (blurred vision, color vision changes), and mental status changes (confusion, delirium, psychosis). The potential for complications with digitalis is increased in patients with hypokalemia, hypercalcemia, and hypomagnesemia. Pain and local irritation occur with extravasation of digitalis preparations. Adverse reactions to digitalis are more common and severe when the drug is administered by the intravenous route.

3. Ephedrine. Ephedrine is a mixed direct- and indirect-acting alpha- and beta-adrenergic receptor agonist with adverse effects similar to but much less frequent and severe than those of epinephrine.[192] Ephedrine does cross the blood-brain barrier and may cause agitation and tremors.

4. Mephentermine. Like ephedrine, this is a mixed-acting drug with alpha- and beta-adrenergic receptor–stimulating properties and similar side effects. In contrast to ephedrine, mephentermine mildly decreases uterine blood flow.[193]

5. Metaraminol. The drug metaraminol produces more intense vasoconstriction than ephedrine and may cause a reflex bradycardia.[184] Metaraminol is stored in postganglionic sympathetic nerve terminals as a false transmitter, and abrupt discontinuation of this drug after a few hours may result in hypotension. It significantly decreases uterine blood flow in pregnancy.[193]

C. Selective beta$_2$ receptor agonists

Used mainly as bronchodilators and to halt contractions in premature labor, selective beta$_2$-adrenergic receptor agonist drugs are less likely to cause cardiac stimulation than the nonselective beta agonists. Selective beta$_2$ agonists in common use include terbutaline, metaproterenol, albuterol, isoetharine, and ritodrine. Adverse effects can include tachycardia, cardiac dysrhythmias, and hypokalemia caused by a shift of potassium into cells.[184,194] When used in the management of premature labor, beta$_2$ agonists may also induce hypertension, pulmonary edema, and deterioration of glucose control in diabetic mothers.[195]

D. Vasopressors

1. Phenylephrine. The drug phenylephrine increases blood pressure caused mainly by direct alpha-adrenergic stimulation. Complications include reflex bradycardia with a resultant decrease in cardiac output and the potential for hypertension if administered in too large a dose.[196] Renal, splanchnic, and uterine blood flow is decreased by phenylephrine.

2. *Methoxamine.* Like phenylephrine, methoxamine is a direct-acting alpha-adrenergic agonist and induces similar side effects.[57] Methoxamine reduces renal blood flow to a greater extent than norepinephrine in equipotent doses.

E. Vasodilators

1. *Nitroprusside.* Nitroprusside is an arterial dilator and venodilator and may rapidly induce hypotension and reflex tachycardia. Such effects can produce myocardial ischemia, infarction, or stroke.[197] Nitroprusside inhibits hypoxic pulmonary vasoconstriction, and hypoxemia may occur.[198] Other adverse effects of nitroprusside include nausea, restlessness, intracranial hypertension,and rarely methemoglobinemia.[197] The degradation of nitroprusside in the body produces cyanide, which is converted by hepatic and renal rhodanase to thiocyanate. Hypothermia does not interfere with the nonenzymatic liberation of cyanide from nitroprusside, but the enzymatic conversion of cyanide to thiocyanate is slowed.[199] Both cyanide and thiocyanate in sufficient concentrations produce toxicity, though the latter is somewhat less dangerous. Features of thiocyanate toxicity include nausea, tinnitus, mental status changes, hyperreflexia, skeletal muscle spasms, and convulsions. Cyanide binds to cytochrome c, thus blocking aerobic metabolism, and cyanide toxicity may be recognized first by resistance to the drug, progressive metabolic acidosis, and increased mixed venous oxygen saturation. Dosage of nitroprusside should be limited to 8 μg/kg/min acutely, or 0.5 mg/kg/hr for infusions over 3 hours to minimize toxicity.[200] In addition to supportive care, hemodialysis may be required for the management of thiocyanate toxicity. Treatment of cyanide toxicity includes both stopping the nitroprusside and administration of thiosulfate (150 mg/kg IV), which acts as a sulfur donor for the rhodanase system to bind cyanide. If cyanide toxicity is imminently life threatening, sodium nitrite (5 mg/kg IV) may be given to convert hemoglobin to methemoglobin, which binds cyanide to form cyanmethemoglobin. Hydroxycobalamin has also been advocated because it combines with cyanide to form cyanocarbalamin. Hydroxycobalamin infusion (25 mg/hr) has been used for the prevention of cyanide toxicity during nitroprusside therapy.[201]

2. *Nitroglycerin.* Although a more prominent venodilator than arterial dilator, intravenous nitroglycerin may induce significant hypotension[202] and may cause hypoxemia because of ventilation-perfusion mismatch.[203] Headache is a frequent complication of nitroglycerin, and rarely methemoglobinemia can occur. In contrast to nitroprusside, reflex tachycardia is not a problem with nitroglycerin therapy.

3. *Hydralazine.* As a direct arteriolar smooth muscle dilator, hydralazine causes a decrease in systemic vascular resistance and blood pressure, which induces reflex tachycardia and increases myocardial work. This effect may exacerbate angina pectoris in susceptible patients, and it has been recommended that hydralazine be used with a beta-adrenergic blocking drug to blunt the reflex tachycardia. The onset of maximal action of hydralazine is 20 to 30 minutes and overshoot hypotension sometimes occurs. Other adverse effects of hydralazine include headache, cutaneous flushing, and after prolonged therapy a lupus-like syndrome.[204,205]

4. *Minoxidil.* Minoxidil is an arterial vasodilator with complications similar to hydralazine, though no lupus-like syndrome has been described.[205] Pericardial effusion has been described with minoxidil therapy. Hair growth occurs with minoxidil, which may be viewed as a complication or more recently as a therapeutic effect.

5. *Diazoxide.* A potent vasodilator chemically related to the thiazide diuretics,[204] diazoxide may cause a reflex tachycardia and precipitate anginal symptoms in patients with coronary artery disease. Other complications may include fluid retention, hyperglycemia, orthostatic hypotension, and pain if the drug is extravasated.

6. *Adenosine.* Used as a vasodilator and also to treat supraventricular tachycardias, adenosine may cause hypotension and heart block.[206]

F. Beta-adrenergic receptor blockers

Propranolol is the prototypical beta-blocking drug. Other common nonselective beta blockers include timolol, pindolol, and nadalol. Propranolol competitively antagonizes both beta$_1$ (cardiac) and beta$_2$ (noncardiac) receptors, and its adverse effects are largely predictable on that basis. Propranolol may induce hypotension, bradycardia, bronchospasm, and congestive heart failure in susceptible patients.[207] Raynaud's phenomenon may be precipitated in patients with peripheral vascular disease caused by blockade of the vasodilatory effect of beta$_2$ receptors. Abrupt cessation of beta-blocker therapy is associated with a rebound sympathetic nervous system hyperactivity with worsening of the patient's underlying disorder (such as angina pectoris or hypertension). In diabetic patients, beta blockers may mask the adrenergically mediated signs of hypoglycemia such as tremor and sweating and may prolong the hypoglycemia by interfering with epinephrine-induced glycogenolysis. Timolol may produce bradycardia and increased airway resistance even when administered as eye drops.[208] Propranolol crosses the blood-brain barrier and may produce depression, lethargy, and rarely psychotic reactions.[207] Nadolol does not readily enter the central nervous system and is much less likely to cause these central nervous system complications. Pindolol is a nonselective beta antagonist with some intrinsic beta agonist activity. It is less likely to cause bradycardia and can produce increases in blood pressure at higher doses.[209]

The selective beta$_1$-adrenergic receptor antagonist drugs include metoprolol, atenolol, and esmolol. It should be recognized that these compounds are only relatively beta$_1$ selective, and may exhibit beta$_2$ adrenergic receptor blocking effects at higher doses.[210] These drugs are much less likely to cause peripheral, metabolic, and bronchospastic complications than the nonselective beta blockers.

General anesthesia in patients receiving beta antagonist drugs is usually well tolerated and the beta antagonist drugs should be continued to the time of surgery because rebound phenomena occur with abrupt withdrawal.[211] Additive cardiac depressant effects when volatile anesthetics are administered to patients receiving beta blockers are less prominent with isoflurane than with enflurane or halothane.[26] Timolol eye drops have been reported to cause significant intraoperative bradycardia.[212]

G. Alpha-adrenergic receptor blockers

1. Phentolamine. As a nonselective alpha-adrenergic receptor antagonist, phentolamine produces peripheral vasodilatation and decreases in blood pressure with a reflex sympathetic cardiac stimulation. Complications may include tachycardia, cardiac dysrhythmias, exacerbation of angina, abdominal pain, and diarrhea.[213]

2. Phenoxybenzamine. Like phentolamine, phenoxybenzamine is a nonselective alpha-adrenergic receptor antagonist with similar adverse effects. Orthostatic hypotension may be prominent with this drug.[213]

3. Prazosin. The drug prazosin is a selective alpha$_1$-adrenergic antagonist that also decreases blood pressure by peripheral vasodilatation. Since alpha$_2$ receptor-mediated inhibition of norepinephrine release remains intact, prazosin causes less reflex tachycardia than phentolamine does.[57] Other complications of prazosin include dry mouth, lethargy, vertigo, orthostatic hypotension, and syncope. Syncope most frequently occurs upon initiation of therapy.[213]

H. Mixed adrenergic antagonist: labetalol

Labetalol acts as a selective alpha$_1$-adrenergic receptor antagonist and a nonselective beta-adrenergic receptor antagonist. Peripheral resistance, cardiac output, and usually heart rate are decreased.[214] Complications include orthostatic hypotension, fatigue, and nausea. Bronchospasm with labetalol appears to be less of a problem than with the other nonselective beta antagonists. Clinical experience indicates that anesthetized patients are somewhat more sensitive to the hypotensive effects of labetalol and that 5 to 10 mg IV avoids overshoot hypotension.

I. Ganglionic blockers: trimethaphan

Trimethaphan is the only ganglionic blocking drug in common clinical use for blood pressure control in the United States.[215] It decreases peripheral vascular tone, cardiac preload, and cardiac output. Tachycardia may occur because of parasympathetic ganglionic blockade. Urinary retention and decreases in gastrointestinal motility to the point of ileus may be produced. Trimethaphan does not increase intracranial pressure as may occur with nitroprusside, but cerebral blood flow is decreased. Plasma cholinesterase is inhibited by trimethaphan, and this effect may prolong the action of succinylcholine.[216] At large doses, trimethaphan may cause histamine release.

J. Central sympatholytics

1. Clonidine. Adverse effects of clonidine include dry mouth, skin rashes, and constipation.[204] Sedation is a common side effect, and the minimum alveolar concentration of volatile anesthetics is reduced in the presence of clonidine.[23] Abrupt discontinuation of clonidine can result in significant rebound hypertension.[217]

2. Methyldopa. Sedation with a reduction in the minimum alveolar concentration is also an effect of therapy with methyldopa.[24] Hepatic dysfunction with fever and malaise may complicate therapy, and fatal hepatic necrosis attributable to methyldopa has been described. A Coombs'-positive hemolytic anemia and orthostatic hypotension may also occur.[204] Like clonidine, abrupt discontinuation of methyldopa is associated with rebound hypertension.[217]

3. Reserpine. Dry mouth, sedation, orthostatic hypotension, and bradycardia are complications of reserpine therapy.[205] Reserpine depletes CNS catecholamines and increases sensitivity to direct-acting sympathomimetics while blunting the response to indirect-acting ones.

XII. CALCIUM-CHANNEL BLOCKING DRUGS

The calcium-channel blocking drugs differ in their relative effects on the heart and peripheral vasculature. Their potential complications differ accordingly.

Patients should have their calcium-channel blockers continued preoperatively when used for treatment of cardiovascular disorders. It might be predicted that abrupt discontinuation of these drugs could produce exacerbation of the patient's underlying condition, and in fact this has been reported. The sudden withdrawal of nifedipine has been associated with hypertensive crisis and exacerbation of rest angina.[218,219] Nonetheless, there are potentially adverse dry interactions of specific relevance to anesthesia. As myocardial depressants and vasodilators, calcium-channel blockers when administered to patients receiving volatile anesthetics should be carefully titrated particularly in the presence of preexisting cardiac disease.[220] Calcium-entry blockers may potentiate the effects of neuromuscular blocking agents.[221] Verapamil has been reported to enhance the toxicity of several other drugs, including digoxin, carbamazepine, and the oral hypoglycemics.[222]

A. Verapamil

The adverse effects of verapamil are mainly extensions of its therapeutic actions. Myocardial depression and hypotension may occur, particularly in patients with preexisting myocardial dysfunction.[223] Atrioventricular heart block can be produced, especially in the presence of underlying sick-sinus syndrome.[224] Verapamil may speed the ventricular response rate in patients with a preexcitation syndrome such as Wolff-Parkinson-White.[225] Caution is advised if verapamil is used in the presence of a beta-blocking drug because complete heart block can occur.[226] Dizziness, nausea, headache, constipation, and hepatic dysfunction are other possible side effects of verapamil. Verapamil has been reported to induce respiratory failure when administered intravenously to a patient with Duchenne's muscular dystrophy, possibly because of a neuromuscular blocking effect.[227]

B. Nifedipine

Unlike verapamil, nifedipine produces little effect on cardiac conduction and has a greater effect in decreasing peripheral vascular tone.[228] This may cause hypotension with a reflex tachycardia. Nifedipine can induce myocardial depression in patients with aortic stenosis or preexisting ventricular dysfunction.

C. Diltiazem

The cardiovascular effects of diltiazem are intermediate between those of nifedipine and verapamil.[229] Reflex tachycardia is not a problem, but bradycardia may occur.

XIII. HISTAMINE BLOCKERS

Histamine blockers may be classified according to whether they antagonize primarily H_1 or H_2 receptors. The potential adverse effects of these two drug classes differ substantially.

A. H_1 blockers

The H_1 receptor antagonists represent a chemically diverse group of compounds, of which diphenhydramine and promethazine are probably of most interest to anesthesiologists. In general, adverse effects of these antihistamines include sedation, dizziness, and the anticholinergic effects of dry mouth and increased heart rate.[230] Rapid intravenous injection may cause a decrease in blood pressure. Antihistaminic poisoning may lead to seizures, coma, and cardiovascular collapse. Promethazine enhances the sedative effects of opioids.[231]

B. H_2 blockers

Cimetidine is the model H_2 blocking drug. Blockade of H_2 receptors decreases gastric acidity as a desired therapeutic effect, though this breakdown of the gastric acid barrier has been alleged to predispose to infection.[232] Cimetidine crosses the blood-brain barrier and can produce sedation, confusion, and even coma, especially in elderly patients.[233] Rapid intravenous administration of cimetidine frequently induces a decrease in blood pressure and has been reported to cause bradycardia, heart block, and cardiac arrest.[234] A reversible interstitial nephritis with an increase in serum creatinine occurs in about 3% of chronically treated patients. Mild increases in serum transaminases and alkaline phosphatase are also described. Gynecomastia may be induced in some male patients. Neutropenia and thrombocytopenia occur rarely with cimetidine and are usually reversible upon discontinuation of the drug.[235] Cimetidine reduces hepatic blood flow and decreases the elimination of drugs metabolized by cytochrome P-450–related enzymes (such as lidocaine, propranolol, and diazepam).[230]

Ranitidine and famotidine are two newer H2 blockers which may have fewer side effects than cimetidine.[236] Ranitidine is less likely to cause sedation than cimetidine, and neither ranitidine nor famotidine appear to alter hepatic metabolism of drugs. Bradycardia has been reported with the intravenous administration of raniti-dine.[237]

XIV. ANTACIDS

Although the use of antacids is remarkably safe, complications can occur.[238] Antacids increase gastric fluid volume[239] and delay gastric empty-ing,[240] and all except aluminum hydroxide may produce a metabolic alkalosis in patients with renal failure. Particulate antacids if aspirated produce a granulomatous pulmonary reaction, which may be as damaging as acid aspira-tion.[241]

A. Aluminum hydroxide

The most common complication of aluminum hydroxide administration is constipation. Hy-pophosphatemia may occur as aluminum binds with phosphates in the intestinal tract, and since these aluminum phosphates are not ab-sorbed, phosphate loss ensues. With this hy-pophosphatemia, calcium absorption increases and hypercalciuria with nephrolithiasis may fol-low.[242] Hypomagnesemia is another potential adverse effect of aluminum hydroxide therapy. In patients with renal failure, the accumulation of aluminum to toxic levels has been re-ported.[243]

B. Calcium carbonate

Hyperphosphatemia and hypercalcemia may oc-cur with calcium carbonate, especially in the presence of renal failure. Acid rebound is com-mon as calcium promotes increased secretion of gastric acid.[244] Hypercalcemic alkalosis with an increase in serum creatinine and blood urea ni-trogen (milk-alkali syndrome) may rarely occur after prolonged calcium carbonate therapy.

C. Sucralfate

Sucralfate, though not itself an antacid, is a complex of aluminum hydroxide and sucrose sulfate. Like aluminum hydroxide, its main complication is constipation.

D. Sodium bicarbonate

Although a very potent acid-neutralizing agent, sodium bicarbonate's effect on gastric pH is short lived, and the large amount of sodium ab-sorbed may cause significant difficulty for pa-tients with hypertension or congestive heart failure.

E. Sodium citrate

Sodium citrate is associated with few adverse effects. Aspiration of 0.3 M sodium citrate causes less pulmonary damage than that caused by particulate antacids. The "complication" of poor palatability is lessened considerably in commercial preparations containing citric acid (such as Polycitra, Bicitra).

XV. DIURETICS
A. Loop diuretics

Loop diuretics (furosemide, ethacrinic acid) are potent drugs that may significantly alter the body's fluid and electrolyte balance. Hypovole-mia, hyponatremia, and hypokalemia can be problems with these drugs.[217] The volume de-pletion caused by the loop diuretics can be se-vere and even result in death.[245] Uric acid con-centrations are increased and precipitation of acute attacks of gout are possible in susceptible persons. Ototoxicity occurs with high peak blood levels of these drugs and rapid injection should be avoided. Ethacrinic acid may be more ototoxic than furosemide. Furosemide has a chemical structure similar to the sulfonamides, and cross-allergic responses occur. Blood pres-sure may decrease after intravenous administra-tion of furosemide because of increased venous capacitance with a decrease in cardiac preload. Interstitial nephritis has been reported occur-ring after furosemide.[246] Lithium clearance is decreased by the loop diuretics, and elevation of lithium levels may occur with the periopera-tive use of furosemide.[247] Furosemide may en-hance the relaxant effect of nondepolarizing neuromuscular blockers.[248]

B. Thiazides

Thiazide diuretics may cause a hypochloremic, hypokalemic metabolic alkalosis, and like loop diuretics may increase serum uric acid levels.[217] These drugs decrease carbohydrate tolerance and can elevate serum glucose levels in diabetic patients. Rashes are common. Other reported complications of thiazide therapy have included purpura, photosensitive dermatitis, antibody-induced thrombocytopenia, bone marrow de-pression, and necrotizing vasculitis.[246]

C. Potassium-sparing diuretics

The potassium-sparing diuretics can seriously elevate serum potassium levels, especially in re-nal failure. In addition, spironolactone may produce nausea and gynecomastia in men.[246]

D. Osmotic diuretics

The osmotic diuretics (mannitol, urea) tran-siently increase extracellular fluid volume[249] and may exacerbate congestive heart failure. Hyponatremia can occur because of the so-dium-losing diuresis of these drugs. Urea pro-duces a significant incidence of venous thrombosis, and tissue necrosis may occur with extravasation of urea solutions.

E. Carbonic anhydrase inhibitors

Carbonic anhydrase inhibitors (such as acetazolamide) may cause paresthesias and drowsiness in large doses.[246] Acetazolamide is teratogenic in animals and has been associated with osteomalacia when combined with phenytoin.

XVI. ANTICOAGULANTS AND THROMBOLYTICS

The chief danger from the use of any of the anticoagulants and thrombolytic agents is hemorrhage.[250] Although the incidence of this complication with these drugs may be minimized by appropriate hematologic monitoring, bleeding may occur despite maintenance of coagulation studies within the desired therapeutic range. Hemorrhagic complications appear to be more frequent in elderly women.

A. Heparin

An acute small decrease in platelet count may accompany heparin therapy in up to one third of patients.[251] This is of little clinical significance; however a severe thrombocytopenia may occur in less than 1% of heparin-treated patients. Platelet counts usually return toward normal levels upon discontinuation of the drug. Paradoxically, some patients may display a thrombotic diathesis during heparin therapy because of a decrease in antithrombin III activity.[252] Necrosis of the skin and subcutaneous tissues has been attributed to heparin.[253] Serum transaminases increase in many patients during heparin therapy.[254] Hyperkalemia may occur, especially in patients with diabetes or renal insufficiency.[255] Heparin is highly protein bound and may displace other drugs (such as diazepam, propranolol) from protein-binding sites thereby increasing their free plasma concentrations.[256]

B. Coumarin derivatives (oral anticoagulants)

Coumarin derivatives are associated with significant teratogenic effects when administered to pregnant women in the first trimester and also cross the placenta to produce a high risk of fetal hemorrhage.[257] Like heparin, coumarin may cause skin necrosis.[253] Concomitant administration of salicylates or phenylbutazone significantly increases the risk of hemorrhagic complications.[258]

C. Thrombolytics

In contrast to the traditional anticoagulants, which prevent formation of new clot, the thrombolytic agents (streptokinase, urokinase, and tissue plasminogen activators) enhance the conversion of plasminogen to plasmin and thus the lysis of existing clot.[250] This pharmacologic action explains the greater risk of hemorrhage with these drugs than with heparin therapy.[259] Fever is a common side effect of these drugs, and allergic responses are more prevalent with streptokinase than with urokinase or tissue plasminogen activators. Aminocaproic acid antagonizes the thrombolytic effect of these drugs and may be used to treat thrombolytic drug overdose.[250]

D. Protamine

Although usually administered to neutralize the effects of heparin, protamine has intrinsic anticoagulant properties.[260] Intraoperative bleeding has been attributed to protamine excess when used to reverse heparin anticoagulation, possibly attributable to inhibition of platelet aggregation.[261] Protamine may be associated with significant histamine release especially if administered rapidly, producing cutaneous flushing, bronchoconstriction, hypotension, and tachycardia.[260] Patients with limited cardiac reserve may be more susceptible to protamine-induced hypotension.[262] Protamine has been reported to increase pulmonary vascular resistance.[263] Allergic reactions to protamine appear to be more likely in patients receiving protamine-containing insulin preparations[264] and possibly in patients allergic to fish because protamine is a fish-derived product.

XVII. ANTIPLATELET AGENTS
A. Aspirin

Aspirin's antiplatelet effect may prolong bleeding time values for several days and may cause excessive intraoperative bleeding.[265] Salicylate toxicity includes symptoms of headache, tinnitus, confusion, drowsiness, nausea, and hyperventilation.[266]

B. Dipyridamole

Complications of dipyridamole therapy include dizziness, abdominal distress, headache, and rashes.[250]

C. Dextrans

Used as volume expanders as well as antiplatelet agents, dextran 40 and dextran 70 have been associated with severe anaphylactoid reactions.[267] Dextran 40 may cause acute renal failure,[268] especially if administered to hypovolemic patients, because it is filtered by the kidney and may increase urine viscosity to the point of tubular obstruction. Dextran 70 may produce a bleeding diathesis.[269]

XVIII. ANTIDYSRHYTHMIC AGENTS

The complications of lidocaine, calcium-channel blockers, digitalis, adenosine, and beta-adrenergic antagonists are covered elsewhere in this chapter.

A. Procainamide

In addition to its membrane-stabilizing effects, procainamide has ganglionic blocking properties. Vasodilatation and hypotension may occur after procainamide administration, particularly after rapid intravenous injection.[269] Procainamide slows impulse conduction through the heart causing widening of the QRS complex and prolongation of the PR and QT intervals on the ECG, which may be premonitory signs of heart block or cardiac arrest. Negative inotropic effects of procainamide can be pronounced in patients with preexisting myocardial dysfunction.[270] Fever, agranulocytosis, and a lupus-like syndrome may also complicate procainamide therapy. Procainamide may enhance the neuromuscular blockade of nondepolarizing muscle relaxants[271] and may induce significant muscle weakness in myasthenic patients.[272]

B. Quinidine

Gastrointestinal upset (nausea, vomiting, diarrhea) are the most frequent side effects of quinidine. On the ECG, prolongation of the QRS complex and QT interval occur with higher blood levels of drug, and serious ventricular dysrhythmias including ventricular tachycardia (torsade de pointes) and ventricular fibrillation may result. Quinidine has alpha-adrenergic blocking properties and can cause hypotension, which can be severe if the drug is administered intravenously. Hypokalemia exacerbates quinidine-induced cardiac dysrhythmias. A high blood concentration of quinidine may produce tinnitus and vertigo similar to salicylate toxicity. Fever, hepatic dysfunction, and thrombocytopenia are immunologically mediated complications of quinidine therapy.[270] Quinidine enhances the muscle-relaxant effects of the depolarizing and nondepolarizing neuromuscular blockers[273] and also increases the plasma concentration of digoxin.[270]

C. Bretylium

Release of endogenous norepinephrine caused by administration of bretylium may cause an initial tachycardia and hypertension; however, bretylium subsequently produces an adrenergic block, which can lead to hypotension and bradycardia.[274] Nausea and vomiting may also occur with bretylium.[186]

D. Phenytoin

Phenytoin (diphenylhydantoin) is a drug with anticonvulsant as well as antidysrhythmic properties. When administered by rapid intravenous infusion, transient high blood levels may induce nystagmus, dizziness, hypotension, heart block, and asystole. Chronic therapy is associated with gingival hyperplasia, peripheral neuropathy, hyperglycemia, skin rashes, megaloblastic anemia, and hepatitis.[270]

E. Disopyramide

The complications of disopyramide include anticholinergic effects (dry mouth, urinary retention), myocardial depression, and conduction abnormalities.[270] Congestive heart failure can be induced by disopyramide when administered in the presence of preexisting myocardial dysfunction.[275]

F. Amiodarone

Administration of the antidysrhythmic drug amiodarone may be accompanied by bradycardia and a lengthening of the QT interval on the ECG.[276] Vasodilatation, hypotension, heart block, and sinus arrest can complicate amiodarone therapy,[277] and severe bradycardia with sinus arrest has occurred under general anesthesia.[278] Bradycardia with amiodarone appears to be resistant to atropine and may require beta-adrenergic therapy with isoproterenol or artificial pacemaker insertion. Chronic therapy with amiodarone can be associated with hyperthyroidism or hypothyroidism, photosensitivity, neuropathies, and hepatotoxicity. Plasma concentrations of digoxin may be significantly elevated by amiodarone.[279]

XIX. ANTIBIOTICS

A complete review of the adverse effects of all available antibiotics is beyond the scope of this chapter. Since anesthesiologists may frequently administer these drugs at the request of the surgeon, however, the antibiotic-induced complications of greatest importance to the practice of anesthesia are presented.

A. Penicillins and cephalosporins

The most common adverse reactions to penicillins and cephalosporins are allergy related.[280] The majority of these reactions are skin rashes, but bronchospasm, angioedema, and anaphylaxis also occur. Despite the common beta-lactam structure, the cross-sensitivity between penicillins and cephalosporins is not absolute but is estimated to occur in up to 10% of patients with a penicillin allergy.[281] Anaphylaxis to a cephalosporin in penicillin-allergic patients can certainly occur.[282] In light of this incidence of cross-sensitivity, the administration of a cephalosporin to a patient with a history of a life-threatening reaction to a penicillin must be done cautiously.[281]

B. Aminoglycosides

The aminoglycosides are associated with several potential complications relevant to anesthetic practice. These agents may cause ototoxicity and nephrotoxicity, especially with high blood levels.[283,284] Rapid intravenous administration of these drugs is best avoided to prevent high peak blood levels, which may induce demonstrable ototoxicity with a single aminoglycoside injection.[285] Skeletal muscle weakness can occur and may be pronounced in patients with myasthenia gravis.[286,287] Systemic absorption resulting in neuromuscular blockage has occurred after intraperitoneal irrigation with solutions containing aminoglycoside antibiotics.[287] Potentiation of the effects of the nondepolarizing neuromuscular blockers can occur.

C. Vancomycin

Rapid intravenous infusion (less than 60 minutes) of vancomycin can be associated with cutaneous flushing, bronchospasm, and profound hypotension caused by histamine release and possibly direct myocardial depression. Skin rashes, ototoxicity, and rarely nephrotoxicity are other complications of vancomycin.[288]

D. Amphotericin B

Significant adverse effects are common with this antifungal agent. During the infusion of amphotericin, fever, chills, and malaise occur frequently, and hypotension is not uncommon. Renal toxicity is common. Anemia, thrombocytopenia, hypokalemia, and seizures can also occur with amphotericin.[289]

XX. MISCELLANEOUS DRUGS
A. Metoclopramide

Metoclopramide stimulates upper gastrointestinal motility and can cause abdominal pain and cramping.[290] The drug should not be used in patients with bowel obstructions or perforations because increases in intraluminal gastrointestinal pressures might cause or increase intraperitoneal spillage of bowel contents. Extreme restlessness (akathisia) can occur with higher blood levels of metoclopramide,[291] especially in children, the elderly, and patients with renal failure. Metoclopramide may cause extrapyramidal reactions and sedation and may increase the extrapyramidal and sedative effects of other drugs. Other complications of metoclopramide therapy occur mainly with long-term

therapy and include dysphoria, agitation, oral or periorbital edema, dry mouth, and cutaneous rashes.

B. Theophylline

Adverse effects seen with theophylline include nausea and vomiting, headache, restlessness, agitation, seizures, tachycardia, and cardiac dysrhythmias.[292,293] Cardiac dysrhythmias may be more frequent or severe when theophylline is combined with beta agonists or halothane anesthesia.[28,293] Avoidance of administration of intravenous theophylline through a central line has been suggested to minimize the exposure of the heart to high drug concentrations.[294] Monitoring the blood concentration of theophylline is useful in avoidance of toxicity.

C. Pentoxifylline

Used in patients with peripheral vascular disease to improve capillary blood flow, pentoxifylline has rare complications, but they include cardiac dysrhythmias, hypotension, and angina.[295]

D. Doxapram

Doxapram may induce hypertension, tachycardia, vomiting, sweating, fever, and convulsions.[296]

E. Dantrolene

Dantrolene sodium administered for prophylaxis against malignant hyperthermia can induce dizziness, nausea, blurred vision, diarrhea, and sedation.[297] Skeletal muscle weakness is a common subjective complaint and can be of clinical significance in patients with preexisting muscular disorders.[298] Hepatitis after chronic therapy with dantrolene is not uncommon;[299] however, hepatic dysfunction with acute administration has not been reported.

REFERENCES

1. Kavan EM and Juliene RM: Central nervous system effects of isoflurane (Forane), Can Anaesth Soc J 21:390-402, 1974.
2. Eger EI, Stevens WC, and Cromwell TH: The electroencephalogram in man anesthetized with Forane, Anesthesiology 35:504-508, 1971.
3. Neigh JL, Garman JK, and Harp JR: The electroencephalographic pattern during anesthesia with Ethrane: effects of depth of anesthesia, PaCO$_2$, and nitrous oxide, Anesthesiology 35:482-487, 1971.
4. Sprague DH and Wolf S: Enflurane seizures in patients taking amitriptyline, Anesth Analg 61:67-68, 1982.
5. Eger EI: Isoflurane (Forane): a compendium and reference, Madison, Wisc, 1984, Ohio Medical Products.
6. Adams RW, Cucciara RF, Gronert GA, et al: Isoflu-

rane and cerebrospinal fluid pressure in neurosurgical patients, Anesthesiology 54:97-99, 1981.

7. Grosslight K, Foster R, Colohan AR, et al: Isoflurane for neurosurgical anesthesia: risk factors for increases in intracranial pressure, Anesthesiology 63:533-536, 1985.

8. Johnston RR, Eger EI, and Wilson, C: A comparative interaction of epinephrine with enflurane, isoflurane, and halothane in man, Anesth Analg 55:709-712, 1976.

9. Reiz S and Ostman M: Regional coronary hemodynamics during isoflurane–nitrous oxide anesthesia in patients with ischemic–heart disease, Anesth Analg 64:570-576, 1985.

10. Tarnow J, Markschies-Hornung A, and Schulte-Sasse U: Isoflurane improves tolerance to pacing-induced myocardial ischemia, Anesthesiology 64:147-156, 1986.

11. Moffit EA, Barker RA, Glenn JJ, et al: Myocardial metabolism and hemodynamic responses with isoflurane anesthesia for coronary artery surgery, Anesth Analg 63:252, 1984.

12. Tuman KJ, McCarthy RJ, Spiess BD, et al: Does choice of anesthetic agent significantly alter outcome after coronary artery surgery? Anesthesiology 70:189-198, 1989.

13. Berman ML and Holaday DA: Inhalation anesthetic metabolism and toxicity. In Barash PG, Cullen BF, and Stoelting RK, editors: Clinical anesthesia, Philadelphia, 1989, JB Lippincott Co.

14. Mazze RI, Calverley RK, and Smith NT: Inorganic fluoride nephrotoxicity: prolonged enflurane and halothane anesthesia in volunteers, Anesthesiology 46:265-271, 1977.

15. Cousins MJ, Greenstein LR, Hitt BA, et al: Metabolism and renal effects of enflurane in man, Anesthesiology 44:44-53, 1976.

16. Mazze RI, Cousins MJ, and Barr GA: Renal effects and metabolism of isoflurane in man, Anesthes 40:536-542, 1974.

17. Munson ES and Embro WJ: Enflurane, isoflurane, and halothane and isolated uterine muscle, Anesthes 46:11-14, 1977.

18. Warren TM, Datta S, Ostheimer GW, et al: Comparison of the maternal and neonatal effects of halothane, enflurane, and isoflurane for cesarean delivery, Anesth Analg 62:516-520, 1983.

19. Murphy MR and Hug CC: The enflurane sparing effect of morphine, butorphanol, and nalbuphine, Anesthes 57:489-492, 1982.

20. Perisho JA, Buechel DR, and Miller RD: The effect of diazepam (Valium) on minimum alveolar anesthetic requirement (MAC) in man, Can Anaesth Soc J 18:536-540, 1971.

21. Saidman LJ and Eger EI: Effect of nitrous oxide and of narcotic premedication on the alveolar concentration of halothane required for anesthesia, Anesthesiology 25:302-306, 1964.

22. DiFazio CA, Niederlehner JR, and Burney RG: The anesthetic potency of lidocaine in the rat, Anesth Analg 55:818-821, 1976.

23. Bloor BC and Flacke WE: Reduction in halothane anesthetic requirements by clonidine, an alpha adrenergic agonist, Anesth Analg 61:741-745, 1982.

24. Miller RD, Way WL, and Eger EI: The effects of alpha-methyldopa, reserpine, guanethidine, and iproniazid on minimum alveolar anesthetic requirement (MAC) Anesthesiology 29:1153-1158, 1968.

25. Thiagararajah S, Grynsztejn M, Lear E, et al: Ventricular arrhythmias after terbutaline administration to patients anesthetized with halothane, Anesth Analg 65:417-418, 1986.

26. Foex P: Alpha- and beta-adrenoceptor antagonists, Br J Anaesth 56:751-765, 1984.

27. Reves JG, Kissin I, Lell WA, et al: Calcium entry blockers: uses and implications for the anesthesiologist, Anesthesiology 57:504-518, 1982.

28. Roizen MF and Stevens VC: Multiform ventricular tachycardia due to the interaction of aminophylline and halothane, Anesth Analg 58:259-260, 1978.

29. Edwards RP, Miller RD, Roizen MF, et al: Cardiac effects of imipramine and pancuronium during halothane and enflurane anesthesia, Anesthesiology 50:421-425, 1979.

30. Navalgund AA, Alifimoff JK, Jakymec AJ, et al: Amiodarone-induced sinus arrest successfully treated with ephedrine and isoproterenol, Anesth Analg 65:414-416, 1986.

31. Liberman BA and Teasdale SJ: Anaesthesia and amiodarone, Can Anaesth Soc J 32:629-638, 1985.

32. Eger EI: Respiratory effects of nitrous oxide. In Eger EI, editor: Nitrous oxide, New York, 1985, Elsevier Science Publishing Co, Inc.

33. Nelson TE and Flewellen EH: The malignant hyperthermia syndrome, N Engl J Med 309:416-418, 1983.

34. Knill RL and Clement JL: Variable effects of anaesthetics on the ventilatory response to hypoxaemia in man, Can Anaesth Soc J 29:93-99, 1982.

35. Hendriksen HT and Jörgensen PB: The effect of nitrous oxide on intracranial pressure in patients with intracranial disorders, Br J Anaesth 45:486-492, 1973.

36. Smith NT, Eger EI, Stoelting RK, et al: The cardiovascular and sympathomimetic responses to the addition of nitrous oxide to halothane in man, Anesthesiology 32:410-412, 1970.

37. Dolan WM, Stevens WC, Eger EI, et al: The cardiovascular and respiratory effects of isoflurane–nitrous oxide anaesthesia, Can Anaesth Soc J 21:557-568, 1974.

38. Smith NT, Calverly RK, Prys-Roberts C, et al: Impact of nitrous oxide on the circulation during enflurane anesthesia in man, Anesthesiology 48:345-349, 1978.

39. McDermott RW and Stanley TH: The cardiovascular effects of low concentrations of nitrous oxide during morphine anesthesia, Anesthesiology 41:89-91, 1974.

40. Eisele JH, Reitan JA, Massumi RA, et al: Myocardial performance and N_2O analgesia in coronary artery disease, Anesthesiology 44:16-20, 1976.

41. Schulte-Sasse U, Hess W, and Tarnow J: Pulmonary vascular responses to nitrous oxide in patients with normal and high pulmonary vascular resistance, Anesthesiology 57:9-13, 1982.

42. Koblin DD, Watson JE, Deady JE, et al: Inactivation of methionine synthetase activity by nitrous oxide in mice, Anesthesiology 54:318-324, 1981.

43. Nunn JF, Weinbren HK, Royston D, et al: Rate of inactivation of human and rodent hepatic methionine synthetase by nitrous oxide, Anesthesiology 68:213-216, 1988.

44. O'Sullivan H, Jennings F, Ward K, et al: Human bone marrow biochemical function and megaloblastic hematopoesis after nitrous oxide anesthesia, Anesthesiology 55:645-649, 1981.

45. Ames JAL, Burman JF, Rees GM, et al: Megaloblastic hematopoesis in patients receiving nitrous oxide, Lancet 2:339-342, 1978.

46. Layzer RB, Fishman RA, and Schafer JA: Neuropathy following abuse of nitrous oxide, Neurology 28:504-506, 1978.

47. Lane GA, DuBoulay PM, Tait AR, et al: Nitrous ox-

ide is teratogenic, halothane is not, Anesthesiology 55:A252, 1981.

48. Crawford JS and Lewis M: Nitrous oxide in early human pregnancy, Anaesthesia 41:900-905, 1986.

49. Aldridge LM and Tunstall ME: Nitrous oxide and the fetus: a review and the results of a retrospective study of 175 cases of anaesthesia for insertion of Shirodkar suture, Br J Anaesth 58:1469-1470, 1986.

50. Eger EI: Anesthetic uptake and action, Baltimore, 1974, Williams & Wilkins.

51. Eger EI and Saidman LJ: Hazards of nitrous oxide in bowel obstruction and pneumothorax, Anesthesiology 26:61-66, 1965.

52. Munson ES and Merrick HC: Effect of nitrous oxide on venous air embolism, Anesthesiology 27:783-787, 1966.

53. Casey WF and Drake-Lee AB: Nitrous oxide and middle ear pressure, Anaesthesia 37:896-900, 1982.

54. Owens WD, Gustave F, and Scaroff A: Tympanic membrane rupture with nitrous oxide anesthesia, Anesth Analg 57:283-286, 1978.

55. Wood MW: Intravenous anesthetic agents. In Wood MW and Wood AJJ, editors: Drugs and anesthesia: pharmacology for anesthesiologists, ed 2, Baltimore, 1990, Williams & Wilkins.

56. Stoelting RK, Dierdorf SF, and McCammon RL: Metabolism and nutrition. In Anesthesia and co-existing disease, ed 2, New York, 1988, Churchill Livingstone, Inc.

57. Durrett LR and Lawson NW: Autonomic nervous system physiology and pharmacology. In Barash PG, Cullen BF, and Stoelting RK, editors: Clinical anesthesia, Philadelphia, 1989, JB Lippincott Co.

58. Sonntag H, Helborg K, Schenk HD, et al: Effects of thiopental on coronary blood flow and myocardial metabolism in man, Acta Anaesth Scand 19:69-78, 1975.

59. Graves CL: Management of general anesthesia during hemorrhage, Int Anesth Clin 12:1-49, 1974.

60. O'Donnell JF, Hewitt JC, and Dundee JW: Clinical studies of induction agents. XXVIII: A further comparison of the venous complications following thiopentone, methohexitone, and propanidid, Br J Anaesth 41:681-683, 1969.

61. Stone HH and Donnelly CC: The accidental intra-arterial injection of thiopental, Anesthesiology 22:995-1006, 1961.

62. Dundee JW and Wyant GM: Intravenous anesthesia, Edinburgh, 1974, Churchill Livingstone Inc.

63. Helrich M, Eckenhoff JE, and Jones RE: Influence of opiates on the respiratory response of man to thiopental, Anesthesiology 17:459-467, 1956.

64. Harrison GA: The influence of different anesthetic agents on the response to respiratory tract irritation, Br J Anaesth 34:804-811, 1962.

65. Power SJ, Morgan M, and Chakrabarti MK: Carbon dioxide response curves following midazolam and diazepam, Br J Anaesth 55:837-841, 1983.

66. Greenblatt DJ, Allen MD, Noel BJ, et al: Acute overdosage with benzodiazepine derivatives, Clin Pharmacol Ther 4:497-514, 1977.

67. Reves JG, Fragen RJ, Vinik HR, et al: Midazolam: pharmacology and uses, Anesthesiology 62:310-324, 1985.

68. Rao S, Sherbaniuk RW, Prasad K, et al: Cardiopulmonary effects of diazepam, Clin Pharmacol 14:182-189, 1973.

69. McCammon RL, Hilgenberg JC, and Stoelting RK: Hemodynamic effects of diazepam and diazepam–nitrous oxide in patients with coronary artery disease, Anesth Analg 59:438-441, 1980.

70. Falk RB, Denlinger JK, Nahrwold ML, et al: Acute vasodilation following induction of anesthesia with intravenous diazepam and nitrous oxide, Anesthesiology 49:149-150, 1978.

71. Samuelson PN, Reves JG, Kouchoukos NT, et al: Hemodynamic responses to anesthetic induction with midazolam or diazepam in patients with ischemic heart disease, Anesth Analg 60:802-809, 1981.

72. Adams P, Gelman S, Reves JG, et al: Midazolam pharmacodynamics and pharmacokinetics during acute hypovolemia, Anesthesiology 63:140-146, 1985.

73. Korttila K and Aromaa U: Venous complications after intravenous injection of diazepam, flunitrazepam, thiopentone, and etomidate, Acta Anaesth Scand 24:227-230, 1980.

74. McClure JH, Brown DT, and Wildsmith JAW: Comparison of the i.v. administration of midazolam and diazepam as sedation during spinal anesthesia, Br J Anaesth 55:1089-1093, 1983.

75. Camman W, Cohen MB, and Ostheimer GW: Is midazolam desirable for sedation in parturients? Anesthesiology 65:441, 1985.

76. Saxen I and Saxen L: Association between maternal intake of diazepam and oral clefts, Lancet 2:498, 1975.

77. Gyermek L: Clinical effects of diazepam prior to and during general anesthesia, Curr Ther Res 17:175-188, 1975.

78. Stanley TH, Bennett GM, Loeser EA, et al: Cardiovascular effects of diazepam and droperidol during morphine anesthesia, Anesthesiology 44:255-258, 1976.

79. White PF: Propofol: pharmakokinetics and pharmacodynamics, Semin Anesth VII:1(suppl):4-20, 1988.

80. Profeta JP, Guffin A, Mikula S, et al: The hemodynamic effects of propofol and thiamylal sodium for induction in coronary artery surgery, Anesth Analg 66:S142, 1987.

81. James MFM, Reyneke CJ, and Whiffler K: Heart block following propofol: a case report, Br J Anaesth 62:213-215, 1989.

82. Tarnow J, Hess W, and Klein W: Etomidate, alfathesin, and thiopentone as induction agents for coronary artery surgery, Can Anaesth Soc J 27:338-344, 1980.

83. Schou Olesen A, Huttel MS, and Hole P: Venous sequelae following the injection of etomidate or thiopentone i.v., Br J Anaesth 56:171-173, 1984.

84. Moss E, Powell D, Gibson W, et al: Effect of etomidate on intracranial pressure and cerebral perfusion pressure, Br J Anaesth 51:347-352, 1979.

85. Wauquier A: Profile of etomidate, Anaesthesia 38S:26-33, 1983.

86. Gancher S, Laxer KD, and Krieger W: Activation of epileptogenic activity by etomidate, Anesthesiology 61:616-618, 1984.

87. Daehlin L and Gran L: Etomidate and thiopentone: a comparative study of their respiratory effects, Curr Ther Res 27:706-713, 1980.

88. Wagner RL, White PF, Kan PB, et al: Inhibition of adrenal steroidogenesis by the anesthetic etomidate, N Engl J Med 310:1415-1421, 1984.

89. Horrigan RW, Moyers JR, Johnson BH, et al: Etomidate versus thiopentone with and without fentanyl: comparative study of awakening in man, Anesthesiology 52:362-364, 1980.

90. Schwartz DA and Horwitz LD: Effects of ketamine on left ventricular performance, J Pharmacol Exp Ther 194:410-414, 1975.

91. Tweed WA, Minuck MS, and Mymin D: Circulatory

response to ketamine anesthesia, Anesthesiology 37:613-619, 1972.

92. Pedersen T, Engback J, Klausen NO, et al: Effects of low-dose ketamine and thiopentone on cardiac performance and myocardial oxygen balance in high risk patients, Acta Anaesth Scand 26:235-239, 1982.

93. White PF, Way WL, and Trevor AJ: Ketamine — its pharmacology and therapeutic uses, Anesthesiology 56:119-136, 1982.

94. Taylor PA and Towey RM: Depression of laryngeal reflexes under ketamine anesthesia, Br Med J 2:688-689, 1971.

95. Takeshita H, Okuda Y, and Sari A: The effects of ketamine on cerebral circulation and metabolism in man, Anesthesiology 36:69-75, 1972.

96. Bidwai AV, Stanley TH, Graves CL, et al: The effects of ketamine on cardiovascular dynamics during halothane and enflurane anesthesia, Anesth Analg 54:588-592, 1975.

97. Drugs for psychiatric disorders, Med Letter Drugs Ther 25:45-47, 1983.

98. Stoelting RK, Dierdorf SF, and McCammon RL: Psychiatric illness. In Anesthesia and co-existing disease, ed 2, New York, 1988, Churchill Livingstone, Inc.

99. Lee CM and Yeakel AE: Patients refusal of surgery following Innovar premedication, Anesth Analg 54:224-226, 1975.

100. Shader RI and DiMascio A: Psychotropic drug side effects: chemical and theoretical perspectives, Baltimore, 1970, Williams & Wilkins Co.

101. Itil TM: Effects of psychotropic drugs on qualitatively and quantitatively analyzed human EEG. In Clark WG and del Giudice J, editors: Principles of psychopharmacology, ed 2, New York, 1978, Academic Press, Inc.

102. Kaufman JS: Drug interactions involving psychotherapeutic agents. In Simpson LL, editor: Drug treatment of mental disorders, New York, 1976, Raven Press.

103. Caroff SN: The neuroleptic malignant syndrome, J Clin Psychiatry 41:79-83, 1980.

104. Guze BH and Baxter LR: Neuroleptic malignant syndrome, N Engl J Med 313:163-166, 1985.

105. Kosanin R: Anesthetic considerations in patients on tricyclic antidepressant therapy, Anesth Rev 8(12):38-41, 1981.

106. Vohra J and Burrows GD: Cardiovascular complications tricyclic antidepressant overdosage, Drugs 8:432-437, 1974.

107. Jaffe JH and Martin WR: Opioid analgesics and antagonists. In Gilman AG, Goodman LS, Rall TW, et al: The pharmacological basis of therapeutics, New York, 1985, Macmillan Publishing Co.

108. Jenkins LC and Graves HB: Potential hazards of psychoactive drugs in association with anaesthesia, Can Anaesth Soc J 23:334-335, 1976.

109. Baldessarian RJ: Chemotherapy in psychiatry: principles and practice, rev ed, Cambridge, 1985, Harvard University Press.

110. Janowsky EC, Risch C, and Janowsky DS: Effect of anesthesia on patients taking psychotropic drugs, J Clin Psychopharmacol 1:14-20, 1981.

111. Bodley PO, Halwax K and Potts L: Low pseudocholinesterase levels complicating treatment with phenelzine, Br Med J 3:510-512, 1969.

112. Brown TCK and Cass NM: Beware — the use of MAO inhibitors is increasing again, Anaesth Intensive Care 7:65-68, 1979.

113. Boakes AJ, Laurence DR, Teoh PC, et al: Interactions between sympathomimetic amines and antidepressant agents in man, Br Med J 1:311-315, 1973.

114. Hirshman CA and Lindeman K: MAO inhibitors: must they be discontinued before anesthesia? JAMA 260:3507, 1988.

115. Martin WR: Pharmacology of opioids, Pharmacol Rev 35:283-323, 1983.

116. Hilgenberg JC: Intraoperative awareness during high dose fentanyl-oxygen anesthesia, Anesthesiology 54:341-343, 1981.

117. Rosow CE, Moss I, Philbin DM, et al: Histamine release during morphine and fentanyl anesthesia, Anesthesiology 56:93-96, 1982.

118. Wood M: Opioid agonists and antagonists. In Wood MW and Wood AJJ, editors: Drugs and anesthesia: pharmacology for anesthesiologists, ed 2, Baltimore, 1990, Williams & Wilkins.

119. Radnay PA, Brodman E, Mankikar D, et al: The effect of equianalgesic doses of fentanyl, morphine, meperidine, and pentazocine on common bile duct pressure, Anaesthetist 29:26-29, 1980.

120. Murphy MR: Opioids. In Barash PG, Cullen BF, and Stoelting RK, editors: Clinical anesthesia, Philadelphia, 1989, JB Lippincott Co.

121. Stanley TH and Liu WS: Cardiovascular effects of meperidine-N_2O anesthesia before and after pancuronium, Anesth Analg 56:669-673, 1977.

122. Flacke JW, Flacke WE, Bloor BC, et al: Histamine release by four narcotics: a double-blind study in humans, Anesth Analg 66:723-730, 1987.

123. Becker L, Paulson B, Miller R, et al: Biphasic respiratory depression after fentanyl-droperidol or fentanyl alone used to supplement nitrous oxide anesthesia, Anesthesiology 44:291-296, 1976.

124. Moldenhauer CC and Hug CC Jr: Use of narcotic analgesics as anaesthetics, Clin Anaesthesiol 2(1):107-138, 1984.

125. Bennet GM and Stanley TH: Comparison of the cardiovascular effects of morphine-N_2O and fentanyl-N_2O balanced anesthesia in man, Anesthesiology 51:S102, 1979.

126. Monk JP, Beresford R, and Ward A: Sufentanil: a review of its pharmacological properties and therapeutic use, Drugs 36:286-313, 1988.

127. Chang J and Fish KJ: Acute respiratory arrest and rigidity after anesthesia with sufentanil: a case report, Anesthesiology 63:710-711, 1985.

128. Miller DR, Wellwood M, Teasdale SJ, et al: Effects of anaesthetic induction on myocardial function and metabolism: a comparison of fentanyl, sufentanil, and alfentanil, Can J Anaesth 35:219-233, 1988.

129. Cousins MJ and Mather LE: Intrathecal and epidural administration of opioids, Anesthesiology 61:276-310, 1984.

130. Smith G and Pinnock C: Naloxone — paradox or panacea? Br J Anaesth 57:547-549, 1985.

131. Longnecker DE, Grazis PA, and Eggers GWN: Naloxone for antagonism of morphine induced respiratory depression, Anesth Analg 52:447-453, 1973.

132. Jasinski DR: Human pharmacology of narcotic antagonists, Br J Clin Pharmacol 7:287S-290S, 1979.

133. Vandam LD: Drug therapy: butorphanol, N Engl J Med 302:381-384, 1980.

134. Popio KA, Jackson DH, Ross AM, et al: Hemodynamic and respiratory effects of morphine and butorphanol, Clin Pharmacol Ther 23:281-287, 1978.

135. Errick JK and Heel RC: Nalbuphine: a preliminary review of its pharmacological properties and therapeutic efficacy, Drugs 26:191-211, 1983.

136. Lee G, Low RI, Amsterdam EA, et al: Hemodynamic

effects of morphine and halbuphine in acute myocardial infarction, Clin Pharmacol Ther 29:576-581, 1981.

137. Brogden RN, Speight TM, and Avery GS: Pentazocine: a review of its pharmacological properties, therapeutic efficacy, and dependence liability, Drugs 5:6-91, 1973.

138. Lee G, DeMaria A, Amsterdam EA, et al: Comparative effects of morphine, meperidine and pentazocine on cardiocirculatory dynamics in patients with acute myocardial infarction, Am J Med 60:949-955, 1976.

139. Heel RC, Brogden RN, Speight TM, et al: Buprenorphine: a review of its pharmacological properties and therapeutic efficacy, Drugs 17:81-110, 1979.

140. Stoelting RK: Opioid agonists and antagonists. In Pharmacology and physiology in anesthetic practice, Philadelphia, 1987, JB Lippincott Co.

141. Mather LE and Cousins MJ: Local anesthetics and their current clinical use, Drugs 18:185-205, 1979.

142. Matsuo S, Rao DBS, Chaudry I, et al: Interaction of muscle relaxants and local anesthetics at the neuromuscular junction, Anesth Analg 57:580-587, 1978.

143. Brown DT, Beamish D, and Wildsmith JAW: Allergic reaction to an amide local anaesthetic, Br J Anaesth 53:435-437, 1981.

144. Nagel JE, Fuscaldo JT, and Fireman P: Paraben allergy, JAMA 237:1594-1595, 1977.

145. Aldrete JA and Johnson DA: Allergy to local anesthetics, JAMA 207:356-357, 1969.

146. Edouard A, Berdeaux A, Langloys J, et al: Effects of lidocaine on myocardial contractility and baroreflex control of heart rate in conscious dogs, Anesthesiology 64:316-321, 1986.

147. Collinsworth KA, Kalman SM, and Harrison DC: The clinical pharmacology of lidocaine as an anti-arrhythmic drug, Circulation 50:1217-1230, 1974.

148. Gross JB, Caldwell CB, Shaw LM, et al: The effect of lidocaine infusion on the ventilatory response to hypoxia, Anesthesiology 61:662-665, 1984.

149. Avery P, Redon D, Schaenzer G, et al: The influence of serum potassium on the cerebral and cardiac toxicity of bupivacaine and lidocaine, Anesthesiology 61:134-138, 1984.

150. Scanlon JW, Brown WU, Weiss JB, et al: Neurobehavioral responses of newborn infants after maternal epidural anesthesia, Anesthesiology 40:121-128, 1974.

151. deJong RH, Ronfeld RA, and DeRosa R: Cardiovascular effects of convulsant and supraconvulsant doses of amide local anesthetics, Anesth Analg 61:3-9, 1982.

152. Morishima HO, Pedersen H, Finster M, et al: Bupivacaine toxicity in pregnant and nonpregnant ewes, Anesthesiology 54:182-186, 1981.

153. Climie CR, McLean S, Starmer GA, et al: Methaemoglobinaemia in mother and foetus following continuous epidural analgesia with prilocaine, Br J Anaesth 39:155-160, 1967.

154. Scott DB and Cousins MJ: Clinical pharmacology of local anesthetic agents. In Cousins MJ and Bridenbaugh PO, editors: Neural blockade in clinical anesthesia and management of pain, Philadelphia, 1980, JB Lippincott Co.

155. Tucker GT: Pharmacokinetics of local anesthetics, Br J Anaesth 58:717-731, 1986.

156. Wang BC, Hillman DE, Spielholz NI, et al: Chronic neurological deficits and Nesacaine-CE—an effect of the anesthetic, 2-chloroprocaine, or the antioxidant, sodium bisulfite? Anesth Analg 63:445-447, 1984.

157. Cregler LL and Mark H: Medical complications of cocaine abuse, N Engl J Med 315:1495-1500, 1986.

158. Severinghaus JW, Xu, F-D, and Spellman MJ Jr: Benzocaine and methemoglobin: recommended actions, Anesthesiology 74:385-386, 1991.

159. Durant NN and Katz RL: Suxamethonium, Br J Anaesth 54:195-209, 1982.

160. Stoelting RK and Peterson C: Adverse effects of increased succinylcholine dose following d-tubocurarine pretreatment, Anesth Analg 54:282-288, 1975.

161. Lebowitz PW and Ramsey FM: Muscle relaxants. In Barash PG, Cullen BF, and Stoelting RK, editors: Clinical anesthesia, Philadelphia, 1989, JB Lippincott Co.

162. Mitchell MM, Ali HH, and Savarese JJ: Myotonia and neuromuscular blocking agents, Anesthesiology 49:44-48, 1978.

163. Ryan JF, Kagen LJ, and Hyman AI: Myoglobinemia after a single dose of succinylcholine, N Engl J Med 285:824-827, 1971.

164. Katz RL and Ryan JF: The neuromuscular effects of suxamethonium in man, Br J Anaesth 41:381-390, 1969.

165. Mecca RS: Postanesthesia recovery. In Barash PG, Cullen BF, and Stoelting RK, editors: Clinical anesthesia, Philadelphia, 1989, JB Lippincott Co.

166. Stoelting RK: The hemodynamic effects of pancuronium and d-tubocurarine in anesthetized patients, Anesthesiology 36:612-615, 1972.

167. Stoelting RK: Hemodynamic effects of dimethyltubocurarine during nitrous oxide–halothane anesthesia, Anesth Analg 53:513-515, 1974.

168. Bartolone RS and Rao TLK: Dysrhythmias following muscle relaxant administration in patients receiving digitalis, Anesthesiology 58:567-569, 1983.

169. Stoelting RK: Hemodynamic effects of gallamine during nitrous oxide–halothane anesthesia, Anesthesiology 39:645-647, 1973.

170. Basta SJ, Ali HH, Savarese JJ, et al: Clinical pharmacology of atracurium besylate (BW33A): a new nondepolarizing muscle relaxant, Anesth Analg 61:723-729, 1982.

171. Starr NJ, Sethna DH, and Estafanous FG: Bradycardia and asystole following the rapid administration of sufentanil with vecuronium, Anesthesiology 64:521-523, 1986.

172. Payne JP, Hughes R, and Azawi SA: Neuromuscular blockade by neostigmine in anaesthetized man, Br J Anaesth 52:69, 1980.

173. Sunew KY and Hicks RG: Effects of neostigmine and pyridostigmine on duration of succinylcholine action and pseudocholinesterase activity, Anesthesiology 49:188-191, 1978.

174. Bidwai AV, Stanley TH, Rogers C, et al: Reversal of diazepam-induced post-anesthetic somnolence with physostigmine, Anesthesiology 51:256-259, 1979.

175. Weiner N: Atropine, scopolamine and related antimuscarinic drugs. In Goodman AG and Gilman A, editors: The pharmacologic basis of therapeutics, New York, 1980, Macmillan Publishing Co.

176. Cooper MJ and Abinader EG: Atropine-induced ventricular fibrillation: case report and review of the literature, Am Heart J 97:225-228, 1979.

177. Gross NJ and Skorodin MS: Anticholinergic, antimuscarinic bronchodilators, Am Rev Respir Dis 129:856-870, 1984.

178. Garde JF, Aston R, Endler GC, et al: Racial mydriatic response to belladonna preparations, Anesth Analg 57:572-576, 1978.

179. Flacke WE and Flacke JW: Cholinergic and anticholinergic agents. In Smith NT and Corbascio AN, editors: Drug interaction in anesthesia, Philadelphia, 1986, Lea & Febiger.

180. Zaritsky AL and Chernow B: Catecholamines and sympathomimetics. In Chernow B and Lake CR, editors: The pharmacologic approach to the critically ill patient, Baltimore, 1983, Williams & Wilkins.

181. Packer M, Gottlieb SJ, and Kessler PD: Hormone-electrolyte interactions in the pathogenesis of lethal cardiac arrhythmias in patients with congestive heart failure, Am J Med 80(4A):23-29, 1986.

182. Tarazi RC: Sympathomimetic agents in the treatment of shock, Ann Intern Med 81:364-371, 1974.

183. Sobel BE and Braunwald E: The management of acute myocardial infarction. In Braunwald E, editor: Heart disease: a textbook of cardiovascular medicine, Philadelphia, 1984, WB Saunders Co.

184. Weiner N: Norepinephrine, epinephrine, and the sympathomimetic amines. In Gilman AG, Goodman LS, Rall TW, et al: The pharmacological basis of therapeutics, New York, 1985, Macmillan Publishing Co.

185. Golbranson FL, Lurie L, Vance RM, et al: Multiple extremity amputations in hypotensive patients treated with dopamine, JAMA 243:1145-1146, 1980.

186. Anderson JL: Bretylium tosylate: profile of the only available class III antiarrhythmic agent, Clin Ther 7:205-224, 1985.

187. Bivins JA, Rapp RP, Griffin WO, et al: Dopamine-phenytoin interaction: a cause of hypotension in the critically ill, Arch Surg 113:245-249, 1978.

188. Rutman HI, LeJemtel TH, and Sonnenblick EH: Newer cardiotonic agents: implications for patients with heart failure and ischemic heart disease, J Cardiothorac Anesth 1:59-70, 1987.

189. Young RA and Ward A: Milrinone: a preliminary review of its pharmacological properties and therapeutic use, Drugs 36:158-192, 1988.

190. Chung EK: Digitalis intoxication, Baltimore, 1969, Williams & Wilkins.

191. Smith TW, Antman EM, Freidman PL, et al: Digitalis glycosides: mechanisms and manifestations of toxicity, Prog Cardiovasc Dis 26:495-540, 1984.

192. Smith NT and Corbascio AN: The use and misuse of pressor agents, Anesthesiology 33:58-101, 1970.

193. Ralston DH, Shnider SM, and deLorimer AA: Effects of equipotent ephedrine, metaraminol, mephentermine and methoxamine on uterine blood flow in the pregnant ewe, Anesthesiology 40:354-370, 1970.

194. Hurlbert BJ, Edelman JD, and David K: Serum potassium levels during and after terbutaline, Anesth Analg 60:723-725, 1980.

195. Spielman FJ and Herbert WN: Maternal cardiovascular complications of drugs that alter uterine activity, Obst Gynecol Surv 43:516-522, 1988.

196. Hug CC and Kaplan JA: Pharmacology—cardiac drugs. In Kaplan JA, editor: Cardiac anesthesia, New York, 1979, Grune & Stratton.

197. Cohn JN and Burke LP: Nitroprusside, Ann Intern Med 91:752-757, 1979.

198. Mookherjee S, Warner R, Keighley J, et al: Worsening of ventilation perfusion relationship in the lungs in the face of hemodynamic improvement during nitroprusside infusion, Am J Cardiol 39:282, 1977.

199. Moore RA, Geller EA, Gallagher JD, et al: Effect of hypothermic cardiopulmonary bypass on nitroprusside metabolism, Clin Pharmacol Ther 37:680-683, 1985.

200. Tinker JH and Michenfelder JD: Sodium nitroprusside: pharmacology, toxicology, and therapeutics, Anesthesiology 45:340-354, 1976.

201. Cotrell JE, Casthely P, Brodie JD, et al: Prevention of nitroprusside-induced cyanide toxicity with hydroxycobalamin, N Engl J Med 298:809-811, 1979.

202. Hill NS, Antman EM, Green LH, et al: Intravenous nitroglycerin: review of pharmacology, indications, therapeutic effects and complications, Chest 79:69-73, 1981.

203. Weygandt GR, Kopman EA, Bauer S, et al: The cause of hypoxemia induced by nitroglycerin, Am J Cardiol 43:427, 1979.

204. Ziegler MG: Antihypertensives. In Chernow B and Lake CR, editors: The pharmacologic approach to the critically ill patient, Baltimore, 1983, Williams & Wilkins.

205. Husserl FE and Messerli FH: Adverse effects of antihypertensive drugs, Drugs 22:189-210, 1981.

206. Owall A, Gordon E, Lagerkranser M, et al: Clinical experience with adenosine for controlled hypotension during cerebral aneurysm surgery, Anesth Analg 66:229-234, 1987.

207. Shand DG: Drug therapy: propranolol, N Engl J Med 293:280-285, 1975.

208. Zimmerman TJ, Kooner JS, and Morgan KS: Safety and efficacy of timolol in pediatric glaucoma, Surv Ophthalmol 28:262-264, 1983.

209. Frishman WH: Pindolol: a new β-adrenoceptor antagonist with partial agonist activity, N Engl J Med 308:940-944, 1983.

210. Koch-Weser J: Drug therapy: metoprolol, N Engl J Med 301:698-703, 1979.

211. Miller RR, Olsen HG, Amsterdam EA, et al: Propranolol-withdrawal rebound phenomenon, N Engl J Med 293:416-418, 1975.

212. Mishra P, Calvey TN, Williams NE, et al: Intraoperative bradycardia and hypotension associated with timolol and pilocarpine eye drops, Br J Anaesth 55:897-899, 1983.

213. Weiner N: Drugs that inhibit adrenergic nerves and block adrenergic receptors. In Gilman AG, Goodman LS, Rall TW, et al: The pharmacological basis of therapeutics, ed 7, New York, 1985, Macmillan Publishing Co.

214. Wilson DJ, Wallin JD, Vlachakis ND, et al: Intravenous labetalol in the treatment of severe hypertension and hypertensive emergencies, Am J Med 75:95-102, 1983.

215. Vickers MD, Schneiden H, and Wood-Smith FG: Cardiovascular drugs (trimethaphan camsylate). In Drugs in anaesthesia practice, ed 6, London, 1984, Butterworth & Co.

216. Wilson SL, Miller RN, Wright C, et al: Prolonged neuromuscular blockade associated with trimethaphan, Anesth Analg 55:353-356, 1976.

217. Some oral antihypertensive drugs, Med Lett Drugs Ther 29:1-10, 1987.

218. Bursztyn M, Tordjman K, Grossman E, et al: Hypertensive crisis associated with nifedipine withdrawal, Arch Intern Med 146:397, 1986.

219. Gottlieb SO, Ouyang P, Baughman KL, et al: Acute nifedipine withdrawal: consequences of preoperative and late cessation of therapy in patients with prior unstable angina, J Am Coll Cardiol 4:382-388, 1984.

220. Merin RG: Calcium channel blocking drugs and anesthetics: Is the drug interaction beneficial or detrimental? Anesthesiology 66:111-113, 1987.

221. Durant NN, Nguyen N, and Katz R: Potentiation of neuromuscular blockade by verapamil, Anesthesiology 60:298-303, 1984.

222. Verapamil for hypertension, Med Lett Drugs Ther 29:37-39, 1987.

223. Chew CY, Hecht HS, Collet JT, et al: Influence of severity of ventricular dysfunction on hemodynamic responses to intravenously administered verapamil in ischemic heart disease. Am J Cardiol 47:917-922, 1981.

224. McGoon MD, Vlietstra RE, Holmes DR, et al: The clinical use of verapamil, Mayo Clin Proc 57:495-510, 1982.

225. Gulamhusein S, Ko P, Carruthers SG, et al: Acceleration of the ventricular response during atrial fibrillation in the Wolf-Parkinson-White syndrome after verapamil, Circulation 65:348-354, 1982.

226. Singh BN, Ellrodt G, and Peter CT: Verapamil: a review of its pharmacological properties and therapeutic use, Drugs 15:169-197, 1978.

227. Zalman F, Perloff JK, Durant NN, et al: Acute respiratory failure following intravenous verapamil in Duchenne's muscular dystrophy, Am Heart J 105:510-511, 1983.

228. Reves JG, Kissin I, Lell WA, et al: Calcium entry blockers: uses and implications for the anesthesiologist, Anesthes 57:504-518, 1982.

229. Chaffman M and Brogden RN: Diltiazem: a review of its pharmacological properties and therapeutic efficacy, Drugs 29:387-454, 1985.

230. Stoelting RK: Histamine and histamine receptor antagonists. In Pharmacology and physiology in anesthetic practice, Philadelphia, 1987, JB Lippincott Co.

231. Keats AS, Telford J, and Kurosu Y: "Potentiation" of meperidine by promethazine, Anesthesiology 22:34-41, 1961.

232. Cristiano P and Paradisi F: Can cimetidine facilitate infections by the oral route? Lancet 2:45, 1982.

233. Schentag JJ, Cerra FB, Calleri G, et al: Pharmacokinetic and clinical studies in patients with cimetidine associated mental confusion, Lancet 1:177-181, 1979.

234. Shaw RG, Mashford ML, and Desmond PV: Cardiac arrest after intravenous injection of cimetidine, Med J Aust 2:629-630, 1980.

235. McGuigan JE: A consideration of the adverse effects of cimetidine, Gastroenterology 80:181-192, 1981.

236. Zedis JB, Friedman LS, and Isselbacher KJ: Ranitidine: a new H$_2$ receptor antagonist, N Engl J Med 309:1368-1373, 1983.

237. Camarri E, Chirone E, Fanteria G, et al: Ranitidine-induced bradycardia, Lancet 2:160, 1982.

238. Stoelting RK. Gastric antacids, stimulants, and antiemetics. In Pharmacology and physiology in anesthetic practice, Philadelphia, 1987, JB Lippincott Co.

239. Schmidt JF, Schierup L, and Banning AM: The effect of sodium citrate on the pH and amount of gastric contents before general anesthesia, Acta Anaesthesiol Scand 28:263-265, 1984.

240. O'Sullivan GM and Bullingham RE: Noninvasive assessment by radiotelemetry of antacid effect during labor, Anesth Analg 64:95-100, 1985.

241. Gibbs CP, Schwartz DJ, Wynne JW, et al: Antacid pulmonary aspiration in the dog, Anesthesiology 51:380-385, 1979.

242. Cooke N, Teitelbaum S, and Avioli LV: Antacid-induced osteomalacia and nephrolithiasis, Arch Intern Med 138:1007-1009, 1978.

243. Alfrey AC, Legendre GR, and Kaehny WS: The dialysis encephalopathy syndrome: possible aluminum intoxication, N Engl J Med 294:184-188, 1976.

244. Clayman CB: The carbonate affair: chalk one up, JAMA 244:2554, 1980.

245. Plumb VJ and James TN: Clinical hazards of powerful diuretics: furosemide and ethacrinic acid, Mod Concepts Cardiovasc Dis 47:91-94, 1978.

246. Weiner IM and Mudge GH: Diuretics and other agents employed in the mobilization of edema fluid. In Gilman AG, Goodman LS, Rall TW, et al: The pharmacological basis of therapeutics, ed 7, New York, 1985, Macmillan Publishing Co.

247. Havadala HS, Borison RL, and Diamond BI: Potential hazards and applications of lithium in anesthesiology, Anesthesiology 50:534-537, 1979.

248. Miller RD, Sohn YJ, and Matteo RS: Enhancement of *d*-tubocurarine neuromuscular blockade by diuretics in man, Anesthesiology 45:442-445, 1976.

249. Warren SE and Blantz RC: Mannitol, Arch Intern Med 141:493-497, 1981.

250. O'Reily RA: Anticoagulant, antithrombotic, and thrombolytic drugs. In Gilman AG, Goodman LS, Rall TW, et al: The pharmacological basis of therapeutics, New York, 1985, Macmillan Publishing Co.

251. Cipolle RJ, Rodovold KA, Seifert R, at al: Heparin-associated thrombocytopenia: a prospective trial in 211 patients, Ther Drug Monit 5:205-211, 1983.

252. Kakkar VV, Bentley PG, Scully MF, et al: Antithrombin III and heparin, Lancet 1:103-104, 1980.

253. Deykin D: Current status of anticoagulant therapy, Am J Med 72:659-664, 1982.

254. Nielsen HK, Husted SE, Koopman HD, et al: Heparin-induced increase in serum levels of aminotransferases: a controlled clinical trial, Acta Med Scand 215:231-233, 1984.

255. Edes TE and Saunderrajan EV: Heparin-induced hyperkalemia, Arch Intern Med 145:1070-1072, 1985.

256. Wood AJJ, Robertson D, Robertson RM, et al: Elevated plasma free drug concentrations of propranolol and diazepam during cardiac catheterization, Circulation 62:1119-1122, 1980.

257. Hall JG, Pauli RM, and Wilson KM: Maternal and fetal sequelae of anticoagulation during pregnancy, Am J Med 68:122-140, 1980.

258. Peterson CE and Kwaan HC: Current concepts of warfarin therapy, Arch Intern Med 146:581-584, 1986.

259. Goldhaber SZ, Buring JE, Lipnick RJ, et al: Pooled analyses of randomized trials of streptokinase and heparin in phlebographically documented acute deep venous thrombosis, Am J Med 76:393-397, 1984.

260. Jaques LB: Protamine—antagonist to heparin, Can Med Assoc J 108:1291-1297, 1973.

261. Ellison N, Edmunds LH, and Colman RW: Platelet aggregation following heparin and protamine administration, Anesthesiology 48:65-69, 1978.

262. Michaels IAL and Barash PG: Hemodynamic changes during protamine administration, Anesth Analg 62:831-835, 1983.

263. Lowenstein E, Johnston WE, Lappas DG, et al: Catastrophic pulmonary vasoconstriction associated with protamine reversal of heparin, Anesthesiology 59:470-473, 1983.

264. Stewart WJ, McSweeney SM, Kellet MA, et al: Increased risk of severe protamine reactions in NPH-insulin–dependent diabetics undergoing cardiac catheterization, Circulation 70:788-792, 1984.

265. Davis DW and Steward DT: Unexplained excessive bleeding during operation: role of acetylsalicylic acid, Can Anaesth Soc J 24:452-462, 1977.

266. Brenner BE and Simon RR: Management of salicylate intoxication, Drugs 24:335-340, 1982.

267. Thompson WL: Rational use of albumin and plasma substitutes, Johns Hopkins Med J 136:220-225, 1975.

268. Feest TG: Low molecular weight dextran: a continuing cause of acute renal failure, Br Med J 2:1300, 1976.

269. Lima JJ, Conti DR, Goldfarb AL, et al: Safety and efficacy of procainamide infusions, Am J Cardiol 43:98-105, 1979.

270. Bigger TJ and Hoffman BF: Antiarrhythmic drugs. In Gilman AG, Goodman LS, Rall TW, et al: The

pharmacological basis of therapeutics, New York, 1985, Macmillan Publishing Co.

271. Roden DM and Woosley RL: Antiarrhythmic drugs. In Wood MW and Wood AJJ, editors: Drugs and anesthesia: pharmacology for anesthesiologists ed 2, Baltimore, 1990, Williams & Wilkins.

272. Kornfeld P, Horowitz SH, and Genkins G: Myasthenia gravis unmasked by antiarrhythmic agents, Mt Sinai J Med 43:10-14, 1976.

273. Miller RD, Way WL, and Katzung BG: The potentiation of neuromuscular blocking agents by quinidine, Anesthesiology 28:1036-1041, 1967.

274. Koch-Weser J: Drug therapy: bretylium, N Engl J Med 300:473-477, 1979.

275. Podrid PJ, Schoenberger A, and Lown B: Congestive heart failure caused by oral disopyramide, N Engl J Med 302:614-617, 1980.

276. Heger JJ, Prystowsky EN, Jackman WM, et al: Amiodarone: clinical efficacy and electro-physiology during long-term therapy for recurrent ventricular tachycardia or ventricular fibrillation, N Engl J Med 305:539-545, 1981.

277. Liberman BA and Teasdale SJ: Anaesthesia and amiodarone, Can Anaesth Soc J 32:629-638, 1985.

278. Navalgund AA, Alifimoff JK, Jakymec AJ, et al: Amiodarone-induced sinus arrest successfully treated with ephedrine and isoproterenol, Anesth Analg 65:414-416, 1986.

279. Moysey JO, Jaggarao NSV, Grundy EW, et al: Amiodarone increases plasma digoxin concentrations, Br Med J (Clin Res) 282:272, 1981.

280. Idsoe O, Guthe T, Wilcox RR, et al: Nature and extent of penicillin side-reactions, with particular reference to fatalities from anaphylactic shock, Bull WHO 38:159-188, 1968.

281. Mandell GL and Sande MA: Penicillins, cephalosporins, and other beta-lactam antibiotics. In Gilman AG, Goodman LS, Rall TW, et al, editors: The pharmacological basis of therapeutics, New York, 1985, Macmillan Publishing Co.

282. Scholand JF, Tennenbaum JI, and Cerilli GJ: Anaphylaxis to cephalothin in a patient allergic to penicillin, JAMA 206:130-132, 1968.

283. Gary NE, Buzzeo L, Solaki RP, et al: Gentamicin-associated acute renal failure, Arch Intern Med 126:1101-1104, 1976.

284. Meyer RD: Amikacin, Ann Intern Med 95:328-332, 1981.

285. Sokoll MD and Gergis SD: Antibiotics and neuromuscular function, Anesthesiology 55:148-159, 1981.

286. Holtzman JL: Gentamicin neuromuscular blockade, Ann Intern Med 84:55, 1976.

287. Wilson P and Ramsden RT: Immediate effects of tobramycin on human cochlea and correlation with serum tobramycin levels, Br Med J 1:259-261, 1977.

288. Geraci JE and Hermans PE: Vancomycin, Mayo Clin Proc 58:88-91, 1983.

289. Bennett JE: Chemotherapy of systemic mycoses (parts 1 & 2), N Engl J Med 290:30-32, 320-322, 1974.

290. Schulze-Delrieu K: Drug therapy: metoclopramide, N Engl J Med 305:28-33, 1981.

291. Bateman DN and Davies DS: Pharmacokinetics of metoclopramide, Lancet 1:166, 1979 [letter].

292. VanDellen RG: Theophylline—practical application of new knowledge, Mayo Clin Proc 54:733-745, 1979.

293. Stirt JA and Sullivan SF: Aminophylline, Anesth Analg 60:587-602, 1981.

294. Wood M: Drugs and the respiratory system. In Wood MW and Wood AJJ, editors: Drugs and anesthesia: pharmacology for anesthesiologists, ed 2, Baltimore, 1990, Williams & Wilkins.

295. Pentoxifylline for intermittent claudication, Med Lett Drugs Ther 26:103-104, 1984.

296. Mark LC: Analeptics: changing concepts, declining status, Am J Med Sci 254:296-302, 1967.

297. Britt BA: Dantrolene, Can Anaesth Soc J 31:61-75, 1984.

298. Watson CB, Reierson N, and Norfleet EA: Clinically significant muscle weakness induced by oral dantrolene sodium prophylaxis for malignant hyperthermia, Anesthesiology 65:312-314, 1986.

299. Davidoff RA: Pharmacology of spasticity, Neurology 28:46-51, 1978.

Chapter 7

Perioperative Nerve Injury

Gale E. Thompson
Anne C. P. Lui

There has been a longtime association of anesthesia with nerve injuries, but the mechanisms of injury are often obscure. Our primary goal in this chapter is to emphasize the great diversity of possible etiologic factors. The subject is certainly far more complex than to reflexly ascribe causation to either a regional anesthetic technique or to a patient positioning problem on the operating room table! An almost imperative corollary to our goal is to emphasize that each case of nerve injury has a temporal perspective. The term "perioperative" must be construed to mean 'preoperative, intraoperative, and postoperative.' The preoperative period may be measured in days, months, or years, and implies that preexistent disease processes may be contributing greatly to what finally becomes overtly manifest as an intraoperative event. Likewise, the postoperative perspective must be days in duration, since nerve injuries may either be induced in that period or become objectively or subjectively apparent only after more acute postsurgical problems are resolved. Careful analysis of any case may reveal multiple possible

etiologic factors playing a role at different times. Such analysis is important from the medical standpoint of prevention as well as the oft-associated legal implications. Although some authors[1] have opined that perioperative nerve injuries should never happen, there is reason to question whether they are indeed always preventable or whether commonly used prophylactic measures are totally rational, scientific, or effective!

From the patient's perspective, there is perhaps nothing more irritating than to come to the hospital for a "successful" surgical procedure and then to go home with a totally unexpected nerve deficit involving a totally separate area of the body. In our experience, the significance of the nerve injury is often compounded by the patient's vocation. For example, an auctioneer who developed a vocal cord paralysis after tracheal intubation or a carpenter who was awarded $60,000 for an ulnar neuropathy of his hammering hand after hernia repair. Similarly distressed was a karate instructor who developed a long thoracic nerve injury after kidney surgery. An even more ominous report is that of a pianist who suffered bilateral ulnar nerve deficits during the course of two separate abdominal operations. Finger contractions developed and ultimately resulted in amputations. The court awarded her roughly $50,000!

The medicolegal scene impacts upon many cases of nerve injury. The doctrine of *res ipsa loquitur* is applied in many instances, and thus defending such a case is a considerable challenge. Dornette has written a good summary of the origins, elements, and pertinent case histories of the *res ipsa* doctrine.[2] The Committee on Professional Liability of the American Society of Anesthesiologists[3,4] found nerve damage to be the second most frequent anesthetic injury (15%) in their review of 1541 closed malpractice claims related to anesthetic care. Even when anesthetic care was judged to be appropriate, payment was made in 45% of claims. The median payment for disabling nerve injury was $56,000 as compared to a median payment of $225,000 for claims for disabling injury not involving nerve damage. Since 92% of these cases occurred between 1975 and 1985, they probably do not reflect current prices. In addition, closed claims analysis is retrospective and provides no information about incidence, since the population of anesthetics from which these claims were drawn is unknown. There are, however, a few historical datum points that would establish the incidence of perioperative nerve injury at about 0.1%. This number is important from the perspective of informed consent, which is another common issue in legal cases.

I. HISTORICAL PERSPECTIVE

It appears that the first association of anesthesiology with nerve injury was a report by Budinger[5] from Vienna in 1894. He described several cases and questioned the role of chloroform as an etiologic agent. Interestingly, both trichloroethylene and nitrous oxide have been other general anesthetic agents that have been considered as inducing metabolic changes that could be neurotoxic. Although these general anesthetic agents have been thus incriminated, the pendulum has now swung far more toward the implication of regional anesthesia as a potential cause of nerve injury. In the first half of this century, some of the problems were obviously attributable to impurities of injected drugs or unsterile techniques in performing nerve blocks. Such problems achieved considerable notoriety and sensationalism, such as the famous *Woolley and Roe*[6] case in England, which cast a pall over the use of spinal anesthe-

sia in that country for many years. Likewise, there were nonanesthesiologist physician critics who wrote articles such as "The Grave Spinal Cord Paralysis Caused by Spinal Anesthesia."[7] Such an inflammatory title did little to promote the use of regional anesthesia and, by implication, accentuated a philosophy that many still have, that is, that regional anesthesia is one of the primary causes of perioperative nerve injury. In 1950, Dhuner[8] authored one of the few available reports of the incidence of nerve injury in a large series of surgical cases. This study, from the Karolinska Institute in Sweden, reported 31 nerve palsies in 30,000 operations for an incidence of 0.1%. Dhuner, too, was prone to be rather critical of spinal anesthesia and wrote, "It is well known that analgesia and even spinal puncture may produce cord or nerve damage." Of 31 neuropathies described by Dhuner, 26 were in the upper extremity. Eleven involved the brachial plexus, seven the radial nerve, and eight the ulnar nerve. There were five cases of lower extremity neuropathy, and each involved the common peroneal nerve. Of the patients with peroneal nerve palsies, four had received subarachnoid block with dibucaine. One of the patients with peroneal nerve palsy received a general anesthetic, and therefore Dhuner was forced to conclude that "other factors may be responsible."

In 1973, Parks[9] reported 72 nerve palsies in a total of 50,000 general surgery patients. Here again, the incidence was about 0.14%. Of these patients, only three out of 72 had received spinal anesthesia. Interestingly, Parks added a new perspective on etiology by suggesting that muscle relaxants may promote the potential for nerve injury. Sixty-three out of the 72 patients did receive muscle relaxants, and the impression was that this sometimes allowed abnormal positioning of extremities with consequent stretching of nerves.

Since 1981, we have been compiling data about nerve injuries through mechanisms of the Quality Assurance Program at Virginia Mason Clinic. Through educational efforts we have gradually increased sensitivity to the problem and devised methods of data collection. During the first 3 years of this study, we were somewhat surprised to find 30 nerve injuries in a series of 26,167 surgical patients (0.11% incidence). By 1988, we had identified a total of 67 perianesthetic neuropathies in 65 patients. One interesting finding was the high incidence of underlying disease in those patients who developed perioperative neuropathy. Of the 65 patients involved, 35 had significant medical problems as depicted in Table 7-1. Thirteen of

Table 7-1. Significant underlying Medical Problems in 65 Neuropathy Patients

Disease	Number of patients
Diabetes mellitus	7
Alcohol abuse	5
Severe peripheral vascular disease	6
Preexisting neuropathy	4
Renal failure	4
Hypothyroidism	2
Morbid obesity	4
Hepatic failure	2
Nelson's disease	1

*From Quality Assurance Program, Virginia Mason Clinic, Seattle, Washington.

our cases did not receive a major anesthetic, and six of these occurred in obstetrical patients. Other cases included a median nerve palsy after intravenous use of vasoactive drugs, a brachial plexus palsy after infiltration of an intravenous catheter through which intravenous pyelogram dye had been injected, median nerve trauma related to angioplasty needle insertion, and a vocal cord paralysis after subclavian venous cannulation.

II. ANATOMIC CONSIDERATIONS

The peripheral nervous system consists of cranial nerves III to XII, spinal roots, autonomic ganglia, nerve plexi, and peripheral nerves in a complex network of efferent and afferent fibers. The neuron is the key conducting unit of the nervous system. It is made up of the cell body (perikaryon) and a cytoplasmic extension called the "axon." The life of the axon depends on continuity with the cell body. Thus axoplasmic transport of macromolecules from the cell body down the entire axon (which can be as much as 1 to 2 meters in length) can pose special problems. This transport system is vital for normal growth and regeneration of the axon, for maintaining the integrity of the axonal membrane and its conducting properties, and for supplying precursors of the cells neurotransmitters. Three kinds of transport are recognized (1) fast axon transport, which is calcium dependent and probably occurs along neurotubules, carrying enzymes, polypeptides, polysaccharides, and neurosecretory granules to the nerve terminals; (2) slow axon transport, which occurs at rates of 1 to 50 mm/day and may correlate with the bulk flow of axoplasm; and (3) retrograde axon transport, which conveys trophic factors back to the cell body. Examples of clinical correlates that illustrate defects in each of these transport systems have been found to support the belief that the transport system dictates the survival and welfare of the axon and to some degree the structures it innervates.[10]

A. Spinal roots

There are 31 pairs of spinal nerves, each formed by a dorsal root and a ventral root that arise from the spinal cord. These spinal nerve roots can be damaged by direct trauma (penetrating injuries, fracture or dislocation of the spine), or by indirect trauma (such as traction injuries of the brachial plexus or lumbosacral plexus), or by lesions encroaching on the intervertebral foramen (osteophytes, tumor of the spine, intervertebral disc disease), or apophyseal joint inflammation.

B. Peripheral nerves

Peripheral nerve fibers originate from sensory, motor, or autonomic cell bodies in the dorsal ganglia or ventral horn of the spinal cord. The cytoplasm of the neuron extends beyond the central nervous system as the axon. Surrounding the axon of many fibers are variable layers of myelin produced by a single Schwann cell. A layer of connective tissue called the "endoneurium" encloses each fiber. Bundles of fibers form fasciles (or funiculi) wrapped in connective tissue known as "perineurium." Several fasciles, encased in more connective tissue called the "epineurium," form the peripheral nerve. Peripheral nerves can be classified by fiber size: larger myelinated A fibers, smaller preganglionic sympathetic myelinated B fibers, and small unmyelinated C fibers (Table 7-2). In addition to nutrient supply from the neuron, blood vessels, along the course of the nerve, also contribute to the fibers' nutrition. These blood vessels called "vasa nervorum," run a longitudinal course with numerous anastomoses and are termed "epineurial, interfascicular perineurial, and intrafascicular arteries, arterioles, and capillaries."

The histologic anatomy of the nerve partly determines the susceptibility to injury. Nerve trunks containing numerous small fibers with abundant perineurim are less vulnerable to compression injuries than those composed of large fibers with little supporting connective tissue. Furthermore, partial injury to a nerve with many small fibers results in less significant deficit than the same injury to a nerve with a few large fibers.[11] Anatomic location is another factor that predisposes certain nerves to injury. Nerves that are superficially located, are in di-

Table 7-2. Classification of peripheral nerve fibers by size and conduction velocity

Type	Diameter (μm)	Conduction velocity (m/sec)
Aα	13-22	80-120
Aβ	8-13	40-80
Aγ	4-8	15-40
Aδ (pain)	2-6	5-30
B	1-3	3-15
C (pain)	1-2	1-2

rect contact with bone, or cross fibrous tissue septa, are liable to damage by compression. Increased tension is placed on a nerve that crosses joints, especially in the extensor aspect. Thus the radial nerve in the spiral groove of the humerus, the common peroneal nerve at the head of the fibula, the ulnar nerve behind the medial condyle, and the supraorbital nerve are all superficial structures that are prone to compression against bone. Extreme flexion, abduction, and external rotation of the thighs in the lithotomy position compresses the femoral nerve against the fibrous inguinal ligament, which may lead to femoral nerve palsy. Chronic friction is another etiologic factor; examples include the ulnar nerve as it crosses the medial intermuscular septum in the forearm, the median nerve in the carpal tunnel, and the lateral femoral cutaneous nerve as it pierces the fascia lata or as it passes through the inguinal ligament.

Even when similar nerves are equally injured, the clinical disability may differ. For example, Sunderland[12] suggests that in injury of the recurrent laryngeal nerve the nerve supply to the adductor and abductor mechanism are often equally damaged. However, the adductor muscle mass, being three times that of the abductor mass, results in relatively greater adductor tone so that there is a tendency to midline drift of the paralyzed vocal cords.

C. Individual nerves

1. Brachial plexus. The brachial plexus is formed by nerve roots from C5 to T1. These roots invaginate the dura in a funnel shape as they leave the spinal cord. The dura continues along each nerve root and eventually blends with the epineurium. The roots can be compressed in the presence of a narrowed intervertebral foramen during hyperextension, lateral flexion, or rotation of the cervical spine. Under increasing tension, the nerve roots fail before the peripheral nerve as a result of a relatively lower tensile strength and lesser amount of

epineurial and perineurial connective tissue. The plexus can also be injured in several ways such as direct trauma, vascular injury, and lesions associated with bone and joint injury[13] (Fig. 7-1) The trunk of the plexus can be compressed between the clavicle and the first rib, or between the scalenus anterior and scalenus medius muscles as in the case of the thoracic outlet syndrome or cervical rib syndrome. Of particular importance to the physician positioning an unconscious patient is that hyperabduction of the arm with the shoulders posteriorly displaced and forced downward reduces the costoclavicular space. In this position, the subclavian artery is also occluded by the costoclavicular compression and the absence of the radial pulse warns of potential nerve compression. Postanesthetic palsies may be attributable to stretch[14] or compression of the plexus for prolonged periods. The plexus is stretched when the neck is extended and flexed to the opposite side, or when the arm is in any extreme position particularly when abducted and externally rotated. This position causes bowing of the cords of the plexus against the head of the humerus. Improperly placed shoulder braces used to support the patient in the Trendelenburg position can force the shoulders downward stretching the plexus or can injure the nerves by direct compression. Similar traction/compression type of injuries are seen in the neuropathies associated with prolonged abnormal positioning in the comatose patient from drug overdose[15] or the asphyxiated patient in the "crowd-crush" disasters[16] (Fig. 7-2).

Nerve palsies in the newborn occur in about 1 in 857 deliveries.[17] Brachial plexus palsies are the most common and are associated with shoulder dystocia or difficult breech with an obstructed aftercoming head. Also in breech deliveries where the arms are fully abducted or conversely when the arms are adducted but forcibly pulled downward to help deliver the head, there is risk of compression and traction injuries to the plexus.

2. Ulnar nerve. The ulnar nerve is particularly susceptible to damage at its superficial position as it passes behind the epicondyle of the humerus. The injury is often the result of either a hyperflexed elbow, which overstretches the nerve in a comatose patient, or to direct compression of the nerve against a hard object such as an armboard or side rail of the operating room table (Fig. 7-3). Supination of the forearm moves the epicondylar area away from direct contact with the hard surface. Tomlinson[18] prospectively studied 335 patients undergoing cardiac surgery and found an incidence of 4.8%

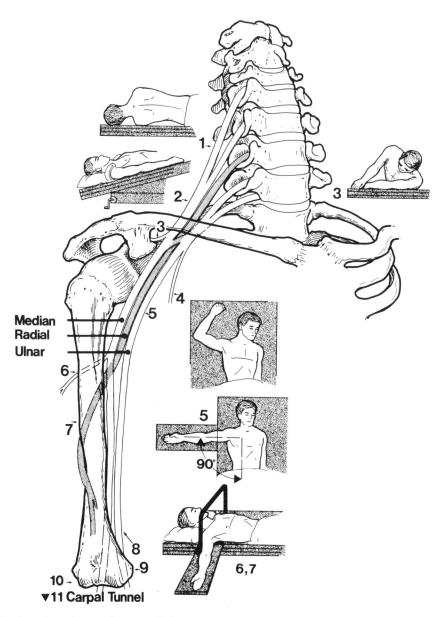

Median
Radial
Ulnar

Carpal Tunnel

Fig. 7-1. Locations and causes of injury to brachial plexus and nerves of the upper extremity. *1,* Impingement or traction of nerve roots; *2,* impingement of brachial plexus between clavicle and first rib; *3,* traction of supraclavicular nerve; *4,* traction of long thoracic nerve; *5,* traction or compression of brachial plexus by head of humerus in abduction; *6,* compression of axillary nerve against humerus; *7,* compression of radial nerve against humerus; *8,* compression of ulnar nerve against medial supracondylar ridge; *9,* traction or compression of ulnar nerve across medial epicondyle; *10,* median neuropathy from intravenous infiltration or direct needle trauma; *11,* carpal tunnel syndrome caused by hyperextension of wrist.

of brachial plexus injury related to traction from the median sternotomy. Specifically the ulnar nerve is the most common clinically identifiable site of nerve injury after use of a sternal retractor. Merchant[19] reported ulnar neuropathy with clinical changes in 15% and subclinical changes in 40% of patients having coronary ar-

tery bypass surgery. Interestingly, there were subclinical changes in 33% of limbs studied preoperatively with electrophysiologic methods. Sy[20] reported 3 cases of ulnar neuropathy associated with the use of automatically cycled blood pressure cuffs. Krolls' closed claim case analysis found that ulnar neuropathy repre-

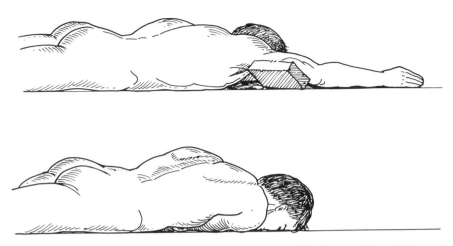

Fig. 7-2. The trauma or drug-overdose patient may have suffered nerve injury before arrival in the operating room. A compressed extremity may experience compartmental pressures up to 225 mm Hg from body weight alone.

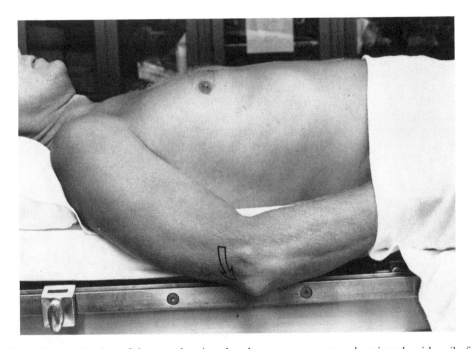

Fig. 7-3. Positioning of the arm showing the ulnar nerve compressed against the side rail of the operating room table, *arrow*.

sented one third of all injuries and that the file contained information specifically stating that the arm was padded in 18% of these patients!

3. Radial nerve. Radial nerve damage is usually the result of prolonged, unyielding pressure on the arm where the nerve spirals around the humerus. There are many specific causes of radial nerve palsy in this region: injection injuries, tourniquet palsy, crutch palsy, Saturday night palsy, drug overdose, birth palsy. There

has also been a report of radial nerve palsy from the use of an automatic blood pressure monitor.[21]

4. Lumbosacral plexus. The lumbosacral plexus is well protected in the psoas muscle and indirect traction injury on the plexus is very unlikely. Because there is limited movement of the lumbar vertebral column, this usually poses little threat to adjacent nerve roots. At the ala of the sacrum, however, the trunk of the plexus is in direct contact with bone against which it can be compressed. The posterior division of L4-L5 and S1 is in proximity to the bony pelvis. Compression of the plexus in this region can result in exclusive involvement of the common peroneal component and a clinical picture of foot drop with accompanying sensory changes. The lumbosacral trunk may be injured in the mother during difficult forceps delivery or may be compressed by the fetal head or buttocks. The lumbosacral plexus is often affected in diabetic radiculo-plexus neuropathy and idiopathic lumbosacral plexus neuropathy.[22] The sacral roots can also be compressed by space-occupying lesions such as tumor or aneurysms in the sacral hollow where the nerves are minimally protected by a thin layer of piriformis muscle.

5. Sciatic nerve. The sciatic nerve is relatively superficial as it passes beneath the lower border of the gluteus maximus before it continues underneath the long head of the biceps femoris. It is vulnerable to direct compression when seated on a firm surface. Furthermore, flexion of the hip stretches the nerve as it comes around between the ischial tuberosity and the greater trochanter of the femur. This bony relationship places the nerve at risk to injury with trauma to the hip joint as well as in certain surgical operations on the hip and femur. The mechanism of injury may be a result of manipulation of the hip joint to facilitate surgery,

leakage of methylmethacrylate (particularly from the acetabular component), or hematoma or postoperative scarring involving the sciatic nerve. The lithotomy position may also overstretch and damage the sciatic nerve, with the common peroneal component being the more vulnerable. Injection injuries may occur anywhere along the gluteal area where the sciatic nerve lies.

a. Peroneal nerve. The superficial branch of the common peroneal nerve is prone to injury where it lies superficially and in direct contact with bone as it wraps around laterally to the head and neck of the fibula. This nerve can be damaged by pressure from a tight plaster cast, or by forcing it against leg braces used for the lithotomy position (Fig. 7-4), or by crossing the leg in the seated position and compressing the nerve against the lower knee. The Japanese kneeling position can compress the nerve between the tendon of the biceps femoris, the lateral head of the gastrocnemius, and the head of the fibula. A case of peroneal nerve palsy after sequential pneumatic compression of prophylaxis of deep venous trombosis has been reported.[23]

6. Femoral nerve. The femoral nerve lies between the psoas and iliacus muscle. Compression injuries by retractors during pelvic surgery are the result of direct pressure or indirect compression of the nerve within the iliopsoas fur-

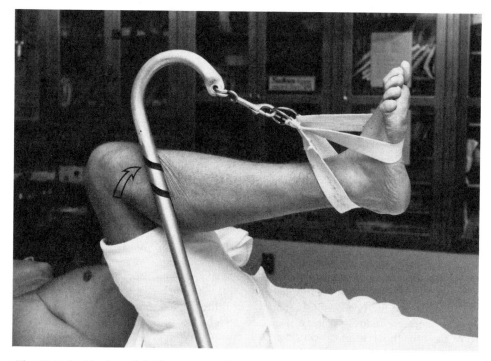

Fig. 7-4. Positioning of the lower extremity showing the superficial branch of the common peroneal nerve compressed against the leg braces used for the lithotomy position, *arrow.*

row from a laterally displaced psoas. The lithotomy position places the nerve at risk for compression under the inguinal ligament. The degree of compression can be estimated by palpation of the femoral artery below the inguinal ligament.

7. Lateral femoral cutaneous nerve. The lateral femoral cutaneous nerve may also be compressed in the lithotomy position. More common is idiopathic meralgia paresthetica, a condition that is rarely disabling. Interesting though is its appearance during pregnancy—perhaps factors yet unknown can increase the susceptibility to entrapment neuropathies. Other sources of injury include soft-tissue contusion medial to the anterior superior iliac spine from seat-belt injury, braces, corsets, or various diseases involving the pelvis or gut such as appendicitis, diverticulitis, or tumors.

8. Long thoracic nerve. Long thoracic nerve palsies that develop after anesthetics for surgical procedures have been recently reviewed by Martin.[24] Mechanisms of injury include direct trauma to the posterior triangle of the neck, compression by shoulder braces in the Trendelenburg position, or traction injuries where the angle of the neck and shoulder is increased or where the shoulder is displaced downward as by a fully loaded knapsack. Prolonged exertion at the shoulder can also selectively injure the long thoracic nerve, as after practice at grenade throwing, archery, or tennis. There is a high incidence of idiopathic onset, and Foo[25] used the term "neuralgic amyotrophy" to describe cases of isolated long thoracic nerve palsy.

9. Optic and facial nerves. The optic nerve may be damaged in the presence of ocular compression by an improperly placed horseshoe headrest in the prone position. The superficial orbital nerves are not protected by soft-tissue padding and can easily be compressed against the orbital rim by underlying or overlying objects such as the endotracheal tube connector. The facial nerve can be compressed against the ramus of the mandible during maneuvers to maintain a patent airway or by a mask strap.

III. ETIOLOGIC FACTORS
A. Pressure changes, ischemia of nerves, and position-related injuries

The normal function and viability of the nerve fiber is dependent on the availability of oxygen and nutrients supplied through the vasa nervorum as previously described. Oxygen supply to the nerve can be compromised by hypoxia or by pressure on the nerve trunk because of compression, traction, stretch, or friction injuries.

1. Compression neuropathy. Compression neuropathy is the result of nerve damage caused by mechanical pressure. A classic example is prolonged external compression of the radial nerve against the humerus resulting in "Saturday night palsy." Other external forces include tourniquet compression, crush injuries, obstetrical nerve injuries, and a tight plaster cast compressing the peroneal nerve against the fibular neck. Nerves may also be compressed by adjacent internal structures such as callus around a healing fracture site; fibrous bands, tumors, or displaced bone; edema, blood extravasation, or hematoma. The type of nerve damage from mechanical injury ranges from transient reversible changes to chronic pain syndromes and permanent paralysis. One classification of localized nerve injuries proposed by Seddon[26] introduced the terms "neuropraxia," "axonotmesis," and "neurotmesis." Neuropraxia is a clinical entity that correlates with mild nerve injury associated with motor paralysis and only partial sensory loss. Spontaneous and rapid recovery usually ensues within days or weeks. Axonotmesis is best illustrated by the injury caused when a nerve is crushed with forceps resulting in axonal interruption but intact neuronal stroma. Wallerian degeneration follows with distal denervation, and finally recovery occurs by axonal regeneration. Neurotmesis refers to partial and complete transection of the nerve.

Sunderland[27] based his classification of nerve injuries on the anatomy of the nerve trunk in relation to the endoneurium, perineurium, and epineurium. Thus he arrived at five degrees of injury: conduction abnormality in the axon, interruption of the axon alone, loss of endoneural continuity, disruption of the perineurium and funiculi, and complete loss of continuity of the nerve trunk.

The pathologic condition of a pressure-induced nerve lesion depends on the magnitude, duration, and rate of application of the compressive force. An acute, transient, deforming force can result in a temporary characteristic pattern of conduction block corresponding to a first-degree injury (or neurapraxia) at one end of the injury scale to a fifth-degree injury with complete nerve transection (neurotmesis) at the other end. The former represents the mildest degree of compression lesion and correlates with studies using sphygmomanometer cuff pressures sufficient to obliterate arterial flow without damage to the nerve fibers. More persistent compression results in focal demyelination caused by local ischemia, and recovery occurs by remyelination. This is consistent with the time to clinical recovery of the Saturday night palsy of 6 to 8 weeks.[28] However, recovery may be delayed for up to 5 months as a result of axonal compression by adjacent cellular edema. A slowly applied persistent deforming force on a nerve fiber leads to axonal thinning, segmental demyelination, wallerian degeneration, and characteristic bulbous paranodal swellings such as that seen in the median nerve in the carpal tunnel syndrome. The pathophysiologic mechanism involved in these lesions remains controversial. Fullerton and Gilliatt[29] believed that direct mechanical damage is the primary cause. Ochoa,[30] on the other hand, suggested that chronic ischemia is the cause.

2. Traction and stretch injury. Traction and stretch injury has been the subject of research for over one and a half centuries. The peripheral nerve behaves as plastic material with individual variations in elasticity, ability to withstand maximum elongation, tensile strength, and susceptibility to breaking forces. These variations are attributable to the different tissue components that make up the nerve. Extension of any nerve involves a primary elongation, but further stretching is resisted by the perineurium with the resultant decrease in cross-sectional area, raising of intraneural pressure, and compression of the vasa nervorum. Lundborg[31,32] has shown that circulatory compromise occurs with as little as 8% elongation, and complete ischemia at 15% elongation.

3. Ischemia. Ischemia is the common end point to both compressive and stretch injuries. When ischemia is the sole etiologic factor in nerve injury, pathologic changes appear later than injury arising from compressive-ischemic mechanism.[33] Fink[34] studied the action potential of A and C fibers under various oxygen tensions and found that the A potential declines progressively with reduction in oxygen tension below 20 mm Hg, whereas C potential remains almost unaffected even at zero oxygen tension. These results show that myelinated A fibers are dependent on aerobic metabolism whereas the C fibers are relatively resistant to hypoxemia and rely on glycolytic metabolism for energy source. This is consistent with observations on ischemic nerve injury where motor function and tactile sensations are lost long before pain transmission is affected.

Peripheral vascular diseases that are associated with neuropathies may involve either large arteries or small arteries. Large arteries can be occluded by emboli (associated with cardiac disease, subacute endocarditis, air, tumor, and so on), thromboangiitis obliterans, arteriosclerosis, Volkmann's ischemia, and vasospasm. Diseases of the arteriae nervorum include polyarteritis nodosa, amyloid, diabetes, and typhus. Various hematologic disorders such as sickle cell disease, polycythemia, macroglobu-

linemia, cryoglobulinemia, thrombocytopenia, hemophilia, and the use of anticoagulants can also lead to nerve ischemia. Common sites for these neuropathies are in the watershed areas in the midarm and midthigh. The pathologic condition is one of patchy nerve fiber degeneration, with a centripetal distribution.

B. Injection injury

Injection, as a route for therapeutic agents or for regional anesthesia, may result in nerve damage by several mechanisms including direct needle trauma, intraneural injection, deposition of toxic material in the perineural space, vasospasm, or thrombosis of nutrient artery.

1. Needle trauma. Needle trauma occurs with passage of the needle through the nerve fascicle. The extent of the injury possibly depends on whether the needle bevel enters parallel or transverse to the nerve fibers.[35] When the needle is inserted parallel to the nerve fibers, only slit-like fiber separation is seen. Transverse insertion of the needle results in more extensive fascicular injury, larger puncture sites, stretch, distortion, and herniation of nerve fibers. Not only is there damage to diffusion barriers because of puncture of nerve fascicles by the needle insertion, but also damage to neural blood vessels and resultant hematoma, edema, degeneration, and finally disruption of the nerve fiber can cause delayed recovery or even permanent deficits. Multiple injections can puncture and herniate the nerve at several levels.[36]

2. Intraneural injection. Intraneural injection causes a rise in intrafascicular pressure[37] and initiates a compression-ischemia type of injury. The anoxic nerve fiber may then be vulnerable even to agents with low neurotoxicity.[38] The pathologic condition appears as fragmentation and swelling of the axon, swelling of the fascicles with separation of fibers, endoneural edema, and hemorrhage.

C. Chemical toxicity

A prudent guideline is that just about any drug has the potential to produce neurotoxicity. Each of the following parenteral agents can result in nerve damage: antimicrobials (sulfa drugs, penicillin, methicillin, tetracycline, erythromycin, streptomycin, chloramphenicol, ethambutol, metromidazole, nitrofurantoin, isoniazid), salicylates, vitamin K, alcohol, paraldehyde, promazine, barbiturates, magnesium sulfate, colchicine, typhoid vaccine, vincristine, vinblastine, cisplatin,[39] phenytoin, perhexilene, hydralazine, amiodarone, clioquinol, dapsone, disulfiram, methaqualone, glutethimide, and thalidomide.

Although local anesthetics are extensively used for peripheral nerve blockade, there are in reality little data on the neurotoxicities of these agents.[40] Neurologic sequelae from the toxic effects of pure local anesthetics at the concentrations used clinically is very rare.[41] However, nerve damage can occur when the local anesthetic is carried in a medium containing neurotoxic additives such as sodium bisulfite[42] at an acid pH or with higher concentrations of local anesthetic injected intraneurally. The injury may be further exacerbated by the presence of epinephrine in the solution. Work from Myers[43,44] laboratory has demonstrated altered perineural permeability and endoneural edema after extraneural injection of many local anesthetics (3% 2-chloroprocaine, 10% procaine, 1% tetracaine, 2% mepivacaine, 1.5% etidocaine, 2% lidocaine, 0.75% bupivacaine). The extent of nerve injury appeared to be dose dependent, and there was no injury produced from injection of the vehicle for these local anesthetic agents.

1. Drug-induced arterial spasm. Drug-induced arterial spasm occurs after intravenous vasoactive substance. Chronic use of drugs such as amphetamine results in necrotizing angiitis and mononeuritis multiplex.

2. Household and industrial poisons. Household and industrial poisons associated with peripheral neuropathy include acrylamide, hexacarbons, carbon disulfide, organophosphates, arsenic, lead, mercury, thallium, and ethylene oxide. Kuzuhara[45] reported three cases of sensorimotor polyneuropathy in workers exposed to ethylene oxide sterilizers.

3. Anesthetic agents
a. Nitrous oxide. Whether nitrous oxide has neuropathic potential, as used in anesthesia, is unclear. There have been clinical reports of neuropathy associated with abuse of nitrous oxide; however a contaminant may have been the etiologic agent. Dyck[46] was unable to demonstrate nitrous oxide neurotoxicity in rats.

b. Trichloroethylene. Trichloroethylene is not neurotoxic, but its metabolite, dichloroacetylene, causes a neuropathy mainly affecting the fifth cranial nerve.[47] This usually becomes evident 8 to 48 hours after exposure and may take 18 months to recover. The pathology of the lesion has not been studied.

D. Neuronutrition

1. Metabolic disorders. In *diabetes mellitus* up to 50% of insulin-dependent diabetics have symptomatic neuropathy. Nerve biopsies of patients with neuropathy reveal prominent intraneural microangiopathy and endothelial hyperplasia.[48] This is consistent with a reduction in intraneural oxygen tension as found by Newrick[49] in his in vivo study of the sural nerve. The exact pathogenesis of this nerve lesion remains controversial, but ischemia is likely one of the mechanisms. Other proposed mechanisms include disturbed lipid and carbohydrate metabolism, which alters cellular composition, accumulation of sorbitol, and deficiency of myoinositol.

Uremic neuropathy is associated with longstanding severe renal failure. The exact pathogenesis is unknown and is probably multifactorial. Main features of this neuropathy include axonal degeneration with segmental demyelination.

2. Nutritional deficiencies. Alcoholic neuropathy is one of the commonest neuropathies in North America and is invariably associated with high alcohol intake and dietary deficiency. Thiamine deficiency plays a major role, but the direct toxic effects of alcohol, as well as multiple nutritional deficiencies, cannot be excluded.

Hypovitaminosis of the B and E groups are well known causes of neuropathy. Deficiencies of thiamine, vitamin B_{12}, nicotinamide, and pyridoxine (as in isoniazid-induced neuropathy) have been well documented to cause peripheral nerve damage.

Starvation after gastric bypass for morbid obesity can result in a demyelinating polyneuropathy with severe sensory ataxia.[50]

E. Congenital neuropathy

Hereditary liability to pressure palsies is an autosomal dominant disorder, affecting mainly those of German or Dutch descent.[51] The condition becomes manifest in the second or third decade. The nerves involved are the usual ones susceptible to compression injury. Neuropathy, with delayed recovery, develops after apparently minor insult, or may develop spontaneously. Other congenital neuropathies may affect the autonomic, sensory, or motor neurons.

F. Occupational palsies

Certain posturing of the limb or recurrent use can result in nerve injuries such as the tailor's crossed-leg palsy. Occupations that require the use of a tool repeatedly pressed into the palm of the hand can result in median nerve paralysis or damage the ulnar nerve in the hypothenar eminence. Occupations at risk include cyclists, gardeners, bulldozer drivers, and ditch diggers. Intense repeated pronation of the forearm can precipitate a friction injury of the median nerve as it passes between the two heads of the pronator teres. A "psuedoneuroma" of the digital nerve is the result of "bowler's thumb" where the edge of the hole of the bowling ball impinges on the thumb. Vocational stress is the most common cause of carpal tunnel syndrome. Compression of the ulnar nerve at the cubital fossa is the cause of the occupational palsy in telephone operators, radio-valve testers, and television addicts who watch TV while leaning on their elbows for prolonged periods.

IV. DIAGNOSIS AND EVALUATION

The initial presentation of a patient's nerve injury may be dramatic or subtle. At times, it is acutely obvious that a patient is suffering from a nonfunctional limb, loss of sensation, or pain. In other situations, it is apparent that the neuropathy either develops slowly or goes unrecognized in the midst of more dominating signs and symptoms that prevail on the postoperative scene. Whatever the situation, it behooves every physician and nurse to be as objective as possible in their written descriptions. A record is being formed with each comment, and the medicolegal implications are great. Truth and objectivity are to be greatly desired, but there is no room for implication, innuendo, and snap defensive or offensive judgments! If the site of nerve trauma or disease is obvious, it is quite likely that some of the initial pain symptoms will arise from nerve endings of pain fibers in adjacent tissues. However, there is no known mechanism for an axon to announce its own site of injury. In many instances, the site of nerve trauma is unclear and sometimes can never be precisely defined despite an array of potentially diagnostic tests. In general, the sites of more peripheral lesions can be identified with greater precision than more central lesions, since simple tests or neuroexamination will provide sufficient evidence. More involved tests must be used to document spinal cord, nerve root, or proximal plexus injury sites, and sometimes the patient may be reluctant to allow further probing into what is already a frustrating, unexpected, and irritating new event in life. Likewise, the physician must recognize that almost every diagnostic measure can also produce its own morbidity, and a judgment must be made about the ultimate value of precise localization. For instance, will it be helpful to therapy, to future prophylaxis, or to identifying causation?

One might wonder why pain should so often be a component of the symptom complex after isolated peripheral nerve injury. Shouldn't there really be a loss of sensation or motor function? In reality, the genesis of pain is a complex matter. Loeser[52] has defined four general mechanisms under the categories of sensitization of peripheral terminals, pathophysiology of primary afferent fibers, cross talk between fibers, and dorsal horn physiologic changes. These concepts are fascinatingly revealing of contemporary neuroscience research, but thus far there is no simple explanation to offer most patients about the cause, management, or future course of their pain.

The initial evaluation of any perioperative neuropathy should entail a careful history and physical examination. Ideally, this should be done by a neurologist who can bring totally objective evidence to bear upon the scene. Follow-up examinations are equally important to define the time course and morbidity from the injury. Specific diagnostic tests may also be indicated at various times. If the differential diagnosis should include epidural or other hematoma, a computerized tomographic scan or magnetic resonance imaging examination should be performed immediately. The electromyogram[53] should also be considered early if there is any hint of preexistent nerve damage, since degeneration potentials are unlikely until 3 weeks after injury. Therefore, if present, they would signify that the nerve lesion existed before the operation. Nerve conduction studies are helpful in localizing the precise site of injury along the course of a nerve. Some nerves are more easily mapped than others, and therefore the site of injury can be predicted with greater certainty. Nerve conduction studies are difficult with deep or paravertebral segments of the nerve. There is also some debate about what constitutes "abnormal," though a motor nerve conduction velocity below 40 meters per second would generally be of concern. The amplitude of the compound muscle action potential can be determined from surface electrodes over certain muscles, and this potential can be quantified and compared with an opposite extremity. It may also be quantified as one moves the stimulating electrode farther and farther away from the muscle along the course of the nerve in an "inching" technique. This is obviously another way in which the precise site of a nerve lesion may be determined. Sensory evoked responses may also give comparative data between the same nerve in opposite extremities or between different nerves in one extremity. The latency and form of these evoked responses can be quantified.

V. PREVENTION AND TREATMENT

As with many diseases, peripheral nerve injuries are better prevented than treated. However, as we understand more about preexistent, subclinical neuropathies and mechanisms of injury, this seemingly obvious precept may not be true or practical in application. With regard to surgical positioning, some operations become increasingly complex during their course and may force intraoperative changes in the patient's body position. Previously cushioned areas of the body may then become vulnerable to pressure from the table, armboards, surgical retraction devices, or previously applied, but now crumpled, pads. In fact, some pads sold as "protective" devices (as for the elbow) have little scientific background to support their use, and one might even wonder if their constricting properties might even contribute to ischemia. Perhaps the best prophylaxis for surgical positioning injuries is for the anesthesiologist (and, one would hope, the surgeon and operating room nurses) to periodically imagine themselves as the patient and then ask, "Would I be comfortable in this position?" It is certainly appropriate to periodically reassess pressure points and perhaps rearrange cushions or body position within reasonable and tolerable limits.[54] While the anesthesiologist is doing this to nonsurgical areas, the surgeon must likewise reevaluate the duration and application of pressures applied to the surgical wound. It is obvious that the diabetic, uremic, alcoholic, or cachectic patient might require a special degree of awareness. Optimal metabolic control of the diabetic, alcoholic, or uremic patient will likely contribute to restoration of normal nerve function if a clinical neuropathy does occur. Steroid therapy may facilitate healing if there is associated connective tissue disease such as rheumatoid arthritis, lupus erythematosus, scleroderma, or any of various vasculitides. Carcinomatous neuropathy might be treated by chemotherapy, radiation therapy, tumor removal, or decompression in some instances. Pyridoxine can reverse isoniazid-induced neuropathy, and beriberi and pellagra (50% incidence of neuropathy) are responsive to dietary thiamine, niacin, trytophan, or other essential amino acids. Other than these specific conditions, one might anticipate that good nutrition might contribute to the resolution of any type of nerve injury.

Frustratingly simple is the counsel that time will be a major contributor to healing. However, neither time nor other treatment will cure all neuropathies, and dogmatic statements about "appropriate" therapy must be viewed with some degree of skepticism. To the patient, it often seems that forced motion of the affected limb will somehow serve to restore function. The medical counterpart of this is to enlist the assistance of a physical therapist who can assist with both passive and active exercises to minimize contracture deformities.[55] Occupational and physical therapists can also encourage and advise the patient about compensatory ways to accomplish basic tasks such as walking, eating, or buttoning a shirt. Attention to such details will certainly serve to enhance rapport! Surgical intervention is sometimes indicated in the treatment of perioperative neuropathies. This is obvious in the case of an epidural hematoma and is probably indicated where other postsurgical or anticoagulant-induced hematoma has produced ischemic nerve injury. For other lesions, some have touted neurolysis or surgical decompression of surrounding tissues. If that is done and a "cure" results, there is still reason to question cause and effect. Likewise, surgery itself may lead to abnormal scarring, intraneural fibrosis, or impairment of nerve blood supply. Miller and Camp[56] report a disturbing persistence of neurologic deficit in eight patients followed for postoperative ulnar neuropathy. Whether treated medically or surgically, every patient had persistent weakness and pain for periods of 6 to 96 months after the time of injury. There is obviously still much to be learned about mechanisms of injury,[57] appropriate and effective preventive measures, as well as appropriate and effective therapeutic modalities.

REFERENCES

1. Britt BA and Gordon RA: Peripheral nerve injuries associated with anaesthesia, Can Anaesth Soc J 11:514, 1964.
2. Dornette WHL: Compression neuropathies: medical aspects and legal implications, Int Anesth Clin 24(4):201, 1986.
3. Cheney FW, Posner K, Caplan RA, and Ward RJ: Standard of care and anesthesia liability, JAMA 261:1599-1603, 1989.
4. Kroll DA, Caplan RA, Posner K, et al: Nerve injury associated with anesthesia, Anesthesiology 73:202-207, 1990.
5. Budinger K: Über Lähmungen nach Chloroformnarkosen, Arch Klin Chir 47:121-145, 1894.
6. Cope RW: The *Woolley and Roe* case, Anaesthesia 9:249-270, 1954.
7. Kennedy F, Effron AS, and Perry G: The grave spinal cord paralysis caused by spinal anesthesia, Surg Gynecol Obstet 91:385, 1950.
8. Dhuner KG: Nerve injuries following operations: a survey of cases occurring during a six year period, Anesthesiology 11:289, 1950.
9. Parks BJ: Postoperative peripheral neuropathies, Surgery 74(3):348, 1973.
10. Dyck PJ, Low PA, and Stevens JC: Diseases of peripheral nerves. In Joynt RJ, editor: Clinical neurology, Philadelphia, 1988, JB Lippincott Co.
11. Sunderland S: Nerves and nerve injuries, ed 2, Edinburgh, 1978, Churchill Livingstone.
12. Sunderland S and Swaney WE: The intraneural topography of the recurrent laryngeal nerve in man, Anat Rec 114:411, 1952.

13. Leffert RD: Brachial plexus injuries, Edinburgh, 1985, Churchill-Livingstone.

14. Jackson L and Keats AS: Mechanism of brachial plexus palsy following anesthesia, Anesthesiology 26:190, 1965.

15. Laforce FM: Crush syndrome after ethanol, N Engl J Med 284:1104, 1971.

16. Leech P and Cuthbert H: Brachial plexus lesions associated with traumatic asphyxia, Br J Surg 59:539, 1972.

17. Rubin A: Birth injuries: incidence, mechanism and end results, Obstet Gynecol 23:218, 1964.

18. Tomlinson D, Hirsch I, Kodali S, and Slogoff S: Protecting the brachial plexus during median sternotomy, J Thorac Cardiovasc Surg 94:291, 1987.

19. Merchant RN, Brown WF, and Watson BV: Peripheral nerve injuries in cardiac anesthesia, Can J Anaesth 37:S152, 1990.

20. Sy WP: Ulnar nerve palsy possibly related to use of automatically cycled blood pressure cuff, Anesth Analg 60:687, 1981.

21. Bickler PE, Schapera A, and Bainton CR: Acute radial nerve injury from use of automatic blood pressure monitor, Anesthesiology 73:186, 1990.

22. Evans BA, Stevens JC, and Dyck PJ: Lumbosacral plexus neuropathy, Neurology 31:1327, 1981.

23. Pittman GR: Peroneal nerve palsy following sequential pneumatic compression, JAMA 261:2201, 1989.

24. Martin JT: Postoperative isolated dysfunction of the long thoracic nerve: a rare entity of uncertain etiology, Anesth Analg 69:614, 1989.

25. Foo CL and Swann M: Isolated paralysis of the serratus anterior: a report of 20 cases, J Bone Joint Surg 65B:552, 1983.

26. Seddon HJ: Three types of nerve injury, Brain 66:237, 1943.

27. Sunderland S: A classification of peripheral nerve injuries producing loss of function, Brain 68:56, 1951.

28. Trojaborg W: Rate of recovery in motor and sensory fibers of the radial nerve: clinical and physiological aspects, J Neurol Neurosurg Psychiatry 33:625, 1970.

29. Fullerton PM and Gilliatt RW: Pressure neuropathy in the hind foot of the guinea pig, J Neurol Neurosurg Psychiatry 30:18, 1967.

30. Ochoa J and Marotte L: The nature of the nerve lesion caused by chronic entrapment in the guinea-pig, J Neurol Sci 19:491, 1973.

31. Lundborg G and Rydevik B: Effects of stretching the tibial nerve of the rabbit, J Bone Joint Surg 55B:390, 1973.

32. Lundborg G: Structure and function of the intraneural microvessels as related to trauma, edema formation and nerve function, J Bone Joint Surg 57A:938, 1975.

33. Lundborg G: Limb ischemia and nerve injury, Arch Surg 104:631, 1972.

34. Fink BR and Cairns AM: A bioenergetic basis for peripheral nerve fiber dissociation, Pain 12:307, 1982.

35. Selander D, Dhuner KG, and Lundborg G: Peripheral nerve injury due to injection needles used for regional anesthesia, Acta Anaesthesiol Scand 21:182, 1977.

36. Hirasawa Y, Katsumi Y, Kusswetter W, and Sprotte G: Experimentelle Untersuchungen zur peripheren Nervenverletzung durch Injektionsnadeln, Reg Anaesth 13:11, 1990.

37. Selander D and Sjöstrand J: Longitudinal spread of intraneurally injected local anesthetics, Acta Anaesthesiol Scand 22:622, 1978.

38. Selander D, Brattsand R, Lundborg G, et al: Local anesthetics: importance of mode of application, concentration and adrenaline for the appearance of nerve lesions, Acta Anaesthesiol Scand 23:127, 1979.

39. Woodhall B, Mahaley S, Boone S, and Huneycutt H: The effect of chemotherapeutic agents upon peripheral nerves, J Surg Res 11:373, 1962.

40. Fink BR: Acute and chronic toxicity of local anaesthetics, Can Anaesth Soc J 20:5, 1973.

41. Covino B: Clinical pharmacology of local anesthetic agents. In Cousins MJ and Bridenbaugh PO, editors: Neural blockade, ed 2, Philadelphia, 1988, JB Lippincott Co.

42. Wang BC, Hillman DE, Spielholtz NI, and Turndorf H: Chronic neurologic deficits and Nesacaine-CE — an effect of anesthetic, 2-chloroprocaine, or the antioxidant, sodium bisulfite? Anesth Analg 63:445, 1984.

43. Myers RR, Kalichman MW, Reisner L, and Powell HC: Neurotoxicity of local anesthetic: altered perineurial permeability, edema, and nerve fiber injury, Anesthesiology 64:29, 1986.

44. Kalichman MW, Powell HC, and Myers RR: Pathology of local anesthetic–induced nerve injury, Acta Neuropathol 75:583, 1988.

45. Kuzuhara S, Kanazawa I, Nakanishi T, and Egashira T: Ethylene oxide polyneuropathy, Neurology 33:377, 1983.

46. Dyck PJ, Grina LA, Lambert EH, et al: Nitrous oxide neurotoxicity studies in man and rat, Anesthesiology 53:205, 1980.

47. Buxton PH and Hayward M: Polyneuritis cranialis associated with industrial trichloroethylene poisoning, J Neurol Neurosurg Psychiatry 30:511, 1967.

48. Dyck PJ, Karns JL, Daube J, et al: Clinical and neuropathological criteria for the diagnosis and staging of diabetic polyneuropathy, Brain 108:861, 1985.

49. Newrick PG, Wilson AJ, Jakabowski J, et al: Sural nerve oxygen tension in diabetes, Br Med J 293:1053, 1986.

50. Feit H, Glasberg M, Ireton C, et al: Peripheral neuropathy and starvation after gastric partitioning for morbid obesity, Ann Intern Med 96:453, 1982.

51. Meier C and Mull C: Hereditary neuropathy with liability to pressure palsies, J Neurol 228:73, 1982.

52. Loeser JD: Peripheral nerve disorders. In Bonica JJ, editor: The management of pain, Philadelphia, 1990, Lea & Febiger.

53. Bralliear F: Electromyography: its use and misuse in peripheral nerve injuries, Orthop Clin North Am 12(2):229, 1981.

54. Martin JT: Positioning in anesthesia and surgery, ed 2, Philadelphia, 1987, WB Saunders Co.

55. Mubarak SJ and Hargens AR: Compartment syndromes and Volkmann's contracture, Philadelphia, 1981, WB Saunders Co, pp 168-171.

56. Miller RG and Camp RE: Postoperative ulnar neuropathy, JAMA 242:1636, 1989

57. Dawson DM and Krarup C: Perioperative nerve lesions, Arch Neurol 46:1355-1360, 1989.

Chapter 8

Why Monitoring During Anesthesia has Unintended and Undesirable Consequences

Nathan Leon Pace

A monitor is more than a box of motors, video tube, and electronics; it has an associated collection of interfacing cables, cords, couplings, hoses, sensors, and transducers. This monitoring ensemble produces numbers and graphics that describe the physiologic state of a patient and the body's response to the trespasses of surgery and to anesthesia care activities (drugs, fluids, breathing, and so forth). This monitoring ensemble can also abrade, burn, constrict, compress, crush, fibrillate, incise, infarct, obstruct, perforate, and shock human tissues. Such injuries can result not only from a defective machine (electrical shock from an improperly grounded electrocardiograph), but also from one without malfunction (transcutaneous gas electrode burn). The injuries can be the consequence of the placement or insertion of a sensor (nosebleed from a nasopharyngeal temperature probe) or coupling tubing (radial artery thrombosis after arterial catheterization). Since many monitor boxes are rather heavy, injuries can also result from a monitor falling onto a patient. Although these complications are important, it is not the task of this chapter to explore in detail complications from defective machines, from monitors improperly secured, or from the associated vascular access procedures to place interfacing devices. Neither will the function or operation of monitors be discussed at length.

Another answer to the question of what perioperative monitoring complications are is suggested by some of the lore of "war" stories of operating room anesthesia.

> *Story 1. A toddler is anesthetized with halothane for lengthy ear surgery. After induction, mechanical ventilation is started with an inhaled halothane concentration of greater than 2%. Monitors include an automatic oscillometric blood pressure cuff and a big-toe pulse oximeter probe. Five minutes later the oximeter fails to display oxygen-saturation readings. The resident spends the next 10 minutes repositioning the oximeter probe without success. Controlled ventilation and the inspired halothane concentration are continued unchanged. The attending anesthesiologist returns and recognizes the impending cardiovascular collapse; pulse oximetry readings and measurable blood pressure return as halothane concentration is rapidly lowered.*

> *Story 2. In the midst of abdominal aortic resection, the anesthesia resident draws an arterial blood sample from an indwelling arterial catheter but omits resetting the stopcock to reestablish circulation to transducer continuity. A few minutes later the sudden discovery of a normal electrocardiograph wave form and an absent pressure pulse prompt the diagnosis of electromechanical dissociation. Increasing doses of vasoactive drugs are administered and simultaneously the surgeons notices increasing blood leak through the aortic-graft suture line.*

> *Story 3. Several recovery room nurses spend 20 minutes exchanging electrocardiograph cables, leads, and skin patches before recognizing cardiac arrest as the cause of a flat line pattern. These stories indicate a broader class of medical mishaps or unintended consequences that could just as well be considered a perioperative complication such as a burn from a pulse oximeter probe.*

A brief list of the broad groupings of perioperative complications would thus be quite inclusive (List 8-1). The wide scope of perioperative complications reinforces the axiom that the risk of monitoring is merited if and only if the control of the monitored variable improves patient care. There are other consequences of a monitor purchase. Most monitors usually require disposable supplies, which can be quite costly. Also, the purchase of monitors that pro-

---

List 8-1. General Categories of Monitoring Complications

1. Monitors and their interfacing devices can directly damage human tissues.
2. Time and attention spent collecting and contemplating variables only tenuously or ambiguously related to patient physiology and pathophysiology is time and awareness taken away from useful physiologic variables.
3. Anesthesiologists are already confronted with an overload of data. Additional monitors may decrease vigilance.[1]
4. Complex or tedious monitor operations and apparent or real monitor malfunctions can distract attention from patient status.
5. The drugs and procedures of anesthesia each have a set of risks; one must consider the harmful consequences of therapies chosen to control and manipulate variables that are either erroneous or uninterpretable.

---

vide useless information leaves less capital available to buy useful monitors.

I. THE INVESTIGATION OF MONITORS AND UNDESIRABLE PERIOPERATIVE CONSEQUENCES

Since the addition of the first devices to aid the anesthesiologist's primary senses, there have been arguments about the merits of monitoring. This debate continues today and usually focuses on the improvement in patient care to be expected.[2,3] However, as forcefully argued by Keats, increased use of monitoring is not synonymous with better patient care and may in fact impair care.[4]

Technology assessment is the attempt to establish formal, structured means of resolving the uncertainty about the technology, new and old, of medicine.[5-7] The arguments to resolve the role of anesthesia monitoring is thus part of a larger effort encompassing all of medicine.[8] In turn, the question, "What are the complications of monitoring?" is part of the debate about the merits of monitoring and awaits technology assessment. The methods of technology assessment should be applied to all aspects of anesthesia monitoring, from the most complex device to the simplest esophageal stethoscope.[9]

The goal of this chapter is to make a examination of the types of evidence used to judge monitor performance and then review the evidence concerning commonly used monitors and their complications. The management of complications of monitoring are not discussed. Although incomplete, there is already some evidence in published reports of the journals of medicine and engineering to answer these questions. These reports can be grouped into three broad categories of evidence concerning the data produced by a monitor.

A. Data reliability

Monitors are for measuring physiologic variables. A patient is the signal generator of these variables. The signals are of two types, electrical potentials and everything else. Electrical potentials include the electrocardiogram, the electroencephalogram, electromyogram, and evoked potentials. The others include pressures, gas tensions, flows, saturations, and displacements. Monitor function proceeds from data (signal) acquisition to data processing and finally to data presentation and display.[10] The electrical potentials can be acquired directly by electrodes; the other signals require transducers to generate an electrical potential. The principles

of measurement incorporated within transducers are in general well engineered and are very rugged and robust; the same can be said for the electronics of the monitor box. However, the signal can always be corrupted with noise by the improper interfacing of patient to sensor (electrode or transducer). The universal use of microprocessor-based monitors has provided extensive data processing and has powerfully improved the data display. Yet this same number crunching can yield displays and numbers whose origin in the raw variable is not clear. For example, the preparation of data for presentation often includes an averaging of the signal over real time; there are many algorithms available for this averaging.[11] These different algorithms applied to the same signal do not produce the same displayed values. With the ever greater degree of variable processing, it is important to confirm the reasonableness of the raw data transformations.

Some monitors are developed with the expec-

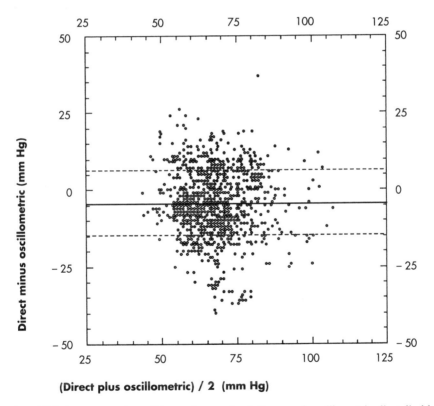

Fig. 8-1. This is a comparison (bias and scatter) of direct and oscillometric diastolic blood pressure measurements. To compare the two measurement methods, one makes a scatter plot of the difference versus average value for each pair of direct and oscillometric values. The mean of the differences is the bias or offset between the two methods; for this plot the mean difference is −4.3 mm Hg and is represented by the *solid horizontal line*. The two *dashed lines* are the upper and lower bounds of the 95% limits of agreement (−14.9 to 6.3 mm Hg). For data within this range, the values of the two monitors are considered indistinguishable. The width of the limits of agreement determines the interchangeability of the standard and alternative measurement method.

tation that their readings will be interchangeable with data provided by an existing monitor; the hope of the monitor developer is to provide a monitor that is less expensive or has more timely results or has less risk. To prove the interchangeability of the new and old monitor data, simultaneous measurements from old and new are obtained in patients. Until recently researchers have mistakenly analyzed these numbers by "calibration" statistical techniques (linear regression and correlation). Statisticians have now convinced researchers that "comparison" statistical techniques (mean difference and variability) should be used.[12-15]

Understanding the variation between measurements focuses in succession on several key points. First, we need to know the repeatability of a measurement over a short period of time in the same subject. With most of the variables obtained by our monitors, successive measurements cannot be obtained with a sufficiently short interval to eliminate physiologic variation. Only the combined physiologic variation and measurement error can be estimated. Bland and Altman recommend calculating a coefficient of repeatability that is the 95% range for the difference in two repeated measurements[13]; numerically it is $2\sqrt{2}\cdot$(pooled within-subject standard deviation). A change from one occasion to another in a subject should be greater to be attributed to a real alteration in patient state.

Next, comparison between devices is specified by a measure of accuracy and a measure of precision. The mean difference, also known as bias, between new and old values shows whether the new method overestimates or underestimates values obtained by the old method. This is accuracy. A statistical test for a nonzero bias uses the standard error of bias. One uses the standard deviation of the individual differences to specify the precision of agreement by calculating the 95% range for the limits of agreement (bias $\pm$ 2·standard deviation). If the difference between a paired old monitor and a new monitor determination lies within this range, the values are considered *indistinguishable*. If this range is sufficiently small as to have no clinical importance and biologic relevance, the values of new and old are *interchangeable*.[13] Graphically, accuracy and precision can be revealed by a regression plot. Instead of plotting new values versus old values, two new derived variables and a new data set are created. For each pair of new and old values, the difference and the mean are calculated. This difference and mean is plotted, and the accuracy and precision are also included (Fig. 8-1).

B. Data interpretability

Monitoring is more than just measuring.[10] Monitoring implies the analysis and interpretation of data. This interpretation can proceed only with a firm grasp of physiology. One way to interpret the variable is by comparing its value with an expected range of acceptable values. How to derive this acceptable range is not a trivial matter. Even when the variable is measured properly, there are variables that may not be interpretable; this occurs if the clinical state of the patient violates the assumptions necessary for understanding the variable.

Each of our clinic's monitors is a diagnostic system; it should provide diagnoses about a patient such as shock, ischemia, and hypoxia. A monitor uncovers undesirable conditions that call for corrective action. Diagnostic systems are usually not perfect and sometimes confuse "noise" with the particular signal that reveals disease or organ dysfunction.[16] The performance of a monitor is established by its application to a group of test patients; a standard method is used to confirm or refute the diagnosis. The selection of patients and the standard method are critical for this performance test.[17] This set of performance data (observed frequencies of each cell) is tabulated in a two-way contingency table (Table 8-1). Several diagnostic measures can be derived from this two-way table (Table 8-2). The measures of test efficacy that are usually chosen are the sensitivity and specificity. The proportion of diseased patients who are correctly classified is called the "sensitivity," or "true-positive ratio," and the proportion of nondiseased patients correctly classified is the "specificity," or "true negative ratio." The ideal diagnostic test would have a sensitivity and specificity of 1.0. These two measures are independent of the prevalence of the disease being identified. Two other measures, the positive and negative predictive values (Table 8-2), are used to calculate the accuracy of the test in a particular patient group. The positive predictive value is the proportion of patients who test positive who actually have the disease. The predictive values depend explicitly on the prevalence of disease and the performance measures of the test:

Positive predictive value =

$$\frac{\text{Prevalence} \times \text{Sensitivity}}{\begin{array}{c}\text{Prevalence} \times \text{Sensitivity} + \\ (1 - \text{Prevalence}) \times (1 - \text{Specificity})\end{array}}$$

Negative predictive value =

$$\frac{(1 - \text{Prevalence}) \times \text{Specificity}}{\begin{array}{c}(1 - \text{Prevalence}) \times \text{Specificity} + \\ \text{Prevalence} \times (1 - \text{Sensitivity})\end{array}}$$

Table 8-1. Truth table

		Disease (reality)		
		Positive = D+ = Disease	Negative = D− = No disease	ROW TOTALS
Test result	Yes = R+ = Positive	TP (true positive)	FP (false positive)	TP + FP
	No = R− = Negative	FN (false negative)	TN (true negative)	FN + TN
	COLUMN TOTALS	TP + FN	FP + TN	TP + FP + FN + TN = N

Table 8-2. Derivation of diagnostic measures

Diagnostic measure	Alternative name	Probability notation	Formula
True-positive ratio	Sensitivity	$P(R+ \mid D+)$	$=\dfrac{TP}{TP+FN}$
False-positive ratio	1 − Specificity	$P(R+ \mid D-) = \alpha$	$=\dfrac{FP}{FP+TN}$
False-negative ratio	1 − Sensitivity	$P(R- \mid D+) = \beta$	$=\dfrac{FN}{TP+FN}$
True-negative ratio	Specificity	$P(R- \mid D-)$	$=\dfrac{TN}{FP+TN}$
Positive predictive value		$P(D+ \mid R+)$	$=\dfrac{TP}{TP+FP}$
Negative predictive value		$P(D- \mid R-)$	$=\dfrac{TN}{FN+TN}$

It is an obvious oversimplification to consider a diagnostic system (including anesthesia monitors) as providing only a binary yes-or-no answer. The millimeters of ST-segment depression necessary to assert the existence of myocardial ischemia is an obvious example. The value to be exceeded may be judged either leniently, a small amount of depression, or strictly, a large amount of depression. The measures of the diagnostic test (sensitivity and specificity) will obviously change depending on the diagnostic cut point. A test measure that accommodates alternative diagnostic cut points is the ROC, or relative operating characteristics, curve.[16] This is a plot of the true-positive ratio versus the false-positive ratio for all possible diagnostic cut points (Fig. 8-2). The area under the curve is the measure of performance. If the curve follows the line of identity (diagonal line), the area is 0.5; such a test has no discriminating ability. An area of 1.0 indicates perfect discrimination; the curve follows the left and upper axes. Although calculations of sensitivity and specificity are common in reports on monitors, ROC curves have been used infrequently, except in studies of medical imaging.[16]

C. Data efficacy and effectiveness

The downstream consequences of using an anesthesia monitor is the ultimate test of that monitor.[18] How does the monitor influence subsequent patient management? Can intermediate variables be manipulated by therapeutic changes? Does the change in patient management alter patient morbidity and mortality? How often does it harm the patient? Statisticians have recommended that the importance of clinical reports be ranked or weighted by the experimental design used (List 8-2). The multiple-center randomized controlled trial (RCT) of patient outcome is the standard for proving the efficacy of a monitor. A distinction is made between efficacy and effectiveness. Efficacy is the monitor at its best under ideal circumstances; effectiveness is the monitor used under ordinary clinical circumstances. Even if efficacy is demonstrated, effectiveness is not assured. Some monitors are just too temperamental or just too risky to be used as other than a research device.

An almost universal problem in discussing the complications of monitors is the inability to calculate an incident rate. Some organizations, such as the ECRI (Technology for Anesthesia, ECRI, Plymouth Meeting, Pennsylvania), maintain databases of complications reported in journals, to the Food and Drug Administration, and to equipment manufacturers. Observational studies are published for selected series of patients at self-reporting institutions. The

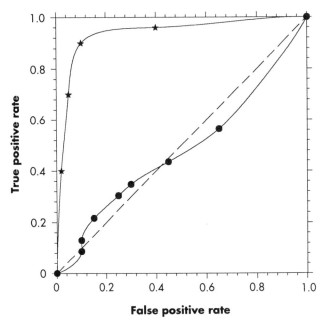

Fig. 8-2. Receiver operating characteristics (ROC) curve is a plot of the true-positive ratio versus the false-positive ratio for all possible diagnostic cut points of a diagnostic test. In this figure, three curves are drawn. The area under the curve is the measure of performance. If the curve follows the line of identity *(diagonal line),* the area is 0.5; such a test has no discriminating ability. An area of 1.0 indicates perfect discrimination; the curve follows the left and upper axes. The top curve *(stars)* reflects a very good test; its area is above 0.9. The third curve *(closed circles)* essentially follows the line of identity. Such a curve would reflect a test or monitor with essentially no diagnostic power.

List 8-2.   Clinical Report Ranking

MOST VALUABLE
1. Multiple-center randomized controlled trial
2. Single-center randomized controlled trial
3. Nonrandomized trial with concurrent controls
4. Nonrandomized trial with historical controls
5. Case series
6. Case report
LEAST VALUABLE

---

generalizability of these reports, usually from academic medical centers, is difficult to assess. Some complications are obviously difficult to define (List 8-1). For all complications, there is no database that maintains a comprehensive record of such. Medical journals will publish only the first few case reports of each type of complication associated with a monitor. Just as hard is to determine patient exposure. There is no inventory of what monitors are used in all the operating rooms of the country. One is dependent on cross-sectional sample surveys to determine how widespread monitor use is. Neither the numerator (number of incidents of complications) nor the denominator (tally of patient exposures to the monitor) are in general available.

One of the choices when one is designing a randomized controlled trial (RCT) of anesthesia monitors is whether the experimenter should prescribe the manner in which the data are used. One could depend on the clinical wisdom of the attending physician, derived from accepted principles of physiology and practice experience, to appropriately interpret and use the monitor data; this allows clinical decisions helped by multiple variates. Such decision making may also be amorphous, without focus, difficult to explicitly formulate, and difficult to replicate consistently. Alternatively the care of patients could be constrained by strict predetermined algorithms for interpretation of the monitor data and changes in therapy; this method is precise but ignores and proscribes alternative multivariate reasoning and unarticulated decisions. Both choices present difficulties in planning, accomplishing, and interpreting the study.

Since RCTs of outcome are so difficult to accomplish, other alternatives have been sought. Surrogate variables or end points can be the focus of the RCT. An example might be blood pressure as a surrogate for stroke. A surrogate end point correlates with the end point of interest (death, stroke, and so forth) but can be measured with less expense or at an earlier time. Other alternatives being attempted as a replacement for large scale RCTs are meta-analyses of existing, usually smaller reports.[19,20] Another is to examine existing databases collected for other purposes such as hospital mortalities or insurance claims.[21] This is being attempted within anesthesia by the review of closed malpractice claims of United States insurance carriers.[22]

The importance of actually demonstrating an improvement in outcome is being reaffirmed by examples of failed monitors. Intrapartum fetal heart-rate monitoring became common in the United States during the past 20 years. It was anticipated that an early warning of the presence of fetal hypoxia by changes in the fetal heart-rate pattern would allow immediate intervention to save the fetus. Neither fetal wastage nor neonatal salvage has been improved by this monitor, which prompted a dramatic increase in the incidence of caesarean delivery.[23] Anesthesia researchers must overcome the inertia and difficulties that through the middle of the last decade prevented the accomplishment of any definitive studies of patient outcome versus anesthesia monitors.[24]

II. COMMONLY USED MONITORS

In a chapter that can offer only some of the highlights of the evidence concerning anesthesia monitors, not all monitors can be discussed. The main emphasis is on commercially available, commonly used devices. Electrocardiography and anesthesia machines with their failure-detection devices are discussed elsewhere. The narrative proceeds variable by variable rather than monitor by monitor.

A. Vascular pressure

In addition to providing anesthesia, our ultimate concern is maintaining homeostasis by assuring the transport of oxygen and substrate to tissues. Blood pressure is measured in the hope that it is an indicator of this flow. Actually two types of pressure are monitored: those pressures that distend and fill the heart and those pressures generated by the heart to cause flow. The true driving force for flow is the difference in fluid energy between the aorta and the right atrium and between the pulmonary artery and

the left atrium. Fluid energy is the summation of pressure energy, gravitational potential energy, and kinetic energy:

$$E = P + \rho gh + \tfrac{1}{2}\rho v^2$$

where P is pressure energy, ρ = fluid density, g = acceleration caused by gravity, h = height above reference point, and v = fluid velocity. In systemic arteries, kinetic energy ($\tfrac{1}{2}\rho v^2$) is a negligible fraction of total fluid energy; in the atria and pulmonary artery, kinetic energy can be a large fraction of total fluid energy. The importance of kinetic energy is illustrated by Bernoulli's principle in which fluid flows against a pressure gradient, but not against the total energy gradient.

The first recorded vascular pressures were obtained invasively by a fluid-filled manometer. Today fluid-filled catheters are used to measure both driving and filling pressures but are attached to transducers. Pressure wave forms are essentially low-frequency sound with most energy in the frequency range below 10 to 20 cycles per second (Hz). To transduce or "hear" and display this pressure wave form faithfully, the intravascular catheter, connecting tubing, stopcocks, transducer, and monitor amplifier must have certain characteristics that describe the dynamic response. The fluid-filled catheter/transducer system is idealized by a model of a mass hooked to a spring. Derived from this model are differential equations with parameters, the natural frequency, f_n, and the damping coefficient zeta, ζ, describing model behavior. Measurements of the real physical system can be made to calculate these parameters; such parameter estimators have been used very successfully in understanding catheter/transducer system performance.[25,26]

If any of the frequencies of fluid vibrations in the catheter/transducer system is close to f_n, the amplitude of the vibrations increases and the peaks and valleys (systolic and diastolic) of the pressure pulse will be exaggerated. As long as the natural frequency is above 20 Hz there will be little distortion. The fluid vibrations die away with time similar to a bouncing ball rebounding less with each bounce. Damping describes the bouncing of the ball. For the catheter/transducer system ζ describes how long the vibrations reverberate. Either excessively high or low damping will distort the pulse pressure. The continuous-flush device may be used to determine if adequate fidelity exists in the catheter/transducer system by the "flush test." The 300 mm Hg pressure at which the flush fluid is maintained is directed against the transducer membrane as almost a square-wave pulse by activating momentarily the rapid-flush mechanism. An adequate pressure wave form is present if the termination of the square wave results in one undershoot on the pressure trace followed by a small overshoot.[27]

1. Invasive driving pressures[28]. The arterial pressure pulse is very complex, being composed of both a pressure wave that is propagated from the heart at a velocity of 5 to 10 m/sec and a flow element that travels more slowly at a velocity of 0.3 to 0.5 m/sec in the aorta. It is generated by the contraction of the ventricle and sustained by the viscoelastic properties of the arteries. The pressure pulse is greatly changed as it travels distally, being both amplified and modified; the flow velocity drops dramatically.

Systemic arterial pressure is obtained from catheters placed in an artery, usually in an extremity and most often in the radial artery. Arterial catheters are end-hole tubes and always placed with the catheter tip facing upstream. The measured pressure is thus a summation of both pressure and kinetic energy. However, even if flow is tripled or more, kinetic energy is still a very small percentage of pressure energy. Catheters advanced through the right side of the heart into the pulmonary artery are also end-hole catheters, but the tip is facing downstream. The measured pressure is the pressure energy minus some fraction of the kinetic energy. Within the pulmonary artery the total driving energy has a large kinetic component; as cardiac output increases threefold, kinetic pressure is one half of total systolic energy. Pulmonary artery pressure so measured is not necessarily an adequate estimator of driving energy.

a. Reliability. Reliability of invasive pressures is largely dependent on the fidelity of the catheter/transducer system.[29] With the now near universal availability of single-use transducers, one can rely on the transducer being within 1% of the transducer sensitivity, which has been fixed at 5.0 μV/V/mm Hg; calibration tests of transducers are no longer necessary. Before one interprets the pressure, the transducer must also be referenced to zero. By convention, pressures are referenced to atmosphere at the atrial level.

The more complicated the plumbing connecting catheter and transducer, the more it is likely that the dynamic system response will be degraded. Long, narrow connecting tubing and the pulmonary arterial catheter itself decrease f_n and increase ζ. On the other hand, if tubing is short and stiff and there are no air bubbles, f_n will increase and ζ will decrease. Improper damping and a low natural frequency do not impair measurement of mean pressure, only systolic and diastolic pressure.

b. Interpretability. Although there are published normal ranges of systemic and pulmonary arterial pressures, the use and interpretation of pressure and pressure changes depends on the patient, the surgery, and the clinical circumstances. Other uses of invasive blood pressure have been attempted. The arterial and pulmonary arterial pressure pulse has been integrated to derive cardiac output. This has always proved less reliable than standard methods of cardiac-output determination. The systemic arterial wave form has been analyzed to obtain systemic vascular resistance; ratios of systolic and diastolic pressure have been integrated over time to predict endocardial ischemia. It seems pointless to attempt such derivations from radial arterial pressure wave forms because there is too much variability and distortion of the pressure pulse as it travels from the aortic arch to the periphery. As one example, the dicrotic notch seen in the pressure wave form in a peripheral artery is probably not related to aortic closure.[30] In fact, even the mean pressure in the radial arterial may be unreliable after cardiopulmonary bypass; there can be a large discrepancy of 10 to 30 mm Hg between central and peripheral mean pressure for 30 or more minutes.[31]

c. Usefulness. Despite the widespread use of the radial arterial catheterization, nearly universally used for all critically ill patients and for all patients having cardiac, vascular, and neurologic surgery, no formal study of the usefulness of invasive systemic pressures is available. The same is true for pulmonary arterial pressures. Radial artery catheters have become such an integral part of anesthesia care that is difficult to conceive of circumstances that would motivate the initiation of a formal randomized controlled trial. Radial artery catheters are also inserted to allow frequent, repetitive sampling of arterial blood. The consequences of this phlebotomy and proof of the usefulness of such sampling is beyond the scope of this review.

What is available are summarized patient experiences compared to historical controls. Rao et al. compared the myocardial reinfarction rate in patients anesthetized between 1977 to 1982 with similar patients treated from 1973 to 1976.[32] The reinfarction rate for those anesthetized within the first 3 months after the primary infarction fell from 36% to about 6%. In the earlier period only a small minority of patients had radial arterial catheterization and almost none had pulmonary arterial catheterization; in the later period these monitors were used almost universally. But there were other differences as well. The increase in the use of β-ad-

List 8-3. Side Effects and Complications of Arterial and Pulmonary Arterial Catheterization

Arrhythmias
Bacteremia
Disconnection hemorrhage
Embolism
Local hematoma
Nerve damage
Pain
Pulmonary artery rupture
Pulmonary infarction
Sepsis
Valve damage
Vascular thrombosis

renergic receptor blocking drugs and the decrease in the use of vasopressors were just as dramatic. Which, if any, of these differences was responsible for the change in outcome is fundamentally unknowable from this report. Studies of pulmonary artery catheter filling pressures are discussed below.

d. Complications. Arterial and pulmonary arterial catheterization produces nontrivial complications (List 8-3). These are discussed in detail elsewhere in this book. This form of monitoring is one for which a variety of reports provide reasonable estimation of rates. Overall, serious complications occur at low rate for both types of catheterization.[33,34] Since it is relatively easy to obtain artifactual pressure readings, the potential for making adverse therapeutic choices is great. These choices would include all those activities used to influence hemodynamics: fluid infusion, blood transfusion, diuresis, vasoconstrictor or vasodilator infusion, sympathomimetic and sympatholytic administration, ventilatory changes, and administration of anesthetic drugs. Mistakes in therapy choices involving erroneously measured pressures or misinterpreted pressures are a common part of the anesthesia experience. It is the hope of anesthesiologists that therapy mistakes are usually soon recognized and corrected.

2. Filling pressures[35,36]. Filling pressures are of two kinds, those reflecting right ventricular end-diastolic (RVEDP) and those reflecting left ventricular end-diastolic pressure (LVEDP). These two pressures are ordinarily obtained by intravascular catheters terminating in either ventricle. Rather, RVEDP and LVEDP are estimated from pressures measured elsewhere. Central venous catheters (tip advanced to the region of the right atrium) have been placed frequently in operative patients for

the last three decades; central venous pressure (CVP) is measured and used to estimate RVEDP. However, most central venous catheters are not now placed primarily for pressure measurements but for other purposes such as fluid administration (parenteral alimentation, cancer chemotherapy, vasoactive drugs, and so on) and blood access (hemodialysis, phlebotomy).

Before 1970 LVEDP could be estimated only by retrograde catheterization of the aorta or by direct placement during open chest surgery of a catheter into the left atrium to measure left atrial pressure (LAP). Since that time a practical balloon-flotation pulmonary arterial catheter has been used to obtain estimates of LVEDP. When an pulmonary arterial catheter is advanced into the pulmonary artery, eventually the tip will wedge and occlude a small arterial branch stopping blood flow. The motionless blood beyond the catheter tip becomes an extension of the fluid column within the catheter lumen. This stationary column of blood terminates at the confluence of small pulmonary veins coming from adjacent lung segments. If the patency of the fluid column is assured, the catheter tip pressure will be in equilibrium with the downstream pressure. The advantage of the balloon catheter is the possibility of inflating the balloon and allowing blood flow to temporarily advance the catheter tip occluding an artery; catheter manipulation (advancement and withdrawal) is avoided. This measurement has been named the "pulmonary artery occlusion pressure" (PAOP) and is an estimate of left atrial pressure (LAP) and LVEDP.

a. Reliability. The initial motivation in measuring central venous pressure was the hope that CVP would allow estimation of RVEDP and that RVEDP and LVEDP would change in parallel; thus a variable of the right side of the heart was expected to describe events in the left side of the heart. Numerous studies have confirmed that although RVEDP and LVEDP might be similar in health there is frequently little agreement during critical illness or surgery. It was this poor correlation that incited the rapid growth in the use of balloon-flotation catheters. The actual measurement of PAOP requires considerable attention because many artifacts are possible (List 8-4). Most of these can be minimized by strict attention to details of measurement. Particularly important is the elimination of respiratory artifact, which can usually be easily eliminated during anesthesia by a momentary interruption of ventilation. Strictly speaking, three criteria should be met to assert that a true PAOP has been obtained: (1)

List 8-4. Artifacts in Pulmonary Arterial
Occlusion Pressure Measurements[37]

Rapidly varying intrathoracic respiratory pressure
changes
Inconsistent maintenance of zero reference level
Patient position [38]
Overwedging (herniation of balloon to cover cathe-
ter tip)
Incomplete wedging
Slow response and update times of monitor digital
displays

a change in the phasic pulmonary artery wave
form, (2) a fall in mean pressure, and (3) the
Pao_2 of a blood sample drawn through a
wedged catheter should be higher than that of
mixed venous blood. Anesthesiologists usually
skip the third criterion.

b. Interpretability. Although there are good
reasons to challenge the validity of the Starling
law of the heart in clinical medicine,[39] clinicians
usually do work with the assumption that the
greater the ventricular filling, the greater is the
flow produced. Clinicians use filling pressure to
estimate ventricular filling. The use of PAOP to
estimate LVEDP has the further hidden assumptions that the following pressures are
nearly identical: PAOP, pulmonary venous
pressure (PVP), LAP, and LVEDP. Although
this is likely to be true during health, altered
physiology resulting from critical illness and the
interventions to maintain homeostasis, for example, mechanical ventilation and positive end-
expiratory pressure (PEEP), makes their relationship tenuous. There are several studies that
found substantial discrepancies between PAOP
and LAP.[40,41] Explanations for these observations are not obvious.

PEEP can make interpretation of PAOP difficult in two ways. First, the actual distending
pressure of a cardiac chamber is the inside pressure minus the outside pressure, also called
the "transmural pressure." With PEEP the true
transmural filling pressure is reduced to the extent that lung parenchyma transmits airway
pressure to the juxtacardiac region. There is basically no feasible clinical method to measure
juxtacardiac pressure. PAOP during PEEP produces an overestimation of transmural filling
pressure. Second, since the pulmonary capillaries are flaccid and collapsible, PAOP equals
PVP only if PVP exceeds alveolar pressure; otherwise PAOP reflects alveolar pressure. This
is an example of the vascular-waterfall phenom-

enon.[42,43] The relationship between PVP and
alveolar pressure is complex and depends on hydrostatic pressure gradients in the lung and the
level of alveolar pressure (PEEP). The measurement of PAOP will also depend on the random
migration of the catheter tip during balloon inflation to dependent or less dependent lung
segments. PAOP will be in equilibrium with
PVP and LAP only if the catheter tip lodges in
the West functional zone III.[44] Although some
pragmatic rules have been given to interpret
PAOP in the face of PEEP, ultimately the presence of a PAOP to PVP discrepancy or the effect of PEEP on transmural pressure cannot be
determined by common clinical measurements.
A temporary removal of PEEP is also not a solution; removal of PEEP causes its own
changes in left ventricular events.

The near equality of LAP and LVEDP does
not always exist. Mitral valve stenosis and insufficiency will make LAP exceed LVEDP. LAP
may also underestimate LVEDP. With conditions impairing left ventricular distensibility,
atrial contraction contributes a much greater
fraction to diastolic filling. LVEDP becomes
greater than LAP, sometimes by as much as 10
mm Hg.[45]

Even if PAOP perfectly reflects LVEDP,
there are reasons to be suspicious of an easy interpretation. The Starling law as usually expressed relates ventricular volume, not pressure,
to the force of contraction. To use PAOP to estimate left ventricular end-diastolic volumes
(LVEDV) requires that the pressure-volume relationship be reasonably linear and fairly constant. An elevated PAOP that reflects overdistension of a healthy heart may indicate normal
or reduced filling in a ventricle stiffened by hypertrophy or injury. There is considerable evidence that during and after cardiopulmonary
bypass,[46,47] abdominal aortic surgery,[48] and
sepsis and acute myocardial disease[49] PAOP is
unreliable. It is likely that even changes in
PAOP are fundamentally ambiguous in those
or similar situations. There has been some attempt to use increases in PAOP during anesthesia to diagnose myocardial ischemia. This was
interpreted to be a reflection of ischemia-induced myocardial wall stiffening. Others have
found a PAOP increase to have little (15%)
positive predictive value of myocardial ischemia
during anesthesia.[50]

Fluid flux into the lung through the pulmonary microvascular is modeled by the Starling
equation; one of the four variables in this equation is the pulmonary capillary pressure. It is
obvious that pulmonary capillary pressure
(PCP) is intermediate between pulmonary ar-

tery pressure (PAP) and PVP; PAOP must be an underestimation of PCP. Attempts have been made to look at the initial PAOP waveform decay during occlusion to estimate PCP; there appear to be many confounding factors preventing this from being a clinically useful measurement.[51]

c. Usefulness. Many skeptical voices have been raised against the common use of balloon-flotation catheters. One went so far as to write that the overuse of these catheters had become a cult.[52] There are even more defenders of their use.[53] This debates continues within anesthesia as well.[54,55] It is clear that the sicker the patient becomes, the less accuracy the clinician will have in estimating PAOP from signs and symptoms; the rate for correctly predicting PAOP was only 30% in one study of critically ill patients.[56] In this same study, therapy was altered in half of the patients after pulmonary arterial catheterization. The more important question always remains whether outcome changes.

Two trials of the intraoperative use of such catheterizations have been performed.[57,58] Both studies were performed in patients having cardiac surgery, but the total number of patients for the two studies combined was only about 1300. The control group received central venous pressure monitoring. Neither study constrained the interpretation of PAOP and the therapeutic choices of the physicians. Neither study showed any difference in morbidity or mortality and did show higher costs with balloon-flotation catheters. Although the lack of any difference may be attributable to the moderate sample size, there is considerable historical experience performing cardiac surgery without balloon-flotation catheters and having enviably low morbidity and mortality.[59] A definitive clinical trial of use versus nonuse does not seem likely. Even less likely is a trial with a focused protocol for use of PAOP information.

d. Complications. Tissue damage from balloon-flotation catheters is briefly listed in List 8-3. The variety of suboptimal or erroneous treatment decisions possible seems endless. Most revolve around the administration or diuresis of fluids and the administration of inotropic drugs. Any positive effects on outcome from valid PAOP data can be easily negated by the all-too-common invalid PAOP data.

3. Noninvasive driving pressures. The oldest noninvasive or indirect method of obtaining blood pressure is direct palpation of an artery. Direct palpation is a continuous measurement, but it cannot easily be quantitated or replicated between observers. Nevertheless, a quick touch-

---

List 8-5. Detection of Arterial Opening with Occlusive Cuff Methods

Palpation
Skin flushing
Doppler changes in flow
Korotkoff sounds
Oscillometry
Plethysmography

---

ing of an artery can provide one with a reality check in deciding whether a monitor or a patient is in trouble. Other methods for noninvasive blood pressure measurement can be grouped together by principle of measurement.

All occlusive cuff methods employ an inflatable cuff wrapped around an extremity to collapse large blood vessels. It is believed that cuff and arterial transmural pressure are equal at the point at which the vessel's lumen just opens. Lumen opening during cuff deflation can be determined in numerous ways (List 8-5). Until 10 or so years ago auscultatory detection was the standard noninvasive method in the operating room. Low-frequency Korotkoff sounds produced by flow turbulence are auscultated through their five phases during cuff deflation. The first and last audible sounds mark systolic and diastolic pressure.[60] Oscillometric methods actually predate the use of Korotkoff sounds, but the purely mechanical devices available till a decade ago had no great popularity. Automatic oscillometric monitors became successful because of built-in inflation pumps and software to control, measure, and display repeated blood-pressure determinations.

Fundamentally different are transcutaneous pulse–recording methods. These attempt to provide continuous, directly calibrated pulse recordings. The Penaz method (Finapres) places a small cuff around a finger; incorporated within the cuff is a photoplethysmograph.[61] The photoplethysmograph measures finger volume; a computer software–driven pump applies varying amounts of cuff pressure (counterpulsation) to keep finger volume constant and allow maximal arterial pulsation. The varying cuff pressure is a continuous measure of arterial pressure. Another transcutaneous pulse–recording method is arterial tonometry.[62] This requires an adequately sized, superficial artery overlaying a bony structure. The principle is similar to ocular tonometry. A special transducer is applied over the center of the artery with sufficient force to distort the vessel. If this position is

List 8-6. Occlusive Cuff Blood Pressure Errors

Cause
Effect
Cuff loosely applied
High reading
Cuff too narrow
High reading
Cuff too wide
Low reading

carefully maintained, the normal contract stress between transducer and skin in the small area directly over the artery approximates arterial pressure. Automated tonometers that intelligently locate the transducer skin contact point are now becoming available.

a. Reliability. An array of difficulties cause artifact in noninvasive blood pressure measurement. All occlusive cuff methods are susceptible to a mismatch of cuff and extremity[63] (List 8-6); a cuff of insufficient width will produce overestimation of pressure by 5 mm Hg or more. A mismatch of cuff and finger is also possible with the Finapres. Auscultatory measurement is very dependent on observer hearing, sight, and skill.[60] Arterial tonometry is exquisitely sensitive to body motion misaligning transducer and artery.

There are more troubling difficulties about the basic meaning of occlusive blood pressures. It has been determined that the cuff pressure at the time of maximum oscillations corresponds with mean pressure.[64] Yet none of the algorithms for derivation of oscillometric pressures has been made public; the user does not know the exact meaning of the displayed pressures.

For 50 years, comparisons of invasive and noninvasive measurements have been published. Bruner et al.[65] summarized these efforts in stating that "the values yielded by direct and indirect measurement did not necessarily correlate. Different investigators found different degrees of noncorrelation; the variations were unpredictable and defied easy rationalization.." All noninvasive methods have been compared with invasive pressures. The relationships are sometimes marvelously precise and other times very tenuous.[66]

b. Interpretability. See the discussion of invasive driving pressures, p. 180.

c. Usefulness. Inspired by the turn-of-the-century competition between the two medical students Codman and Cushing to give the best anesthesia care, repetitive auscultatory blood pressure determinations as a standard practice spread throughout the community of anesthesiologists at the turn of this century.[67,68] This practice seems so reasonable that it has never been seriously questioned. This practice still seems plausible when one considers the dramatic effects on hemodynamics of current anesthetic drugs and the devastating possible trespasses of surgical tissue manipulation. Yet the recently published Multicenter Study of General Anesthesia provides an interesting prospective about the usefulness of blood pressure.[69,70] About 17,000 patients were randomly assigned to receive one anesthetic, which was either halothane, enflurane, isoflurane, or fentanyl, for elective surgery. Hypertension was more common and hypotension less common with fentanyl compared to the three inhalational drugs, but there was no difference in death or other severe morbidity (stroke, myocardial infarction) between these anesthetics. Do we really know if and when blood pressure makes a difference?

Cooper has argued that the automated devices should replace auscultatory measurements because they would be more reliable in detecting problems.[71] An interesting study of anesthesia residents showed that the use of automatic noninvasive blood pressure devices during the maintenance phase of anesthesia appeared to decrease vigilance.[72] If monitors do in fact decrease vigilance, no matter what their convenience and continual data production, their use might not be desirable. This point awaits clarification.

d. Complications. All occlusive cuff measurements have the potential of leaving an extremity ischemic for long periods if cuff inflation is too frequent or cuff deflation is too slow. This ischemia may produce nerve palsy[73] and an acute compartment syndrome with muscle necrosis.[74] The small finger cuff used by the Penaz method remains constantly inflated above venous pressure and produces fingertip venous stasis, swelling, hypoxemia and acidemia; transient finger numbness and fingertip pressure blisters have been noted.[75,76] Direct tissue injury is certainly rare compared to that seen with invasively obtained driving pressures. Since it is very easy to obtain artifactual pressure readings, the potential for making adverse therapeutic choices is as great as or greater than with invasive pressures.

B. Gas partial pressure

1. Respiratory gas monitoring.[77] Intraoperative capnography is encouraged by the American Society of Anesthesiologists and is now commonplace. Besides CO_2, other respiratory and anesthetic gases are routinely measured. A variety of methods are available for gas mea-

Table 8-3. Properties of respiratory gas monitors

Analyzer type	Sampling	Gases	Volatile agent specificity
Infrared absorption	Sidestream/ in line	CO_2, N_2O, volatile anesthetics	No (pending?)
Mass spectroscopy	Sidestream	O_2, CO_2, N_2, N_2O, volatile anesthetics	Yes
Photoacoustic spectroscopy	Sidestream	O_2, CO_2, N_2O, volatile anesthetics	No
Piezoelectric microbalance	Sidestream	Volatile anesthetics	No
Raman spectroscopy	Sidestream	O_2, CO_2, N_2, N_2O, volatile anesthetics	Yes

List 8-7. Physical Principles of Gas Monitors

1. *Infrared absorption:* Infrared analyzers emit one or more wavelengths of infrared light and measure light absorption.
2. *Mass spectroscopy:* The mass spectrometer uses electrostatic and magnetic fields to spread gases into a spectrum according to their mass-to-charge ratios for measurement by ion-current detectors.
3. *Photoacoustic spectroscopy:* Acoustic gas measurement involves pulsing the gas sample with several wavelengths of infrared light; the absorbed light heats the molecules, increases pressure, and creates sound detected by a microphone.
4. *Piezoelectric microbalance:* Gas molecules adhering to the coated surface of a oscillating piezoelectric crystal changes the resonant mass of the crystal and induces a proportional change in the crystal's resonant frequency.
5. *Raman spectroscopy:* The gas sample is illuminated by coherent photons that interact and excite the molecules; some photons are reemitted at a lower energy and frequency. The frequency shift between incident and scattered light is specific for each gas.

surement (Table 8-3). Their physical principles can be briefly summarized (List 8-7). The respiratory gas is usually drawn from the breathing circuit by a pump and sent to the analyzer (sidestream); some infrared analyzers have been sufficiently miniaturized to mount the detector directly in the ventilatory gas stream (in line). Originally mass spectrometers, which were too costly, were installed at a central site and sequentially sampled the operating suites by long sampling lines. All types of analyzers are now available as solo units. All capnometers have software with breath-detection algorithms to detect inspired and expired peak values.

a. Reliability. Gas monitors in general have an enviable record of providing reliable data. Their accuracy is satisfactory, being within a few tenths of a percent to standard reference samples for all measured gases when using frequent automatic self-calibration to compensate for drift and maintain an excellent repeatability. Precision is also good for all measured gases. The time-shared mass spectrometers cannot provide continuous monitoring of all patients; the most recent data may be several minutes old. The in line analyzers have optical windows in the sensor for the transmission of light through the gas stream; being close to the endotracheal tube, these windows are easily coated with secretions. There is a degradation in performance of all infrared analyzers, sidestream and in line, when the optics are contaminated. All sidestream analyzers may be disabled by water drops or secretions in the sampling line preventing aspiration of sample gas. All sidestream analyzers are susceptible of providing factitious values if inspired gas can be entrained and mixed with expired gas near the sampling port; end-tidal CO_2 ($P_{ET}CO_2$) will be underestimated.

The 10% to 90% rise time, the response of the sensor to a change in gas concentration, varies from about 50 to 500 msec for different analyzers. This is preceded by a delay phase of several seconds for sidestream analyzers as gas flows from the patient to the sensor. The maximum breathing rate that can be accurately measured depends on the rise time. As rise time becomes greater than 600 msec, respiratory rates above 20 breaths per minute will have artifactually high inspired CO_2 (P_ICO_2) and low $P_{ET}CO_2$.[78]

b. Interpretability. In health, arterial CO_2 (P_aCO_2) is kept in a carefully controlled range near 40 mm Hg. Under anesthesia, (P_aCO_2) may be allowed to vary from 25 to 65 mm Hg or higher with little apparent consequence as long as coexisting hypoxemia is prevented. There is no clear $P_{ET}CO_2$ cutoff point at which ventilation should be increased or decreased. Since $P_{ET}CO_2$ is used to estimate P_aCO_2, the P_aCO_2-to-$P_{ET}CO$ difference (gradient) is of great importance. Unfortunately this gradient increases with increasing dead space secondary to any increased mismatching of ventilation to perfusion. Induction of anesthesia by itself without any pulmonary disease worsens ventilation-to-perfusion matching. The degree of dead space cannot be determined from the $P_{ET}CO_2$ alone.

The $P_{ET}CO_2$ does have an interesting potential as a predictor of the restoration of a spontaneous heart beat during resuscitation from cardiac arrest. CO_2 delivery to the lung depends on cardiac output; an increasing $P_{ET}CO_2$ is consistent with improving cardiac output by external chest compression or internal cardiac massage. In a human study those who were resuscitated had a higher $P_{ET}CO_2$ in the early phases of advanced cardiac life support than that of those who could not be resuscitated. A cutoff point of 15 mm Hg of $P_{ET}CO_2$ had a very high positive and negative predictive value.[79]

The gases O_2 and N_2O are measured principally to detect failure of gas delivery to or within the anesthesia machine. Since nitrogen (N_2) is so insoluble, it is quickly washed out of the body during anesthesia with the common use of mixtures of O_2 and N_2O. Detection of N_2 during anesthesia thus has a straightforward interpretation; either air has entered the breathing circuit through a leak or venous air embolism is occurring.

Volatile anesthetics (currently halothane, enflurane, and isoflurane) are given by titration; the minimum alveolar concentration (MAC) provides only an estimate of the appropriate anesthetizing concentration for any given patient. The low therapeutic index of volatile anesthetics and their severe myocardial depression require constant vigilance. Nevertheless, within the range of 0 to 2.5%, no inspired concentration is absolutely contraindicated for all patients. Even higher inspired concentrations may be used temporarily to decrease the time to achieve anesthetizing concentrations in the brain. The agent-specific analyzers can certainly detect the misfilling of a vaporizer; all analyzers can identify a vaporizer that is out of calibration.

c. Usefulness. Capnography seems to be used for two purposes: to detect catastrophes and to adjust ventilation. The former seems the most important. Catastrophes are usually episodes of hypoventilation signaled by absent CO_2 in the capnogram and result from esophageal intubation, tracheal extubation, anesthesia circuit disconnection, endotracheal tube obstruction, ventilator malfunction, and patient apnea. No better way of detecting these catastrophes is available.[80,81] The sudden appearance of a falling $P_{ET}CO_2$ during constant minute ventilation may warn of massive dead-space effect from venous embolism (air, fat, thrombus, amniotic fluid) to the pulmonary artery. Although no randomized controlled trial has been performed, the fact that efficacy of capnography is likely is suggested by the review of closed malpractice claims.[22] About 30% of the negative outcomes were believed preventable by additional monitoring; in one half of that 30%, capnography and pulse oximetry were deemed the monitors of greatest likely use. Arguments about the degree of usefulness of capnography for more than catastrophe detection continues.[82,83]

Inspiratory O_2 and N_2O from the gas analyzers provide a redundancy for the machine-mounted in-circuit O_2 sensor. The usefulness of N_2 measurements to detect venous air embolism is confirmed in animal studies, but its clinical results has been discussed only in case reports.[84] Detection of breathing circuit leaks and disconnections is also claimed feasible.

Again, no randomized controlled trial has confirmed the efficacy of using intraoperative measurements of the volatile anesthetics. Large surveys of patient outcome do indicate that they may have a role. In one such report of over 150,000 anesthetic cases, half of the cardiac arrests were identified as being from an overdose of volatile anesthetics.[85]

d. Complications. There are almost no reports of direct patient injury from respiratory gas monitors though the mainstream analyzers can become sufficiently hot to cause burns. Since respiratory gas monitoring requires the interposition of a sampling port near the mask or endotracheal tube, there is an increased chance for a breathing circuit disconnection. Of course, the gas monitor will apprehend its own disconnection. Misapplication of monitoring data also seems most unlikely to harm the patient. Sudden changes in $P_{ET}CO_2$ will only increase vigilance. The analyzers cannot develop a failure state in which normal CO_2 wave forms are displayed unless there is gas movement.

C. Blood flow[86,87]

The measurement of cardiac output is an integral part of the anesthesia care of many patients. Historically, measurement of flow by the Fick principle came first and is still considered the standard. Derived from conservation of mass considerations, the basic relationship states that arterial oxygen transport equals mixed venous oxygen transport plus oxygen consumption. Formally this is written

$$\dot{Q} \times C_aO_2 = \dot{Q} \times C_{\bar{v}}O_2 + \dot{V}O_2$$

where $\dot{Q}$ is cardiac output, $\dot{V}O_2$ is oxygen consumption, and C_aO_2 and $C_{\bar{v}}O_2$ are arterial and mixed venous oxygen content. Algebraic manipulation produces the solution for cardiac output

$$\dot{Q} = \frac{\dot{V}O_2}{(C_aO_2 - C_{\bar{v}}O_2)}$$

Because expired gases must be collected for several minutes to obtain an average oxygen consumption, this is a steady-state determination in which $\dot{Q}$ represents an average flow during the time of expired gas collection. The difficulty of the oxygen-consumption measurement and the need for obtaining a mixed venous blood sample has kept Fick determinations a research tool.

Several rapid-injection indicator-dilution methods derive flow by the conservation of mass or energy principle. Initial use of this measurement technique used the actual intravenous injection of a green dye. It is now most commonly implemented by the addition of a thermistor to a pulmonary artery catheter and the use of a bolus of cool or cold fluid (usually 10 ml of normal saline) as the injectate; negative calories (temperature decrease) are the indicator. Temperature at the catheter tip after bolus injection exhibits a temperature fall and then a return to a base-line value. The conservation of heat principle, analogous to conservation of mass, allows derivation of the Stewart-Hamilton equation, which can be written as

$$\dot{Q} = \frac{K \times M}{\int_0^T C(t)dt}$$

where K is an empirical constant, M is the mass of indicator (quantity of negative calories), and $C(t)$ is the time-varying indicator concentration (temperature changes). A dedicated microprocessor integrates the temperature change over time and calculates cardiac output. The terminal portion of integration is an extrapolation. Temperature measurement is truncated or stopped before return to base-line temperature is complete; this is done to avoid recirculation artifacts and minimize the effect of pulmonary artery temperature fluctuations. The derived flow is an averaged $\dot{Q}$ over the several heart beats of temperature integration. Clinical use of thermodilution methods mandates an average of

triplicate determinations obtained over a several-minute period.

Two other techniques of flow measurement are also available, thoracic bioimpedance, and various types of continuous-wave and pulsed Doppler ultrasonography. Both are less invasive than Fick and indicator dilution methods and offer the promise of continuous cardiac output. With each heart beat the volume of blood within the thorax varies temporally with the cardiac cycle. Blood has the highest conductivity of any body tissue (lowest impedance, denoted Z, to the flow of electricity), and thus the conductivity of the entire thorax varies with the cardiac cycle; conductivity also varies with blood-flow velocity. Four pairs of surface electrocardiogram electrodes are placed on the neck and chest. Two of the electrodes inject an alternating milliampere current into the body; the other two measure changes in electrical potential and impedance. Stroke volume is a quadratic or cubic function of an idealized thoracic dimension, maximum rate of change of impedance, base-line impedance, and ventricular ejection time; several different functional relationships for estimating stroke volume are in used. A typical equation is of the following form:

$$\dot{Q} = HR \times SV_{bioimpedance} = HR \times \frac{f(L) \times T \times dZ/dt}{Z_{baseline}}$$

Bioimpedance monitors average a string of heart beats and display the cardiac output.

High frequency, inaudible sound (above 2 MHz) can be aimed through the body by ultrasound transducers, which are combined transmitters and receivers. As the sound is reflected back toward the transducer by the internal structures of the body, those objects that are moving change the frequency of the reflected sound in proportion to the velocity of the moving object; this is called the "Doppler effect." If the velocity of aortic blood flow is measured, cardiac output can be determined from the equation:

$$\dot{Q} = HR \times SV_{Doppler} = HR \times CSA \times \int V(t)dt$$

where the heart rate (HR) and aortic cross-sectional area (CSA) are multiplied by the time integral of aortic root blood velocity. There are many variations on the implementation of this monitor. The transducer is usually placed in the suprasternal notch, but esophageal probes have been developed. Both continuous and pulsed Doppler scanners are used. The number of heart beats averaged to calculate cardiac output also varies. In some systems CSA is measured; in others nomograms adjust CSA values for gender, age, height, and weight.

a. Reliability. To obtain thermodilution cardiac output, one must use an empirical constant (K, see above) that adjusts for the injectate volume, injectate temperature, catheter size, and the particular monitor. Error is added if actual injectate temperature and volume vary from the predetermined values. Numerous studies have show little difference between using room temperature and cold injectate.[86] Automatic injectors to consistently deliver the solution over a fixed interval also does not reduce variability.[88] Intracardiac shunts and valvular regurgitation of the right side of the heart may prevent accurate thermodilution measurement because the injectate may not properly mix or even pass the thermistor.

A thermodilution value varies somewhat depending on when in the respiratory cycle the injection is made. The usual convention is to start injection during the end-expiratory pause; this improves the precision of repeated determinations.[89] Since blood flow varies during the respiratory cycle because of complex interactions between intrathoracic pressure, ventricular filling, and ventricular emptying,[90,91] the values from end expiration, though precise, are biased. They would not necessarily reflect a time-weighted average over the several beats of a complete respiratory cycle.

In general the reproducibility of thermodilution values is good; Stetz et al. summarized nine studies of the thermodilution method.[92] The average triplicate value has to change only about 6% to 15% between measurement sessions to imply a change in patient hemodynamics. Stetz et al. also compiled 11 studies that compared thermodilution cardiac outputs to the Fick or dye dilution method.[92] Although these reports did not use proper accuracy and precision measures, the overall impression claimed an interchangeability of thermodilution with older methods.

The biggest reliability issue for Doppler cardiac outputs is the value of aortic cross-sectional area used in the calculation. The aorta is not a cylinder, its shape and area changes with every heart beat, and its area depends on aortic pressure. Error is added by the assumption that cross-sectional area is constant. Many refinements of empirical bioimpedance equations have been attempted. All such equations are empirically derived and make simplifying assumptions of a symmetric thorax and constancy of blood resistivity among the various circulatory parts.[93] Reports on these two methods have not generally included reproducibility data. After the initial enthusiastic reports for each new variation of Doppler and bioimpedance methods, other authors conduct comparison trials versus thermodilution methods. Certainly for perioperative use, these follow-up studies have failed to validate the interchangeability of these noninvasive methods with the thermodilution method.[94-96]

b. Interpretability. As with most physiologic variables, cardiac output can vary widely during anesthesia without apparent adverse consequences. Cardiac output is one of those variables that reflects the balance between ongoing surgical trauma, "stress," and the suppression by anesthetic drugs of the hormonal and metabolic response to that "stress." During and after anesthesia is the stress response good or bad? If it is good, under what circumstances? If bad, how bad? This issue has not been resolved.[97] Until it is, one will have difficulty deciding whether any particular cardiac output value is too high, too low, or just right.

Certain variables are derived from cardiac output and vascular pressures. Systemic (SVR) and pulmonary vascular resistance (PVR) are calculated by a variation on Ohm's law; driving pressure minus filling pressure is divided by flow. Since left ventricular systolic performance is inversely related to the force opposing ventricular fiber shortening, a clinically obtainable measure of this opposition, called "left ventricular afterload," is desirable. Clinicians have used SVR to adjust vasodilator drug infusion in hopes that they were rationally manipulating afterload. Unfortunately, SVR is basically not related to ventricular afterload.[98] SVR does reflect peripheral vasomotor tone. Blood ejection from the heart is pulsatile; Ohm's law is inappropriate. The real afterload is a complex mixture of ventricular geometry, pressure changes, flow acceleration, and the elasticity and viscosity of the aorta. Similar problems interfere with the interpretation of PVR. Changes in PVR cannot easily distinguish among vasodilatation, vascular recruitment, or rheologic changes.[99] Some researchers have advocated the abandonment of PVR as now calculated.[100]

c. Usefulness. There have been no clinical trials in the operating room focused on whether the availability of blood flow monitoring changes patient outcome. There are two studies that have focused on the wider perioperative period and have made such comparisons. In both studies cardiac output was by thermodilution; the control group had central venous pressure (CVP) monitoring only. Schultz et al. studied 70 nutritionally depleted, underprivileged, chronically ill elderly patients with hip fractures.[101] All patients required several or more days of medical management before surgical reduction and internal fixation. The specifics of how flow measurement were interpreted were not given. The death rate was about 30% in the control group and 3% in the monitored group. Shoemaker et al. studied 88 high-risk general surgery patients.[102] Three groups were created; one received CVP monitoring and the other two had thermodilution balloon-flotation catheters placed. In one of the thermodilution groups, a detailed protocol to create a hyperdynamic circulatory state by the transfusion of blood and the use of vasoactive drugs was followed. This latter group had a 4% death rate; the other two lost 23% and 33% of their patients. One question about both studies is whether the aggressive management in fact requires flow measurements. Nevertheless, these results are impressive. These results prove nothing for lower risk surgical patients but are suggestive for any group of high-risk surgical patients.

d. Complications. For thermodilution outputs the risks are those of the balloon-flotation catheter with one addition. The repetitive injection of aliquots of saline presents opportunities for contamination and bacterial growth in the injectate. Patients may unexpectedly be inoculated with microbes. If prefilled syringes of injectate or bags or bottles of injectate are kept for 24 hours at room temperature, about 15% have positive cultures for skin organisms.[103] There seem to be no reports of complications with the two noninvasive output methods. The Doppler method as implemented in an esophageal probe would seem to have the potential for oral, pharyngeal, and esophageal trauma.

Whether clinicians are giving frequent unnecessary fluid challenges and inotrope infusions because of erroneous flow measurements is not known because no one reports such information. Considering the disparity between the usual clinical interpretations and the real meaning of SVR and PVR, one must conclude that patients benefit from therapies chosen to manipulate resistance despite the measurement and not because of it. Do other clinical clues really provide the basis for the therapies?

D. Hemoglobin oxygen saturation

Two forms of in vivo oximetry have been incorporated as anesthesia monitors: pulse oximetry and mixed venous oximetry. The principle of measurement is spectrophotometry; the extinction (absorbance) of red and near-infrared light (600 to 1000 nanometers) transmitted through blood and tissues is proportional to the concentration of the hemoglobins. Each hemoglobin species (reduced [HHb], oxyhemoglobin [O_2Hb], methemoglobin [MetHb], carboxyhemoglobin [COHb], and so forth) has a unique extinction pattern. If a blood specimen is transilluminated with one distinct wavelength for each hemoglobin present and the intensity of transmitted light is measured, the Lambert-Beer law allows the calculation of the concentration of each hemoglobin species. By assuming that methemoglobin and carboxyhemoglobin are present in negligible quantities, one can simplify in vivo oximeters to include light emitters and detectors for only two wavelengths (usually 660 [red] and 940 [near infrared] nm). A specific, calibrated light-emitting diode is used to generate each wavelength.[104-107]

1. Pulse oximetry.[104-107] The light transmitted through any tissue is mostly absorbed by skin, soft tissue, bones, and venous and capillary blood; since this extinction is constant, it can be called the "constant component" of extinction. The hemoglobin in arterial blood makes only a small contribution to light extinction. Serendipitously it was noted that there are pulsatile variations in light transmission that are caused by pulsatile arterial blood volume changes. This pulsatile change in extinction is also a function of arterial saturation and can be called the "pulsatile component." For each wavelength (660 and 940 nm), the ratio of constant to pulsatile extinction is calculated; this is called the "pulse-added absorbance." The pulse oximeter determines the ratio of pulsatile change in light extinction at the two wavelengths to allow estimation of saturation (pulse-added absorbance$_{660}$/pulse-added absorbance$_{940}$). Because the optics of the tissue between emitter and detector are not ideal (do not satisfy all the conditions of the Lambert-Beer law), this estimation is derived from empirical calibration curves obtained in human volunteers. Pulse oximetry saturation is denoted S_PO_2 and represents the functional saturation of hemoglobin available for oxygen binding $100 \cdot O_2Hb/(O_2Hb + HHB)$. Clearly S_PO_2 might be different from the oxyhemoglobin percentage obtained from a multiwavelength spectrometer that equals $100 \cdot O_2Hb/(O_2Hb + HHB + MetHb + COHb)$.

a. Reliability. Considering the number of assumptions inherent in oximetry, one might expect limitations. There are many studies that have compared pulse oximetry with in vitro oximetry; unfortunately, most have used calibration statistical methods. Kelleher[105] and Tremper and Barker[106] have very usefully tabulated the results of these numerous studies, including bias and precision when it has been derived. In the range of oxygen saturations from 70% to 100%, the bias is generally small (1%

to 2%) as is the range of agreement (±4% to 5%); this bias and precision are compatible with the manufacturer's claims.

Although the presence or absence of other hemoglobins cannot be determined by pulse oximetry, COHb and MetHb can interfere with S_pS_2 accuracy because both species absorb light in the red to near-infrared spectrum. With increasing COHb, S_pO_2 falls much more slowly than the oxyhemoglobin percentage falls. The presence of COHb is treated by the pulse oximeter as if it were a mixture of 90% O_2Hb and 10% Hb.[108] MetHb can cause both an overestimation and an underestimation of S_pO_2; as MetHb increases, S_pO_2 settles toward 85% regardless of the actual oxyhemoglobin percentage.[109] Accuracy at very low saturations (less than 70%) is problematic; this is understandable, since S_pO_2 is estimated from empirical calibrations during which severe hypoxemia is not induced. In general, saturation is underestimated, and precision deteriorates at values below 70%.[110]

Users of pulse oximeters are familiar with many other circumstances in which S_pO_2 is unavailable or cannot be trusted (List 8-8). It is also important to remember that the response time of the monitor to actual changes in saturation is mostly a function of the circulation time to the sensor site. Although probes on the ear can respond in 10 seconds, finger and toe locations will take 20 to 30 and 40 to 80 seconds respectively.

b. Interpretability. Assuring adequate oxygen transport, especially to the brain and heart, is one of the anesthesiologist's primary concern. S_pO_2 is monitored to avoid and correct hypoxic hypoxia. Whether S_pO_2 is interpretable depends on the exact expectations placed on S_pO_2. If the

---

List 8-8. Other Limitations of Pulse Oximetry Causing Absent or Low S_pO_2 Reading

---

1. Low pulse-amplitude states[111]
   a. Hypotension
   b. Ischemia
   c. Vasoconstriction
   d. Hypothermia
2. Dyes
   a. Methylene blue
   b. Indigo carmine
   c. Nail polish
3. Other
   a. Motion artifact
   b. Shivering
   c. Electrocautery
   d. Excessive ambient light

---

detection of a large, relatively rapid fall in saturation from the 90% range is the goal, S_pO_2 serves well as a catastrophe alarm. If instead the goal is to determine the safety of mild hypoxemia after anesthesia at discharge from the PACU (postanesthesia care unit), S_pO_2 is of little help.[112] Although there are research devices capable of measuring tissue oxygen status (high-energy phosphate concentrations by magnetic resonance spectroscopy and cytochrome redox state by near-infrared spectroscopy), there has been no systematic clinical study of the minimum level of S_pO_2 associated with maintenance of sufficient cerebral tissue oxygen delivery.

c. Usefulness. There are several well-conducted studies that show that low saturation is often missed without the aid of pulse oximetry. This may occur during preinduction placement of monitoring catheters,[113] anesthesia,[114] transport to the PACU,[115] and care within the PACU.[116] These reports have changed anesthesia and postanesthesia care unit practices. For example, continuous postoperative O_2 therapy is now common in the PACU and this O_2 therapy is frequently continued upon transfer from the PACU to the hospital ward. Nevertheless, there are no controlled clinical trials that reveal an improvement in outcome. With the greater recognition of the frequency of desaturation and the change in practice management, it is doubtful that any study of sufficient size is now possible. Other attempts to justify pulse oximetry have included economic analysis of the cost of operating room catastrophes (death and brain damage) versus the cost of oximeters.[117,118] Finally, it is being claimed that since the adoption of monitoring standards in Massachusetts there have been few or no anesthesia deaths and hypoxic brain injuries as a result of better monitoring including pulse oximetry.[119]

d. Complications. Remarkably few patient injuries have been reported from pulse oximeters. These have consisted of burns and ischemic skin necrosis.[120,121] Also pulse oximetry does not seem to decrease overall vigilance or produce distractions. If desaturation is noticed, the treatment is ordinarily straightforward and includes one or more of the following (List 8-9). Even if this desaturation is fictitious, these routine patient care activities, as usually instituted during anesthesia, have little associated risk.

2. Mixed venous oximetry.[122,123] Fiberoptic bundles have been implanted in pulmonary artery catheters, terminating at the catheter tip, to provide mixed venous oximetry. This is a reflectance spectrophotometry. Red and near-infrared light is transmitted through part of the

---

List 8-9. Treatment Categories for Arterial Desaturation

Increase inspired oxygen
Increase ventilation
Correct equipment failure
Increase functional residual capacity
Lower oxygen consumption

---

bundles, and the reflected light is conducted back to light detectors through the remaining bundles. Mixed venous oxygen saturation is displayed continuously by the monitor. Since less than four wavelengths of light are used, assumptions about the absence of other hemoglobin species must be made. There are two mixed venous oximeters available, one using two wavelengths and the other using three wavelengths. Because the catheter tip is embedded in flowing blood, pulse oximetry methods are not necessary. The derived saturation is empirically calculated because it depends on Hb concentration, blood velocity, and other factors. An in vitro calibration before insertion and repeated in vivo recalibrations are necessary because the monitor performance drifts over time.

a. Reliability. Compared to pulse oximetry, far fewer studies comparing in vivo mixed venous saturations to bench oxygen saturations have been performed. These studies have not generally included comparison statistics. There does appear to be a difference in the stability of accuracy and precision between the two- and three-wavelength catheters. In one study the initial bias and precision, compared to bench oximetry, for both oximeter catheters was less than 2% and 3% respectively, similar to pulse oximeter performance; over time the two-wavelength catheter showed a large increase in bias, to 6% with a very poor precision greater than 5%.[124] In vivo oximetry certainly appears to face the same problems as pulse oximeters in the presence of MetHb and COHb.[109]

b. Interpretability. A rewriting of the Fick equation is the usual method for interpreting mixed venous saturation ($S_{\bar{v}}O_2$):

$$S_{\bar{v}}O_2 \propto C_{\bar{v}}O_2 = C_aO_2 - \frac{\dot{V}O_2}{\dot{Q}}$$

Assuming that C_aO_2 is constant , $S_{\bar{v}}O_2$ is proportional to the balance of oxygen uptake and cardiac output. Sometimes there is the further assumption that $\dot{V}O_2$ is constant; then $S_{\bar{v}}O_2$ is hyperbolically proportional to $\dot{Q}$. Since $S_{\bar{v}}O_2$ is about 75% in healthy persons, values less than that are said to reflect failing physiologic com-

pensations for maintaining oxygen delivery during anemia, hypovolemia, sepsis, fever, and so on. It is particularly hoped that $S_{\bar{v}}O_2$ will provide an early warning of hemodynamic changes.

A careful examination of these and other assumptions reveal that interpretation of mixed venous oxygen is fraught with uncertainty. The use of $S_{\bar{v}}O_2$ is an example of the use of arteriovenous concentration differences with the assumption that arterial concentration is constant.[125] Oxygen transport should probably be modeled as a nonlinear, nonstationary system. Mixed venous blood is the combined flow of venous blood from all parts of the body; mixed venous oxygen content is the average of oxygen content of these flows, averaged in proportion to the amount of blood from an organ as expressed by the equation:

$$C_{\bar{v}}O_2 = \frac{\sum_i \dot{Q}_i \times C_{\bar{v}i}O_2}{\sum_i \dot{Q}_i}$$

Any $C_{\bar{v}}O_2$ and by extension any $S_{\bar{v}}O_2$ can be derived from an infinite number of combinations of flows and oxygen consumptions within and between organs, flows and oxygen consumptions that can change dramatically and quickly with anesthesia and critical illness. No particular $S_{\bar{v}}O_2$ value is proof of adequate oxygen transport to any specific organ. These objections to facile interpretation are not merely theoretical but are based on empirical observations. Threshold values of $S_{\bar{v}}O_2$ that result in death or organ failure have not been demonstrated.[126,127] Changes in $S_{\bar{v}}O_2$ correlate poorly with changes in $\dot{Q}$.[128]

c. Usefulness. In the debate about efficacy, enthusiasts of the use of mixed venous pulmonary arterial balloon catheters have published testimonials to their clinical applicability.[129] The high cost of this technology have prompted several clinical trials. In one case series (coronary artery surgery) compared to historical controls at the same institution[130] and in two randomized controlled clinical trials (coronary artery surgery and critical illness),[58,131] the availability of $S_{\bar{v}}O_2$ did not improve outcome but did increase the cost of care. These studies suffer from their small size and the lack of a firm protocol for the interpretation and use of the data. Considering the basic ambiguity of $S_{\bar{v}}O_2$, one is skeptical that there will ever be such a successful demonstration. Perhaps, when real-time oxygen consumption is available, $S_{\bar{v}}O_2$ monitoring can become effective.

d. Complications. There seem to be no tissue injuries other than those from any pulmonary arterial catheter.

E. The neuromuscular function: mechanical displacement[132,133]

In 1954 Beecher and Todd reviewed deaths during 600,000 anesthetic sessions, concluded that the use of curare increased mortality six-fold, and recommended that it not be used for trivial reasons.[134] Since then the complexity of the neuromuscular junction and the potent actions of neuromuscular blocking drugs has been richly explored. Seventy to 80% of the acetylcholine receptors of the neuromuscular junction must be occupied before loss of neuromuscular function is detected.[135] The neuromuscular junction has both prejunctional and postjunctional acetylcholine receptors; this explains differential effects of neuromuscular blocking drugs.[136] There is great individual variation in the response to neuromuscular blocking drugs.[137] Muscles have different sensitivity to neuromuscular blocking drugs (from least to most: respiratory < facial < thenar < pharyngeal.[138,139]

A few years after the report of Beecher and Todd, equipment to objectively test neuromuscular function during anesthesia was created and recommended.[140] A supramaximal electrical stimulus (50 to 60 milliamps) is applied to a peripheral nerve; the muscle enervated is observed for the evoked contraction. The stimulus is applied by needle electrodes, disposable skin pads, or direct contact. The most commonly used nerves are the ulnar and a branch of the facial with observation of the abductor pollicis and orbicularis oculi respectively. The stimulation is most commonly applied as a single burst at 0.1 Hz, four consecutive bursts at 2 Hz (train-of-four), or repetitive 5-second bursts at 50 to 100 Hz. The contraction can be evaluated by visual examination, tactile examination, forced transduction (thenar muscles), accelerometry (piezoelectric transducer on thumb), and electromyography (thenar or facial muscles). A single stimulation is observed for the strength of twitch; the ratio of the fourth twitch to the first twitch is calculated for the train-of-four; with tetanic stimulation, the re-sulting tetany is observed for fade with time. Nerve stimulation is applied to allow one to judge and titrate the onset and continuation of paralysis and the restoration of neuromuscular function at the termination of anesthesia.

a. Reliability. Two aspects of reliability are important: the function of the nerve stimulator and the method of contractile assessment. Nerve stimulators are rugged, compact, well-packaged instruments. Most offer a variety of preprogrammed stimulation patterns; some are now incorporated with assessment and recording devices. It is hard to find a systematic comparison of nerve stimulators. The forced transduction mechanomyogram is the standard measurement of contraction, but the equipment requires excessive care and attention to be a useful clinical monitor. Visual and tactile examination are the most common methods of evaluation, but quantification is difficult; tactile assessment has been shown to lack accuracy.[141] Electromyography requires the amplification of very low level electrical signals, needs considerable signal processing, and is vulnerable to electrical surgical interference; but in some studies it appears interchangeable with forced transduction mechanomyograms.[142] Accelerometry is an easily applied new method not requiring special positioning of the thumb and showing very good precision with the forced transduction method.[143]

Several circumstances produce unreliable data. Direct placement of the stimulating electrodes over the muscle must be avoided. Direct muscle stimulation is possible even with total acetylcholine receptor blockade. Immediately after a tetanic stimulation the single or multiple twitch responses will be increased (posttetanic facilitation) for 10 or so minutes. The degree of blockade increases with falling temperature; if a temperature differential exists between the extremities and the core, misleading information is obtained.[144]

b. Interpretability. The evaluation of neuromuscular block after succinylcholine is relatively simple, with all responses being abolished for 5

Table 8-4. Correlation of nerve stimulator responses, receptor occupancy, and clinical relaxation with nondepolarizing neuromuscular blocking drugs

Receptor occupancy (%)	0.1 Hz single twitch (% control)	2 Hz train-of-four ratio (%)	5 sec 50 Hz tetanic stimulation	Clinical consequences
50	100	100	Sustained	Sustained head lift
70-75	100	~70	Sustained	Normal vital capacity
80	20-80	0-40	Fade	Normal tidal volume
90-95	0	0	Minimal response	Surgical skeletal muscle relaxation

to 20 minutes with the usual intubating dosage. Use of nondepolarizing drugs is more complicated. Waud and Waud,[135] Ali and Savarese,[132] and Viby-Mogensen[133] have synthesized animal and clinical studies to relate stimulus response and clinical consequences; a compilation of their findings roughly indicates the patterns of response (Table 8-4). Because of the differential sensitivity of skeletal muscles, these tests on peripheral muscles may not at all times allow adequate prediction of abdominal relaxation; clinical observation of the surgical field is still necessary. The greatest controversy remains; that is, one should consider what test performance should be achieved to allow one to predict safe extubation at the termination of induced paralysis.[145] A typical criterion has been the achievement of a train-of-four ratio of 70%.[146] Some recent work has suggested that a train-of-four ratio of 80%[147] or even a sustained head lift may be necessary to allow one to predict successful airway maintenance and airway protection.[138] The latter is obviously difficult to consistently assess in patients emerging from anesthesia.

c. Usefulness. It is well documented that patients who have been paralyzed during anesthesia with nondepolarizing neuromuscular blocking drugs show a high frequency of clinically significant residual paralysis if a nerve stimulator is not used to allow assessment of neuromuscular function.[148] The use of nerve stimulators has become quite common over the last 20 years. But, as with other monitors, no clinical trials have been performed to prove greater patient safety. However, large epidemiologic surveys no longer identify patients receiving paralyzing drugs as having a higher mortality.[149] The American Society of Anesthesiologists Closed Claim Study does not identify residual paralysis as a cause of respiratory complications[150] or identify nerve stimulators as a monitor that might have prevented a mishap.[22] Is this evidence that nerve stimulators are of no use? Or is the more likely explanation that their use is already sufficiently widespread to have removed this source of complications? The latter seems more plausible.

d. Complications. Although nerve stimulators inject electrical current into the body, their complications are rarely mentioned. A small full-thickness burn under a disposable skin electrode has occurred.[151] The balance between information and complications is very favorable.

F. Temperature[152]

Being a homeotherm, man maintains his body temperature near 37° Celsius (C) by muscular activity, changes in metabolism, sweating, vasomotor redistribution, and behavioral activities. This thermoregulation is controlled from the hypothalamic region. During general anesthesia thermoregulation is dramatically degraded and body temperature depends much more on environmental conditions.

Body temperature is measured by contact and noncontact methods. The former methods include glass thermometers, thermistors, thermocouples, and liquid crystals. The radiant heat (infrared photons) emitted by the body can give temperature without contact. Temperature is measured in the nose, mouth, rectum, tympanic membrane, bladder, heart, pulmonary artery and muscle, and at multiple skin sites including the axilla, big toe, and forehead.

a. Reliability. All methods available are accurate to ±0.3 Celsius degree or better. Most physiologic monitors now incorporate temperature monitoring by thermistor or thermocouple methods and provide digital displays with precision to 0.1 Celsius degree. Their response time to temperature change is quite rapid and depends mostly on the heat mass of the temperature probe itself. Self-contained liquid crystal strips applied to the skin are the least accurate and slowest responding method used during anesthesia.

b. Interpretability. Most temperature change, up or down, during anesthesia is an unnecessary and undesirable consequence of surgical conditions (exposure, skin preparation solutions, and open body cavities) and environmental changes (cool rooms and multiple layers of insulating covers). Specialized surgery (cardiopulmonary bypass and rarely neurosurgical techniques) may require the induction of a hypothermic state. Anesthesia may be requested to allow patients to tolerate the deliberate production of hyperthermia. And of course the rare genetic disorder malignant hyperthermia is always possible.

The interpretation is simple. If temperature is up, so is body heat content and vice versa. The solutions are also simple: reduce heat production and increase heat loss, or reduce heat loss and add heat. The separation of passive warming causing hyperthermia from the active process of malignant hyperthermia is suggested when one considers the rate of temperature increase, slowly for the former and quickly for the latter. Additional diagnostic methods are used if malignant hyperthermia is suspected.

Not totally resolved in clinical monitoring is the question of which temperature is the best to monitor. Tympanic membrane temperature is probably the temperature that best allows prediction of thermoregulatory activity of the body.[153,154] And there are temperature gradients throughout the body, the central heat core of the body being the brain, thorax, and abdomen.[155] Tympanic, nasopharyngeal, and esophageal are usually considered to be the best estimates of core temperature. Yet on occasion core temperature can be misleading about the heat content of the body. During the rewarming of cardiopulmonary bypass these core temperatures rapidly return to 37° C whereas rectal and bladder temperature recover more sluggishly. Complicated surgical procedures require temperature monitoring at multiple sites.

Skin temperature (skin liquid crystals or temperature probes placed on the skin) can be useful, but because of temperature gradients between core and periphery, it cannot provide the same information as other temperatures can.

c. Usefulness. The well-known effects of hypothermia on anesthetic requirements, volatile anesthetic uptake and elimination, and drug metabolism provide very convincing inspiration to monitor every patient's temperature. Also the devastating consequences of unrecognized malignant hyperthermia require 100% recognition of this condition.

d. Complications. All temperature probes can abrade or puncture the tissue into or against which they are placed. Since temperature probes are usually reusable, cross infection between patients is possible if the probe is not cleaned properly. Epistaxis is common with nasopharyngeal temperature monitoring but is usually a self-limiting injury. Of particular concern is the perforation of the tympanic membrane, which occurs on occasion with tympanic thermometry during anesthesia.[156] Since the probe is usually inserted after anesthesia is induced, the patient cannot complain when the probe is inserted too deeply. The risk of tympanic perforation discourages most anesthesiologists from the use of this monitoring site. Considering the minimal morbidity evident in published reports, the existing near-universal use of temperature monitoring, and the great importance of temperature control, temperature monitoring seems assured to continue.

G. Esophageal contractility

In man, the lower half of the esophagus consists solely of smooth muscle innervated by the vagus nerve. Besides the esophageal contractions related to swallowing (primary), there are spontaneous contractions (tertiary) of the lower esophagus apparently related to stress. Contractions can also be provoked by esophageal distension (secondary). It was proposed by Evans et al. that esophageal contractility, both secondary and tertiary, would be a guide to the adequacy of anesthesia.[157] Esophageal contractions are counted by an esophageal probe with two balloons. One balloon connects to a pressure transducer; the other balloon can be distended by an air pump to provoke secondary contractions. There are no reported complications from using this probe.

Indeed, the frequency of spontaneous and provoked contractions or the weighted average of both spontaneous and provoked contractions is related to the inspiratory concentration of halothane and isoflurane and signs of light anesthesia.[158,159] However, the predictive ability of esophageal contractility has not been confirmed by other researchers. During narcotic-infusion anesthesia spontaneous contractions had poor sensitivity and positive predictive value for signs of light anesthesia.[160] In another report, spontaneous contractions could not predict movement at the moment of skin incision in children breathing halothane and nitrous oxide;[161] by relative operating characteristics (ROC) analysis, esophageal contractions had no predictive ability.[162] The role of esophageal contractility in routine monitoring remains to be established.

H. Transcutaneous gas measurements

In the midnineteenth century the existence of transcutaneous respiration was discovered; CO_2 and O_2 diffuse across the skin.[163] Over 100 years later transcutaneous sensors that used either a Clark polarographic Po_2 electrode for the O_2 measurement (P_SO_2)[164] or a Severinghaus type of Pco_2 electrode for the CO_2 measurement (P_SCO_2) were developed.[165] The skin is heated to increase and make blood flow uniform in the skin and to lower skin resistance to gas diffusion. Burns are possible; their incidence is unknown. Later a combined electrode to measure both O_2 and CO_2 was invented.[166] Use of such electrodes is not simple, requiring sensor calibration, skin cleaning, application to the skin of an adhesive mounting ring and contact liquid, insertion of the electrode into the mounting ring, and stabilization of the skin and electrode temperature at about 44° C.

Transcutaneous gases are not equivalent to arterial blood gases; P_SCO_2 and P_SO_2 are a function of O_2 consumption by skin and electrode and CO_2 production by skin, oxygen delivery to and carbon dioxide removal from the skin, and gas transfer through the skin. Especially for oxygen, there is considerable inhomogeneity in the delivery of oxygen to the skin. P_SO_2 has been found in multiple reports to produce an underestimation of P_aO_2 and to have inconstant and unpredictable errors in use on adults.[167] Attempts to derive useful information from the P_SO_2 include the calculation a P_SO_2 index (the ratio of P_SO_2 to P_aO_2); low values were found in patients with poor peripheral perfusion.[168] Unfortunately there remains a fundamental ambiguity with P_SO_2 in separating P_aO_2 and perfusion changes. P_SCO_2 appears to be more consistently related to P_aCO_2.[169] A large multicenter study has confirmed these findings for P_SO_2 and P_SCO_2 and has encouraged the continued use of skin CO_2 monitoring.[170] The unreliability of skin-oxygen measurement, the apparent universal acceptance of routine capnography, and the awkwardness of using skin electrodes seem to have caused the abandonment of transcutaneous monitoring in adults.

III. MORE SPECIALIZED MONITORS

The previously discussed monitors are accessible to essentially every anesthesiologist. Many are used universally; others have or have had proponents arguing for standard use in all patients. The invasive pressure methods have been taught routinely by training programs for at least 15 years. The cost of equipment is within the budget capabilities of most hospitals; the insertion and application of interfacing devices and monitor use are common skills.

There are two other monitoring methods that are much more specialized; these are imaging of the heart and recording of cerebral electrical activity. Although all have emerged from pure research use, clinical use is not universal. The use of these monitors is not a common skill; there is a real concern about the training process. Equipment costs can be from $30,000 to $200,000, several orders of magnitude higher than some of the previously discussed monitors. Most institutions have found it effective to provide full-time technician support for the devices; this is not the case for other perioperative monitoring technologies. There is a very extensive literature for these methods. Only limited comments are presented here to highlight a few aspects of their perioperative role.

A. Cerebral electrical activity[171]

For the last 30 years recording of central nervous system activity has gradually moved from the physiology laboratory and the electroencephalographer's office to the operating room. This move was conditional on the development of better electronics, microprocessors, and signal-averaging software. The operating room is a hostile environment for the detection, amplification, and processing of the very low voltage scalp potentials; there are numerous sources of electrical noise that can overwhelm the detection of physiologic signals. Since most intraoperative monitoring uses processed rather than raw electroencephalograms (EEGs), it is vital to remember that the computer software can process junk signals just as well as the real thing. The monitoring environment process is also hostile because three clinical events, cerebral hypoxia, hypothermia, and deep anesthesia, produce much the same result—a decreased frequency and a decreased amplitude of cerebral electrical potentials.

In general terms there are two potential applications for intraoperative EEGs: (1) determination of anesthetic depth and (2) detection of cerebral ischemia. There is a third application, seizure recognition during epilepsy surgery, which is superspecialized and actually uses electrocorticography; a fully trained electroencephalographer performs this monitoring. Analog EEG (strip-chart recorder) has proved too difficult for use by anesthesiologists in the operating room for those first two purposes. Processed EEGs showing the amplitudes of bands of frequency activity are now available by a variety devices that use several algorithms to extract analog EEG features. Good electrode placement with low impedance pathways is always critical.

Interest in anesthetic depth would be to avoid light anesthesia with awareness, to prevent needless deep anesthesia, and to titrate deep anesthesia to increase brain resistance to ischemia or hypoxia. The analog EEG has been extensively used to uncover EEG patterns associated with inhalation and intravenous anesthetics; there is a great diversity of patterns by dose, within inhalation and intravenous drugs, and between inhalation and intravenous drugs.[172] Many of the individual patterns can no longer be recognized with a processed EEG. There are EEG patterns for restricted circumstances (certain drugs, certain patients) that allow identification of light anesthesia, but these patterns have no universality for all patients and all the possible drug combinations. The basic problem is the inability to relate consciousness mechanistically to electrical activity; only empirical correlations are available.[173]

Sufficiently deep anesthesia will produce electrical silence. It is hoped that this suppression of EEG would reflect a condition of brain protection, the ability of the central nervous system to tolerate longer periods of hypoxia with full recovery.[174] Some attempts have been successful; others have not. After successful resuscitation from cardiac arrest some patients remained in coma; an attempt to improve survival by using a high-dose barbiturate therapy was not successful.[175] Nussmeier et al. titrated barbiturate therapy during cardiopulmonary bypass by EEG monitoring and reduced neuropsychiatric complications.[176] The use of routine EEG monitoring during heart surgery to detect cerebral hypoxia and ischemia remains controversial.[177,178] Some centers report routine EEG use during carotid artery surgery to determine the necessity of shunting during carotid artery cross clamping.[179]

Event-related activity of the central nervous system can be detected by repeated stimulation of a sensory system and averaging of the EEG to show pathway-specific electrical activity. Evoked potentials (EVPs) are very low voltage signals produced by somatosensory, auditory, or visual-field stimulation. Five hundred to 1000 stimuli are required to generate an evoked potential. Somatosensory EVPs are the most commonly used during anesthesia. Anesthetic agents can considerably modify these EVPs, hampering interpretation. The evidence for their usefulness has been extensively reviewed by Gugino and Chabot.[180] The use of somatosensory EVPs in spinal surgery is now routine though questions remain about their sensitivity and specificity. Their use in aortic and carotid surgery remains controversial.

If needle electrodes are used, EEGs and EVPs would have the risk of cross infection. Other complications are not reported. Improperly obtained or interpreted cerebral electrical signals have obvious possibilities for prompting mistakes. For example, the failure to recognize loss of dorsal column pathway function during surgical distraction of the spinal column could leave a patient paraplegic.

B. Cardiac imaging[181-184]

Echocardiography uses sound waves in the 2.5 to 5 MHz range to penetrate tissue. Piezoelectric crystals emit these high-frequency sound waves; the same or another set of crystals receive the reflected sound waves. The time delay of the echo specifies the distance of a structure from the emitter; the intensity of the echo is proportional to tissue density; any Doppler shift in the reflected signal provides information about velocity. By mechanical or electronic means echo probes now scan a 90-degree sector; computer software generates a two-dimensional image or tomographic slice through tissue from the reflected sound. By repeated imaging (30 Hz) of the heart, a series of images can be displayed to provide a real-time slice of the

beating heart. If Doppler measurement is used, color-flow mapping of blood velocity can be superimposed on the two-dimensional image.

Initial cardiac imaging used a transthoracic approach. This provided diagnostic images of valve lesions, heart size, and so on; intraoperative use was not practical. With the miniaturization of electronic components, the Doppler probe was mounted on a flexible gastroscope and advanced blindly down the esophagus to provide a transesophageal retrocardiac view of the heart. The depth of the probe down the esophagus and its angulation provide three distinct views: (1) a basal short-axis view of the outflow tracts and valves, (2) a long-axis view of all four chambers, and (3) a short-axis cross section of the left ventricle. The main emphasis of intraoperative use has been continuous visualization of the left ventricle short axis for assessment of global ventricular function, contractile indices, left ventricular filling, and regional ventricular function. Only the last topic is further discussed as an example of the development of intraoperative echocardiography.

Great interest is being expressed in observations of regional wall motion for the early detection of myocardial ischemia.[185] As a segment of ventricular wall becomes ischemic, the contraction of that segment progressively changes within seconds from normal motion to hypokinesis, akinesis, and dyskinesis. The sudden development of regional wall motion abnormalities is the earliest and most sensitive detector of ischemia.[186] New regional wall motion abnormalities after cardiopulmonary bypass in patients receiving coronary artery bypass grafts was predictive of postoperative myocardial infarction and death.[187] Yet this issue is not fully resolved. A debate continues as to whether echocardiography or electrocardiography should be the main tool for the detection of intraoperative myocardial ischemia.[188,189] A recent editorial raised questions about the reliability, interpretability, and usefulness of this technology for detection of ischemia.[190] These questions and others are still in the process of investigation (List 8-10).

Reports of complications with intraoperative transesophageal echocardiography are rare but should be similar to those associated with flexible gastroscopy. Esophageal perforation secondary to a difficult esophageal intubation would be the most feared event.[181] An esophageal tear has now been reported in a patient despite the easy passage of the gastroscope.[192] Temporary unilateral vocal cord paralysis was observed in two patients monitored during sitting craniotomy.[193] It is unknown how often

---

List 8-10. Questions Concerning Transesophageal Echocardiography Detection of Regional Wall Motion Abnormalities

---

1. What training is necessary for one to be an intraoperative echocardiographer?[191]
2. What is the reproducibility of the images? Is the current short-axis left ventricular view sufficiently representative of the entire muscle mass?
3. What criteria should be established for asserting the diagnosis of ischemia? Can these criteria be consistently applied to real-time images?
4. What patient groups have a sufficiently high preoperative probability of the development of intraoperative ischemia for the ischemia criteria to have a useful positive predictive value?
5. What type of studies are possible to demonstrate that the detection of regional wall motion abnormalities will change therapy and change patient outcome?
6. Is this technology sufficiently robust to be used in common clinical practice?

---

erroneous interpretations lead to mistaken therapy changes. This monitoring method is still in its youth, but its proponents are rapidly reporting answers to the many questions.

IV. CONCLUSIONS

There is a clear dilemma for anesthesiologist with respect to the complications caused by perioperative monitoring. The tissue injuries produced by most monitors are well understood. The immediate consequences of therapy chosen mistakenly because of a monitored variable are more or less predictable. Yet it is hard to pin down with assurance the benefits of monitoring in terms of patient morbidity and mortality. One must be skeptical about one's clinical impressions about monitors because of the enormous variability in patient physiologic behavior. Formal studies using rigorous methods are necessary. Without a firm estimate of benefits, no reasonable model can be written to balance risks and benefits.

Albert Einstein offered the following insight about science:[194] "Science is the attempt to make the chaotic diversity of our sense-experience correspond to a logically uniform system of thought. In this system single experiences must be correlated with the theoretic structure in such a way that the resulting coordination is unique and convincing. The sense-experiences are the given subject-matter. But the theory that shall interpret them is man-made. It is the result of an extremely laborious process of ad-

aptation: hypothetical, never completely final, always subject to question and doubt." The specialty of anesthesiology in particular and medicine in general lack such models at present to provide certitude in choices about monitoring and its complications.

REFERENCES

1. Gaba DM: Human error in anesthetic mishaps, Int Anesthesiol Clin 27:137-147, 1989.
2. Moyers J: Monitoring instruments are no substitute for careful clinical observation, J Clin Monit 4:107-111, 1988.
3. Pierce EC Jr: Monitoring instruments have significantly reduced anesthetic mishaps, J Clin Monit 4:111-114, 1988.
4. Keats AS: Anesthesia mortality in perspective, Anesth Analg 71:113-119, 1990.
5. Fuchs VR and Garber AM: The new technology assessment, N Engl J Med 323:673-677, 1990.
6. Banta HD and Thacker SB: The case for reassessment of health care technology: once is not enough, JAMA 264:235-240, 1990.
7. Mosteller F and Burdick E: Current issues in health care technology assessment, Int J Technol Assess Health Care 5:123-136, 1989.
8. Pace NL: Technology assessment of anesthesia monitors, J Clin Monit (Accepted).
9. Cooper JO and Cullen BF: Observer reliability in detecting surreptitious random occlusions of the monaural esophageal stethoscope, J Clin Monit 6:271-275, 1990.
10. Hope CE and Morrison DL: Understanding and selecting monitoring equipment in anaesthesia and intensive care, Can Anaesth Soc J 33:670-679, 1986.
11. Ream AK: Mean blood pressure algorithms, J Clin Monit 1:138-144, 1985.
12. Altman DG and Bland JM: Measurement in medicine: the analysis of method comparison studies, Statistician 32:307-317, 1983.
13. Bland JM and Altman DG: Statistical methods for assessing agreement between two methods of clinical measurement, Lancet 1:307-310, 1986.
14. Chinn S: The assessment of methods of measurement, Stat Med 9:351-362, 1990.
15. LaMantia KR, O'Connor T, and Barash PG: Comparing methods of measurement: an alternative approach, Anesthesiology 72:781-783, 1990.
16. Swets JA: Measuring the accuracy of diagnostic systems, Science 240:1285-1293, 1988.
17. Begg CB: Biases in the assessment of diagnostic tests, Stat Med 6:411-423, 1987.
18. Jaeschke R and Sackett DL: Research methods for obtaining primary evidence, Int J Technol Assess Health Care 5:504-519, 1989.
19. Eddy DM, Hasselblad V, and Shachter R: A Bayesian method for synthesizing evidence: the confidence profile method, Int J Technol Assess Health Care 6:31-55, 1990.
20. Laird NM and Mosteller F: Some statistical methods for combining experimental results, Int J Technol Assess Health Care 6:5-30, 1990.
21. Moses LE: Framework for considering the role of data bases in technology assessment, Int J Technol Assess Health Care 6:183-193, 1990.
22. Tinker JH, Dull DL, Caplan RA, et al: Role of monitoring devices in prevention of anesthetic mishaps: a closed claim analysis, Anesthesiology 71:541-546, 1989.

23. Freeman R: Intrapartum fetal monitoring—a disappointing story, N Engl J Med 322:624-626, 1990.

24. Pace NL: But what does monitoring do to patient outcome? Int J Clin Monit Comput 1:197-200, 1985.

25. Kleinman B: Understanding natural frequency and damping and how they relate to the measurement of blood pressure, J Clin Monit 5:137-147, 1989.

26. Fry DL: Physiologic recording by modern instruments with particular reference to pressure recording, Physiol Rev 40:753-788, 1960.

27. Gardner RM: Direct blood pressure measurement: dynamic response requirements, Anesthesiology 54:227-236, 1981.

28. Bruner JMR: Handbook of blood pressure monitoring, Littleton, Mass, 1978, PSG Publishing Co, Inc, p 174.

29. Gardner RM: System concepts for invasive pressure monitoring. In Civetta JM, Taylor RW, and Kirby RR, editors: Critical care, Philadelphia, 1988, JB Lippincott Co, pp 303-310.

30. Schwid HA, Taylor LA, and Smith NT: Computer model analysis of the radial artery pressure waveform, J Clin Monit 3:220-228, 1987.

31. Pauca AL, Hudspeth AS, Wallenhaupt SL, et al: Radial artery-to-aorta pressure difference after discontinuation of cardiopulmonary bypass, Anesthesiology 70:935-941, 1989.

32. Rao TLK, Jacobs KH, El-Etr AA: Reinfarction following anesthesia in patients with myocardial infarction, Anesthesiology 59:449-505, 1983.

33. Shah KB, Rao TLK, Laughlin S, and El-Etr AA: A review of pulmonary artery catheterization in 6,245 patients, Anesthesiology 61:271-275, 1984.

34. Slogoff S and Keats AS: On the safety of radial artery cannulation, Anesthesiology 59:42-47, 1983.

35. O'Quin R and Marini JJ: Pulmonary artery occlusion pressure: clinical physiology, measurement, and interpretation, Am Rev Respir Dis 128:319-326, 1983.

36. Tuman KJ, Carroll GC, and Ivankovich AD: Pitfalls in interpretation of pulmonary artery catheter data, J Cardiothorac Anesth 3:625-641, 1989.

37. Schmitt EA and Brantigan CO: Common artifacts of pulmonary artery and pulmonary artery wedge pressures: recognition and interpretation, J Clin Monit 2:44-52, 1986.

38. Groom L, Frisch SR, and Elliott M: Reproducibility and accuracy of pulmonary artery pressure measurement in supine and lateral position, Heart Lung 19:147-151, 1990.

39. Altschule MD: Invalidity of using so-called Starling curves in clinical medicine, Perspect Biol Med 26:171-187, 1983.

40. Mammana RB, Hiro S, Levitsky S, et al: Inaccuracy of pulmonary capillary wedge pressure when compared to left atrial pressure in the early postsurgical period, J Thorac Cardiovasc Surg 84:420-425, 1982.

41. Walston A and Kendall MD: Comparison of pulmonary wedge and left atrial pressure in man, Am Heart J 86:159-164, 1973.

42. Permutt S, Bromberger-Barnea B, and Bane HN: Alveolar pressure, pulmonary venous pressure, and the vascular waterfall, Med Thorac 19:239-260, 1962.

43. Permutt S and Riley RL: Hemodynamics of collapsible vessels with tone: the vascular waterfall, J Appl Physiol 18:924-932, 1963.

44. West JB, Dollery CT, and Naimark A: Distribution of blood flow in isolated lung: relation to vascular and alveolar pressures, J Appl Physiol 19:713-724, 1964.

45. Rahimtolla SH, Ehsani A, Sinn MZ, et al: Left atrial transport function in myocardial infarction: importance of the booster pump function, Am J Med 59:686-694, 1975.

46. Hansen RM, Viquerat CE, Matthay MA, et al: Poor correlation between pulmonary arterial wedge pressure and left ventricular end-diastolic volume after coronary artery bypass graft surgery, Anesthesiology 64:764-770, 1986.

47. Ellis RJ, Mangano DT, and VanDyke DC: Relationship of wedge pressure to end-diastolic volume in patients undergoing myocardial revascularization, J Thorac Cardiovasc Surg 78:605-613, 1979.

48. Kalman PG, Wellwood MR, Weisel RD, et al: Cardiac dysfunction during abdominal aortic operation: the limitations of pulmonary wedge pressures, J Vasc Surg 3:773-781, 1986.

49. Calvin JE, Driedger AA, and Sibbald WJ: Does the pulmonary capillary wedge pressure predict left ventricular preload in critically ill patients? Crit Care Med 9:437-443, 1981.

50. van Daele MERM, Sutherland GR, Mitchell MM, et al: Do changes in pulmonary capillary wedge pressure adequately reflect myocardial ischemia during anesthesia? a correlative preoperative hemodynamic, electrocardiographic, and transesophageal echocardiographic study, Circulation 81:865-871, 1990.

51. Dawson CA, Bronikowski TA, Linehan JH, et al: On the estimation of pulmonary capillary pressure from arterial occlusion, Am Rev Respir Dis 140:1228-1236, 1989.

52. Robin ED: The cult of the Swan-Ganz catheter: overuse and abuse of pulmonary flow catheters, Ann Intern Med 103:445-449, 1985.

53. Matthay MA and Chatterjee K: Beside catheterization of the pulmonary artery: risks compared with benefits, Ann Intern Med 109:826-834, 1988.

54. Keats AS: The Rovenstein Lecture, 1983: cardiovascular anesthesia—perceptions and perspectives, Anesthesiology 60:467-474, 1984.

55. Lowenstein E and Teplick R: To (PA) catheterize or not to (PA) catheterize—that is the question, Anesthesiology 53:361-353, 1980 [editorial].

56. Eisenberg PR, Jaffe AS, and Schuster DP: Clinical evaluation compared to pulmonary artery catheterization in the hemodynamic assessment of critically ill patients, Crit Care Med 12:549-553, 1984.

57. Tuman KJ, McCarthy RJ, Spiess BD, et al: Effect of pulmonary artery catheterization on outcome in patients undergoing coronary artery surgery, Anesthesiology 70:199-206, 1989.

58. Pearson KS, Gomez MN, Moyers JR, et al: A cost/benefit analysis of randomized invasive monitoring for patients undergoing cardiac surgery, Anesth Analg 69:336-341, 1989.

59. Bashein G, Johnson PW, Davis KB, and Ivey TD: Elective coronary bypass surgery without pulmonary artery catheter monitoring, Anesthesiology 63:451-454, 1985.

60. Frohlich ED, Grim C, Labarthe DR, et al: Recommendations for human blood pressure determination by sphygmomanometers: report of a special task force appointed by the steering committee, American Heart Association, Circulation 77:502A-514A, 1988.

61. Boehmer RD: Continuous, real-time, noninvasive monitor of blood pressure: Penaz methodology applied to the finger, J Clin Monit 3:282-287, 1987.

62. Drzewiecki GM, Melbin J, and Noordergraaf A: Arterial tonometry: review and analysis, J Biomech 16:141-152, 1983.

63. Manning DM, Kuchirka C, and Kaminski J: Miscuffing: inappropriate blood pressure cuff application, Circulation 68:763-766, 1983.

64. Geddes LA, Voelz M, Combs C, et al: Characterization of the oscillometric method for measuring indirect blood pressure, Ann Biomed Eng 10:271-280, 1982.

65. Bruner JMR, Krenis LJ, Kunsman JM, and Sherman AP: Comparison of direct and indirect methods of measuring arterial blood pressure I, II, III, Med Instrum 14:11-21, 97-101, 182-188, 1981.

66. Pace NL and East TD: A simultaneous comparison of intra-arterial, oscillometric and Finapres monitoring during anesthesia, Anesth Analg 1991 (In press).

67. Beecher HK: The first anesthesia records (Codman, Cushing), Surg Gynecol Obstet 71:689-693, 1940.

68. Neuhauser D: Ernest Amory Codman, M.D., and end results of medical care, Int J Technol Assess Health Care 6:307-325, 1990.

69. Forrest JB, Rehder K, Goldsmith CH, et al: Multicenter study of general anesthesia. I. Design and patient demography, Anesthesiology 72:252-261, 1990.

70. Forrest JB, Cahalan MK, Rehder K, et al: Multicenter study of general anesthesia. II. Results, Anesthesiology 72:262-268, 1990.

71. Cooper JB: Toward prevention of anesthetic mishaps, Int Anesthesiol Clin 22:167-183, 1984.

72. Kay J and Neal M: Effect of automatic blood pressure devices on vigilance of anesthesia residents, J Clin Monit 2:148-150, 1986.

73. Bickler PE, Schapera A, and Bainton CR: Acute radial nerve injury from use of an automatic blood pressure monitor, Anesthesiology 73:186-188, 1990.

74. Celoria G, Dawson JA, and Teres D: Compartment syndrome in a patient monitored with an automated blood pressure cuff, J Clin Monit 3:139-141, 1987.

75. Northwood D: Morbidity after use of the Finapres blood pressure monitor, Anaesthesia 44:1010-1011, 1989.

76. Gravenstein JS, Paulus DA, Feldman J, and McLaughlin G: Tissue hypoxia distal to a Penaz finger blood pressure cuff, J Clin Monit 1:120-125, 1985.

77. Gravenstein JS, Paulus DA, and Hayes TJ: Capnography in clinical practice, Boston, Mass, 1989, Butterworth J.

78. Brunner JX and Westenskow DR: How the rise time of carbon dioxide analysers influences the accuracy of carbon dioxide measurements, Br J Anaesth 61:628-638, 1988.

79. Callaham M and Barton C: Prediction of outcome of cardiopulmonary resuscitation from end-tidal carbon dioxide concentration, Crit Care Med 18:358-362, 1990.

80. Birmingham PK, Cheney FW, and Ward RJ: Esophageal intubation: a review of detection and techniques, Anesth Analg 65:886-891, 1986.

81. Cote CJ, Liu LMP, Szyfelbein SK, et al: Intraoperative events diagnosed by expired carbon dioxide monitoring in children, Can Anaesth Soc J 33:315-320, 1986.

82. Polaheimo MPJ: A carbon dioxide monitor that does not show the waveform has value, J Clin Monit 4:210-212, 1988.

83. Block FE: A carbon dioxide monitor that does not show the waveform is worthless, J Clin Monit 4:213-214, 1988.

84. Matjasko J, Petrozza P, and Mackenzie CF: Sensitivity of end-tidal nitrogen in the detection of venous air embolism in the dog, Anesthesiology 63:418-423, 1985.

85. Keenan RL and Boyan CP: Cardiac arrest due to anesthesia: a study of incidence and causes, JAMA 253:2372-2377, 1985.

86. Banner T and Banner MJ: Cardiac output measurement technology. In Civetta JM, Taylor RW, and Kirby RR, editors: Critical care, Philadelphia, 1988, JB Lippincott Co, pp 361-376.

87. Levett JM and Replogle RL: Thermodilution cardiac output: a critical analysis, J Surg Res 27:392-404, 1979.

88. Nelson LD: Automatic vs manual injections for thermodilution cardiac output determinations, Crit Care Med 10:190-192, 1982.

89. Stevens JH, Raffin TA, Mihm FG, and Rosenthal MH: Thermodilution cardiac output measurement: effects of the respiratory cycle on its reproducibility, JAMA 253:2240-2242, 1985.

90. Peters J, Kindred MK, and Robotham JL: Transient analysis of cardiopulmonary interactions: II. Systolic events, J Appl Physiol 64:1518-1526, 1988.

91. Peters J, Kindred MK, and Robotham JL: Transient analysis of cardiopulmonary interactions: I. Diastolic events, J Appl Physiol 64:1506-1517, 1988.

92. Stetz CW, Miller RG, Kelly GE, and Raffin TA: Reliability of the thermodilution method in the determination of cardiac output in clinical practice, Am Rev Respir Dis 126:1001-1004, 1982.

93. Handelsman H: Public health service assessment: cardiac output by electrical bioimpedance, National Center for Health Services Research and Health Care Technology Assessment, Public Health Service, US Department of Health and Human Services, 1989.

94. Spahn DR, Schmid ER, Tornic M, et al: Noninvasive versus invasive assessment of cardiac output after cardiac surgery: clinical validation, J Cardiothorac Anesth 4:46-59, 1990.

95. Siegel LC, Shafer SL, Martinez GM, et al: Simultaneous measurements of cardiac output by thermodilution, esophageal Doppler, and electrical impedance in anesthetized patients, J Cardiothorac Anesth 2:590-595, 1988.

96. Wong DH, Tremper KK, Stemmer EA, et al: Noninvasive cardiac output: simultaneous comparison of two different methods with thermodilution, Anesthesiology 72:784-792, 1990.

97. Roizen MF: Should we all have a sympathectomy at birth? Or at least preoperatively? Anesthesiology 68:482-484, 1988.

98. Lang RM, Borow KM, Neumann A, and Janzen D: Systemic vascular resistance: an unreliable index of left ventricular afterload, Circulation 74:1114-1123, 1986.

99. Borback MS: Problems associated with the determination of pulmonary vascular resistance, J Clin Monit 6:118-127, 1990.

100. McGregor M and Sniderman A: On pulmonary vascular resistance: the need for more precise definition, Am J Cardiol 55:217-221, 1985.

101. Schultz RJ, Whitfield GF, LaMura JJ, et al: The role of physiologic monitoring in patients with fractures of the hip, J Trauma 25:309-316, 1985.

102. Shoemaker WC, Appel PL, Kram HB, et al: Prospective trial of supranormal values of survivors as therapeutic goals in high-risk surgical patients, Chest 94:1176-1186, 1988.

103. Burke KG, Larson E, Maciorowski L, and Adler DC: Evaluation of the sterility of thermodilution room-temperature injectate preparations, Crit Care Med 14:503-504, 1986.

104. Prologe JA: Pulse oximetry: technical aspects of machine design, Int Anesthesiol Clin 25:137-153, 1987.

105. Kelleher JF: Pulse oximetry, J Clin Monit 5:37-62, 1989.

106. Tremper KK and Barker SJ: Pulse oximetry, Anesthesiology 70:98-108, 1989.

107. Wukitsch MW, Petterson MT, Tobler DR, and Prologe JA: Pulse oximetry: analysis of theory, technology, and practice, J Clin Monit 4:290-301, 1988.

108. Barker SJ and Tremper KK: The effect of carbon monoxide inhalation on pulse oximeter signal detection, Anesthesiology 67:599-603, 1987.

109. Barker SJ, Tremper KK, and Hyatt J: Effects of methemoglobinemia on pulse oximetry and mixed venous oximetry, Anesthesiology 70:112-117, 1989.

110. Severinghaus JW, Naifeh KH, and Koh SO: Errors in 14 pulse oximeters during profound hypoxia, J Clin Monit 5:72-81, 1989.

111. Severinghaus JW and Spellman MJ Jr: Pulse oximeter failure thresholds in hypotension and ischemia, Anesthesiology 73:532-537, 1990.

112. Fairley HB: Changing perspectives in monitoring oxygenation, Anesthesiology 70:2-4, 1989.

113. Hensley FA Jr: Oxygen saturation during preinduction placement of monitoring catheters in the cardiac surgical patient, Anesthesiology 66:834-836, 1987.

114. Raemer DB, Warren DL, Morris R, et al: Hypoxemia during ambulatory gynecologic surgery as evaluated by the pulse oximeter, J Clin Monit 3:244-248, 1987.

115. Tyler IL, Tantisira B, Winter PM, and Motoyama EK: Continuous monitoring of arterial oxygen saturation with pulse oximetry during transfer to the recovery room, Anesth Analg 64:1108-1112, 1985.

116. Morris RW, Buschman A, Warren DL, et al: The prevalence of hypoxemia detected by pulse oximetry during recovery from anesthesia, J Clin Monit 4:16-20, 1988.

117. Whitcher C, Ream AK, Parsons D, et al: Anesthetic mishaps and the cost of monitoring: a proposed standard for monitoring equipment, J Clin Monit 4:5-15, 1988.

118. Caplan RA, Ward RJ, Posner K, and Cheney FW: Unexpected cardiac arrest during spinal anesthesia: a closed claims analysis of predisposing factors, Anesthesiology 68:5-11, 1988.

119. Brahams D: Anaesthesia and the law: monitoring, Anaesthesia 44:606-607, 1989.

120. Murphy KG, Secunda JA, and Rockoff MA: Severe burns from a pulse oximeter, Anesthesiology 73:350-352, 1990.

121. Sloan TB: Finger injury by an oxygen saturation monitor probe, Anesthesiology 68:936-938, 1988.

122. Kupeli IA and Satwicz PR: Mixed venous oximetry, Int Anesthesiol Clin 27:176-183, 1989.

123. Schweiss JF: Mixed venous hemoglobin saturation: theory and application, Int Anesthesiol Clin 25:113-136, 1987.

124. Karis JH and Lumb PD: Clinical evaluation of the Edwards Laboratories and Oximetrix mixed venous oxygen saturation catheters, J Cardiothorac Anesth 2:440-444, 1988.

125. Zierler KL: Theory of the use of arteriovenous concentration differences for measuring metabolism in steady and non-steady states, J Clin Invest 40:2111-2125, 1961.

126. Schlichtig R, Cowden WL, and Chaitman BR: Tolerance of unusually low mixed venous oxygen saturation: adaptions in the chronic low cardiac output syndrome, Am J Med 80:813-818, 1986.

127. Astiz ME, Rackow EC, Kaufman B, et al: Relationship of oxygen delivery and mixed venous oxygenation to lactic acidosis in patients with sepsis and acute myocardial infarction, Crit Care Med 16:655-658, 1988.

128. Magilligan DJ Jr, Teasdall R, Eisinminger R, and Peterson E: Mixed venous oxygen saturation as a predictor of cardiac output in the postoperative cardiac surgical patient. Ann Thorac Surg 44:260-262, 1987.

129. Norfleet EA and Watson CB: Continuous mixed venous oxygen saturation measurement: a significant advance in hemodynamic monitoring? J Clin Monit 1:245-258, 1985.

130. Larson LO and Kyff JV: The cost-effectiveness of Oximetrix pulmonary artery catheters in the postoperative care of coronary artery bypass graft patients, J Cardiothorac Anesth 3:257-259, 1989.

131. Jastremski MS, Chelluri L, Berney KM, and Bailly RT: Analysis of the effects of continuous on-line monitoring of mixed venous oxygen saturation on patient outcome and cost-effectiveness, Crit Care Med 17:148-153, 1989.

132. Ali HH and Savarese JJ: Monitoring of neuromuscular function, Anesthesiology 45:216-249, 1976.

133. Viby-Mogensen J: Clinical assessment of neuromuscular transmission, Br J Anaesth 54:209-223, 1982.

134. Beecher HK and Todd DP: A study of the deaths associated with anesthesia and surgery, Springfield, Ill, 1954, Charles C Thomas, publisher, p 66.

135. Waud BE and Waud DR: The relation between response to "train-of-four" stimulation and receptor occlusion during competitive neuromuscular block, Anesthesiology 37:413-416, 1972.

136. Bowman WC: Prejunctional and postjunctional cholinoreceptors at the neuromuscular junction, Anesth Analg 59:935-943, 1980.

137. Matteo RS, Spector S, and Horowitz PE: Relation of serum d-tubocurarine concentration to neuromuscular blockade in man, Anesthesiology 41:440-443, 1974.

138. Pavlin EG, Holle RH, and Schoene RB: Recovery of airway protection compared with ventilation in humans after paralysis with curare, Anesthesiology 70:381-385, 1989.

139. Paloheimo MPJ, Wilson RC, Edmonds HL Jr, et al: Comparison of neuromuscular blockade in upper facial and hypothenar muscles, J Clin Monit 4:256-260, 1988.

140. Christie TH and Churchill-Davidson HC: The St. Thomas's Hospital nerve stimulator in the diagnosis of prolonged apnoea, Lancet 1:775-778, 1958.

141. Dupuis JY, Martin R, Tessonnier JM, and Tetrault JP: Clinical assessment of the muscular response to tetanic nerve stimulation, Can J Anaesth 37:397-400, 1990.

142. Kopman AF: The dose-effect relationship of metocurine: the integrated electromyogram of the first dorsal interosseous muscle and the mechanomyogram of the adductor pollicis compared, Anesthesiology 68:604-607, 1988.

143. May O, Nielsen K, and Werner MU: The acceleration transducer: an assessment of its precision in comparison with a force displacement transducer, Acta Anaesthesiol Scand 32:239-243, 1988.

144. Thornberry EA and Mazumdar B: The effect of change of temperature on neuromuscular monitoring in the presence of atracurium blockade, Anaesthesia 43:447-449, 1988.

145. Miller RD: How should residual neuromuscular blockade be detected? Anesthesiology 70:379-380, 1989.

146. Brand JB, Cullen DJ, Wilson NE, and Ali HH: Spontaneous recovery from nondepolarizing neuromuscular blockade: correlation between clinical and evoked responses, Anesth Analg 56:55-58, 1977.

147. Engbaek J, Ostergaard D, Viby-Mogensen J, and Skovgaard LT: Clinical recovery and train-of-four ratio measured mechanically and electromyographically following atracurium, Anesthesiology 71:391-395, 1989.

148. Viby-Mogensen J, Jørgensen BC, and Ording H: Residual curarization in the recovery room, Anesthesiology 50:539-541, 1979.

149. Cohen MM, Duncan PG, and Tate RB: Does anesthesia contribute to operative mortality? JAMA 260:2859-2863, 1988.

150. Caplan RA, Posner KL, Ward RJ, and Cheney FW: Adverse respiratory events in anesthesia: a closed claims analysis, Anesthesiology 72:828-833, 1990.

151. Cooper JB, DeCesare R, and D'Ambra MN: An engineering critical incident: direct current burn from a neuromuscular stimulator, Anesthesiology 73:168-172, 1990.

152. Holdcroft A: Body temperature control in anaesthesia, surgery and intensive care, London, 1980, Bailliere Tindall, p 179.

153. Benzinger M: Tympanic thermometry in surgery and anesthesia, JAMA 209:1207-1211, 1969.

154. Benzinger TH: Clinical temperature: a new physiological basis, JAMA 209:1200-1206, 1969.

155. Cork RC, Vaughan RW, and Humphrey LS: Precision and accuracy of intraoperative temperature monitoring, Anesth Analg 62:211-214, 1983.

156. Wallace CT, Marks WE Jr, Adkins WY, and Mahaffey JE: Perforation of the tympanic membrane, a complication of tympanic thermometry during anesthesia, Anesthesiology 41:290-291, 1974.

157. Evans JM, Davies WL, and Wise CC: Lower oesophageal contractility: a new monitor of anaesthesia, Lancet 1:1151-1154, 1984.

158. Maccioli GA, Kuni DR, Silvay G, et al: Response of lower esophageal contractility to changing concentrations of halothane or isoflurane: a multicenter study, J Clin Monit 4:247-255, 1988.

159. Evans JM, Bithell JF, and Vlachonikolis IG: Relationship between lower oesophageal contractility, clinical signs and halothane concentration during general anaesthesia and surgery in man, Br J Anaesth 59:1346-1355, 1987.

160. Schwieger IM, Hug CC Jr, Hall RI, and Szlam F: Is lower esophageal contractility a reliable indicator of the adequacy of opioid anesthesia? J Clin Monit 5:164-169, 1989.

161. Watcha MF and White PF: Failure of lower esophageal contractility to predict patient movement in children anesthetized with halothane and nitrous oxide, Anesthesiology 71:664-668, 1989.

162. Pace NL: Evaluation of new medical devices, Anesthesiology 72:952, 1990.

163. Lubbers DW: Theory and development of transcutaneous oxygen pressure measurement, Int Anesthesiol Clin 25:31-65, 1987.

164. Tremper KK: Transcutaneous P_{O_2} measurement, Can Anaesth Soc J 31:664-677, 1984.

165. Severinghaus JS, Stafford M, and Bradley AF: tcP_{CO_2} electrode design calibration and temperature gradient problems, Acta Anaesthesiol Scand 68:118-122, 1978.

166. Severinghaus JW: A combined transcutaneous P_{O_2}-P_{CO_2} electrode with electrochemical HCO_3 stabilization, J Appl Physiol 51:1027-1032, 1981.

167. Tremper KK and Barker SJ: Transcutaneous oxygen measurement: experimental studies and adult applications, Int Anesthesiol Clin 25:67-96, 1987.

168. Tremper KK and Shoemaker WC: Transcutaneous oxygen monitoring of critically ill adults, with and without low flow shock, Crit Care Med 9:706-709, 1981.

169. Phan CQ, Tremper KK, Lee SE, and Barker SJ: Noninvasive monitoring of carbon dioxide: a comparison of transcutaneous and end-tidal carbon dioxide with the partial pressure of arterial carbon dioxide, J Clin Monit 3:149-154, 1987.

170. Palmisano BW and Severinghaus JW: Transcutaneous P_{CO_2} and P_{O_2}: a multicenter study of accuracy, J Clin Monit 6:189-195, 1990.

171. Moller AR: Evoked potentials in intraoperative monitoring, Baltimore, 1988, Williams & Wilkins, p 224.

172. Muzzi D and Cucchiara RF: Brain monitoring with the electroencephalogram, Semin Anesth 8:93-101, 1989.

173. Mori K: The EEG and awareness during anaesthesia, Anaesthesia 42:1153-1155, 1987.

174. Michenfelder JD: A valid demonstration of barbiturate-induced brain protection in man—at last, Anesthesiology 64:140-142, 1986 [editorial].

175. Abramson NS: Randomized clinical study of thiopental loading in comatose survivors of cardiac arrest, N Engl J Med 314:397-403, 1986.

176. Nussmeier NA, Arlund C, and Slogoff S: Neuropsychiatric complications after cardiopulmonary bypass: cerebral protection by a barbiturate, Anesthesiology 64:165-170, 1986.

177. Lin C-Y: Con: the EEG should not be monitored during cardiopulmonary bypass, J Cardiothorac Anesth 3:124-126, 1989.

178. Zablocki AD and Albin MS: Pro: the EEG should be monitored during cardiopulmonary bypass, J Cardiothorac Anesth 3:119-123, 1989.

179. Chemtob GA and Kearse LA Jr: The use of electroencephalography in carotid endarterectomy, Int Anesthesiol Clin 28:143-146, 1990.

180. Gugino V and Chabot RJ: Somatosensory evoked potentials, Int Anesthesiol Clin 28:154-164, 1990.

181. Seward JB, Khandheria BK, Oh JK, et al: Transesophageal echocardiography: technique, anatomic correlations, implementation, and clinical applications, Mayo Clin Proc 63:649-680, 1988.

182. Nishimura RA, Miller FA Jr, Callahan MJ, et al: Doppler echocardiography: theory, instrumentation, technique, and application, Mayo Clin Proc 60:321-343, 1985.

183. Mitchell MM, Sutherland GR, Gussenhoven EJ, et al: Transesophageal echocardiography, J Am Soc Echocardiography 1:362-377, 1988.

184. Cahalan MK, Litt L, Botvinick EH, and Schiller NB: Advances in noninvasive cardiovascular imaging: implications for the anesthesiologist, Anesthesiology 66:356-372, 1987.

185. Clements FM and de Bruijn NP: Perioperative evaluation of regional wall motion by transesophageal two-dimensional echocardiography, Anesth Analg 66:249-261, 1987.

186. Smith JS, Cahalan MK, Benefiel DJ, et al: Intraoperative detection of myocardial ischemia in high-risk patients: electrocardiography versus two-dimensional transesophageal echocardiography, Circulation 72:1015-1021, 1985.

187. Leung JM, O'Kelly B, Browner WS, et al: Prognostic importance of postbypass regional wall-motion abnormalities in patients undergoing coronary artery bypass graft surgery, Anesthesiology 71:16-25, 1989.

188. Cahalan MK: Pro: transesophageal echocardiography is the "gold standard" for detection of myocardial ischemia, J Cardiothorac Anesth 3:369-371, 1989.

189. McCloskey G: Con: transesophageal echocardiography is not the "gold standard" for detection of myocardial ischemia, J Cardiothorac Anesth 3:372-374, 1989.

190. Vandenberg BF and Kerber RE: Transesophageal

echocardiography and intraoperative monitoring of left ventricular function, Anesthesiology 73:799-801, 1990.

191. Popp RL and Winters WL Jr: Clinical competence in adult echocardiography: a statement for physicians from the ACP/ACC/AHA task force on clinical privileges in cardiology, Circulation 81:2032-2035, 1990.

192. Dewhirst WE, Stragand JJ, and Fleming BM: Mallory-Weiss tear complicating intraoperative transesophageal echocardiography in a patient undergoing aortic valve replacement, Anesthesiology 73:777-778, 1990.

193. Cucchiara RF, Nugent M, Seward JB, and Messick JM: Air embolism in upright neurosurgical patients: detection and localization by two dimensional transesophageal echocardiography, Anesthesiology 60:353-355, 1984.

194. Einstein A: The fundamentals of theoretical physics, Science 91:487-492, 1940.

PART TWO

The Causes of Systemic Complications

Chapter 9

Causes and Consequences of Impaired Gas Exchange

Thomas J. Gal

Abnormalities of gas exchange are reflected by the gas composition of the arterial blood. Such a composition represents a weighted average of all the gas-exchanging units in the lungs. In the blood leaving each alveolus, the O_2 and CO_2 tensions depend on the composition of the alveolar gas and the efficiency with which the incoming pulmonary blood flow is able to equilibrate. Anesthetic drugs and techniques appear to significantly alter this process, and the effects are often further compounded by preexisting disease and other acute events. The purpose of this discussion is to provide some insight into the nature and mechanism of anesthesia-induced alterations in normal gas exchange and to examine the important physiologic consequences.

I. OVERALL GAS EXCHANGE
A. Carbon dioxide elimination

1. Fundamental determinants of CO_2 tensions. The carbon dioxide that is removed by alveolar ventilation is constantly added to the alveolar gas from the pulmonary circulation. The CO_2 tension in the arterial blood (Pa_{CO_2}) is the net result of the balance between the metabolic rate of CO_2 production by body tissues ($\dot{V}_{CO_2}$) and the rate at which the lungs excrete CO_2 by alveolar ventilation $\dot{V}_A$. The Pa_{CO_2} is directly proportional to $\dot{V}_{CO_2}$ and inversely

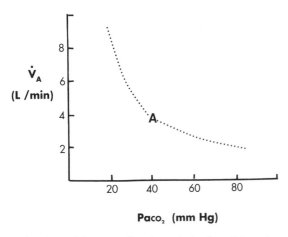

Fig. 9-1. CO_2 excretion hyperbola describing the reciprocal relationship between alveolar ventilation ($\dot{V}_A$) and arterial CO_2 tension ($Paco_2$). The curve assumes a constant CO_2 production. Under normal resting conditions the relationship lies at point *A*. (From Gal TJ: Respiratory physiology during anesthesia. In Kaplan JA, editor: Thoracic anesthesia, ed 2, New York, 1990, Churchill Livingstone.)

proportional to $\dot{V}_A$. This relationship can be expressed as:

$$Paco_2 = K \times \frac{\dot{V}_{CO_2}}{\dot{V}_A}$$

The proportionally constant (K) is equal to 0.863 when $\dot{V}_{CO_2}$ is expressed in milliliters per minute as a dry gas at standard temperature and pressure (STPD) and $\dot{V}_A$ is expressed in liters per minute as a saturated gas at body temperature and pressure (BTPS). The K value allows simultaneous conversion of concentration to partial pressure and corrects for units that conventionally express the gas volumes.

This equation simply states that under the ideal conditions of a steady state, the CO_2 output is matched by the alveolar ventilation. If $\dot{V}_A$ is depressed for some reason, $Paco_2$ must rise in proportion to this decrease in V_A and $Paco_2$ as is described by a rectangular hyperbola (Fig. 9-1), but in many clinical settings this simple relationship is modified by other factors that result in hypercapnia ($Paco_2$ >46 mm Hg).

2. Causes of hypercapnia

a. Normal lung function. Endogenous CO_2 production may increase with such conditions as fever, sepsis, seizures, hyperthyroidism, and total parenteral nutrition with a very high glucose intake.[1] Unless ventilation is increased accordingly, CO_2 elevations may occur in such patients.

Occasionally nonmetabolic sources for CO_2 may be present. For example, an increase in $Paco_2$ may be observed after CO_2 installation for laparoscopy. Similarly, transient elevations in $Paco_2$ occur after administration of sodium bicarbonate if the ventilation is not allowed to increase.[2] More common and perhaps more dangerous is an increased CO_2 in the inspired gas. Whether this results from anesthetic mishaps such as failure of soda lime absorber, incompetent values in the circle system, or merely breathing in confined spaces, a new steady state will be achieved. This new level of $Paco_2$ will be defined by the quantity of CO_2 in the inspired air, the CO_2 generated by metabolism, and the relative changes in alveolar ventilation.

How the system responds to an increase in alveolar ventilation is a crucial determinant of how adequately CO_2 is eliminated. Alveolar hypoventilation may result in hypercapnia whether respiratory system disease is present. The responsiveness of the respiratory control system to CO_2 is an important determinant of $Paco_2$. This respiratory controller is affected by a wide variety of disease states and drugs. These are discussed in more detail later in the chapter. Signals arising in the respiratory controller must produce a response in the respiratory system bellows. If the respiratory muscles are weak or easily fatigued, the respiratory drive will not be translated into adequate levels of ventilation. Similarly, if the muscles must overcome an increased mechanical work load because of decreased compliance or increased resistance of the respiratory system, CO_2 retention may occur also.

b. Impaired lung function. Retention of carbon dioxide occurs more commonly when there is disturbance of the gas exchange function of the lung. In abnormal lungs, net effective alveolar ventilation can be decreased even if total ventilation is increased. This situation results either because significant portions of the lung are not perfused and function as a dead space or disease is severe enough to significantly affect the matching of ventilation and perfusion.

The alveolar ventilation, which influences the level of $Paco_2$, cannot be measured directly but must be derived from another volume, the minute volume ($\dot{V}_E$). The alveolar ventilation differs from this volume of air, which moves in and out of the lungs each minute by an amount of gas that does not participate in the exchange of CO_2 with the blood. This volume of gas is usually referred to as the "physiologic dead space." However, some have preferred to term this "wasted ventilation," since this portion of each breath is literally wasted with respect to its contribution to gas exchange.

A portion of this dead space gas is contained within the conducting airways from the mouth and nose down to the terminal bronchioles and is termed the "anatomic dead space." In a normal adult, this consists of about one third the volume of each breath. The anatomic dead space (V_D) is larger in males than in females presumably because of body size and lung volume. The anatomic V_D is larger in older men than in younger men because of the increase in end-expiratory lung volume (FRC, functional residual capacity) seen with advancing age. In general, the anatomic V_D is affected by changes in airway caliber and is increased with increasing lung volume. The average increase appears to be 2 to 3 ml per 100 ml lung volume increase.[3] Other factors that influence the size of the upper airway affect V_D. These include positioning of neck and jaw and the presence of artificial oral airways. Finally tracheal intubation, which decreases the volume of the upper airway, and tracheostomy, which bypasses the upper airway, also serve to decrease anatomic V_D.

The other portion of the physiologic dead space, the alveolar dead space, may be defined as the part of the inspired gas that passes through the conducting airways to mix with gas at the alveolar level but does not actively participate in gas exchange. The alveolar dead space results from a lack of effective perfusion of the air spaces to which inspired gas is distributed. Factors such as reduced cardiac output, hypovolemia, hypotension, and pulmonary embolism reduce pulmonary blood flow. Thus they increase the alveolar dead-space fraction and impair CO_2 excretion.

The sum of the combined anatomic and alveolar components, the physiologic dead space, cannot be measured directly but can be calculated from CO_2 tensions in simultaneously collected samples of mixed expired air (P_ECO_2) and arterial blood ($PaCO_2$). The formula utilized to calculate the fraction of wasted ventilation per breath, or more specifically, the ratio of physiologic dead space (V_D) to tidal volume (V_T) is a modification of the classic Bohr equation proposed by Enghoff. In this equation, alveolar CO_2 tension (P_ACO_2) is replaced by $PaCO_2$. The expired gas is a mixture of dead-space gas and that from the gas-exchanging compartment. Since dead-space gas contains essentially no CO_2, the quantity of CO_2 expired should come entirely from the gas-exchanging compartment.

$$V_T \times P_ECO_2 = (V_T - V_D) \times PaCO_2$$

Amount of	**Amount expired**
CO_2 expired	**from gas-**
	exchanging
	compartment

By solving for V_D/V_T one can express it as:

$$\frac{V_D}{V_T} = \frac{PaCO_2 - P_ECO_2}{PaCO_2}$$

Typical values for V_D/V_T in healthy subjects are about 0.30 such that nearly one-third of the inspired V_T does not participate in gas exchange. In diseased lungs, V_D/V_T increases and values greater than 0.75 may be observed.

The concept of dead space (V_D) and ventilation perfusion ($\dot{V}_A/\dot{Q}$) mismatch involve a continuum in which V_D implies the most extreme mismatch in which the $\dot{V}_A/\dot{Q}$ ratio reaches infinity. If such a large increase in $\dot{V}_A/\dot{Q}$ mismatch cannot be compensated for by increasing ventilation, $PaCO_2$ will of necessity rise. A less common malfunction of CO_2 excretion results when large areas of right-to-left shunt areas or low $\dot{V}_A/\dot{Q}$ areas are present. Here the CO_2 in mixed venous blood enters the arterial system without the opportunity for excretion via a ventilated alveolus. Again, ventilation must increase to compensate for this inefficiency in CO_2 excretion.

In patients with chronic obstructive pulmonary disease, hypercapnia appears to be more the result of this $\dot{V}_A/\dot{Q}$ mismatch than the result of actual decreases in total ventilation.[4] Such patients who remain normocapnic must compensate for this mismatch by increasing total minute ventilation to very high levels. Such increased levels of ventilation may achieve normocapnia but invariably do so at the expense of an excessively increased work of breathing in the presence of airflow obstruction.

3. Physiologic consequences of abnormal CO_2 levels

a. Hypercapnia. There are no specific clinical diagnostic signs of hypercapnia. The varied signs and symptoms include headache, nausea, sweating, flushing, restlessness, tachypnea, and with pronounced hypercapnia (greater than 90 mm Hg) unconsciousness. These reflect the actions of CO_2 on the respiratory, cardiovascular, and central nervous system functions.

(1) RESPIRATORY EFFECTS. As $PaCO_2$ rises to produce hypercapnia, CO_2 excretion is less than its production. As a steady state arises, excretion must equal production. Thus the ventilatory response to CO_2 (increased $\dot{V}_E$) must take place or $PaCO_2$ will continue to rise further until severe hypercapnia ($PaCO_2 > 90$ mm Hg) ensues and depresses respiration. The ventilatory response to CO_2, so characteristic in the awake patient, is blunted though not completely eliminated during general anesthesia.

Hypercapnia may affect respiratory gas exchange by its mild effect on pulmonary vasoconstriction,[5] or by depression of diaphragmatic function.[6] In addition, the reduced alveolar ventilation associated with increased Pa_{CO_2} may also be inadequate to deliver oxygen to the alveoli to replace that taken up by the pulmonary blood flow. Thus the oxygen tension in the alveoli ($P_{A_{O_2}}$) decreases and in turn produces a reduction in Pa_{O_2}. This secondary effect of hypercapnia is also associated with a shift of the oxyhemoglobin dissociation curve to the right. The rightward shift further decreases oxygen saturation at any given level of Pa_{O_2}. However, this decreased affinity of hemoglobin for oxygen does facilitate unloading of oxygen from blood to tissues at a higher Pa_{O_2}.

(2) CARDIOVASCULAR EFFECTS. Many of the circulatory effects of hypercapnia appear to enhance oxygen delivery and CO_2 removal at the tissue level. The direct effect of CO_2 and the accompanying acidosis on the heart and blood vessels is to depress function of smooth and cardiac muscle. The result is decreased cardiac contractility and in most vascular beds, vasodilatation. The one exception of course is the pulmonary circulation, which tends to constrict.

In healthy persons the direct effects of CO_2 are modified by those of central sympathetic stimulation, which result in tachycardia, mild hypertension, and increased myocardial contractility. With disease states that depress autonomic responsiveness and with most anesthetics, most of this sympathetic stimulation is obtunded and the direct depressant effects of acidosis on the tissues are manifest.

(3) CENTRAL NERVOUS SYSTEM EFFECTS. Hypercapnia affects central nervous system function by its stimulating effect on breathing. The excess CO_2 also acts on the cerebral vascular bed to produce vasodilatation. In the presence of a cerebral disorder, the vasodilatation within the closed cranial space may produce dangerous increases in intracranial pressure. Higher CO_2 tensions depress general neuronal activity and produce a state of unconsciousness not unlike that of general anesthesia.

b. Hypocapnia. Alveolar hyperventilation from any cause will result in decreased CO_2 tension (hypocapnia). This hypocapnia may decrease cardiac output by decreasing sympathetic activity, ionized calcium, or coronary blood flow. At the same time a leftward shift of the oxyhemoglobin dissociation curve (increased affinity for O_2) will result in reduced ability to give up O_2 at the tissue level. This necessitates an increased cardiac output to maintain the same rate of O_2 delivery. Vasoconstriction of cerebral and spinal cord vessels may also have undesirable effects. To add to this, hypocapnia may further increase oxygen consumption in the face of a decreased tissue oxygen supply.

Hypocapnia also decreases ionized calcium and serum potassium concentrations. The latter, for example, changes about 1.5 mEq/L with each 10 mm Hg change in Pa_{CO_2}[7] as a result of altered potassium distribution between intracellular and extracellular spaces.

Further abnormalities in gas exchange may occur in response to reductions in CO_2 tension. Disturbances in $\dot{V}/\dot{Q}$ matching may develop if hypocapnia inhibits hypoxic pulmonary vasoconstriction. Local increases in airway resistance may also occur in normal patients and those with lung disease.[8] This bronchoconstriction appears to be a response to the reduction in alveolar CO_2 tension, which in a sense is analogous to the vascular response to reduced alveolar O_2 tension.

Some of the physiologic impact of hypocapnia relates to the difference in time for CO_2 levels associated with acute hyperventilation to change as opposed to those of hypoventilation. The Pa_{CO_2} tends to decrease far more rapidly during hyperventilation than it increases during hypoventilation. After hyperventilation 50% of the decrease in Pa_{CO_2} occurs in 3 minutes, whereas 50% increase in Pa_{CO_2} takes nearly 20 minutes to occur after a decrease in ventilation.[9] During complete apnea, Pa_{CO_2} rises 8 to 15 mm Hg in the first minute or so and exhibits a subsequent linear increase of about 3 mm Hg/min.[10]

B. Oxygenation

Whenever the supply of oxygen to the tissues is unable to meet metabolic demands, hypoxia results. Hypoxia has been variously subdivided into (1) hypoxic, (2) stagnant, (3) anemic, and (4) histotoxic types. Stagnant hypoxia is produced when blood flow to the tissues is reduced, whereas anemic hypoxia results from a decreased oxygen-carrying capacity because of low hemoglobin or binding of hemoglobin with other substances (such as carbon monox-

Table 9-1. Typical partial pressures (mm Hg) for respiratory gases during normal air breathing ($F_{I_{O_2}} = 0.2$)

Gas*	Atmosphere	Trachea	Alveoli
O_2	150	150	100
CO_2	0	0	40
H_2O	20	47	47
N_2	590	563	573
TOTAL	760	760	760

*Water vapor pressure varies with relative humidity and ambient temperature. Partial pressures of oxygen (P_{O_2}) and nitrogen (P_{N_2}) change accordingly.

ide). If the cell is unable to utilize oxygen to produce energy, the term "histotoxic hypoxia" is applied. Such hypoxia can result from cyanide toxicity and, unlike the other forms of hypoxia, is characterized by an increase in mixed venous oxygen tension, since tissues cannot utilize the oxygen presented to them.

By far, the most common variant of hypoxia encountered clinically is hypoxic hypoxia. This is associated with an abnormally low arterial oxygen tension (Pa_{O_2}), which is referred to as "hypoxemia." The causes of hypoxemia are many and varied and must take into account factors such as inspired O_2 concentration, alveolar CO_2 tension, barometric pressure, patient age, and the presence of lung disease.

1. Alveolar gas composition. The alveolar gas content is influenced by the matching of ventilation and blood flow and by the composition of the mixed venous blood. First and foremost, however, the composition of gas in the alveoli depends on the content of the gas that is inspired. The partial pressure of each gas in this inspired mixture is proportional to the fractional concentration of the gas. As gases enter the respiratory tract, they are warmed to body temperature and humidified. Thus it is necessary to take into account the partial pressure exerted by water vapor (PH_2O) at body temperature, which is usually 47 mm Hg. Thus, the fractional concentration of oxygen in the inspired air ($F_{I}O_2$), which is expressed as a dry gas, can be used to calculate the inspired oxygen tension ($P_{I}O_2$) within the trachea:

$$P_{I}O_2 = F_{I}O_2 (P_B - 47) \text{ mm Hg}$$

For clinical purposes, it is sufficient to use the standard barometric pressure (P_B) at sea level, 760 mm Hg, to calculate. Thus in a subject breathing room air:

$$P_{I}O_2 = 0.21 (760 - 47) = 150 \text{ mm Hg}$$

The differences in gas composition between ambient air and that in the trachea are listed in Table 9-1. The total pressure of gas in the trachea and alveoli is equal to the atmospheric pressure (Table 9-1). Since there is no exchange of nitrogen within the respiratory tract, the partial pressure of nitrogen is the same in the alveoli as it is in the trachea. The oxygen tension in the alveoli ($P_{A}O_2$), however, will be less than the $P_{I}O_2$ in the trachea because CO_2 is added to the alveoli from mixed venous blood. The $P_{A}O_2$ therefore will differ from the $P_{I}O_2$ by an amount directly related to the quantity of CO_2 added. If the CO_2 volume added by the blood equals the oxygen taken up by the blood, $P_{A}O_2$ may be calculated simply as:

$$P_{A}O_2 = P_{I}O_2 - P_{A}CO_2$$

Usually the ratio of CO_2 produced to the O_2 consumed, the respiratory exchange ratio (R), is less than 1.0. If one assumes that R approximates 0.8 and also assumes that ideal $P_{A}CO_2$ can be estimated by arterial CO_2 tension (Pa_{CO_2}), the alveolar gas equation can be simplified for clinical uses as:

$$P_{A}O_2 = P_{I}O_2 - Pa_{CO_2}/0.8$$

2. Causes of hypoxemia
a. Normal lung function. When there is no impairment of lung function, hypoxemia may result from a variety of factors, which include low fractional inspired O_2 concentration ($F_{I}O_2$), hypoventilation, decreased cardiac output, increased oxygen consumption, a shift in the O_2 hemoglobin dissociation curve, and decreased hemoglobin concentration. By far, the most dangerous but easily correctable causes of hypoxemia is a low $F_{I}O_2$. Any decreases in inspired O_2 concentration below that of normal ambient air will result in a decreased alveolar oxygen tension and hypoxemia. The alveolar to arterial O_2 difference ($A-aD_{O_2}$) however, will not be increased.

The $P_{A}O_2$ can also be decreased by a diminished alveolar ventilation whether because of airway obstruction or drug-induced depression of breathing. The simplified alveolar air equation indicates that as CO_2 tension increases $P_{A}O_2$ will decrease by a similar amount. Thus, unless $F_{I}O_2$ is increased above 0.21 hypoxemia can result from hypoventilation. Again, as in the case of decreased $F_{I}O_2$, the $A-aD_{O_2}$ will not be increased.

The effect of increasing $F_{I}O_2$ from 0.21 to 0.30 is shown in Fig. 9-2. The improvement in $P_{A}O_2$ at any level of ventilation or $P_{A}CO_2$ is about 64 mm Hg. Thus at the high levels of $P_{A}CO_2$ associated with pronounced hypoventilation, an $F_{I}O_2$ of 0.30 appears to be the maximum O_2 concentration required to correct the hypoxemia present with the ambient air.

The $P_{A}O_2$ can be influenced by a decrease in cardiac output, which, in the absence of other changes, may temporarily increase $P_{A}O_2$ because less blood flows through the lungs to remove O_2 from the alveolar gas. More important, the reduced cardiac output is associated with increased tissue O_2 extraction, which results in a reduced O_2 content in the mixed venous blood. As the blood passes through whatever shunt pathways exist in the lungs with its reduced O_2 content, the resultant Pa_{O_2} is decreased compared to that with a normal cardiac output. Abnormal O_2 transport because of decreased hemoglobin concentration or rightward shifts of the oxyhemoglobin dissociation curve

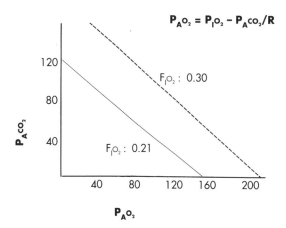

$$P_{A_{O_2}} = P_{I_{O_2}} - P_{A_{CO_2}}/R$$

Fig. 9-2. O_2-CO_2 diagram based on the simplified alveolar air equation for ambient air ($F_{I}O_2 = 0.21$) at sea level (atmospheric pressure = 760 mm) is indicated by the *solid line*, whereas that for an enriched O_2 mixture ($F_{I}O_2 = 0.30$) is indicated by the *dotted line*. An R value of 0.8 was used to calculate both lines. (From Gal TJ: Respiratory physiology in anesthetic practice, Baltimore, 1991, Williams & Wilkins.)

of increased oxygen consumption also can lead to increased O_2 extraction by tissues and a similar reduction in mixed venous and arterial oxygen tensions.

b. Abnormal lung function. When hypoxemia occurs in the presence of a normal or increased $P_{A}O_2$, it can result only from disturbances in the normal gas exchange function of the lung. This interference with the lung's ability to oxygenate blood consists in three basic abnormalities:

1. *Diffusion*—an impaired movement of gas (O_2) from alveolus to capillary.
2. *Shunt*—the presence of channels (extrapulmonary and pulmonary) that allow venous blood to bypass the normal gas exchange units in the lung.
3. *Ventilation-perfusion mismatch*—poor matching of blood and gas at the alveolar level.

(1) DIFFUSION ABNORMALITY. Normally O_2 and CO_2 equilibrate between blood and gas phases in far less time than it takes the red blood cell to traverse the pulmonary capillary network. Thus diffusion limitation plays very little role in normal gas exchange at rest unless the $F_{I}O_2$ is reduced, as at high altitude. During vigorous exercise, however, some patients can develop a decreased PaO_2 because the increased velocity of blood flow through the pulmonary capillaries shortens the time available for diffusion equilibrium. Although this abnormal diffusion can be caused by thickening of the air-blood interface (alveolar-capillary block), it

more commonly results from a reduction in pulmonary capillary blood volume. The latter state differs from the thickened membrane in that, as capillaries are destroyed or obstructed, others are recruited, and the flow velocity through these remaining vessels increases. Thus with severe disease such as emphysema the time available for gas exchange at rest may be as short as with exercise and equilibration of gas fails to occur adequately. Of course, one can offset this easily by increasing the driving pressure for O_2 (that is, the $P_{A}O_2$) by oxygen-enriched mixtures.

(2) SHUNTS. Another interference with ideal gas exchange occurs in the form of right-to-left shunts. Normally, a small amount of venous blood bypasses the right ventricle and empties directly into the left atrium. The "anatomic shunt" represents venous return from pleural, bronchial, and thebesian veins, which comprises as much as 5% of total cardiac output. Right-to-left shunts of greater magnitude occur with cyanotic congenital heart disease.

In addition to these discrete anatomic pathways, a shunt effect may be produced by normal vessels that perfuse areas of lung that are not ventilated because the airways are closed or the conducting airways are obstructed. The term "shunt effect," or "venous admixture," is generally applied to these lung units whose ventilation is maximally decreased compared to the amount of perfusion. The venous admixture is manifest clinically by hypoxemia, which is responsive to increased inspired O_2 concentrations. In diseases associated with major areas of lung without ventilation (absolute shunt) or in the case of the anatomic shunts, the hypoxemia is refractory to O_2 administration.

(3) VENTILATION-PERFUSION ($\dot{V}/\dot{Q}$) IMBALANCE. The distribution of ventilation and pulmonary blood flow is neither uniform nor proportionate even in normal lungs. This nonuniform distribution or $\dot{V}_A/\dot{Q}$ results in impaired gas exchange. The primary effect of $\dot{V}_A/\dot{Q}$ mismatch is an impairment of oxygenation. The high PaO_2 of lung regions with high $\dot{V}_A/\dot{Q}$ ratios are able to produce only a minimal increase in the O_2 content of the blood because of the relatively flat oxyhemoglobin dissociation curve in that range of partial pressures. Hence these areas are unable to compensate for regions with low $\dot{V}_A/\dot{Q}$ values. CO_2 elimination is also impaired by $\dot{V}_A/\dot{Q}$ mismatching, but the elevated CO_2 stimulates ventilation. Because the CO_2 dissociation curve is nearly linear in the physiologic range, this increased ventilation is able to compensate for low $\dot{V}_A/\dot{Q}$ areas and maintain CO_2 near normal. With severe $\dot{V}_A/\dot{Q}$ mismatch

or impaired ability to increase ventilation, this compensation is inadequate to avoid an increase in CO_2.

3. Physiologic consequences of hypoxemia. Foremost among the clinical manifestations of hypoxemia is cyanosis, which marks the presence of a significant amount of desaturated hemoglobin (usually greater than 5 g/dl). Although rather subjective, cyanosis usually is observed with hemoglobin saturations less than 85%. This is usually associated with a PaO_2 of 45 to 50 mm Hg in the adult, whereas, in the infant, because of the leftward shift of the oxyhemoglobin dissociation curve, it may correspond to a PaO_2 of 35 to 40. Cyanosis may be apparent without actual hypoxemia as in methemoglobinemia and sulbhemoglobinemia and, on the other hand, may not be apparent in the presence of anemia or intense peripheral vasoconstriction. Thus the diagnosis of hypoxemia is established only with certainty when O_2 saturation or PaO_2 are measured.

Hypoxemia is associated with an increased minute ventilation largely through an increased respiratory rate. This brisk response to low PaO_2 resides in the carotid bodies and is very sensitive to the depressive effects of the volatile anesthetics. These anesthetics exert a similar blunting effect on the circulatory responses to hypoxia. The latter responses also appear to be mediated through the carotid bodies. The circulatory compensation to hypoxia acts to redistribute blood flow and maintain arterial pressure. The aim is to increase the quantity of O_2 carried to important tissues and consists largely in an increased heart rate and cardiac output with vasodilatation in brain and heart while the muscle beds and splanchnic circulation undergo constriction.

Ultimately the consequences of hypoxia manifest themselves by a disruption of the function of all major organ systems. The cerebral cortex, which begins to cease function after about 30 seconds of hypoxia, may suffer irreversible damage after 5 minutes. Cardiac function takes about 5 minutes to cease functioning and experiences tissue death after about 10 minutes.

II. IMPAIRED GAS EXCHANGE ASSOCIATED WITH ANESTHESIA

The abnormal pulmonary gas exchange associated with general anesthesia is manifested by an increased alveolar-arterial O_2 tension difference and an increase in arterial end-tidal CO_2 tension gradient. The impaired oxygenation and to some extent the CO_2 elimination appear to be a reflection of an increased $\dot{V}_A/\dot{Q}$ mismatch, right-to-left intrapulmonary shunting, and an in-

increase in alveolar dead space. All these changes tend to be increased substantially in the presence of preexisting lung disease. Some theories have been proposed to account for these changes, many based on the changes in respiratory mechanics associated with general anesthesia. Foremost among these are the reduction in functional residual capacity and alterations in the distribution of ventilation.

A. Alterations in respiratory mechanics

1. Decrease in functional residual capacity (FRC). General anesthesia affects the static (pressure-volume) and the dynamic (pressure-flow) behavior of the respiratory system. These mechanical effects have interested clinicians and investigators because of their potential contribution to the impaired gas exchange so characteristic in anesthetized patients. Perhaps no facet of respiratory system behavior has received as much attention as the change in the functional residual capacity (FRC). A decrease in FRC with induction of general anesthesia was first noted by Bergman.[11] Subsequent observations in supine anesthetized humans indicate that the FRC is reduced an average of about 500 ml or 15% to 20/% of the awake value.[12] The decreased volume is similar in magnitude to that observed when subjects go from erect to recumbent position as noted earlier. The magnitude of FRC reduction appears to be related to age and body habitus (that is, the weight-to-height ratio). In fact, morbidly obese patients demonstrate a much larger decrease in the FRC to about 50% of their preanesthetic values.[13]

The changes in FRC occur within a minute after induction of anesthesia,[14] do not appear to progress with time,[15] and are not further affected by addition of muscle paralysis.[16] Several factors may contribute to the FRC reduction, but the underlying mechanisms are complex and as yet not totally clear. Some of these possibilities include atelectasis, increased expiratory muscle activity, trapping of gas in distal airways, cephalad displacement of the diaphragm, decreased outward chest wall recoil, increased lung recoil, and increases in thoracic blood volume. These are discussed in detail elsewhere.[12]

In supine subjects the induction of general anesthesia reduces FRC such that end-expiratory volume decreases close to residual volume. This FRC may lie below the closing capacity, that is, the volume associated with dependent airway closure or, more precisely, dynamic flow limitation.[17] Early observations with halothane anesthesia indicated a possible correlation between the degree of impaired oxygenation and the reduction in FRC[18] and led to the hypothesis that airway closure and atelectasis were the consequences of a reduced FRC.

One important aspect of the theory of airway closure lies in the assumption that the closing capacity (CC) remains the same in both anesthetized and awake states. The decrease in lung compliance in the anesthetized state reflects an increased elastic recoil. Airway closure to a great extent is attributable to an increase in lung elastic recoil. As a result one might expect a decrease in closing capacity (that is, an increase in airway closure) with general anesthesia. Initial reports suggested no difference in closing capacity between awake and anesthetized states.[19,20] Subsequent work, however, provided evidence that both FRC and CC are proportionately reduced with anesthesia.[21] These authors utilized the foreign gas bolus technique as opposed to the resident gas (N_2) technique utilized in the previous study and suggested that the latter might not adequately measure CC when lung volumes are restricted. However, an additional study found no difference when the two techniques were compared.[22] Therefore the issue of whether awake control CC values are the same as those in anesthetized subjects is not resolved.

The degree of intrapulmonary shunting does appear to correlate with the reduction in FRC[23] and with the degree of atelectasis that develops in dependent lung regions.[24] It is thus tempting to attribute such atelectasis simply to the reduced FRC. However, a study in awake supine subjects with thoracoabdominal restriction argues against this simple mechanism.[25] The restriction in these subjects reduced lung volume and altered pulmonary mechanics in a fashion similar to that seen with general anesthesia. The FRC decreased by more than 20% and was matched by a reduction of CC as measured by the resident gas (N_2) technique. No atelectasis was observed with computerized tomographic scanning and $\dot{V}_A/\dot{Q}$ distribution, and arterial blood gases were unchanged from the control state. Thus gas exchange in these awake subjects with chest restriction differed from anesthetized subjects though they both had some relative decrement in FRC. The authors concluded that the development of compression atelectasis in the anesthetized patients cannot be ascribed solely to a decrease in FRC, nor can the changes in pulmonary mechanics with restriction be attributed solely to the development of atelectasis.

2. Alternated intrapulmonary gas distribution. Ventilation is not normally uniform throughout the lung. The effects of gravity on

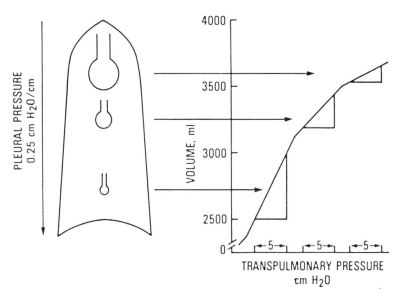

Fig. 9-3. Pleural pressure gradient increases down the lung such that the dependent alveoli are small and nondependent ones are relatively large. A change in transpulmonary pressure of 5 cm H_2O produces a greater change in volume (or ventilation) of the small dependent air spaces because they lie on a steeper portion of the compliance or pressure-volume curve. The large nondependent alveoli lie on a flatter portion of the curve and thus undergo less volume change. (From Benumof JL: Respiration physiology and respiratory function during anesthesia. In Miller RD, editor: Anesthesia, ed 3, New York, 1990, Churchill Livingstone.)

the lung and the forces necessary to allow it to conform to the shape of the thorax result in a vertical gradient of pleural pressure.[26] The pleural pressure acting on the upper (nondependent) areas of the lung is more subatmospheric (negative) than that acting on the lower (dependent) portions. As a result, the nondependent areas are more inflated than the dependent ones (Fig. 9-3). The gradient of pleural pressure up and down the lung changes about 0.25 cm H_2O per each centimeter of lung height. Thus, in a lung 30 cm high, a 7.5 cm H_2O pressure difference exists from apex to base. In the supine position, the dorsal areas become dependent. The height of the lungs is reduced by nearly one third, and thus the gravitational effect is diminished somewhat.

Although the nondependent lung areas are more distended at FRC, a transpulmonary pressure of 5 cm generated during a normal breath produces a greater volume change or ventilation to the dependent areas (Fig. 9-3). This is because of the sigmoid shape of the pressure-volume curve. The larger nondependent areas have a lower regional compliance; that is, they lie on a less steep portion of the pressure-volume curve.

These regional differences in ventilation are important in matching ventilation to perfusion. The dependent or basal areas tend to be better perfused because of gravitational effects. Since the bases are also better ventilated, there is good matching of ventilation and perfusion (Fig. 9-4); that is, both higher ventilation and blood flow are delivered to the bases. In supine anesthetized paralyzed humans, the ventilation or distribution of inspired gas becomes more uniform from top to bottom lung areas (Fig. 9-4), largely because basal lung units undergo further reduction in size to a point that reduces their regional compliance. Anesthetics, meanwhile, produce a decrease in pulmonary artery pressure, which impedes perfusion of nondependent lung regions. Increased alveolar pressures with mechanical ventilation further interfere with perfusion of nondependent areas. Thus dependent lung areas are well perfused but rather poorly ventilated. In contrast, nondependent areas receive more ventilation but considerably less perfusion.

In addition to changes in static lung mechanics, the overall $\dot{V}_A/\dot{Q}$ inhomogeneity may also be increased during anesthesia because of changes in dynamics, that is, the pressure-flow relationships in the airways. The smooth-muscle relaxation associated with anesthetics may be useful in preventing the increased bronchial tone associated with bronchospasm. However, reductions in normal bronchomotor tone may interfere with the normal $\dot{V}_A/\dot{Q}$ matching and thus impair gas exchange.[27]

In addition, local decreases in alveolar CO_2 tension tend to improve the normal $\dot{V}_A/\dot{Q}$ matching by producing local increases in bronchomotor tone. In a sense, this hypocapnic bronchoconstriction is analogous to hypoxic pulmonary vasoconstriction. Whether the inhalation anesthetics as a group block this bronchoconstriction induced by hypocapnia is not known. Thus far, only halothane has been shown to reduce this bronchoconstrictive effect of hypocapnia.[28,29]

3. Further alterations in distribution of ventilation in the lateral position. Subjects in the lateral decubitus position exhibit a greater blood flow to the dependent lung, largely because of gravitational effects. In the awake state,

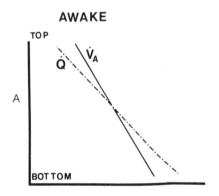

AWAKE

TOP

$\dot{Q}$ $\dot{V}_A$

A

BOTTOM

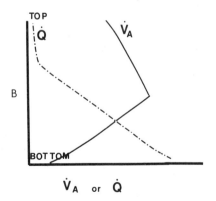

ANESTHESIA/PARALYSIS

TOP

$\dot{Q}$ $\dot{V}_A$

B

BOTTOM

$\dot{V}_A$ or $\dot{Q}$

Fig. 9-4. Diagram of the distribution of ventilation ($\dot{V}_A$) and perfusion ($\dot{Q}$) between nondependent *(top)* lung areas and dependent *(bottom)* areas. Notice that $\dot{V}_A$ tends to be distributed more uniformly from top to bottom in the anesthetized paralyzed state, **B.** (From Gal TJ: Respiratory physiology during anesthesia. In Kaplan JA, editor: Thoracic anesthesia, ed 2, New York, 1990, Churchill Livingstone.)

the normal vertical gradient of pleural pressure also allows for greater ventilation of the same dependent lung and maintenance of normal $\dot{V}_A/\dot{Q}$ distribution. This is more true in the case of the larger right lung, which is not subject to compression by an enlarged heart. In fact, in relatively normal persons with unilateral lung disease, respiratory gas exchange is optimal if the good lung is dependent.[30,31] Exceptions to this appear to occur in infants and with patients with chronic obstructive pulmonary disease. In these groups, the nondependent lung appears to be better ventilated.[32,33]

Radiographic and bronchospirometric studies show that the dependent lung normally receives a greater ventilation and has a higher O_2 uptake in the lateral position. Although its functional residual capacity is lower than the nondependent lung, N_2 washout is also more rapid.[34] When patients are anesthetized in the lateral position as for thoracic surgery, distribution of the pulmonary blood flow is similar to the awake state; that is, the dependent lung receives greater perfusion. The greater portion of ventilation, however, is switched from the dependent to the nondependent lung. In a sense, the ventilation is more uniform, and this is reflected in more equal N_2 clearance for each lung.[34] This shift in distribution of ventilation results from a loss of lung volume (decreased FRC) that is shared but unequally by both lungs. The dependent lung, which undergoes a greater decrease in FRC (because the abdominal contents as well as the mediastinum impede dependent lung expansion), moves to a less steep portion near the bottom of the pressure-volume curve (Fig. 9-3), whereas the nondependent lung moves from a relatively flat portion to a steeper one. Thus the anesthetized patient in the lateral position has a nondependent lung that is well ventilated but poorly perfused. In contrast, the well-perfused dependent lung is poorly ventilated. Opening the chest may only serve to increase the overventilation of the nondependent lung.

In summary, the increased $\dot{V}_A/\dot{Q}$ mismatching that accompanies anesthesia and paralysis whether in the supine or lateral positions appears to be largely a result of altered distribution of ventilation with a relative failure of intrapulmonary perfusion to adjust.[35] Although some of this failure of blood flow to adjust for the altered ventilation may relate to inhibition of hypoxic pulmonary vasoconstriction by the inhalation anesthetics, the altered pattern of expansion of the lung with anesthesia and paralysis may also effect the distribution of blood flow along with ventilation.

B. Inhibition of hypoxic pulmonary vasoconstriction

In the systemic vascular beds, hypoxia causes vasodilatation, which aids oxygen delivery and carbon dioxide removal. The pulmonary vessels, on the other hand, respond to acute hypoxia by constricting. This unique behavior in response to hypoxia is called "hypoxic pulmonary vasoconstriction" (HPV). This HPV response is an important compensatory mechanism that serves to divert flow away from hypoxic alveoli. Blood flow thus shifts from poorly ventilated alveoli to better ventilated ones to match ventilation and perfusion and minimize arterial hypoxemia.

The physiologic manifestations of HPV depend heavily on the size of the lung area that is hypoxic. If the segment of hypoxic lung is small, HPV will result in diversion of flow away from the hypoxic area and little or no change in pulmonary artery pressure (Fig. 9-5, A). If, on the other hand, the hypoxic area is very large or more so if the alveolar hypoxia is diffuse and generalized, flow cannot be diverted and the vasoconstriction results in an increased pulmonary artery pressure (Fig. 9-5, B). Thus for flow diversion to occur the hypoxic segment must comprise a small fraction of the total lung; that is, flow diversion is inversely related to the size of the hypoxic segment. The increases in pulmonary artery pressure therefore are directly related to the fraction of total lung that is hypoxic. Thus the proportion of flow changes to pressure change decreases as the size of the hypoxic lung segment increases. This distinction between localized and the more generalized or diffuse hypoxia is essential to understanding the nature of HPV.

The major segment of the vascular system at which HPV occurs appears to be at the level of the precapillary arterioles (30 to 50 μm).[36] These small muscular vessels are closely related to alveoli and are in an ideal position to respond to changes in alveolar oxygen concentration. Indeed, the most important stimulus to HPV appears to be the alveolar oxygen tension ($P_{A_{O_2}}$). Constriction occurs as $P_{A_{O_2}}$ decreases below normal, and the response reaches a maximum at about 30 mm Hg. The oxygen tension in the mixed venous blood ($P_{\bar{v}_{O_2}}$) also plays a role in the HPV response. The $P_{\bar{v}_{O_2}}$ becomes increasingly important at very low levels of $P_{A_{O_2}}$ and in an atelectatic lung may be the only stimulus for HPV. At alveolar oxygen tensions above 60 mm Hg, $P_{\bar{v}_{O_2}}$ appears to have only a minor effect.[37]

The HPV response is attenuated in many diverse clinical situations and by many classes of drugs, foremost of which are the anesthetic

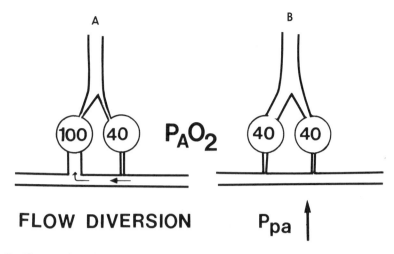

Fig. 9-5. Changes in pulmonary artery pressure (P_{pa}) and diversion of blood flow are depicted for localized hypoxia, **A,** and for diffuse or generalized hypoxia, **B.** (**A** and **B** from Gal TJ: Respiratory physiology in anesthetic practice, Baltimore, 1991, Williams & Wilkins.)

drugs. Intravenous drugs of most classes utilized in anesthesia (opioids, barbiturates, benzodiazepine, ketamine) do not appear to have a detectable effect on the HPV response. In vitro and in vivo experiments have shown that the pulmonary vasoconstrictive response to hypoxia is maintained at blood concentrations of these drugs sufficient to produce analgesia and anesthesia.[38,39]

In vitro experiments utilizing isolated perfused lungs have generally shown that the current halogenated inhalation agents halothane, enflurane, and isoflurane all inhibit HPV in a dose-related manner. In vitro observation with nitrous oxide shows that it produces little or no effect on HPV.[38] Studies in intact animals, however, suggest that 70% nitrous oxide moderately diminishes the HPV response.[39,40] The halogenated anesthetics also appear to antagonize the HPV response in intact animals and humans but widely divergent results have been reported in contrast to the in vitro experiments. The Marshalls[41] have provided a unifying concept for these findings based on the proportion of the lung that is made hypoxic. They suggest that the differences in most studies arise from the size of the lung segment used. The larger the hypoxic segment studied, the less effective will be the vasoconstriction and flow diversion away from the hypoxic site. They have also suggested that the antagonism of HPV by inhalation anesthetics may be obscured by other hemodynamic effects. The anesthetics depress myocardial function and produce a decrease in cardiac output. The latter is associated with decreased $P_{\bar{v}}O_2$ and pulmonary artery pressures,

both of which tend to intensify HPV. Thus, unless such effects are considered, the anesthetic actions on HPV may be subtle or misinterpreted.

The hypothesis that antagonism of HPV by inhalation anesthetics is important in the cause of abnormal gas exchange during anesthesia is indeed an attractive one. However, blunting of the HPV response does not appear to sufficiently account for the impaired oxygenation observed. Inappropriately low PaO_2 values are often seen in patients breathing hyperoxic mixtures that would be expected to provide all open alveolar units with an oxygen tension far above that at which HPV comes into play. Therefore other factors such as altered lung mechanics may play a more significant role in the impaired gas exchange.[42]

C. Alterations in the control of breathing

Although the analysis of the system that controls breathing can be subdivided into chemical and neural elements, clinical appraisal of the neural control system is much more difficult and hazardous. The chemical control system that is profoundly affected by anesthesia has been extensively studied and responds to three basic physiologic stimuli: increases in the partial pressure of CO_2, increases in hydrogen-ion concentration (decreased blood pH), and decreases in arterial PO_2.

1. CO_2 sensitivity. Metabolically produced carbon dioxide relies on ventilation for its removal. If ventilation is reduced, $PaCO_2$ will rise. Similarly, if ventilation is voluntarily or reflexly increased, $PaCO_2$ will decrease. The reciprocal relationship between ventilation and CO_2 is described by a rectangular hyperbola. For CO_2 excretion (Fig. 9-1) it is apparent from the diagram that a doubling of alveolar ventilation ($\dot{V}_A$) results in halving of CO_2 tension, whereas CO_2 tension doubles if ventilation is halved. An average normal man has an alveolar ventilation of about 4 liters per minute and a resting Pa_{CO_2} near 40 mm Hg as shown in the figure as the set point.

In the same normal person, inhalation of CO_2 increases ventilation, which rises in nearly linear fashion with changes in Pa_{CO_2}. Stimulation to breathe depends on the hydrogen-ion concentration in the extracellular fluid surrounding the central nervous system chemoreceptors near the ventral-lateral surface of the medulla. The changes in hydrogen-ion concentration as a result of inhalation CO_2 depend somewhat on the concentration of bicarbonate in the extracellular fluid. Alterations of bicarbonate levels in blood or cerebrospinal fluid from metabolic disturbances can therefore modify the ventilatory response to CO_2. The central chemoreceptors account for about 80% of the total increase in ventilation during inhalation of CO_2. The remaining 20% increase seems to arise from stimulation of peripheral chemoreceptors in the carotid body.

2. Sensitivity to hypoxia. The ventilatory response to decreases in inspired oxygen tension tends to be hyperbolic (Fig. 9-6) such that decreases in oxygen tension exert a greater effect on ventilation when hypoxemia is severe as opposed to mild reductions in oxygen supply. This curvilinear relationship can be conveniently converted to a straight line when one plots ventilation against the reciprocal of arterial oxygen tension ($1/Pa_{O_2}$) or, as is more common, against arterial O_2 saturation. The nice linear relationship with O_2 saturation indicates that ventilation may be influenced by the oxygen content primarily. Most studies, however, point to oxygen tension or partial pressure (Pa_{O_2}) rather than O_2 saturation as the stimulus to the peripheral chemoreceptors. This is underscored by the effect of inhaling carbon monoxide, which greatly affects O_2 content but has little or no effect on ventilation because Pa_{O_2} is not affected.

The hypoxic ventilatory response is mediated by the peripheral chemoreceptors in the carotid body. In their absence, the hypoxic ventilatory drive is lost, and hypoxia may exert a depressant action on the central chemoreceptors. The carotid bodies exert only a subtle influence on resting ventilation when Pa_{O_2} is greater than 60 mm Hg. Below this, ventilation increases dramatically in hyperbolic fashion, whereas at a Pa_{O_2} of 200 mm Hg or more the carotid body discharge diminishes to a minimal level.

An important interaction occurs between the two major ventilatory stimulants of hypoxia and hypercapnia. The presence of hypoxia en-

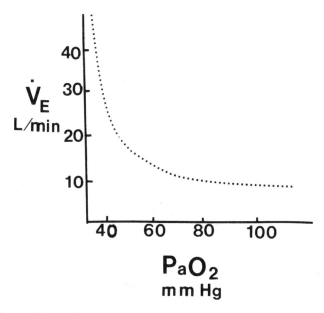

Fig. 9-6. Effects of decreasing arterial oxygen tension ($P_{A_{O_2}}$) on minute ventilation ($\dot{V}_E$). The hyperbolic plot can be linearized by plotting of $\dot{V}_E$ against the reciprocal of Pa_{O_2} or against O_2 saturation. (From Gal TJ: Respiratory physiology during anesthesia. In Kaplan JA, editor: Thoracic anesthesia, ed 2, New York, 1990, Churchill Livingstone.)

hances the ventilatory response to CO_2. Similarly, an increase in CO_2 results in a greater sensitivity to hypoxia. These interactive effects require an intact central as well as peripheral chemoreceptor function.

3. Response to acidosis. A decrease in arterial pH from metabolic acidosis with normal Pao_2 and $Paco_2$ stimulates ventilation primarily by the effect of the acidemia on the peripheral chemoreceptors (carotid bodies). This arises from the concept that neither hydrogen nor bicarbonate ions readily cross the blood-brain barrier and is supported by observations in dogs that carotid body denervation attenuates and delays the response.[43] Biscoe et al.[44] demonstrated in cats that a change of 0.20 pH units (7.45 to 7.25) increased carotid body neural output two to three times. This doubling of ventilation is roughly equivalent to that seen when Pao_2 decreases from normal to about 40 or 50 mm Hg.

In normal volunteers, Knill and Clement noted approximately a doubling of ventilation in normoxic normocarbic volunteers[45] as the hydrogen-ion concentration was increased about 13 nmol/L (about 0.12 unit pH decrease). This response was attenuated by hyper-oxia and enhanced by hypoxia, again attesting to the interaction of these stimuli at the peripheral chemoreceptor.

All in all, for the same degree of acidemia or pH change, the addition of CO_2 evokes a larger increment in ventilation than the addition of fixed acid does. The initial response to acute metabolic acidosis is weak because as $Paco_2$ decreases from carotid body stimulation, CO_2 tension in the cerebrospinal fluid decreases and pH increases. Thus the strong peripheral stimulation of the hydrogen ion is offset by a central alkalosis and reduced stimulus to the medullary chemoreceptors. Gradually after several hours, bicarbonate levels decrease and permit cerebrospinal fluid pH to decrease back toward its normal value and thus restore central chemoreceptor activity to normal.

4. Ventilatory indices of chemosensitivity

a. Carbon dioxide response. The two basic variables of ventilatory control, that is, resting ventilation and $Paco_2$, may be highly variable and only slightly affected when the ventilatory control system is significantly altered.[46] Nevertheless, they have been advocated as indices of ventilatory control.[47]

Conventional means of expressing CO_2 sensi-

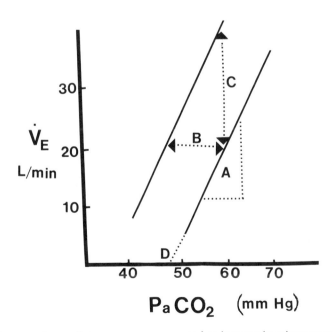

Fig. 9-7. Hypercapnic ventilatory response expressed as increase in minute ventilation ($\dot{V}$) as a function of increased arterial CO_2 tension ($Paco_2$). *A,* Slope of the response; *B,* displacement of the response (that is, a change in the abscissa at a constant ordinate value); *C,* change in ordinate at a constant abscissal value; *D,* apneic threshold. (From Gal TJ: Respiratory physiology during anesthesia. In Kaplan JA, editor: Thoracic anesthesia, ed 2, New York, 1990, Churchill Livingstone.)

tivity utilize a plot of the CO_2 load or stimulus on the abscissa and ventilation on the ordinate. The latter values are obtained from actual data points with steady-state techniques, whereas least-squares linear regression determines the plot with rebreathing data. The carbon dioxide stimulus on the abscissa has included inspired CO_2 concentration, but end-tidal tension is most often utilized. However, arterial tension (Pa_{CO_2}) may be the most accurate reflection of the CO_2 stimulus, particularly if pulmonary disease is present. The ordinate on the carbon dioxide ventilation plot is provided by respiratory minute volume, ($\dot{V}_E$). The hyperoxic carbon dioxide sensitivity is expressed as the increment in $\dot{V}_E$ (L/min) per increment in Pa_{CO_2} (mm Hg). This can be quantitated by the equation:

$$\dot{V}_E = S\,(Pa_{CO_2} - B)$$

where S is the slope of the relationship between $\dot{V}_E/Pa_{CO_2}$ and B is the intercept on the x-axis. The steeper the slope, the more vigorous is the response to CO_2 (Fig. 9-7). As such it provides a measure of the gain of the control system.

In most normal young adults, the slope of the CO_2 response ranged from 1.5 to 5 L/min/ mm Hg CO_2.[48] Much of the interindividual differences in the response relates to the tidal-volume response during rebreathing. In general, the lowest ventilatory responses tend to occur in individuals whose tidal volumes are small.

Changes in CO_2 sensitivity can be indicated by slope changes in the response. However, some factors such as pharmacologic intervention may alter CO_2 sensitivity without changing slope. In this case the shift of the CO_2 response can be characterized by a term referred to as "displacement" (Fig. 9-7). This is the shift across the x-axis in mm Hg CO_2 at a constant ordinate $\dot{V}_E$) value, usually 20 or 20 L/min. Another expression for the shift of the CO_2 response curve utilizes a change in ordinate ($\dot{V}_E$) at a constant CO_2 value (Fig. 9-7). Often 60 mm Hg is used, and the term referred to as the "$\dot{V}_E 60$." Another interesting term represents an extrapolation of the CO_2-response curve to zero ventilation on the CO_2 axis (Fig. 9-7). This "apneic threshold" represents the CO_2 level at which apnea should occur from hyperventilation. This value is not easily obtainable in awake man and may not provide any more information than the resting Pa_{CO_2}.

b. Hypoxic response. Ideally the hypoxic ventilatory response should be expressed as a change in ventilation for a change in the stimulus (decreased O_2). However, the curvilinear nature of the relationship renders it complex and not eas-

ily characterized by a single index. One early index compared the ratio of the slopes of two CO_2-response curves, one performed in the presence of hypoxia ($P_{A_{O_2}} = 40$ mm Hg) and the other normoxia ($P_{A_{O_2}} = 150$ mm Hg). This dimensionless ratio has little physiologic meaning and is highly dependent on the hypercapnic response.

Severinghaus[49] introduced an index termed "$\Delta\dot{V}_{40}$," which was expressed in liters per minute. This represented the increase in minute ventilation that occurred as oxygen tension was reduced from above 200 to 40 mm Hg with normocapnia. At an oxygen tension of 40, the ventilatory response is rather steep (Fig. 9-8). Thus the potential for error exists in estimating the actual ventilation value, since small decreases in P_{O_2} are associated with rather large increases in ventilation. The $\Delta\dot{V}_{40}$ can also be estimated from the two CO_2-response curves, one performed with normoxia and the other at hypoxic level ($Pa_{O_2} = 40$ mm Hg). Ventila-

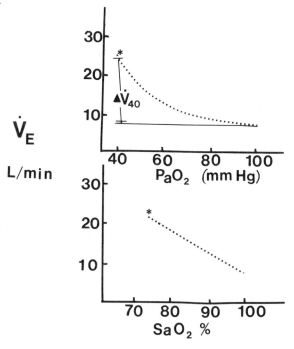

Fig. 9-8. The hyperbolic response to hypoxia can be quantitated as $\dot{V}_{40}$, the increase in ventilation ($\dot{V}_E$) at a hypoxic level ($Pa_{O_2} = 40$ mm Hg) compared to normoxia. Notice that the increased $\dot{V}_E$ is linearly related to arterial O_2 saturation ($Sa_{O_2}\%$). At $Pa_{O_2} = 40$, the blood is roughly 25% desaturated ($Sa_{O_2} = 75$). Thus ventilation at this point and at $Pa_{O_2} = 40$ are nearly identical (*). (From Gal TJ: Respiratory physiology during anesthesia. In Kaplan JA, editor: Thoracic anesthesia, ed 2, New York, 1990, Churchill Livingstone.)

tions measured at an isocapnic point ($Paco_2$ = 40 mm Hg) can thus be compared.

The ventilatory response to hypoxia can be linearized when one plots the reciprocal of ventilation against Po_2 or more conveniently when one relates the change in ventilation to arterial oxyhemoglobin saturation (Fig. 9-8). Thus the hypoxic response can be quantitated as $\Delta\dot{V}/\%$ desaturation. Although the latter index is the simplest means of quantitating the hypoxic response, a more complex description of the hyperbolic relationship between ventilation ($\dot{V}_E$) and oxygen tension (Pao_2) is equally popular. Parameter "*A*" is utilized to characterize the shape of the curve that is expressed mathematically by the equation:

$$\dot{V} = \dot{V}_0 + \frac{A}{Pao_2 - 32}$$

where $\dot{V}_0$ is the asymptote for ventilation; *32* is the asymptote for Pao_2 at which ventilation is assumed to be infinite. The magnitude for *A* is related to the briskness of the response.

In normal subjects the ventilatory response to hypoxia appears to be more variable than the hypercapnic response. For example, while the mean value for parameter *A* was 186, the range of values was from 69 to 410.[50] In terms of desaturation, hypoxic sensitivity ranged from 0.16 to 1.35 L/min per 1% desaturation (mean = 0.6)[51] while $\Delta\dot{V}_{40}$ values ranged from 5.4 to 64.8 L/min.[52] Certain mathematical interrelationships can be constructed for these three indices. For example, since normal blood undergoes a 25% desaturation at a Pao_2 of 40 mm Hg, the $\Delta\dot{V}/1\%$ desaturation and $\dot{V}_{40}$ are related by a factor of 25 to 1 such that $\Delta\dot{V}_{40}/25 = \dot{V}1\%$ desaturation. Also, if "Pao_2 is 40 mm Hg" is substituted into the equation containing parameter *A*, the following relationship results:

$$A = \Delta\dot{V}_{40} \times 8$$

5. Effects of anesthetics on respiratory control. Most drugs utilized in the practice of anesthesiology including the intravenous and volatile anesthetic agents have as their principle side effect an alteration of respiratory control. This is manifest as a depressed desire to breathe, which assumes great clinical relevance, since these drug effects may seriously impair ventilation and thus gas exchange in the perioperative period.

a. Inhalation anesthetics

(1) CO₂ RESPONSES. Each of the present-day halogenated inhalation agents (halothane, enflurane, and isoflurane) produce profound respiratory depression in a dose-related manner.

This respiratory depression is far greater than that associated with older outmoded agents (ether, cyclopropane, or fluroxene). At concentrations that produce loss of consciousness and surgical anesthesia, tidal volume is reduced. Although respiratory rate increases, minute ventilation decreases and an elevation of CO_2 occurs in proportion to the depth of anesthesia (expressed as multiples of the minimum alveolar concentration, MAC). The extent of this hypoventilation and CO_2 retention varies with each agent. At 1.0 MAC halothane produces a modest increase in CO_2 to about 45 mm Hg. By comparison, the same level of isoflurane increases CO_2 to about 50 mm Hg, whereas enflurane produces even more pronounced hypercapnia to above 60 mm Hg.[53] Although the effects of surgical stimulation tend to counteract this rise in CO_2, the hypercapnia tends to worsen in patients with COPD in proportion to their degree of airway obstruction.[54] In the face of the added mechanical load such patients are unable to achieve adequate gas exchange with the rapid shallow breathing pattern associated with halothane.

The normal increase in ventilation with increasing CO_2 (that is, the slope of the response) is blunted by the inhalation anesthetics in a dose-dependent manner. Whereas sedating halothane doses (0.1 MAC) produce little or no change in the slope of the response, anesthetizing doses (greater than 1.0 MAC) produce significant decreases in slope. The observations of Tusiewicz et al.[55] show that that much of this ventilatory depression may be attributable to a reduction of rib-cage recruitment that occurs at higher levels of ventilation in the awake state. The latter may also help to explain the effects of surgical stimulation, which produces a decrease in resting CO_2 but no change in the slope of the CO_2 response.[56]

The absence of wakefulness with the inhalation anesthetics results in a complete dependence on the chemical regulation of ventilation. Thus passive hyperventilation, which removes the CO_2 stimulus, results in apnea. Such apnea is difficult if not impossible to elicit in conscious subjects but easy to achieve during anesthesia. This CO_2 level, which is 5 to 9 mm Hg below the normal awake resting value or resting CO_2 tension while one is anesthetized, is referred to as the "apneic threshold." One can estimate the apneic threshold by linear extrapolation of the CO_2-response curve to zero ventilation (Fig. 9-7).

(2) RESPONSE TO HYPOXIA. Traditional views of the peripheral chemoreceptors considered them the body's last defense and resistant to

Table 9-2. Ventilatory responses with inhalation anesthetics

	0.1 MAC			1.1 MAC			2.0 MAC		
	H	E	I	H	E	I	H	E	I
CO_2 response ($\Delta\dot{V}_E/CO_2$, % of awake)	100	77	130	37	37	33	—	—	17
Hypoxic response (ΔV_{45}, % of awake)	30	42	45	0	3	3	—	—	—

Data are summarized from the studies of Knill et al.[58-60]
MAC, Minimum alveolar concentration; *H*, halothane; *E*, enflurane; *I*, isoflurane.

drug depression. Present knowledge, however, recognizes that these structures are profoundly depressed in humans by even sedating levels of anesthesia. The initial studies in dogs by Weiskopf and associates demonstrated blunting of the hypoxic response with 1.1% halothane.[57] Knill and Gelb[58] noted that the response in humans was even more profound. Similar effects were seen with enflurane[59] and isoflurane.[60] Noteworthy is the relatively profound depression of the response in contrast to the hypercapnic response (Table 9-2). At levels that minimally affect the CO_2 response, the hypoxic response is nearly abolished. This also appears to be true for nitrous oxide, which at concentrations of 30% to 50% has no effect on the CO_2 response and depresses the ventilatory response to hypoxia.[61] Furthermore, it has been shown in humans[59] and dogs[58] that the normal synergistic interaction between hypoxia and hypercapnia is eliminated. Rather than acting to increase ventilation, the two stimuli act to depress ventilation in anesthetized subjects.

Like the response to hypoxia, the response to added $[H^+]$ metabolic acidemia is mediated by peripheral chemoreceptors. Knill and associates[62] have shown that halothane sedation and anesthesia in humans greatly attenuates the response to acidemia and its attendant interaction with hypoxemia. Thus any patient compensation for these derangements must arise from measures instituted by the physician.

b. Intravenous agents

(1) BARBITURATES. Among the various central nervous system depressants utilized to achieve sedation, the barbiturates do not appear to have a significant effect on resting ventilation when used in doses that produce sedation or drowsiness. Intramuscular pentobarbital (2 mg/kg) reduced the ventilatory response to hypoxia in 5 out of 10 healthy volunteers for a period of about 90 minutes.[63] Sedative doses of thiopental did not significantly affect resting ventilation or the response to isocapnic hypoxia and hyperoxic hypercapnia.[64] However, hypnotic or anes-

thetic levels of thiopental depressed both hypoxic and hypercapnic responses to nearly the same extent (35% to 45% of control). In this respect, the barbiturates differ from inhalation anesthetics, since the latter agents depress hypoxic response far in excess of their effects on hypercapnic responses.

(2) OPIOIDS. The prototype of the pure opioid agonists, morphine, depresses ventilation in the usual analgesic doses (10 to 20 mg). This is manifest by a decrease in respiratory frequency, a small decrease in tidal volume, and a resultant increase in resting CO_2. The CO_2 response with such doses is altered primarily by a rightward displacement with little or no change in slope (Fig. 9-9). Larger doses of morphine (0.5 mg/kg) begin to depress CO_2-response slope in a fashion that appears to be related to the depression in the state of consciousness. Indeed, sleep has been shown to enhance the ventilatory depression of morphine.[65] Other opioids consistently demonstrate the same pattern and degree of respiratory depression when given in equianalgesic doses. Much of the depression is mediated by depression of the contribution of the rib cage to ventilation.[66] This phenomenon is similar but less pronounced than that observed with halothane anesthesia.[55] However, the decrease in respiratory rate, in contrast to the tachypnea noted with halothane, results in a disproportionate decrease in minute ventilation.

The hypoxic response, much like with the inhalation anesthetics, was originally believed to be unaffected by opioids. However, depressed hypoxic responses have been demonstrated to occur after morphine (7.5 mg given subcutaneously)[67] and meperidine (1.2 mg/kg given orally).[68] Much like the benzodiazepines and barbiturates but unlike the inhalation anesthetics, the magnitude of depression with opioids is approximately the same for both hypoxic and hypercapnic responses.

The safety of parenteral opioids is limited by the risk of severe ventilatory depression with increasing doses. Intrathecal and epidural admin-

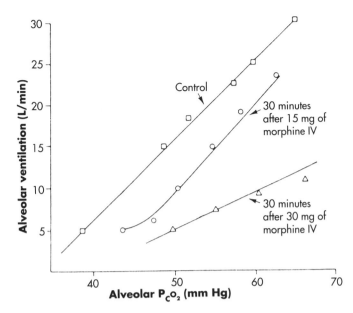

Fig. 9-9. Effects of morphine on the ventilatory response to CO_2. A typical premedication dose (15 mg) is compared with a larger more sedating dose (30 mg) likely to be associated with greater decrease in the level of consciousness. (From Bailey PL and Stanley TH: Pharmacology of intravenous narcotic anesthetics. In Miller RD, editor: Anesthesia, ed 3, New York, 1990, Churchill Livingstone.)

istration of opioids was initially believed to be free of such risks because relatively small doses are required to achieve high concentrations at the dorsal spinal roots, thereby obviating systemic toxicity. However, there is evidence that epidural morphine produces respiratory depression of slightly greater magnitude than that of the same dose of drug administered parenterally.[69] The ventilatory depression is delayed and prolonged with the epidural administration and has been attributed to rostral spread of the drug along the neuraxis. With fentanyl the respiratory effects were also greater with epidural administration.[70] Since plasma fentanyl levels were lower in the epidural group, the authors also ascribed the effects to rostral spread despite the highly lipid-soluble character of fentanyl. In contrast, observations with another more lipid-soluble opioid, sufentanil, indicate that an important part of the analgesic and respiratory effects of that drug may also be mediated centrally but only after systemic absorption occurs.[71]

(3) BENZODIAZEPINES. The benzodiazepines have become increasingly popular as sedating agents and have virtually replaced barbiturates as preoperative medications, amnestic agents, and adjuvants to opioids. Intravenous doses of diazepam (0.1 to 0.4 mg/kg) have been shown to depress the slope of the CO_2 response.[72] This respiratory depression has not appeared to

be consistent in several other studies. Gross et al.[73] have clarified the transient nature of the response and have demonstrated that the depressant effect peaks in about 3 minutes and lasts for 30 minutes. More importantly, they showed that the ventilatory depression correlated with the subject's state of consciousness. The effects of another benzodiazepine, midazolam, were qualitatively similar to diazepam with perhaps a slightly briefer duration of effect.[74]

The ventilatory response to hypoxia appears to be blunted by diazepam in a transient fashion and to a similar extent as the hypercapnic response. Lakshinarayan et al.[75] observed a decrease in parameter A to about one half of control values in eight healthy volunteers. The effect was consistently demonstrated for 30 minutes after 10 mg of intravenous diazepam.

(4) KETAMINE. The dissociative anesthetic ketamine appears to have minimal depressant actions on respiratory control. Early observations indicated that intravenous doses of 2.2 mg/kg did not affect resting ventilation or the response to CO_2 challenge.[76] In a study of dogs anesthetized with ketamine the hypercapnic response appeared to be increased,[77] and this finding led to speculation that ketamine may be a respiratory stimulant by virtue of the increased sympathetic nervous system activity. However, another more precisely controlled study in dogs demonstrated that ketamine produced slight

but significant depressions of both hypoxic and hypercapnic responses.[78] In healthy human volunteers, 3 mg/kg intravenously administered ketamine appears to produce respiratory depression similar to that observed with premedicant doses of morphine (0.2 mg/kg).[79] In children, an intravenous bolus dose of ketamine produced nearly a 40% decrease in the CO_2-response slope.[80] This transient response disappeared in 30 minutes, whereas a continuous infusion was maintained. The respiratory depression in the latter "steady-state" infusion period was similar to that observed in adults,[79] that is, a rightward shift of the CO_2-response curve but no change in slope. Again these changes are characteristic of premedicant doses of morphine (Fig. 9-9).

III. CLINICAL CONDITIONS ASSOCIATED WITH IMPAIRED GAS EXCHANGE CLINICAL CONDITIONS

A. Pulmonary edema

By far the most common clinical cause of pulmonary edema is one in which the forces that drive fluid across the vessel wall are increased. Such increased intravascular pressures are the hallmark of cardiogenic pulmonary edema, that is, those associated with congestive heart failure. Early in the development of pulmonary edema, well in advance of fluid accumulation in the air space, interstitial fluid has been shown to accumulate around arterioles and bronchioles.[81] This "cuffing" action serves to increase both airway and pulmonary vascular resistance at the lung bases. Both ventilation and perfusion are redistributed away from these lower lung zones to more apical areas, and an imbalance in the $\dot{V}_A/\dot{Q}$ relationship results. The immediate consequence of this $\dot{V}_A/\dot{Q}$ mismatch is arterial hypoxemia with average PaO_2 values of 50 to 55 mm Hg commonly observed.[82] Hypercapnia is not usually considered a usual consequence of pulmonary edema; however, elevated $PaCO_2$ values have been reported.[82] The mechanism for hypercapnia is not entirely clear but may be related to the severity of the ventilation-perfusion imbalance. Normally hyperventilation can compensate for hypercapnia, since the CO_2-dissociation curve is linear. However, if work of breathing is significantly increased, as it may be in a congested stiff lung with increased airway resistance, ventilation may not be able to increase sufficiently to restore $PaCO_2$ to normal. Furthermore, with extremely high work of breathing the metabolic load of CO_2 produced by the increased ventilation may offset the exhaled CO_2 and worsen hypercapnia.

Other noncardiac varieties of pulmonary edema basically consist of conditions in which fluid movement to the outside of vessels is increased because of increased permeability usually from loss of the integrity of the vessel wall. This group includes such states as the adult respiratory distress syndrome, neurogenic pulmonary edema, and the pulmonary edema associated with heroin overdose or exposure to high altitude. The major abnormality of gas exchange in such patients results from large degrees of intrapulmonary shunting. The arterial hypoxemia in these states is also quite vulnerable to any factors that alter $P_{\bar{v}}O_2$, in particular, cardiac output.

One other variant of pulmonary edema with transient failure of gas exchange in the form of an increased alveolar-arterial O_2 difference is that associated with the development and relief of acute upper airway obstruction. Many factors play a role in the pathogenesis of such pulmonary edema. However, the fact that it is often referred to as "negative pressure pulmonary edema" simplistically implies that a pronounced negative inspiratory pressure is the predominant if not the only cause. Lloyd et al.[83] demonstrated that negative inspiratory pressures associated with breathing through inspiratory resistances promoted lung lymph formation in sheep in a fashion similar to that resulting from elevated intravascular pressures. On the other hand, Hansen et al.[84] were unable to show any effect of inspiratory obstruction on steady-state lung lymph flow. Since they utilized supplemental O_2, they postulated that a key to development of edema is the presence of alveolar hypoxia, which mediates pulmonary vasoconstriction and may cause capillary leak. This is an attractive explanation, since patients with upper airway obstruction are usually not receiving O_2 and are likely to experience severe hypoxia. Other interesting evidence that casts some doubt on the dominant role of negative pressure in the genesis of pulmonary edema is the abundance of studies in which human subjects[85] or animals[86] have breathed against severe extrinsic inspiratory obstructions and developed inspiratory pressures more than 10 times those of quiet breathing and yet have not developed pulmonary edema.

B. Pulmonary embolism

Abnormal gas exchange inevitably accompanies acute pulmonary embolism. Abnormalities are influenced by the size and extent of the vascular occlusion, the presence of underlying cardiovascular disease, and the time since the acute embolization. Arterial hypoxemia is frequently though not universally found. However, the patients in whom significant arterial hypoxemia does not develop with ambient air do exhibit an increased alveolar-to-arterial oxygen gradient. The failure of these patients to develop hypoxemia results from the hyperventilation that usually accompanies the embolism. In most of these patients the increased ventilation is associated with some hypocapnia.

The other significant consequence of the embolism is an increased alveolar dead space because the occlusion is associated with absent flow to distal lung areas. The occlusion may not be total, and thus regions of high $\dot{V}_A/\dot{Q}$ ratios may prevail. These zones of lung with vascular obstruction develop "pneumoconstriction," which may be the result of airway hypocapnia and the release of bronchoconstrictive amines.

This pneumoconstriction teleologically reduces the extent of the alveolar dead space and high $\dot{V}_A\dot{Q}$ areas but may contribute to development of low $\dot{V}_A/\dot{Q}$ zones. Such zones may preexist in many patients. They can increase acutely from hyperperfusion of the vascular bed in unaffected areas and from the development of atelectasis distal to areas of vascular obstruction.

Another important contributor to the abnormal oxygenation is a reduction in cardiac output because of right ventricular failure. This generally requires massive vascular obstruction (greater than 50%). As cardiac output falls, $P_{\bar{v}O_2}$ also decreases and amplifies the effect of right-to-left shunting and low $\dot{V}_A/\dot{Q}$ areas.[87]

C. Bronchospasm

Episodes of bronchoconstriction in asthmatics, whether spontaneous or induced by bronchial provocation testing, are associated not only with increased airflow resistance, but also with changes in gas exchange. The most prominent manifestation is hypoxemia, and most current evidence points to $\dot{V}_A/\dot{Q}$ abnormalities as the major cause. There appears to be a considerable broadening of $\dot{V}_A/\dot{Q}$ relationships with a preponderance for very low but finite $\dot{V}_A/\dot{Q}$ ratios, but no absolute shunt.[88]

Inhalation of aerosolized isoproterenol is associated with worsening of hypoxemia and $\dot{V}_A/\dot{Q}$ inequality, presumably from an increased perfusion of lung units with low $\dot{V}_A/\dot{Q}$ ratios. This apparent decrease in pulmonary vascular resistance and increased perfusion of low $\dot{V}_A/\dot{Q}$ areas indicates that isoproterenol may be inhibiting hypoxic pulmonary vasoconstriction (HPV). However, this may not be the entire mechanism, since breathing pure oxygen does not seem to increase flow to these low $\dot{V}_A/\dot{Q}$ areas.[88]

Patients with severe acute asthma requiring mechanical ventilation exhibit qualitatively the same pattern of $\dot{V}_A/\dot{Q}$ abnormalities seen in less sever severe disease. They do, however, have a high degree of preexisting HPV that responds to pure oxygen breathing with a significant amount of shunt.[89] Although the latter may also reflect the development of absorption atelectasis,[90] it is most likely attributable to increased perfusion of these previously insignificant shunt areas.

D. Pulmonary aspiration of gastric contents

The initial response to aspiration of acidic gastric contents is one of intense bronchoconstriction. This irritative reaction is rapidly followed by transudation of large amounts of fluid from the respiratory epithelium into the air spaces. The result is profound arterial hypoxemia ($Pa_{O_2} <50$) as in severe cardiogenic pulmonary edema. Increased $F_{I}O_2$ will offset the hypoxemia, but a large alveolar-arterial O_2 difference persists as a reflection of the severe ventilation-perfusion mismatch. As in cardiogenic pulmonary edema this mismatch may be severe enough, given the increased work of breathing, to also impair CO_2 removal. The degree of respiratory acidosis will depend on the ability to produce adequate alveolar ventilation, whereas metabolic acidosis may result from concomitant tissue hypoxia.

E. Pneumothorax

The clinical presentation of pneumothorax may be confused with bronchospasm because of the presence of increased airway pressure, wheezing, diminished breath sounds, and hypoxemia. This picture is further complicated by the fact that pneumothorax is more frequent in patients with obstructive airway disease. Progressive expansion of the pneumothorax compresses lung parenchyma and creates more and more areas with low $\dot{V}_A/\dot{Q}$ ratios and thus hypoxemia. The limited ability to increase ventilation and the cardiac depression may be associated with hypercapnia as well.

F. Influence of chronic disease states on gas exchange

1. Cardiac disease. Cardiac function has its most obvious effect on gas exchange by its effect on the oxygen content of mixed venous blood. If cardiac function is inadequate to match demands of peripheral O_2 consumption, arterial-venous O_2 differences increase and have an eventual effect on Pa_{O_2}. Mild degrees of cardiac failure, in contrast to the already-discussed effects of pulmonary edema, are associated with minimal effects on gas exchange and little or no alteration in $\dot{V}_A/\dot{Q}$ distributions.

2. Renal disease. Patients with renal disease often exhibit hypocapnia as a result of attempts to compensate for systemic acidosis by hyperventilation. The presence of coexistent lung disease or cardiac failure may result in hypoxemia. Arterial hypoxemia is also observed during and after hemodialysis. Both the acetate and bicarbonate dialysates are associated with hypoxemia, which appears to be related to a transient hypoventilation.[91] The acetate removes some of the CO_2 load presented, whereas with bicarbonate dialysis it appears that respiratory drive is suppressed by a gain in bicarbonate. Ventilation-perfusion abnormalities appear to contribute somewhat to this postdialysis hypoxemia, which is similar in patients with and without lung disease.[92] Another contributing factor may be the reduction in cardiac output that so commonly occurs with dialysis.[93] However, the principal cause of the reduced arterial O_2 tension appears to be a decrease in alveolar O_2 tension ($P_{A}O_2$) because of hypoventilation.[94] Thus the $A-aDo_2$ does not change and Pao_2 is reduced concomitantly with $P_{A}O_2$. This is somewhat analogous to the posthyperventilation hypoxia seen after general anesthesia.[95]

3. Liver disease. In patients with hepatic cirrhosis who have relatively normal lung mechanics, arterial hypoxemia is a frequent finding. In patients with mild hypoxemia the abnormal gas exchange is primarily attributable to $\dot{V}_A/\dot{Q}$ mismatch.[96] Patients with severe hypoxemia have exhibited considerable right-to-left shunting as well.[97] Clinically, such patients demonstrate decreased oxygenation in the upright compared to recumbent positions (orthodeoxia) as well as dyspnea in the upright position that was relieved by recumbency (platypnea).

4. Obesity. The reduced respiratory system compliance and other mechanical ventilatory consequences of obesity would allow prediction that abnormal gas exchange is likely. Indeed there is hypoxemia usually unaccompanied by hypercapnia. This is most likely a reflection of "closed" peripheral lung units with low $\dot{V}_A/\dot{Q}$ ratios and increased shunting.[98]

Of considerable importance are the added derangements of cardiovascular and respiratory function imposed by changes in posture in the obese patient.[99] Movement from upright to recumbent and Trendelenburg positions would have progressively more adverse consequences on lung volumes and oxygenation during and after anesthesia. In the immediate postoperative period the semirecumbent positioning seems to

be associated with better oxygenation than the supine position.[100]

5. Pulmonary disease

a. Restrictive disease. The common element in the many forms of restrictive lung disease is a loss of volume. This is a result of alterations in one of the major structural components of the thorax: (1) skeletal, (2) neuromuscular, (3) pleural, (4) lung parenchymal (interstitial and alveolar). The reduction in lung volume is associated with a decreased lung compliance, the major consequences of which are increased work of breathing and maldistribution of ventilation. This maldistribution produces low $\dot{V}_A/\dot{Q}$ areas whose major impact on arterial blood gases is a pattern of hypoxemia, hypocapnia, and an increase in $A-aDo_2$. The hypocapnia indicates that hyperventilation is effective in maintaining CO_2 excretion. If hypercapnia occurs, it usually indicates advanced terminal disease in restrictive illness.

b. Obstructive disease. Chronic obstructive disease spans the spectrum between airflow obstruction (bronchitis) and overinflation or air trapping (emphysema). The maldistribution of ventilation that impairs gas exchange results from abnormally long time constants ($R \times C$). In the case of bronchitis, resistance (R) is increased, whereas compliance (C) is increased in emphysema. In emphysematous patients ("pink puffers") high ($\dot{V}_A/\dot{Q}$) areas or areas of relative "wasted ventilation" are prominent. Such patients tend to exhibit some mild hypoxemia and are usually normocapnic despite high levels of resting ventilation. In contrast, the more bronchitic types ("blue bloater") characteristically exhibit more low $\dot{V}_A/\dot{Q}$ areas and present with moderate to severe hypoxemia (Pao_2 <50 mm Hg) and significant hypercapnia ($Paco_2$ >50 mm Hg).

REFERENCES

1. Askanazi J, Weissman C, Rosenbaum SH, et al: Nutrition and the respiratory system, Crit Care Med 10:163-172, 1982.
2. Kaplan JA, Bush GL, Lecky JH, et al: Sodium bicarbonate and systemic hemodynamics in volunteers anesthetized with halothane, Anesthesiology 42:550-558, 1975.
3. Shepard RH, Campbell EJM, Martin HB, and Enns T: Factors affecting the pulmonary dead space as determined by single breath analysis, J Appl Physiol 11:241-244, 1975.
4. West JB: Causes of carbon dioxide retention in lung disease, N Engl J Med 284:1232-1236, 1971.
5. Figueras J, Stein L, Diez V, et al: Relationships between pulmonary hemodynamics and arterial pH and carbon dioxide tension in critically ill patients, Chest 70:460-472, 1976.
6. Juan G, Calverley P, Talamo C, et al: Effect of carbon dioxide on diaphragmatic function in human beings, N Engl J Med 310:874-879, 1984.

7. Edwards R, Winnie AP, and Ramamurthy S: Acute hypocapneic hypokalemia: an iatrogenic anesthetic complication, Anesth Analg 56:786-792, 1977.
8. Cutillo A, Omboni E, Perondi R, and Tana F: Effect of hypocapnia on pulmonary mechanics in normal subjects and in patients with chronic obstructive pulmonary disease, Am Rev Respir Dis 110:25-33, 1974.
9. Nunn JF: Applied respiratory physiology, ed 3, Boston, 1987, Butterworth & Co, pp 227-228.
10. Eger EI and Severinghaus J: The rate of rise of P_aCO_2 in the apneic anesthetized patient, Anesthesiology 22:419-425, 1961.
11. Bergman NA: Distribution of inspired gas during anesthesia and artificial ventilation, J Appl Physiol 18:1085-1089, 1963.
12. Rehder K and Marsh HM: Respiratory mechanics during anesthesia and mechanical ventilation. In Macklem PT and Mead J, editors: Handbook of physiology. The respiratory system: mechanics of breathing, Bethesda, Md, 1986, American Physiological Society, pp 737-752.
13. Damia G, Mascheroni D, Croci M, and Tarenzi L: Perioperative changes in functional residual capacity in morbidly obese patients, Br J Anaesth 60:574-578, 1988.
14. Bergman NA: Reduction in resting end-expiratory position of the respiratory system with induction of anesthesia and neuromuscular paralysis, Anesthesiology 57:14-17, 1982.
15. Hewlett AM, Hulands GH, Nunn JF, and Milledge JS: Functional residual capacity during anesthesia. II. Spontaneous respiration, Br J Anaesth 46:486-494, 1974.
16. Westbrook PR, Stubbs SE, Sessler AD, et al: Effects of anesthesia and muscle paralysis on respiratory mechanics in normal man, J Appl Physiol 34:81-86, 1973.
17. Rehder K, Marsh HM, Rodarte JR, and Hyatt RE: Airway closure, Anesthesiology 47:40-52, 1977.
18. Hickey RF, Visick WD, Fairley HB, and Fourcade HE: Effects of halothane anesthesia on functional residual capacity and alveolar-arterial oxygen tension difference, Anesthesiology 38:20-24, 1973.
19. Gilmour I, Burnham M, and Craig DB: Closing capacity measurement during general anesthesia, Anesthesiology 45:477-482, 1976.
20. Hedenstierna G, McCarthy G, and Bergström M: Airway closure during mechanical ventilation, Anesthesiology 44:114-123, 1976.
21. Juno P, Marsh HM, Knopp TJ, and Rehder K: Closing capacity in awake and anesthetized paralyzed man, J Appl Physiol 44:238-244, 1978.
22. Hedenstierna G and Santesson J: Airway closure during anesthesia: a comparison between resident gas and argon bolus techniques, J Appl Physiol 47:874-881, 1979.
23. Dueck R, Prutow RJ, Davies NJH, et al: The lung volume at which shunting occurs with inhalation anesthesia, Anesthesiology 69:854-861, 1988.
24. Hedenstierna G, Tokics L, Strandberg A, et al: Correlation of gas exchange impairment to development of atelectasis during anesthesia and muscle paralysis, Acta Anaesthesiol Scand 30:183-191, 1986.
25. Tokics L, Hedenstierna G, Brismar BO, et al: Thoracoabdominal restriction in supine men: CT and lung function measurements, J Appl Physiol 64:599-604, 1988.
26. Agostoni E: Mechanics of the pleural space, Physiol Rev 52:57-128, 1972.
27. Crawford ABH, Makowska M, and Engel LA: Effect of bronchomotor tone on static mechanical properties of lung and ventilation distribution, J Appl Physiol 63:2278-2285, 1987.
28. McAslan C, Mima M, Norden I, and Norlander O: Effects of halothane and methoxyflurane on pulmonary resistance to gas flow during lung bypass, Scand J Thorac Cardiovasc Surg 5:193-197, 1971.
29. Coon RL and Kampine JP: Hypocapnic bronchoconstriction and inhalation anesthetics, Anesthesiology 43:635-641, 1975.
30. Remolina C, Kahn AU, Santiago TV, and Edelman NH: Positional hypoxemia in unilateral lung disease, N Engl J Med 304:523-525, 1981.
31. Fishman AF: Down with the good lung, N Engl J Med 304:537-538, 1981.
32. Davies H, Kitchman R, Gordon I, and Helms P: Regional ventilation in infancy: reversal of adult pattern, N Engl J Med 313:1626-1628, 1985.
33. Shim C, Chun K, Williams MH, and Blaufox MD: Positional effects on distribution of ventilation in chronic obstructive pulmonary disease, Ann Intern Med 105:346-350, 1986.
34. Rehder K, Hatch DJ, Sessler AD, and Fowler WS: The function of each lung of anesthetized and paralyzed man during mechanical ventilation, Anesthesiology 37:16-26, 1972.
35. Landmark SJ, Knopp TJ, Rehder K, and Sessler AD: Regional pulmonary perfusion and V/Q in awake and anesthetized paralyzed man, J Appl Physiol 43:993-1000, 1977.
36. Nagasaka Y, Bhattacharya J, Nanjo S, et al: Micropuncture measurements of lung microvascular pressure profile during hypoxia in cats, Circ Res 54:90-95, 1984.
37. Marshall C and Marshall B: Influence of perfusate Po_2 on hypoxic pulmonary vasoconstriction in rats, Circ Res 52:691-696, 1983.
38. Bjertnaes LJ: Hypoxia-induced vasoconstriction in isolated perfused lungs exposed to injectable or inhalation anesthetics, Acta Anaesthesiol Scand 21:133-147, 1977.
39. Benumof JL and Wahrenbrock EA: Local effects of anesthetics on regional hypoxic pulmonary vasoconstriction, Anesthesiology 43:525-532, 1975.
40. Mathers J, Benumof JL, and Wahrenbrock EA: General anesthetics and regional hypoxic pulmonary vasoconstriction, Anesthesiology 46:111-114, 1977.
41. Marshall BE and Marshall C: Continuity of response to hypoxic pulmonary vasoconstriction, J Appl Physiol 49:189-196, 1980.
42. Marshall BE and Marshall C: Anesthesia and the pulmonary circulation. In Covino BG, Fozzard HA, Rehder K, and Stricharz GR, editors: Effects of anesthesia, Bethesda, Md, 1985, American Physiological Society, pp 121-136.
43. Mitchell RA: The regulation of respiration in metabolic acidosis and alkalosis. In Brooks CMC, Kao FF, and Lloyd BB, editors: Cerebrospinal fluid and the regulation of ventilation, Oxford, 1965, Blackwell Scientific Publishers, pp 109-131.
44. Biscoe TJ, Purves MJ, and Sampson SR: The frequency of nerve impulses in single carotid body chemoreceptor afferent fibers recorded in vivo with intact circulation, J Physiol (London) 208:121-131, 1970.
45. Knill RL and Clement JL: Ventilatory responses to acute metabolic acidemia in humans awake, sedated, and anesthetized with halothane, Anesthesiology 62:745-753, 1985.
46. Gross JB: Resting ventilation measurements may be misleading, Anesthesiology 61:110, 1984.

47. Knill RL: Wresting or resting ventilation, Anesthesiology 59:599-600, 1983.

48. Stremel RW, Huntsman DJ, Casaburi R, et al: Control of ventilation during intravenous CO_2 loading in the awake dog, J Appl Physiol 44:311-316, 1978.

49. Severinghaus J, Bainton CR, and Carcelen A: Respiratory insensitivity to hypoxia in chronically hypoxic man, Resp Physiol 1:308-334, 1966.

50. Hirshman CA, McCullough RE, and Weil JV: Normal values for hypoxic and hypercapnic ventilatory drives in man, J Appl Physiol 38:1095-1098, 1975.

51. Rebuck AS and Woodley WE: Ventilatory effects of hypoxia and their dependence on P_{CO_2}, J Appl Physiol 38:16-19, 1975.

52. Kronenberg RS, Hamilton FN, Gabel R, et al: Comparison of three methods for quantitating respiratory response to hypoxia, Respir Physiol 16:109-125, 1972.

53. Hickey RF and Severinghaus JW: Regulation of breathing: drug effects. In Hornbein TF, editor: Lung biology in health and disease: regulation of breathing, New York, 1978, BC Dekker, Inc, pp 1251-1312.

54. Pietak S, Weenig CS, Hickey RF, and Fairley HB: Anesthetic effects on ventilation in patients with chronic obstructive pulmonary disease, Anesthesiology 42:160-166, 1975.

55. Tusiewicz K, Bryan AC, and Froese AB: Contributions of changing rib cage—diaphragm interactions to the ventilatory depression of halothane anesthesia, Anesthesiology 47:327-337, 1977.

56. Lam AM, Clement JL, and Knill RL: Surgical stimulation does not enhance ventilatory chemoreflexes during enflurane anesthesia in man, Can Anaesth Soc J 27:22-28, 1980.

57. Weiskopf RB, Raymond LW, and Severinghaus JW: Effects of halothane on canine respiratory responses to hypoxia with and without hypercarbia, Anesthesiology 41:350-360, 1974.

58. Knill RL and Gelb AW: Ventilatory responses to hypoxia and hypercapnia during halothane sedation and anesthesia in man, Anesthesiology 49:244-251, 1978.

59. Knill RL, Manninen PH, and Clement JL: Ventilation and chemoreflexes during enflurane sedation and anaesthesia in man, Can Anaesth Soc J 26:353-360, 1979.

60. Knill RL, Kieraszewicz HT, and Dodgson BG: Chemical regulation of ventilation during isoflurane sedation and anaesthesia in humans, Can Anaesth Soc J 30:607-614, 1983.

61. Yacoub O, Doell D, Kryger MH, and Anthonisen NR: Depression of hypoxic ventilatory response by nitrous oxide, Anesthesiology 45:385-389, 1976.

62. Knill RL and Clement JL: Ventilatory responses to acute metabolic acidemia in humans awake, sedated, and anesthetized with halothane, Anesthesiology 62:745-753, 1985.

63. Hirshman CA, McCullough RE, Cowen PJ, and Weil JV: Effect of pentobarbitone on hypoxic ventilatory drive in man, Br J Anaesth 47:963-968, 1975.

64. Knill RL, Bright S, and Manninen P: Hypoxic ventilatory responses during thiopentone sedation and anesthesia in man, Can Anaesth Soc J 25:366-372, 1978.

65. Forrest WH Jr and Belleville JW: The effect of sleep plus morphine on the respiratory response to carbon dioxide, Anesthesiology 25:137-141, 1964.

66. Rigg JRA and Rondi P: Changes in rib cage and diaphragm contribution to ventilation after morphine, Anesthesiology 55:507-514, 1981.

67. Weil JV, McCullough RE, Kline JS, and Sodal IE: Diminished ventilatory response to hypoxia and hypercapnia after morphine in normal man, N Engl J Med 292:1103-1106, 1975.

68. Kryger MH, Yacoub O, Dosman J, et al: Effect of meperidine on occlusion pressure responses to hypercapnia and hypoxia with and without external inspiratory resistance, Am Rev Respir Dis 114:333-340, 1976.

69. Knill RL, Clement JL, and Thompson WR: Epidural morphine causes delayed and prolonged ventilatory depression, Can Anaesth Soc J 28:537-543, 1981.

70. Negre I, Gueneron J-P, Ecoffey C, et al: Ventilatory response to carbon dioxide after intramuscular and epidural fentanyl, Anesth Analg 66:707-710, 1987.

71. Koren G, Sandler AN, Klein J, et al: Relationship between the pharmacokinetics and the analgesic and respiratory pharmacodynamics of epidural sufentanil, Clin Pharmacol Ther 46:458-462, 1989.

72. Forster A, Gardaz J-P, Suter PM, and Gemperle M: Respiratory depression by midazolam and diazepam, Anesthesiology 53:494-497, 1980.

73. Gross JB, Smith L, and Smith TC: Time course of ventilatory response to carbon dioxide after intravenous diazepam, Anesthesiology 57:18-21, 1982.

74. Gross JB, Zebrowski ME, Carel WD, et al: Time course of ventilatory depression after thiopental and midazolam in normal subjects and in patients with chronic obstructive pulmonary disease, Anesthesiology 58:540-544, 1983.

75. Lakshminarayan S, Sahn SA, Hudson LD, and Weil JV: Effect of diazepam on ventilatory responses, Clin Pharmacol Ther 20:178-183, 1976.

76. Virtue RW, Alanis JM, Mori M, et al: An anesthetic agent: 2-orthochlorophenyl, 2-methylamino cyclohexanone, HCl (CI-581), Anesthesiology 28:823-833, 1967.

77. Soliman MG, Brindle GF, and Kuster G: Response to hypercapnia under ketamine anesthesia, Can Anaesth Soc J 22:486-494, 1975.

78. Hirshman CA, McCullough RE, Cohen PJ, and Weil JV: Hypoxic ventilatory drive in dogs during thiopental, ketamine, or pentobarbital anesthesia, Anesthesiology 43:628-634, 1975.

79. Bourke DL, Malit LA, and Smith TC: Respiratory interactions of ketamine and morphine, Anesthesiology 66:156-157, 1987.

80. Hamza J, Ecoffey C, and Gross JB: Ventilatory response to CO_2 following intravenous ketamine in children, Anesthesiology 70:422-425, 1989.

81. Staub NE, Nagand H, and Pearce ML: Pulmonary edema in dogs, especially the sequence of fluid accumulation in lungs, J Appl Physiol 22:227-240, 1967.

82. Aberman AD and Fulop M: The metabolic and respiratory acidosis of acute pulmonary edema, Ann Intern Med 76:173-184, 1972.

83. Lloyd JE, Nolop KB, Parker RE, et al: Effects of inspiratory resistance loading on lung fluid balance in awake sheep, J Appl Physiol 60:198-203, 1986.

84. Hansen TN, Gest AL, and Landers S: Inspiratory airway obstruction does not affect lung fluid balance in lambs, J Appl Physiol 58:1314-1318, 1985.

85. Roussos CS and Macklem PT: Diaphragmatic fatigue in man, J Appl Physiol 43:189-197, 1977.

86. Bazzy AR and Haddad GG: Diaphragmatic fatigue in unanesthetized adult sheep, J Appl Physiol 57:182-190, 1984.

87. D'Alonzo GE and Dantzker DR: Gas exchange alterations following pulmonary thromboembolism, Clin Chest Med 5:411-419, 1984.

88. Wagner PD, Dantzker DR, Iacovoni VE, et al: Ventilation-perfusion inequality in asymptomatic asthma, Am Rev Respir Dis 118:511-524, 1978.

89. Rodriguez-Roisin R, Ballester E, Roca J, et al: Mechanisms of hypoxemia in patients with status asthmaticus requiring mechanical ventilation, Am Rev Respir Dis 139:732-739, 1989.

90. Dantzker DR, Wagner PD, and West JB: Instability of lung units with low $\dot{V}_A/\dot{Q}$ ratios during O_2 breathing, J Appl Physiol 38:886-895, 1975.

91. Hunt JM, Chappel TR, Henrich WL, and Rubin LJ: Gas exchange during dialysis, Am J Med 77:255-260, 1984.

92. Pitcher WD, Diamond SM, and Henrich WL: Pulmonary gas exchange during dialysis in patients with obstructive lung disease, Chest 96:1136-1141, 1989.

93. Handt A, Farber MO, and Szwed JJ: Intradialytic measurement of cardiac output by thermodilution and impedance cardiography, Clin Nephrol 7:61-64, 1977.

94. Patterson RW, Nissenson AR, Miller J, et al: Hypoxemia and pulmonary gas exchange during hemodialysis, J Appl Physiol 50:259-264, 1981.

95. Sullivan SF, Patterson RW, and Papper EM: Post hyperventilation hypoxia, J Appl Physiol 22:431-435, 1967.

96. Melot C, Naeije R, Dechamps P, et al: Pulmonary and extrapulmonary contributors to hypoxemia in liver cirrhosis, Am Rev Respir Dis 139:632-640, 1989.

97. Edell ES, Cortese DA, Krowka MJ, and Rehder K: Severe hypoxemia and liver disease, Am Rev Respir Dis 140:1631-1635, 1989.

98. Rochester DF and Enson Y: Current concepts in the pathogenesis of obesity-hypoventilation syndrome: mechanical and circulatory factors, Am J Med 57:402-420, 1974.

99. Paul DR, Hoyt JL, and Boutros AR: Cardiovascular and respiratory changes in response to change of posture in the very obese, Anesthesiology 45:73-78, 1976.

100. 100. Vaughn RW and Wise L: Postoperative arterial blood gas measurement: effect of position on gas exchange, Ann Surg 182:705-709, 1975.

Chapter 10

Causes and Consequences of Arrhythmias

Roger L. Royster

The monitoring of cardiac rate and rhythm in the operating room during anesthesia and surgery has been a routine standard of care in this country for many years. A retrospective study suggests that electrocardiographic monitoring may be lifesaving in 1 of 3500 cases and shows through a risk-benefit analysis that electrocardiographic monitoring is indicated in all patients.[1] Thus monitoring abnormalities of cardiac rate and rhythm are an important indicator of either primary or secondary changes in cardiopulmonary function during the operative period.

For most patients, monitoring of cardiac rate and rhythm on a continuous basis first occurs during anesthesia and postanesthesia care. Anesthesiologists must be aware of the normal base-line variability in cardiac rate and rhythm in healthy unanesthetized persons to understand and recognize significant rate and rhythm changes that occur during anesthesia. Moreover, these changes (in cardiac rate and rhythm) may occur during anesthesia secondary to changes in the depth of anesthesia; to changes in autonomic balance; to direct effects of anesthetics, analgesics, muscle relaxants, and reversal agents; and to mechanical stimulation secondary to invasive procedures and surgical manipulation.

Frequently, patients with a history of cardiac arrhythmias require anesthesia and surgery. The number of patients with arrhythmias presenting for surgery is increasing because of a multitude of factors; the general population is aging, there is longer survival after myocardial infarction, improved emergency medical services increase out-of-hospital survival of sudden death, technologic advances provide surgical procedures for older and sicker patients, and improved monitoring techniques allow physicians greater ability to recognize and diagnose rhythm disturbances. Management of these patients during the preoperative, intraoperative, and postoperative periods requires basic knowledge of arrhythmia electrophysiology and antiarrhythmic pharmacology. Awareness of toxic side effects of antiarrhythmic therapy is of tremendous importance and may affect anesthetic management. Potential cofactors involved in arrhythmogenesis during anesthesia include electrolyte abnormalities, acid-base disturbances, hemodynamic alterations, and myocardial ischemia.

This chapter is a discussion of the incidence of cardiac arrhythmias during the unanesthetized and anesthetized states, the effects of anesthetic agents on arrhythmia generation, and the management of patients with a history of preoperative arrhythmias during the perioperative period.

I. INCIDENCE OF ARRHYTHMIAS
A. Healthy unanesthetized persons

Arrhythmias are common in normal, unanesthetized patients (Table 10-1). They occur frequently in healthy children,[2] women,[3,4] and men.[5,6] A study of 50 male medical students with 24-hour Holter monitoring during various activities revealed a 56% incidence of premature atrial contractions (PACs), 50% incidence of premature ventricular contractions (PVCs), with 12% having multifocal PVCs and 2% having ventricular tachycardia.[6] In a study of 80 healthy runners all under 40 years of age, 24-hour Holter monitoring revealed PVCs in 41 (50%) and PACs in 33 (41%).[7] There were two episodes of paired PVCs and one episode of nonsustained ventricular tachycardia (5 beats). There was no relationship between distances run and incidence of arrhythmias. Kantelip et al.[8] found in subjects over 80 years of age without cardiac disease that at least one PAC/hour occurred in 76% and at least one PVC/hour in 72%. The number of PVCs exceeded 10/hour in 32% and were multifocal in 18% of subjects. The frequency of arrhythmias in these older subjects surpassed the frequency found in other studies of younger subjects. Others have shown that PVCs increase with age,[3,9] with risk factors for coronary artery disease,[5] and with underlying myocardial disease.[5,10] The long-term prognosis in asymptomatic healthy subjects with frequent complex ventricular ectopy is similar to that of the general healthy population.[11]

B. Anesthetized patients

Arrhythmias are common during anesthesia and surgery (Table 10-2). Publications as early as 1911 have reported cardiac irregularities occurring during chloroform anesthesia.[12] Other

Table 10-1. Incidence of premature atrial and ventricular complexes in healthy, unanesthetized patients

Study	Year	Number (sex)	Age range (years)	Monitoring (hours)	PACs (percent)	PVCs (percent)
Scott et al.[2]	1980	131 (M)	10-13	48	13	26
Romhilt et al.[3]	1984	200 (F)	20-59	24	28	34
Sobotka et al.[4]	1981	50 (F)	22-28	24	64	54
Hinkle et al.[5]	1969	301 (M)	55 (median)	6	76	62
Brodsky et al.[6]	1977	50 (M)	23-27	24	56	50
Pilcher et al.[7]	1983	80 (MF)	31 (mean)	24	41	50
Kantelip et al.[8]	1986	50 (MF)	80-100	24	100	96
Kostis et al.[9]	1981	101 (MF)	16-68	24	—	39
Poblete et al.[10]	1978	30 (?)	47 (mean)	24	—	40

Table 10-2. Incidence of arrhythmias during anesthesia and surgery

Study	Year	Number	Arrhythmia (%)	Monitoring	Highest incidence related to
Dodd et al.	1961	569	29.9	Intermittent	Heart disease Intra-abdominal surgery
Vanik and Davis	1968	5013	17.9	Intermittent	Age Intubation Heart disease
Kuner et al.	1967	154	61.7	Holter	Neurologic, head and neck, thoracic surgery Intubation Surgery >3 hours
Bertrand et al.	1971	100	84.0	Holter	Intubation Extubation Heart disease

studies during the 1920s and 1930s documented cardiac arrhythmias during anesthesia and surgery.[13-15] More recent studies using visual inspection of continuous electrocardiographic monitoring (the most common type of clinical monitoring) have documented a high incidence of arrhythmias during anesthesia.[16,17] Vanik and Davis[16] reported that 901 of 5013 patients (18%) developed an arrhythmia. There was an increased incidence with increasing age, intubation, cyclopropane anesthesia, preoperative digitalis therapy, and anesthetic induction. Only 47 (1%) were considered serious. Dodd et al.[17] reported an incidence of arrhythmias of 29.9% in 569 patients. Incidence was higher in patients with preexisting heart disease and intra-abdominal surgery.

In studies of patients monitored with continuous electrocardiographic recordings (Holter monitoring) during anesthesia (Table 10-2), the incidence of arrhythmias is higher, between 60% and 80%. Kuner et al.[18] found an incidence of arrhythmias of 61.7% in 154 patients. Arrhythmias were more frequent in neurologic, thoracic, and head and neck procedures lasting 3 hours or longer. This analysis included any abnormality of cardiac rhythm including minor abnormalities, such as PACs, wandering atrial pacemaker, sinus bradycardia, and atrioventricular dissociation, and more severe arrhythmias, such as PVCs, atrial fibrillation, and ventricular tachycardia. However, the incidence of clinically significant cardiac arrhythmias was low. In their study of 100 patients, Bertrand et al.[19] found 84 patients had either a supraventricular or a ventricular arrhythmia. Arrhythmias were more common at the time of intubation and extubation, and ventricular arrhythmias were more common in patients with cardiac disease.

In summary, clinical studies have shown an increased incidence of cardiac arrhythmias in anesthetized patients who are tracheally intubated, breathing spontaneously, or treated with digitalis; who have a history of heart disease or preexisting arrhythmias; or whose surgery lasts longer than 3 hours. The incidence of clinically significant arrhythmias in these studies was less than 5%. However, the recognition and evaluation of patients with preexisting arrhythmia and organic heart disease, the knowledge of precipitating and aggravating factors during anesthesia and surgery, and the necessity of initiating therapy are important components of the perioperative anesthetic plan.

II. ARRHYTHMIC EFFECTS OF ANESTHETIC AGENTS
A. Mechanisms of arrhythmia generation*

The specific mechanisms involved in the generation of cardiac rhythm disturbances are fundamental to the development of specific antiarrhythmic therapy (List 10-1). Basic scientists have gained greater knowledge in understanding mechanisms of cardiac rhythm disturbances over the past several years, especially in the areas of abnormal automaticity and triggered activity.[20] Determination of the mechanism is helpful in the therapy of supraventricular arrhythmias; for example, sinus node and AV-node reentry are responsive to calcium-channel blockers, whereas automatic rhythms from the atrial and AV nodal are not so responsive to calcium-channel blockers. Moreover, definite

---

*Adapted from Royster RL and Robertie PG: Recognition and treatment of ectopic beats. In Thomas S, editor: Diagnosis and management of intraoperative arrhythmias, Anesthesiol Clin North Am 7:315-336, Philadelphia, 1989, WB Saunders Co.

Adapted from Royster RL and Robertie PR: Recognition and treatment of ectopic beats. In Thomas S, editor: Diagnosis and management of intraoperative arrhythmias, Anesthesiol Clin North Am 7:315-336, Philadelphia, 1989, WB Saunders Co.

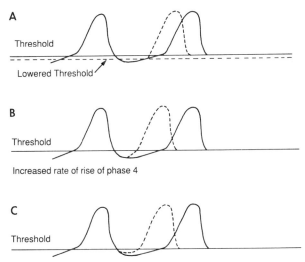

Fig. 10-1. Basic changes in normal electrophysiology of cardiac conducting cells such as lowered threshold potential, **A,** increased rate of rise of phase 4 of the action potential, **B,** and the presence of a less negative resting membrane potential, **C,** may result in the generation of an ectopic impulse. (From Royster RL and Robertie PG: Recognition and treatment of ectopic beats. In Thomas S, editor: Diagnosis and management of intraoperative arrhythmias, Anesthesiol Clin North Am 7:315, Philadelphia, 1989, WB Saunders Co.)

electrocardiographic clues help the anesthesiologist differentiate supraventricular reentry from automaticity. Determination of the mechanism in ventricular arrhythmias is difficult clinically, and therapy remains largely empirical. However, knowledge of likely clinical settings that correspond to certain mechanisms may lead to proper therapy for that mechanism (that is, early afterdepolarization—overdrive pacing). For the more serious student of arrhythmias, Atlee and Bosnjak[21] recently published a comprehensive review of the probable mechanisms of arrhythmias during anesthesia and surgery.

1. Normal automaticity. Normal automaticity with inherent diastolic depolarization is a property of the sinus node, atrial conduction fibers, areas of the AV nodal complex, and the His-Purkinje system. The rate of automatic depolarization decreases from the sinus node to the Purkinje system; thus all lower automatic cells are generally suppressed and are usually not responsible for ectopic beats but for escape rhythms. However, at lower heart rates and with enhanced intrinsic or extrinsic sympathetic stimulation, it is possible for a normal automatic cell to depolarize before overdrive suppression by a higher automatic focus, resulting in an ectopic complex. An extremely anxious or maximally sympathetically stimulated patient receiving a high-dose narcotic anesthetic that resulted in bradycardia would fulfill these criteria for normal automaticity–induced ectopic beats.

2. Abnormal automaticity. The characteristics of the action potential can be changed by cardiac disease, drug effect, or electrolyte ef-

fects. Theoretically, reduction in the threshold potential to a more negative value, increasing the rate of rise of phase 4 (spontaneous diastolic depolarization), and increasing the maximum diastolic potential (resting membrane potential) to a less negative value may lead to enhanced automaticity[22] (Fig. 10-1). It appears that a less negative resting membrane potential may be the most important of these effects. Less negative membrane potentials have been found in atrial cells, in patients with rheumatic and congenital heart disease, and in ventricular cells in areas of ischemia and infarction.[22] When the membrane potential reaches -60 mV, spontaneous depolarization may occur in atrial or ventricular fibers or Purkinje cells, probably through activation of the slow Ca^{++} channels.

3. Triggered automaticity (activity). A triggered ectopic beat differs from a truly automatic beat by requiring a preceding action potential for its generation.[23] This activity, occurring after depolarization is complete, may occur during phase 3 of repolarization and is called an "early afterdepolarization," or it may occur after repolarization is complete during phase 4,

Early Afterdepolarization

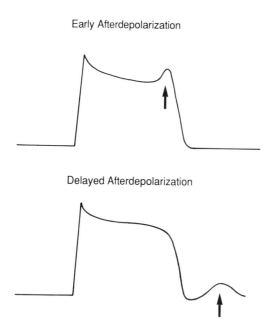

Delayed Afterdepolarization

Fig. 10-2. Triggered activity. The top action potential shows an abnormal stimulus, *arrow,* during phase 3 of repolarization. This depolarizing stimulus is called an "early afterdepolarization." The bottom action potential demonstrates a depolarizing current *arrow,* after repolarization is complete, a "late afterdepolarization." Etiology of these afterdepolarizations is discussed in the text. (From Royster RL and Robertie PG: Recognition and treatment of ectopic beats. In Thomas S, editor: Diagnosis and management of intraoperative arrhythmias, Anesthesiol Clin North Am 7:315, Philadelphia, 1989, WB Saunders.)

when it is called a "delayed afterdepolarization" (Fig. 10-2).

a. Early afterdepolarizations. Early afterdepolarizations are believed to occur because of a change in K^+ movement out of the cell during repolarization or to a permeability change to Na^+ or Ca^{++} movement into the cell. These action potential changes have been induced under a variety of conditions including hypokalemia, high concentrations of catecholamines, acidosis, hypoxia, and drugs that prolong repolarization like quinidine and procainamide.[24] Early afterdepolarizations also appear more likely during slow heart rates and are probably responsible for ventricular arrhythmias in the prolonged Q-T syndrome (that is, torsade de pointes).[25]

b. Delayed afterdepolarizations. Delayed afterdepolarizations appear primarily mediated by increases in intracellular Ca^{++}.[23] This can occur by inhibition of the Na^+-K^+ pump[26] (digitalis and hypomagnesemia), an increased serum Ca^{++} level,[27] stimulation of receptor-operated channels[28] (catecholamines), and failure to

pump Ca^{++} out of the cell (ischemia).[29] Delayed afterdepolarizations have been demonstrated in normal canine coronary sinus tissue[30] and in atrial tissue and ventricular specialized conducting tissue from normal and diseased hearts exposed to toxic concentrations of digitalis.[31]

4. Reentry. Reentry is the classic mechanism of ectopic beat formation. Prerequisites for reentry are an available circuit, a difference in refractory periods of two limbs of the circuit, and conduction somewhere in the circuit sufficiently slow to allow the remainder of the circuit to recover responsiveness.[32]

Normally, the conducting impulse of the heart driven by sinus rhythm dies out after sequential activation of the atria and ventricles because it is surrounded by refractory tissue that it has recently excited. But in disease states, differences in refractoriness of tissue and slow conduction may be present, setting up a perfect substrate for reentry formation. This is especially true in Purkinje fibers because of their arborization in the distal conducting system of the ventricle, which sets up a suitable anatomic network for reentry.[32]

Larger anatomic circuits may exist in the sinus node, AV node, accessory pathways, venae cavae, and ventricular aneurysms and may lead to reentry. The prototypical example of reentry is patients with preexcitation syndromes, using atrial muscle, the AV node, ventricular muscle, and the accessory pathway for the reentry circuit. The AV node also demonstrates dual pathways with different refractory periods and conduction velocities, which may lead to AV nodal reentry arrhythmias.[33]

5. Reflection. Reflection is a form of reentry that occurs in a single fiber and does not require a distinct, circuitous loop as in classic reentry.[34] Reflection may occur because of abnormal refractoriness of adjacent areas in an individual Purkinje fiber. This process, termed "longitudinal dissociation," essentially isolates areas of conducting tissue with different refractoriness, potentially allowing recovered tissue to reexcite.[34] Reflection is also believed to occur in areas of ischemic and possibly infarcted conducting tissue, which can transmit depolarizing current (functioning as a passive conduit) without depolarizing.[35] When excitable tissue is reached, depolarization may again occur, with a return of the depolarizing current across this inexcitable segment to reexcite the conducting tissue that originated the depolarizing current.[35]

6. Parasystole. A parasystole is usually a ventricular automatic focus possibly caused by either normal automaticity, abnormal automatic-

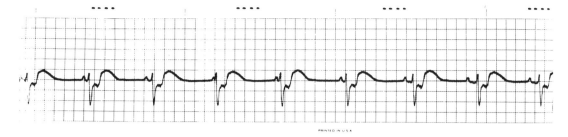

Fig. 10-3. Isorhythmic atrioventricular dissociation. This arrhythmia frequently occurs during inhalational anesthesia and is attributable to an autonomic imbalance resulting in similar intrinsic rates of the sinus rhythm and an AV escape nodal rhythm. Although usually benign, this arrhythmia may result in hemodynamic compromise in patients with reduced ventricular compliance. Modes of therapy include (1) reduction of the inhalational anesthetic, (2) atropine, (3) succinylcholine, 10 to 20 mg, and (4) small doses of beta-adrenergic receptor blockers.

ity, or triggered activity.[36] This ectopic focus resists overdrive suppression from higher pacemaker cells with faster intrinsic rates. This requires some form of protection surrounding the parasystolic focus, possibly caused by a unidirectional entrance block but not exit block.[37] This allows the parasystole to exit and depolarize the ventricles without allowing depolarization currents to enter and suppress it. Occasionally there may be forms of exit block that cause the parasystole to be intermittent.[38] Therefore a parasystole represents both abnormal impulse generation and abnormal conduction.

B. Inhalational anesthetics (halothane, enflurane, isoflurane)

All inhalational anesthetics have significant electrophysiologic effects. Although the presently used inhalational agents generally decrease sinus rate in awake and anesthetized animals,[39] the effect in humans may be altered by autonomic reflexes. In patients, isoflurane and enflurane generally increase the sinus rate, whereas halothane causes no change or mild depression of the sinus rate. In animals, halothane and enflurane significantly prolong AV nodal conduction with minimal prolongation, if at all, by isoflurane.[40] Also in this study, His-Purkinje conduction with all three agents was minimally prolonged but statistically significant. Recently, Scheffer et al.[41] reported the first study of the basic electrophysiologic effects of halothane in humans. In patients breathing 2 MAC halothane and oxygen, the sinus rate decreased, AV nodal conduction times were prolonged, and the His-Purkinje conduction time did not change.

A very common rhythm disturbance with these agents is isorhythmic AV dissociation (Fig. 10-3), which occurs when an AV nodal pacemaker assumes control of the heart rhythm at a slightly faster rate than the sinus node.[42] This probably occurs because of a greater autonomic effect (vagal) on the sinus node by the inhalation agents as catecholamine stimulation increases the automatic rate of the latent pacemaker in the AV node. Isorhythmic AV dissociation is generally a benign rhythm disturbance, but in patients with noncompliant hypertrophied ventricles who are more dependent on atrial contraction for ventricular filling, this rhythm can cause severe hemodynamic compromise.[43] Reduction of the level of anesthesia, or administration of atropine,[43] small doses of succinylcholine,[44] or small doses of beta-adrenergic receptor blockers[45,46] are reported to convert AV dissociation back to sinus rhythm.

Many clinical events and pharmacologic agents may interact with inhalation agents to produce arrhythmias (List 10-2). The inhala-

---

List 10-2. Precipitating Events and Agents Associated with Halothane-Induced Arrhythmias

---

Clinical events
  Hypoxia   Tachycardia
  Hypercapnia   Hypertension
  Fasting
Agents
  Thiopental   Cocaine
  Ketamine   Exogenous catecholamines and
  Succinylcholine   mines and
  Atropine   vasopressors
  Pancuronium and   Aminophylline
    tricyclics   Nitrous oxide

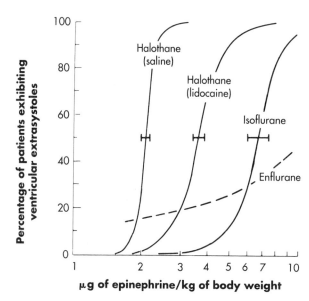

Fig. 10-4. Inhalational anesthetic-epinephrine interaction. The number of patients having premature ventricular contractions (PVCs) versus the submucosal epinephrine dose during inhalational anesthesia. The submucosal dose of epinephrine required to elicit three or more PVCs in 50% of patients was 2.1 μg/kg for halothane, 6.7 μg/kg for isoflurane, and 10.9 μg/kg for enflurane. When lidocaine was added to the epinephrine, the arrhythmic dose was greater in halothane-anesthetized patients. It is suggested that the safe dose of epinephrine during inhalational anesthesia is 1 μg/kg; this may be higher in children. (From Johnston RR, Eger EI II, and Wilson C: Anesth Analg 55:709, 1976.)

tional agents themselves are probably not arrhythmogenic, but when combined with increased catecholamine stimulation (from hypercapnia,[47] hypoxia,[48] hypertension and tachycardia,[49] light anesthesia, and so forth) or the administration of exogenous catecholamines[50,51] or aminophylline,[52,53] arrhythmias, especially PVCs, may result. In a frequently quoted study, Johnston et al.[54] found that the submucosal dose of epinephrine needed to produce ventricular arrhythmias in 50% of adult patients was 2.1 μg/kg with halothane, 3.7 μg/kg halothane with lidocaine, 6.7 μg/kg with isoflurane, and 10.9 μg/kg with enflurane (Fig. 10-4). Children may be more resistant to catecholamine-induced arrhythmias[55] and may tolerate 10 μg/kg epinephrine subcutaneously during halothane anesthesia without arrhythmias.

C. Intravenous anesthetics

1. Thiopental. Thiopental may result in no change or slight reduction in the heart rate because it does not completely suppress baroreceptor reflexes.[56] Thiopental potentiates epi-

nephrine-induced arrhythmias with halothane, enflurane, and isoflurane in animal studies.[57,58] However, thiopental does not appear to produce clinically significant arrhythmias in humans.

2. Ketamine. Ketamine may increase the heart rate based on its sympathomimetic effects. Ketamine also potentiates epinephrine-induced arrhythmias during halothane administration in animal studies[59] but makes digitalis-toxic arrhythmias less likely in animals.[60] Ketamine, like thiopental, does not produce clinically significant arrhythmias in man. The arrhythmogenic effects of other intravenous anesthetic agents, such as etomidate, the benzodiazepines, and propofol, also appear clinically insignificant. However, propofol is reported to cause bradycardia in some patients.[61]

D. Local anesthetics

1. Bupivacaine cardiotoxicity. Although most local anesthetics possess antiarrhythmic activity because of sodium-channel blocking effects, bupivacaine and etidocaine in toxic doses have apparent clinical ventricular arrhythmogenic activity.[62] Animal studies demonstrate multiple arrhythmic effects, including PR and Q-T interval prolongation, QRS widening, AV block, and ventricular tachycardia and fibrillation[63] (Fig. 10-5). The cause of bupivacaine-induced ventricular arrhythmias is unclear. The recovery time of blocked sodium channels with bupivacaine is almost 10 times that of lidocaine.[64] This prolongation of repolarization may lead to a long Q-T interval syndrome; torsade de pointes is reported in animals given toxic doses of bupivacaine.[63] Bupivacaine causes a 50% prolongation of the Q-T interval at a lower concentration than any other local anesthetic.[65] Successful resuscitation with CPR, epinephrine, and lidocaine for arrhythmia control in humans has been reported.[66,67] Animal studies suggest that bretylium may be more effective than lidocaine and may raise the ventricular tachycardia threshold lowered by bupivacaine.[68] Recently, magnesium sulfate suppressed bupivacaine-induced cardiac arrhythmias in an animal study.[69] Acidosis and hypoxia enhance the arrhythmogenic effects and increase the mortality of sheep given intravenous bupivacaine[70] and should be especially avoided in patients likely to have high serum levels of bupivacaine.

E. Opioids

All the opioids slow the heart rate by central vagal stimulation[71,72] or suppression of sympathetic activity,[73] except for meperidine,[74] which

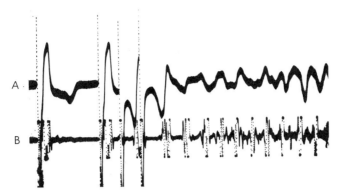

Fig. 10-5. Bupivacaine-induced ventricular fibrillation. **A,** Surface ECG. **B,** Intra-aortic electrogram during programed stimulation of PVCs in the dog. Programed stimulation did not produce ventricular fibrillation in 7 dogs before bupivacaine but did produce ventricular fibrillation in 4 dogs after 2 mg/kg bupivacaine given intravenously.

has anticholinergic effects. Fentanyl, besides slowing the rate of sinus node discharge, also prolongs AV nodal conduction and AV nodal and ventricular refractoriness.[75] There are case reports of AV nodal block and asystole with fentanyl and sufentanil.[76,77] This generalized depression of the conducting system is supported by a canine study that revealed that the incidence of ventricular tachyarrhythmias in fentanyl-anesthetized dogs was less than that in dogs anesthetized with inhalational agents.[78] Additionally, fentanyl increases the ventricular fibrillation threshold in dogs by sympathetic inhibition rather than by vagotonic effects.[79] On the other hand, morphine significantly raises ventricular fibrillation thresholds by increased vagal activity.[72] The suppression of PACs elicited by programmed stimulation by fentanyl has also been reported.[80] All these studies suggest that opioid-based anesthesia may be advantageous in patients with significant cardiac arrhythmias.

F. Neuromuscular relaxants

1. Succinylcholine. Most muscle relaxants, except succinylcholine and pancuronium, have little effect on cardiac rhythm. Succinylcholine causes a bradycardia secondary to vagotonic effects probably induced by succinylmonocholine,[81] especially after repeated doses in children. It can precipitate ventricular fibrillation (List 10-3) secondary to increases in serum K^+ in burn patients, neurologically injured patients, denervated patients, and patients with multiple trauma.[82] Also, succinylcholine has been reported to cause many other rhythm disturbances, including AV dissociation.[83] Succinylcholine reportedly decreases the threshold of

---

List 10-3. Succinylcholine-Associated Arrhythmias

Sinus bradycardia (repeated doses)
Atrioventricular dissociation
Atrioventricular block and asystole (combined with intravenous induction agents and narcotics)
Ventricular arrhythmias (acute hyperkalemia)
  Burns
  Multiple trauma
  Quadriplegia, paraplegia (spinal cord injury)
  Muscular dystrophy
  Hemiparesis (stroke)
  Closed head injury
  Multiple sclerosis
  Prolonged bed confinement?
    (Muscle disuse, such as Guillain-Barré syndrome, critically ill patients)

---

catecholamine-induced ventricular arrhythmias. Several cases of AV nodal block and asystole have also been reported with combinations of sufentanil and alfentanil with succinylcholine.[76,84] However, all these case reports involved the addition of barbiturates or benzodiazepines to the anesthetic induction sequence. Others have shown that rapid-sequence techniques with *only* sufentanil and succinylcholine result either in no change or in increased heart rate.[85]

2. Pancuronium. Pancuronium increases heart rate and shortens AV nodal conduction time[86] because of vagolysis[87] and possible catecholamine release.[88] Pancuronium has been reported to cause PACs and severe ventricular arrhythmias in combination with halothane and

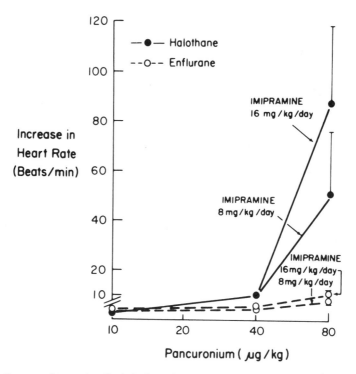

Fig. 10-6. Pancuronium, tricyclic, halothane interaction. In animals fed imipramine (a tricyclic antidepressant compound), extreme increases in heart rate occurred during halothane anesthesia, *closed circles,* after 0.08 μg/kg pancuronium compared to minimal changes in heart rate during enflurane anesthesia, *open circles,* and pancuronium. (From Edwards RP, Miller RD, Roizen MF, et al: Anesthesiology 50:421, 1979.)

tricyclic antidepressants.[89] In an important study stimulated by two patients with severe tachyarrhythmias, pancuronium and halothane in dogs given tricyclics caused worse tachycardia and ventricular arrhythmias than in other dogs receiving pancuronium, enflurane, and tricyclics[89] (Fig. 10-6). In the animals that developed arrhythmias, there was a pronounced increase in serum norepinephrine levels. The pancuronium-halothane combination should be avoided in patients receiving these antidepressant drugs. The mechanism of pancuronium-associated arrhythmias was addressed by Jacobs et al.,[90] who demonstrated delayed afterdepolarizations and abnormal automaticity in isolated papillary muscle fibers exposed to concentrations of pancuronium and epinephrine.

3. Vecuronium. Vecuronium has been reported to cause bradycardia requiring treatment when combined with high dose opioids.[91] Other cases of transient asystole[92] and even cardiac arrest[93,94] after vecuronium administration have been reported when vecuronium was combined with pharmacologic agents or intraoperative reflexes that increase vagal tone.

Table 10-3. Incidence of arrhythmias after muscle relaxant reversal with atropine-edrophonium in fentanyl-based (group 1) or isoflurane-based (group 2) anesthesia

Arrhythmias	Group 1	Group 2
None	8*	19
Severe	8*	3
Second and third degree AV block	6*	
Ventricular dysrhythmia	1	1
Heart rate <40 bpm	1	1
Moderate	7	4
Sinus bradycardia	4	3
First-degree AV block	3	1
Mild	3	3
Junctional rhythm	2	3
P-wave change	1	0

Adapted from Urquhart ML, Ramsey FM, Royster RL, et al: Anesthesiology 67:561-565, 1987.
*P <0.01 between group 1 and group 2.

G. Reversal agents

1. Naloxone. Naloxone has caused ventricular tachycardia and fibrillation,[95] in addition to myocardial ischemia, tachycardia, hypertension, and pulmonary edema, during reversal of nonoverdose, opioid-induced sedation and respiratory depression. A sudden increase in sympathomimetic stimulation after opioid withdrawal is hypothesized as the cause. If naloxone is required, very small doses (1 $\mu g/kg$ IV) should be titrated to effect to avoid the surge in sympathetic tone that may cause the arrhythmias.

2. Muscle-relaxant reversal. Arrhythmias with atropine-edrophonium reversal of neuromuscular blockade are reported to occur in 36% to 57% of patients.[96,97] Atropine-glycopyrrolate reversal induced arrhythmias in 53% of patients.[96] In a study of 55 patients after atropine-edrophonium reversal in either fentanyl-based or isoflurane-based anesthesia, there was a significantly higher incidence of arrhythmias in the fentanyl group (mainly transient AV nodal block).[98] Five patients required therapy. However, all types of atrial, nodal, and ventricular arrhythmias occurred, but none were of clinical consequence (Table 10-3).

Cholinesterase inhibitors without anticholinergics cause slowing of SA node and AV node conduction and may result in sinus arrest and AV nodal block.[99] Small doses of edrophonium have been used in treatment of sinus tachycardia and paroxysmal supraventricular tachycardia. Physostigmine administration has reportedly caused atrial fibrillation in a patient recovering from general anesthesia.[100] Small and large doses of atropine have caused AV dissociation.[101] Ventricular arrhythmias with atropine administration have occurred during inhalational anesthesia.[102]

H. Arrhythmias induced by anesthetics and surgical procedures

Cardiac arrest may occur during spinal anesthesia. Caplan et al.[102] reported that in 14 healthy patients who sustained cardiac arrest central nervous system depression and cyanosis resulting in respiratory compromise was the likely cause of cardiac arrest and not cardiac arrhythmias. High spinal anesthesia may also block sympathetic input to the heart and result in bradycardia. Asystole has been reported during spinal anesthesia in a patient with sick sinus syndrome.[103]

As previously mentioned, endotracheal intubation is associated with arrhythmias because of reflex sympathetic stimulation.[104] One report found PVCs in 18% of patients[105] during intubation. Very anxious patients with high catecholamine levels who present for anesthetic induction may be especially sensitive to the stimulus of intubation. Intravenous narcotics, lidocaine, or beta-adrenergic receptor blockers blunt the cardiovascular responses to intubation and may decrease the incidence of arrhythmias.

Insertion of central vascular catheters may also cause arrhythmias. The process of gaining venous access for central venous catheter insertion with the use of an intravenous guidewire may cause arrhythmias[106] if the guidewire is inserted too far into the heart. Furthermore, pulmonary artery catheter insertion frequently causes atrial and ventricular arrhythmias.[107] These mechanically stimulated ectopic beats generally are not suppressed with antiarrhythmics.[108] Manipulation of the catheter to prevent coiling in a cardiac chamber and repositioning is the proper response. The sudden onset of arrhythmias at any time after insertion should also arouse one's suspicions of a malpositioned catheter.[109]

Numerous surgically induced reflexes and manipulations may cause cardiac arrhythmias. An intrathoracic noncardiac procedure with manual cardiac irritation by the surgeon may lead to arrhythmias. Peritoneal traction, tracheal traction, brainstem compression, and compression of the eye (oculocardiac reflex) may result in either sympathetic- or parasympathetic-mediated arrhythmias. The proper response is to alert the surgeon to discontinue the surgical manipulation, which usually controls the arrhythmia.

III. PATIENTS WITH ARRHYTHMIAS PRESENTING FOR ANESTHESIA AND SURGERY

A. Preoperative evaluation

Patients with a preoperative history of cardiac arrhythmias require a thorough cardiac preoperative evaluation including specific discussion of the arrhythmia history and the type of antiarrhythmic medication. Precipitating or aggravating factors should be discussed. Relief or lack of relief of symptoms such as palpitations, dizziness, or syncope may be a sign of successful therapy or failure of therapy. Other cardiac symptoms such as dyspnea, angina, or syncope may indicate worsening of associated cardiac disease. Goldman et al.[110] have demonstrated that any cardiac rhythm other than sinus rhythms, PACs, and greater than 5 PVCs per minute on preoperative evaluation are directly related to perioperative cardiac morbidity. Arrhythmias are frequently a marker of associated cardiac disease (ischemic, valvular, cardiomyopathic, and so forth) and treatment of decompensated cardiac disease preoperatively frequently aids in arrhythmia control in the perioperative period.

All patients should have an electrocardiogram with rhythm strip before surgery. The electrocardiogram can yield information about worsening ischemic disease (ST-segment analysis, new Q waves), possible electrolyte abnormalities, and Q-T interval changes secondary to antiarrhythmic therapy (proarrhythmic effects). A prolonged rhythm strip will give some base-line information on arrhythmia frequency before surgery. Occasionally, preoperative 24-hour Holter monitoring is indicated, especially if symptoms worsen, to allow one to assess adequacy of therapy and stabilization of arrhythmic events. For example, a patient has previously controlled bursts of nonsustained ventricular tachycardia every 2 minutes before surgery; this is a sign of electrical instability that may warrant further antiarrhythmic therapy or additional therapy of underlying cardiac disease. A more recent electrographic technique developed for patients with arrhythmias is signal-averaged electrocardiography.[111] This electrocardiogram is a computer-based process that eliminates nonrepeating random noise and averages multiple samples of repetitive wave forms to demonstrate periods of late depolarization occurring through slowly conducting tissue at the terminal end of the QRS complex.[112] These "late potentials" have been demonstrated in patients with ventricular tachycardia, and the elimination of late potentials correlates with successful antiarrhythmic therapy.[112] Lastly, lack of arrhythmia control and electrical instability preoperatively may require electrophysiologic testing with intravenous drug trials and programed stimulation. Most of these questions can be addressed by a thought-provoking cardiology consultation with arrhythmia specialists.

Other preoperative laboratory evaluations should include measurement of serum K^+ and Mg^{++} concentrations, antiarrhythmic drug concentration if available, and a chest roentgenogram when structural cardiac disease is present. Many patients with arrhythmias and congestive heart failure require diuretics and digitalis preparations. Diuretic-induced hypokalemia and hypomagnesemia are common.[113] Diuretic therapy in hypertensive disease is associated with a higher mortality secondary to diuretic-induced electrolyte disturbances and arrhythmias.[113] However, since K^+ and Mg^{++} are the two major intracellular ions, normal serum concentrations may not correlate with total body or tissue concentrations of these ions.[114] Digitalis-induced arrhythmias are also more likely in the presence of hypokalemia and hypomagnesemia.[114] Digitalis levels before surgery may be helpful to prevent digitalis-toxic arrhythmias and symptoms in the postoperative period. Digitalis toxicity is common in hospitalized patients.[115] Other drug concentrations of antiarrhythmics such as procainamide and its active metabolite (N-acetyl procainamide) are helpful in the assessment of adequate therapeutic or toxic concentrations before surgery.

The continuation of all cardiac antiarrhythmic medication until the time of surgery is important for perioperative arrhythmia control. An increase in arrhythmia frequency and difficulties in arrhythmia control because of the stress of the perioperative period caused by release of catecholamines should be anticipated. Thus adequate preoperative anxiety control with or without sedative-hypnotic agents as indicated is of utmost importance as with any preoperative preparation.

B. Causes and consequences of supraventricular arrhythmias

1. Premature atrial contractions. The causes of premature atrial contractions (PACs) during anesthesia and surgery may include any of the mechanisms previously discussed involving any of the supraventricular structures (SA node, atrial tissue, AV node). However, atrial tissue ectopic activity itself accounts for most premature supraventricular beats. Clinical causes of PACs include ischemic heart disease, congestive heart failure from ischemic or valvular heart disease increasing left atrial dimensions, electrolyte abnormalities, acid-base problems, hypoxemia, drug effects, autonomic imbalance, stress primarily from catecholamine stimulation, surgical manipulations, and central line insertion. In patients with AV nodal reentry and accessory pathways connecting atrial to ventricular, premature atrial depolarization may occur secondary to retrograde conduction depolarizing the atria from an AV nodal to SA nodal direction, which creates an inverted P wave on the electrocardiogram.[116] This may precipitate sustained paroxysmal supraventricular tachycardia (PSVT). The PAC is the primary stimulus for most supraventricular arrhythmias such as PSVT, atrial fibrillation, atrial flutter, and multifocal atrial tachycardia[116] (Fig. 10-7). Thus preventing the PAC from occurring provides preventive therapy for supraventricular arrhythmias.

The key to diagnosis of PACs is locating the P wave.[117] Lead II or V_1 is usually best for P-wave determination. Depending on the degree of prematurity of the atrial contraction, the P

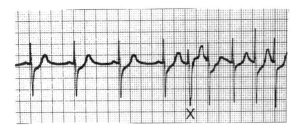

Fig. 10-7. Premature atrial contraction (PAC) resulting in atrial fibrillation. Notice the changes in T-wave morphology from the normal T-waves before and after QRS X, representing PACs in the T-waves. The premature QRS X has a different morphology from the normal QRS complexes illustrating aberrant ventricular conduction. (From Royster RL and Robertie PG: Recognition and treatment of ectopic beats. In Thomas S, editor: Diagnosis and management of intraoperative arrhythmias, Anesthesiol Clin North Am 7:315-336, Philadelphia, 1989, WB Saunders.)

Table 10-4. Differences in aberrantly conducted premature atrial complexes and premature ventricular complexes.

Aberrant conduction (PACs)	PVCs
Preceding P waves	P waves absent
RBBB* pattern common	RBBB* pattern uncommon
Initial deflection of QRS identical to normal QRS	Initial QRS deflection may differ from normal QRS
QRS width >0.12 sec	QRS width >0.14 sec
Noncompensatory pause	Compensatory pause
In atrial fibrillation, varying coupling intervals	In atrial fibrillation, constant coupling intervals

Adapted from Royster RL and Robertie PR: Recognition and treatment of ectopic beats. In Thomas S, editor: Diagnosis and management of intraoperative arrhythmias, Anesthesiol Clin North Am 7:315-336, Philadelphia, 1989, WB Saunders Co.
*RBBB, Right bundle branch block.

wave may occasionally be located within the T wave, slightly altering the basic T wave morphology (Fig. 10-4). The shape of the P wave is usually different from that of the sinus P wave, being almost identical when the premature focus is near the sinus node, or being inverted when the focus is near the atrioventricular groove. The origin of PACs may be either right or left atrial tissue, and because the spread of atrial depolarization proceeds in all direc-

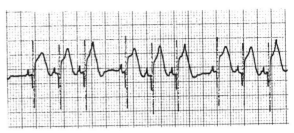

Fig. 10-8. Blocked premature atrial contractions (PACs). Notice the peaked T-wave configuration before the pauses compared to the preceding T-wave morphology. PACs are blocked at the AV node because of their severe prematurity causing depolarization to enter the AV node during its effective refractory period.

tions, the sinus node is usually depolarized prematurely and reset to the intrinsic sinus rate. Therefore, the interval after the PAC is equal to the intrinsic P-P interval of the sinus rhythm.

The QRS complex with PACs usually appears normal; however, as the degree of prematurity of a PAC increases, the pathway taken through the intraventricular conduction system may become abnormal or *aberrant*[118] because areas of the distal conducting system have yet to repolarize. The most proximal portion of the right bundle branch is usually the last part of the ventricular conduction system to repolarize; therefore the conduction will proceed down the left bundle, yielding a QRS complex resembling a right bundle branch block. Aberrantly conducted PACs are also common in atrial fibrillation. It is important to distinguish aberrancy from the wide QRS complex of premature ventricular complexes. Table 10-4 lists some distinguishing features of aberrantly conducted premature supraventricular complexes and premature ventricular complexes. Very premature atrial contractions may block at the level of the AV node and fail to conduct to the ventricle, creating a pause in the QRS cycle (Fig. 10-8).

The class IA antiarrhythmics have atrial electrophysiologic properties suitable for the treatment of premature supraventricular beats. Intravenous procainamide is suitable for the perioperative period to suppress ectopic atrial foci. Additionally, procainamide is effective in converting atrial fibrillation to sinus rhythm, further supporting its antiarrhythmic properties on atrial tissue.[119] Digitalis has been classically used in suppressing atrial arrhythmias; however, its major benefit is slowing AV node conduction and fast ventricular response after supraventricular tachyarrhythmias arise.[120] Beta-adrenergic receptor blockers also may aid in the therapy of premature atrial beats associated with high autonomic states or increased catecholamine levels.[121] Verapamil may be especially helpful in preventing premature nodal beats that result from AV nodal reentry, since verapamil is effective in converting AV nodal reentry supraventricular tachycardia to sinus rhythm.[122]

2. Paroxysmal supraventricular tachycardia. Paroxysmal supraventricular tachycardias (PSVTs) originate suddenly in the anatomic structures of the supraventricular area: the sinus node, atrial muscle, AV node, and accessory AV connection.[116] Sinus node, AV node, and accessory AV connection tachycardias are usually attributable to a reentry mechanism, whereas primary atrial tachycardias may be either reentry or some form of automaticity.[116] The QRS complexes may be narrow or wide, and wide complex supraventricular tachycardia must be differentiated from ventricular tachycardia.[123] A basic approach to diagnosis of supraventricular tachyarrhythmias is shown in List 10-4. An adequate 12-lead electrocardiogram with an accompanying rhythm strip compared to preceding electrocardiograms is essential for diagnosis of supraventricular arrhythmias. An esophageal lead or intracardiac electrogram may give additional valuable information for diagnosing supraventricular arrhythmias.

a. Sinus node reentry. Sinus node reentry is an uncommon form of PSVT, occurring in less than 2% of patients.[116,117] P-wave morphology is *identical* to sinus P-wave morphology (List 10-5), with the important differential factor being the sudden onset of tachycardia. Carotid sinus massage may terminate the tachycardia because the sinus node is under vagal innervation. In addition, sinus node depolarization is primarily calcium dependent; verapamil, 75 μg/kg given slowly, or beta blockers may be effective in conversion (Fig. 10-9). Sinus node reentry primarily occurs in patients with ischemic heart disease.

b. Atrial tachycardia. Atrial tachycardias, comprising approximately 8% of PSVTs, result from either an ectopic automatic focus or a reentry pathway.[116,117] Atrial tachycardias have a P-wave morphology *different* from that of the P wave in sinus rhythm (List 10-5). This arrhythmia is true paroxysmal "atrial" tachycardia, which previously was the common term to describe all PSVTs. Like multifocal atrial tachycardia (a variant), atrial tachycardia can be very difficult to treat. Carotid sinus massage and verapamil may slow the ventricular response and cause AV nodal block, but conversion is rare. Therapy is aimed at the underlying process,

---

List 10-4. Basic Approach to Diagnosis of Tachyarrhythmias

What is the rate?
1. Ventricular rates of 150 beats/min frequently represent atrial flutter with 2:1 AV block.
2. Any ventricular rate greater than 200 beats/min in an adult patient is suggestive of an accessory AV connection.

Rhythm: regular or irregular?
1. An irregular ventricular response is highly suggestive of atrial fibrillation.
2. Atrial flutter with variable AV conduction or atrial tachycardias with variable AV block also cause an irregular rhythm (such as multifocal atrial tachycardia).

P waves: present or absent?
1. The presence of P waves indicates a supraventricular tachycardia.
2. P-wave morphology is compared to sinus P-wave morphology (see List 10-5).
3. The absence of P waves is consistent with a supraventricular tachycardia or ventricular tachycardia.
4. If P waves are not visible on a rhythm strip, then an esophageal lead, a saline bridge, or an intracardiac electrogram may give further information on atrial activity.

QRS complex: narrow or wide?
1. A narrow QRS complex (<0.12 sec) is indicative of a supraventricular tachyarrhythmia.
2. A wide QRS (>0.12 sec) complex indicates either a supraventricular or a ventricular tachycardia.
3. Wide QRS complexes occur with a supraventricular tachycardia when a preexisting bundle branch block, aberrant ventricular conduction, or an accessory AV connection resulting in preexcitation of the ventricle is present.
4. Ventricular tachycardia is suggested by a QRS complex duration >0.14 sec.

QRS axis: normal or abnormal?
1. A severe left-axis deviation (−60° to −120°) during the tachycardia is suggestive of a ventricular origin.
2. Supraventricular tachycardias usually maintain a normal axis.

Ventricular tachycardia is distinguished from supraventricular tachycardia by the following criteria: a QRS duration >0.14 sec, left-axis deviation, a monophasic positive QRS complex in lead V_1, and AV dissociation.

1. P waves are absent (usually within QRS)

   AV node reentry

2. P waves are positive, inferior leads, preceding the QRS
   a. Identical morphology to sinus node P waves

      SA node reentry

   b. Morphology different from that of sinus P waves

      Intra-atrial reentry or automaticity

3. P waves inverted, before or after the QRS

   AV node reentry or
   AV accessory connection

PSVT   HR = 153

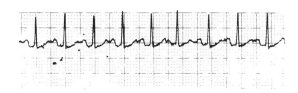

Post Esmolol   100 mg IV, HR = 110

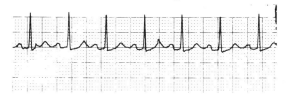

Fig. 10-9. Sinoatrial (SA) node reentry tachycardia. The sudden (paroxysmal) onset of a supraventricular tachyarrhythmia (PSVT) at a heart rate (HR) of 153 beats/min that suddenly converted to a heart rate of 110 after intravenous administration of 100 mg of esmolol. P-wave analysis reveals similar P morphology during the tachycardia and sinus rhythm, indicating SA node reentry as the most likely cause.

such as myocardial ischemia, congestive heart failure, chronic obstructive pulmonary disease with hypoxemia and hypercapnia, or electrolyte disturbances. Electrical cardioversion may be required for termination. Type IA antiarrhythmics (quinidine, procainamide, and disopyramide) are beneficial in preventing the recurrence of the premature atrial focus. Intravenous

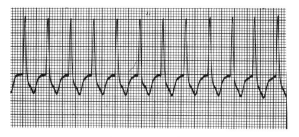

Fig. 10-10. Atrioventricular (AV) nodal reentry. A narrow complex tachycardia at a heart rate of approximately 160 beats/min without evidence of atrial activity is strongly suggestive of AV nodal reentry.

procainamide is preferable in critically ill patients.

c. Atrioventricular node reentry. AV node reentry is the most common PSVT, occurring in 60% of patients.[122] Reentry may occur in the AV node because of dual AV nodal pathways. These AV nodal pathways have different conduction velocities and refractory periods, which present an ideal substrate for the development of a reentrant arrhythmia. Most commonly, P waves are not present on the electrocardiogram because of almost simultaneous retrograde activation of the atria and antegrade activation of the ventricle from the AV nodal focus (Fig. 10-10). Occasionally, inverted P waves in leads II, III, and aV_F may occur either before or after the QRS complex (List 10-5). Carotid sinus massage may convert AV nodal reentry, and verapamil, 75 µg/kg, repeated in several minutes if no effect is seen, is the drug of choice and is very effective in conversion to sinus rhythm[124] (Fig. 10-11). Hypotension can be avoided with slow administration. Recently, adenosine was released for clinical use in this country. Adenosine, 6 to 12 mg intravenously, appears effective in the treatment of this arrhythmia.[124] The main advantage of adenosine is an extremely short half-life of a few seconds, which avoids side effects.

d. Accessory AV connections. Electrophysiologic studies have demonstrated the second most frequent cause (approximately 30%) of PSVT is accessory AV connections.[116,117] These connections, along with the AV node, form a reentry pathway between atria and ventricle that can sustain a PSVT. These tachycardias most frequently have a narrow QRS complex; however, in patients with the preexcitation syndrome (that is, Wolff-Parkinson-White, WPW) the QRS complex may be wide.[125] This early depolarization of the ventricle creates a slurred upstroke (delta wave) of the QRS complex and a short PR interval, both classic manifestations of

PSVT

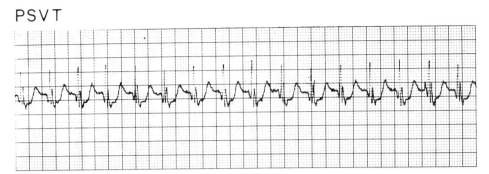

Post 2.5 mg VP

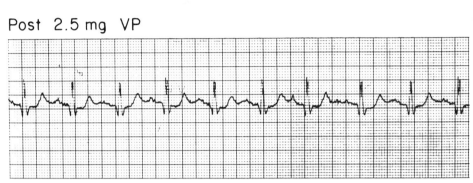

Fig. 10-11. Conversion of AV nodal reentry (PSVT) with verapamil (VP) 2.5 mg intravenously. Again notice the absence of atrial activity present on the surface electrocardiogram.

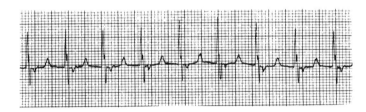

Fig. 10-12. Paroxysmal supraventricular tachyarrhythmia (PSVT) with retrograde P waves. Inverted P waves following the narrow QRS (rate = 140 beats/min) complex occur with either AV nodal reentry or accessory AV connections.

the WPW syndrome. During the tachycardia, P waves are frequently inverted after the QRS complex, an indication of retrograde activation of the atria (Fig. 10-12).

Approximately 50% of patients with the electrocardiographic manifestations of preexcitation have no symptoms, whereas 50% have symptoms of palpitations, dizziness, and syncope, indicating an arrhythmia problem. The most common arrhythmia associated with WPW is PSVT,[125] occurring in about 80% of patients, whereas atrial fibrillation and atrial flutter occur in the remainder of patients. Because of the potential fast conduction velocity and short refractory period of the accessory pathway, atrial fibrillation or atrial flutter may result in ex-

tremely fast ventricular rates (more than 300 beats/min), which can lead to sudden death (Fig. 10-13). These patients conducting at fast ventricular rates should have catheter or surgical ablation of their accessory pathways. In patients with slower ventricular rates, with atrial flutter, fibrillation, or PSVT, pharmacologic therapy is usually beneficial.

If the QRS complex is *wide,* demonstrating preexcitation, intravenous procainamide,[126] 100 mg IV q 5 min until conversion, is the drug of choice (Figs. 10-14 and 10-15). Intravenous lidocaine[127] is also successful; however, one report demonstrated that an increased heart rate could occur in some patients.[128] Continuous infusions are usually not necessary or beneficial if loading doses fail. Intravenous verapamil[129] and digoxin[130] have been shown to increase the tachycardia rate in atrial fibrillation with wide QRS complexes and therefore are relatively contraindicated in WPW. However, electrophysiologic studies may demonstrate that verapamil or digoxin is suitable for treatment in some patients. Adenosine also has been effec-

tive in patients with accessory pathways.[124] Most anesthetic agents have little effect on accessory pathway function, except droperidol,[131] which has been shown to slow conduction across the pathway. Chronic oral therapy includes the type IA antiarrhythmics or newer oral agents such as amiodarone and encainide. The treatment of a PSVT with a *narrow* QRS complex with the reentry pathway proceeding down the AV node across ventricular muscle and conducting retrograde up the accessory pathway to the atria is identical to treatment for most AV nodal reentry supraventricular tachycardias: carotid sinus massage, verapamil, or adenosine.

3. Atrial fibrillation. Atrial fibrillation is an oscillating base line on the electrocardiogram, best seen in lead II, with conducted ventricular complexes having a totally irregular rhythm. This irregularity is from the constant bombardment of the AV node by impulses that traverse the AV node in a competing and variable fashion creating periods of physiologic block. The ventricular rate in untreated patients may vary between 120 and 200 beats/min and frequently results in decreases in cardiac output that are detrimental to the anesthetized or critically ill patient. Occasionally, untreated patients may present for surgery in atrial fibrillation with an intrinsically slow ventricular response due to underlying conducting system disease. These patients do not need preoperative therapy; however, the anesthesiologist should be prepared to treat increases in the ventricular response should it occur during the stress of surgery. Cardiac problems predisposing to atrial fibrillation include congestive heart failure, rheumatic heart disease, coronary artery disease, and pericarditis. Noncardiac conditions include thyrotoxicosis, pulmonary embolus, chronic obstructive lung disease, consumption of alcohol or caffeine, and electrolyte disturbances. Paroxys-

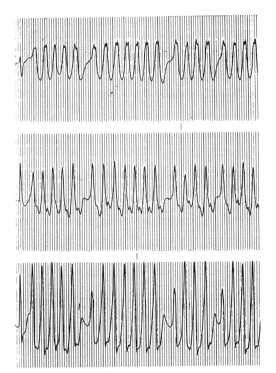

Fig. 10-13. Atrial fibrillation with an accessory pathway. Three different leads show the extremely fast rate (300 beats/min), irregular rhythm, and wide QRS complexes exhibiting preexcitation. These are classic findings of atrial fibrillation in adult patients with accessory pathways (see Fig. 10-14 and 10-15).

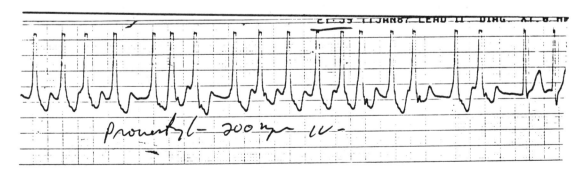

Fig. 10-14. Procainamide slowing of atrial fibrillation in patient with accessory pathway in Fig. 10-13. The patient converted to sinus rhythm after 200 mg of procainamide administered intravenously (see Fig. 10-15).

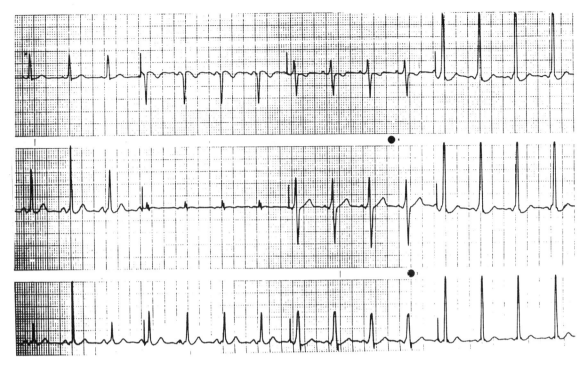

Fig. 10-15. Twelve-lead electrocardiogram after conversion of atrial fibrillation demonstrating short PR interval and delta waves in most leads of the patient with an accessory pathway (see Figs. 10-13 and 10-14).

mal atrial fibrillation may occur intermittently in patients without any associated underlying disease. Anesthesiologists should assume that the patient with intermittent atrial fibrillation will likely have the arrhythmia occur during his anesthetic period.

Verapamil, 75 μg/kg, is usually very effective in reducing the ventricular rate in atrial fibrillation within several minutes, but conversion to sinus rhythm is rare.[132] An intravenous bolus of verapamil may result in hypotension, which may be prevented by the slow administration of verapamil 1 mg/min or by pretreatment with an intravenous dose of calcium.[133] Calcium therapy reverses the hemodynamic effects of verapamil but does not reverse the electrophysiologic effects. A 30% reduction in the ventricular rate can be expected with the initial dose of verapamil, but maximal clinical effects last only 30 to 45 minutes. To maintain heart rate reduction, intravenous digoxin is given after successful rate reduction with verapamil. However, digoxin is as effective as verapamil in rate control during the stress of exercise and may lack effectiveness in rate control during the stress of the perioperative period.[134] Esmolol, 0.5 to 1 mg/kg loading dose with a 50 μg/kg/min infusion with repeat loading doses before 50 μg/kg/min increments in infusion up to 250 μg/kg/min, is effective in slowing the ventricular response in atrial fibrillation and also in conversion to sinus rhythm[135] (Fig. 10-16). This short-acting, cardioselective beta blocker may prove effective in rate control during the stress of the perioperative period.

If the conversion of atrial fibrillation is not accomplished with pharmacologic therapy or treatment of the underlying disease, cardioversion may be necessary. Anesthesiologists are frequently asked to provide anesthesia for electrical cardioversion of atrial fibrillation and flutter. Patients who are successfully cardioverted usually have atrial fibrillation of less than 1 year's duration, have a left atrial dimension of less than 45 mm by echocardiography, have no ventricular enlargement, and have successful treatment of the precipitating cardiac or noncardiac factors. Anticoagulation for several weeks is considered before elective cardioversion in patients with atrial fibrillation longer than 4 to 5 days and is maintained for several weeks after establishment of sinus rhythm to prevent systemic embolization.[136]

4. Atrial flutter. Atrial flutter is much less common than atrial fibrillation but shares the same predisposing factors. Atrial flutter is cate-

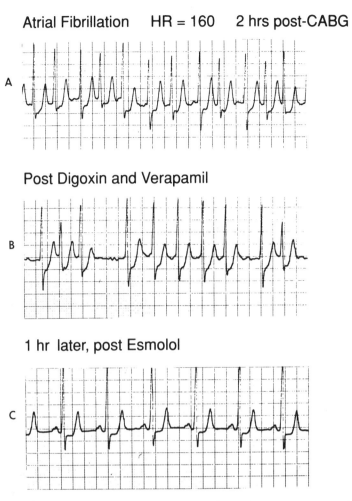

Fig. 10-16. Conversion of atrial fibrillation with esmolol after coronary artery bypass grafting (CABG), **A.** Digoxin and verapamil slowed the ventricular response as demonstrated in **B,** but the rate remained unacceptably fast. After 1 hour to allow verapamil levels to decrease, esmolol, 0.5 mg/kg × 2, followed by a 100 μg/kg/min infusion, converted the patient to sinus rhythm, **C.**

gorized into two types[137] (Fig. 10-17). *Type I,* or classic, atrial flutter usually occurs at a rate of 300 beats/min with a ventricular rate of 150 beats/min. The flutter waves are of a typical sawtooth or biphasic appearance in the inferior leads, and type I flutter may be converted by rapid atrial pacing. *Type II* atrial flutter exhibits a flat base line with a positive flutter wave in the inferior leads, with a rate usually greater than 350 beats/min. Type II atrial flutter frequently cannot be converted by rapid atrial pacing. Electrophysiologic studies have demonstrated flutter and fibrillation existing in the atria at the same time.

Atrial flutter compared to fibrillation is usually more difficult to treat. However, rapid atrial pacing in type I atrial flutter is effective.[138] Rapid atrial pacing involves pacing the atria with an atrial pacemaker at a rate approximately 20% faster than the flutter rate (360 for type I) from a site high in the right atrium.[138] In the operating room this can be accomplished with atrial electrodes placed during cardiac surgery, through an atrial electrode inserted through a paceport pulmonary artery catheter, by insertion of a temporary transvenous pacing electrode, or by an esophageal atrial pacing probe. During rapid atrial pacing, a change in the morphology of the flutter pattern is a sign of overdrive suppression. In addition, there is a critical duration of rapid atrial pacing required to convert atrial flutter.[138] After interruption of atrial flutter, pacing should proceed for approximately 30 seconds; pacing for shorter amounts of time may not be successful. Because atrial thresholds are usually higher in atrial flutter[139]

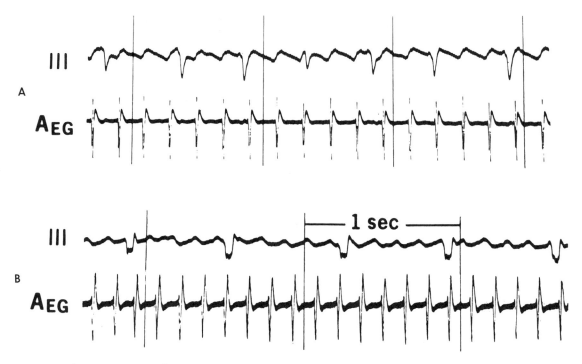

Fig. 10-17. Atrial flutter subtypes. **A,** Type I atrial flutter with the classic sawtooth pattern in lead III and an atrial rate of 300 beats/min on an atrial electrogram (A_{EG}). **B,** Type II flutter with positive flutter waves in lead III and an atrial rate of 400 beats/min. (From Waldo AL et al: Circulation 50:665, 1979, American Heart Association.)

than sinus rhythm and determination of capture is difficult, maximal current (usually 20 mA) should be used on all temporary pacemakers for overdrive suppression. If suppression does not occur in type I flutter, it is usually because of inadequate rate, pacing time, or current.

5. Multifocal atrial tachycardia. The arrhythmia multifocal atrial tachycardia (MAT) usually occurs in the seriously ill, elderly patient, frequently in the setting of decompensated chronic obstructive lung disease.[140] However, coronary artery disease, congestive heart failure, and the postoperative state may be associated with this arrhythmia.[141] MAT is diagnosed with the following criteria: three or more P waves with varying morphology and varying PP-cycle lengths, an atrial rate usually between 100 and 200 beats/min with irregular RR intervals, and varying PR intervals with varying degrees of AV block.[140] In most cases of MAT, the ventricular rate is between 100 and 150 beats/min. The ectopic P waves are often large and peaked and resemble the P waves seen in chronic pulmonary disease. Aberrant ventricular conduction may also occur, and this arrhythmia is frequently misdiagnosed as atrial fibrillation.

The classic treatment for MAT has been the improvement of the underlying chronic lung disease. Correction of hypoxemia, acidemia, and electrolyte disturbances will aid in management. Digoxin and many other antiarrhythmics, including cardioversion, are ineffective.[140] Several reports have suggested that the theophylline drugs are highly associated with the development of this arrhythmia[142] and that discontinuation of theophylline agents should result in return to sinus rhythm (Fig. 10-18). Both verapamil[143] and metoprolol[144] will decrease the atrial and ventricular rates and convert the arrhythmia to sinus rhythm in some patients.

C. Causes and consequences of ventricular arrhythmias

Treatment of premature ventricular depolarizations requires the anesthesiologist to have an adequate knowledge of arrhythmia history, underlying organic heart disease, and prior antiarrhythmic therapy, as discussed in the preoperative evaluation. Patients with ventricular arrhythmias can be divided into three classes based on their associated risk for sudden death.[145] Most of these patients, especially those with malignant ventricular arrhythmias, need preoperative cardiology consultation. Ap-

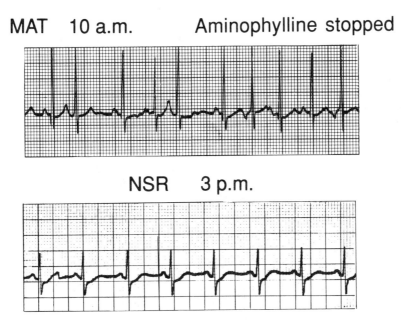

MAT   10 a.m.   Aminophylline stopped

NSR   3 p.m.

Fig. 10-18. Multifocal atrial tachycardia (MAT). This arrhythmia occurred in an ICU patient with decompensated chronic lung disease and converted to normal sinus rhythm, *NSR*, with discontinuation of an aminophylline infusion.

propriate questions to ask include: "What are the risks of the patient developing his ventricular arrhythmia during the increased sympathetic stress of the perioperative period?" and "What antiarrhythmic or other therapy do you recommend if the patient develops his ventricular arrhythmia during surgery?"

1. Benign ventricular arrhythmias. Benign ventricular arrhythmias occur in patients without structural heart disease whose risk of sudden death is minimal.[145] These patients usually have no hemodynamic symptoms and frequently are not treated; although if palpitations and dizziness are bothersome to the person, therapy may be elected. These patients may or may not have a history of ventricular arrhythmias. As previously discussed, ventricular arrhythmias are common in the normal general population and increase with age.[5,6] During surgery the anesthesiologist may be the first physician to monitor the patient for any prolonged length of time and may uncover these common benign arrhythmias. Therapy is usually not indicated; however, the prudent anesthesiologist should use these cardiac electrical problems as a warning that a noncardiac cause may exist, including myocardial ischemia, hypoxemia, hypercarbia, acidemia, light anesthesia, sympathetic stimulation, electrolyte abnormalities, or drug effects. If intraoperative problems arise associated with ventricular arrhythmias, antiarrhythmic therapy may be justified

until the cause of these problems can be determined.

2. Potentially malignant ventricular arrhythmias. Potentially malignant ventricular arrhythmias occur in patients with structural heart disease,[145] with severe coronary artery disease and history of myocardial infarction, and with congestive or hypertrophic cardiomyopathy. All these patients have a higher risk of sudden death than patients with no known heart disease and ventricular arrhythmias. These patients usually are receiving antiarrhythmic therapy before their anesthetic, and if arrhythmias arise during anesthesia and surgery, they should be treated. Once again, after noncardiac causes are ruled out, therapy is based on the patient's organic heart disease and any previous antiarrhythmic therapy. Any patient with ischemic heart disease with new ventricular arrhythmias must have ischemia ruled out. Intravenous nitroglycerin has frequently eliminated premature ventricular depolarizations without antiarrhythmic therapy.[146] Patients with congestive heart failure or congestive cardiomyopathy may have worsening failure with a dilated heart, which should be managed appropriately. Worsening obstruction in hypertrophic cardiomyopathy may require volume loading, pure vasopressors like phenylephrine (Neo-Synephrine), beta blockade, or calcium-entry blockade to help relieve the obstruction.

3. Malignant ventricular arrhythmias. The

final classification, malignant ventricular arrhythmias, is associated with severe structural heart disease with associated hemodynamic abnormalities.[145] These patients have symptoms of dizziness and syncope and may have a history of cardiac arrest. Some of these patients may have automatic implantable cardioverter defibrillator units or have had invasive or noninvasive ablative therapy for their arrhythmia. The management of patients with malignant ventricular arrhythmias is basically the same as for potentially malignant ventricular arrhythmias, except that the anesthesiologist and cardiologist must be more aggressive in documenting adequate therapy and in considering prophylactic therapy. When a patient with potentially malignant ventricular arrhythmia is receiving antiarrhythmic therapy before surgery, the patient should be questioned to see if any symptoms have been relieved. Drug levels, if available, should be obtained to verify adequate therapeutic levels. Most of these patients will benefit from intravenous antiarrhythmic therapy during the stress of the perioperative

---

List 10-6. Intravenous Ventricular Antiarrhythmic Therapy*

Class I

Procainamide (IA), 100 mg IV loading dose every 5 minutes until arrhythmia subsides or total dose of 15 mg/kg (rarely needed) with continuous infusion of 2 to 6 mg/min.

Lidocaine (IB), 1.5 mg/kg in divided doses given twice over 20 minutes with continuous intravenous infusion of 1 to 4 mg/min.

Class II

Propranolol, 0.5 to 1 mg given slowly up to a total beta-blocking dose of 0.1 mg/kg. Repeat bolus as needed.

Metoprolol, 2.5 mg given slowly up to a total beta-blocking dose of 0.2 mg/kg. Repeat bolus as needed.

Esmolol, 0.5 to 1 mg/kg loading dose with each 50 µg/kg/min increase in infusion, with infusions of 50 to 300 µg/kg/min. Hypotension and bradycardia are limiting factors.

Class III

Bretylium, 5 mg/kg loading dose given slowly with a continuous infusion of 1 to 5 mg/min. Hypotension may be a limiting factor with infusion.

Overdrive pacing is effective in conversion of ventricular tachycardia. The procedure is the same as that for atrial flutter: set rate at 20% faster than ventricular rate, set current at 20 mA, pace for 30 seconds, slowly decrease rate.

period. The cardiologist should be asked what intravenous antiarrhythmic agent is appropriate for each individual patient should ventricular arrhythmias occur in the operating room. The most commonly used intravenous agents for control of ventricular arrhythmias are shown in List 10-6.

Intravenous antiarrhythmic therapy begins with lidocaine, which remains a very effective agent against PVCs with minimal side effects.[147] If lidocaine is not effective, the substitution or addition of intravenous procainamide may prove effective.[147,148] Procainamide is also an excellent antiarrhythmic for PVCs with efficacy similar to lidocaine and, when combined with lidocaine (class IA and IB), may be more effective than with single-drug therapy.[149] Theoretically, combination therapy with drugs with different electrophysiologic effects (from different classes) may be successful in patients with refractory ventricular arrhythmias when a single agent fails.[149] For refractory PVCs during the perioperative period, beta-adrenergic receptor blockers (class II) are useful because they antagonize the increased catecholamine levels that occur during stress and cause PVCs.[121] Intravenous lidocaine and bretylium (class IB and III) also is a potentially beneficial combination for therapy of PVCs in the perioperative period.[149]

The most common organic heart problem in patients with malignant ventricular arrhythmias is coronary artery disease, and ischemia is a likely precipitating cause. Ischemia during the perioperative period secondary to increases in myocardial demands or decreases in oxygen supply including coronary vasospasm may result in atrial or ventricular arrhythmias. Therapy with anti-ischemic drugs may eliminate the ischemic arrhythmic event. Maseri et al. showed that in patients with ventricular arrhythmias secondary to coronary vasospasm, anti-ischemic therapy was more effective in arrhythmia management than antiarrhythmics.[146] In animal studies, nitroglycerin reverses the decrease in ventricular fibrillation thresholds caused by ischemia and prolongs ventricular refractoriness that was shortened by ischemia.[150] Prophylactic nitroglycerin with intravenous antiarrhythmic therapy and beta blockade with the usual precautions for anesthetic induction and maintenance in these patients are entirely appropriate.

D. Complications of antiarrhythmic therapy

The important complications of pharmacologic therapy for arrhythmias are best understood by a discussion of the classification of antiarrhythmic agents by Vaughan-Williams (List 10-7).

List 10-7. Classification of Antiarrhythmic Agents with Associated Significant Side Effects

Class I
These drugs have local anesthetic or Na⁺-channel blocking properties and are subdivided into categories A, B, and C.
IA drugs slow conduction velocity and prolong repolarization.
Quinidine—Hepatic toxicity, prolongs Q-T interval
Procainamide—Negative inotropy
Disopyramide—Significant negative inotropy
Moricizine—Mild negative inotropy
IB drugs slow conduction velocity and shorten repolarization.
Lidocaine—Seizures
Mexiletine—Hepatic toxicity
Tocainide—Negative inotropy, pulmonary fibrosis, hepatitis
Phenytoin—Drug interactions
IC drugs slow conduction velocity and have variable effects on repolarization. Recent studies show increased mortality after myocardial infarction.
Flecainide—Negative inotropy, proarrhythmia
Encainide—Proarrhythmia
Propafenone—Negative inotropy

Class II
These drugs block beta-adrenergic receptors, *propanolol, esmolol, metoprolol*-negative inotropy, and hypotension.

Class III
These drugs prolong the action potential duration and effective refractory period.
Bretylium—Hypotension
Amiodarone—Negative inotropy, pulmonary fibrosis

Class IV
These drugs block calcium entry into the cells.
Verapamil—Hypotension, contraindicated in wide QRS tachycardia (if ventricular tachycardia, ventricular fibrillation may result) and in neonates (apnea, hypotension, asystole)
Diltiazem—Negative inotropy, conduction system slowing

The most important toxic effects of each drug are also listed. Preoperative assessment of the toxicity of the appropriate organ system is of obvious importance to the anesthesiologist. Patients receiving negative inotrope antiarrhythmics may require a less myocardium-depressant anesthetic. Agents that cause pulmonary toxicity may require more definitive preoperative pulmonary tests and anticipated problems with gas exchange during anesthesia and surgery. The more conservative anesthesiologist may desire to avoid inhalational agents in patients who receive potentially hepatotoxic antiarrhythmics. Drug interactions are important because of altered serum levels of various pharmacologic agents and of altered hemodynamic responses during anesthesia.

1. Myocardial depression. Negative inotropic effects of the antiarrhythmics are common, with disopyramide (Norpace) having the most significant effect. Acute pulmonary edema may occur with intravenous therapy. One study demonstrated new or worse congestive failure in 50% of patients with a history of previous congestive failure receiving disopyramide.[151] Anticholinergic effects of acute urinary retention, blurred vision, and dry mouth are other common side effects of disopyramide, with severe hypoglycemia rarely reported. Amiodarone may also cause clinically significant myocardial depression during anesthesia.[152] Thyroid dysfunction, corneal microdeposits, and bluish skin discoloration are other side effects associated with amiodarone.

2. Pulmonary toxicity. Adverse pulmonary effects, including pulmonary infiltrates and pulmonary fibrosis, have been reported with amiodarone[153] and tocainide.[154] However, the pulmonary complications with amiodarone may occur in as many as 5% to 15% of patients, and autopsy studies indicate that this complication may be underdiagnosed.[155] Propafenone and other antiarrhythmics with beta-blocking effects may precipitate bronchospasm.

3. Hepatic toxicity. Many antiarrhythmics may induce mild elevations in liver enzymes; however, quinidine[156] may cause a hypersensitivity reaction involving the liver, and tocainide may cause hepatitis. Most antiarrhythmics are hepatically metabolized, and reduced drug administration may be required in patients with hepatic disease. Serum levels are helpful preoperatively.

4. Proarrhythmias. All antiarrhythmics have

the potential to increase the frequency of arrhythmias and cause clinically significant worsening of arrhythmias (proarrhythmic effect). The class IC drugs (flecainide and encainide) are especially prone to cause proarrhythmic events.[157] Verapamil will quickly slow the ventricular response in atrial fibrillation but may cause delayed conversion of atrial fibrillation to sinus rhythm. Verapamil is also contraindicated in wide complex tachycardias because it may convert ventricular tachycardia to ventricular fibrillation and cardiac arrest.

5. Drug interactions. Other adverse reactions of particular importance to anesthesiologists are drug interactions. Amiodarone,[158] quinidine,[158] propafenone,[159] and verapamil[160] may increase digitalis levels. Phenytoin (Dilantin), by inducing liver microsomal enzymes, may reduce the serum levels of quinidine,[161] disopyramide,[162] and mexilitine.[159] Amiodarone also increase warfarin, quinidine, procainamide, and phenytoin levels.[163] Immediate therapy with intravenous beta blockers after intravenous verapamil may result in second- or third-degree AV block. Bretylium (alpha), amiodarone (alpha, beta), and propafenone (alpha, beta) and other antiarrhythmics with antiadrenergic effects of alpha- or beta-receptor blocking properties may alter hemodynamic responses during anesthesia.

IV. PATIENTS WITH MISCELLANEOUS DISEASE STATES ASSOCIATED WITH ARRHYTHMIAS
A. Mitral valve prolapse

The mitral valve prolapse syndrome is estimated to occur in 5% of the general population and in 10% to 20% of young, healthy females[164] and is accompanied by anxiety, tachycardia, neurasthenia, arrhythmias, and chest pain. More serious complications include acute mitral regurgitation from chordae tendineae rupture, infective endocarditis, stroke, and sudden death.[165] Mitral valve prolapse is associated with autonomic dysfunction, with high serum levels of catecholamines present in many patients.[166] Myxomatous degeneration of one or both mitral leaflets has been reported, with atrial muscle–like muscle fibers occasionally seen on pathologic analysis.[165] Atrial and ventricular arrhythmias may occur and are more common in patients with resting ST-segment and T-wave abnormalities.[167] PSVT is the most common tachyarrhythmia[168] caused by AV nodal reentry or accessory AV connections (more common with mitral valve prolapse). Q-T interval prolongation is also associated with mitral valve prolapse.[169]

Adequate preoperative preparation that provides anxiety relief and antibiotic prophylaxis for infective endocarditis is important. Hemodynamic alterations during anesthesia may make the prolapsing worse. Vasodilatation, hypovolemia, or head-up position reduces the size of the left ventricle and allow the leaflets of the mitral valve to prolapse more into the left atrium.[170,171] Maintaining adequate volume and using phenylephrine (Neo-Synephrine) for hypotension may prevent or treat arrhythmias initiated by the prolapse.[171] One study of patients with adrenergic hypersensitivity in mitral valve prolapse showed greater increases in heart rate to catecholamine stimulation than in control patients.[166] Beta blockers are frequently effective antiarrhythmics,[172] though other antiarrhythmic agents may be needed for suppression of refractory atrial and ventricular arrhythmias.

B. Prolonged Q-T syndrome

1. Congenital. Patients presenting for anesthesia and surgery with a prolonged Q-T interval have either a congenitally prolonged Q-T interval or an acquired long Q-T interval secondary to electrolyte disturbances, drug therapy, or cardiac disease.[173] The congenital syndrome is important to anesthesiologists because of the numerous case reports of ventricular tachyarrhythmias occurring during anesthesia and surgery.[174,175] An imbalance or increase in left sympathetic cardiac input through the sympathetic chain is a possible cause of the congenitally prolonged Q-T interval.[176] These children with refractory arrhythmias may present for left stellate sympathectomy, which frequently corrects the prolonged Q-T interval.[177] Sympathetic stimulation caused by the stress of the perioperative period is a precipitating factor in these patients.[173] Beta blockers shorten the congenital long Q-T syndrome,[178] and this therapy should be maintained during the perioperative period[174] (Fig. 10-19). Adequate premedication, deep levels of anesthesia during induction and extubation, and postoperative pain relief are important features of the anesthetic plan.[173] Although no specific type of anesthetic has been proved in controlled studies to be beneficial, isoflurane in several case reports appears not to cause worsening of the Q-T interval.[174,179] Drugs with sympathomimetic effects, such as pancuronium and ketamine, should be avoided.[180]

2. Acquired. In the acquired long Q-T interval, polymorphic ventricular tachycardia (torsade de pointes) may result[181] (Fig. 10-20).

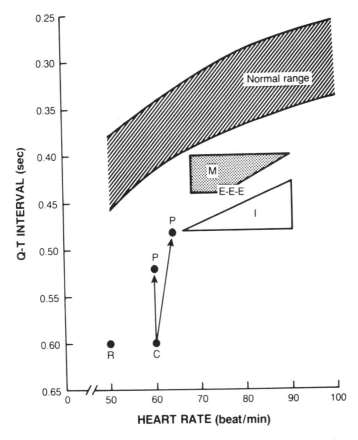

Fig. 10-19. Changes in the Q-T interval during anesthesia with isoflurane in a patient who had an arrest during a previous anesthetic without propranolol pretreatment. The control, *C,* Q-T shortens after propranolol, *P.* The Q-T intervals during anesthesia are denoted by *I,* intubation, *M,* maintenance, and *E,* emergence. The return point Q-T interval, *R,* after surgery is similar to the control, *C,* Q-T interval. Beta-adrenergic receptor blockers are indicated in all patients perioperatively with the congenitally long Q-T interval. (From Medak R and Benumof JL: Br J Anaesth 55:361, 1983.)

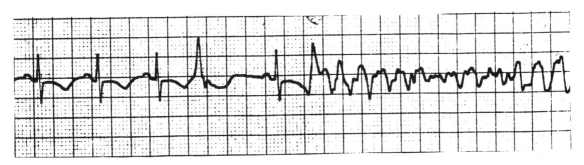

Fig. 10-20. Ventricular tachycardia (torsade de pointes) occurring in a patient with an acquired long Q-T interval secondary to quinidine toxicity. Notice the second premature ventricular contraction occurring on the inverted T-wave, precipitating the ventricular arrhythmia.

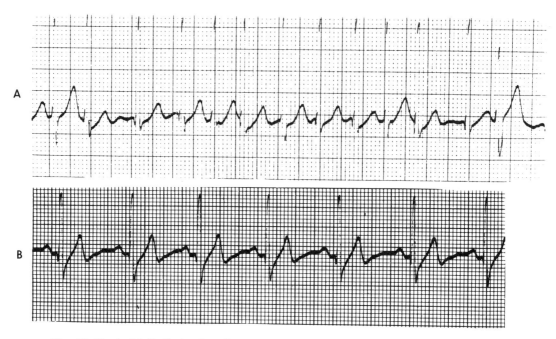

Fig. 10-21. Atrial fibrillation in a 50-year-old man after craniotomy for atrioventricular malformation (AVM) repair, **A,** and after therapy with esmolol, **B,** which converted the atrial fibrillation to sinus rhythm. Esmolol, 500 μg/kg × 4 and a 200 μg/kg/min infusion, was required.

Treatment of hypokalemia, hypomagnesemia, myocardial ischemia, or discontinuation of drugs prolonging the Q-T interval should be performed before surgery.[173,182] In contrast to therapy for the congenital syndrome, beta-receptor stimulation is beneficial in the acquired syndrome.[183,184] Increasing the heart rate with isoproterenol or overdrive pacing prevents the early afterdepolarizations[183,184] that occur during the prolonged period of repolarization. Bradycardia should be avoided. No anesthetic technique appears to have any advantages over others, though inhalational agents that prolong His-Purkinje conduction theoretically may prolong repolarization and the Q-T interval. However, a recent abstract comparing isoflurane anesthesia with opioid anesthesia found no difference between the two techniques and the ultimate effect on the Q-T interval.[185] Some antiarrhythmic agents that prolong refractoriness and the Q-T interval are associated with torsade de pointes (quinidine),[186] and some are not (amiodarone).[187] Drugs prolonging the Q-T interval not associated with torsade de pointes have Ca^{++}-antagonistic properties,[188] as the inhalational anesthetic agents do. This finding indicates, though does not prove, that the inhalational agents may be safe to use in the acquired syndrome, as supported by the case reports.

C. Central nervous system disease

Cardiac arrhythmias have been known for years to be associated with various central nervous system (CNS) diseases. Both supraventricular and ventricular arrhythmias secondary to closed head injury, subarachnoid hemorrhage, and stroke are reported in the literature.[189-191] But few prospective studies of arrhythmias and CNS disease were performed until recently. Di Pasquale et al.[192] found arrhythmias in 90% of 107 patients with subarachnoid hemorrhage, with a high incidence of PVCs, PACs, and sinus arrhythmia. Nine patients had atrial fibrillation (Fig. 10-21) or PSVT, and 6 had ventricular tachycardia or fibrillation. Of these 6, 4 patients had torsade de pointes associated with a long Q-T interval, which is known to occur with subarachnoid hemorrhage.[193] Other human and animal studies have demonstrated that acute increases in intracranial pressure, brainstem compression, blood injected into the subarachnoid space, and blood irritating the brainstem or other intracranial structures may precipitate cardiac arrhythmias.[194-197] The neuroanesthesiologist must be aware of this relationship and be prepared to treat associated arrhythmias.

D. Valvular heart disease

There is a high incidence of ventricular arrhythmias occurring in aortic stenosis. Von Olshausen et al.[198] found 84% of patients with aortic valve disease to have PVCs, with 73% having multifocal PVCs, couplets, or longer runs of ventricular tachycardia. There appears to be a relationship between left ventricular wall stress, increased pressure gradients, lower ejection fractions, and the more complex ventricular arrhythmias.[198] Some studies have shown a reduction in these complex ventricular arrhythmias after valve replacement, and some have not.[199,200] Considering the reduction of ventricular fibrillation thresholds after ischemic periods of cardiac surgery and this high incidence of ventricular arrhythmias, one should give serious consideration to instituting ventricular antiarrhythmic therapy in patients having aortic valve replacement.

Loss of atrial contraction in atrial fibrillation or junctional rhythm may cause severe hemodynamic problems in aortic stenosis because of the increased importance of atrial contraction on ventricular filling. Atrial fibrillation may occur during intravenous guidewire insertion, pulmonary artery catheterization, or venous cannulation before cardiopulmonary bypass. Electrical cardioversion is necessary if hemodynamic collapse occurs. If time and hemodynamics permit, esmolol is very efficacious in converting atrial fibrillation to sinus rhythm. Avoiding inhalational anesthetics in aortic stenosis is wise because junctional rhythms causing AV dissociation commonly occur with these agents.

Tachycardia worsens mitral stenosis by decreasing diastolic filling time, decreasing blood flow across the valve, and increasing the transvalvular gradient. Tachycardia in atrial fibrillation worsens symptoms in patients with mitral stenosis and not the fibrillation itself.[201] Atrial fibrillation does not affect mitral regurgitation as significantly because increased heart rate does not usually increase the left atrial pressure, and atrial contraction is not effective because of the usually giant atrial size.

E. Arrhythmias in children

Junctional ectopic tachycardia (JET) is one of the most dangerous arrhythmias encountered by physicians who care for children, and mortalities are extremely high.[202] There are two forms of junctional ectopic tachycardia, congenital and postsurgical. Anesthesiologists are exposed to children with this arrhythmia who have congenital heart disease after cardiac or noncardiac surgery. JET is caused by an enhanced automatic mechanism of the distal conducting system in the area of the His bundle.[203] This arrhythmia may have ventricular rates greater than 300 beats/min, and a cardiomyop-

athy with congestive heart failure may develop.[202] Postoperative JET occurs most commonly in infants who have congenital cardiac defects repaired.[204] Most infants have low cardiac output, are maintained on ventilators, and are receiving drugs such as meperidine, barbiturates, and pancuronium bromide. Inotropic agents are frequently required, and many children are mildly acidemic.[204] Thus the causal factors are multifactorial. Therapy is aimed at reducing adrenergic tone, increasing vagal tone, and maintaining hemodynamic and normal metabolic function.[204] Mild hypothermia also is suggested to be helpful in reducing the tachycardia.[205]

Medical therapy with digoxin or beta blockers, or both, is rarely successful.[206,202] Verapamil, as in other supraventricular tachycardias in infants, should not be given because of reports of apnea, bradycardia, severe hypotension, and death.[207] Overdrive pacing and electrical cardioversion are not effective.[202] Recently, Villain et al.[208] reported amiodarone to restore the heart rate to below 150 beats/min in 8 of 14 patients with congenital JET. Flecainide, encainide, and propafenone have been reported to be successful in this arrhythmia.[209,210] Because mortality may approach 35%,[208] catheter and surgical ablative therapy should be considered in refractory cases.[202]

F. Electrolyte abnormalities

All physicians are aware of the arrhythmogenic effects of hypokalemia, which increases the automaticity and excitability of the myocardial cell membrane.[211] Controversy exists in the relationship of PVCs to hypokalemia in clinical studies.[211,212] However, there are clear data indicating that hypokalemia is associated with the development of ventricular tachycardia and fibrillation, especially during stressful situations with increased catecholamine levels and acute myocardial ischemia.[213]

Patients presenting for anesthesia and surgery who are receiving diuretics are prone to hypokalemia and potassium depletion.[214] In patients with arrhythmias, serum K^+ concentrations should be maintained greater than 4.0 mEq/L before surgery.[210] Further K^+ decreases may occur during surgery because of hyperventilation, which shifts K^+ into cells and stress-induced epinephrine secretion, which stimulates beta$_2$-adrenergic receptors, promoting an uptake of potassium into cells.[215] The arrhythmogenic electrophysiologic effects of hypokalemia may oppose the antiarrhythmic effects of antiarrhythmic medication.[216]

In contrast to the well-known electrophysiologic effects of hypokalemia, the electrophysiologic effects of hypomagnesemia are less clear.[217] Watanabe and Dreifus[218] demonstrated in perfused rabbit hearts that the effects on transmembrane potentials of hypomagnesemia were entirely dependent on extracellular potassium, with minor changes occurring when extracellular potassium was normal. Magnesium is required as a cofactor for the Na^+-K^+ pump and Ca^{++}-ATPase pump, which maintains low intracellular calcium levels. Low serum magnesium levels reduce Na^+-K^+ pump activity, which increases Na^+-Ca^{++} exchange, increases intracellular Ca^{++}, and reduces intracellular K^+ concentrations.[219] Reduced intracellular Mg^+ also decreases Ca^{++} extrusion via the Ca^{++}-ATPase pump, resulting in increased intracellular Ca^{++} currents, which are arrhythmogenic in triggered automaticity models.[220]

Well-controlled clinical studies have not proved a relationship between hypomagnesemia and PVCs.[221,222] In many of the clinical studies suggesting that hypomagnesemia is arrhythmogenic, concurrent hypokalemia was present.[223-225] However, hypomagnesemia has definite electrophysiologic effects in humans of prolonging SA and AV node recovery times and increasing atrial-His intervals,[226] and such prolongation supports magnesium's effectiveness in treating supraventricular arrhythmias.[227,228] Magnesium is also beneficial in digitalis-toxic arrhythmias,[229] in torsade de pointes,[230] and in managing refractory ventricular arrhythmias.[231]

Chronic Mg^{++} depletion occurs in diuretic usage, aminoglycoside therapy, alcohol abuse, secondary aldosteronism, and malabsorption syndromes.[232] Serum Mg^{++} levels do not reflect intracellular Mg^{++} levels, especially in chronic depletion,[233] and treatment is indicated despite normal serum levels. Iseri et al.[234] recommend 2 g of $MgSO_4$ intravenously given over 2 to 3 min when ventricular arrhythmias are refractory to lidocaine and procainamide. A continuous infusion is begun with 10 g given over 5 hours and, especially if arrhythmias subside, a second 10 g given over 10 hours to restore intracellular magnesium levels. Hypotension is a side effect that can be reversed easily with small doses of calcium. Serum K^+ and Mg^{++} levels are monitored during Mg^{++} therapy.

REFERENCES

1. Hur D and Gravenstein JS. Is ECG monitoring in the operating room cost effective? Biotelemetry Patient Monitoring 6:200-206, 1979.
2. Scott O, Williams GJ, and Fiddler GI: Results of 24 hour ambulatory monitoring of electrocardiogram in 131 healthy boys aged 10 to 13 years, Br Heart J 44:304-308, 1980.
3. Romhilt DW, Chaffin C, Choi SC, et al: Arrhythmias on ambulatory electrocardiographic monitoring in women without apparent heart disease, Am J Cardiol 54:582-586, 1984.
4. Sobotka PA, Mayer JH, Bauernfeind RA, et al: Arrhythmias documented by 24-hour continuous ambulatory electrocardiographic monitoring in young women without apparent heart disease, Am Heart J 101:753-759, 1981.
5. Hinkle LE Jr, Carver ST, and Stevens M: The frequency of asymptomatic disturbances of cardiac rhythm and conduction in middle-aged men, Am J Cardiol 24:629-650, 1969.
6. Brodsky M, Wu D, Denes P, et al: Arrhythmias documented by 24 hour continuous electrocardiographic monitoring in 50 male medical students without apparent heart disease, Am J Cardiol 39:390-395, 1977.
7. Pilcher GF, Cook AJ, Johnston BL, et al: Twenty-four-hour continuous electrocardiography during exercise and free activity in 80 apparently healthy runners, Am J Cardiol 52:859-861, 1983.
8. Kantelip J-P, Sage E, Duchene-Marullaz P: Findings on ambulatory electrocardiographic monitoring in subjects older than 80 years, Am J Cardiol 57:398-401, 1986.
9. Kostis JB, McCrone K, Moreyra AE, et al: Premature ventricular complexes in the absence of identifiable heart disease, Circulation 63:1351-1356, 1981.
10. Poblete PF, Kennedy HL, and Caralis DG: Detection of ventricular ectopy in patients with coronary heart disease and normal subjects by exercise testing and ambulatory electrocardiography, Chest 74:402-407, 1978.
11. Kennedy HL, Whitlock JA, Sprague MK, et al: Long-term follow-up of asymptomatic healthy subjects with frequent and complex ventricular ectopy, N Engl J Med 312:193-197, 1985.
12. Levy AG and Lewis T: Heart irregularities resulting from the inhalation of low percentages of chloroform vapor and their relationship to ventricular fibrillation, Heart 3:99-108, 1911-1912.
13. Lennox WG, Graves RC, and Levine SA: An electrocardiographic study of fifty patients during operation, Arch Intern Med 30:57-72, 1922.
14. Marvin HM and Paston RB: The electrocardiogram and blood pressure during operation and convalescence, Arch Intern Med 35:768-781, 1925.
15. Kurtz CM, Bennett JH, and Shapiro H: Electrocardiographic studies during surgical anesthesia, JAMA 106:434-441, 1936.
16. Vanik PE and Davis HS: Cardiac arrhythmias during halothane anesthesia, Anesth Analg 47:299-307, 1968.
17. Dodd RB, Sims WA, and Bone DJ: Cardiac arrhythmias observed during anesthesia and surgery, Surgery 51:440-447, 1962.
18. Kuner J, Enescu V, Utsu F, et al: Cardiac arrhythmias during anesthesia, Dis Chest 52:580-587, 1967.
19. Bertrand CA, Steiner NV, Jameson AG, et al: Disturbances of cardiac rhythm during anesthesia and surgery, JAMA 216:1615-1617, 1971.
20. Wit AL and Rosen MR: Pathophysiologic mechanisms of cardiac arrhythmias, Am Heart J 106:798-811, 1983.
21. Atlee JL and Bosnjak ZJ: Mechanisms for cardiac dysrhythmias during anesthesia, Anesthesiology 72:347-374, 1990.
22. Hoffman BF and Rosen MR: Cellular mechanisms

for cardiac arrhythmias, Circ Res 49:1-15, 1981.

23. Cranefield PF: Action potentials, afterpotentials and arrhythmias, Circ Res 41:415-423, 1977.

24. Damiano BP and Rosen MR: Effects of pacing on triggered activity induced by early afterdepolarizations, Circulation 69:1013-1025, 1984.

25. Sasyniuk BI, Valois M, and Toy W: Recent advances in understanding the mechanisms of drug-induced torsades de pointes arrhythmias, Am J Cardiol 64:29J-32J, 1989.

26. Ferrier GR: The effects of tension on acetylstrophanthidin-induced transient depolarizations and after contractions in canine myocardial and Purkinje tissue, Circ Res 38:156-162, 1976.

27. Cranefield PF and Aronson RS: Initiation of sustained rhythmic activity by single propagated action potentials in canine cardiac Purkinje fibers exposed to sodium-free solution or to ouabain, Circ Res 34:477-481, 1974.

28. Hewett KW and Rosen MR: Alpha and beta adrenergic interactions with ouabain-induced delayed after depolarizations, J Pharmacol Exp Ther 229:188-192, 1984.

29. Ferrier GR, Moffat MP, and Lukas A: Possible mechanisms of ventricular arrhythmias elicited by ischemia followed by reperfusion, Circ Res 56:184-194, 1985.

30. Wit AL and Cranefield PT: Triggered and automatic activity in the canine coronary sinus, Circ Res 44:435-445, 1977.

31. Ferrier GR: Digitalis arrhythmias: role of oscillatory after potentials, Prog Cardiovasc Dis 19:459-474, 1977.

32. Rosen MR: Mechanisms for arrhythmias, Am J Cardiol 61:2A-8A, 1988.

33. Wu D: Supraventricular tachycardias, JAMA 249(24):3357-3360, 1983.

34. Wit AL, Hoffman BF, and Cranefield PF: Slow conduction and reentry in the ventricular conducting system: I. Return extrasystole in canine Purkinje fibers, Circ Res 30:1-10, 1972.

35. Antzelevitch C, Jalife J, and Moe GK: Characteristics of reflection as a mechanism of reentrant arrhythmias and its relationship to parasystole, Circulation 61:182-191, 1980.

36. Kinoshita S: Mechanisms of ventricular parasystole, Circulation 58:715-722, 1978.

37. Scherf D, Choi KY, Bahadori A, et al: Parasystole, Am J Cardiol 12:527-538, 1963.

38. Cohen H, Langendorf R, and Pick A: Intermittent parasystole: mechanism of protection, Circulation 48:761-774, 1973.

39. Bosnjak ZJ and Kampine JP: Effects of halothane, enflurane and isoflurane on the SA node, Anesthesiology 58:314-321, 1983.

40. Atlee JL III, Brownlee SW, and Burstrom RE: Conscious-state comparisons of the effects of inhalation anesthetics on specialized atrioventricular conduction times in dogs, Anesthesiology 64:703-710, 1986.

41. Scheffer GJ, Jonges R, Holley HS, et al: Effects of halothane on the conduction system of the heart in humans, Anesth Analg 69:721-726, 1989.

42. Sethna DH, Deboer GE, and Millar RA: Observations on "junctional rhythms" during anaesthesia, Br J Anaesth 56:924-925, 1984 (Letter).

43. Boba A: Significant effects on the blood pressure of an apparently trivial atrial dysrhythmia, Anesthesiology 48:282-283, 1978.

44. Galindo A, Wyte SR, and Wetherhold JW: Junctional rhythm induced by halothane anesthesia—treatment with succinylcholine, Anesthesiology 37:261-262, 1972.

45. Breslow MJ, Evers AS, and Lebowitz P: Successful treatment of accelerated junctional rhythm with propranolol: possible role of sympathetic stimulation in the genesis of this rhythm disturbance, Anesthesiology 62:180-182, 1985.

46. Hill RF: Treatment of isorhythmic A-V dissociation during general anesthesia with propranolol, Anesthesiology 70:141-144, 1989.

47. Black GW, Linde HW, Dripps RD, et al: Circulatory changes accompanying respiratory acidosis during halothane (Fluothane) anesthesia in man, Br J Anaesth 31:238-246, 1959.

48. Downing SE, Mitchell JH, and Wallace AG: Cardiovascular responses to ischemia, hypoxia and hypercapnia of the central nervous system, Am J Physiol 204:881-887, 1963.

49. Zink J, Sasyniuk BI, and Dresel PE: Halothane-epinephrine–induced cardiac arrhythmias and the role of heart rate, Anesthesiology 43:548-555, 1975.

50. Katz RL and Katz GJ: Surgical infiltration of pressor drugs and their interaction with volatile anaesthetics, Br J Anaesth 38:712-718, 1966.

51. Catenacci AJ, DiPalma JR, Anderson JD, et al: Serious arrhythmias with vasopressors during halothane anesthesia in man, JAMA 183:662-665, 1963.

52. Stirt JA, Berger JM, Ricker SM, et al: Arrhythmogenic effects of aminophylline during halothane anesthesia in experimental animals, Anesth Analg 59:410-416, 1980.

53. Roizen MF and Stevens WC: Multiform ventricular tachycardia due to the interaction of aminophylline and halothane, Anesth Analg 57:738-741, 1978.

54. Johnston RR, Eger EI II, and Wilson C: A comparative interaction of epinephrine with enflurane, isoflurane and halothane in man, Anesth Analg 55:709-712, 1976.

55. Karl HW, Swedlow DB, Lee KW, et al: Epinephrine-halothane interactions in children, Anesthesiology 58:142-145, 1983.

56. Bristow JD, Prys-Roberts C, Fisher A, et al: Effects of anesthesia on baroreflex control of heart rate in man, Anesthesiology 31:422-428, 1969.

57. Atlee JL III and Malkinson CE: Potentiation by thiopental of halothane-epinephrine–induced arrhythmias in dogs, Anesthesiology 57:285-288, 1982.

58. Atlee JL and Flaherty MP: Thiopental and epinephrine arrhythmias with enflurane and isoflurane in dogs, Anesthesiology 59:A84, 1983 (Abstract).

59. Roberts FL, Burstrom RE and Atlee JL: Effects of ketamine and etomidate on epinephrine-induced ventricular dysrhythmias in dogs anesthetized with halothane, Anesthesiology 61:A36, 1984 (Abstract).

60. Ivankovich AD, El-Etr AA, Janeczko GF, et al: The effects of ketamine and Innovar anesthesia on digitalis tolerance in dogs, Anesth Analg 54:106-111, 1975.

61. Thomson SJ and Yate PM: Bradycardia after propofol infusion, Anaesthesia 42:430, 1987.

62. Albright GA: Cardiac arrest following regional anesthesia with etidocaine or bupivacaine, Anesthesiology 51:285-287, 1979 (Editorial).

63. Kasten GW: High serum bupivacaine concentrations produce rhythm disturbances similar to torsades de pointes in anesthetized dogs, Reg Anaesth 11:20-26, 1986.

64. Clarkson C and Hondeghem L: Mechanism for bupivacaine depression of cardiac conduction: fast block of sodium channels during the action potential with slow recovery from block during diastole, Anesthesiology 62:396-405, 1985.

65. Block A and Covino BG: Effect of local anesthetic

agents on cardiac conduction and contractility, Reg Anaesth 6:55-61, 1981.

66. Conklin KA and Ziadlou-Rad F: Bupivacaine cardiotoxicity in a pregnant patient with mitral valve prolapse, Anesthesiology 58(6):596, 1983 (Letter).

67. Davis NL and de Jong RH: Successful resuscitation following massive bupivacaine overdose, Anesth Analg 61:62-64, 1982.

68. Kasten GW and Martin ST: Bupivacaine cardiovascular toxicity: comparison of treatment with bretylium and lidocaine, Anesth Analg 64:911-916, 1985.

69. Soloman D, Buneqin L, and Albin M: The effect of magnesium sulfate administration on cerebral and cardiac toxicity of bupivacaine in dogs, Anesthesiology 72:341-346, 1990.

70. Rosen M, Thigpen J, Shnider S, et al: Bupivacaine-induced cardiotoxicity in hypoxic and acidotic sheep, Anesth Analg 64:1089-1096, 1985.

71. Loeb JM, Lichtenthal PR, and de Tarnowsky JM: Parasympathomimetic effects of fentanyl on the canine sinus node, J Auton Nerv Syst 11:91-94, 1984.

72. de Silva RA, Verrier RL, and Lown B: Protective effect of the vagotonic action of morphine sulphate on ventricular vulnerability, Cardiovasc Res 12:167-172, 1978.

73. Daskalopoulos NT, Laubie M, and Schmitt H: Localization of the central sympatho-inhibitory effect of a narcotic analgesic agent, fentanyl, in cats, Eur J Pharmacol 33:91-97, 1975.

74. Tammisto T, Takki S, and Toikka P: A comparison of the circulatory effects in man of the analgesics fentanyl, pentazocine, and pethidine, Br J Anaesth 42:317-324, 1970.

75. Royster RL, Keeler KD, Haisty WK, et al: Cardiac electrophysiologic effects of fentanyl and combinations of fentanyl and neuromuscular relaxants in pentobarbital anesthetized dogs, Anesth Analg 67:15-20, 1988.

76. Sherman EP, Lebowitz PW, and Street WC: Bradycardia following sufentanil-succinylcholine, Anesthesiology 66:106, 1987 (Letter).

77. Latson TW and Lappas DG: Use of a pacing catheter to control heart rate in a patient with aortic insufficiency and coronary artery disease, Anesthesiology 63:712-715, 1985.

78. Puerto BA, Wong KC, Puerto AX, et al: Epinephrine-induced dysrhythmias: comparison during anaesthesia with narcotics and halogenated inhalational agents in dogs, Can Anaesth Soc J 26:263-268, 1979.

79. Saini V, Carr DB, and Hagestad EL: Antifibrillatory action of the narcotic agonist fentanyl, Am Heart J 115:598-605, 1988 (Review).

80. Royster RL, Keeler DK, Prough DS, et al: Fentanyl attenuates stimulation of atrial premature depolarizations and prolongs atrioventricular and ventricular refractoriness in dogs, Anesthesiology 63(suppl 3A):A77, 1985 (Abstract).

81. Yasuda I, Hirano T, Amaha K, et al: Chronotropic effects of succinylcholine and succinyl monocholine on the sinoatrial node, Anesthesiology 57:289-292, 1982.

82. Cooperman LH: Succinylcholine-induced hyperkalemia in neuromuscular disease, JAMA 213: 1867-1871, 1970.

83. Stoelting RK and Peterson C: Heart-rate slowing and junctional rhythm following intravenous succinylcholine with and without intramuscular atropine preanesthetic medication, Anesth Analg 54:705-709, 1975.

84. Maryniak JK and Bishop VA: Sinus arrest after alfentanil, Br J Anaesth 59:390-391, 1987.

85. Butterworth JF, Bean VE, and Royster RL: Premedication determines the circulatory responses to rapid

sequence induction with sufentanil for cardiac surgery, Br J Anaesth 63:351-353, 1989.

86. Geha DG, Rozelle BC, Raessler KL, et al: Pancuronium bromide enhances atrioventricular conduction in halothane-anesthetized dogs, Anesthesiology 46:342-345, 1977.

87. Son SL and Wand BE: Potencies of neuromuscular blocking agents at the receptors of the atrial pacemaker and the motor endplate of the guinea pig, Anesthesiology 47:34-36, 1977.

88. Domenech JS, Garcia RC, Sastain JMR, et al: Pancuronium bromide: an indirect sympathomimetic agent, Br J Anaesth 48:1143-1148, 1976.

89. Edwards RP, Miller RD, Roizen MF, et al: Cardiac responses to imipramine and pancuronium during anesthesia with halothane or enflurane, Anesthesiology 50:421-425, 1979.

90. Jacobs HK, Lim S, Salem MR, et al: Cardiac electrophysiologic effects of pancuronium, Anesth Analg 64:693-699, 1985.

91. Gravlee GP, Ramsey FM, Roy RC, et al: Rapid administration of a narcotic and neuromuscular blocker: a hemodynamic comparison of fentanyl, sufentanil, pancuronium, and vecuronium, Anesth Analg 67:39-47, 1988.

92. Starr NJ, Sethna PH, and Estafanous FG: Bradycardia and asystole following the rapid administration of sufentanil with vecuronium, Anesthesiology 64:521-523, 1986.

93. Pollok AJP: Cardiac arrest immediately after vecuronium, Br J Anaesth 58:936-937, 1986 (Letter).

94. Milligan KR and Beers HT: Vecuronium-associated cardiac arrest, Anaesthesia 40:385, 1985 (Letter).

95. Andree RA: Sudden death following naloxone administration, Anesth Analg 59:782-784, 1980.

96. Azar I, Pham AN, Karambelkar DJ, et al: The heart rate following edrophonium-atropine and edrophonium-glycopyrrolate mixtures, Anesthesiology 59:139-141, 1983.

97. Cronnelly R, Morris RB, and Miller RO: Edrophonium: duration of action and atropine requirement in humans during halothane anesthesia, Anesthesiology 57:261-266, 1982.

98. Urquhart ML, Ramsey FM, Royster RL, et al: Heart rate and rhythm following an edrophonium/atropine mixture for antagonism of neuromuscular blockade during fentanyl/N_2O/O_2 or isoflurane/N_2O/O_2 anesthesia, Anesthesiology 67:561-565, 1987.

99. Sprague DH: Severe bradycardia after neostigmine in a patient taking propranolol to control paroxysmal atrial tachycardia, Anesthesiology 42:208-210, 1975.

100. Maister AH: Atrial fibrillation following physostigmine, Can Anaesth Soc J 30:419-421, 1983.

101. Dauchot P and Gravenstein JS: Effects of atropine on the electrocardiogram in different age groups, Clin Pharmacol Ther 12:274-280, 1971.

102. Caplan RA, Ward RJ, Posner K, et al: Unexpected cardiac arrest during spinal anesthesia: a closed claims analysis of predisposing factors, Anesthesiology 68:5-11, 1988.

103. Cohen LI: Asystole during spinal anesthesia in a patient with sick sinus syndrome, Anesthesiology 68:787-788, 1988.

104. King BD, Harris LC Jr, Greifenstein FE, et al: Reflex circulatory responses to direct laryngoscopy and tracheal intubation performed during general anesthesia, Anesthesiology 12:556-566, 1951.

105. Saanivaara L and Kentala E: Comparison of electrocardiographic changes during microlaryngoscopy under halothane anaesthesia induced by Althesin® or thiopentone, Acta Anaesthesiol Scand 21:71-79, 1977.

106. Royster RL, Johnston WE, Gravlee GP, et al: Arrhythmias during venous cannulation prior to pulmonary artery catheter insertion, Anesth Analg 64:1214-1216, 1985.

107. Damen J and Bolton D: A prospective analysis of 1400 pulmonary artery catheterizations in patients undergoing cardiac surgery, Acta Anaesthesiol Scand 30:386-392, 1986.

108. Salmenperä M, Peltola K, and Rosenberg P: Does prophylactic lidocaine control cardiac arrhythmias associated with pulmonary artery catheterization? Anesthesiology 56:210-212, 1982.

109. Kasten GW, Owens E, and Kennedy D: Ventricular tachycardia resulting from central venous catheter tip migration due to arm position changes: report of two cases, Anesthesiology 62:185-187, 1985.

110. Goldman L, Caldera DL, Southwick FS, et al: Cardiac risk factors and complications in non-cardiac surgery, Medicine (Baltimore) 57:357-370, 1978.

111. Berbari EJ and Lazzara R: An introduction to high-resolution ECG recordings of cardiac late potentials, Arch Intern Med 148:1859-1863, 1988.

112. Cain ME, Ambros D, Witkowski FX, et al: Fast-Fourier transform analysis of signal-averaged electrocardiograms for identification of patients prone to sustained ventricular tachycardia, Circulation 69:711-720, 1984.

113. Hollifield JW: Electrolyte disarray and cardiovascular disease, Am J Cardiol 63:21B-26B, 1989 (Review).

114. Cohen L and Kitzes R: Magnesium sulfate and digitalis-toxic arrhythmias, JAMA 249:2808-2810, 1983.

115. Shapiro S, Slone D, Lewis PG, et al: The epidemiology of digoxin: a study of three Boston hospitals, J Chronic Dis 22:361-371, 1979.

116. Josephson ME and Kastor JA: Supraventricular tachycardia: mechanisms and management, Ann Intern Med 87:346-358, 1977 (Review).

117. Wu D: Supraventricular tachycardias, JAMA 249:3357-3360, 1983.

118. Singer DH and Ten Eick RE: Aberrancy: electrophysiologic aspects, Am J Cardiol 28:381-401, 1971.

119. Fenster PE, Comess KA, Marsh R, et al: Conversion of atrial fibrillation to sinus rhythm by acute intravenous procainamide infusion, Am Heart J 106:501-504, 1983.

120. Watanabe AM: Digitalis and the autonomic nervous system, J Am Coll Cardiol 5(suppl A):35A-42A, 1985 (Review).

121. Venditti FJ Jr, Garan H, and Ruskin JN: Electrophysiologic effects of beta blockers in ventricular arrhythmias, Am J Cardiol 60:3D-9D, 1987.

122. Littman L, Tenczer J, and Fenyvesi T: Atrioventricular nodal reentrant paroxysmal supraventricular tachycardia, Arch Intern Med 144:129-131, 1984.

123. Wellens HJ, Bar FW, and Lie KI: The value of the electrocardiogram in the differential diagnosis of a tachycardia with a widened QRS complex, Am J Med 64:27-33, 1978.

124. Garratt C, Linker N, Griffith M, et al: Comparison of adenosine and verapamil for termination of paroxysmal junctional tachycardia, Am J Cardiol 64:1310-1316, 1989.

125. Richardson JM: Ventricular preexcitation: practical considerations, Arch Intern Med 143:760-764, 1983.

126. Mandel WJ, Laks MM, Obayashi K, et al: The Wolff-Parkinson-White syndrome: pharmacologic effects of procaine amide, Am Heart J 90:744-754, 1975.

127. Josephson ME, Kastor JA, and Kitchen JG III: Lidocaine in Wolff-Parkinson-White syndrome with atrial fibrillation, Ann Intern Med 84:44-45, 1976.

128. Akhtar M, Gilbert CJ and Shenasa M: Effect of lidocaine on atrioventricular response via the accessory pathway in patients with Wolff-Parkinson-White syndrome, Circulation 63:435-441, 1981.

129. McGovern B, Garan H, and Ruskin JN: Precipitation of cardiac arrest by verapamil in patients with Wolff-Parkinson-White syndrome, Ann Intern Med 104:791-794, 1986.

130. Sellers TB Jr, Bashore TM, and Gallagher JJ: Digitalis in the pre-excitation syndrome: analysis during atrial fibrillation, Circulation 56:260-267, 1977.

131. Gómez-Arnau J, Márquez-Montes J, and Avello F: Fentanyl and droperidol effects on the refractoriness of the accessory pathway in the Wolff-Parkinson-White syndrome, Anesthesiology 58:307-313, 1983.

132. Rinkenberger RL, Prystowsky EN, Heger JJ, et al: Effects of intravenous and chronic oral verapamil administration in patients with supraventricular tachyarrhythmias, Circulation 62:996-1010, 1980.

133. Haft JI and Habbab MA: Treatment of atrial arrhythmias: effectiveness of verapamil when preceded by calcium infusion, Arch Intern Med 146:1085-1089, 1986.

134. Goldman S, Probst P, Selzer A, et al: Inefficacy of "therapeutic" serum levels of digoxin in controlling the ventricular rate in atrial fibrillation, Am J Cardiol 35:651-655, 1975.

135. Platia EV, Michelson EL, Porterfield JK, et al: Esmolol versus verapamil in the acute treatment of atrial fibrillation or atrial flutter, Am J Cardiol 63:925-929, 1989.

136. Dunn M, Alexander J, de Silva R, et al: Antithrombotic therapy in atrial fibrillation, Chest 89:68S-74S, 1986 (Review).

137. Wells JL Jr, Maclean WA, James TN, et al: Characterization of atrial flutter: studies in man after open heart surgery using fixed atrial electrodes, Circulation 50:665-673, 1979.

138. Waldo AL, Wells JL Jr, Cooper TB, et al: Temporary cardiac pacing: applications and techniques in the treatment of cardiac arrhythmias, Prog Cardiovasc Dis 23:451-474, 1981 (Review).

139. Plumb VJ, Karp RB, James TN, et al: Atrial excitability and conduction during rapid atrial pacing, Circulation 63:1140-1149, 1981.

140. Shine KI, Kastor JA, and Yurchak PM: Multifocal atrial tachycardia: clinical and electrocardiographic features in 32 patients, N Engl J Med 279:344-349, 1968.

141. Scher DL and Arsura EL: Multifocal atrial tachycardia: mechanisms, clinical correlates, and treatment, Am Heart J 118:574-580, 1989 (Review).

142. Levine JL, Michael JR, and Guarnieri T: Multifocal atrial tachycardia: a toxic effect of theophylline, Lancet 1:12-14, 1985.

143. Levine JH, Michael JR, and Guarnieri T: Treatment of multifocal atrial tachycardia with verapamil, N Engl J Med 312:21-25, 1985.

144. Hazard PB and Burnett CR: Treatment of multifocal atrial tachycardia with metoprolol, Crit Care Med 15:20-25, 1987.

145. Bigger JT Jr: Identification of patients at high risk for sudden cardiac death, Am J Cardiol 54:3D-8D, 1984.

146. Maseri A, L'Abbate A, Chierchia S, et al: Significance of spasm in the pathogenesis of ischemic heart disease, Am J Cardiol 44:788-792, 1979 (Review).

147. Bigger JT Jr and Giardina EGV: The pharmacology and clinical use of lidocaine and procainamide, Medical College of Virginia Quarterly 9:65-76, 1973.

148. Giardina EGV, Heissenbuttel RH, and Bigger JT Jr: Intermittent intravenous procaine amide to treat ventricular arrhythmias: correlation of plasma concentration with effect on arrhythmia, electrocardiogram, and blood pressure, Ann Intern Med 78:183-193, 1973.

149. Levy S: Combination therapy for cardiac arrhythmias, Am J Cardiol 61:95A-101A, 1988 (Review).

150. Levites R, Bodenheimer MM, and Helfant RH: Electrophysiologic effects of nitroglycerin during experimental coronary occlusion, Circulation 52:1050-1055, 1975.

151. Podrid PJ, Schoeneberger A, and Lown B: Congestive heart failure caused by oral disopyramide, N Engl J Med 302:614-617, 1980.

152. Gallagher JD, Lieberman RW, Meranze J, et al: Amiodarone-induced complications during coronary artery surgery, Anesthesiology 55:186-188, 1981.

153. Marchlinski FE, Gansler TS, Waxman HL, et al: Amiodarone pulmonary toxicity, Ann Intern Med 97:839-845, 1982.

154. Perlow GM, Jain BP, Pauker SG, et al: Tocainide-associated interstitial pneumonitis, Ann Intern Med 94:489-490, 1981.

155. Dunn M and Glassroth J: Pulmonary complications of amiodarone toxicity, Prog Cardiovasc Dis 31:447-453, 1989 (Review).

156. Koch MJ, Seef LB, Crumley CE, et al: Quinidine hepatotoxicity: a report of a case and review of the literature, Gastroenterology 70:1136-1140, 1976.

157. Falk RH: Flecainide-induced ventricular tachycardia and fibrillation in patients treated for atrial fibrillation, Ann Intern Med 111:107-111, 1989.

158. Hager WD, Fenster P, Mayersohn M, et al: Digoxin-quinidine interaction: pharmacokinetic evaluation, N Engl J Med 300:1238-1241, 1979.

159. Bigger JT Jr: The interaction of mexiletine with other cardiovascular drugs, Am Heart J 107:1079-1085, 1984.

160. Klein HO, Lang R, Weiss E, et al: The influence of verapamil on serum digoxin concentration, Circulation 65:998-1003, 1982.

161. Data JL, Wilkinson GR, and Nies AS: Interaction of quinidine with anticonvulsant drugs, N Engl J Med 294:699-702, 1976.

162. Aitio ML, Mansury L, Tala E, et al: The effect of enzyme induction on the metabolism of disopyramide in man, Br J Clin Pharmacol 11:279-285, 1981.

163. Vrobel TR, Miller PE, Mostow ND, et al: A general overview of amiodarone toxicity: its prevention, detection, and management, Prog Cardiovasc Dis 31:393-426, 1989 (Review).

164. Procacci PM, Savran SV, Schreiter SL, et al: Prevalence of clinical mitral-valve prolapse in 1,169 young women, N Engl J Med 294:1086-1088, 1976.

165. Mills P, Rose J, Hollingsworth BA, et al: Long-term prognosis of mitral-valve prolapse, N Engl J Med 297:13-18, 1977.

166. Boudoulas H, Reynolds JC, Mazzaferri E, et al: Mitral valve prolapse syndrome: the effect of adrenergic stimulation, J Am Coll Cardiol 2:638-644, 1983.

167. Savage DD, Devereux RB, Garrison RJ, et al: Mitral valve prolapse in the general population: I. Epidemiologic features: the Framingham Study, Am Heart J 106:571-576, 1983.

168. Kramer HM, Kligfield P, Devereux RB, et al: Arrhythmia in mitral valve prolapse: effect of selection bias, Arch Intern Med 144:2360-2364, 1984.

169. Puddu PE, Pasternac A, Tubau JF, et al: QT interval prolongation and increased plasma catecholamine levels in patients with mitral valve prolapse, Am Heart J 105:422-428, 1983.

170. Thiagarajah S and Frost EA: Anaesthetic considerations in patients with mitral valve prolapse, Anaesthesia 38:560-566, 1983.

171. Krantz EM, Viljoen JF, Schermer R, et al: Mitral valve prolapse, Anesth Analg 59:379-383, 1980.

172. Barlow JB and Pocock WA: The mitral valve prolapse enigma—two decades later, Mod Concepts Cardiovasc Dis 53:13-17, 1984.

173. Galloway PA and Glass PSA: Anesthetic implications of prolonged QT interval syndromes, Anesth Analg 64:612-620, 1985 (Review).

174. Medak R and Benumof JL: Perioperative management of the prolonged QT interval syndrome, Br J Anaesth 55:361-364, 1983.

175. Wig J, Bali IM, Singh RG, et al: Prolonged QT interval syndrome: sudden cardiac arrest during anaesthesia, Anaesthesia 34:37-40, 1979.

176. Yanowitz F, Preston JB, and Abildskov JA: Functional distribution of right and left stellate innervation to the ventricles: production of neurogenic electrocardiographic changes by unilateral alteration of sympathetic tone, Circ Res 18:416-428, 1966.

177. Moss AJ and McDonald J: Unilateral cervicothoracic sympathetic ganglionectomy for the treatment of the long QT syndromes, N Engl J Med 285:903-904, 1971.

178. Schwartz PJ, Periti M, and Malliani A: The long QT-syndrome, Am Heart J 89:378-390, 1975.

179. Carlock FJ, Brown M, and Brown EM: Isoflurane anaesthesia for a patient with long QT syndrome, Can Anaesth Soc J 31:83-85, 1984.

180. Ponte J and Lund J: Prolongation of the QT interval (Romano-Ward syndrome): anaesthetic management, Br J Anaesth 53:1347-1350, 1981.

181. Bardy GH, Ungerleider RM, Smith WM, et al: A mechanism of torsades de pointes in a canine model, Circulation 67:52-59, 1983.

182. Tzivoni D, Banai S, Schuger C, et al: Treatment of torsade de pointes with magnesium sulfate, Circulation 77:392-397, 1988.

183. Milne JR, Ward DE, Spurrell AJ, et al: The long QT syndrome: effects of drugs and left stellate ganglion block, Am Heart J 104(2 Pt 1):194-198, 1982.

184. Kahn MM, Logan KR, McComb JM, et al: Management of recurrent ventricular tachyarrhythmias associated with QT prolongation, Am J Cardiol 47:1301-1308, 1981.

185. Roizen MF, Lampe GH, Benefiel DJ, et al: Change in QT interval with anesthesia: should it determine whether to use a narcotic or inhalational agent? Anesthesiology 69(3A):A53, 1988 (Abstract).

186. Roden DM, Woosley RL, and Primm PK: Incidence and clinical features of the quinidine-associated long QT syndrome: implications for patient care, Am Heart J 111:1038-1093, 1986.

187. Singh BN and Vaughan-Williams EM: The effect of amiodarone, a new anti-anginal drug, on cardiac muscle, Br J Pharmacol 39:357-367, 1970.

188. Singh BN: When is QT prolongation antiarrhythmic and when is it proarrhythmic? Am J Cardiol 63:867-869, 1989 (Editorial).

189. Rotem M, Constantini S, Shir Y, et al: Life-threatening torsade de pointes arrhythmia associated with head injury, Neurosurgery 23:89-92, 1988.

190. Marion DW, Segal R, and Thompson ME: Subarachnoid hemorrhage and the heart, Neurosurgery 18:101-106, 1986.

191. Mikolich JR, Jacobs WC, and Fletcher GF: Cardiac arrhythmias in patients with acute cerebrovascular accidents, JAMA 246:1314-1317, 1981.

192. Di Pasquale G, Pinelli G, Andreoli A, et al: Holter detection of cardiac arrhythmias in intracranial subarachnoid hemorrhage, Am J Cardiol 59:596-600, 1987.

193. Hust MH, Nitsche K, Hohnloser S, et al: Q-T prolongation and torsades de pointes in a patient with subarachnoid hemorrhage, Clin Cardiol 7:44-48, 1984.

194. Stober T, Sen S, Anstatt T, et al: Correlation of cardiac arrhythmias with brainstem compression in patients with intracerebral hemorrhage, Stroke 19:688-692, 1988.

195. Smith M and Ray CT: Cardiac arrhythmias, increased intracranial pressure, and the autonomic nervous system, Chest 61(suppl):125-133, 1972.

196. Estanol BV, Loyo MV, Mateos JH, et al: Cardiac arrhythmias in experimental subarachnoid hemorrhage, Stroke 8:440-449, 1977.

197. Lacy PS and Earle AM: A small animal model for electrocardiographic abnormalities observed after an experimental subarachnoid hemorrhage, Stroke 14:371-377, 1983.

198. von Olshausen K, Amann E, Hofmann M, et al: Ventricular arrhythmias before and late after aortic valve replacement, Am J Cardiol 54:142-146, 1984.

199. von Olshausen K, Schwarz F, Apfelbach J, et al: Determinants of the incidence and severity of ventricular arrhythmias in aortic valve disease, Am J Cardiol 51:1103-1109, 1983.

200. Schilling G, Finkbeiner T, Elberskirch P, et al: Incidence of ventricular arrhythmias in patients with aortic valve replacement, Am J Cardiol 49:894, 1982 (Abstract).

201. Parris TM, Mintz GS, Ross J, et al: Importance of atrial contraction to left ventricular filling in mitral stenosis, Am J Cardiol 61:1135-1136, 1988.

202. Gillette PC: Evolving concepts in the management of congenital junctional ectopic tachycardia, Circulation 81:1713-1714, 1990 (Editorial).

203. Garson A Jr and Gillette PC: Junctional ectopic tachycardia in children: electrocardiography, electrophysiology and pharmacologic response, Am J Cardiol 44:298-302, 1979.

204. Gillette PC: Diagnosis and management of postoperative junctional ectopic tachycardia, Am Heart J 118:192-194, 1989 (Editorial).

205. Bash SE, Shah JJ, Albers WH, et al: Hypothermia for the treatment of post-surgical greatly accelerated junctional ectopic tachycardia, J Am Coll Cardiol 10:1095-1099, 1987.

206. Grant JW, Serwer GA, Armstrong BE, et al: Junctional tachycardia in infants and children after open heart surgery for congenital heart disease, Am J Cardiol 59:1216-1218, 1987.

207. Porter CJ, Gillette PC, Garson A Jr, et al: Effects of verapamil on supraventricular tachycardia in children, Am J Cardiol 48:487-491, 1981.

208. Villain E, Vetter VL, Garcia JM, et al: Evolving concepts in the management of congenital junctional ectopic tachycardia: a multicenter study, Circulation 81:1544-1549, 1990 (Review).

209. Kunze KP, Kuck KH, Schluter M, et al: Effect of encainide and flecainide on chronic ectopic atrial tachycardia, J Am Coll Cardiol 7:1121-1126, 1986.

210. Garson A Jr, Moak JP, Smith RT Jr, et al: Usefulness of intravenous propafenone for control of postoperative junctional ectopic tachycardia, Am J Cardiol 59:1422-1424, 1987.

211. Podrid PJ: Potassium and ventricular arrhythmias, Am J Cardiol 65:33E-44E, 1990.

212. Papademetriou V, Fletcher R, Khatri IM, et al: Diuretic-induced hypokalemia in uncomplicated systemic hypertension: effect of plasma potassium correction on cardiac arrhythmias, Am J Cardiol 52:1017-1022, 1983.

213. Hulting J: In hospital ventricular fibrillation and its relation to serum potassium, Acta Med Scand 647(suppl):109-116, 1981.

214. Hollifield JW: Thiazide treatment of hypertension: effects of thiazide diuretics on serum potassium, magnesium, and ventricular ectopy, Am J Med 80(suppl 4A):8-12, 1986.

215. Struthers AD, Reid JL, Whitesmith R, et al: Effect of intravenous adrenaline on electrocardiogram, blood pressure and serum potassium, Br Heart J 49:90-93, 1983.

216. Watanabe Y, Dreifus LS, and Likoff W: Electrophysiologic antagonism and synergism of potassium and antiarrhythmic agents, Am J Cardiol 12:702-710, 1963.

217. Surawicz B: Is hypomagnesemia or magnesium deficiency arrhythmogenic? J Am Coll Cardiol 14:1093-1096, 1989.

218. Watanabe Y and Dreifus LS: Electrophysiological effects of magnesium and its interactions with potassium, Cardiovasc Res 6:79-88, 1972.

219. Skou JC: The influence of some actions on an ATPase from peripheral nerves, Biochim Biophys Acta (Amst.) 23:394-401, 1957.

220. January CT and Fozzard HA: Delayed afterdepolarizations in heart muscle: mechanisms and relevance, Pharmacol Rev 40:219-227, 1988.

221. Abraham AS, Rosenman D, Meshulam Z, et al: Serum, lymphocyte, and erythrocyte potassium, magnesium, and calcium concentrations and their relation to tachyarrhythmias in patients with acute myocardial infarction, Am J Med 81:983-988, 1986.

222. Bunton RW: Value of serum magnesium estimation in diagnosing myocardial infarction and predicting dysrhythmias after coronary artery bypass grafting, Thorax 38:946-950, 1983.

223. Ragnarsson J, Hardarson T, and Snorrason SP: Ventricular dysrhythmias in middle-aged hypertensive men treated either with a diuretic agent or a β-blocker, Acta Med Scand 221:143-148, 1987.

224. Hollifield JW and Slaton PE: Thiazide diuretics, hypokalemia and cardiac arrhythmias, Acta Med Scand, suppl 647:67-73, 1981.

225. Dyckner T: Serum magnesium in acute myocardial infarction: reaction to arrhythmias, Acta Med Scand 207:59-66, 1980.

226. DiCarlo LA Jr, Morady F, de Buitleir M, et al: Effects of magnesium sulfate on cardiac conduction and refractoriness in humans, J Am Coll Cardiol 7:1356-1362, 1986.

227. Rasmussen HS, McNair P, Norregard P, et al: Intravenous magnesium in acute myocardial infarction, Lancet 1:234-236, 1986.

228. Boyd LJ and Scherf D: Magnesium sulfate in paroxysmal tachycardia, Am J Med Sci 206:43-48, 1943.

229. French JH, Thomas RG, Siskind AP, et al: Magnesium therapy in massive digoxin intoxication, Ann Emerg Med 13:562-566, 1984.

230. Tzivoni D, Banai S, Schuger C, et al: Treatment of torsade de pointes with magnesium sulfate, Circulation 77:392-397, 1988.

231. Iseri LT, Chung P, and Tobis J: Magnesium therapy for intractable ventricular tachyarrhythmias in hormomagnesemic patients, West J Med 138:823-828, 1983.

232. Wester PO: Magnesium, Am J Clin Nutr 45:1305-1312, 1987.

233. Reinhart RA: Magnesium metabolism: a review with special reference to the relationship between intracellular content and serum levels, Arch Intern Med 148:2415-2420, 1988 (Review).

234. Iseri LT: Role of magnesium in cardiac tachyarrhythmias, Am J Cardiol 65:47K-50K, 1990.

Chapter 11

Hypotension, Hypertension, Perioperative Myocardial Ischemia, and Infarction

Philip K. Kraker
Charles J. Kopriva

The continuous supply of oxygenated blood is an absolute necessity for normal human existence. The kinetic and potential energy generated, stored, and distributed by the cardiovascular system provides the vital forces to ensure the constant delivery of nutrient-laden blood. The cardiovascular system is endowed with considerable compensatory capabilities allowing adaptations to variability in normal human activities as well as compensations for pathophysiologic states. Although remarkably efficient within their limits, these compensatory mechanisms can be overwhelmed by the ravages of disease. The administration of anesthesia can also cause complications that are deleterious to both function and structure. In this chapter we focus upon hypotension, hypertension, perioperative myocardial ischemia, and perioperative myocardial infarction listing the major causes of these abnormalities and suggesting appropriate treatment.

I. PERIOPERATIVE HYPOTENSION

Hypotension is probably the most commonly observed and feared complication during anesthesia. The widespread use of continuous arterial manometry and the more recent introduction of automated "cuff" blood pressure methods have further focused our attention upon hypotension.

Generically defined, the term "hypotension" means abnormally low blood pressure. As is commonly known, blood pressure can be low in the systemic circuit or in the pulmonary circuit and can involve either systolic, diastolic, or both systolic and diastolic values. However, in common usage the word "hypotension" refers to an abnormally low systemic systolic blood pressure. Although the systemic systolic blood pressure is certainly not the only pressure affecting critical blood flow, nevertheless lowering of the systolic pressure serves as a "red flag" for critical examination of cardiovascular functional status.

The physical dynamics of systolic blood pressure generation and detection are beyond the scope of this chapter. However, any factor that seriously lowers cardiac output or peripheral vascular resistance or both can significantly lower systolic blood pressure and mean arterial blood pressure. A generalized classification of the causes of systemic arterial hypotension mirrors the classifications of "shock," including hypovolemic shock, cardiogenic shock, septic shock, and neurogenic shock. Each of these abnormalities are considered separately.

A. Hypovolemic hypotension

The word "hypovolemia" refers to a reduction in the intravascular blood volume. Hypovole-

mia may result from losses of whole blood, reductions in red cell volume, reductions in plasma volume, or reductions in free water.

Hemorrhage is often an obvious cause of hypotension because the anesthesiologist may easily detect massive bleeding. However, it can be difficult to observe pelvic bleeding or bleeding into the chest cavity during thoracic surgery. In trauma cases one must keep in mind that bleeding into an unsuspected area of injury remote from the operative site can occur. Likewise, hemorrhage can be hidden as in the large retroperitoneal hematomas seen with pelvic fractures or the large blood loss into the thigh that can accompany hip or femur fractures.

Early diagnosis of hemorrhagic hypotension is extremely important in minimizing morbidity and mortality especially in patients with compromised cardiovascular systems. The classical signs of hemorrhagic hypotension are often enumerated as tachycardia, vasoconstriction, low systolic blood pressure, and sometimes low urinary output. To the novice in anesthesia these are the signs of hypovolemic hypotension. However, seasoned clinicians recognize that these abnormalities are not the first signs of hemorrhagic hypotension. Long before these signs occur the astute clinician will appreciate that suctioning of blood from the operative field is occurring much more frequently and there will be a change in the demeanor of the surgeons. The most competent surgeons faced with acute hemorrhage will often become quiet, serious, and directed toward an organized plan. The emotional outbursts of the less competent are easy to detect.

Hypovolemic hypotension during anesthesia can also result from decreases in plasma volume. Preoperative or intraoperative use of potent diuretics are common causes of intraoperative hypovolemic hypotension. Decreases in plasma volume can occur intraoperatively secondary to handling of bowel and mesentery. Even more extensive losses can occur during the retroperitoneal operative dissections done during abdominal aortic aneurysm repair or pancreaticoduodenectomy.[1]

The specific treatment of hypovolemic hypotension is to restore adequate circulating intravascular volume. This can be done with whole blood, packed red blood cells, albumin or hetastarch, or a balanced electrolyte solution such as lactated Ringer's solution. The resistance to fluid flow through an intravenous cannula is directly proportional to cannula length and inversely proportional to the diameter of the cannula. Consequently, if rapid fluid administration is necessary, short, large-bore cannulas (14 or 16 gauge) are very desirable. However, even with optimal intravenous cannulas and pressure-infusion devices, rapid volume repletion is sometimes too slow in restoring systemic blood pressure. The judicious use of a vasoconstrictor such as phenylephrine or a "mixed-action" drug such as epinephrine will allow restoration of improved arterial blood pressure while volume deficits are replaced.

Adjunctive supportive measures are often necessary during the treatment of severe hypovolemic hypotension. Administration of 100% oxygen will help to promote optimal peripheral oxygen delivery. Volatile anesthetic agents often must be discontinued and reliance placed on muscle relaxants to provide an immobile patient. In this setting, intra-anesthetic recall can occur easily unless one administers an amnesic agent with minimal circulatory effects. We have found intravenous scopolamine to be especially useful. Acute renal failure can develop during or after hypotension. Clinicians have commonly administered potent intravenous diuretics such as furosemide in an attempt to minimize renal damage. However, at least two studies have indicated that diuretics do not decrease renal damage resulting from hypotension.[2,3]

B. Cardiogenic hypotension

Many different conditions can cause the left ventricle to pump inadequate volumes of blood. When this occurs, the peripheral circulation may attempt to compensate by vasoconstriction, but if impairment of left ventricular ejection is severe enough, hypotension will result. This can be appropriately called "cardiogenic hypotension" and can be caused by several conditions, which are considered separately.

1. Pharmacologic causes. All modern inhalation agents and many intravenous agents are capable of depressing myocardial contractility.[4-8] The cardiogenic hypotension seen with inhalation anesthetics can result from frank overdoses of the agents but more commonly arises when clinically acceptable dosages are given. Previous deficiencies in myocardial contractility or the presence of "relative" hypovolemia may accentuate cardiogenic hypotension. In the majority of cases, one can treat cardiogenic hypotension associated with volatile agents by decreasing or perhaps temporarily discontinuing the administration of the agent while administering 250 to 500 ml of fluid. Patients with healthy cardiovascular systems will tolerate such maneuvers very well, but those with preexisting severe cardiovascular disease may require estimation of left ventricular filling pressures using a pulmonary artery catheter. The use of pulmonary artery pressures to estimate left ventricular pre-

load is the most commonly used method in 1990. It must be recognized, however, that changes in pulmonary capillary wedge pressure do not necessarily correlate well with changes in left ventricular end-diastolic volume, which is the true index of adequate preload.[9,10] Two-dimensional transesophageal echocardiography provides a method for estimation of left ventricular end diastolic volume. It is quite possible that this methodology will come into more widespread use in the future. At the present time, however, transesophageal echocardiography equipment is expensive and requires significant training before the anesthesiologist or cardiologist can make proper accurate use of this method.

2. Mechanical compression. Mechanical compression of the heart can impair diastolic filling of the left ventricle resulting in inadequate stroke volume and cardiogenic hypotension. Pericardial tamponade is a classic cause. Trauma, cardiac surgery, and intracardiac catheterization all may lead to pericardial tamponade. The condition can be life threatening requiring pericardiocentesis using an 18-gauge spinal needle. If this fails, emergency subxiphoid thoracostomy is indicated.[11] Mechanical displacement of the heart during cardiac surgery and during esophagogastrectomy can also cause hypotension. Tension pneumothorax shifts the mediastinum and kinks the great veins as they enter the thorax. This leads to severe hypotension, which may require emergency decompression using a 16-gauge needle followed by tube thoracostomy.[11] In supine obstetric patients the gravid uterus may compress the inferior vena cava leading to impaired preload and severe hypotension. This can be treated using intravenous fluids, left uterine displacement, and intravenous ephedrine.[12]

3. Poor myocardial function. Systemic arterial hypotension can result when left ventricular muscle cannot contract adequately. Very severe myocardial contusion can result in transmural myocardial infarction with attendant hypotension.[13] This condition can also cause severe ventricular arrhythmias. Both antiarrhythmic and inotropic agents may be required for effective treatment.

"Stunned" myocardium refers to postischemic depression of the left ventricle, reduced high-energy phosphate stores, and an abnormal ultrastructure.[14,15] Stunned myocardium may be encountered immediately after cardiopulmonary bypass and in other cases in which severe hypotension has persisted for at least 15 to 20 minutes. The resultant left ventricular dysfunction may be clinically significant. Ischemia causes poor cardiac contraction, incomplete ventricular emptying (systolic failure), and impaired ventricular relaxation (diastolic failure). Fortunately, "stunned" myocardium can be stimulated by infusion of sympathomimetics, which can "buy time" until the biochemical abnormalities are reversed.[16,17]

Intraoperative myocardial infarction can cause hypotension. This is especially true of transmural infarction involving a large amount of myocardium. Intraoperative infarcts can be "silent," but if a significant amount of myocardium is destroyed, there will be systolic failure with poor stroke volume, low cardiac output, and systemic arterial hypotension. Failure of ventricular relaxation leads to high filling pressures. The seven-lead electrocardiogram may help to establish the diagnosis, particularly if the standard leads are diagnostic as in an inferior infarct. MB-CPK levels are not helpful in diagnosing most intraoperative infarcts, since the enzyme levels may not become elevated until 12 to 24 hours after the infarct.[18] Most patients who sustain an intraoperative myocardial infarct will benefit from radial artery and pulmonary artery blood pressure monitoring. Judicious fluid management is important. The use of inotropic and vasoactive drugs may be necessary to support systemic blood pressure. An intra-aortic balloon can be helpful in cases with severe circulatory compromise. It is possible that thrombolytic therapy could benefit patients with intraoperative infarcts especially those occurring during operations with minimal bleeding potential. However, at this time this is conjecture. Myocardial infarction is considered in greater depth later in this chapter.

C. Hypotension secondary to decreased peripheral resistance

The contractile state of smooth muscles in small arterioles determines peripheral vascular resistance. Even small changes in arteriolar diameter can have profound effects on peripheral vascular resistance because it is inversely related to the fourth power of the vessel radius.

1. Premedication. Preoperative hypotension may occasionally be caused by an overdose or a "relative" overdose of premedicant drugs such as barbiturates, narcotics, and benzodiazepine derivatives. This is most likely to occur in patients who are relatively hypovolemic. Often a small bolus of lactated Ringer's solution will restore satisfactory blood pressure. If a serious circulatory derangement such as myocardial ischemia or pulmonary embolus can be ruled out, anesthesia can often be induced after the fluid administration.

2. Inhalational agents. All modern inhalation agents may cause some decrease in peripheral resistance, which may be partly responsible for intraoperative hypotension. Reduction in the inhaled concentration of the agent, a small bolus of fluids, and judicious use of inotropes or vasoconstrictors can rapidly treat this type of hypotension.

3. Spinal and epidural anesthesia. Administration of spinal or epidural anesthesia can cause blockade of the sympathetic nervous system followed by decreased peripheral vascular resistance and severe hypotension. Severe hypotension is most likely to occur in patients with high levels of blocks or in patients who are hypovolemic. Bradycardia secondary to blockade of the cardioaccelerator fibers further accentuates the hypotension. Usually, hypotension is easily detected after spinal or epidural anesthesia and can be treated with fluid infusion, oxygen administration, and appropriate doses of a vasoconstrictor such as phenylephrine. In very high levels of spinal or epidural anesthesia attention must also be directed toward provision of adequate ventilation, which may sometimes require intubation.

4. Vasodilator adjuncts. Intravenous vasodilators are widely used during anesthetic care. Sodium nitroprusside, trimethaphan (Arfonad), nitroglycerin, and prostaglandins are well known causes of severe hypotension. Hypotension secondary to these agents is easily anticipated and can be treated when one discontinues the agent and administers a fluid bolus. If the hypotension is very severe or persistent, the judicious use of an alpha-adrenergic agent such as phenylephrine may be required. Hypotension secondary to sodium nitroprusside is especially prevalent in hypovolemic patients. Judicious fluid administration will often allow for satisfactory control of blood pressure with sodium nitroprusside.

5. "Antibiotic" hypotension. Intravenously administered vancomycin can produce life-threatening hypotension. The predominant mechanism is peripheral vascular dilatation, which led to its description as the "red man syndrome." The administration of vancomycin may cause an erythematous rash over the face, neck, upper trunk, and upper arms. This is often accompanied by pruritus (in awake patients) and angioedema.[19] The incidence of "vancomycin hypotension" has been shown to be related to the rate of administration.[20,21] Profound hypotension has been reported when 1000 mg of the drug is given over 30 minutes or less.[22] Rapid infusion has been shown to cause increased plasma histamine levels, and it has been suggested that the hypotension is mediated through a histaminergic response. Dogs pretreated with methapyrilene (an antihistamine) do not have hypotension after rapid administration of vancomycin.

Prevention is the best cure for vancomycin hypotension. Administering the drug slowly over 45 minutes definitely minimizes the incidence of hypotension. However, hypotensive episodes have been reported even at very slow rates.[23] Severe vancomycin hypotension can be life threatening, and we have seen one case in which the systolic arterial pressure decreased to 38 mm Hg. The return toward normal was extremely slow and was accomplished after several minutes of infusion of epinephrine up to 0.15 µg/kg/min. The use of a "mixed-action" drug such as epinephrine may be rational, since Cohen has shown that cardiac depression is part of the syndrome.[24] Administration of large volumes of lactated Ringer's may also be helpful. If the syndrome does not respond to epinephrine and fluids, the addition of bolus doses of phenylephrine may be appropriate.

6. Methylmethacrylate hypotension. Severe hypotension, hypoxemia, and cardiac arrest have been reported after the introduction of the bone cement methylmethacrylate into the marrow cavities of long bones, especially the femoral shaft. Investigations have shown that methylmethacrylate monomer does not produce hypotension.[25,26] It seems probable that the reaction is caused by fat and gas embolization resulting when high pressure is generated in the marrow cavity during implantation of a prosthesis. Venting the femoral shaft appears to reduce the amount of embolization.[27] The use of high oxygen tensions during implantation may minimize hypoxemia, and careful attention to the pulse oximeter may allow one to identify the reaction early. Effective bone venting should prevent the majority of these reactions, but occasionally a severe reaction requiring epinephrine or phenylephrine (Neo-Synephrine) may be still be encountered.

7. Carcinoid syndrome. Severe hypotension can occur during the anesthetic care of patients with carcinoid tumors. These tumors, which frequently occur in the jejunum or ilium, arise from enterochromaffin tissues and may release vasoactive substances including histamine, prostaglandins, kallikreins, and serotonin. Approximately 5% of patients with carcinoid tumors develop carcinoid syndrome.[28] Carcinoid tumors may metastasize to heart valves causing tricuspid regurgitation or pulmonary stenosis, or both. Severe bronchospasm can result in air trapping and increased intrathoracic pressures,

which may impair venous return and further accentuate hypotension.

The best treatment for hypotension of the carcinoid syndrome is to make every effort to prevent it. H_1 and H_2 receptor blockers may minimize the effects of histamine. Preoperative administration of cyproheptadine (Periactin) may also block the effects of intraoperative histamine release and can also block the effects of serotonin.[29] Morphine, *d*-tubocurarine, atracurium, metocurine, and succinylcholine should probably be avoided because they can release histamine. Many different anesthetic techniques have been used in patients with carcinoids, and none has been proved to be superior. However, a general anesthetic consisting of nitrous oxide, short-acting opioids, and pancuronium would appear to be a reasonable choice.[30] Monitoring both central venous pressure and pulmonary artery pressures to allow assessment of cardiovascular status is recommended. If hypotension develops, catecholamines should be avoided because they activate kallikreins. Rather one should give intravascular fluids and be guided by central venous and pulmonary artery pressures. Angiotensin 1.5 mg/kg may also reverse the hypotension.[31]

8. Protamine hypotension. Protamine sulfate given to reverse heparin anticoagulation can produce ominous hypotension secondary to its profound vasodilating properties.[32,33] The noticeable decrease in peripheral vascular resistance is most apparent in patients with poor ventricular function who can compensate only partially for the decreased peripheral resistance.[34] Temporary discontinuation of protamine infusion, increasing intravascular volume, and calcium chloride 1 to 2 g will usually successfully reverse this type of protamine hypotension. Occasionally, in the highest-risk patients, inotropic support with epinephrine or vasoconstriction using phenylephrine may be necessary.

Far more serious are anaphylactic reactions to protamine. Several groups of patients including those taking protamine zinc insulin, vasectomized men, and patients allergic to finned fish may be especially prone to anaphylactic reactions, though good controlled studies are lacking. Lowenstein described catastrophic pulmonary vasoconstriction occurring during protamine reversal of heparin.[35] Pulmonary arterial hypertension, right ventricular dilatation, decreased left ventricular filling pressure, and systemic hypotension characterized this serious reaction, which has been reported after only 10 mg of protamine. In a later study by the same group Morel described the mediator profile of patients with catastrophic postprotamine pulmonary reactions. Protamine was injected into the right atrium in a dose of 20 mg for mitral valve patients and 100 mg for coronary artery bypass graft patients. Of the 48 patients studied, 3 patients sustained pulmonary vasoconstrictive reactions.[36] The first sign was an increase in peak airway pressure followed immediately by an acute increase in pulmonary artery pressure and subsequent systemic hypotension requiring treatment with calcium chloride and phenylephrine. Thromboxane B_2 (TxB_2) increased greatly after protamine in all pulmonary reactors but remained normal in the nonreactors. Plasma C5a levels also increased greatly in the pulmonary reactors. Acute leukopenia and a significant decrease in the platelet count in systemic blood also occurred in patients who received 100 mg of protamine. Morel concluded that in the patients who developed catastrophic pulmonary increases in C5a anaphylatoxin led to thromboxane generation, which in turn caused the pulmonary vasoconstriction and bronchoconstriction. It is important to remember that this reaction involves bronchoconstriction and that an increase in peak airway pressure was the very first sign.

Protamine-induced hypotension can result from other, complex mechanisms and can range in severity from mild hypotension to total cardiovascular collapse. In an excellent review article Horrow has classified the adverse responses to protamine into three types. Type 1 is hypotension related to rapid administration, type 2 includes anaphylactoid responses, and type 3 is catastrophic pulmonary vasoconstriction.[37]

The best treatment for protamine reactions is prospective planning to prevent them whenever possible. However, it can be difficult to predict which patients will develop protamine hypotension. Patients who have a history of having developed severe hypotension in the cardiac catheterization lab after receiving protamine should certainly be suspect. Any patient who has had cardiac surgery and reports difficulty after protamine should be managed with a special care. Patients with finned fish (not shellfish) allergies should be suspect. Occasionally, patients who have received NPH insulin may have severe reactions, but we simply cannot predict this reaction with accuracy. Consequently, our approach is as follows: Protamine is always considered to be potentially dangerous. It is diluted to a concentration of 4 mg/ml and administered in low dead-space lines to preclude inadvertent bolus injection. A test dose of 4 to 8 mg of protamine is administered slowly with an automated cassette infusion device. The infusion is then stopped, and during the next 1 to 2 minutes we closely follow peak airway pressure, systemic arterial pressure, and pulmonary artery diastolic pressure. If no change occurs in any of these, the calculated protamine dose is slowly administered over 10 minutes by the automatic infusion pump. If a pronounced increase in airway pressure and pulmonary hypertension occurs after the test dose, we may elect not to administer the drug. At any rate, if a frank catastrophic pulmonary vasoconstrictive reaction occurs, pulmonary artery diastolic pressure will increase greatly. At this point, one might be tempted to administer intravenous nitroglycerin to lower the pulmonary artery diastolic pressure before continuing with the infusion of protamine. In our opinion this is ill advised because lowering right ventricular preload will cause extremely serious decreases in the stroke volume of the right ventricle, which is already struggling against a very high afterload. It is probably much better to stop the infusion and treat the hypotension with epinephrine, calcium chloride, or possibly isoproterenol. Since the prostaglandin PGE_1 is a pulmonary vasodilator, one might also consider its use.

9. Vascular graft material. Dacron vascular graft material has generally been assumed to be inert. However, Roizen et al.[38] recently reported five cases in which severe vasodilatation and disseminated intravascular coagulation developed shortly after blood flow began through aortic grafts. Blood samples from two of the patients demonstrated activation of complement and of the kinin system. The graft was urgently replaced in three patients. Two of those made a full recovery and one died. In two patients the graft was not replaced. Both died. Roizen et al. postulate that plasticizers in the grafts caused the abnormalities. Although this problem has not been widely recognized, it is worth considering if severe vasodilatation and a bleeding diathesis develops shortly after an aortic graft is placed. Definitive therapy appears to be replacement of the Dacron graft with a graft made from a different material.

D. Septic hypotension

Hypotension occurring in a patient with known or suspected infection should always raise the diagnostic possibility of septic shock. Sepsis-associated hypotension is a complex and very serious condition with a mortality somewhere between 50% and 90%.[39] Septic shock has been recognized since 1831 when Laënnec published his early report.[40] The anesthesiologist may encounter septic hypotension in association with a wide variety of surgical conditions (List 11-1).

List 11-1.   Surgical Conditions That May Be Associated With Septic Shock

1. Urinary tract infections
2. Pelvic abscess
3. Intraperitoneal abscess
4. Necrotizing fasciitis
5. Respiratory tract infection (particularly in patients with a tracheostomy)
6. Ascending cholangitis
7. Infected burns
8. Septic abortions
9. Postpartum infections
10. Subphrenic abscess

Hypotension is a prominent feature of septic shock. The occurrence of other hemodynamic derangements depends on whether the patient is euvolemic or hypovolemic. Euvolemic patients in septic shock are hypotensive, are vasodilated, and have high cardiac outputs and warm pink extremities. Hypovolemic septic patients, on the other hand, are hypotensive, have low cardiac outputs, are vasoconstricted, and have cold extremities.[41]

Septic hypotension is a complex disease. Specific treatment necessitates surgical drainage of the infected area and administration of antibiotics. However, one must also deal with the "toxic" aspects of the disease. These are particularly apparent in gram-negative shock. In the future, it is possible that specific monoclonal antibodies can be used to eradicate endotoxins. However, at the present time, supportive care is extremely important to "buy time" while the surgical infection is eradicated and antibiotic treatment started.

Rational supportive care of the cardiovascular system during septic hypotension necessitates assessment of ventricular filling pressures, cardiac outputs, and peripheral vascular resistance. Use of a pulmonary artery catheter and radial artery blood-pressure measurement facilitates diagnosis and guides therapy. Appropriate fluid therapy is extremely important in patients with septic hypotension. Patients with low filling pressures should receive fluids until cardiac output increases or pulmonary artery diastolic or pulmonary artery wedge pressures increase to approximately 18 torr. If cardiac output does not improve with increasing fluid infusion, it is important to use an inotropic agent and to treat metabolic acidosis. Dopamine at 2 to 5 μg/kg/min is often recommended as an initial choice. The dose can be increased to 20 μg/kg/min if necessary. If this fails to elevate blood pressure

to satisfactory levels, levarterenol is added and dopamine is reduced to "renal" doses (2 to 5 μg/kg/min). If the patient remains hypotensive despite this therapy, the prognosis is extremely poor.[42] Steroid therapy is no longer advocated because prospective controlled studies have shown that they offer no benefit.[43-45]

II. PERIOPERATIVE HYPERTENSION

Hypertension can be a significant complication in the preoperative, intraoperative, and postoperative care of surgical patients. The term "hypertension" denotes an elevated systemic systolic arterial pressure. Abnormally high systolic arterial pressure is often accompanied by increases in the diastolic and mean arterial pressure.

Hypertension commonly exists in elderly patients and can represent a substantial anesthetic risk. Known complications of severe perioperative hypertension include cerebrovascular accident, cerebral changes of "malignant" hypertension, myocardial ischemia, left ventricular failure, malignant cardiac arrhythmias, and rupture of preexisting aneurysms or atherosclerotic vessels.

A. Preoperative hypertension

Preoperative hypertension can be associated with a wide variety of clinical conditions. Essential hypertension is probably the most common cause. In the early phases of essential hypertension, blood pressure may be normal during nonstressed conditions but may rise abnormally in response to stresses such as preoperative pain or preoperative anxiety. These conditions can be treated with opioids and anxiolytics. In chronic hypertension the blood pressure will be consistently above 140/90 and requires treatment. Although antihypertensive therapy is usually continued until the time of operation, the clinician may occasionally encounter a patient whose antihypertensive medications have been discontinued in preparation for operation. This can be seen in patients receiving many different types of drugs including clonidine.[46] Other less-common causes of preoperative hypertension are pheochromocytoma, Conn's syndrome, coarctation of the aorta, renal artery stenosis, and increased intracranial pressure. Occasionally, preoperative hypertension may be seen in a trauma patient who has received excessive fluid during resuscitation.

B. Intraoperative hypertension

1. Verifying hypertension. Severe intraoperative hypertension is a substantial risk to the patient. On the other hand, treatment with potent vasodilators also carry substantial risks making it necessary to eliminate errors in diagnosis. If systemic hypertension is diagnosed from an arterial line, it is important to establish that the zero point and the calibration are both accurate. This can be done very rapidly. Another method for verifying arterial blood pressure is to inflate a blood pressure cuff on the catheterized arm until the arterial tracing disappears. The cuff is slowly deflated. The systemic arterial pressure is roughly equivalent to the point at which arterial pulsations reappear. It is also axiomatic that the anesthesiologist must examine the arterial-pressure wave form before accepting the digital readout. This is important because detection of spikes at peak arterial pressure indicate systolic overshoot, an error in measurement attributable to resonance in the system.[47]

Once the diagnosis of intraoperative hypertension has been firmly established, the cause must be persued. Hypertension can be caused by many different factors during anesthesia, which are considered separately.

2. Intubation hypertension. Laryngoscopy and endotracheal intubation are known causes of hypertension during anesthesia. Intubation hypertension is most likely to occur during administration of a general anesthetic induced with the hypnotic such as pentothal followed rapidly by the administration of a muscle relaxant for intubation. The reaction does not occur frequently in patients who have received a high-dose fentanyl or sufentanil induction. Intubation hypertension is most severe when laryngoscopy is prolonged and can be minimized by preadministration of lidocaine 1.5 mg/kg, or sodium nitroprusside.[48] In healthy patients intubation hypertension is usually not harmful, but during anesthesia for aneurysm surgery or in patients with myocardial ischemia or left ventricular failure it can be very significant.

3. Inadequate anesthesia. Surgical stimulation during light anesthesia causes the sympathetic nervous system to respond, and arterial pressure frequently increases. There is no specific monitor to diagnose inadequate anesthesia. However, if the systemic arterial pressure increases rapidly after a surgical incision, exploration of the peritoneum, scraping of periosteal surfaces of bone, or other significant surgical stimuli, one may deduce that the anesthesia is "too light." Correlative findings include tachycardia, sweating, grimacing, tearing, or movement on the operative table. The doses of each agent that has been given must be reviewed and compared to usual amounts. Individual factors such as alcoholism or narcotic addiction may increase anesthetic requirement and must be

considered. Occasionally, hypertension during primarily inhalation anesthesia may result when vaporizers are empty or deliver a concentration of agent lower than that selected. The mass spectrometer can be very useful in documenting that a particular agent is being administered in appropriate doses.

4. Hypercapnia. Intraoperative hypercapnia causes sympathetic stimulation and may result in hypertension.[49-52] During anesthesia intraoperative hypercapnia can result from inadequate tidal volume, inadequate minute volume, depleted soda lime, malfunctioning valves within the anesthetic circle, disconnection of the "inner hose" of a Bain circuit, inadequate fresh gas flow to a Bain circuit, or increased CO_2 production caused by malignant hyperthermia or thyrotoxicosis. Elevated end-tidal carbon dioxide levels detected by infrared capnography or by a mass spectrometer will give suspicion of hypercapnia. However, the conclusive diagnosis is established by arterial blood gases. Proper treatment will depend on which of these factors is causing hypercapnia.

5. Hypoxemia. Severe hypoxemia increases cardiac output to almost every organ. In the early phases of hypoxemia, systolic arterial pressure may be little effected. But in very severe hypoxemia the systolic arterial pressure is greatly elevated. It must be emphasized that systolic hypertension is a very late sign in hypoxemia and is often the harbinger of complete circulatory collapse.[53]

6. Pharmacologic adjuncts. Administration of inotropic and vasoconstrictor agents is an obvious cause of intraoperative hypertension. "Bolus" doses of phenylephrine or epinephrine given in urgent situations can frequently cause severe hypertension. Medication errors resulting from failure to identify ampules or labeled syringes may produce severe hypertension. Another cause is "flushing" an intravenous line that contains a vasopressor or inotropic drug. Hypertension can occur during regional anesthetic blocks if an epinephrine-containing local anesthetic solution is injected intravenously. During ophthalmic surgery, 10% phenylephrine drops may be instilled in the eye to produce mydriasis. Significant amounts of this drug can pass through the nasolacrimal duct to the nasal mucosa where rapid absorption results in hypertension. These reactions can be minimized by limitation of the concentration of phenylephrine to 5%[54] and by application of pressure over the medial canthus to occlude the nasolacrimal duct.[55]

7. Pheochromocytoma. Massive amounts of epinephrine and norepinephrine can rapidly enter the circulation in patients with pheochromocytomas. If the diagnosis is known before operation, intraoperative hypertension is easily explained. However, in the case of occult pheochromocytomas, the cause of severe hypertension may be less obvious. Pheochromocytoma must always be considered in the differential diagnosis of unexplained intraoperative hypertension. In such cases, it is usually impossible to establish the definitive diagnosis until a postoperative workup has been done. Fortunately, the intraoperative control of blood pressure and tachycardia in these patients is nonspecific and involves vasodilators, beta-adrenergic receptor blockers and perhaps calcium-channel blockers.

8. Distension of urinary bladder. Distension of the urinary bladder causes increased sympathetic activity leading to hypertension. This is often diagnosed in the recovery room.[56]

9. Aortic cross-clamping. Cross-clamping the aorta at any of several locations may be required during vascular surgery procedures. Hypertension from this cause is most commonly seen during abdominal aortic aneurysm surgery. It may also be seen during repair of coarctation of the aorta and during operations for thoracic aortic aneurysms. Hypertension from cross-clamping is usually obvious, occurring almost immediately after placement of an aortic clamp. Good communication between surgical and anesthetic teams is essential in minimizing cross-clamping hypertension and preventing hypertensive crises.

10. Aortic valve replacement. Patients with longstanding aortic stenosis develop a concentrically hypertrophied left ventricle capable of generating very high systolic pressures. During aortic valve replacement the stenotic area in the left ventricular outflow tract is removed, allowing the full peak systolic left ventricular pressure to be transmitted to the vascular tree. This can result in severe hypertension. This cause is obvious and well known to most cardiac anesthesiologists.

11. Hypertension after carotid endarterectomy. Baroreceptor dysfunction is a common cause of hypertension after carotid endarterectomy.[57] Surgical dissection renders the carotid sinus less sensitive to increases in blood pressure, thereby permitting development of significant arterial hypertension. Knowledge of this fact will prevent an unnecessary search for the cause of hypertension in these patients. Treatment usually necessitates antihypertensive agents.

12. Hypertension after extubation. Removal of an endotracheal tube may cause significant sympathetic stimulation with resultant hypertension. Usually extubation hypertension is relatively short lived. However, if prevention is necessary, a bolus dose of lidocaine given several minutes before extubation can minimize extubation hypertension.[58]

13. Postpartum hypertension. A vasoconstrictor administered before delivery can lead to severe postpartum hypertension. After delivery, the normal uterine autotransfusion causes an increased cardiac output. If this increased output faces an increased afterload because of the administration of a vasoconstrictor, severe hypertension occurs. This should be a rare event in obstetrics, since potent vasoconstrictors such as methoxamine and phenylephrine decrease uterine blood flow and are usually avoided in modern obstetric anesthesia.

III. PERIOPERATIVE MYOCARDIAL ISCHEMIA

A. Definition of myocardial ischemia

Myocardial ischemia is a dual state composed of inadequate myocardial oxygenation and accumulation of anaerobic metabolites. It occurs when myocardial oxygen demand exceeds myocardial oxygen supply. A thorough grasp of this complication depends on in-depth understanding of the dynamics of normal coronary blood flow and the deranged flow that occurs in disease.

B. Dynamics of normal myocardial oxygenation

The coronary circulation is far more complex than the circulation to other organs. Large epicardial arteries originate at the aorta and travel across the epicardial surface of the heart. These vessels branch into smaller penetrating vessels that arise approximately at right angles to the surface epicardial coronary arteries. The penetrating or intramural arteries course downward between muscle fibers of the cardiac syncytium. Anastomotic connections without an intervening capillary bed exist between portions of the same coronary artery and between different coronary arteries. Under normal circumstances these collaterals are almost invisible but become apparent only when a major coronary artery is occluded. After passing through a dense capillary bed, cardiac venous blood travels either through the coronary sinus to the right atrial appendage or into the left ventricle. Coronary perfusion pressure is the pressure in a coronary artery minus either the right atrial or left ventricular end-diastolic pressure depending on whether the blood drains into the coronary sinus or into the left ventricle.

Pressure in the proximal coronary arteries

meets major resistances in the penetrating or intramural arteries. These intramural arteries have both an intrinsic and an extrinsic resistance. Intrinsic coronary resistance is the resistance that originates within the substance of the intramural vessels themselves and is influenced by many factors. The coronary arteries contain sympathetic and parasympathetic nerves. Stimulation of the sympathetic nerves causes coronary vasoconstriction. Stimulation of the parasympathetic nerves results in coronary vasodilatation. Myogenic factors refer to the tendency of vascular smooth muscle to contract when perfusion pressure increases. This mechanism is called the "Bayliss effect."[59] Metabolic factors also exert a pronounced effect on intrinsic coronary resistance. When a region of myocardium is hypoperfused, vasodilator metabolites accumulate and dilate the coronary vasculature. Adenosine is an especially powerful coronary vasodilator[60] that blocks a receptor on the surface of vascular smooth muscle cells and prevents entry of calcium into muscle cells.[59] Although adenosine is probably the major metabolic coronary vasodilator, prostaglandins such as PGI_2 and PGE_2 can cause coronary vasodilatation. Several other substances such as acetylcholine, ATP, ADP, bradykinin, and histamine are capable of dilating coronary arteries but must act through an intact endothelium. The endothelium of muscular arteries may have receptors for these vasodilators. When vasodilators bind to these receptors, they cause the endothelial cells to release a substance that causes relaxation of vascular smooth muscle. This substance has been called endothelium-derived relaxant factor (EDRF). EDRF is a labile compound that activates guanylate cyclase in vascular smooth muscle resulting in an increase in intracellular cyclic guanosine monophosphate, causing vascular relaxation.[61-64] Damage to the coronary vascular endothelium can impair this relaxation response.[65]

Extrinsic coronary vascular resistance of the intramural arteries is the factor that clearly distinguishes the coronary circulation. The intramural coronary arteries and arterioles are virtually surrounded by the cardiac muscle synctium. During systole, contraction of cardiac muscle squeezes coronary arteries and at end systole coronary blood flow ceases.[66] As the diastolic period begins, cardiac muscle relaxes, the extrinsic squeezing of the coronary arteries is relieved, and the cardiac muscle receives a "rush" of blood. The diastolic portion of the cardiac cycle is extremely important for adequate coronary perfusion,[66] since approximately 85% of coronary blood flow occurs during diastole in the normal person. Tachycardia decreases diastolic time and thereby decreases coronary flow.

Increases in myocardial oxygen demand occur frequently during exercise and emotion. Persons with normal coronary arteries have the ability to accommodate for increased oxygen demands because their total coronary blood flow can increase five times over the resting level. In addition, regional increases in myocardial blood flow can occur through adenosine-induced decreases in intrinsic coronary vascular tone termed "autoregulation."[67]

C. Major conditions predisposing to myocardial ischemia

The two most common conditions that predispose to myocardial ischemia are coronary artery disease and left ventricular hypertrophy.

1. Coronary artery disease. The fixed and dynamic obstructions encountered in coronary artery disease severely limit myocardial blood flow. Autoregulation is faulty, since the poststenotic coronary vascular bed may be maximally vasodilated in the resting state and cannot dilate further during exercise or stress. Left ventricular dilatation secondary to heart failure may increase ventricular wall tension, particularly in the subendocardial area, leading to poor subendocardial flow and resultant ischemia. A tachycardia may severely limit the time for coronary blood flow.

2. Left ventricular hypertrophy. Left ventricular hypertrophy predisposes to myocardial ischemia because the increased oxygen requirements of the thickened myocardium can easily exceed oxygen supply. Impairment of oxygen supply occurs because abnormal diastolic relaxation increases impedance to coronary flow. Left ventricular hypertrophy leading to myocardial ischemia is most commonly seen in patients with chronic hypertension.

D. Types of myocardial ischemia

Myocardial ischemia may be either symptomatic or "silent."

1. Symptomatic. Symptomatic myocardial ischemia usually refers to ischemia that causes cardiac pain. The presence of typical cardiac pain may lead to thorough preoperative evaluation and treatment and specialized plans for intra-anesthetic and postanesthetic monitoring and treatment. Treatment of patients with symptomatic ischemia can be challenging but at least one can be prepared for it.

2. "Silent." On the other hand, "silent" myocardial ischemia is especially dangerous because of its concealed nature. Two major types of problems can arise from silent ischemia. The first is that a patient with advanced coronary disease and active ischemia may come to anesthesia without our realizing that he is prone to ischemia. Indeed some 2% to 4% of the middle-aged male population have asymptomatic coronary artery disease with silent ischemia.[68] Since the anesthesiologist has no reason to suspect coronary disease, prevision for electrocardiographic *ischemia* monitoring may not be made. Repeated and prolonged ischemic episodes may go unrecognized. This can lead to myocardial infarction[69,70] and intraoperative or postoperative death. In this setting, it is very likely that the infarction or death would be attributed to substandard anesthetic care. It is obviously important to obtain a postmortem examination in such cases because the demonstration of fresh coronary thrombosis or plaque rupture may exonerate the anesthesiologist.

The second major problem posed by "silent" ischemia is that episodes of myocardial ischemia in patients with known coronary artery disease may be missed. This is a real problem, since approximately 70% of ischemic episodes in patients with stable angina are silent.[68] Bouts of silent ischemia are most likely to be missed when the patient is not monitored for *ischemia.* Most elective surgical patients with coronary disease do not have constant electrocardiographic ischemia monitoring in the hours immediately preceding their operation. Ischemia monitoring drug transport to and from the operating room is not often done. And ischemia monitoring in many recovery rooms is certainly not optimal. Thus it is very likely that ischemic events can be easily missed in coronary artery disease patients with silent ischemia.

E. Myocardial ischemia without hemodynamic alterations

The fact that hemodynamic alterations can be valuable in predicting and treating myocardial ischemia is discussed in subsequent paragraphs. However, it must be emphasized that studies done in coronary bypass patients have indicated that the majority of perioperative ischemic episodes are *not* accompanied by hemodynamic changes.[71] Likewise Cheng et al.[72] reported that "good" control of blood pressure and pulse rate do not necessarily *prevent* myocardial ischemia. This perplexing and frustrating observation is explained by the contention that most episodes of preoperative myocardial ischemia are associated with distal coronary vasospasm or reversible platelet aggregation, or both. Neither of these conditions can be detected *directly* by our current monitoring.

F. Myocardial ischemia associated with hemodynamic alterations

1. Tachycardia. Perioperative myocardial ischemia may follow the onset of adverse hemodynamic changes. The occurrence of tachycardia is particularly dangerous because it increases oxygen demand *and* simultaneously decreases myocardial oxygen supply. The decrease in supply is particularly severe, since the time available for coronary flow is drastically and disproportionally reduced. For example, at a heart rate of approximately 60, the total diastolic time is approximately 800 msec. Increasing the heart rate to 90 will decrease coronary flow time to only 200 msec.[73] It is important to emphasize that increases in heart rate that would ordinarily be within the "normal range" can be a serious threat to the patient with coronary vascular disease.

Perioperative tachycardia can result from many causes including light anesthesia, endotracheal intubation, hypovolemia, fever, anemia, congestive heart failure, and postoperative pain. The principle of treating the underlying cause is obviously the sensible thing to do. However, in practicality, if myocardial ischemia clearly accompanies tachycardia, damage to the myocardium may be time dependent, and therefore it may be appropriate to use esmolol to decrease the heart rate while the causal condition is treated. For example, a patient with severe coronary vascular disease who has a temperature of 103° F (39.3° C) may develop tachycardia and myocardial ischemia. In principle, treating the elevated temperature would remove the cause and result in cardiac slowing. However, the process of cooling is so slow that severe myocardial damage could occur while the temperature is being lowered. Alternatively, if tachycardia is caused by an ectopic supraventricular pacemaker, the administration of esmolol, propranolol, verapamil, or adenosine may be important.

2. Tachycardia and hypotension. The combination of tachycardia *and* hypotension is especially likely to precipitate myocardial ischemia, since two supply factors are simultaneously decreased. Hypotension reduces the driving force across the coronary bed, and tachycardia reduces the time available for coronary blood flow. These two hemodynamic derangements are commonly encountered in hypovolemia. Treating the basic cause is always rational, but when evidence of ischemia accompanies these two changes, the time required for appropriate volume replacement may result in prolonged ischemia and possible evolution into myocardial infarction. This is particularly true if the placement of a pulmonary artery catheter or a central venous pressure catheter is required before volume replacement. Consequently, in severe hypotension and tachycardia it may be necessary to "buy time" by increasing coronary perfusion pressure with a potent alpha-adrenergic agent such as phenylephrine. This drug may also decrease cardiac rate by a baroreceptor response.

3. Hypervolemia. Iatrogenic hypervolemia can cause myocardial ischemia. Overzealous fluid administration can easily result in an abnormally large left ventricular end-diastolic volume (LVEDV). As left ventricular volume increases, the left ventricular end-diastolic pressure and the mean myocardial wall tension both increase, leading to an increase in myocardial oxygen consumption. If the coronary vessels are unable to increase flow to match this increased demand, myocardial ischemia can result. Detection of hypervolemia using a single measurement can be difficult. Central venous pressure monitoring often fails to detect changes in LVEDV. An abnormally high pulmonary capillary wedge pressure can correlate with a large left ventricular end-diastolic volume if compliance of the left ventricle is normal. However, it is possible that direct estimation of left ventricular end-diastolic volume obtained with the use of a transesophageal two-dimensional echocardiogram (2-D TEE) may be more accurate. This method also has limitations because transesophageal echocardiography provides a measurement of left ventricular end-diastolic *area* and not a direct measurement of left ventricular end-diastolic *volume*. Accurate diagnosis of hypervolemia can be difficult and may require consideration of changes in several measurements including pulmonary capillary wedge pressure, cardiac output, arterial oxygen tension, and heart size on chest roentgenograms.

4. Postpartum hypervolemia. Hypervolemia-induced myocardial ischemia may also occur in healthy obstetric patients. In a recent paper, Palmer et al. found ST-segment or T-wave changes in 44 of 93 apparently healthy women giving birth through cesarean section under regional anesthesia.[74] Fifteen of these patients developed chest pain, pressure, or dyspnea, and no patient without ECG changes developed chest symptoms. The authors speculate that the ECG changes were caused by myocardial ischemia related to sudden hypervolemia resulting from fluid loading and autotransfusion during delivery. Although it is difficult to believe that half of these healthy women had clinically significant myocardial ischemia, these findings are not easily ignored. Undoubtedly, this report will stimulate further research in parturients.

The treatment of myocardial ischemia secondary to hypervolemia involves preload reduction, diuretics, and occasionally phlebotomy. Endotracheal intubation, controlled ventilation, and oxygen supplementation are also frequently required to maintain adequate arterial oxygenation.

5. Hypertension. Hypertension is another adverse condition in patients with coronary artery disease. Systemic arterial hypertension increases myocardial oxygen consumption. In the presence of coronary artery disease, the increased myocardial oxygen consumption may exceed myocardial oxygen supply resulting in acute ischemia. This is particularly true if tachycardia coexists with hypertension. Although the role of hypertension as a predictor for the onset of ischemia has been questioned,[68,75] some studies have suggested that acute hypertensive episodes precede as many as 50% of intraoperative ischemic episodes.[76,77]

G. Myocardial ischemia associated with other conditions

1. Coronary spasm (Prinzmetal's angina). Coronary artery spasm can produce severe transmural myocardial ischemia. Coronary spasm that accompanies Prinzmetal's (variant) angina occurs at rest, is usually not precipitated by physical or emotional exertion, and is accompanied by ST-segment elevations on the electrocardiogram.[78] This type of myocardial ischemia results from a transient abrupt decrease in the diameter of an epicardial or large septal coronary artery. The spasm can be clearly demonstrated by coronary arteriography.[79] Prinzmetal's angina may be associated with myocardial infarction, serious cardiac arrhythmias, including ventricular tachycardia and fibrillation, and even sudden death.[80] Ganz et al. have suggested that the abnormality in Prinzmetal's angina is a hypercontractility of the arterial wall related to the atherosclerotic process.[81] Others have suggested that endothelial damage reverses the dilator response associated with endothelium-derived relaxation factor (EDRF).[82] Unless a history of Prinzmetal's angina is known, its occurrence under anesthesia, including the pronounced ST-segment elevation, can mimic an acute myocardial infarction.

2. Handling the heart. Direct handling of the heart may cause ischemia particularly in patients with coronary artery disease. Lifting, twisting, and compressing the heart all may "kink" atherosclerotic coronary arteries, which may predispose to spasm, plaque rupture, and even thrombosis and occlusion. Hyduke recently reported severe intraoperative myocardial ischemia after manipulation of the heart in a patient undergoing esophagogastrectomy.[83] It may be impossible to totally avoid cardiac manipulation during certain surgical procedures. However, the incidence of attendant myocardial ischemia may be lessened by gentle handling of the heart and minimizing the degree and duration of cardiac displacement.

3. Carbon monoxide exposure. Carbon monoxide exposure may predispose the patient with coronary artery disease to myocardial ischemia. Allred et al. found that, during incremental exercise testing, patients with coronary artery disease who were exposed to carbon monoxide had a reduction in the time to a threshold ischemic ST-segment change.[84] The stressed surgical patient might have a similar response. For example, burned patients who have suffered smoke inhalation may be particularly prone to myocardial ischemia. Likewise, a period of heavy cigarette smoking before surgery in an ambulatory setting might predispose the patient with coronary disease to myocardial ischemia.

4. Cocaine abuse. Numerous reports have indicated that cocaine abuse can cause myocardial ischemia and myocardial infarction. It is well known that cocaine inhibits the reuptake of norepinephrine, increases cardiac rate, elevates blood pressure, and increases myocardial oxygen consumption. Additionally, cocaine given intranasally in modest amounts was shown by Lange to produce coronary artery vasoconstriction.[85] Cocaine withdrawal may lead to asymptomatic episodes of ST-segment changes. This has been demonstrated by Holter monitoring of a group of known cocaine addicts.[86] Chronic cocaine addiction has also been shown to accelerate coronary atherosclerosis.[87] Thus young cocaine addicts may be more prone to perioperative myocardial ischemia.

H. Diagnosing myocardial ischemia

With the onset of myocardial ischemia, a series of events that can have diagnostic implications occur. Ischemia may result in cardiac pain, myocardial lactate production, regional wall-motion abnormalities, decreased myocardial contractility, decreased ejection fraction, increased left ventricular end-diastolic pressure, and ST-segment abnormalities. Although each of these sequelae can accompany myocardial ischemia, some of these abnormalities are highly useful in the "state-of-the-art" diagnosis in the early 1990s. Others hold promise for the future and some such as lactate production require sampling methodology, which is simply impractical for day-to-day use. Although new methods such as transesophageal echocardiog-

raphy and cardiokymography present exciting possibilities for the future, it is important to fully utilize state-of-the-art monitoring as it exists in the early 1990s.

1. New cardiac pain. The onset of new cardiac pain can be extremely important when one is diagnosing myocardial ischemia preoperatively, during surgery under local or regional anesthesia, and postoperatively in the recovery room. One should certainly be aware that chest pressure, chest pain, and a sense of chest constriction are symptoms of myocardial ischemia. Cardiac pain may also be referred to either arm, the neck, the jaws, the teeth, and even the posterior scapular areas. The onset of any of these symptoms should not be ignored. Cardiac pain is extremely useful as a diagnostic aid when it occurs. It is important to remember, however, that the absence of cardiac pain does not rule out myocardial ischemia.[88] Diabetic patients may have myocardial ischemia without perceiving pain because pain pathways may be impaired by diabetic neuropathy.[89] "Silent" myocardial ischemia can also occur in nondiabetic patients. In fact, many authorities agree that approximately 70% of ischemic episodes in patients with symptomatic coronary artery disease are not associated with angina.[90] Since 70% of myocardial ischemic episodes in fully awake man are asymptomatic, it is sobering to consider that the elderly, sedated patient receiving regional anesthesia probably will have no symptoms even if he develops myocardial ischemia!

2. Electrocardiography: anachronism or a standard? Contemporary literature contains many reports emphasizing the limitations of electrocardiography relative to futuristic monitors such as echocardiography and cardiokymography. Despite these, electrocardiography is an extremely important method for detecting myocardial ischemia. It can be utilized preoperatively, intraoperatively, and postoperatively. It can be utilized in patients undergoing regional anesthesia and with general anesthesia with or without endotracheal intubation. Electrocardiographic leads can be applied to the patient without pain and at minimal cost. Deviations in the ST-segment can be easily recognized, recorded, and measured. The proper frequency band width for diagnostic electrocardiography and the criteria for proper voltage standardization have been established. Postoperative electrocardiograms can be easily compared to preoperative tracings. The ST-segment can be analyzed by computer, recorded, and "trended" both during and after anesthesia. Because of its practicality, the electrocardiogram remains the standard for the diagnosis of myocardial ischemia in the 1990s.

The value of electrocardiography depends on its proper use. The electrocardiogram must be calibrated to give a pen deflection of 10 mm for 1 mV potential. This is extremely important, since excessive gain can produce false ST-segment depression and inadequate gain can mask such depression. The proper frequency band width must be used. Most modern operating room ECG monitors contain both a diagnostic and a monitor mode. The monitoring mode is designed to "filter out" electrical interference. However, ischemia monitoring using the monitor mode may produce false T-wave and ST-segment changes. Proper diagnosis of ischemia from the electrocardiogram depends on the use of the "diagnostic" mode, which brackets a frequency band width of 0.05 to 100 Hz.

The standard electrocardiogram consists of 12 leads. Inclusion of all 12 leads gives the best overall assessment and can be used preoperatively and postoperatively. However, during anesthesia, monitoring is usually limited to seven leads. Selection of the best leads is important. Blackburn demonstrated that 89% of significant ST-segment depression after exercise was found in precordial lead V_5.[91] He also demonstrated that 100% of ST-segment changes can be detected by recording leads V_3-V_6 and leads II and aV_F.[92] The seven-lead system allows the standard leads and lead V_5 to be monitored. Any of these seven leads can be recorded when necessary. In routine practice, leads II and V_5 are continuously monitored giving views of the inferior and lateral myocardium. Continuous scanning of several leads would seem to improve the detection of myocardial ischemia. Kotrly described the use of a modified microcomputer-based ECG that continuously monitors leads I, II, and V_5 and gives a summation of ST-segment deviations.[93] Many commercial monitors are available with computer analysis and automatic ST-segment trending.

Whether one uses computerized ST-segment trending, it is still important to have a working knowledge of critical ST-segment analysis. In the normal ECG, the ST-segment is isoelectric. Elevations or depressions are fairly easy to recognize. Depressions of 1 mm or greater are usually indicative of subendocardial ischemia, and upsloping depression of this magnitude may be the first sign of myocardial ischemia. Horizontal or downsloping ST-segment depression of 1 mm or more indicates significant subendocardial ischemia. ST-segment elevation greater than 1 mm indicates severe transmural ischemia.[94] ST-segment depression is usually measured 80 msec after the J-point, which is the junction of the S-wave and the ST-segment.

However, the ST-segment may be distorted by the preoperative presence of a left bundle branch block, left ventricular hypertrophy, digitalis effect, and ventricular pacing. These conditions make the ECG diagnosis of ischemia extremely difficult.

3. Pulmonary artery catheter measurements during ischemia. With the onset of myocardial ischemia, myocardial compliance decreases leading to a "stiff" heart. Theoretically this stiffness should result in an increased pulmonary capillary wedge pressure. Kaplan and Wells reported that increases in pulmonary capillary wedge pressure (PCWP) could be used to diagnose early myocardial ischemia.[95] Other studies have indicated an increase in PCWP during ischemia induced by cardiac pacing[96-98] and during coronary angioplasty.[99-101] However, these observations do not necessarily mean that increases in pulmonary capillary wedge pressure can be used as an *early* and *reliable* indicator of myocardial ischemia during anesthesia. In order to examine the value of increases in pulmonary capillary wedge pressure as an early indicator of myocardial ischemia detected by electrocardiography and echocardiography, van Daele et al. studied 100 patients undergoing coronary artery bypass grafting. Increases in wedge pressure frequently did not occur during ischemia.[102] From these results it appears that increases in pulmonary capillary wedge pressure are neither a sensitive nor a specific indicator of the onset of myocardial ischemia during anesthesia.

4. Echocardiography: futuristic standard? During normal cardiac systole the myocardium thickens. Within seconds after total interruption of circulation to a region, systolic thickening decreases and other aspects of wall motion are impaired. Both systolic thickening and wall motion can be monitored by use of two-dimensional transesophageal echocardiography (2-D TEE). Studies done during coronary angioplasty have shown that echocardiography is more sensitive than electrocardiography in the detection of myocardial ischemia.[101] Other experimental data and clinical studies have suggested that regional wall-motion abnormalities are more sensitive than ST-segment changes for the early detection of myocardial ischemia.[103-106] Continuous on-line images provide the anesthesiologist with beat-to-beat observations of the heart. The recent introduction of "quad screen" technology allows the anesthesiologist to "freeze" previous cardiac images for comparison with the on-line measurements. Color-flow Doppler technology gives the potential for detection of acute mitral regurgitation secondary to ischemic papillary muscle dysfunction. Left ventricular end-diastolic area can be measured and recorded during rapid volume infusion, which may help in the early detection of overdistension of the left ventricle. The transesophageal echo probe is a modified gastroscope that can be easily inserted after endotracheal intubation. Complications associated with the use of the esophageal probe have been infrequent. And ultrasound has no known medical complications.

All the foregoing facts plus prominent exposure at national anesthesia meetings have contributed to enthusiasm for the use of transesophageal echo as an extremely sensitive monitor of myocardial ischemia. However, this must be viewed in perspective. The studies were done by investigators who had extensive training *and* experience in transesophageal echocardiography. In their hands, transesophageal echocardiography may indeed be a more sensitive indicator of myocardial ischemia than the electrocardiogram. However, the majority of readers in the early 1990s will not have had this training and experience, and therefore use of transesophageal echocardiography by an untrained person may result in inadequate or less sensitive diagnosis. It is also important to emphasize that transesophageal echocardiography has serious limitations. Preoperative images would require preoperative passage of the probe, which is time consuming and uncomfortable for the awake patient. Transesophageal echocardiography cannot be used easily in the awake patient undergoing regional anesthesia. Its use as an ischemia detector in the recovery room is limited unless the patient is still sedated and intubated. When one is monitoring for myocardial ischemia, the most commonly utilized short-axis view is at the mid–left ventricular level. Ischemia confined to the right ventricle or to the base or apex of the left ventricle may be missed. Rotation or translation of the entire heart can make segmental contraction difficult to evaluate. Discoordinated contraction may not be attributable to ischemia if a patient has a preexisting bundle branch block or is undergoing ventricular pacing. Other wall-motion abnormalities may represent "stunned," or "hibernating," myocardium instead of acutely ischemic myocardium. Quantitative methods for wall-thickening analysis are tedious and frequently limited by inadequate visualization of the epicardium.[107] And finally, because of biologic differences, not all normal hearts contract "normally" and not all parts of the same heart contract to the same degree.[108] In summary, if the anesthesiologist has the training, experi-

ence, and equipment to do transesophageal echocardiography, it may be very helpful in the early detection of myocardial ischemia. However, unbridled enthusiasm for new methods must not overlook the fact that echocardiography has serious limitations. London recently reported very interesting work done in a department of experienced echocardiographers. As a part of a study, these investigations compared echocardiography to electrocardiography as an ischemia monitor.[109] They reported that many ischemic episodes detected by electrocardiography were missed by echocardiography. The authors concluded that "the discordant relation between TEE and ECG changes observed here necessitates careful monitoring of the *ECG* when TEE is used clinically." Although transesophageal echocardiography holds much promise as a futuristic detector of myocardial ischemia, it is still in developmental stages and therefore cannot be the standard for ischemia detection for most clinicians at this time.

5. Cardiokymography. The cardiokymograph (CKG) is an electronic device that can noninvasively detect an analog representation of regional wall motion. It has been used to augment exercise electrocardiography. Two recent reports suggest that it is a highly sensitive monitor for myocardial ischemia.[110,111] The cardiokymograph may be a futuristic monitor of myocardial ischemia. However, fairly serious limitations may preclude its practical use. It requires accurate placement of a precordial transducer, is difficult to use in spontaneously ventilating patients, and is insensitive to changes in motion of the inferior, posterior, and lateral left ventricular walls.

I. Treatment of perioperative myocardial ischemia

1. Prevention of myocardial ischemia. The best treatment for perioperative myocardial ischemia is prevention of its occurrence. This can be a very difficult task, since many factors are simply not under the control of the anesthesiologist. Careful preoperative histories and appropriate preoperative workup will do much to identify susceptible patients. However, these conscientious efforts will not result in identification of all patients at risk. Some patients will have "silent" myocardial ischemia. Others will simply deny serious cardiac symptoms. However suspicion of coronary artery disease in the elderly, in patients with noticeable truncal obesity, in heavy smokers, and in those with a family history of coronary artery disease will help in preoperative identification.

Careful attention to prevention of tachycardia during anesthesia is extremely important, and it must be remembered that seemingly normal heart rates (such as 80 beats/min) may precipitate myocardial ischemia in patients with coronary artery disease. Judicious use of appropriate levels of anesthesia, particularly if it includes fentanyl will do much to prevent tachycardia. Judicious use of ultra–short acting beta blockers can also be very beneficial in preventing tachycardia. In perspective, the perceived dangers of beta blockers are probably more imaginary than real. Although beta blockers do have serious side effects, the majority of cardiac side effects can be very rapidly reversed using common drugs such as atropine or calcium chloride.

Coriat has demonstrated that the prophylactic administration of intravenous nitroglycerin 1 μg/kg/min will significantly decrease the incidence of intraoperative myocardial ischemia in patients with coronary artery disease.[112] Seitelberger et al. have shown that the intravenous infusion of nifedipine after coronary artery bypass grafting decreases the incidence of myocardial ischemia.[113] Although nifedipine is not available as an intravenous preparation in the United States, other calcium-channel blockers might have similar prophylactic effects.

Despite our best preventive efforts, perioperative myocardial ischemia may still occur. Since myocardial ischemia may be secondary to complex and interrelated causes, the specifics of treatment in any given case depend on the details of that case. However, it is possible to draw some useful generalities.

2. Establishment of temporal relationships. Myocardial ischemia can occur with or without significant hemodynamic aberrations. If hemodynamic aberrations are associated with myocardial ischemia, they may proceed and be the cause of the ischemia. On the other hand, ischemia may precede and may cause the hemodynamic aberrations. Close monitoring and *establishment of a temporal relationship* may be extremely important. For example, if an anesthetized patient has normal ST-segments and then develops tachycardia followed by ST-segment depression, it is reasonable to assume that tachycardia caused the ischemia, and therefore efforts should be directed at reduction of the pulse rate. If hypovolemic hypotension precedes the onset of ST-segment depression, perhaps the hypotension and decrease in myocardial oxygen supply may be the cause. Details of treatment in any given case will also depend on the urgency of the situation and whether appropriate monitoring lines are in place when ischemia occurs.

3. Ischemia without hemodynamic alterations. In susceptible patients, myocardial ischemia manifested by ST-segment depression will often occur without attendant hemodynamic aberrations. In these cases the administration of nitroglycerin can be extremely helpful. Nitroglycerin will decrease preload, decrease wall tension, dilate epicardial coronary arteries, and increase subendocardial flow. Intravenous administration is preferred in acute situations. However, if the intravenous preparation is not immediately available, a 400 μg tablet can be placed sublingually or be dissolved in 1 ml of saline solution and administered intranasally.[114] Because intranasal administration of 400 μg of dissolved nitroglycerin can occasionally produce hypotension, we recommend an initial dose of 200 μg. However, even with careful dose selection, intranasal administration is less predictable than intravenous.

4. Ischemia accompanied by tachycardia and hypertension. A combination of tachycardia and hypertension can lead to myocardial ischemia. Hypertension increases myocardial oxygen demand, and tachycardia decreases oxygen supply. After satisfactory ventilation, oxygenation, and anesthetic administration have been quickly verified, esmolol or propranolol should be administered to decrease the pulse rate. In many cases moderate hypertension will decrease to normal levels as the pulse rate slows. If hypertension and electrocardiographic evidence of ischemia continue after the pulse rate is decreased to approximately 70 beats/min, sodium nitroprusside is recommended in small titrated doses guided by radial artery blood pressure monitoring.

5. Ischemia: hypotension and tachycardia. The combination of hypotension and tachycardia is particularly likely to produce myocardial ischemia because both derangements can drastically reduce myocardial oxygen supply. A common cause of this combination is hypovolemia. Treatment of hypovolemia as the first priority would appear logical. However, in the face of hypotension and myocardial ischemia, volume replacement as the *only* treatment may be too slow. Certainly we would begin volume replacement as rapidly as possible, but in the interim it is critical to restore coronary perfusion pressure and slow the pulse rate. Phenylephrine is extremely useful in this situation. In critical cases we would administer phenylephrine using a 1 ml syringe. A small syringe facilitates the accurate administration of a reasonable first dose of 20 to 50 μg. The response can be rapidly assessed and more drug can be given easily if necessary. Judicious administration of phenylephrine may "buy time" while intravascular volume is restored.

6. Coronary spasm and ischemia. Coronary spasm may produce acute, severe transmural myocardial ischemia manifested by ST-segment *elevation*. This might easily be confused with the early stages of a transmural myocardial infarction. However, with a history of atypical angina or knowledge that the patient has recently been taking cocaine or is a withdrawing cocaine addict, one might suspect the diagnosis. If coronary spasm is suspected, it can be treated with sublingual nifedipine or intravenous verapamil.

7. Ectopic supraventricular tachycardia. The sudden onset of a supraventricular tachycardia may precipitate myocardial ischemia. In this case, slowing the pulse rate is extremely important and drugs such as esmolol, propranolol, verapamil, propranolol, verapamil, and adenosine[115] should be considered. One may rapidly terminate the myocardial ischemia by restoring normal sinus rhythm at a slow rate.

8. Severe resistant myocardial ischemia. Occasionally the anesthesiologist will encounter severe myocardial ischemia resistant to reasonable doses of all antianginal drugs. In this setting, the intra-aortic balloon can be invaluable. Counterpulsation provided by an intra-aortic balloon will acutely decrease myocardial oxygen requirements and may increase myocardial oxygen supply. The balloon can be quickly inserted percutaneously by a cardiac surgeon or an invasive cardiologist. It is important that a radial artery line also be inserted to establish the correct timing of the balloon and also to assure that it is not advanced into the arch of the aorta.

IV. PERIOPERATIVE MYOCARDIAL INFARCTION
A. Significance of infarction

Myocardial infarction occurring before, during, or after anesthesia and operation is a major complication with significant morbidity and mortality. This is especially true in patients who have suffered a myocardial infarction sometime in the 6 months immediately preceding an operation. Older data have indicated that between 27% and 37% of these patients will sustain a perioperative reinfarction and of these approximately 50% will die before leaving the hospital.[116-118] Although inconclusive, newer studies have suggested that the use of aggressive invasive hemodynamic monitoring and prompt treatment of hemodynamic abnormalities can greatly decrease the reinfarction and mortality.[119,120] Despite these apparent improvements, perioperative myocardial infarction still

occurs and can lead to major problems such as pulmonary edema, low cardiac output, severe intractable cardiac arrhythmias, cerebral and renal damage, and even death.

B. Factors associated with infarction

The overwhelming majority of perioperative infarctions occur in patients with significant preexisting coronary vascular disease. However, hypertensive patients with left ventricular hypertrophy and patients with left ventricular hypertrophy secondary to aortic valve disease are also very susceptible to perioperative myocardial infarction.

Perioperative myocardial infarction can occur after many pathophysiologic processes. Slogoff et al. have demonstrated that myocardial ischemia occurring during coronary artery bypass operations leads to an increased incidence of postoperative myocardial infarction.[121,122] Although this relationship has been established in patients undergoing coronary artery bypass grafting, conclusive studies establishing the relationship during other operations have not been done. However, it is the authors' firm opinion that significant myocardial ischemia during many different types of operations will lead to an increased incidence of postoperative myocardial infarction especially if the ischemic episode is severe and prolonged.

Coronary atherosclerotic plaques may undergo sudden changes resulting in perioperative myocardial infarction. It must be emphasized that these changes can occur without apparent precipitating factors and at any time. When a sudden myocardial infarction occurs, surgeons and anesthesiologists are likely to ask, "Why did this happen now?" This may not always be easily answered. It has been shown that the majority of myocardial infarctions in unanesthetized patients follow a circadian variation with an increase beginning about 7 A.M. and reaching the zenith of the peak at approximately 8 A.M. This is the time when anesthesia is being induced in many patients. There is also an evening peak beginning around 6 P.M. reaching the zenith at about 10 P.M.[123] The cause for these peaks is unknown. We do know that sudden acute myocardial infarction can result from plaque rupture leading to an occlusive intimal flap. Hemorrhage into an existing plaque is another mechanism. The development of a fissure in an atherosclerotic plaque can expose platelets to collagen, which leads to thrombus formation. Prolonged or repetitive coronary artery spasm may also lead to coronary thrombosis.[124] Withdrawing cocaine addicts may develop coronary spasm with silent myocardial ischemia demonstrated by Holter monitoring. These episodes occur spontaneously and may not be associated with stress.[87] Chronic cocaine addicts have accelerated coronary atherogenesis, making it especially likely that a withdrawing addict could develop a perioperative infarction. It has recently been demonstrated that cocaine use can lead to acute coronary spasm, making it probable that cocaine abusers arriving for surgery may develop perioperative coronary artery spasm and infarction.[86] Chest injury can also lead to trauma of coronary arteries with laceration and thrombosis. Other numerous conditions not involving coronary atherosclerosis can be associated with acute myocardial infarction (List 11-2).

C. Diagnosing perioperative myocardial infarction

1. Preoperative diagnosis. All myocardial infarctions occurring in the 3 months immediately before an operation must be considered as perioperative myocardial infarctions because they can lead to major perioperative morbidity and mortality. In some cases a preoperative infarct will be associated with a discrete event characterized by hospitalization, a thorough workup, and a complete description of therapy and complications. Perusal of hospital records will substantiate the diagnosis and document the severity of the infarct. In other cases, a patient may come to the preoperative holding area and experience crushing substernal chest pain radiating to the left arm and appear dyspneic and cyanotic. Acute myocardial infarction will clearly be the most likely cause. But pain does not always accompany myocardial infarction, particularly in the diabetic patient or in the aged patient.[125] Studies have indicated that between 20% and 60% of nonfatal myocardial infarcts are completely unrecognized by the patient and are discovered on subsequent electrocardiogram or postmortem examinations.[126] Other patients will have clear-cut cardiac symptoms for which they seek medical advice but will nevertheless subsequently deny them! Preoperative myocardial infarctions may be detected occasionally by the new appearance of Q-waves on the preoperative electrocardiogram or by the appearance of a new left bundle branch block (LBBB). The new onset of atrial fibrillation may be another marker for preoperative infarction, particularly in the elderly patient. The very early stage of an acute myocardial infarction may be indicated by tall narrow T-waves, a phenomena referred to as peaked or "hyperacute" T-waves. The new appearance of tall R-waves in lead V_1 may indicate a true posterior

List 11-2. Myocardial Infarction Not Associated With Coronary Atherosclerosis

Congenital coronary anomalies
Coronary artery aneurysms
Left coronary artery arising from anterior sinus of Valsalva
Coronary arteriovenous fistulas
Origin of left coronary artery from pulmonary artery

Hematologic
Thrombocytosis
Hypercoagulability
Disseminated intravascular coagulation
Thrombocytopenic purpura
Polycythemia vera

Coronary artery emboli
Left atrial or ventricular mural thrombus
Prolapse of mitral valve
Prosthetic valve emboli
Papillary fibroelastoma of the aortic valve
Cardiac myxoma
Paradoxic emboli

Arteritis
Ankylosing spondylitis
Rheumatoid arthritis
Disseminated lupus erythematosus
Kawasaki's syndrome
Takayasu's disease
Polyarteritis nodosa
Luetic aortitis

Miscellaneous
Carbon monoxide poisoning
Thyrotoxicosis
Aortic insufficiency
Mucopolysaccharidosis
Fabry's disease
Amyloidosis
Pseudoxanthoma elasticum

myocardial infarct, particularly if there is ST-segment depression in lead I.[127] It may be tedious to consider all these alternatives preoperatively, but the benefits in minimizing morbidity and mortality and promoting good risk management will pay the anesthesiologist a hundredfold for his efforts!

2. Intraoperative diagnosis. Diagnosing a myocardial infarct that occurs during the administration of an anesthetic can be difficult for several reasons. Many intraoperative infarcts are subendocardial and will not cause hypotension or arrhythmias. Complete electrocardiographic tracings usually cannot be done during an operation, and evolutionary electrocardiographic changes often occur after the operation is completed. Diagnostic increases in MB-CPK levels usually occur postoperatively. Because of these diagnostic limitations, it is important for the anesthesiologist to maximally utilize the information he does have.

Intraoperative myocardial infarction is probably easier to diagnose in patients undergoing local or regional anesthetics than it is in patients undergoing general anesthesia. Although the onset of cardiac pain does not always accompany myocardial infarction, nevertheless when it does occur it can be extremely useful. The astute clinician will not only consider chest pain or chest pressure, but will also carefully consider the new onset of pain in either the right or left arm, the neck, jaws, teeth, or posterior scapular regions. The most obvious infarcts will be glaringly apparent, and occasionally an unfortunate patient will die soon after experiencing cardiac pain. In less severe infarcts, findings from a seven-lead intraoperative electrocardiogram may be helpful. The seven-lead electrocardiogram includes leads II, III, and aV_F, which allow a good "look" at the inferior surface of the heart and also lead V_5, which gives a good view of the lateral aspect of the heart. T-wave inversions, ST-segment depressions, or ST-segment elevations in any of these leads may indicate a developing myocardial infarct. Those infarcts associated with extensive myocardial damage will probably be associated with hypotension and cardiac arrhythmias.

Patients receiving general anesthetics will obviously not complain of pain but may have hypotension, arrhythmias, signs of congestive heart failure, and electrocardiographic changes of either subendocardial or transmural ischemia. The sudden appearance of severe wall-motion abnormalities in patients being monitored with transesophageal echocardiography may also indicate myocardial infarction though the differential diagnosis between acute ischemia, evolving infarction, "stunned" myocardium, and "hibernating" myocardium may be difficult to distinguish using echocardiographic findings.[128] Increased levels of the MB fraction of creatinine phosphokinase (CPK) are not useful intraoperatively, since the leakage of these enzymes into the circulation can require 8 to 24 hours after a myocardial infarct. Indeed, some investigators have indicated that peak MB-CPK levels occur at highly variable times after an infarct, with a range of 12 to 24 hours.[18] Although the MB-CPK level cannot be expected to increase in the first few hours after an infarct, nevertheless if an infarct is suspected it may be useful to draw blood for levels to establish a "base-line" value. Additionally, if the operation is still proceeding 8 hours after the onset of what appears to be an infarct, the anesthesiologist should draw MB-CPK levels. Serial MB-CPK levels in the postoperative period for up to 24 hours after the first signs and symptoms of the infarct will obviously be very important.

Serial postoperative electrocardiograms play a major role in documenting a probable intraoperative or early postoperative myocardial infarction. The initial 12-lead electrocardiogram is frequently nondiagnostic. Therefore a series of electrocardiograms is necessary to determine whether evolution of the electrocardiographic changes of infarction has occurred. The earliest ECG changes in myocardial infarction involve T-wave peaking followed by symmetric inversion of the T-waves. Later, ST-segment elevation is seen, and finally new Q-waves appear. It is important to distinguish true pathologic Q-waves from the normal Q-waves caused by septal depolarization. Pathologic Q-waves are greater than 0.04 sec in duration, and the depth of the Q-wave must be at least one third of the height of the R-wave in the same QRS complex. (An exception to this rule applies to lead aV_R, which normally has a very deep Q-wave). New pathologic Q-waves appear within hours to days after an onset of a myocardial infarction, and in most patients they persist for their lifetime.[129]

In most cases, the diagnosis of intraoperative or postoperative myocardial infarction will be established by clinical signs and symptoms, elevation of cardiac isoenzymes, and evolutionary ECG changes. However, a small number of infarcts may be missed by these methods. Infarct-avid technetium pyrophosphate scanning using single-photon emission computerized tomography may be helpful in diagnosing elusive postoperative myocardial infarcts.[72] However, it is possible that this type of scanning may overestimate the incidence and size of postoperative myocardial infarcts, since technetium pyrophosphate is known to bind not only to infarcted tissue but also to severely damaged but nonetheless viable myocardium.

Magnetic resonance imaging can be used to detect, localize, and establish the size of an acute myocardial infarction. It can also assess perfusion of infarcted and noninfarcted tissues and can help identify areas of jeopardized but nevertheless viable myocardium. Magnetic resonance imaging can also reveal myocardial edema, myocardial fibrosis, wall thinning, and hypertrophy.[130] Although magnetic resonance appears to have many advantages in diagnosing myocardial infarcts, the need to move the patient to the magnetic resonance scanner places a practical limitation on its widespread use in this disease.

D. Treatment of perioperative myocardial infarction

Treatment of patients who have sustained an acute preoperative or postoperative myocardial infarct is usually done by cardiologists or surgeons. However, the anesthesiologist has a major *intraoperative* role in caring for patients who develop myocardial infarction during anesthesia. The specific treatment plan for any patient depends on the details of the case. However, broad treatment guidelines are useful.

If the diagnosis of myocardial infarct seems probable, it is obviously important to monitor the patient closely. Attention to the pulse oximeter will allow very early detection of hypoxemia and may give early warning of significant decreases in pulse volume. If blood pressures have been determined using the Riva-Rocci method, a rapid change to an automated blood pressure cuff will provide more frequent blood pressures. However, beat-to-beat direct arterial manometry is superior. Therefore a radial arterial line should be inserted as soon as possible in the contralateral arm. If radial artery pulses are weak, one should consider cannulating the brachial artery. Hypotension should be treated rapidly in order to restore coronary perfusion pressure and perhaps to "open up" collateral vessels. Hypotension in the patient anesthetized with potent volatile anesthetic agents should be treated by decreasing or discontinuing administration of these agents as appropriate. Administration of 100% oxygen should always be considered. Moderate hypotension in the patient experiencing an acute myocardial infarct will often respond to volume expansion consisting of a 300 to 500 ml rapid infusion of crystalloid. If systolic pressures of 60 to 80 mm Hg persist after conservative volume expansion, we believe vasoactive or inotropic drugs should be given to elevate coronary perfusion pressure to buy time while a method for intravascular volume estimation is established. Although it is true that vasoactive or inotropic agents will increase myocardial oxygen consumption, it is also true that a critical coronary perfusion pressure must exist or the patient will certainly die! Use of inotropes will maximize the contractile power of myocardium uneffected by the infarct. We do not advocate prolonged administration of these agents unless absolutely necessary, but they do serve well to help support the patient through very critical short periods.

Pulmonary artery catheterization may be helpful if conservative volume replacement does not restore adequate blood pressure. This procedure can be done in both awake and asleep patients from several peripheral sites. We prefer the internal jugular route. If operative considerations preclude this, the left medial basilic vein is another alternative as is the femoral vein. Because of the possibility of pneumothorax and laceration of major vessels, we prefer to avoid the subclavian route whenever possible. If pulmonary artery wedge pressures are 12 mm Hg or below, we would continue volume expansion with a crystalloid if hematocrit levels will allow moderate hemodilution without impairing arterial oxygen content. If pulmonary wedge pressures are high, use of an inotropic agent such as dopamine 3 to 5 µg/kg/min should be considered. If a fairly rapid response to dopamine is seen, the drug may be continued. However, if severe hypotension persists after 5 µg/kg/min, we prefer to change to a more potent inotrope such as epinephrine. Although many clinicians cringe at the thought of infusing epinephrine, this emotional reaction is usually unwarranted. Epinephrine can be lifesaving if used properly. It is potent and rapid acting. We have found infusions of epinephrine in the range of 0.01 to 0.15 µg/kg/min to be extremely helpful in critically ill patients.

In some patients, increased afterload during epinephrine infusion can be detrimental to the newly infarcted heart. The cautious addition of sodium nitroprusside will attenuate the increased afterload associated with epinephrine.

Amrinone is a phosphodiesterase inhibitor that may be useful if inotropic support is needed during intraoperative myocardial infarction. Amrinone is an inotrope and a peripheral vascular dilator. After a bolus dose of 0.75 to 3 mg/kg, cardiac output and blood pressure will often increase within a few minutes. Although not a first-line drug, it may be useful in selected patients.

Some patients with intraoperative myocardial infarct will not respond adequately to pharmacologic therapy. In some of these patients the use of an intra-aortic balloon can be lifesaving. The balloon can be inserted percutaneously and can almost immediately decrease myocardial oxygen requirements and may possibly increase myocardial oxygen supply. Early use of the balloon in severe intraoperative infarctions may help to decrease the size of the resultant infarct.

Metabolic acidosis may result from low cardiac output. This can lead to a vicious cycle in which the acidosis further depresses cardiac function and limits the effectiveness of inotropic drugs. Early treatment of metabolic acidosis may help to restore cardiac function in a patient with an intraoperative infarct. Hypoxemia also frequently follows acute myocardial infarction. Measures to increase arterial oxygen tension may help to limit the size of an intraoperative infarct.

A wide variety of cardiac arrhythmias can accompany acute myocardial infarction. Sinus bradycardia occurs commonly in inferior and posterior infarctions.[131-133] Sinus tachycardia may be the result of pain, anxiety, or congestive heart failure. Atrial fibrillation can occur especially in those patients with cardiac failure and increased left atrial pressure. Ventricular arrhythmias ranging from premature ventricular beats to ventricular fibrillation are also seen in acute infarctions. Unifocal or multifocal premature ventricular contractions can usually be controlled with intravenous lidocaine. However, an occasional patient may require procainamide or propranolol. Ventricular fibrillation will necessitate electrical defibrillation.

Some patients with severe bradycardia will require cardiac pacing. Noninvasive temporary ventricular pacing can be done using the Zoll external pacer.[134] This requires the application of large conductive pregelled pacing electrodes to the front and back of the left chest. Transcutaneous pacing may be uncomfortable for the awake patient, but under general anesthesia discomfort from external pacing is not felt. One can also accomplish emergency intraoperative cardiac pacing by passing a straight pacer wire through a 7 French introducer in the internal jugular vein. One may also accomplish pacing by using the Chandler pace-port pulmonary artery catheter. This is a modification of a standard pulmonary artery catheter that has a right ventricular port through which a small pacing wire can be passed.[135]

After acute hemodynamic aberrations have been treated, we should consider myocardial salvage to minimize the damage caused by an intraoperative infarct. Intravenous thrombolysis using tissue thromboplastic activator (t-PA) or streptokinase has revolutionized care of patients with acute myocardial infarction. To be effective the drugs must be given within 4 hours of onset of symptoms. The major limitation of thrombolysis in surgical patients is that it will cause excessive bleeding and is therefore contraindicated in patients with fresh surgical wounds. However thrombolysis may be valuable in selected patients. For example, the patient who has sustained a myocardial infarct during a cystoscopy or diagnostic laryngoscopy may be a very good candidate for thrombolysis. If radial and pulmonary artery monitoring appear to be necessary, the catheters should be inserted *before* thrombolytic drugs are administered. Patients who receive t-PA should also be given a sustained infusion of heparin.[136]

In addition to thrombolysis, medical therapy with nitrates, beta blockers, calcium antagonists, and antiplatelet drugs can also be important components of maximum myocardial salvage.

V. SUMMARY

Severe hemodynamic derangements can lead to unfavorable outcome after anesthesia and surgery. However, it would be naïve and unrealistic to propose that adverse hemodynamic changes can be eliminated completely. Rather, the goals of the anesthesiologist should be to prevent these complications whenever possible and to recognize and treat them *early* when they do occur. We hope that the material presented in this chapter will advance those goals.

REFERENCES

1. Proctor HJ: Fluid and electrolyte management. In Hardy JD, editor: Hardy's Textbook of surgery, Philadelphia, 1983, JB Lippincott Co.
2. Kleinknecht D, Ganeval D, González-Duque LA, et al: Furosemide in acute oliguric renal failure: a controlled trial, Nephron 17:51, 1976.
3. Brown CB, Ogg CS, and Cameron JS: High dose furosemide in acute renal failure: a controlled trial, Clin Nephrol 15:90, 1981.
4. Johnstone M: Human cardiovascular response to Fluothane anesthesia, Br J Anaesth 28:392, 1954.
5. Stevens WC and Eger EI II: Comparative evaluation of new inhalation anesthetics, Anesthesiology 35:125, 1971.
6. Dobkin AB, Nisioka K, Gengaje DB, et al: Ethrane (compound 347) anesthesia: a clinical and laboratory review of 700 cases, Anesth Analg 48:477, 1969.
7. Stevens WC, Cromwell TH, Halsey MJ, et al: The cardiovascular effects of a new inhalation anesthetic, Forane, in human volunteers at constant arterial carbon dioxide tension, Anesthesiology 35:3, 1971.
8. Calverley RK, Smith NT, Jones CW, et al: Ventilatory and cardiovascular effects of enflurane during spontaneous ventilation in man, Anesth Analg 57:610, 1978.
9. Beaupre PN, Cahalan MK, Kremer PF, et al: Does pulmonary artery occlusion pressure adequately reflect left ventricular filling during anesthesia and surgery? Anesthesiology 59:A3, 1983.
10. Ellis RJ, Mangando, PT, and VanDyke DC: Relationship of wedge pressure to end-diastolic volume in patients undergoing myocardial revascularization, J Thorac Cardiovasc Surg 78:605, 1979.
11. Trunkey DD and Holcroft JW: Trauma: general survey in synoposis of management of specific injuries. In Hardy JD, editor: Hardy's Textbook of surgery, Philadelphia, 1983, JB Lippincott Co.
12. Pregnant patients, Chapter 34 in Stoelting RK, Dierdorf SF, and McCammon RL, editors: Anesthesia and co-existing disease, ed 2, Edinburgh and New York, 1988, Churchill Livingstone, Inc.
13. Jones FL Jr: Transmural myocardial necrosis after nonpenetrating cardiac trauma, Am J Cardiol 26:419, 1970.

14. Braunwald E and Kloner RA: The stunned myocardium: prolonged post-ischemic ventricular dysfunction, Circulation 66:1146, 1982.

15. Vatner SF, Heyndrickx GR, and Fallon JT: Effects of brief periods of myocardial ischemia on regional myocardial function and creatine kinase release in conscious dogs and baboons, Can J Cardiol, Suppl A: 19A-24A, July 1986.

16. Arnold JMO, Braumwald E, Sandor T, and Kloner RA: Inotropic stimulation of reperfused myocardium with dopamine: effects on infarct size and myocardial function, J Am Col Cardiol 6:1026, 1985.

17. Ellis G, Wynne J, Braunwald E, et al: Response of reperfused-salvaged stunned myocardium to inotropic stimulation, Am Heart J 107:13, 1984.

18. Lee T and Goldman L: Serum enzyme assays in the diagnosis of acute myocardial infarction: recommendations based on a quantitative analysis, Ann Intern Med 102:221, 1986.

19. Rothenberg HJ: Anaphylactoid reaction to vancomycin, JAMA 171:1101-1102, 1959.

20. Schaad UB, McCraken GH Jr, and Nelson JD: Clinical pharmacology and efficacy of vancomycin in pediatric patients, J Pediatr 96:119-126, 1980.

21. Wold JS and Turnipseed SA: Toxicology of vancomycin in laboratory animals, Rev Infect Dis 3(suppl):S224-S229, 1981.

22. Southorn PA, Plevak EJ, Wright AAJ, et al: Adverse effects of vancomycin administered in the perioperative period, Mayo Clin Proc 61:721-724, 1986.

23. Pau AK and Kahakoo R: "Red-neck syndrome" with slow infusion of vancomycin, N Engl J Med 313:576-577, 1985.

24. Cohen LS, Wechsler AS, Mitchell JH, and Glick G: Depression of cardiac function by streptomycin and other antimicrobial agents, Am J Cardiol 26:505-511, 1970.

25. Modig J, Busch C, and Waernbaum G: Effect of graded infusions of monomethylmethacrylate on coagulation, blood lipids, respiration and circulation, Clin Orthop 113:187, 1975.

26. Modig J, Busch C, Olerud S, et al: Arterial hypotension and hypoxemia during total hip replacement: the importance of thromboplastic products, fat embolism and acrylic monomers, Acta Anaesthesiol Scand 19:28, 1975.

27. Kallos T: Impaired arterial oxygenation associated with use of bone cement in the femoral shaft, Anesthesiology 42:210, 1975.

28. Weidner FA and Zieter FMH: Carcinoid tumors of the gastrointestinal tract, JAMA 245:1153-1155, 1981.

29. Stone CA, Wenger HC, Ludden CT, et al: Antiserotonin-antihistamine properties of cyproheptadine, J Pharmacol Exp Ther 131:73-84, 1961.

30. Stoelting RK, Dierdorf SF, and McCammon RL: Anesthesia and coexisting disease, ed 2, New York, 1988, Churchill Livingstone, Inc, pp 404.

31. Barash PG, Cullen BF, and Stoelting RK: Clinical anesthesia Philadelphia, 1989, JB Lippincott Co, pp 1129.

32. Houghie C: Anticoagulant action of protamine sulfate, Proc Soc Exp Biol Med 98:130-133, 1958.

33. Fadali MA, Ledbetter M, Papacostas CA, et al: Mechanism responsible for the cardiovascular depression effect of protamine sulfate, Ann Surg 180:232-235, 1974.

34. Michaels I and Barash PG: Hemodynamic changes during protamine administration, Anesth Analg 62:831-835, 1983.

35. Lowenstein E, Johnston WE, Lappas DG, et al: Catastrophic pulmonary vasoconstriction associated with protamine reversal of heparin, Anesthesiology 59:470-473, 1983.

36. Morel DR, Zapol WM, Thomas SJ, et al: C5a and thromboxane generation associated with pulmonary vaso- and broncho-constriction during protamine reversal of heparin, Anesthesiology 66:597-604, 1987.

37. Horrow JC: Protamine: a review of its toxicity, Anesth Analg 64:348-361, 1985.

38. Roizen MF, Rodgers GM, et al: Anaphylactoid reactions to vascular graft material presenting with vaso-dilatation and subsequent disseminated intravascular coagulation, Anesthesiology 71:331-338, 1989.

39. Shoemaker WC et al: Textbook of critical care, ed 2, Philadelphia, 1989, WB Saunders Co, p 1020.

40. Laënnec RTH: Traité de l'auscultation médiate et des maladies des poumons et du cœur, Paris, 1831, JS Chaude, pp 138.

41. MacLean LD, Mulligan WG, McLean APH, et al: Patterns of septic shock in man: a detailed study of 56 patients, Ann Surg 166:543, 1967.

42. Shoemaker WC et al: Textbook of critical care, ed 2, Philadelphia, 1989, WB Saunders Co, p 1021.

43. Bone RG, Fisher CJ, Clemmer TP, et al: A controlled clinical trial of high-dose methylprednisolone in the treatment of severe sepsis and septic shock, N Engl J Med 317:653, 1987.

44. Veterans Administration: Systemic Sepsis Cooperative Study Group: Effects of high-dose glucocorticoid therapy on mortality in patients with clinical signs of systemic sepsis, N Engl J Med 317:659, 1987.

45. Parrillo JE: High dose glucocorticoid therapy: two prospective randomized, controlled trials find no efficacy: update, Crit Care Med 2:1, 1987.

46. Brodsky JB and Brabo JJ: Acute postoperative clonidine withdrawal syndrome, Anesthesiology 44:519-520, 1976.

47. Bruner JMR: Handbook of blood pressure monitoring, Littleton, Mass, 1978, PSG Publishing Co, Inc, pp 78-79.

48. Stoelting RK: Attenuation of blood pressure response to laryngoscopy and tracheal intubation with sodium nitroprusside, Anesth Analg 58:116, 1979.

49. Collen BF, Eger EI, Smith NT, et al: The circulatory response to hypercapnia during fluroxene anesthesia in man, Anesthesiology 34:415, 1971.

50. Hornbein TF, Martin WE, Bonica JJ, et al: Nitrous oxide effect on the circulatory and ventilatory responses to halothane, Anesthesiology 31:250, 1969.

51. Marshall BE, Cohen PJ, Klingenmaier CH, et al: Some pulmonary and cardiovascular effects of enflurane (Ethrane) anesthesia with varying $Paco_2$ in man, Br J Anaesth 43:996, 1971.

52. Cromwell TH, Stevens WC, Eger EI II, et al: The cardiovascular effects of compound 469 (Forane) during spontaneous ventilation and carbon dioxide challenge in man, Anesthesiology 35:17, 1971.

53. Collins VJ: Principles of anesthesiology, ed 2, Philadelphia, 1976, Lea & Febiger, pp 305.

54. Haddad NJ, Moyer NJ, and Riley FC: Mydriatic effects of phenylephrine hydrochloride, Am J Ophthalmol 70:729-733, 1970.

55. Zimmerman J, Konner AS, Kandarakis AS, et al: Improving the therapeutic index of topically applied ocular drugs, Arch Ophthalmol 102:551-553, 1984.

56. Barash PG, Collen BF, and Stoelting RK: Clinical anesthesia, Philadelphia, 1989, JP Lippincott Co, pp 1043.

57. Bove EL, Fry WJ, Gross WS, et al: Hypotension and hypertension as consequences of baroreceptor dysfunction following carotid endarterectomy, Surgery 85:633, 1979.

58. Bidwai AV, Bidwai VA, and Rogers CA: Blood pressure and pulse rate responses to endotracheal extuba-

tion with and without prior injection of lidocaine, Anesthesiology 51:171-173, 1971.

59. Berne RM and Rubio R: Coronary circulation. In Burne RM, Sperelakis N, and Geiger SR, editors: Handbook of physiology. Section 2, The cardiovascular system, Bethesda, Md, 1979, American Physiological Society, p 897.

60. Rubio R and Berne RM: Release of adenosine by the normal myocardium and its relationship to the regulation of coronary resistance, Circ Res 25:407, 1969.

61. Furchgott RF and Zawadski JB: The obligatory role of endothelial cells in the relaxation of arterial smooth muscle by acetylcholine, Nature 288:373, 1980.

62. Deboer LWV, Rude RE, Davis RF, et al: Extension of myocardial necrosis into normal epicardium following hypotension during experimental coronary occlusion, Cardiovasc Res 16:423, 1982.

63. Peach MJ, Loeb AL, Singer HA, and Saye JA: Endothelium-derived vascular relaxing factor, Hypertension 7(suppl 1):94, 1985.

64. Peach MJ, Singer HA, Izzo NJ Jr, and Loeb AL: Role of calcium in endothelium-dependent relaxation of arterial smooth muscle, Am J Cardiol 59:35A, 1987.

65. Freiman PC, Mitchell GG, Heistad DD, et al: Atherosclerosis impairs endothelium-dependent vascular relaxation to acetylcholine and thrombin in primates, Circ Res 58:783, 1986.

66. Braunwald E: Heart disease: a textbook of cardiovascular medicine, ed 3, Philadelphia, 1988, WB Saunders Co, p 1194.

67. Braunwald E: Heart disease: a textbook of cardiovascular medicine, ed 3, Philadelphia, 1988, WB Saunders Co, p 1198.

68. Parmley WW: Prevalence and clinical significance of silent myocardial ischemia, Circulation 80(6; suppl IV):66-73, 1989.

69. Geft IL, Fishbein MC, Ninomiya K, et al: Intermittent brief periods of ischemia have a cumulative effect and may cause myocardial necrosis, Circulation 66:1150-1153, 1982.

70. Cohn PF: Total ischemic burden: pathophysiology and prognosis, Am J Cardiol 59:3C-6C, 1987.

71. Knight AA, Hollenberg M, and London MJ: Perioperative myocardial ischemia: importance of the preoperative ischemic pattern, Anesthesiology 68:681-688, 1988.

72. Cheng DC, Chung F, Burns RJ, et al: Postoperative myocardial infarction documented by technetium pyrophosphate scan using single photon emission computed tomography: significance of intraoperative myocardial ischemia and hemodynamic control, Anesthesiology 71:818-826, 1989.

73. Boudoulas H, Lewis RP, Rittgers SE, et al: Increased diastolic time: a possible important factor in the beneficial effect of propranolol in patients with coronary artery disease, J Cardiovasc Pharmacol 1:503, 1979.

74. Palmer CM, Norris MC, Giudici MC, et al: Incidence of electrocardiographic changes during caesarean delivery under regional anesthesia, Anesth Analg 70:36-43, 1990.

75. Mangano DJ: Perioperative cardiac morbidity, Anesthesiology 72:170, Jan 1990.

76. Roy WL, Edelist G, and Gilbert B: Myocardial ischemia during non-cardiac surgical procedures in patients with coronary artery disease, Anesthesiology 51:393-397, 1979.

77. Coriat P, Harari A, Daloz M, and Viars P: Clinical predictors of intraoperative myocardial ischemia in patients with coronary artery disease undergoing noncardiac surgery, Acta Anaesthesiol Scand 26:287-290, 1982.

78. Prinzmetal M, Kennamer R, Merliss R, et al: A variant form of angina pectoris, Am J Med 27:375, 1959.

79. Oliva PB, Potts DE, and Pluss RG: Coronary arterial spasm in Prinzmetal angina: documentation by coronary arteriography, N Engl J Med 288:745, 1973.

80. Braunwald E: Heart disease: A textbook of cardiovascular medicine, ed 3, Philadelphia, 1988, WB Saunders Co, p 1360.

81. Ganz P and Alexander RW: New insights into the cellular mechanisms of vasospasms, Am J Cardiol 56:11E, 1985.

82. Lundmer PL, Celwyn AP, Shook TL, et al: Paradoxical vasoconstriction induced by acetylcholine in atherosclerotic coronary arteries, N Engl J Med 315:1046, 1986.

83. Hyduke JF, Pineda JJ, Smith CE, and Rice TW: Severe intraoperative myocardial ischemia following manipulation of the heart in a patient undergoing esophagogastrectomy, Anesthesiology 71:154-158, 1989.

84. Allred EN, Bleecker ER, Chaitman DR, et al: Short-term effects of carbon monoxide exposure on the exercise performance of subjects with coronary artery disease, N Engl J Med 321:1426-1432, 1989.

85. Lange RA, Cigarroa RG, Yancy CW, et al: Cocaine induced coronary artery vasoconstriction, N Engl J Med 321(23):1557-1562, 1989.

86. Nademanee K, Gorelick DA, Josephson MA, et al: Myocardial ischemia during cocaine withdrawal, Ann Intern Med 111:876-888, 1989.

87. Dressler FA, Malekzadeh S, and Roberts WC: Quantitative analysis of amounts of coronary arterial narrowing in cocaine addicts, Am J Cardiol 65:303-308, 1990.

88. Parmley WW: Prevalence and clinical significance of silent myocardial ischemia, Circulation 80(6; suppl IV):S68-S73, 1989.

89. Margolis JR, Kannel WS, Feinleib M, et al: Clinical features of unrecognized myocardial infarction—silent and symptomatic: eighteen year follow-up: the Framingham Study, Am J Cardiol 32:1-7, 1973.

90. Epstein SE, Quyyumi AA, and Bonow R: Myocardial ischemia: silent or asymptomatic, N Engl J Med 318:1038-1042, 1988.

91. Blackburn H and Katigbak R: What electrocardiographic leads to take after exercise? Am Heart J 67:184, 1964.

92. Blackburn H, Taylor HL, Okamato N, Et al: Standardization of the exercise electrocardiogram: a systematic comparison of chest lead configurations employed for monitoring during exercise. In Karoonen MJ and Barry AJ, editors: Physical activity and the heart, Springfield, Ill, 1967, Charles C Thomas, Publisher, p 101.

93. Kotrly KJ, Kotter GS, Mortara D, et al: Intraoperative detection of myocardial ischemia with an ST-segment trend monitoring system, Anesth Analg 63:343, 1984.

94. Kaplan JA: Electrocardiographic monitoring. In Kaplan JA, editor: Cardiac anesthesia, New York, 1979, Grune & Stratton, p 117.

95. Kaplan JA and Wells PH: Early diagnosis of myocardial ischemia using the pulmonary arterial catheter, Anesth Analg 60:789-793, 1981.

96. Aroesty JM, McKay RG, Heller GB, et al: Simultaneous assessment of left ventricular systolic and diastolic dysfunction during pacing-induced ischemia, Circulation 71:889-900, 1985.

97. Iskandrian AS, Bemis CE, Hakki AH, et al: Ventricular systolic and diastolic impairment during pacing-induced myocardial ischemia in coronary artery disease: simultaneous hemodynamic electrocardiographic and

radionuclide angiographic evaluation, Am Heart J 112:382-391, 1986.
98. Bourdillon PD, Lorell BH, Mirsky I, et al: Increased regional myocardial stiffness of the left ventricle during pacing-induced angina in man, Circulation 67:316-323, 1983.
99. Wyns W, Serruys PW, Slager C, et al: Effects of coronary occlusion during percutaneous transluminal angioplasty in humans on left ventricular chamber stiffness and regional diastolic pressure-radius relations, J Am Coll Cardiol 7:455-463, 1986.
100. Serruys PW, van den Brand M, Wijns W, et al: Systolic and diastolic left ventricular function during transluminal acute occlusion, Circulation 68(suppl III):237, 1983.
101. Bowman LK, Cleman MW, Cabin HS, et al: Dynamics of early and late left ventricular filling determined by Doppler 2-dimensional echocardiography during percutaneous transluminal coronary angioplasty, Am J Cardiol 61:541-545, 1988.
102. van Daele M, Sutherland GR, Mitchell MM, et al: Do changes in pulmonary capillary wedge pressure adequately reflect myocardial ischemia during anesthesia? A correlative preoperative hemodynamic, electrocardiographic, and transesophageal echocardiographic study, Circulation 81(3):865-871, 1990.
103. Smith JS, Cahalan MK, Benefiel CJ, et al: Intraoperative detection of myocardial ischemia in high-risk patients: electrocardiography versus 2-dimensional transesophageal echocardiography, Circulation 72(5):1015-1021, 1985.
104. Hauser AM, Gangadharn V, Ramos RG, et al: Sequence of mechanical electrocardiographic and clinical effects of repeated coronary artery occlusion in human beings: echocardiographic observations during coronary angioplasty, J Am Coll Cardiol 5:193-197, 1985.
105. Wohlgelerter D, Cleman M, Higman HA, et al: Regional myocardial dysfunction during coronary angioplasty: evaluation by 2-dimensional echocardiography and 12-lead electrocardiography, J Am Coll Cardiol 7:1245-1254, 1986.
106. Leung J, O'Kelly MB, Browner W, et al: Are regional wall motion abnormalities detected by transesophageal echocardiography triggered by acute changes in supply and demand? Anesthesiology 69:A901, 1988.
107. Cahalan MK: Intraoperative evaluation of left ventricular function with transesophageal echocardiography: problems and pitfalls, Monograph of 1990 Workshops "Update on Intraoperative Echo," Orlando, Fla, 1990, Society of Cardiovascular Anesthesiologists (Richmond, Va), 12th annual meeting, pp 142-145.
108. Pandian NG, Skorton DJ, Collins SM, et al: Heterogenicity of left ventricular segmental wall motion thickening and excursion in 2-dimensional echocardiograms of normal human subjects, Am J Cardiol 51:1667-1673, 1983.
109. London MJ, Tubau TF, Wong MG, et al: The "natural history" of segmental wall motion abnormalities in patients undergoing non-cardiac surgery, Anesthesiology 73:644-655, 1990.
110. Weiner DA: Accuracy of cardiokymography during exercise testing: results of a multicenter study, J Am Coll Cardiol 6(3):502-509, 1985.
111. Bellows WH, Bode RH, Levy JH, et al: Noninvasive detection of peri-induction ischemic ventricular dysfunction by cardiokymography in humans: preliminary experience, Anesthesiology 60:155-158, 1984.
112. Coriat P, Daloz M, Bousseau D, et al: Prevention of intraoperative myocardial ischemia during noncardiac surgery with intravenous nitroglycerin, Anesthesiology 61:193-196, 1984.

113. Seitelberger R, Zwölfer W, Binder TM, et al: Infusion of nifedipine after coronary artery bypass grafting decreases the incidence of early postoperative myocardial ischemia, Ann Thorac Surg 49:61-67, 1990.
114. Hill AB, Bowley CJ, and Nahrwold ML: Intranasal administration of nitroglycerin, Anesthesiology 51(35):567, 1979.
115. DiMarco JP, Miles W, Akhtar M, et al: Adenosine for paroxysmal supraventricular tachycardia: dose ranging and comparison with verapamil, Ann Intern Med 113:104-110, 1990.
116. Arkins R, Smessaert AA, and Hicks RG: Mortality and morbidity in surgical patients with coronary artery disease, JAMA 190(6):93-96, 1964.
117. Steen PA, Tinker JH, and Tarhan S: Myocardial reinfarction after anesthesia and surgery, JAMA 239(24):2566-2570, 1968.
118. Topkins MJ and Artusio JF: Myocardial infarction and surgery, a five year study, Anesth Analg 43:716-720, 1964.
119. Wells PH and Kaplan JA: Optimal management of patients with ischemic heart disease for non-cardiac surgery by complementary anesthesiologist and cardiologist interaction, Am Heart J 102:102-109, 1981.
120. Rao TLK, Jacobs KH, and El-Etr AA: Reinfarction following anesthesia in patients with myocardial infarction, Anesthesiology 59:499-505, 1983.
121. Sloghoff S and Keats AS: Does perioperative myocardial ischemia lead to postoperative myocardial infarction? Anesthesiology 62:107-114, 1985.
122. Sloghoff S and Keats AS: Further observations on perioperative myocardial ischemia, Anesthesiology 65:539-542, 1986.
123. Muller JE et al: Circadian variation in the frequency of onset of acute myocardial infarction, N Engl J Med 313:1315, 1985.
124. Benacerraf A, Scholl JM, Achard F, et al: Coronary spasm and thrombosis associated with myocardial infarction in a patient with nearly normal coronary arteries, Circulation 67:1147, 1983.
125. Norris RM: Myocardial infarction, Edinburgh and New York, 1982, Churchill Livingstone, p 322.
126. Roseman MD: Painless myocardial infarction: a review of the literature and analysis of 220 cases, Ann Intern Med 41:1, 1954.
127. Thaler MS: The only EKG book you'll ever need, Philadelphia, 1988, JB Lippincott Co, pp 209-211.
128. Braunwald E and Kloner RA: The stunned myocardium: prolonged post-ischemic ventricular dysfunction, Circulation 66:1146-1149, 1982.
129. Thaler MS: The only EKG book you'll ever need, Philadelphia, 1988, JB Lippincott Co, p 202.
130. Braunwald E: Heart disease: a textbook of cardiovascular medicine, ed 3, Philadelphia, 1988, WB Saunders Co, p 1242.
131. Adgey AAJ, Alley JD, Geddes JS, et al: Acute phase of myocardial infarction, Lancet 2:501, 1971.
132. Graner LE, Gershen BJ, Orlando MM, and Epstein SE: Bradycardia and its complications in pre-hospital phase of acute myocardial infarction, Am J Cardiol 32:607, 1973.
133. Zipes DP: The clinical significance of bradycardic rhythms in acute myocardial infarction, Am J Cardiol 24:814, 1969.
134. Zoll PM, Zoll RH, Falx RH, et al: External non-invasive temporary cardiac pacing: clinical trials, Circulation 71:937, 1985.
135. Product information: Baxter Healthcare Corp, Santa Ana, CA 92711-1150.
136. Braunwald E: Heart disease: a textbook of cardiovascular medicine, ed 3, Philadelphia, 1988, WB Saunders Co, p 1257.

Chapter 12

Complications Related to Cardiopulmonary Bypass

Nancy A. Nussmeier
Anthony M. Mills

I. **Neurologic Complications**
  A. Cerebral Infarction Resulting in Overt Neurologic Sequelae
    1. Macroembolization of air and particulate material
      a. Incidence and etiology of macroembolic phenomena
      b. Prevention of macroembolic phenomena
      c. Minimizing effects of macroembolic phenomena
    2. Massive air embolism and other pump problems
    3. Role of concomitant cerebrovascular disease
  B. Subtle Neuropsychologic Dysfunction
    1. Incidence and etiology of neuropsychologic dysfunction
    2. Prevention of neuropsychologic dysfunction
      a. Microembolism
      b. Perfusion techniques during cardiopulmonary bypass (CPB)
  C. Profound Hypothermia and Circulatory Arrest (PHCA)
    1. Incidence and types of neurologic complications after PHCA
    2. Prevention of neurologic complications
      a. Hypothermia itself
      b. Circulatory arrest versus low perfusion flow
      c. Glucose
  D. Peripheral Nerve Injury
II. **Cardiovascular Complications**
  A. Problems with Cannulation and Systemic Perfusion During CPB
    1. Improper cannulation
      a. Aortic and arterial dissection
      b. Inadvertent entry of aortic arch vessels
      c. Improper connection to CPB circuit (reversed cannulation)
    2. Obstruction of venous return
    3. Massive air embolism
    4. Inadequate anticoagulation
  B. Low Cardiac Output and Hypotension/Hypertension After CPB
    1. Acute myocardial ischemia
    2. Acute myocardial depression
    3. Unrecognized cardiac valve dysfunction
    4. Protamine reactions and anaphylaxis
    5. Pericardial tamponade
    6. Monitoring artifact
    7. Hypertension
    8. Right ventricular failure
  C. Arrhythmias
    1. Supraventricular tachydysrhythmias
    2. Bradydysrhythmias and atrioventricular conduction defects
    3. Ventricular irritability
III. **Pulmonary Complications**
  A. Bronchospasm
  B. Postperfusion ARDS and Pulmonary Edema
IV. **Renal Complications—Acute Renal Insufficiency**
V. **Gastrointestinal Complications**
VI. **Infectious Complications**
VII. **Immunologic Complications**
  A. Complement Activation
  B. Changes in Leukocytes and Immunoglobulins
VIII. **Hematologic Complications**
  A. Inadequate Surgical Hemostasis
  B. Residual Heparin Activity
  C. Thrombocytopenia and Platelet Dysfunction
  D. Fibrinolysis and Decreased Fibrinogen
  E. Other Causes of Coagulopathy
  F. Hemolysis and Shortened Erythrocyte Survival
IX. **Metabolic and Systemic Derangements**
  A. Metabolic Acidosis
  B. Hypokalemia
  C. Hyperkalemia
  D. Hypocalcemia
  E. Hypomagnesemia
  F. Hyperglycemia
  G. Hypothermia

I. NEUROLOGIC COMPLICATIONS

A. Cerebral infarction resulting in overt neurologic sequelae

1. *Macroembolization of air and particulate material*

a. Incidence and etiology of macroembolic phenomena. Despite improvements in cardiac surgical techniques and extracorporeal apparatus, overt as well as subtle neurologic complications still occur. The risk of overt sequelae varies with the type of cardiac operation. Historically, *intracardiac* operations such as valve replacements carried a greater risk (4.1% to 14%),[1-6] compared to *extracardiac* operations, that is, coronary artery bypass grafting (0.3% to 5.4%).[7-17] The reported incidence of neurologic complications also varies according to differences in study design. For example, the incidence is less in studies examining only major insults such as stroke, compared to studies reporting both major and minor insults, such as postoperative psychiatric dysfunction or retinal infarction. Also the incidence of cerebral damage is less in studies that include only permanent damage, as opposed to those that include temporary dysfunction as well. Most importantly, the incidence in retrospective studies is less than that in prospective studies.[18]

Macroembolization from the surgical field is believed to be the most common cause of overt neurologic complications.[1-3,7-9,19-25] The risk of intraoperative macroembolism of air or particulate matter is greater during intracardiac surgery compared to coronary artery bypass grafting (CABG).[2,24-26] Intracardiac procedures (such as valve replacement or repair, ventricular aneurysm resection, or closure of a septal defect) require opening of a cardiac chamber. Certainly, air embolism is more common after such open-chamber operations because large intracardiac bubbles can remain trapped after the heart is closed.[25,27-32] Also, macroembolism of particulate debris from the surgical field (such as calcium fragments,[3,24] valve vegetations,[19] intraventricular thrombus,[9] or fat[22]) is more common after open chamber surgery and may be the cause of most permanent or severe dysfunction. Studies demonstrating that severe neurologic complications occur most frequently after replacement of extensively calcified valves support this view.[1,3,24]

Despite the historically higher incidence of overt cerebral dysfunction after *intracardiac* procedures, factors such as extreme age and the coexisting presence of diffuse arteriosclerotic disease are exerting an unfavorable influence on patients undergoing CABG.[12,15-17] Several studies have noted a low risk of neurologic sequelae, less than 2%, after CABG in patients less than 70 years of age (Fig. 12-1).[12-17,33] However, in these same studies, the risk is considerably greater, 6% to 8%, in patients older than 70 years. Furthermore, some investigators have noted an initial decrease in incidence of stroke after CABG during an earlier period (1975 to 1979), followed by a progressive rise in incidence in more recent years.[12,17] Data analysis demonstrated that the risk of stroke had increased concomitantly with patient age.[12,17] Older patients have more extensive peripheral vascular disease and higher risk of macroembolism during CABG.[2,8,34] Cannulation or cross-clamping of the ascending aorta, necessary for anastomosis of the proximal end of a vein graft, or aortotomy alone, may liberate cholesterol or calcific plaque debris and result in cerebral infarction.[9,21,34,35] Frequently, there are yellow plaque areas in the aorta and regions of aortic stiffness that can be palpated by the surgeon[9,34] or delineated with intraoperative ultrasound techniques.[35] Another source of emboli during CABG may be large left ventricular clots formed in infarcted areas.[9] Also, older patients have more extensive cerebrovascular disease, which may result in greater likelihood of decreased regional cerebral perfusion.[12,14,36] Since the average age of patients undergoing coronary surgery is increasing, the risk of major neurologic complications in such patients may now be greater than previous reports had indicated.

b. *Prevention of macroembolic phenomena*

(1) TECHNICAL ASPECTS. Prevention of air and particulate macroemboli during intracardiac surgery depends primarily on meticulous surgical technique.[3,28,37] The success of conscientious efforts to minimize embolization, particularly the elimination of air and particulate debris from the left side of the heart before termination of cardiopulmonary bypass (CPB), has been documented by serial studies in two institutions.[2,3,24,38] Eventual reduction in the incidence of neuropsychiatric complications was attributed to a heightened awareness among surgeons of the risk of emboli, resulting directly from data collected and communicated at these institutions.[2,24] However, *total* elimination of air is rarely possible, and fragments of particulate matter can occasionally remain undetected in the left atrium or ventricle. Thus, despite careful surgical technique, a persistent though decreased incidence of debilitating cerebral complications is present after high-risk intracardiac operations.

Macroembolization is most likely during aortic cannulation (before initiation of CPB) and

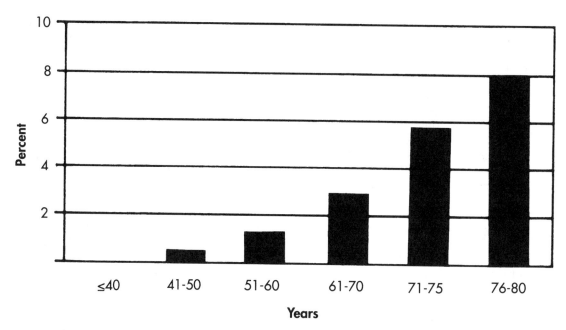

Fig. 12-1. The incidence of stroke after coronary artery bypass grafting increased according to the age of the patient, from 0.42% for patients 41 to 50 years of age to 7.14% for patients older than 75 years (*p* <0.001). (From Gardner TJ, Horneffer PJ, Manolio TA, et al: Ann Thorac Surg 40:574-581, 1985.)

during the initial cardiac ejections (upon weaning from bypass) because the heart is not excluded from the circulation by the aortic cross-clamp during these periods.[2,3,39] Before initiation of CPB, all air must be eliminated from the aortic cannula, which is primed with fluid from the CPB circuit. The anesthesiologist and surgeon should examine the cannula just before insertion to detect any residual air bubbles. After initiation of CPB, the ascending aorta routinely is clamped before any chamber of the heart is opened, thereby excluding air from the systemic circulation. Cardiac contractions, which would eject air, are subsequently eliminated when the heart is arrested with cold cardioplegia solution or ventricular fibrillation is induced. During intracardiac repair, diligent surgical attention is required to ensure removal of all tiny fragments of valve tissue, calcific debris, and so forth from the field. After completion of the repair, an effort to eliminate all air, especially from the left side of the heart, is essential (Fig. 12-2). This should be accomplished before termination of bypass and before the first ventricular ejections.

Intracardiac air and debris can remain trapped in atrial, ventricular, or aortic cul-de-sacs, such as those in the left atrial appendage, in the left ventricular apex, between the chordae tendineae, in crevices between the papillary muscles, within the irregularities of the trabeculae carneae, and beneath the mural leaflet of the mitral valve.[40] Eventual embolization may oc-

cur at any time during the postbypass period. Some surgeons prefer to keep the patient in Trendelenburg's position for at least 5 to 10 minutes after release of the aortic cross-clamp in order to keep the carotid arteries in the most dependent position. Ejected residual air is then likely to traverse the inside of the aortic arch rather than the carotid arteries, thus avoiding embolism to the brain.[41] The use of nitrous oxide should be avoided during and after CPB because this gas would dramatically expand any retained air bubbles. Although some clinicians advocate carotid compression during the initial cardiac ejections accompanying weaning from CPB (when embolization is most likely to occur), this technique may reduce cerebral blood flow. An alternative preventive measure would be to provide cerebral *protection* against the resultant neurologic sequelae, an approach discussed later in this chapter.

Another challenging surgical problem is the heavily calcified aorta, which must be managed to prevent embolization of atherosclerotic plaque. Barzilai and colleagues, using intraoperative Doppler ultrasound to assess the ascending aorta, found that 8 of 33 patients had sufficient atherosclerotic disease at the originally intended site of cannulation or cross-clamping to necessitate choosing an alternative site.[35] Occasionally, femoral arterial cannulation with retrograde perfusion may be necessary. Deep hypothermia and circulatory arrest also enable exten-

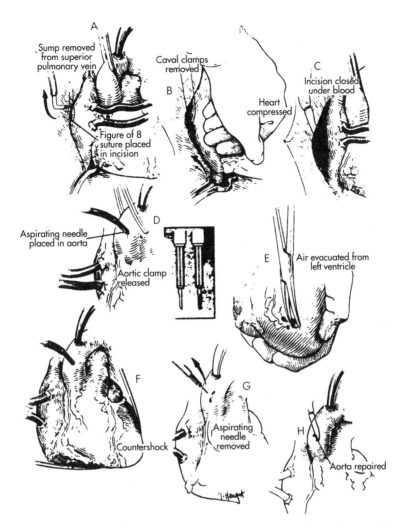

Fig. 12-2. Evacuation of air from the cardiopulmonary system. (From Cooley DA: Cannulation for temporary bypass. In Cooley DA, editor: Techniques in cardiac surgery, Philadelphia, 1984, WB Saunders Co, p 88.)

sive aortic surgery when aortic clamping may be undesirable.[42,43]

(2) DETECTION. Recently, echocardiography has been used to detect air retained in cardiac chambers after intracardiac repair.[25,29-32,44,45] With M-mode transesophageal echocardiography (TEE), Oka and associates found a large incidence of air emboli after completion of standard air evacuation maneuvers.[25,31] Seventy-nine percent of patients ($n = 15$) undergoing intracardiac procedures and 11% ($n = 18$) of patients undergoing CABG had detectable air emboli. Central nervous system dysfunction occurred in 23% of the patients with air emboli and in none of those without air emboli. Topol et al. also detected intracavitary left ventricular microbubbles during cardiac operations, more often in valvular (intracardiac) surgery than in coronary revascularization.[30] These

authors attempted to quantitate the presence of microbubbles using a graded scale based on the number of bubbles per stop frame. However, they did not find the presence of high-grade microbubbles to be predictive of postoperative neurologic complications.[30]

Although precise quantification of the amount of retained air is not possible using TEE, the qualitative estimates obtained may be clinically useful. For example, recurrent showers of air emboli may be prevented when maneuvers are repeated to evacuate air detected by TEE. Oka et al. reported that the addition of several maneuvers to the surgical team's routine air evacuation methods allowed nearly complete elimination of air before termination of CPB.[31] These maneuvers included positive cardiac chamber filling accompanied by echocardiographic demonstration of left atrial stretching, vigorous chamber ballottement, and specific echo-directed chamber aspiration before release of the aortic cross-clamp. The authors emphasized that CPB was maintained until TEE indicated no retained air.

During CPB, measurement of cerebral electrical activity may detect potentially disastrous cerebral events. Widespread use of the multichannel EEG has been limited because of problems with electrical interference in the operating room and the need for additional personnel to interpret the massive quantity of data generated by traditional polygraph recorders.[46] More recently, advances in automated EEG processing techniques have enhanced clarity of display and achieved compression of otherwise voluminous data, thus facilitating interpretation. Ideally, an instrument displaying processed EEG data will also display at least one channel of raw EEG data for comparison, in order to assist the observer in recognizing an artifact.

There are anecdotal reports describing use of the processed EEG to detect potentially disastrous events causing cerebral ischemia during CPB. El-Fiki and Fish noted an episode of severe bilateral abnormality in the density spectral array EEG, which occurred because of a perfusion accident during CPB (disconnection of the arterial return tubing from the pump). This event resulted in total loss of arterial blood pressure and, within 10 seconds, nearly total loss of EEG activity (Fig. 12-3).[47] The EEG was also used to monitor recovery from this episode. Sixty seconds after perfusion was restored, EEG activity began to return, and after a further 4 minutes the EEG had recovered to the pre-event level of activity. Later in the same case, these authors noted an abrupt bilateral decrease in EEG activity coincident with coronary air embolization and, presumably, simultaneous air embolization to the cerebral circulation, with recovery over a 1-hour period. Postoperatively the patient showed no signs of focal injury. However, neuropsychologic testing showed some deterioration, and the patient reported some intellectual change.[47] Similarly, Michaels and Sheehan noted unilateral decreased EEG activity on the left, occurring shortly after initiation of CPB, because of aortic dissection (Fig. 12-4).[48] Steele et al. reported left-sided loss of power and spectral edge, indicating unilateral cerebral ischemia caused by

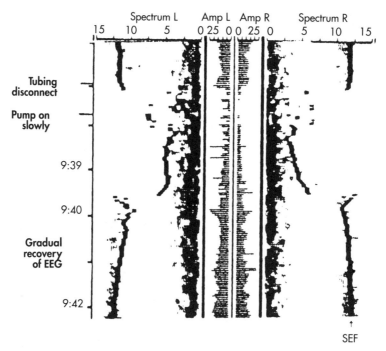

Fig. 12-3. Density spectral array recording of the EEG. The density of the dots correspond to those frequencies making the largest contribution to the EEG. Frequency is shown at the top from 0 to 15 Hz for the two cerebral hemispheres; amplitude (μV) is shown in the center by the horizontal bars. The time markers on left indicate 1-minute intervals. At the pump tubing disconnection, immediate loss of EEG spectral edge frequency (SEF) and amplitude can be seen. Recovery occurred slowly over a 5-minute period. (From El-Fiki M and Fish KJ: Anesthesiology 67:575-578, 1987.)

vertebrobasilar artery insufficiency (Fig. 12-5).[49] Finally, Bolsin reported three cases of neurologic damage, presumably occurring during CPB, detected by changes in the frequency distribution recorded by a cerebral function analyzing monitor.[50]

c. Minimizing effects of macroembolic phenomena.

(1) HYPOTHERMIA. The traditional form of cerebral protection during CPB is hypothermia. Hypothermia is most commonly used when global complete ischemia is expected, such as elective circulatory arrest for extensive repair of congenital lesions in infants or aortic arch repair in adults. Although the benefit of hypothermia is well established in circulatory arrest, as described later in this chapter, it is important

to remember that CPB does not usually include circulatory arrest. Therefore the utility of hypothermia in reducing postoperative central nervous system deficits during routine cardiac operations is limited and currently unproved. First, it is not known whether hypothermia reduces CNS injuries in patients subjected to regional ischemia. Second, it must be remembered that normothermia is restored before the end of CPB. Embolization to the CNS is unlikely during the hypothermic period, since the heart and surgical field are excluded from circulation by the aortic cross-clamp throughout that period. At the suspected time of greatest risk of embolization, that is, when the aorta is declamped, the CNS is unprotected by hypother-

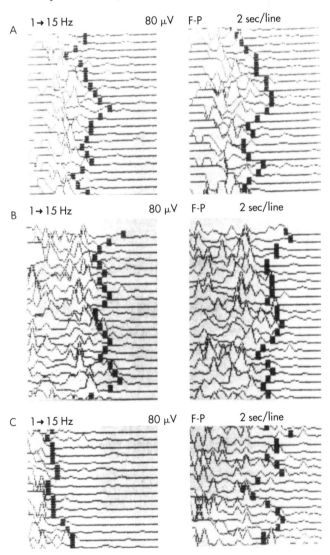

Fig. 12-4. Compressed spectral array (CSA) EEG of left and right cerebral hemispheres: **A,** after induction; **B,** immediately after initiation of cardiopulmonary bypass; **C** after 40 minutes of cardiopulmonary bypass. (From Michaels I and Sheehan J: Anesth Analg 63:946-948, 1984.)

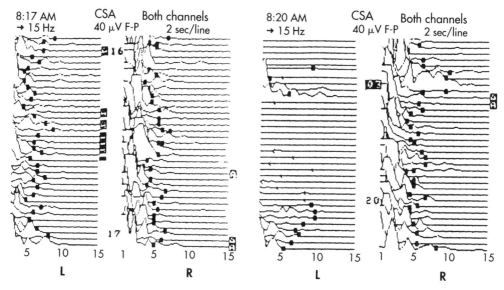

Fig. 12-5. Postinduction left, *L,* and right, *R,* cerebral hemispheric compressed spectral array (CSA) EEG recording demonstrating symmetric activity of the two hemispheres. Moments later, the head is extended and there is a loss of power and spectral edge in the left hemisphere, indicating cerebral ischemia. (From Steele ER, Albin MS, Monts JL, and Harman PK: Anesth Analg 66:271-273, 1987.)

mia. During these critical normothermic periods of CPB, only pharmacologic cerebral protective options are possible.

(2) BARBITURATES. Of the pharmacologic agents that have been investigated as cerebral protectants, barbiturates have received the most extensive study. Animal studies using various forms of *incomplete* ischemia consistently indicate improved outcome with barbiturate therapy.[51-60] Lower morbidity and mortality in animal models is associated with measurable barbiturate-induced reduction in the mass of infarcted brain tissue.[54-57] However, this form of protection is effective only when the barbiturate is administered before, during, or very shortly after the ischemic event.[58,59] Furthermore, the protective effect of barbiturates is dose dependent. For example, dose is correlated with improved neuropathologic outcome in stroke models, indicating a cerebral protective effect.[56,60] Also, barbiturates reduce the cerebral metabolic rate of oxygen consumption ($CMRO_2$) in a dose-dependent manner, with maximal reduction occurring at doses that abolish cortical electrical activity.[60,61] Additional barbiturate administration increases cardiac and respiratory depression but produces no further reduction in cerebral metabolic rate.[61] Since both $CMRO_2$ reduction and cerebral protection are dependent on barbiturate dose, it has long been assumed that the mechanism of barbiturate-induced protection is cerebral metabolic suppression, but this mechanism has not been unequivocally established. Other mechanisms may contribute to protection, including a "reverse steal effect" like that occurring with hypocapnia,[62-64] reduction in intracranial blood volume and pressure,[65,66] free-radical scavenging activity,[67] or properties that prevent accumulation of free fatty acids[68] and seizures.[69] A combination of these actions may prevent or reduce the effects of cerebral ischemia in specific disease states.

Slogoff and associates were the first to study barbiturate protection in patients undergoing intracardiac and extracardiac procedures during normothermic CPB.[2] Neuropsychiatric outcome was not significantly improved with thiopental administration in this study, though the incidence of abnormalities was less in the treatment group than in the control group. The authors suggested that they were unable to demonstrate a protective effect with thiopental because of the relatively low dose they had chosen (15 mg/kg) and the timing of thiopental administration (during the prebypass period only). Neuropsychiatric complications were more frequent after intracardiac procedures, as expected.[2]

The suggestion of improved outcome with barbiturate pretreatment in the first study prompted revisions in experimental design and execution of a second prospective randomized study at the same institution.[3] Only patients undergoing intracardiac procedures during normothermic CPB were included. In addition, the dose of thiopental was adjusted to maintain a nearly isoelectric EEG throughout cannulation and CPB. Specifically, thiopental was administered to maintain a burst-suppression pattern having an interval of more than 60 seconds between bursts. The mean dose required to achieve this degree and duration of EEG suppression during normothermic CPB was nearly 40 mg/kg, almost three times that used in the earlier study. The results of the second study demonstrated significant barbiturate protection. On the first postoperative day, 5 of 89 patients in the thiopental group and 8 of 93 patients in the control group exhibited clinical neuropsychiatric abnormalities.[3] By the tenth postoperative day, all neuropsychiatric dysfunction had resolved in the thiopental group but persisted in 7 (7.5%) of the 8 patients in the control group. The authors theorized that barbiturate therapy could not decrease the frequency of embolization but rather reduced its permanent expression, presumably by decreasing the size of the resulting infarct. Administration of thiopental in such large dose during CPB was not entirely without negative consequence. Although all thiopental patients were successfully weaned from CPB, they required more frequent inotropic support than the control group did. Also the large doses of thiopental led to a longer recovery period for both arousal and extubation.

Because of these side effects, a third study at the same institution was instituted.[70] The investigators wished to test the hypothesis that properly timed and titrated administration of a lower thiopental dose would be effective. Therefore, 100 patients undergoing intracardiac surgery during moderate hypothermia (28° to 30° C) were randomized so that 52 received standard treatment, having thiopental titrated to maintain a nearly isoelectric EEG throughout CPB, whereas the other 48 patients received only a single bolus of thiopental just before removal of the aortic cross-clamp (titrated to produce transient EEG burst suppression with greater than 60 seconds between bursts). The mean thiopental dose in the standard group was 36 mg/kg, compared to 16 mg/kg in the single-bolus group. The results of this study showed no difference between the treatment groups. There were 3 of 52 (6%) patients in the standard group and 2 of 48 (4%) in the single-bolus group who exhibited postoperative neuropsychiatric dysfunction. By the tenth postoperative day, only one patient (in the standard group) exhibited persistent dysfunction, characterized by disorientation and lethargy. The authors concluded that the low incidence of neuropsychiatric dysfunction in both groups indicated equally efficacious protection with either method of thiopental administration.[70] However, side effects were not much changed by administration of the lower thiopental dose. The transient use of inotropic support was equally frequent in both groups, and there was no significant difference in the recovery period for awakening. There was a significantly shorter period until extubation could be accomplished (16 versus 18 hours). A possible weakness of this study is the absence of a control group of patients receiving no thiopental. The investigators chose not to include a control group because it is the practice in their institution to provide cerebral protection with thiopental to all patients undergoing intracardiac surgery.

A group of investigators at another institution has asked whether thiopental administration would be effective in preventing overt neurologic complications occurring after *extracardiac* (CABG) surgery.[71] Presumably, in these operations, air emboli would not occur under usual circumstances. Therefore protective efforts would be directed against particulate emboli, or perhaps against regional hypoperfusion caused by the higher incidence of cerebrovascular disease in this population. Zaidan and colleagues studied 300 patients undergoing CABG surgery during hypothermic (28° C) CPB. Again, the end point of thiopental titration was near-isoelectricity of the EEG throughout CPB (burst suppression with bursts occurring no more often than every 30 seconds). These investigators found no significant difference between thiopental and control groups with respect to transient or persistent neuropsychiatric outcome. In the thiopental group, 13 of 149 patients exhibited transient neuropsychiatric dysfunction, compared to 7 of 151 patients in the control group.[71] By the tenth postoperative day, 5 of 149 patients in the thiopental group had persistent neuropsychiatric dysfunction compared to 7 of 151 patients in the control group. These authors concluded that thiopental administration is not effective in this population of patients undergoing extracardiac surgery, perhaps because large particulate emboli occur, rather than the air emboli that are more likely during intracardiac surgery. Indeed, CT scans revealed single or multiple infarcts in each of the patients who had an overt stroke. Side effects were similar in this study to those previously reported (more frequent use of inotropic agents to achieve weaning from CPB and increased time to postoperative awakening and extubation).

To summarize, the use of thiopental during *intracardiac* surgery, administered either as an infusion throughout CPB or as a bolus injected shortly before release of the aortic cross-clamp, appears to be effective as a pharmacologic means of reducing the incidence of overt postoperative neuropsychiatric dysfunction. Apparently, however, this therapy is not effective during *extracardiac* surgery.[72] Also it should be emphasized that barbiturates are *not* equivalent to hypothermia, even though the mechanism for barbiturate protection is, at least in part, attributable to the metabolic suppression. Barbiturates affect the metabolic rate of only an actively functioning brain, a brain generating EEG activity.[51] Hypothermia, on the other hand, affects all the energy-consuming processes of the brain. It is this difference that explains why hypothermia will prolong the brain's tolerance for *complete* ischemia (as from cardiac arrest) whereas barbiturates cannot. Therefore there is no role for barbiturates in situations of cardiac arrest, either prophylactically before elective arrest (which is appropriately performed under conditions of profound hypothermia) or as a resuscitative agent after unexpected cardiac arrest. The key is that the complete ischemia itself almost instantly produces an isoelectric EEG; therefore barbiturates have nothing to add in this setting.[51]

(3) OTHER AGENTS. As noted above, the side effects of a large thiopental dose administered to provide protection from *incomplete* ischemia during CPB are not insignificant. An alternative drug or drug combination with lesser cardiac effects or a shorter duration of action, if as effective as thiopental, would be desirable. Isoflurane has been suggested as a cerebral protective agent in circumstances of incomplete ischemia or hypoxemia.[73] The rapid recovery possible with isoflurane would be advantageous because it would avoid the prolonged postoperative sedation noted with large doses of thiopental. Like the barbiturates, isoflurane produces a dose-related decrease in $CMRO_2$ because of suppression of cortical electrical activity. An isoelectric EEG can be produced at isoflurane concentrations of approximately 2 MAC.[73] Isoflurane prolongs hypoxic survival in mice,[73] minimizes changes in cerebral high-energy phosphates and lactate during profound hemorrhagic hypotension in dogs,[73] and reduces the "critical" regional cerebral blood flow (that is, that flow below which EEG signs of ischemia appear) during carotid occlusion for carotid

endarterectomy in humans.[74] Thus some evidence indicates that isoflurane may be effective in protecting the brain during periods of low perfusion pressure. However, it is not certain that isoflurane provides cerebral protection in situations of focal ischemia, comparable to that provided by barbiturates.[75] Certain properties of barbiturates are probably not shared by isoflurane, such as reduction in intracranial blood volume and pressure and prevention of seizures. In contrast to barbiturates, isoflurane has cerebral vasodilating properties that may redistribute cerebral blood flow away from ischemic regions. Furthermore, it is possible that the protective effect of a large dose of thiopental is attributable, in part, to ongoing cerebral effects of the drug after termination of CPB. This would not be true with isoflurane, if administration were discontinued upon full emergence from CPB.

Several other agents, including calcium-entry blocking drugs, free-radical scavengers, and excitotoxin antagonists, are currently clinically available or will be available in the near future. For example, nimodipine, a calcium-entry blocking drug, has been shown to improve outcome if administered before[76] or shortly after[77] complete cerebral ischemia in animals. In humans, nimodipine has been administered shortly after subarachnoid hemorrhage[78] and acute stroke,[79] with improved outcome compared to control groups receiving standard therapy for these clinical situations. However, in humans, nimodipine did not improve outcome after resuscitation from cardiac arrest.[80] Recently, another group of drugs, the excitatory amino acid antagonists, have received considerable attention. There is some evidence to indicate that dizocilpine maleate (MK-801), a glutamate antagonist active at the N-methyl-D-aspartate (NMDA) receptor site, may attenuate neuronal damage.[81,82] However, in a canine model, this drug failed to improve neurologic outcome.[83] Once such potentially valuable cerebral protection agents have received further study, the neurologic dysfunction that occurs after CPB might provide an appropriate model for testing their clinical efficacy.[3,84]

(4) INTRAOPERATIVE GLUCOSE. Another issue is whether the use of glucose in the maintenance fluids or in the CPB prime may aggravate the effects of cerebral ischemia. An important determinant of outcome after cerebral ischemia appears to be the blood (and brain) glucose concentrations at the time of the injury.[85,86] The presumed explanation for the glucose effect is that increased glucose permits increased lactic acid production secondary to anaerobic metab-

olism, and this, in turn, is reflected by a lower pH and increased neuronal damage. It has been postulated that prevention of hyperglycemia in patients at risk for central nervous system injury, including patients undergoing CPB, can reduce morbidity.[87-89]

In adult patients undergoing CABG, Metz and Keats performed a randomized prospective study comparing patients receiving lactated Ringer's ($n = 53$) to those receiving 5% dextrose in lactated Ringer's ($n = 54$) for volume maintenance and priming of the CPB circuit.[90] Patients in the group who received glucose produced more urine and required less crystalloid volume during and after CPB. Five days after operation, patients who received glucose weighed 2 kg less than their cohorts who received no glucose. No patients who received glucose exhibited postoperative neuropsychiatric dysfunction, whereas two patients in the group receiving glucose-free solutions had overt postoperative neurologic or psychiatric deficits, a difference that was not significant. These authors recommended adding glucose to the priming solution in patients undergoing CABG, since there is a demonstrated benefit (reduction in perioperative fluid requirements) and no documented neurologic risk.[90]

It has been emphasized that even in the setting of acute stroke, no definite recommendations can be made about the use of glucose or glucose-lowering therapies at this time.[91] Some models of permanent focal ischemia fail to demonstrate an adverse effect of hyperglycemia (and a few models actually demonstrate improvement in outcome with hyperglycemia).[91] Many centers do avoid administration of glucose-containing solutions during CPB. However, as yet, there are no prospective outcome studies demonstrating a detrimental effect of glucose in this setting. Therefore this issue remains quite controversial.

2. Massive air embolism and other problems.
As always, any surgery requiring extracorporeal circulation bears some risk of iatrogenic massive air embolism resulting from technical mishap.[37,92] A survey of 350 cardiac surgeons that canvassed 375,000 operations during a 6-year period revealed that a pump oxygenator accident serious enough to cause patient injury or death occurred once per 1000 procedures.[92] The most common cause of massive air embolism was a ruptured arterial tubing or connector.[92] In other reviews, massive embolism usually resulted from a lapse in attention to oxygenator blood level, leading to reservoir depletion and pumping of air instead of blood via the aortic cannula.[37,93,94] Other reported causes

include reversed ventricular vent suction tubing[37,92] and oxygenators that have clotted, pressurized, burst, leaked, or accidentally fallen.[92] Also, runaway pump heads,[95] reversed direction of the arterial pump,[96] and rupture of an air-driven pulsatile assist device[97] have produced massive air embolism.

Although there are ongoing improvements in perfusion technology, the mainstay of prevention of massive air embolism lies in meticulous attention to detail.[37] Nearly continuous observation of the blood level in the oxygenator is mandatory throughout the bypass procedure. Blood level alarm sensors should be used. Sudden pharmacologic vasodilatation during CPB may result in a drastic change in the oxygenator blood level, which, unless the perfusionist is advised, may lead to a low level in the reservoir. Because detachment of the oxygenator may lead to instantaneous pumping of air, surgical team "traffic" around perfusion tubing should be minimized. To avoid accidental reversal of the vent tubing and consequent pumping of air, one should test vents and cardiotomy suckers in a sterile solution at the operating table to ensure suction and not pressure. In addition, the integrity of the perfusion tubing and the direction of flow should be checked by the perfusionist before CPB is initiated. One can control a runaway pump head by unplugging the bypass machine and manually rotating the pump head. If slow rotation of the arterial pump head is continued once CPB is complete, the perfusionist should carefully avoid emptying the oxygenator and perfusing air into the arterial circuit.

Once it occurs, management of massive arterial air embolism must be immediate. The pump is stopped to prevent further air embolization. The patient is placed in steep Trendelenburg's position. Air is rapidly evacuated from aortic perfusion tubing. Many authors recommend reversal of circulation in order to take back as much air as possible from the aorta.[93,94] Others recommend cooling the patient (if the accident occurs during normothermia),[37,93,96-99] administration of barbiturates,[37,93,96,98,99] or use of large doses of steroids.[37,93,94,96,97,99,100] Some unique suggestions appear in anecdotal case reports.[37,93,94,96-102] For example, retrograde perfusion of the superior vena cava with oxygenated blood at a pressure of 40 mm Hg has been recommended to flush air bubbles out of the cerebral circulation.[37,96,99,100,102] During retrograde perfusion, the aortic cannula is divided and opened to the atmosphere as a vent. Also, transfer to a hyperbaric chamber has been suggested.[97,101] Positive results in each of these anecdotal reports are difficult to evaluate because of the small number of cases involved, the uncertain quantity of embolized air in each case, and a reasonable probability of good outcome, since air rather than particulate matter was embolized.

3. Role of concomitant cerebrovascular disease. Patients with carotid atherosclerosis who must undergo a procedure requiring CPB present another difficult management problem. Preexisting cerebrovascular disease is a known risk factor associated with a higher incidence of overt neurologic injury[12,36,103] but is not predictive of the incidence of subtle neuropsychologic deficit.[104] It is believed that carotid disease may simply be a marker for severe generalized atherosclerotic disease, suggestive of a higher probability of macroembolization of atherosclerotic debris from the aorta or perhaps from the carotid artery itself.[34,105] There is general agreement that there is no benefit to subjecting patients with an asymptomatic carotid bruit to prophylactic carotid endarterectomy, either before or at the time of their cardiac operation.[103,105-111] In patients with ocular or hemispheric symptoms of carotid artery disease, the decision to opt for prophylactic or concurrent carotid endarterectomy must be individualized to the patient. Factors such as the severity or instability of the patient's cardiac disease should be considered.[105-107]

A common recommendation is that perfusion pressure should be maintained above 50 mm Hg during CPB in patients with significant occlusive carotid disease.[110] This is accomplished by an increase in the pump flow or by administration of alpha-adrenergic receptor agonists. In a recent study, von Reutern and colleagues used transcranial Doppler ultrasound of the middle cerebral artery during CPB to demonstrate that blood-flow velocity was not reduced in 16 patients with severe unilateral carotid stenosis or occlusion when mean arterial pressure was maintained greater than 60 mm Hg.[111] However, there are no controlled prospective studies to support the practice of maintaining high perfusion pressures in such patients. In fact, measurement of CBF using xenon-133 clearance methodology in a single patient with significant (greater than 80%) bilateral carotid stenoses demonstrated similar values at a mean arterial pressure of 35 mm Hg compared to 85 mm Hg.[112] Furthermore, Brusino and colleagues examined CBF during hypothermic CPB in a group of patients over 65 years of age.[113] Cerebral blood flow in these elderly patients was not different from that of patients aged less than 50 years, whereas autoregulation was intact in both age groups.[113] These reports suggest that cerebral autoregulation remains intact over a wide range of pressure, despite old age and severe cerebrovascular disease. However, this theory has not been conclusively proved by outcome studies in patients with known cerebrovascular disease.

B. Subtle neuropsychologic dysfunction

1. Incidence and etiology of neuropsychologic dysfunction. Subtle neurobehavioral impairment is much more common than overt postoperative neurologic complications after CPB.[18,114-119] It is widely recognized that some cardiac surgical patients who lack any positive findings on careful postoperative neurologic examination may still have subtle changes in mentation or behavior, noted by themselves or by family members. Such neuropsychologic impairment is more noticeable in patients undergoing surgery requiring CPB than that in patients having noncardiac surgery.[38,116-119]

Psychometric testing is required to detect and measure subtle neuropsychologic dysfunction. A group of selected tests is administered in the preoperative period and at least once in the postoperative period. Ideally, such tests would include assessment of general level of ability (intelligence), memory, complex problem-solving, receptive understanding and expressive language, efficiency of information processing, motor and visual motor functions, and psychosocial adjustment.[46] In practice, the tests are often limited by the need to keep the testing period short (approximately 20 to 60 minutes) in order to obtain optimal patient cooperation.

Controversy exists concerning the degree and duration of subtle brain dysfunction. For example, Goy et al. found that 55% of patients demonstrated deterioration in problem solving and memory in the immediate postoperative period, with 25% continuing to show deficits 6 months later.[120] In contrast, Ellis et al. found transient memory impairment 4 weeks postoperatively in 83% of patients undergoing CABG, with little deficit remaining after 1 year.[121] Other investigators have found impairment in the immediate postoperative period, with no impairment at re-evaluation after 2 or 6 months.[122,123] Most recently, using an extensive battery of tests, Townes et al. found that cardiac surgical patients showed generalized impairment on all tests at the time of discharge from the hospital compared to a nonsurgical control group.[119] At follow-up testing 7 months later, there was no evidence of residual impairment in 87% of these patients. However, the performance of the remaining patients (13%) declined between preoperative and final follow-up testing. Interestingly, neuropsychologic outcome was not related to the type of operation (intracardiac versus CABG). The only predictor of negative outcome was advanced age.

Another method of measuring subtle brain damage is examination of cerebrospinal fluid (CSF) for biochemical markers of injury. This method has not been used extensively, since it requires lumbar puncture in the postoperative period and, ideally, in the preoperative period as well. Aberg et al. measured changes in CSF adenylate kinase (AK) in 38 patients undergoing CPB compared to 8 patients undergoing thoracic surgery without CPB.[124] Twenty-four hours after surgery there were no changes in AK in the patients having thoracic surgery, whereas significant increases occurred in all patients undergoing CPB. In a subsequently published study, these same authors found that the postoperative AK in cerebrospinal fluid was significantly correlated with a decrement in neuropsychologic examination scores but not with abnormalities in the CT scan.[23] Other investigators have noted a lack of correlation between abnormal biochemical markers of cerebral injury and *overt* postoperative neurologic deficits.[9,125]

Several theories have been advanced to account for development of subtle cerebral dysfunction after CPB. These include diffuse particulate microemboli such as platelet aggregates, fibrin, and foreign particles taken up by the cardiotomy suction,[24,126,127] diffuse gaseous microemboli from bubble oxygenators,[24,127-130] inadequate cerebral perfusion caused by low pressure or low flow during CPB,[117,131,132] hyperperfusion or hypoperfusion related to $Paco_2$ management,[133,134] nonpulsatile perfusion during CPB,[114] and prolonged CPB.[18,24,117] Also, advanced patient age has been consistently associated with development of postoperative cognitive impairment.[1-3,8,9,18,23,25,119] Although the precise cause of neuropsychologic dysfunction is unknown, the following sections discuss various methods proposed to prevent it.

2. Prevention of neuropsychologic dysfunction

a. Microembolism. Apart from macroembolic phenomena, numerous sources of microemboli have been identified, including gaseous microemboli from bubble oxygenators,[129,135-137] release of particulate matter from extracorporeal tubing,[138] as well as platelet aggregates, fat, and fibrin taken up by the cardiotomy suction.[136,139] The use of microfilters in the arterial line and cardiotomy return[130] and the use of membrane instead of bubble oxygen-

ators[128,129,137] might reduce air and particulate microemboli from such sources. However, these measures would have little impact on direct embolization from the surgical field. In fact, several investigations have failed to demonstrate that inclusion of a microfilter in the CPB circuit produces improvement in either measured microembolism or, more importantly, in outcome.[126,140,141]

In a study in which 21 patients were randomized for presence or absence of an arterial line filter, Blauth et al. used fluorescein angiography to quantitate cerebral microembolism in the retinal microvasculature just before termination of CPB.[126] The total microembolic count was not reduced by arterial line filtration with a Pall 40 μm filter. Henriksen et al. measured CBF during CPB and noted that cerebral autoregulation was not affected by inclusion of an arterial filter in the CPB circuit.[140] Aris et al. studied 100 patients randomly assigned to one of two groups: 50 patients underwent CPB with a 20 μm filter in the arterial line and 50 patients had no filter.[141] Preoperative and postoperative neurologic and neuropsychologic examinations were performed in all patients. Postoperatively there were no differences between the filtered and the unfiltered groups in incidence or severity of neurologic or neuropsychologic dysfunction.

In an investigation designed to assess the superiority of membrane oxygenators, Blauth et al. demonstrated retinal microvascular occlusion in 100% of patients undergoing CPB with a bubble oxygenator, an incidence that declined after conversion to membrane oxygenators.[128] However, there is, as yet, no evidence that the use of membrane (instead of bubble) oxygenators during CPB decreases the incidence of either overt or subtle postoperative cerebral dysfunction.

b. Perfusion techniques during cardiopulmonary bypass (CPB)

(1) PERFUSION PRESSURE AND HEMODILUTION. Early studies indicated an increased incidence of cerebral complications in patients with "low" arterial pressures during CPB.[19,131,132,142,143] Some investigators concluded that mean arterial pressure should be maintained at greater than 50 mm Hg to avoid postoperative neuropsychiatric dysfunction, presumably because of inadequate CBF.[131,143] However, in these investigations, hypotension occurring during periods other than CPB was not similarly considered. More importantly, these investigators did not report the degree of hemodilution employed and assumed that low perfusion pressure reflected low perfusion flow. The use of hemodi-

lution with crystalloid priming solution provides a perfusate of much lower viscosity, which causes perfusion pressure to be lower at the same perfusion flow, without change in arteriolar resistance. With perfusion techniques unchanged and the advent of hemodilution, hypotension during CPB rarely reflects low flow, only acutely reduced perfusate viscosity.[144,145] This may explain the absence of an association between CPB pressure and clinically apparent postoperative neurologic or neuropsychologic dysfunction, as demonstrated in all recent studies in which hemodilution was used during CPB.[2,3,9,26,121,145-147]

(2) CO_2 MANAGEMENT. Several studies have demonstrated that cerebral blood flow (CBF) is not affected by perfusion pressures ranging between 30 and 100 mm Hg during CPB, in the absence of exogenous CO_2.[133,146,148-150] Thus autoregulation is preserved. However, it is important to understand that there is a significant correlation between regional CBF and Pa_{CO_2}.[146,150,151,152] Cerebral blood flow does become pressure passive when CO_2 is administered (via the oxygenator) during CPB.[133,149] Most centers now use the alpha-stat method of managing arterial blood gases, maintaining a pH of 7.4 and a Pa_{CO_2} of 40 mm Hg measured at 37° C (temperature-uncorrected values). With this method, CO_2 is not added to the gases supplying the oxygenator, and coupling between cerebral metabolic rate and CBF remains intact. However, some centers utilize the pH-stat method of managing arterial blood gases, maintaining a pH of 7.4 and a Pa_{CO_2} of 40 at the patient's actual body temperature (temperature-corrected values). With this method, exogenous CO_2 must be added to the gases supplying the oxygenator because, as body temperature is reduced, CO_2 becomes more soluble in blood and CO_2 production decreases. Administration of CO_2 produces passive cerebral vasodilatation, uncoupling the flow-to-metabolism relationship and resulting in luxury perfusion.[133] Interestingly, although increasing Pa_{CO_2} during CPB increases cerebral blood flow, cerebral oxygen consumption is decreased.[152]

The influence of CO_2 management upon neuropsychologic outcome has been addressed. Theoretically the enzymes of brain metabolism should function better with alpha-stat management because autoregulation is preserved with this method. In fact, even with alpha-stat management, there is luxury perfusion of the brain (that is, during hypothermia, the reduction of oxygen delivery attributable to hypothermia is less than the reduction of the brain's metabolic

needs).[133,153] Nevertheless, many anesthesiologists practice pH-stat management of Pa_{CO_2}. They argue that hypocapnia might reduce cerebral oxygen delivery because of leftward shift in the oxyhemglobin dissociation curve, with consequent reduction in CBF. However, with pH-stat management, autoregulation is lost, allowing a further excess of CBF over the metabolic requirements.[133,153] It has been suggested that such unregulated CBF could cause a "steal" phenomenon and increase delivery of microemboli to the brain.[133,149,150] To address these issues, Bashein and colleagues randomly assigned 86 patients to alpha-stat or pH-stat management of blood gases during hypothermic CPB.[154] Neuropsychologic function was assessed with a series of tests administered preoperatively, just before hospital discharge, and again 7 months later. At both postoperative testing times, there was no significant difference observed in neuropsychologic performance between the Pa_{CO_2} groups.[154] These data strongly support the hypothesis that CO_2 management during CPB has no important effect upon neuropsychologic outcome. Furthermore, Gravlee and colleagues have shown that higher levels of arterial carbon dioxide tensions, such as those resulting from the pH-stat management technique, are apparently not associated with potentially harmful redistribution of cerebral blood flow (intracerebral steal).[155] Prough and colleagues suggest that the final resolution of this question awaits correlation of neuropsychologic end points with measured circulatory and metabolic changes in individual patients during CPB.[156]

(3) PERFUSION FLOW. The influence of perfusion flow on postoperative neurologic function has been addressed in several studies. Kolkka and Hilberman studied flows of 30 to 50 ml/kg (accompanying mean arterial pressures of 30 to 60 mm Hg).[26] Flow and pressure characteristics of CPB were identical in 35 patients suffering some detectable neurologic or neuropsychologic deficit, as compared to 169 patients without any deficit. Ellis et al. similarly assessed cerebral function in 30 patients undergoing CPB with "reduced flow rate" (less than 40 ml/kg) during cardioplegic arrest and found no correlation between mean flow rate and postoperative dysfunction.[121] More recently, Slogoff et al. did not find "low flow," expressed either in absolute values or in intensity-duration units, to be a predictor of adverse cerebral or renal outcome.[145] Finally, Rebeyka et al. examined the effect of sequential reduction in flow rates on cerebral cortical metabolism and function during hypothermic CPB in dogs.[157] Somato-

sensory neural transmission remained intact until flow was reduced to 0.25 L/min/m^2, at which time loss of the signal occurred. These investigators then subjected 5 patients to brief periods of low-flow CPB (Q = 1.0 L/min/m^2) at 21° to 25° C. Somatosensory evoked potentials remained intact during flow reduction, and postoperative neurologic evaluations were normal in all patients. These authors concluded that the flow rate threshold for incurring functional cerebral injury during hypothermic CPB is less than 1.0 L/min/m^2.[157] It is notable that each of the above studies was performed in patients without known cerebrovascular disease.

(4) PULSATILE FLOW. The issue of whether pulsatile flow has advantages in preserving cerebral function remains controversial.[158-160] Methods of producing pulsatile flow include partial CPB (in which some amount of blood remains in the patient's heart to be ejected), use of an in situ intra-aortic balloon pump to generate pulsations, and pulsations produced by roller pumps specially designed to rotate at varying speeds. There are numerous experimental studies supporting and disputing advantages of pulsatile perfusion for the brain, as well as for other vital organs.[158-164] However, many reports comparing pulsatile and nonpulsatile flow have not employed "pulsation" comparable to that generated by the native heart.[160,164] Clinical studies that demonstrate significant neurologic or subtle neuropsychologic differences between pulsatile versus nonpulsatile flow are lacking.[159]

(5) DURATION OF CPB. Finally, the duration of CPB may be important in determining neuro-

logic or neuropsychologic outcome after cardiac surgery.[3,12,18,24,26,117,165] Intuitively one could expect that the physiologic alterations that occur during CPB would be more likely to result in irreversible damage if the duration of CPB is prolonged. In one study of patients undergoing CABG, the risk of perioperative stroke increased threefold if the duration of CPB exceeded 120 minutes.[12] However, some recent studies have not confirmed this association, either with respect to overt neurologic[145] or neuropsychologic[119,122] outcome.

C. Profound hypothermia and circulatory arrest (PHCA)

1. Incidence and types of neurologic complications after PHCA. Another area of concern is the potentially damaging effects of elective total circulatory arrest during profound hypothermia. The hypothesis underlying the use of total circulatory arrest (global cerebral ischemia) for cardiac surgery is that there is a "safe" duration of this state. Safety is defined by absence of detectable functional or structural organ derangements in the early or late postoperative period. It is generally agreed that the brain has the shortest safe circulatory arrest time of any organ of the body.[166] Data from patients are somewhat conflicting, but there is considerable agreement that arrest times longer than 60 minutes at 16° to 20° C are not safe; after 60 minutes the incidence of postoperative neurologic problems increases significantly (Fig. 12-6).[166-168] Some data indicate the probability that arrest periods longer than 30 minutes may not be safe.[169-171] The length of the

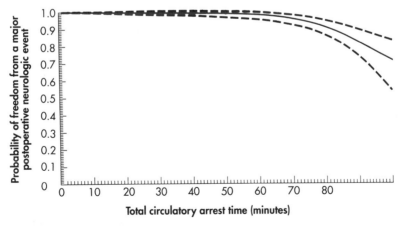

Fig. 12-6. Relationship between the probability of the occurrence of a major postoperative neurologic event and the total circulatory arrest time in 219 patients (8 events) undergoing open intracardiac operations. (From Kirklin JW and Barratt-Boyes BG: Hypothermia, circulatory arrest, and cardiopulmonary bypass. In Kirklin JW and Barratt-Boyes BG, editors: Cardiac surgery, New York, 1986, John Wiley & Sons, p 39.)

safe period for the brain is inversely related to the temperature during the arrest period though temperatures less than 10° C are not used because of potential damage to other organs.[167,172] Nasopharyngeal or tympanic membrane temperatures are measured to approximate cerebral cortex temperature. However, the brain tends to cool unevenly, leaving some areas more susceptible to ischemic damage than others.[173] In fact, even when circulatory arrest is not employed, there may be some microscopic cerebral damage from deep hypothermia.[171,174]

The technique of profound hypothermia and total circulatory arrest (PHCA) is used fairly often in infants undergoing repair of congenital heart lesions. In such patients, postoperative neurologic complications include transient seizures, choreoathetosis, and impaired intellectual development.[166] Transient seizures occur in a significant number of patients (4% to 10%) after PHCA.[175,176] However, the seizures are not necessarily a sign of permanent brain damage; usually they are followed by uneventful convalescence.[175,176] Choreoathetosis occurs early in the postoperative period in 1% to 12% of children undergoing PHCA.[177-179] With time, the movements usually lessen in severity but, if originally severe, may persist to some extent. Choreoathetosis occurs only when the duration of total circulatory arrest exceeds a range of 30 to 45 minutes and is especially likely to occur if duration exceeds 60 minutes.[166,179] Also, profound hypothermia by itself may cause choreoathetosis.[180]

The issue of intellectual impairment in children undergoing PHCA is not yet settled. Studies addressing this issue are difficult because of the very young age of most patients at the time of surgery (and consequent absence of preoperative base-line data), the possible effects of severe congenital heart disease before operation, and frequent concomitant problems such as other congenital abnormalities, prematurity, and low birth weight. Some studies show an eventual decrease in intelligence quotient (IQ) in patients with congenital heart disease who had undergone PHCA compared to control patients who did not have congenital heart disease[178] or compared to control patients who had undergone repair of congenital heart disease without PHCA.[181] Also, data obtained by Wells and colleagues cast doubt upon the idea that 60 minutes of total circulatory arrest at 18° C is safe.[182] They found that late postoperative IQs of patients with arrest times of ≥50 minutes were significantly lower than those of patients with arrest times of less than 50 minutes.

However, other studies show normal IQ distributions after circulatory arrest periods of up to 70 minutes.[183-185]

Profound hypothermia (16° to 24° C) with total circulatory arrest is occasionally used in adults for operations such as aortic arch repair or replacement of aortic aneurysms, ectasia, or dissections.[186-189] Also, adult patients with complex neurosurgical lesions, such as giant aneurysms of the cerebral circulation, are occasionally treated with the aid of this technique.[190,191] In adults, it is difficult to sort out neurologic damage that occurs because of PHCA versus damage that is secondary to preexisting cerebrovascular disease[189] or preexisting central nervous system pathosis.[191] However, it appears that this technique is used with relative safety in adults with rare but severe neurologic damage.[186-188]

2. Prevention of neurologic complications

a. Hypothermia itself. The benefit of hypothermia in reducing central nervous system (CNS) deficits has been demonstrated in animal studies examining global CNS injuries and in some human studies of complete ischemia (such as elective circulatory arrest).[172,186,188,189,192] The protective effect presumably is the result of a decrease in neuronal metabolic activity.[51,193] The consequent reduction in cerebral metabolic rate for oxygen consumption ($CMRO_2$) may permit neurons to tolerate longer periods of nonperfusion before permanent infarction occurs. However, the preservative effects of hypothermia in the central nervous system are greater than would be anticipated from the decreased $CMRO_2$ alone. Apparently, the "no-reflow" phenomenon is prevented.[194] At profoundly hypothermic temperatures (16° to 20° C), the CNS can endure somewhere between 30 and 60 minutes of arrest time with minimal damage, as discussed above. It is important that one minimize inhomogeneity of cooling by using surface cooling, assuring appropriate perfusion flow and temperature gradients (between perfusate and patient), and allowing adequate time for cooling.

The intraoperative EEG can be used to monitor the functional state of the human brain during and after profound hypothermia and total circulatory arrest. During core cooling in humans to 18.5° C, continuous phasic activity in the EEG persists throughout.[195-198] There is a gradual disappearance of fast components and an increase in slow components. Occasionally, repetitive fast discharges occur. It has been suggested that the EEG is the best monitor to determine the ideal brain temperature before circulatory arrest is established.[199,200] Experimental evidence shows a correlation between brain temperature and development of cerebral iso-electricity. In fact, there can be a wide variation in temperature among body sites when cerebral electrical silence occurs (nasopharyngeal, 10.1° to 24.1° C; esophageal, 7.2° to 23.1° C; rectal, 12.8° to 28.6° C).[199,200] However, the EEG provides an objective method of determining when electrical silence occurs; this event may indicate the temperature "safest" for institution of circulatory arrest. If the EEG is not yet flat when circulatory arrest is established, EEG activity disappears within an average time of 109 seconds.[195] The time required for disappearance of EEG activity is inversely related to temperature at the time of arrest (Fig. 12-7).[195]

b. Circulatory arrest versus low perfusion flow. The problem of whether continuous perfusion of the brain (at low or very low perfusion flows) is preferable to a period of elective circulatory arrest is under study. Many centers adopt the strategy of breaking a prolonged period of arrest into two or more shorter periods, separated by an intervening period of normal bypass perfusion, especially for circulatory arrest times that may exceed 60 minutes.[167] After an initial period of arrest that is kept under 60 minutes, CPB is resumed for a period of time, perhaps 15 minutes, though deep hypothermia is maintained. Presumably, reperfusion and reoxygenation of tissues occurs, with washout of acidotic metabolic products. The surgical repair is completed during a subsequent period of circulatory arrest. Using this approach, operations requiring total arrest times of greater than 100 minutes have resulted in successful outcome.[201] Another approach uses low-flow bypass with deep hypothermia, with periods of total circulatory arrest being avoided. These low flows may protect brain viability while providing the surgeon with acceptable if not optimal operating conditions.[161,167] Whether such continuous CPB provides better cerebral protection than circulatory arrest during repair of congenital heart lesions remains controversial.[161,202]

In infants, cerebral blood flow has been studied during hypothermic CPB with and without circulatory arrest.[203] As in adults, CBF is primarily influenced by temperature. Pressure-flow autoregulation is preserved during moderate hypothermic CPB (25° to 32° C).[203] However, under conditions of deep hypothermia (18° to 22° C), pressure-flow autoregulation is lost, and there *is* an association between CBF and mean arterial pressure. In infants undergoing hypothermic CPB without elective circulatory arrest, CBF returns to base-line value during rewarming. However, after a period of circulatory arrest, CBF remains decreased throughout rewarming and even after weaning from CPB.[203] The clinical effect of this apparently impaired cerebral reperfusion is unknown.

c. Glucose. Another issue is whether glucose infusion should be avoided in patients undergo-

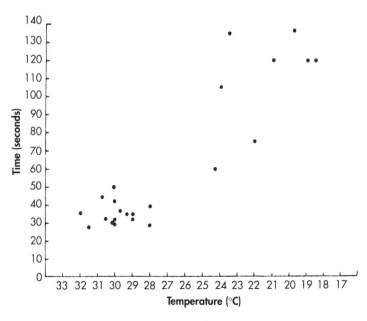

Fig. 12-7. Length of time (in seconds) between the beginning of total circulatory arrest and the appearance of electroencephalographic quiescence, related to nasopharyngeal temperature at the time of circulatory arrest. (Redrawn from Harden A, Pampiglione G, and Waterston DJ: Br Med J 2:1105-1108, 1966.)

ing PHCA. Steward and colleagues retrospectively studied prearrest blood glucose concentration in pediatric patients who underwent elective circulatory arrest under profound hypothermic conditions.[204] Those with high glucose concentration were more likely to have "detectable evidence of neurologic deterioration" (varying in severity from mild seizures to cortical blindness) than those with lower glucose concentration. These authors recommended avoiding unnecessary glucose infusions during pediatric cardiac surgery. On the other hand, Zucker et al. performed a randomized prospective study comparing blood glucose concentrations in two groups of children undergoing elective hypothermic circulatory arrest.[205] One group received glucose-containing solution (*n* = 37); the other group received only non–glucose containing solution (*n* = 60) during the prebypass period. These authors found that avoidance of glucose administration results in *hypo*glycemia in some patients and was ineffective in eliminating the *hyper*glycemia that usually occurs during CPB and hpothermic circulatory arrest.[205] Zucker et al. recommended continuing glucose infusions throughout the prebypass period and obtaining serial intraoperative blood glucose levels.[205] In children, as in adults, this issue remains controversial.

D. Peripheral nerve injury

After cardiac surgery, the incidence of postoperative brachial plexus injury is 5% to 30%.[118,206-208] Typical deficits include paresthesias in the C8-T1 distribution, decreased two-point discrimination, and muscle weakness. Such injuries can remain symptomatic for several months postoperatively.[207,208] The most common hypothesis as to the cause of this problem is that the sternum is excessively retracted, possibly causing displacement of the first rib into the brachial plexus.[118,209] Other explanations include traumatic attempts at cannulation of the internal jugular vein and nerve compression at the elbow.[118,207,210] Avoidance of wide retraction of the sternum or high placement of sternal retractors may best prevent such complications.

Peripheral nerve injuries also occur in the lower extremities during cardiac surgery.[117,206] The most common problem is abnormal sensation in the distribution of the saphenous nerve related to removal of the long saphenous vein during surgery.[117] Peroneal nerve injuries are related to incorrect positioning. External rotation of the thighs and legs, known to stretch the common peroneal nerve, is an unavoidable necessity of positioning for CABG surgery to provide access to the saphenous vein. Thigh pads are used by many cardiac teams to avoid any compression of the peroneal nerve against the fibular head.

Finally the phrenic nerve is occasionally injured during cardiac surgery. Markand and colleagues noted that 11% of their patients demonstrated postoperative diaphragmatic dysfunction.[211] Possible causes include cryogenic injury from iced saline used to bathe the pericardium or stretch injury from tension on the pericardium.

II. CARDIOVASCULAR COMPLICATIONS

Low cardiac output is the most common cardiac complication after CPB.[212] In a review of over 14,000 cardiac surgical patients, 10.6% required some type of pharmacologic support to successfully terminate CPB.[213] An estimated 2000 patients die each year in the United States after unsuccessful attempts to wean them from CPB.[214] Important causes of low cardiac output after CPB include acute myocardial ischemia, acute myocardial depression, and unrecognized cardiac valve dysfunction. In addition, a variety of confounding situations can occur, leading to hypotension and cardiovascular instability.

A. Problems with cannulation and systemic perfusion during CPB

1. Improper cannulation

a. Aortic and arterial dissection. The aortic cannulation site may occasionally become the origin of an aortic dissection. A dissection can be created during the process of cannulation or during perfusion, if the cannula orifice is situated in the arterial wall or in a false lumen.[215] Prevention of this disaster is primarily a surgical responsibility. However, placement of the aortic cannula within the true lumen of the aorta should be documented before one begins extracorporeal circulation. A properly located cannula will bleed back with brisk pulsatile flow. The pressure wave form within the cannula, measured by the perfusionist, should be pulsatile and should correlate with the radial or femoral arterial monitoring line. Once CPB begins, unusual hypotension or zero blood pressure might indicate that the cannula is not in the true aortic lumen. Alternatively the perfusionist might detect inappropriately high arterial cannula pressure. Eventually evidence of organ hypoperfusion (oliguria, pupil asymmetry) would become evident. Once diagnosed, CPB should be discontinued while the surgeon repositions the arterial cannula. Surgical repair of the aortic dissection itself, as well as repair of the coronary or aortic arch vessels, may be necessary.

b. Inadvertent entry of aortic arch vessels. Overperfusion of the patient's head can result from initial malposition or later migration of the aortic cannula into a brachiocephalic vessel, usually the innominate artery.[216-221] Also, the bevel of the perfusion cannula can be inappropriately angled toward either carotid artery, directing a disproportionate flow to the brain. Use of a short aortic cannula with a flange may help prevent this complication. After cannulation of the aorta, the anesthesiologist should check for bilateral carotid pulses. Upon onset of CPB, unilateral facial paleness may occur when the carotid artery is inadvertently cannulated.[218-220] During CPB, cannulation of a brachiocephalic vessel may be heralded by a sudden increase[221] or decrease in measured blood pressure, depending on whether the cannula enters an artery ipsilateral or contralateral to the arterial pressure-monitoring line. If not promptly detected, cerebral edema or rupture of the innominate or carotid arteries because of high perfusion pressure may result. Cerebral edema manifests by conjunctival edema and, eventually, hemifacial swelling.[217,218] Primary treatment is repositioning of the arterial cannula. Measures to reduce cerebral edema (such as head-up position, mannitol) may be helpful.[215]

c. Improper connection to CPB circuit (reversed cannulation). Although extremely rare, it is possible for the surgical team to mistakenly connect the pump circuit's venous drainage tubing to the aorta and the arterial pump line to the right atrium or venae cavae. Also, it is possible for the perfusionist to set the pump roller head on "reverse."[215] Thus blood would be sucked out of the aorta and infused back into the venae cavae at high pressures. Arterial hypotension and high venous pressures result from this reversed CPB flow. Although some organs may receive retrograde perfusion, high pressures may rupture veins.[215] Also, bubble formation within the aorta may cause air embolization when anterograde perfusion is later established.

This problem is routinely prevented when one carefully traces pump tubing onto the field both before and after hookup to the patient. Once CPB begins, diagnosis of reversed cannulation is made after one observes arterial hypotension, conjunctival and facial edema, high central venous pressures, a flaccid aorta, and tense venae cavae.[215] In infants, a bulging fontanelle may also be seen. Once this complication is diagnosed, CPB is immediately discontinued and the tubing connections are corrected. Before one resumes CPB, steps to re-

move air emboli must be taken (see the first section of this chapter dealing with neurologic complications).

2. Obstruction of venous return. On the venous side, impaired venous drainage can result from multiple causes. Large air bubbles within the venous tubing produce an "air lock," which obstructs flow. Often the surgeon must temporarily lift the heart to accomplish portions of the surgical procedure, with resultant impedance of venous drainage. Also, the venous cannulas may kink or be malpositioned against a vessel wall. If flow from the superior vena cava is obstructed, cerebral venous congestion and cerebral edema may occur. This problem is usually indicated by an increase in central venous pressure or by development of conjunctival edema and facial plethora. (However, a CVP catheter with its orifice within the right atrium may show a low CVP if separate superior and inferior vena cava cannulas were inserted and secured with "caval tapes," preventing vena cava blood from entering the right atrium.) CPB must be stopped, or perfusion flow reduced, while the cause of the venous obstruction is sought. An air lock in the venous return line can be "milked" or "tapped" through the line and into the pump reservoir. A kinked or malpositioned cannula can be repositioned. This complication is dangerous, not only because of the possibility of cerebral edema, but also because the pump reservoir of blood may empty (since its venous return is inadequate), introducing the risk of massive arterial air embolism.

3. Massive air embolism. The introduction of air into the arterial tree through the aortic cannula is a feared complication of CPB that may cause instant death or irreversible organ damage. The causes, prevention, and treatment of this complication are discussed in the first section of this chapter dealing with neurologic complications.

4. Inadequate anticoagulation. In its extreme form, inadequate anticoagulation could result in overt thrombosis ("clotting of the pump"). This is an extremely rare catastrophe that probably occurs only if no heparin is administered or if protamine is injected prematurely. For this reason, heparin is administered into a central line, with aspiration of blood before and after administration, while protamine is kept in a physically separate location from other drugs. One can diagnose inadequate anticoagulation by observing clot in the pump reservoir or tubing or high pressure in the arterial cannula, an indication of a partially clotted arterial line filter. Treatment includes reheparinzation and replacement of the oxygenator and CPB circuit.

A less extreme degree of inadequate anticoagulation may result in invisible low-grade coagulation leading to consumption of platelets and procoagulants. Theoretically, this can result in microemboli or in a hemorrhagic diathesis after the termination of CPB. The activated coagulation time (ACT) or protamine titration, or both, are most commonly used to individualize heparin therapy during cardiac surgery.[222] For the activated coagulation time, the minimum values most often used for maintenance of anticoagulation, 480 seconds[223] and 400 seconds,[224] have been considered safe. However, these "standards" are somewhat arbitrary. Recently, Cardoso et al. studied the concentration of coagulation factors II, V, and VIII, fibrinogen, and platelet count in two groups of pigs submitted to hypothermic CPB for 3 hours with membrane oxygenators.[225] In one group, heparin was administered to keep the ACT in excess of 450 seconds, whereas in the other group ACT was maintained between 250 and 300 seconds. No significant difference in any of these coagulation parameters and no difference in oxygenator performance were observed between the groups.[225] These authors concluded that significant reduction in heparin (and protamine) administration can be accomplished without adversely affecting the safety of CPB. Furthermore, in a clinical study, Metz and Keats were unable to detect visible thrombus or predict increased chest tube drainage in patients having relatively low ACT values (ranging from 234 to 400 seconds).[226] In another patient study, Gravlee et al. studied three methods of heparin management.[227] These investigators measured plasma fibrinopeptide A concentrations (to estimate the degree of subclinical plasma coagulation) and chest tube drainage during the first 24 hours after CPB. They concluded that an ACT greater than 350 seconds results in acceptable fibrinopeptide A levels and post-CPB clotting. In fact, patients who received the highest heparin doses had the greatest postoperative mediastinal blood loss in this study.[227] Clearly the minimum safe level of anticoagulation has not yet been identified.

B. Low cardiac output and hypotension/hypertension after CPB

1. Acute myocardial ischemia. Acute myocardial ischemia and perioperative myocardial infarction are serious complications of cardiac surgery, though a causal relationship to CPB is not always certain. The incidence of perioperative myocardial ischemia ranges from 0.6% to 16%.[228-231] This incidence varies depending on the type of operation (CABG versus valve repair and primary procedure versus reoperation) and the criteria used to define infarction (Q waves, elevations in MB creatine phosphokinase, or both). Ischemia can occur immediately after termination of CPB because of several factors. Myocardial protection during CPB may be suboptimal. Also, after a period of elective cardiac arrest to allow performance of the surgical procedure, the heart has to be reperfused. This can lead to a paradoxical extension of the ischemic damage resulting from "reperfusion injury." Furthermore, surgical revascularization may be inadequate, resulting in imperfect restoration of coronary flow. Finally, internal mammary arterial or saphenous vein grafts may be obstructed by kinking, emboli (of either air or particulate debris), or spasm. Coronary spasm often results in abrupt cardiac failure or life-threatening arrhythmias.

Traditionally, diagnosis of these ischemic events is made by direct observation of the heart in the surgical field and by observation of the depression or elevation of ST segments in multiple leads of the ECG or increases in central venous pressure (CVP) or pulmonary capillary wedge pressure(PCWP), an indication of decreased right or left ventricular compliance. More recently, transesophageal echocardiography has been used to detect regional wall motion abnormalities; this technique may be superior to the ECG in allowing one to diagnose acute myocardial ischemia.[232] A recent review of perioperative cardiac morbidity provides an excellent critique of techniques for myocardial ischemia detection.[233]

Treatment is aimed at the cause of the ischemic insult. Surgical repair must be reevaluated, with consideration given to revision of existing coronary grafts or to further revascularization. Reperfusion injury may be lessened by controlled warm reperfusion of the myocardium before removal of the aortic cross-clamp. Also, various drugs, including free-radical scavengers, osmotic agents, coronary vasodilators, and drugs that inhibit platelet aggregation, have been studied in the treatment of reperfusion injury. Coronary embolism may require surgical repair. In the case of air embolism, consideration should be given to coronary massage and a period of rest (that is, a return to CPB) or administration of a vasopressor to raise the perfusion pressure and force bubbles through to the venous side. Treatment of coronary spasm requires coronary vasodilators or calcium-channel blockers, or both types.[234] As discussed later in this section, the arrhythmias that may accompany acute myocardial ischemia are treated with appropriate pharmacologic or electrical therapy.

2. Acute myocardial depression. Postbypass acute myocardial depression may occur, despite recent improvements in myocardial preservation during CPB. The preoperative functional status of the patient's left ventricle is the most important predictor of myocardial depression after CPB. Patients in NYHA (New York Heart Association) class IV, who have preoperative congestive heart failure, have an increased risk of operative mortality because of low cardiac output.[235] Although preoperative cardiac function is integral to postoperative function, the demands of anesthesia and cardiac surgery play vital contributing roles in the development of low cardiac output states.

Braunwald and colleagues have specified syndromes of ischemic myocardial dysfunction and have coined the terms "hibernating" myocardium[236] and "stunned" myocardium.[237] The former refers to chronic reversible resting ischemic dysfunction, which should theoretically improve after surgical reperfusion. The latter refers to a prolonged state of myocardial dysfunction that persists after medical or surgical reperfusion. This prolonged dysfunction may be attributable to a combination of factors, including the washout of metabolic precursors, alterations in calcium flux, and the toxic effects of oxygen free radicals.[238] Recovery of stunned myocardium may require days to weeks. During this period, the circulation must be supported as necessary by pharmacologic means or mechanical support (intra-aortic balloon pump or ventricular assist device).

Prevention of low cardiac output after CPB is the combined responsibility of the surgeon and the anesthesiologist. To ensure against further damage to already compromised myocardium, the delicate balance between myocardial oxygen supply and myocardial oxygen demand must be maintained throughout the perioperative period. In the prebypass period, it is the responsibility of the anesthesiologist to ensure a smoothe and hemodynamically stable induction. Nitroglycerin may be administered to improve coronary blood flow. Left and right end-diastolic volumes and inotropic state are assessed directly by echocardiographic visualization of the ventricles and indirectly by estimation of ventricular filling (such as CVP, PCWP) combined with thermodilution cardiac outputs provided by a pulmonary arterial catheter. It is important to remember certain limitations of the latter approach, that is, that ventricular compliance determines the relationship between pressures and volumes and that regional

myocardial dysfunction is often not evident in measurements of global myocardial function (cardiac output).

During CPB, it is the responsibility of the surgeon to attend to the basic components of myocardial preservation. With adequate myocardial hypothermia to reduce oxygen demand and cardioplegia to chemically induce ventricular asystole, ischemic time has been extended from a few minutes to several hours. Certainly, hypothermia is widely acknowledged to be the fundamental component of myocardial protection during cardiac operations. Although it prolongs the period of ischemic arrest by reducing oxygen demands, hypothermia is associated with several major disadvantages, including its detrimental effects on enzymatic function, energy generation, and cellular integrity. In a provocative recent study, Lichtenstein et al. developed a novel approach to myocardial protection during 121 cardiac operations in which the chemically arrested heart was maintained at 37° C while being perfused continuously with blood (warm cardioplegia).[239] Compared to a historical cohort of 133 patients treated with *hypothermic* cardioplegia, perioperative myocardial infarction was significantly less prevalent in the warm cardioplegic group, as was the use of the intra-aortic balloon pump and the prevalence of low-output syndrome.[239] Clearly, this new approach (or rather revitalization of a historical approach) to the problem of maintaining excellent myocardial preservation during CPB deserves further research. Also the optimal components of cardioplegic solution remains a controversial topic. Potassium, which is used to maintain ventricular standstill, is the most common additive. Other suggested additives include mannitol (as an osmotic agent to prevent myocardial edema), oxygen-carrying substances, metabolic substrates, steroids, and a variety of other pharmacologic agents to further lower cellular energy requirements.[240-246]

Upon completion of the repair and after adequate rewarming and reperfusion of the coronary beds, attempts to separate from extracorporeal circulation may reveal the first signs of acute myocardial depression. These signs include a low systemic blood pressure, small pulse pressure, depressed upstroke, and poor ventricular function upon direct visualization of the surgical field. Therapeutic decisions are aimed at optimizing cardiac output, emphasizing the following five variables: heart rate, heart rhythm, contractility, ventricular preload (end-diastolic volume), and ventricular afterload (impedance to ejection, vascular resistance) (Fig. 12-8). Optimization of heart rate and rhythm is

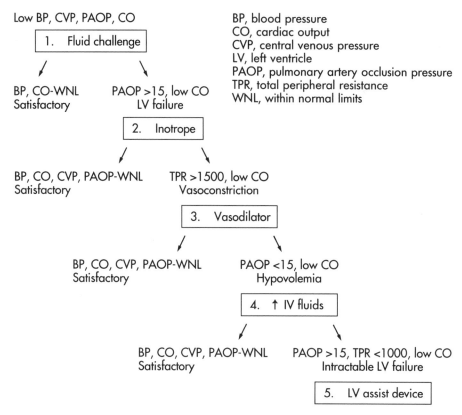

Fig. 12-8. Algorithm for therapy of low perfusion state. (From Hug CC Jr: Hemodynamic resuscitation at the end of cardiopulmonary bypass. In Annual Refresher Course Lectures, Park Ridge, Ill, 1990, American Society of Anesthesiologists.)

discussed later in this section. Adequate preload must be maintained, though it is absolutely critical to avoid ventricular distension. Inotropic support with one or more of a variety of agents (including dopamine, dobutamine, epinephrine, norepinephrine, and amrinone) are selected based on the individual patient's hemodynamic needs. In situations where low output and peripheral vasoconstriction coexist, vasodilators (sodium nitroprusside and nitroglycerin) can improve cardiac output by decreasing afterload.

IABP counterpulsation may be required in cases where pharmacologic manipulation yields only suboptimal cardiac function. Opinions vary regarding the timing of IABP insertion. Many now favor early implementation of balloon counterpulsation in lieu of high-dose drug therapy. In cases where administration of pharmacologic agents and balloon counterpulsation are ineffective in achieving separation from CPB, consideration must be given to mechanical ventricular assist devices.[247] These may assist one or both ventricles and have been used effectively in a substantial number of patients who otherwise could not be weaned from CPB. The majority of patients requiring ventricular assist devices will improve their myocardial function over the ensuing days to weeks. Short-term hospital survival rates of 35% to 45% have been reported.[248] For those whose cardiac function does not return to a level compatible with life, cardiac transplantation may be considered.

3. Unrecognized cardiac valve dysfunction. After coronary surgery, unrecognized mitral regurgitation attributable to mechanical distension of the left ventricle (with overfilling), posterior papillary muscle ischemic dysfunction, or myocardial infarction with rupture of a papillary muscle may make weaning from CPB difficult or impossible. After valve surgery, when the heart appears to be contracting with sufficient vigor but is not ejecting, one should suspect mechanical difficulty with the newly implanted valve. Although rare, surgical malposition or mechanical failure of a prosthetic valve can occur. A prosthetic valve can be sewn in backwards, develop a significant perivalvular leak, or mechanically obstruct flow because of an improperly functioning disc, ball, or valve in the prosthesis. Placement of sutures for either aortic or mitral prostheses incurs the risk of distorting the other valve (or of damaging a portion of the conduction system). Also, too extensive removal of calcium from the mitral anulus may weaken the posterior myocardial wall sufficiently to allow rupture of the atrioventricular (AV) junction, which is usually fatal.[249] The patient may also have dysfunction of one of the remaining valves. For example, after mitral valve replacement, there may be residual tricuspid regurgitation. Valvular function can be assessed utilizing two-dimensional echocardiography with Doppler flow.

4. Protamine reactions and anaphylaxis. In most patients, protamine produces minimal hemodynamic effects if it is administered slowly. However, after rapid administration, precipitous hypotension often occurs.[250] Hypotension is attributable to a decrease in preload and systemic vascular resistance. Histamine is the presumed mediator.[251] There is little evidence to indicate that protamine *directly* depresses contractility of the human heart.[250]

Infrequently an idiosyncratic reaction to protamine occurs. Several different mechanisms are probably responsible.[250] Anaphylactoid responses include true allergic reactions of an immediate hypersensitive nature (anaphylaxis) because of IgE or IgG antibodies. Another type of reation involves an immediate anaphylactoid response without antibody involvement.[250] This probably occurs because the heparin-protamine complex can activate the classic complement pathway, liberating complement fragments that degranulate mast cells or basophils, releasing vasoactive substances into the circulation.[251-255] Finally, a very rare but potentially catastrophic protamine reaction causes intense pulmonary hypertension and bronchoconstriction,[256] probably because of generation of high plasma levels of C5a anaphylatoxins and thromboxane.[251] It has been theorized that patients with prior neutral Hagedorn insulin use, a history of fish allergy, or prior vasectomy are at increased risk for idiosyncratic protamine reactions. However, a recent prospective study failed to confirm these as risk factors.[257] Therapy for idosyncratic protamine reactions is detailed in Table 12-1.

5. Pericardial tamponade. Many surgeons close the pericardium after completion of a cardiac operation to prevent adhesion of the heart to the posterior aspect of the sternum, thus facilitating sternotomy in any subsequent cardiac procedure.[249] In the postbypass or postoperative periods, excessive mediastinal bleeding can

Table 12-1. Therapy for idiosyncratic protamine reactions

Initial therapy
1. Stop administration of protamine.
2. Maintain airway with 100% oxygen.
3. Discontinue all anesthetic agents.
4. Start intravascular volume expansion (2-4 liters of crystalloid with hypotension).
5. Give epinephrine (4-8 µg IV bolus with hypotension, titrate as needed; 0.1-1.0 mg IV with cardiovascular collapse).
6. Reinstitute cardiopulmonary bypass for severe reactions to allow time for drug therapy to take effect.

Secondary treatment
1. Antihistamines (0.5-1 mg/kg diphenhydramine, 300 mg of cimetidine, 20 mg of famotidine, or 50 mg of ranitidine)
2. Catecholamine infusions (starting doses: epinephrine 2-4 µg/min, norepinephrine 2-4 µg/min, *or* isoproterenol 0.5-1.0 µg/min as a drip, titrated to desired effects)
3. Aminophylline (5-6 mg/kg over 20 minutes with persistent bronchospasm) followed by infusion
4. Corticosteroids (0.25-1.00 g of hydrocortisone; alternatively, 1-2 g of methylprednisolone; methylprednisolone may be the drug of choice if the reaction is suspected to be mediated by complement
5. Sodium bicarbonate (0.5-1.0 mEq/kg with persistent hypotension or acidosis)
6. Airway evaluation (before extubation)

Specific treatment for catastrophic pulmonary vasoconstriction
Therapy as above; once diagnosed, treatment of pulmonary hypertension, right-sided heart failure, and bronchoconstriction should include immediate hyperventilation and one or more of the following treatments: nitroglycerin; isoproterenol; aminophylline; prostaglandin E_1; amrinone.

Modified from Levy JH: Anaphylactic reactions in anesthesia and intensive care, Boston, 1986, Butterworth & Co, p 104.

result in pericardial tamponade. Classic diagnostic findings of tamponade include elevation and equalization of the filling pressures (right atrial, pulmonary capillary wedge, left atrial, and ventricular diastolic pressures). Other signs include pulsus paradoxus (a 15 to 20 mm Hg decrease in systolic blood pressure during spontaneous inspiration or exaggerated blood pressure response to positive inspiratory pressure), hypotension, compensatory tachycardia, a widened mediastinal shadow on chest roentgenogram, and decreased voltage on ECG.[258] Previously brisk drainage from the chest tubes that has suddenly slowed or ceased often indicates clotted tubes and pericaridal tamponade.

Adequate surgical hemostasis and adequate drainage via the chest tubes are necessary to prevent this complication. Once it occurs, the primary treatment of acute tamponade is emergent mediastinal reexploration with evacuation of blood and clot from the pericardium and surgical control of residual bleeding. Support of the circulation with volume and intropic or chronotropic drugs may be necessary to allow time to return to the operating room. If transport to the operating suite cannot occur immediately, the inferior aspect of the sternotomy wound can be opened to allow temporary drainage of the pericardium while urgent reexploration is arranged. The clinician should anticipate a sudden and dramatic increase in systemic blood pressure and decrease in filling pressures upon opening of the pericardium.

6. Monitoring artifact. It is important to remember that a radial arterial catheter may not accurately reflect central aortic pressure at the end of CPB.[259-262] For at least 30 minutes after termination of CPB, radial pressure tends to underestimate central aortic pressures.[260] The patient might appear to be severely hypotensive when, in fact, aortic pressure is satisfactory (Fig. 12-9).[261,262] Noninvasive cuff pressure should be checked but may also poorly predict central systemic pressure. Before initiating treatment of clinically significant hypotension, one should obtain confirmation of low pressure by temporarily placing a needle or 18-gauge catheter in the aortic root. Separation from CPB can be accomplished while pressure monitoring via such an aortic root catheter or via a femoral arterial catheter is continuing.

7. Hypertension. Hypertension occurs after CPB in 15% to 60% of patients undergoing coronary artery bypass grafting.[263-265] Patients having chronic hypertension are at increased risk. However, the cause of this complication is probably multifactorial.[264] There is a well-characterized sympathetic nervous system response

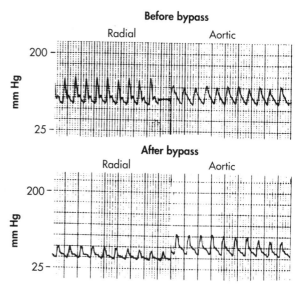

Fig 12-9. Data showing the reversal of usual relationships between simultaneous aortic and radial pressures after cardiopulmonary bypass in one patient. (From Stern DH, Gerson JI, Allen FB, et al: Anesthesiology 62:557-571, 1985.)

to CPB.[266,267] Epinephrine increases ninefold, peaking while patients are being rewarmed from induced hypothermia (Fig. 12-10).[268] Generally, there is a greater rise in epinephrine compared to norepinephrine, an indication that the predominant adrenergic response to the abnormal physiologic state of CPB is a sympathoadrenal (stresslike) response.[268] Frequently, postoperative hypertension is mediated by such a sympathetic mechanism. Patients who develop postoperative hypertension are catecholamine responders both during CPB and during emergence from anesthesia.[269] Although it is not definitely known whether attenuation of the stress response to CPB would decrease the incidence or severity of postoperative hypertension, various anesthetic and other pharmacologic methods to achieve this end have been investigated.[270-273]

Hypertension in the postbypass period can strain recently created anastomoses and areas such as ligatures on saphenous vein graft branches and the aortotomy site.[249] Also, the increased myocardial work necessary to generate such pressures increases myocardial oxygen consumption, risking postbypass ischemia. Obvious causes of hypertension, such as pain, hypoxemia, and hypothermia, should be treated. Persistent postbypass hypertension usually responds to nitroglycerin or nitroprusside.[274] Also, esmolol, labetalol, and clonidine have been useful in this setting.[266,273,275,276]

8. Right ventricular failure. In the last several years, increased attention has been directed toward right ventricular (RV) failure after CPB. Most commonly, this complication has occurred in patients undergoing coronary artery bypass grafting. The cause is usually ischemia. There is evidence that right ventricular myocardium is as sensitive to ischemic and reperfusion injury as left ventricular myocardium is and that metabolic recovery from injury is equally prolonged.[277,278] Inadequate myocardial protection and incomplete right-sided heart revascularization may contribute to postbypass ischemic dysfunction of the RV.[279] This problem may be further exacerbated by pulmonary arterial hypertension, which increases right ventricular afterload. Right ventricular function and metabolism can be experimentally evaluated by methods analogous to methods used in the left ventricle.[278] Clinical findings leading to diagnosis of RV failure include depressed cardiac output, inappropriate elevation of central venous pressure compared to pulmonary capillary wedge pressure (unless biventricular failure exists), and increased pulmonary vascular resistance (PVR) to >200 dynes·sec·cm^{-5} (2.5 Wood units).

The presence of right instead of or in addition to left ventricular failure requires different considerations when one is choosing vasodilators and inotropes. Ischemia, of course, is treated by administration of nitroglycerin. Afterload reduction with nitroprusside can augment cardiac output by decreasing right ventricular afterload, PVR, and left ventricular end-diastolic volume. Preferred inotropes are those that increase contractility of the RV and also decrease PVR (isoproterenol). D'Ambra et al. have described use of prostaglandin E_1 for treatment of refractory heart failure and pulmonary hypertension after mitral valve replacement.[280] Also, nonpharmacologic adjuncts may be helpful, such as increasing preload, or decreasing PVR with a combination of hyperventilation and avoidance of hypoxia and acidemia.

C. Arrhythmias

Cardiac arrhythmias are known to occur in up to 84% of patients undergoing general anesthesia and surgery, regardless of the type of proce-

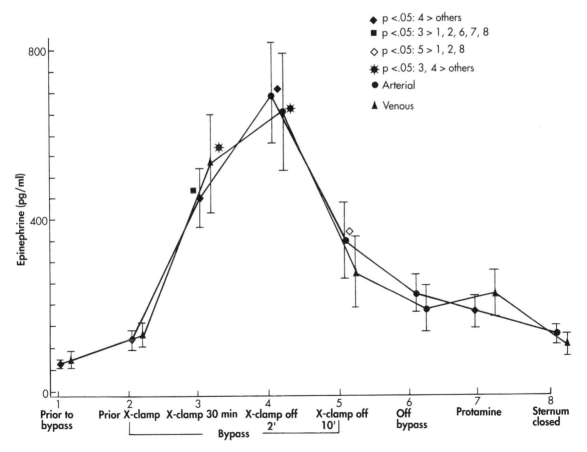

Fig. 12-10. Mean plasma levels of epinephrine during cardiac anesthesia and surgery. Bars indicate SEM. (From Reves JG, Karp RB, Buttner EE, et al: Circulation 66:49-55, 1982.)

dure performed.[281] These arrhythmias should be treated if they are associated with an increase in myocardial oxygen consumption or a decrease in cardiac output, or are likely to deteriorate into potentially lethal dysrhythmias. Patients undergoing cardiac surgery are at an increased risk for specific arrhythmias that may be attributed to extracorporeal circulation and cardioplegia. Supraventricular tachyarrhythmias, atrioventricular conduction defects, and ventricular irritability are the arrhythmias most commonly associated with CPB. The incidence of these arrhythmias may be increasing because of the increasing complexity of the surgical procedures (necessitating a concomitant increase in ischemic time).[282]

1. Supraventricular tachydysrhythmias. The incidence of supraventricular conduction abnormalities after cardiac surgery was noted to increase greatly after the reintroduction of cold potassium cardioplegia in the late 1970s.[283] Theories behind this increase centered initially on the direct effects of the cardioplegic solution on the atria and conduction system.[284] However, Smith et al. demonstrated the role of inadequate atrial hypothermia and subsequent atrial ischemia in the development of supraventricular conduction injury.[285] In addition, decreases in red blood cell deformability and subsequent alterations in the microcirculation supplying the conductive tissue have been believed to contribute to postbypass arrhythmias.[286]

The supraventricular arrhythmias seen most often after CPB include sinus tachycardia, atrial fibrillation, and supraventricular tachycardia (SVT). These dysrhythmias are seen in patients undergoing both CABG and valve procedures, though the incidence of dysrhythmias is greater during and after valve repair.[283,287,288] Michelson et al. found the incidence of atrial dysrhythmias after CABG to be 38%, whereas the incidence after valve repair approached 80%.[283] In more than one study, age has been the most important predictor of atrial fibrillation and flutter after coronary artery bypass grafting.[289,290]

Treatment of postbypass supraventricular conduction disturbances should begin with close attention to myocardial, particularly atrial, protection during CPB. Conversion of atrial fibrillation to sinus rhythm can lead to a substantial increase in cardiac output, especially in the presence of poor ventricular compliance.[291] Poor tolerance of SVT is an indication for immediate electrical countershock. Initial hemodynamic stability allows time for pharmacologic or mechanical therapy of the dysrhythmia. Increasing vagal tone by carotid sinus massage, Valsalva maneuver, sustained lung inflation, or

eyeball pressure can act to break the arrhythmia. Successful termination of SVT may be achieved by administration of phenylephrine to induce a reflex vagal discharge or edrophonium to directly stimulate cardiac muscarinic cholingergic receptors. Overdrive pacing is often effective. Most often, agents such as digoxin, verapamil, and beta-adrenergic receptor blockers, are used to convert supraventricular tachyarrhythmias to sinus rhythm (or to appropriately slow the ventricular response).[290]

2. Bradydysrhythmias and atrioventricular conduction defects. Bradydysrhythmias and AV conduction defects are not infrequent after CPB, often causing serious intraoperative problems by greatly affecting cardiac performance. AV conduction defects can stem either from local trauma to the AV node and the conduction pathway (as can occur in the repair of an atrial septal defect) or from ischemic damage. It is known that atrial and AV nodal conducting systems are very sensitive to ischemia[292] and that these areas are poorly protected by hypothermic cardioplegia.[293,294] Therefore it is logical to conclude that AV nodal dysfunction is primarily ischemic in origin. However, hyperkalemia secondary to potassium-containing cardioplegia may also contribute to conduction system dysfunction.[284] Furthermore, preoperative medications, particularly digoxin, can contribute to AV conduction delay. Although the effects of hemodilution on digoxin levels are small because of its small degree of protein binding, serum concentrations of digoxin increase after CPB because of reequilibration with tissue stores.[294] After CPB, a rebound peak concentration of digoxin associated with an increased risk of AV conduction delay can occur.

Treatment of bradydysrhythmias after bypass most commonly begins with temporary pacemaker placement. Both atrial and ventricular leads are routinely inserted, since synchronized contraction can substantially increase cardiac output. Pharmacologic therapy can include atropine, which acts as a vagolytic agent, and isoproterenol, which acts as a direct beta-adrenergic receptor agonist. Most bradyarrhythmias and conduction delays resolve in the postoperative period, but a few patients require permanent pacemaker insertion.

3. Ventricular irritability. Ventricular ectopic beats are common in patients with coronary artery disease and can be observed throughout the perioperative period. Causes of ventricular irritability include myocardial ischemia, hypoxemia, acidosis, and electrolyte abnormalities ($\uparrow\downarrow K^+$, $\downarrow Mg^{++}$, $\uparrow\downarrow pH$). When increased ectopic activity occurs after CPB, treatable causes should be ruled out. Drugs used to improve myocardial performance, such as iso-proterenol, epinephrine, and dopamine, can prompt increases in ventricular irritability. Ectopic ventricular beats may be an incidental finding, or they may progress to ventricular fibrillation or ventricular tachycardia. Multifocal beats, multiple beats, coupled beats, and R-on-T phenomenon are ominous signs and require treatment. Useful drugs include lidocaine, procainamide, bretylium, beta-adrenergic receptor antagonists, and quinidine.

III. PULMONARY COMPLICATIONS
a. Bronchospasm

Severe bronchospasm occurring after CPB is an unusual but potentially fatal event.[295-298] Usually this problem is detected at the end of the bypass period when initial attempts to inflate the lungs are accompanied by expiratory wheezing, high inflation pressures, and difficulty in deflating the lungs.[297] Upon detection of wheezing, it is essential to rule out mechanical causes.[297] Tracheobronchial obstruction is ruled out by endotracheal tube suctioning and fiberoptic bronchoscopy. Cardiac wheezing would be accompanied by elevated left atrial pressure and pulmonary edema. Pneumothorax would most likely be unilateral and would not cause both lungs to appear overly inflated with crowding of the mediastinum and surgical field. Nonmechanical causes of bronchospasm include severe allergic reactions, usually to antibiotics or protamine. Also, activation of C3a and C5a complement anaphylatoxins, as discussed in the section on immunologic complications, may stimulate the release of mast cell histamine and contraction of bronchial smooth muscle. Finally, beta-adrenergic receptor blocking drugs, which are commonly used to treat tachycardia and arrhythmias during cardiac surgery, occasionally induce bronchospasm.

Separation from CPB is often extremely difficult or impossible until bronchospasm has been adequately treated.[296-298] Epinephrine is the drug of choice when the cause is anaphylaxis. Obviously, administration of betamimetics, methylxanthines, and anticholingergics must be undertaken with care in patients with coronary artery disease. Halothane may be used because of its bronchodilating effects, but its negative inotropic effects must also be considered. It may be necessary to maintain extracorporeal circulation until the bronchoconstriction itself and the side effects of therapy are controlled.

B. Postperfusion ARDS and pulmonary edema

Pulmonary dysfunction after CPB ranges from mild decreases in Pao_2 to respiratory failure resembling the adult respiratory distress syndrome (ARDS).[299,300] Most patients exhibit some widening of the alveolar-to-arterial oxygen tension difference and the arterial-to-end-tidal carbon dioxide tension difference after CPB.[301] Patients who develop serious respiratory insufficiency have progressively increasing $A-aDo_2$ and decreasing Pao_2 in the postoperative period. Pronounced pulmonary interstitial fluid, patchy infiltrates, and small areas of consolidation appear on the chest roentgenogram. The clinical picture continues to worsen with increasing pulmonary shunt, decreasing pulmonary compliance, and radiographically obvious pulmonary edema and confluence of pulmonary infiltrates. Another cause of pulmonary pathosis is trauma to the lungs or to the airways during CPB, especially in the presence of anticoagulation, which causes bleeding into the airway. This leads to alveolar collapse, atelectasis, $\dot{V}/\dot{Q}$ mismatch, and hypoxemia.

The full-blown syndrome of "pump lung" (or ARDS) described in the early CPB literature is seldom seen with current conduct of extracorporeal circulation. However, similar mechanisms are believed to cause mild pulmonary dysfunction.[300,302,303] Both light and electron microscopic studies of lung biopsy samples from patients who have undergone CPB have shown pathologic changes consistent with an acute inflammatory response.[304,305] The pulmonary capillaries are plugged with leukocytes, intracellular edema is present in endothelial cells, and there is noticeable interstitial edema.[303,307] It is known that leukocytes are required for the increased pulmonary microvascular permeability that develops after microembolization.[307] Based on these and other experimental studies, a current hypothesis for postoperative pulmonary dysfunction involves complement activation, leading to release of C3a and C5a anaphylatoxins. C5a is bound to specific sites on polymorphonuclear leukocytes, which are then activated and deposited in the lungs.[308] These activated white blood cells release reactive oxygen species and lysosomal enzymes, which contribute to endothelial injury, alterations in permeability, and accumulation of extravascular fluid.[302,309-311] Leukocyte depletion (with a leukocyte filter incorporated in the bypass circuit) may reduce the pulmonary injury seen after CPB.[312]

Although cardiogenic pulmonary edema is the result of an increase in capillary hydrostatic pressure, noncardiogenic pulmonary edema is the result of an increase in pulmonary capillary permeability. In adults, risk factors for developing postoperative pulmonary edema include preexisting pulmonary disease or pulmonary edema, high bypass flow rates, and prolonged bypass duration.[313] In infants, Kirklin et al. developed an overall index of risk for pulmonary morbidity relating higher levels of C3a anaphylatoxin, longer duration of CPB, and younger age to greater probability of morbidity (Fig. 12-11).[314] Therefore complement activation and the subsequent chain of pathologic events may be minimized when one limits the total duration of CPB. However, in one study of adult patients, complement and neutrophil activation during CPB were not associated with acute pulmonary epithelial injury,[315] a finding indicating that any increase in pulmonary epithelial permeability may be attributable to other factors.

Pronounced elevations of pulmonary venous pressure during CPB can also produce increased extravascular lung water and, eventually, pulmonary edema. One important cause of this problem is malfunction of the left ventricular vent during CPB. Significant amounts of blood may return to the left ventricle during CPB (because of inadequate venous drainage or aortic valvular insufficiency, or through bronchial arterial flow, thebesian drainage, or coronary sinus effluent). Unless the left side of the heart is properly vented during CPB, distension of the left ventricle can occur, with consequent distension of the left atrium and pulmonary veins. Ideally, pulmonary venous pressure should be at zero during total CPB and certainly not above 10 mm Hg. Upon termination of CPB, acute left ventricular dysfunction can result in disastrous increases in pulmonary venous pressure.

Rarely, a dramatic form of noncardiogenic pulmonary edema manifests acutely as an outpouring of proteinaceous edema fluid from the endotracheal tube in the immediate postbypass period.[316-319] Proposed causes of acute noncardiogenic pulmonary edema include white blood cell reactions attributable to antileukocyte antibodies and severe anaphylactoid reactions to protamine.[316-318] White blood cell reactions may be avoided by the use of packed cells rather than whole blood (particularly the whole blood of multiparous donors) and avoidance of fresh-frozen plasma.

The pulmonary lesion of noncardiogenic pulmonary edema is usually completely reversible. When the pulmonary response is acute and severe, CPB should not be terminated until cardiovascular stability is achieved. Epinephrine should be administered to counter hypotension and bronchoconstriction. Some investigators advocate administration of steroids (such as methylprednisolone at 30 mg/kg), though there are no randomized studies demonstrating efficacy of this therapy. Hemodynamic monitoring is helpful. If not already present, a pulmonary artery catheter should be placed for measure-

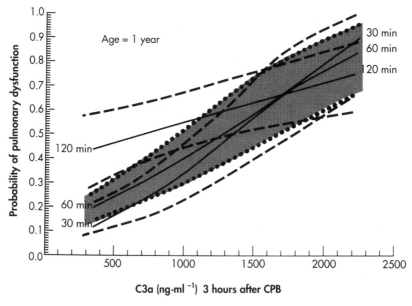

Fig. 12-11. Nomogram from a multivariate analysis of postoperative pulmonary morbidity after cardiac surgery. The nomogram relates C3a levels (obtained 3 hours after cardiopulmonary bypass, CPB) and CPB time to the probability of pulmonary dysfunction, when age is 1 year. *Shaded areas,* 70% confidence limits for 60 minutes of CPB. (From Kirklin JK, Westaby S, Blackstone EH, et al: J Thorac Cardiovasc Surg 86:845-847, 1983.)

ment of pulmonary artery pressures and cardiac output. A direct left atrial pressure measurement is preferred to the pulmonary capillary wedge pressure because of the unpredictable transpulmonary capillary gradient in the acutely impaired pulmonary vascular bed.[316] Respiratory support depends primarily on the use of PEEP to maintain adequate oxygenation.[299] Oxygenation also may be improved by other measures, such as paralysis or sedation of agitated patients.[299] Aggressive tracheobronchial toilet is necessary. With failure of conventional therapy, temporary use of venovenous extracorporeal membrane oxygenation (ECMO) has been reported.[319]

IV. RENAL COMPLICATIONS— ACUTE RENAL INSUFFICIENCY

Although advances in techniques of CPB have reduced the incidence of postoperative renal complications, acute renal failure (ARF) after cardiac surgery remains a significant cause of morbidity and mortality. Although renal dysfunction after cardiac surgery most commonly manifests as mild to moderate elevation in serum creatinine and blood urea nitrogen without significant oliguria, it can be severe and can result in a temporary or permanent need for dialysis. The reported incidence of renal failure after CPB varies depending on the criteria used to define it. Mild renal dysfunction, characterized by a transient decrease in renal function, occurs in 2.5% to 20% of patients undergoing CPB.[145,320-322] The incidence of severe renal dysfunction requiring dialysis ranges from 0.9% to 7.0%.[320-324] Mortality in patients requiring dialysis is extremely high, 27% to 89%.[321-323,325,326]

In the past, many investigations explored the causal relationship between extracorporeal circulation and renal failure after cardiac surgery. Studies have correlated occurrence of renal dysfunction with duration of cardiopulmonary bypass.[320-322,324] Early studies showed that renal plasma flow, glomerular filtration rate, and electrolyte excretion decrease during CPB.[327,328] These data combined with the relatively high incidence of renal dysfunction after CPB led investigators to believe that CPB itself was deleterious to renal function. Recently, however, new issues have come to light that question this causal relationship. Many earlier large-scale studies of renal dysfunction after CPB employed a blood prime of the oxygenator and, if any degree of hemodilution was employed, circulating hematocrit during bypass was usually not reported. Gordon et al. demonstrated the importance of hemodilution in reducing viscos-

ity and thereby lowering perfusion pressure at the same perfusion flows (if one assumes no change in arteriolar resistance).[144] Recent investigations have emphasized the safety of low pressures and low flows with low-viscosity perfusates and has demonstrated a lack of correlation between these variables and postoperative renal dysfunction.[145,320] In the presence of precise hemodilution during CPB, Slogoff et al. found the incidence of even moderate renal dysfunction after CPB to be only 3.0%.[145]

The primary cause of ARF after cardiac surgery is ischemia. Renal ischemia may occur as the result of emboli to the kidney. Sources of emboli during cardiac surgery include atherosclerotic debris, calcium, valvular vegetations, and intracardiac thrombus. Also, aortic dissection can occur (most commonly in association with femoral arterial cannulation for femoral arterial perfusion) and one or both renal arteries may become obstructed, resulting in complete renal failure. Most commonly, however, renal ischemia is believed to be secondary to inadequate perfusion. Low cardiac output is the most common cause of renal dysfunction after CPB.[145,322,329] Although the importance of adequate renal perfusion during CPB is well known, recent emphasis has been placed on the importance of adequate perfusion during the entire perioperative period.[145] Inadequate perioperative perfusion may occur because of myocardial ischemia, congestive heart failure, hypotension, blood loss, or vasopressor requirement, and each of these factors has been associated with an increased incidence of renal failure after cardiac surgery.[145] Perioperative hemodynamic monitoring may provide early detection of conditions causing ARF.

Various pharmacologic agents used in the perioperative period may also adversely affect renal function. Iodinized contrast dye used in patients undergoing cardiac catheterization increases the risk of renal failure because of damage from uric acid precipitation.[329] The use of nephrotoxic agents (particularly antibiotics and immunosuppressive medications) may act synergistically with poor renal perfusion to produce renal dysfunction. Careful monitoring of serum concentrations of nephrotoxic agents is necessary to prevent the development of ARF. In addition to exogenous agents, endogenous toxins may adversely affect renal function. Hemoglobinuria, reflecting intrinsic hemolysis, is well established as a cause of renal dysfunction.

The treatment of ARF should be aimed at its cause. Appropriate monitoring provides the key to diagnosis of perioperative low cardiac output states. Volume administration, inotropic support, and cardiac assist devices should be employed when indicated to support a failing heart. Dopamine in the range of 2 to 5 µg/kg/min has the selective effect of increasing renal blood flow. If hemoglobinuria is present, the urine should be alkalinized to avoid further renal damage. If oliguria persists after hemodynamic problems are corrected, diuretics may be used to stimulate urine production,[330] though this may not alter the long-term course of the renal impairment. Once renal failure is established, dialysis should be instituted promptly to avoid hyperkalemia and other metabolic derangements. Peritoneal dialysis is generally well tolerated in the immediate postoperative period, and hemodialysis may be implemented when cardiovascular stability permits.

V. GASTROINTESTINAL COMPLICATIONS

As the number of procedures requiring cardiopulmonary bypass has increased, the importance of intra-abdominal complications has become increasingly apparent. Although relatively uncommon and difficult to diagnose in patients who are sedated, gastrointestinal complications present challenging management problems during the perioperative period. In several large-scale studies performed in the past decade, the reported incidence of gastrointestinal complications after cardiac surgical procedures ranged from 0.3% to 3.0%.[331-340] The most common complications, in approximate order of decreasing frequency, were gastrointestinal bleeding (with or without the presence of gastroduodenal ulcers), gastroduodenal ulcers (either bleeding or perforated), intestinal obstruction or profound ileus, acute cholecystitis, pancreatitis, intestinal ischemia or infarction, and perforation elsewhere in the gastrointestinal tract (that is, esophagus or intestine). Although the incidence was low, mortality in these studies was 12% to 67%.[331-340] The most dangerous complications were intestinal ischemia, perforated ulcer, and hepatic failure. Mortality from these complications approached 100%.

The probable cause of most gastrointestinal problems after cardiac surgical procedures is visceral hypoperfusion. Moneta et al. found that 75% of their patients who developed gastrointestinal complications had prolonged bypass times or evidence of poor perfusion in the postoperative period.[337] Both Leitman et al. and Krasna et al. found a significant correlation between the duration of bypass and the incidence of gastrointestinal complications.[339,340] Krasna et al. also noted a correlation between gastrointestinal complications and the following factors: valve procedures, age over 70 years, female sex, postoperative low cardiac output, and the use of vasopressors or an intra-aortic balloon pump.[340]

In most series, gastrointestinal bleeding accounted for over 50% of intra-abdominal complications after cardiac surgery. This propensity to bleed may be attributable to a combination of factors, including the physiologic stress of surgery, lack of antacid or histamine blockade prophylaxis, previous history of peptic ulcer disease, and use of anticoagulants in the perioperative period.[341-443] It has been shown that maintenance of gastric pH greater than 4 is effective in prevention of stress erosion of the gastric mucosa.[344,345] Preventive measures have thus been aimed at interventions that increase gastric pH. Lehot et al. noted that with orally administered diazepam premedication alone, gastric pH remained high throughout the perioperative period.[346] Also, Lehot et al. concluded that the addition of an H_2-receptor antagonist (ranitidine) was not necessary to maintain a gastric pH greater than 4. Furthermore, administration of ranitidine led to an increase in bacterial colonization of gastric fluid, which may increase the risk of nosocomial infection.[346]

Hypoperfusion leading to mucosal injury, breakdown of the mucosal barrier, and backdiffusion of acid has been proposed as the common underlying mechanism of intra-abdominal injury.[347] Although no single intervention has been proved effective in preventing these complications, maintenance of adequate cardiac output and tissue perfusion may be the most important factor in improving patient outcome. Treatment of gastrointestinal bleeding once it occurs may begin conservatively, but most authors advocate early surgical intervention for bleeding that fails to respond quickly to appropriate medical therapy.[332-340,348,349]

VI. INFECTIOUS COMPLICATIONS

Infection is a major cause of morbidity and mortality in cardiac surgical patients. Common infectious complications include superficial presternal infections, mediastinitis, endocarditis (of native or prosthetic valves), and septicemia arising from a variety of sources. For several reasons, patients undergoing cardiac surgery with cardiopulmonary bypass are at an increased risk of developing an infection. Many patients are debilitated preoperatively. Their nutritional state, as well as their unstable hemodynamic state, can serve to lower the body's inherent defense mechanisms.[350,351] Cardiopulmonary bypass is known to cause alterations in host defenses by altering phagocytic function[352,353] and both humoral[354] and cellular[355,356] immunity. These alterations have been shown to vary directly with the duration of CPB and return to normal in the first few postoperative days.[357,358] In addition, there appears to be an obligate denaturing of plasma proteins that occurs at the surface interface of nonmembrane oxygenators,[359] which may be eliminated with the use of membrane oxygenators.[360] The CPB apparatus itself is a potential source of infection, though it has been shown not to increase the overall risk of infection after heart surgery.[361] Other factors predisposing cardiac surgical patients to infection include sternotomy itself,[362] a history of previous sternotomy,[363,364] postoperative resternotomy,[365] prolonged operative time,[360] postoperative cardiopulmonary complications including hemorrhage,[366] and the use of the IMA for coronary bypass.[363,367,368]

Prevention is the key to controlling postoperative infection in cardiac surgical patients. Intraoperative surveillance of infection control measures is mandatory. Preoperative preparation of the patient includes optimizing nutrition, respiratory function, and immunologic competence. In addition, any preoperative infection must be thoroughly treated and surgery delayed if necessary. Significant dental problems should be treated, especially if prosthetic material is to be used intraoperatively. Skin preparation before incision should be carefully monitored. Meticulous sterile technique in line placement and careful surgical technique, including attention to hemostasis, is essential. Prophylactic antibiotics are standard and have served to lower the incidence of endocarditis,[369,370] as well as other perioperative infections.[371] Antibiotics must be administered such that serum bactericidal levels are maintained throughout the procedure. Antibiotic prophylaxis must change as the spectrum of postoperative pathogens changes. Postoperatively, any infection must be promptly recognized and appropriately treated. Diligent care of indwelling lines and catheters, including their removal as soon as feasible, is important.

VII. IMMUNOLOGIC COMPLICATIONS
A. Complement activation

The complement system consists of 20 plasma proteins that function as a part of the normal host defense system against traumatic, immunologic, or foreign-body insult. The complement cascade can be activated by antibody molecules through the classical pathway after reaction with a specific antigen or after minor denaturation of antibodies. It can also be activated by an alternative pathway by macromolecules such as endotoxins, thrombin, and plasmin. During CPB, the alternative pathway of complement activation is believed to predominate, though the classical pathway may also play a role.[166,305,372] The complement cascade, once activated, results in the production of powerful anaphylatoxins, C3a and C5a, which increase vascular permeability, cause smooth muscle contraction, mediate leukocyte chemotaxis, and facilitate leukocyte aggregation and enzyme release.[166] The final product of complement activation is a glycoprotein complex, C5b-9, that aids in membrane lysis and phagocytosis.

During CPB, interaction among the patient's blood, the artificial surfaces, and the pump causes complement activation and a systemic inflammatory response (Fig. 12-12).[314] This process eventually results in some degree of direct cellular injury, which, in its most severe form, has been termed the "postperfusion syndrome." Direct evidence of complement activation during CPB was first provided by Chenoweth et al.[308] These investigators demonstrated a progressive increase of C3a concentration throughout CPB, with peak plasma levels more than five times preoperative levels. Maximal generation of C3a apparently occurs during normothermic periods (at initiation of CPB and during rewarming).[373] Further complement activation by the classical pathway occurs after the administration of protamine at the end of CPB, adding to the whole-body inflammatory reaction in some patients.[252-254] Hypothermia, hemodilution, and heparinization attenuate complement activation in vitro and possibly during CPB.[374]

The adverse effects of complement activation are multiple. They include the adverse effects of the anaphylatoxins (C5a and C3a), stimulation of polymorphonuclear leukocytes (resulting in adherence and leukoaggregation), and release of reactive oxygen species and lysosomal enzymes.[166,305] After weaning from bypass and reestablishment of the pulmonary circulation, neutrophils are trapped in the vessels of the lung.[308,310] The extent of pulmonary leukocyte sequestration is apparently related to the degree of complement activation caused by CPB.[375] Furthermore, there is an increase in plasma concentrations of peroxidation products (free radicals) after removal of the aortic cross-clamp, simultaneous with pulmonary sequestration of neutrophils.[310] Therefore it is believed that the peroxidation products are primarily produced by complement-stimulated neutrophils, though

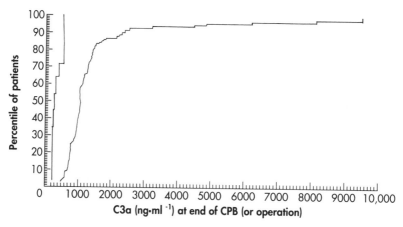

Fig. 12-12. C3a levels (ng/ml) at the end of cardiopulmonary bypass, expressed in a cumulative percentile plot. The steep vertical line on the left represents closed heart patients, 100% of whom had nearly normal or normal levels. The curve on the right represents open cases, virtually all of whom had increased levels. Fifty percent of patients had levels greater than 1000 ng/ml, whereas 25% had levels greater than 1600 ng/ml. (From Kirklin JK, Westaby S, Blackstone EH, et al: J Thorac Cardiovasc Surg 86:845-847, 1983.)

reperfusion of the lungs also may contribute. There is further evidence that neutrophils generate reactive oxygen species during and after CPB.[309,311] Finally, release of lysosomal enzymes from neutrophil granulocytes has been documented during CPB.[376-379]

Although many studies incriminate complement activation as a contributing factor to the postperfusion syndrome, the clinical significance of this response is not yet well characterized.[305] Only a few studies have related the degree of complement activation to outcome. Kirklin et al. reported that increased levels of C3a in 116 patients correlated with an increased possibility of morbidity after CPB, including postoperative pulmonary, renal, and cardiac dysfunction, as well as abnormal bleeding.[314] Moore reported that plasma C3a was greater in 13 patients requiring mechanical ventilation for greater than 24 hours, compared to 67 patients without respiratory complications.[374] However, despite the presence of complement and neutrophil activation in 8 patients undergoing CPB, Tennenberg did not find increased pulmonary epithelial permeability (measured by radioaerosol lung clearance of technetium 99m–labeled diethylenetriamine pentaacetic acid).[315]

Methods to minimize the systemic inflammatory response have been investigated. Studies comparing the degree of complement activation with use of bubble versus membrane oxygenators yield conflicting results.[309,375,372] Another possibility is pharmacologic manipulation of this immune response. Administration of methylprednisolone before institution of CPB may inhibit complement activation.[375,380,381] How-

ever, there are no randomized studies documenting any effect of methylprednisolone on perioperative morbidity. Treatment with calcium-channel blockers to inhibit granulocyte activation[379] or drugs that counteract the deleterious effects of reactive oxygen species, such as superoxide dismutase or catalase, may be tested in the future.[305] Other areas of current and future research include manipulation of the pump-priming solution[382] and development of materials with enhanced biocompatibility for use in extracorporeal circuitry.

B. Changes in leukocytes and immunoglobulins

Another adverse effect of CPB is inhibition of the normal immune response. Shortly after the onset of CPB there is a pronounced decrease in circulating polymorphonuclear leukocytes, largely because of hemodilution but partly because of margination of neutrophils along vessel walls and aggregation.[166,305,383] As CPB progresses, a rebound neutrophilia becomes evident.[166,384] The neutrophilia is more pronounced in patients treated with corticosteroids. Also the ability of neutrophils to orient themselves and move toward an area of infection (chemotaxis) and their phagocytic activity are transiently impaired during CPB.[353,376] Furthermore, reduction in the number of T-lymphocytes, helper T-cells, and suppressor T-cells has been reported to occur after CPB.[384-386] The activity of natural killer cells (a subpopulation of lymphoid cells) is also depressed after CPB, compared with preoperative values.[385,387] Finally, in addition to these effects on various types of leukocytes, there is a reduction in serum levels of immunoglobulins (IgG, IgA, and IgM), though hemodilution may be the major cause of these changes.[388] Such abnormalities may contribute to sepsis and other infectious complications after CPB.[389]

VIII. HEMATOLOGIC COMPLICATIONS

A. Inadequate surgical hemostasis

Continued bleeding after cardiac operations is a significant problem, leading to transfusion with its attendant risks and possibly resulting in hypovolemia or cardiac tamponade. The most common cause of excessive postbypass bleeding is inadequate surgical hemostasis. Prevention of this complication is primarily dependent on fastidious surgical technique. Careful surgical dissection and meticulous control of bleeding sites before sternal closure reduce the risk of postoperative hemorrhage. Common sources of "surgical bleeding," deserving particular attention, include vascular anastomoses and suture lines, as well as sternal wire holes. Recognition of surgical bleeding in the postoperative period is dependent on the surgeon's ability to admit this likelihood and willingness to reexamine his work.

An effort to distinguish bleeding caused by systemic coagulopathy from "surgical bleeding" is warranted. Generalized oozing from previously dry wound edges and vascular cannulation sites, as well as epistaxis or hematuria, indicate the former. Continuing blood loss in excess of 300 ml/hour is suggestive of a surgical bleeding site and mandates a return to the operating suite, particularly if results of coagulation studies are near normal. The presence of a measurable coagulopathy in the postoperative period by no means excludes the possibility that inadequate surgical hemostasis is the primary problem. Excessive bleeding from a surgical site and the transfusion of blood in response to this may result in hypothermia and depletion of coagulation factors, which frequently results in a measurable coagulopathy. This situation is best corrected by prompt reexploration.

Finally, as discussed in the section dealing with pericardial tamponade, one should remember that diminution of chest tube output after a period of excessive bleeding may be the result of chest tube clotting, portending the onset of tamponade, rather than clinical improvement.

B. Residual heparin activity

A relatively uncommon cause of postbypass hemorrhage is residual heparin activity. After protamine administration, it is appropriate to test for residual heparin. The most common screening test for residual unneutralized heparin is the activated coagulation time, performed in the operating room. If the ACT returns to the patient's base-line (preheparin) value ±10%, the presence of residual unneutralized heparin is unlikely. A prolonged ACT and prolonged partial thromboplastin time are suggestive of residual heparin activity.[390] However, pronounced deficiencies in the intrinsic coagulation system or severe thrombocytopenia may also prolong the ACT. Residual heparin activity is more specifically detected when a protamine titration or a direct heparin assay is performed.[390,391] Such a titration is particularly useful when ACT prolongation persists or increases despite additional protamine administration.[390]

The phenomenon of "heparin rebound" should be mentioned. The phenomenon was first described by Kolff et al. as a situation in which "heparin is neutralized by protamine sulfate and the clotting time becomes normal in a matter of minutes. However, protamine seems to be eliminated from the blood before heparin is, thus leaving the heparin uncovered as demonstrated by protamine titration."[392] The reported incidence of heparin rebound varies from 0% to 50% but is probably rare today.[391,393,394] Theoretically this phenomenon occurs because of the pharmacodynamics of an acutely administered drug undergoing redistribution (protamine) titrated against a drug that is completely distributed (heparin).[391] A protamine titration serves to rule out the possibility of heparin rebound.

C. Thrombocytopenia and platelet dysfunction

Thrombocytopenia and platelet dysfunction are among the most predictable complications of CPB.[395-397] The quantitative decrease in platelet number is the result of several key factors. Hemodilution with crystalloid or blood priming solution combined with the addition of crystalloid cardioplegia can lead to a dilutional reduction in the concentration of circulating platelets. Cardiotomy suction, which serves to decrease overall blood loss, significantly damages circulating platelets. Destruction of platelets occurs at the blood-gas interface of bubble oxygenators, and prolonged duration of bypass with these oxygenators can lead to a substantial reduction in platelet numbers. Also, arterial and cardiotomy filters can sequester and destroy platelets. Finally, the use of pulmonary arterial catheters and certain pharmacologic agents (including heparin, protamine, quinidine, and various antibiotics) have been associated with thrombocytopenia.

Likewise, the qualitative impairment of platelet function has several causes. Direct platelet contact with the synthetic surfaces of either membrane or bubble oxygenators is the major source of platelet dysfunction. Platelets adhere to the surfaces, are activated, and are subsequently degraded, leading to greatly inadequate function of these platelets in the hemostatic process. The degree of impairment of platelet function is directly related to the duration of CPB.[398] Also, hypothermia worsens platelet function. Bleeding times have been found to be prolonged when measured at hypothermic skin sites in vivo.[399] In addition, many pharmacologic agents are known to be detrimental to platelet function, including certain anti-inflammatory drugs, antibiotics, psychoactive drugs, cardiovascular drugs, and even some anesthetic agents.

Thrombocytopenia alone rarely decreases platelet number below that required for hemostasis after CPB, and usually the platelet count returns to normal levels within 1 week after surgery. However, platelet *dysfunction* is a major cause of postbypass abnormalities of hemostasis, though it generally resolves within the first 24 hours after uncomplicated surgery. Methods of preventing bleeding secondary to thrombocytopenia and platelet dysfunction include the use of controlled cardiotomy suction and membrane oxygenators for cases with total bypass times exceeding 120 minutes. Also, it is important to avoid postbypass hypothermia and pharmacologic agents that may adversely affect platelet function.

D. Fibrinolysis and decreased fibrinogen

Primary fibrinolysis, defined as the activation of the fibrinolytic system in the absence of active coagulation, has been reported to play a role in hemorrhage after CPB.[400,401] The incidence of primary fibrinolysis varies depending on the criteria used in its definition. Some degree of increased fibrinolytic activity after CPB can be found in nearly all patients when sensitive clot assay techniques are used. Fibrinolytic activity increases during CPB because of intrinsic plasminogen activation by both hypothermia and contact with synthetic surfaces. Characteristically, this activity increases upon initiation of CPB and returns to normal shortly after its termination. Despite this, hyperfibrinolysis and elevated fibrinogen split products are rare after CPB, as is prolonged hemorrhage secondary to primary fibrinolysis.

Although fibrinogen itself decreases after CPB, kinetic measurements of fibrinogen levels are equivalent to levels of clottable fibrinogen, a finding suggestive that fibrinogen dysfunction does not play a major role in abnormal hemostasis.[399] Disseminated intravascular coagulation (DIC), a syndrome of uncontrolled systemic fibrin deposition and concurrent fibrinolysis, has been reported after cardiac surgery.[402] However, standardization of anticoagulation techniques has served to prevent intravascular coagulation, resulting in an extremely low incidence of this complication. As in noncardiac surgical patients, DIC may still occur in the presence of shock, sepsis, hemolytic transfusion reactions, and dissecting aortic aneurysms.

E. Other causes of coagulopathy

As a result of hemodilution, plasma concentrations of nearly all clotting factors decrease during CPB.[403] In general, these reductions in coagulation factor activity are not sufficient to account for postoperative bleeding. For all factors except factor V, plasma levels above 30% of normal are considered adequate for hemostasis; for factor V, a level of only 10% to 15% is adequate.[399] Clinically significant abnormalities in clotting factors can occur in patients in the presence of preexisting clotting factor deficiencies, excessive hemodilution, massive transfusion, excessive use of cell-washing techniques, and hyperfibrinolysis.[404]

Recently, much attention has focused on the importance of the Von Willebrand half of factor VIII (Von Willebrand factor, or VWF) in postbypass hemostatic abnormalities. Mammen and co-workers found a defect in ristocetin-induced platelet aggregation (reflective of a generalized decrease in platelet adhesion) in patients undergoing cardiac surgery, suggestive of the involvement of VWF, which is required for this aggregation.[405] Desmopressin acetate (1-deamino-8-D-arginine, or DDAVP) increases circulating levels of coagulation factors VIII:C and VIII:VWF by a mechanism that is not known. DDAVP has been used to normalize bleeding in a wide variety of situations because of its ability to promote platelet adhesion.[406,407] Studies evaluating the efficacy of DDAVP in preventing hemostatic dysfunction after cardiac surgery have yielded conflicting results.[408-411] Salzman and co-workers found that prophylactic administration of DDAVP substantially decreased early postoperative bleeding, transfusion requirements, and hemorrhagic events requiring reoperation, without detectable adverse effects.[410] However, other studies have not shown any benefit with prophylactic DDAVP therapy, particularly in routine primary CABG operations, in reducing postoperative bleeding or transfusion requirements or in enhancing platelet function.[411] Studies evaluating the efficacy of the drug in correcting existing hemostatic abnormalities are underway. Concerns regarding the empiric use of DDAVP center on its side effects, including hypotension, antidiuresis, plasminogen activation, and the possibility that it may increase the incidence of graft occlusion. Currently, the only indication for DDAVP in cardiac surgery is in the treatment of patients known to be deficient in VWF.

F. Hemolysis and shortened erythrocyte survival

Erythrocytes are damaged during CPB primarily by shear stresses.[166,412] At worst, this damage results in immediate lysis, with release of free hemoglobin. At best, it results in shortened cellular life span. The intracardiac suction systems are particularly deleterious to erythrocytes because of high shear stresses generated under negative pressure. However, during CPB, passage of blood through the oxygenator exacerbates hemolysis, particularly with bubble (instead of membrane) oxygenators.[413] Serum hemoglobin levels during CPB do not accurately reflect the degree of hemolysis because hemoglobin is continuously removed from the circulating blood by the reticuloendothelial system and the kidneys. The plasma hemoglobin may peak several hours after CPB, probably because of ongoing destruction of damaged erythrocytes.[166] When plasma hemoglobin level exceeds 40 mg/dl, casts may form in the renal tubules, though there is little likelihood of acute renal failure unless plasma levels exceed 100 mg/dl.[166] The shortened survival time of surviving erythrocytes results in a progressive loss of red blood cell mass in the first 72 hours after surgery. Certainly, the resulting postoperative anemia is a common complication of CPB.

IX. METABOLIC AND SYSTEMIC DERANGEMENTS
A. Metabolic acidosis

Metabolic acidosis, primarily from lactacidemia, is a well-known complication of CPB. It is attributable, in part, to inhomogeneous perfusion during hypothermic nonpulsatile CPB. Tissues receiving little perfusion may accumulate large quantities of lactic acid that is washed out into the circulation when regional perfusion improves. Metabolic acidosis can also result from acute reductions in systemic perfusion. There is a steady and significant increase in blood lactate concentration during operations requiring CPB, which is minimized by use of adequate

pump flow rates.[414] Usually, metabolic acidosis is corrected simply by reestablishment of adequate cardiac output and systemic perfusion. Vasodilator therapy may speed washout of regional accumulations of lactic acid. In patients with poor postbypass cardiac function, correction of metabolic acidosis (with sodium bicarbonate) may be essential to improve the myocardial response to inotropic therapy.

B. Hypokalemia

Hypokalemia commonly occurs in the postbypass period. Causes include chronic diuretic therapy, hemodilution during CPB, urinary losses during and after CPB, and intracellular shifts caused by abnormalities of the glucose-insulin system or by hyperventilation. Furthermore, there is evidence that the amount and concentration of intracellular potassium is decreased during CPB.[415] The treatment of hypokalemia is potassium replacement, particularly if dysrhythmias occur.

C. Hyperkalemia

Hyperkalemia may be transiently present in the postbypass period because of administration of a large cardioplegic dose. Patients with normal renal function and mild hyperkalemia ($K^+ <6.0$ mEq/L) generally do not need treatment though repeated determinations of potassium concentration should be obtained. If hyperkalemia is severe ($K^+ <7.0$ mEq/L), treatment is essential with or without renal dysfunction. Methods of treatment include diuresis, calcium chloride (10 to 20 mg/kg) to antagonize the effects of potassium on the cardiac cell membranes, sodium bicarbonate (1 to 2 mEq/kg or 1 amp [44.6 mEq] in adults) to produce moderate alkalinity and shift potassium intracellularly, or, to achieve a similar effect, infusion of glucose and insulin (1 to 2 g of glucose/kg with 0.3 units of regular insulin per gram of glucose, or 25 g of glucose combined with 10 units of regular insulin in adults).

D. Hypocalcemia

Calcium chloride is frequently administered to patients during weaning from CPB to provide vasopressor and inotropic support during the immediate postbypass period, though this therapy is controversial.[416,417] Several investigators have reported that CPB can lower plasma ionized-calcium levels, at least transiently, because of hemodilution, inclusion of citrate in the pump priming solution, or the ability of heparin to complex with ionized calcium.[418-420] However, other investigators have not found important changes in ionized calcium during CPB.[421,422] An intravenous calcium chloride dose of 5 to 10 mg/kg just after termination of CPB produces rapid elevation of plasma ionized calcium. Proponents of this therapy argue that the amount of sarcolemmal calcium depends greatly on the amount of ionized calcium in the extracellular fluid and, in turn, on the ionized calcium level in the blood.[417] Furthermore, it is a time-tested therapy for improving hemodynamics, and it may offset the effects of potassium cardioplegic solutions.[417] Studies have confirmed that calcium administration significantly increases blood pressure, cardiac index, stroke volume index, and left ventricular stroke work index, while reducing right atrial pressure.[423,424] Apparently the increase in systemic vascular resistance predominates in the presence of normal or high plasma concentrations of ionized calcium.

Opponents of calcium administration in the postbypass period argue that there is no specific indication for calcium and that increased intracellular calcium is associated with myocardial dysfunction and cell death.[416,425,426] Vitez argues that almost all serious perioperative deficits in myocardial contraction are related to intracellular calcium processes, not low extracellular calcium concentration.[416] Furthermore, high extracellular calcium levels may inhibit diastolic relaxation and actually decrease contractility in some settings. Finally, administration of exogenous calcium may precipitate coronary artery spasm and ischemia. Most anesthesiologists currently use calcium chloride for selected patients at the end of bypass rather than as a routinely administered drug and may avoid calcium altogether if there is a likelihood of persistent myocardial ischemia or reperfusion injury.

E. Hypomagnesemia

Hypomagnesemia may result from dilution with a magnesium-free priming solution for the CPB circuit, from intracellular sequestration during CPB, or from chronic critical illness. Most of the total body magnesium is intracellular. Therefore large losses occur before the serum level is decreased. Magnesium levels usually parallel changes in potassium. Hypomagnesemia, like hypokalemia, causes prolonged

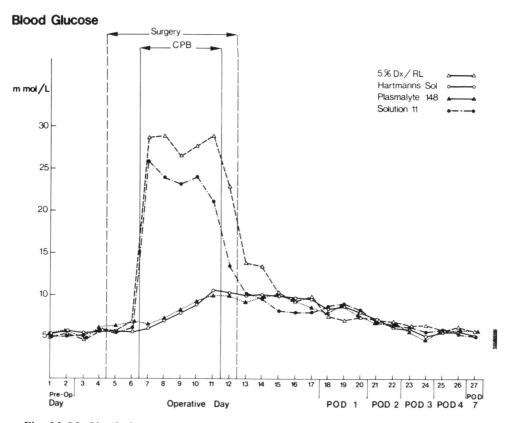

Fig. 12-13. Blood glucose concentrations (mmol/L) during and after cardiopulmonary bypass (CPB) with four different pump-priming solutions. *Dx,* Dextrose; *RL,* lactated Ringer's solution; *POD,* postoperative days. To convert mmol/L to mg/dl, multiply by 18. (From McKnight CK, Elliott MJ, Pearson DT, et al: J Thorac Cardiovasc Surg 90:97-111, 1985.)

PR and QT intervals, widened QRS complexes, and dysrhythmias, which may be refractory to treatment with antiarrhythmic drugs.[427] Also, like hypokalemia, magnesium deficiency predisposes to the development of dysrhythmias produced by the cardiac glycosides. Furthermore, hypomagnesemia may contribute to myocardial depression. Efforts to prevent hypomagnesemia include supplying magnesium in the pump priming solution (approximately 2 to 5 mEq/liter of priming solution). If supplementation is required, 2 to 4 g is administered over 30 to 40 minutes, followed by an infusion of 1 g/hour with frequent monitoring of levels.

F. Hyperglycemia

The implications of hyperglycemia in the presence of cerebral ischemia have been previously discussed in this chapter. Hyperglycemia is common during CPB for several reasons. There is a well characterized and pronounced sympathetic nervous system response to CPB (see Fig. 12-10).[268] High catecholamine concentrations would be expected to increase the rates of both gluconeogenesis and glycogenolysis.[428] Hypothermia inhibits release of insulin during CPB, delaying metabolic response to the stress-induced hyperglycemia.[429] Also, many centers include glucose in the pump priming solution, which results in very high concentrations of glucose during bypass (Fig. 12-13).[87,90,428,429] Furthermore, heparin may interact with insulin receptors and thus alter insulin binding.[430] Finally, adsorption of insulin to polyvinyl chloride surfaces, such as those used in CPB circuitry, is known to occur.[431]

Whether hyperglycemia during CPB is harmful remains a controversial issue.[87,90] In adult patients, recommendations to prevent extreme elevations in plasma glucose include avoidance of glucose-containing pump priming solutions,[87-89,204] administration of insulin infusions to diabetic and possibly even nondiabetic patients,[428,429,432] and use of pulsatile perfusion to minimize the stress response during CPB.[433] However, as discussed in the section on neurologic complications of CPB, there are no prospective outcome studies demonstrating a detrimental effect of hyperglycemia in this setting. In fact, Metz and Keats have emphasized a potential benefit of hyperglycemia during CPB (reduction of perioperative fluid requirements).[90] Furthermore, avoiding glucose administration in children undergoing PHCA may not eliminate hyperglycemia during CPB and, in fact, may result in *hypo*glycemia in the prebypass period.[205] In summary, although many centers avoid administration of glucose-containing solutions during cardiac surgery, the issue remains controversial.

G. Hypothermia

During hypothermic CPB, both core and peripheral temperatures are significantly decreased. Rewarming increases blood and core temperatures to normal. However, several vascular beds, such as muscle and fat, remain severely vasoconstricted. These areas then become vasodilated during the 45 to 90 minutes after the termination of bypass, causing a decrease in core temperature. Usually, patients are hypothermic upon arrival in the intensive care unit, with rectal temperatures approximately 34° C.[434] During and after separation from CPB, measures to minimize postbypass hypothermia are employed. For example, rewarming on CPB is continued until rectal temperature is 35° C, and during rewarming, perfusion flows are increased and vasodilators are administered. Also, a warming blanket is applied, and the ambient temperature, inspired gases, and irrigation fluids for the chest cavity are warmed.

Hypothermia has adverse effects on hemodynamics, oxygen consumption, and coagulability of the blood.[435] Systemic and pulmonary arterial tone increase as temperature decreases, resulting in increased left and right ventricular afterload, which may decrease cardiac output and increase myocardial oxygen consumption. Also, systemic venous tone is increased, thereby decreasing venous capacitance. As the patient rewarms during the initial few hours in the intensive care unit, large abrupt changes occur in systemic vascular resistance (SVR) and venous capacitance. The hypothermic patient who is vasoconstricted may have a normal blood pressure but decreased intravascular volume, low cardiac output, and a high SVR. Abrupt decreases in SVR and increases in venous capacitance during rewarming can produce sudden severe hypotension. Hemodynamic instability during the rewarming period is exacerbated by inadequate sedation and analgesia. Stimulation such as endotracheal tube suctioning can result in pronounced changes in sympathetic tone and sudden hypertension. Therapy during rewarming coordinates volume and vasodilator administration (nitroprusside or nitroglycerin). The goal is maintenance of normal hemodynamics, including cardiac filling pressures (CVP and PCWP), cardiac output, and systemic and pulmonary vascular resistances. Maintenance of adequate sedation with narcotics and hypnotics is equally important.

Another important problem that occurs during the rewarming period is shivering. Shivering increases metabolism, thereby increasing oxygen consumption and myocardial work. This may result in decreased mixed venous oxygen saturation and systemic acidosis, which may be particularly detrimental to patients who have impaired cardiac function after cardiac surgery.[436-438] The effects of shivering can be prevented by the use of muscle relaxants or meperidine.[437,438]

REFERENCES

1. Sotaniemi KA: Brain damage and neurological outcome after open-heart surgery, J Neurol Neurosurg Psychiatry 43:127-135, 1980.
2. Slogoff S, Girgis KZ, and Keats AS: Etiologic factors in neuropsychiatric complications associated with cardiopulmonary bypass, Anesth Analg 61:903-911, 1982.
3. Nussmeier NA, Arlund C, and Slogoff S: Neuropsychiatric complications after cardiopulmonary bypass: cerebral protection by a barbiturate, Anesthesiology 64:165-170, 1986.
4. Heikkinen L, Harjula A, and Mattila S: Neurological events in cardiac surgery, Ann Chir Gynaecol 74:118-123, 1985.
5. Craver JM, Weintraub WS, Jones EL, et al: Predictors of mortality, complications, and length of stay in aortic valve replacement for aortic stenosis, Circulation 78 (suppl I):I-85–I-90, 1988.
6. Rioux C, Leguerrier A, Langanay T, et al: Valvular replacement for aortic stenosis in patients over 70 years: immediate risk and long-term results, Eur Heart J 9(suppl E):121-127, 1988.
7. Gonzalez-Scarano F and Hurtig HI: Neurologic complications of coronary artery bypass grafting: case-control study, Neurology 31:1032-1035, 1981.
8. Martin WRW and Hashimoto SA: Stroke in coronary bypass surgery, Can J Neurol Sci 9:21-26, 1982.
9. Breuer AC, Furlan AJ, Hanson MR, et al: Central nervous system complications of coronary artery bypass graft surgery: prospective analysis of 421 patients, Stroke 14:682-687, 1983.
10. Bojar RM, Najafi H, DeLaria GA, et al: Neurological complications of coronary revascularization, Ann Thorac Surg 36:427-432, 1983.
11. Shaw PJ, Bates D, Cartlidge NEF, et al: Early neurological complications of coronary artery bypass surgery, Br Med J 291:1384-1387, 1985.
12. Gardner TJ, Horneffer PJ, Manolio TA, et al: Stroke following coronary artery bypass grafting: a ten-year study, Ann Thorac Surg 40:574-581, 1985.
13. Acinapura AJ, Rose DM, Cunningham JN, et al: Coronary artery bypass in septuagenarians: analysis of mortality and morbidity, Circulation 78(suppl I):I-179–I-184, 1988.
14. Fuse K and Makuuchi H: Early and late results of coronary artery bypass grafting in the elderly, Jpn Circ J 52:460-465, 1988.
15. Naunheim KS, Fiore AC, Wadley JJ, et al: The changing profile of the patient undergoing coronary artery bypass surgery, J Am Coll Cardiol 11:494-498, 1988.
16. Salomon NW, Page S, Bigelow JC, et al: Cononary artery bypass grafting in elderly patients: comparative results in a consecutive series of 469 patients older than 75 years, J Thorac Cardiovasc Surg 101:209-218, 1991.
17. Jones EL, Weintraub WS, Craver JM, et al: Coronary bypass surgery: Is the operation different today? J Thorac Cardiovasc Surg 101:108-115, 1991.
18. Sotaniemi KA: Cerebral outcome after extracorporeal circulation: comparison between prospective and retrospective evaluations, Arch Neurol 40:75-77, 1983.
19. Gilman S: Cerebral disorders after open-heart operations, N Engl J Med 272:489-498, 1965.
20. Brierly JB: Brain damage complicating open-heart surgery: a neuropathological study of 46 patients, Proc R Soc Med 60:858-859, 1967.
21. McKibbin DW, Bulkley BH, Green WR, et al: Fatal cerebral atheromatous embolization after cardiopulmonary bypass, J Thorac Cardiovasc Surg 71:741-745, 1976.
22. Ghatak NR, Sinnenberg RJ, and DeBlois GG: Cerebral fat embolism following cardiac surgery, Stroke 14:619-621, 1983.
23. Aberg T, Ronquist G, Tyden H, et al: Adverse effects on the brain in cardiac operations as assessed by biochemical, psychometric, and radiologic methods, J Thorac Cardiovasc Surg 87:99-105, 1984.
24. Aberg T and Kihlgren M: Cerebral protection during open-heart surgery, Thorax 32:525-533, 1977.
25. Oka Y, Moriwaki KM, Hong Y, et al: Detection of air emboli in the left heart by M-mode transesophageal echocardiography following cardiopulmonary bypass, Anesthesiology 63:109-113, 1985.
26. Kolkka R and Hilberman M: Neurologic dysfunction following cardiac operation with low-flow, low-pressure cardiopulmonary bypass, J Thorac Cardiovasc Surg 79:432-437, 1980.
27. Taber RE, Maraan BM, and Tomatis L: Prevention of air embolism during open-heart surgery: a study of the role of trapped air in the left ventricle. Surgery 68:685-691, 1970.
28. Lawrence GH, McKay HA, and Sherensky RT: Effective measures in the prevention of intraoperative aeroembolus, J Thorac Cardiovasc Surg 62:731-735, 1971.
29. Rodigas PC, Meyer FI, Haasler GB, et al: Intraoperative 2-dimensional echocardiography: Ejection of microbubbles from the left ventricle after cardiac surgery, Am J Cardiol 50:1130-1132, 1982.
30. Topol EJ, Humphrey LS, Borkon M, et al: Value of intraoperative left ventricular microbubbles detected by transesophageal two-dimensional echocardiography in predicting neurologic outcome after cardiac operations, Am J Cardiol 56:773-775, 1985.
31. Oka Y, Inoue T, Hong Y, et al: Retained intracardiac air: transesophageal echocardiography for definition of incidence and monitoring removal by improved techniques, J Thorac Cardiovasc Surg 91:329-338, 1986.
32. Diehl JT, Ramos D, Dougherty F, et al: Intraoperative, two-dimensional echocardiography-guided removal of retained intracardiac air, Ann Thorac Surg 43:674-675, 1987.
33. Faro RS, Golden MD, Javid H, et al: Coronary revascularization in septuagenarians, J Thorac Cardiovasc Surg 86:616-620, 1983.
34. Parker FB, Marvasti MA, and Bove EL: Neurologic complications following coronary artery bypass: the role of atherosclerotic emboli, Thorac Cardiovasc Surg 33:207-209, 1985.
35. Barzilai B, Marshall WG Jr, Saffitz JE, et al: Avoidance of embolic complications by ultrasonic characterization of the ascending aorta, Circulation 80(suppl I):I-275–I-279, 1989.
36. Coffey CE, Massey EW, Roberts KB, et al: Natural history of cerebral complications of coronary artery bypass graft surgery, Neurology 33:1416-1421, 1983.

37. Mills NL and Ochsner JL: Massive air embolism during cardiopulmonary bypass: causes, prevention and management, J Thorac Cardiovasc Surg 80:708-717, 1980.

38. Aberg T and Kihlgren M: Effect of open heart surgery on intellectual dysfunction, Scand J Thorac Cardiovasc Surg 8(suppl 15):1-63, 1974.

39. Krebber HJ, Hanrath P, Janzen R, et al: Gas emboli during open heart surgery, Thorac Cardiovasc Surg 30:401-404, 1982.

40. Padula RT, Eisenstat TE, Bronstein MH, et al: Intracardiac air following cardiotomy: location, causative factors, and a method for removal, J Thorac Cardiovasc Surg 62:736-742, 1971.

41. Gomes OM, Pereira SN, Castagna RC, et al: The importance of the different sites of air injection in the tolerance of arterial air embolism, J Thorac Cardiovasc Surg 65:563-568, 1973.

42. Cooley DA, Ott DA, Frazier OH, et al: Surgical treatment of aneurysms of the transverse aortic arch: experience with 25 patients using hypothermic techniques, Ann Thorac Surg 32:260-272, 1981.

43. Crawford ES, Stowe CL, Crawford JL, et al: Aortic arch aneurysm: a sentinel of extensive aortic disease requiring subtotal and total aortic replacement, Ann Surg 199:742-752, 1984.

44. Spotnitz HM and Malm JR: Two-dimensional ultrasound and cardiac operations, J Thorac Cardiovasc Surg 83:43-51, 1982.

45. Duff HJ, Buda AJ, Kramer R, et al: Detection of entrapped intracardiac air with intraoperative echocardiography, Am J Cardiol 46:255-260, 1980.

46. Bashein G, Bledsoe SW, Townes BD, et al: Tools for assessing central nervous system injury in the cardiac surgery patient. In Hilberman M, editor: Brain injury and protection during heart surgery, Boston, 1988, Martinus Nijhoff Publishers.

47. El-Fiki M and Fish KJ: Is the EEG a useful monitor during cardiac surgery? a case report, Anesthesiology 67:575-578, 1987.

48. Michaels I and Sheehan J: EEG changes due to unsuspected aortic dissection during cardiopulmonary bypass, Anesth Analg 63:946-948, 1984.

49. Steele ER, Albin MS, Monts JL, et al: Compressed spectral array EEG monitoring during coronary bypass surgery in a patient with vertebrobasilar artery insufficiency, Anesth Analg 66:271-273, 1987.

50. Bolsin SNC: Detection of neurological damage during cardiopulmonary bypass, Anaesthesia 41:61-66, 1986.

51. Michenfelder JD: Brain hypoxia: current status of experimental and clinical therapy, Semin Anesthesia 2:81-90, 1983.

52. Michenfelder JD and Theye RA: Cerebral protection by thiopental during hypoxia, Anesthesiology 39:510-517, 1973.

53. Michenfelder JD and Milde JH: Influence of anesthetics on metabolic, functional and pathological responses to regional cerebral ischemia, Stroke 6:405-410, 1975.

54. Smith AL, Hoff JT, Nielsen SL, et al: Barbiturate protection in acute focal cerebral ischemia, Stroke 5:1-7, 1974.

55. Michenfelder JD, Milde JH, and Sundt TM Jr: Cerebral protection by barbiturate anesthesia: use after middle cerebral artery occlusion in Java monkeys, Arch Neurol 33:345-350, 1976.

56. Corkill G, Sivalingam S, Reitan JA, et al: Dose dependency of the post-insult protective effect of pentobarbital in the canine experimental stroke model, Stroke 9:10-12, 1978.

57. Moseley JI, Laurent JD, and Molinari GF: Barbiturate attenuation of the clinical course and pathologic lesions in a primate stroke model, Neurology 25:870-874, 1975.

58. Corkill G, Chikovani OK, McLeish I, et al: Timing of pentobarbital administration for brain protection in experimental stroke, Surg Neurol 5:147-149, 1976.

59. Selman WR, Spetzler RF, Roski RA, et al: Barbiturate coma in focal cerebral ischemia: relationship of protection to timing of therapy, J Neurosurg 56:685-690, 1982.

60. Hoff JT, Smith AL, Hankinson HL, et al: Barbiturate protection from cerebral infarction in primates, Stroke 6:28-33, 1975.

61. Michenfelder JD: The interdependency of cerebral functional and metabolic effects following massive doses of thiopental in the dog, Anesthesiology 41:231-236, 1974.

62. Feustal PJ, Ingvar MC, and Severinghaus JW: Cerebral oxygen availability and blood flow during middle cerebral artery occlusion: effects of pentobarbital, Stroke 12:858-863, 1981.

63. Branston NM, Hope DT, and Symon L: Barbiturates in focal ischemia of primate cortex: effects on blood flow distribution, evoked potential and extracellular potassium, Stroke 10:647-653, 1979.

64. Kofke WA, Nemoto EM, Hossman KA, et al: Brain blood flow and metabolism after global ischemia and post-insult thiopental therapy in monkeys, Stroke 10:554-560, 1979.

65. Simeone FA, Frazer G, and Lawner P: Ischemic brain edema: comparative effects of barbiturates and hypothermia, Stroke 10:8-12, 1979.

66. Lawner P, Laurent J, Simeone F, et al: Attenuation of ischemic brain edema by pentobarbital after carotid ligation in the gerbil, Stroke 10:644-647, 1979.

67. Flamm ES, Demopoulos HB, Seligman ML, et al: Possible molecular mechanisms of barbiturate-mediated protection in regional cerebral ischemia, Acta Neurol Scand 56(suppl 64):150-151, 1977.

68. Nemoto EM, Shiu GK, Nemmer JP, et al: Free fatty acid accumulation in the pathogenesis and therapy of ischemic-anoxic brain injury, Am J Emerg Med 1:175-179, 1983.

69. Todd MM, Chadwick HS, Shapiro HM, et al: The neurologic effects of thiopental therapy following experimental cardiac arrest in cats, Anesthesiology 57:76-86, 1982.

70. Metz S and Slogoff S: Thiopental by single bolus compared to infusion for cerebral protection during cardiopulmonary bypass, J Clin Anesthesiol 2:226-231, 1990.

71. Zaidan JR, Klochany A, Martin WM, et al: Effect of thiopental on neurologic outcome of coronary artery bypass grafting, Anesthesiology 74:406-411, 1991.

72. Todd MM, Hindman BJ, and Warner DS: Barbiturate protection and cardiac surgery: a different result, Anesthesiology 74:402-405, 1991.

73. Newberg LA and Michenfelder JD: Cerebral protection by isoflurane during hypoxemia or ischemia, Anesthesiology 59:29-35, 1983.

74. Messick JM Jr, Casement B, Sharbrough FW, et al: Correlation of regional cerebral blood flow (rCBF) with EEG changes during isoflurane anesthesia for carotid endarterectomy: critical rCBF, Anesthesiology 66:344-349, 1987.

75. Nehls DG, Todd MM, Spetzler RF, et al: A comparison of the cerebral protective effects of isoflurane and barbiturates during temporary focal ischemia in primates, Anesthesiology 66:453-464, 1987.

76. Steen PA, Newberg LA, Milde JH, et al: Nimodipine

improves cerebral blood flow and neurologic recovery after complete cerebral ischemia in the dog, J Cereb Blood Flow Metab 3:38-43, 1983.

77. Steen PA, Gisvold SE, Milde JH, et al: Nimodipine improves outcome when given after complete cerebral ischemia in primates, Anesthesiology 62:406-414, 1985.

78. Allen GS, Ahn HS, Preziosi TJ, et al: Cerebral arterial spasm: a controlled trial of nimodipine in patients with subarachnoid hemorrhage, N Engl J Med 308:619-624, 1983.

79. Gelmers HJ, Gortem K, de Weerdt CJ,et al: A controlled trial of nimodipine in acute ischemic stroke, N Engl J Med 318:203-207, 1988.

80. Forsman M, Aarseth HP, Nordby NK, et al: Effects of nimodipine on cerebral blood flow and cerebrospinal fluid pressure after cardiac arrest: correlation with neurologic outcome, Anesth Analg 68:436-443, 1989.

81. Foster AC, Gill R, and Woodruff GN: Neuroprotective effects of MK-801 *in vivo:* selectivity and evidence for delayed degeneration mediated by NMDA receptor activation, J Neurosci 8:4745-4754, 1988.

82. Church J, Zeman S, and Lodge D: The neuroprotective action of ketamine and MK-801 after transient cerebral ischemia in rats, Anesthesiology 69:702-709, 1988.

83. Michenfelder JD, Lanier WL, Scheithauer BW, et al: Evaluation of the glutamate antagonist dizocilipine maleate (MK-801) on neurologic outcome in a canine model of complete cerebral ischemia: correlation with hippocampal histopathology, Brain Res 481:228-234, 1989.

84. Prough DS and Mills SA: Should thiopental sodium administration be a standard of care for open cardiac procedures? J Clin Anesthesiol 2:221-225, 1990.

85. Pulsinelli WA, Levy DE, Sigsbee B, et al: Increased damage after ischemic stroke in patients with hyperglycemia with or without established diabetes mellitus, Am J Med 74:540-544, 1983.

86. Lanier WL, Strangland KJ, Scheithauer BW, et al: The effects of dextrose infusion and head position on neurologic outcome after complete cerebral ischemia in primates: examination of a model, Anesthesiology 66:39-48, 1987.

87. McKnight CK, Elliott MJ, Pearson DT, et al: The effects of four different crystalloid bypass pump-priming fluids upon the metabolic response to cardiac operation, J Thorac Cardiovasc Surg 90:97-111, 1985.

88. Sieber FE, Smith DS, Traystman RJ, et al: Glucose: a reevaluation of its intraoperative use, Anesthesiology 67:72-81, 1987.

89. Benzing G, Francis PD, Kaplan S, et al: Glucose and insulin changes in infants and children undergoing hypothermic open-heart surgery, Am J Cardiol 52:133-136, 1983.

90. Metz S and Keats AS: Benefits of a glucose-containing priming solution for cardiopulmonary bypass, Anesth Analg 72:428-434, 1991.

91. Helgason CM: Blood glucose and stroke, Stroke 19:1049-1053, 1988.

92. Stoney WS, Alford WC Jr, Burrus GR, et al: Air embolism and other accidents using pump oxygenators, Ann Thorac Surg 29:336-340, 1980.

93. Spampinato N, Stassano P, Gagliardi C, et al: Massive air embolism during cardiopulmonary bypass: successful treatment with immediate hypothermia and circulatory support, Ann Thorac Surg 32:602-603, 1981.

94. Ghosh PK, Kaplan O, Barak J, et al: Massive arterial air embolism during cardiopulmonary bypass, J Cardiovasc Surg 26:248-250, 1985.

95. Kurusz M, Shaffer CW, Christman EW, et al: Runaway pump head: new cause of gas embolism during cardiopulmonary bypass, J Thorac Cardiovasc Surg 77:792-795, 1979.

96. Toscano M, Chiavarelli R, Ruvolo G, et al: Management of massive air embolism during open-heart surgery with retrograde perfusion of the cerebral vessels and hyperbaric oxygenation, Thorac Cardiovasc Surg 31:183-184, 1983.

97. Tomatis L, Nemiroff M, Riahi M, et al: Massive arterial air embolism due to rupture of pulsatile assist device: successful treatment in the hyperbaric chamber, Ann Thorac Surg 32:604-608, 1981.

98. Diethrich EB, Koopot R, Maze A, et al: Successful reversal of brain damage from iatrogenic air embolism, Surg Gynecol Obstet 154:572-575, 1982.

99. Brown JW, Dierdorf SF, Moorthy SS, et al: Venoarterial cerebral perfusion for treatment of massive arterial air embolism, Anesth Analg 66:673-674, 1987.

100. Stark J and Hough J: Air in the aorta: treatment by reversed perfusion, Ann Thorac Surg 41:337-338, 1986.

101. Steward D, Williams WG, and Freedom R: Hypothermia in conjunction with hyperbaric oxygenation in the treatment of massive air embolism during cardiopulmonary bypass, Ann Thorac Surg 24:591-593, 1977.

102. Hendriks FFA, Bogers AJJC, de la Riviere AB, et al: The effectiveness of venoarterial perfusion in treatment of arterial air embolism during cardiopulmonary bypass, Ann Thorac Surg 36:433-436, 1983.

103. Reed GI III, Singer DE, Picard EH, et al: Stroke following coronary-artery bypass surgery: a case-control estimate of the risk from carotid bruits, N Engl J Med 319:1246-1250, 1988.

104. Harrison MJG, Schneidau A, Ho R, et al: Cerebrovascular disease and functional outcome after coronary artery bypass surgery, Stroke 20:235-237, 1989.

105. Schultz RD, Sterpetti AV, and Feldhaus RJ: Early and late results in patients with carotid disease undergoing myocardial revascularization, Ann Thorac Surg 45:603-609, 1988.

106. Barnes RW: Asymptomatic carotid disease in patients undergoing major cardiovascular operations: Can prophylactic endarterectomy be justified? Ann Thorac Surg 42(suppl):S36-S40, 1986.

107. Brener BJ, Brief DK, Alpert J, et al: The risk of stroke in patients with asymptomatic carotid stenosis undergoing cardiac surgery: a follow-up study, J Vasc Surg 5:269-279, 1987.

108. Furlan AJ and Craciun AR: Risk of stroke during coronary artery bypass graft surgery in patients with internal carotid artery disease documented by angiography, Stroke 16:797-799, 1985.

109. Ivey TD, Strandness E, Williams DB, et al: Management of patients with carotid bruit undergoing cardiopulmonary bypass, J Thorac Cardiovasc Surg 87:183-189, 1984.

110. Gravlee GP, Cordell AR, Graham JE, et al: Coronary revascularization in patients with bilateral internal carotid occlusions, J Thorac Cardiovasc Surg 90:921-925, 1985.

111. von Reutern G-M, Hetzel A, Birnbaum D, et al: Transcranial Doppler ultrasonography during cardiopulmonary bypass in patients with severe carotid stenosis or occlusion, Stroke 19:674-680, 1988.

112. Brusino FG, Reves JG, Prough DS, et al: Cerebral blood flow during cardiopulmonary bypass in a patient with occlusive cerebrovascular disease, J Cardiothorac Anesth 3:87-90, 1989.

113. Brusino FG, Reves JG, Smith LR, et al: The effect of

age on cerebral blood flow during hypothermic cardiopulmonary bypass, J Thorac Cardiovasc Surg 97:541-547, 1989.

114. Hammeke TA and Hastings JE: Neuropsychologic alterations after cardiac operation, J Thorac Cardiovasc Surg 96:326-331, 1988.

115. Shaw PJ, Bates D, Cartlidge NEF, et al: Early intellectual dysfunction following coronary bypass surgery, Q J Med 58:59-68, 1986.

116. Raymond M, Conklin C, Schaeffer J, et al: Coping with transient intellectual dysfunction after coronary bypass surgery, Heart Lung 13:531-539, 1984.

117. Smith PL, Treasure T, Newman SP, et al: Cerebral consequences of cardiopulmonary bypass, Lancet 1:823-825, 1986.

118. Shaw PJH, Bates D, Cartlidge NEF, et al: Neurologic and neuropsychological morbidity following major surgery: comparison of coronary artery bypass and peripheral vascular surgery, Stroke 18:700-707, 1987.

119. Townes BD, Bashein G, Hornbein TF, et al: Neurobehavioral outcomes in cardiac operations: a prospective controlled study, J Thorac Cardiovasc Surg 98:774-782, 1989.

120. Goy M, Schmitt R, Sabatier M, et al: Retentissement des interventions à cœur ouvert sur l'efficience intellectuelle, Arch Mal Cœur 77:167-173, 1984.

121. Ellis RJ, Wisniewski A, Pott R, et al: Reduction of flow rate and arterial pressure at moderate hypothermia does not result in cerebral dysfunction, J Thorac Cardiovasc Surg 79:173-180, 1980.

122. Fish KJ, Helms KN, Sarnquist FH, et al: A prospective randomized study of the effects of prostacyclin on neuropsychological dysfunction after coronary artery surgery, J Thorac Cardiovasc Surg 93:609-615, 1987.

123. Savageau J, Stanton BA, Jenkins CD, et al: Neuropsychological dysfunction following elective cardiac operation: a six-month reassessment, J Thorac Cardiovasc Surg 84:595-600, 1982.

124. Aberg T, Ronquist G, Tyden H, et al: Release of adenylate kinase into cerebrospinal fluid during open-heart surgery and its relation to postoperative intellectual function, Lancet 1:1139-1142, 1982.

125. Arén C, Blomstrand C, Wikkelsö C, et al: Hypotension induced by prostacyclin treatment during cardiopulmonary bypass does not increase the risk of cerebral complications, J Thorac Cardiovasc Surg 88:748-753, 1984.

126. Blauth CI, Arnold JV, Schulenberg WE, et al: Cerebral microembolism during cardiopulmonary bypass: retinal microvascular studies in vivo with fluorescein angiography, J Thorac Cardiovasc Surg 95:668-676, 1988.

127. Taylor KM: Brain damage during open-heart surgery, Thorax 37:873-876, 1982.

128. Blauth CI, Smith PL, Arnold JV, et al: Influence of oxygenator type on the prevalence and extent of microembolic retinal ischemia during cardiopulmonary bypass: assessment by digital image analysis, J Thorac Cardiovasc Surg 99:61-69, 1990.

129. Padayachee TS, Parsons S, Linley RTJ, et al: The detection of microemboli in the middle cerebral artery during cardiopulmonary bypass: a transcranial Doppler ultrasound investigation using membrane and bubble oxygenators, Ann Thorac Surg 44:298-302, 1987.

130. Padayachee TS, Parsons S, Theobold R, et al: The effect of arterial filtration on reduction of gaseous microemboli in the middle cerebral artery during cardiopulmonary bypass, Ann Thorac Surg 45:647-649, 1988.

131. Stockard JJ, Bickford RG, and Schauble JF: Pressure-dependent cerebral ischemia during cardiopulmonary bypass, Neurology 23:521-529, 1973.

132. Stockard JJ, Bickford RG, Myers RR, et al: Hypotension-induced changes in cerebral function during cardiac surgery, Stroke 5:730-746, 1974.

133. Murkin JM, Farrar JK, Tweed WA, et al: Cerebral autoregulation and flow/metabolism coupling during cardiopulmonary bypass: the influence of $Paco_2$, Anesth Analg 66:825-832, 1987.

134. Nevin M, Adams S, Colchester ACF, et al: Evidence for involvement of hypocapnia and hypoperfusion in aetiology of neurological deficit after cardiopulmonary bypass, Lancet 2:1493-1495, 1987.

135. Gallagher EG and Pearson DT: Ultrasonic identification of sources of gaseous microemboli during open heart surgery, Thorax 28:295-305, 1973.

136. Solis RT, Noon GP, Beall AC, et al: Particulate microembolism during cardiac operation, Ann Thorac Surg 17:332-344, 1974.

137. Pedersen TH, Karlsen HM, Semb G, et al: Comparison of bubble release from various types of oxygenators, Scand J Thorac Cardiovasc Surg 21:73-80, 1987.

138. Knopp EA, Baumann G, Pratt D, et al: Release of particulate matter from extracorporeal tubing: ineffectiveness of standard arterial line filters during bypass, J Cardiovasc Surg 23:470-476, 1982.

139. Clark RE, Dietz DR, and Miller JG: Continuous detection of microemboli during cardiopulmonary bypass in animals and man, Circulation 54(suppl III):74-78, 1976.

140. Henriksen L and Hjelms E: Cerebral blood flow during cardiopulmonary bypass in man: effect of arterial filtration, Thorax 41:386-395, 1986.

141. Aris A, Solanes H, Camara ML, et al: Arterial line filtration during cardiopulmonary bypass: neurologic, neuropsychologic, and hematologic studies, J Thorac Cardiovasc Surg 91:525-533, 1986.

142. Javid H, Tufo HM, Najafi H, et al: Neurological abnormalities following open heart surgery, J Thorac Cardiovasc Surg 58:502-509, 1969.

143. Tufo HM, Osfeld AM, and Shekelle R: Central nervous system dysfunction following open heart surgery, JAMA 212:1333-1340, 1970.

144. Gordon RJ, Ravin M, Rawitscher RE, et al: Changes in arterial pressure, viscosity, and resistance during cardiopulmonary bypass, J Thorac Cardiovasc Surg 69:552-561, 1975.

145. Slogoff S, Reul GJ, Keats AS, et al: Role of perfusion pressure and flow in major organ dysfunction after cardiopulmonary bypass, Ann Thorac Surg 50:911-918, 1990.

146. Govier AV, Reves JG, McKay RD, et al: Factors and their influence on regional cerebral blood flow during nonpulsatile cardiopulmonary bypass, Ann Thorac Surg 38:592-600, 1984.

147. Shaw PJ, Bates D, Cartlidge NEF, et al: An analysis of factors predisposing to neurological injury in patients undergoing coronary bypass operations, Q J Med 72:633-646, 1989.

148. Soma Y, Hirotani T, Yozu R, et al: A clinical study of cerebral circulation during extracorporeal circulation, J Thorac Cardiovasc Surg 97:187-193, 1989.

149. Rogers AT, Stump DA, Gravlee GP, et al: Response of cerebral blood flow to phenylephrine infusion during hypothermic cardiopulmonary bypass: influence of $Paco_2$ management, Anesthesiology 69:547-551, 1988.

150. Henriksen L: Brain luxury perfusion during cardiopulmonary bypass in humans: a study of the cerebral

blood flow response to changes in CO_2, O_2, and blood pressure, J Cereb Blood Flow Metab 6:366-378, 1986.

151. Prough DS, Stump DA, Roy RC, et al: Response of cerebral blood flow to changes in carbon dioxide tension during hypothermic cardiopulmonary bypass, Anesthesiology 64:576-581, 1986.

152. Prough DS, Rogers AT, Stump DA, et al: Hypercarbia depresses cerebral oxygen consumption during cardiopulmonary bypass, Stroke 21:1162-1166, 1990.

153. Murkin JM: Cerebral hyperfusion during cardiopulmonary bypass: the influence of Pa_{CO_2}. In Hilberman M, editor: Brain injury and protection during heart surgery, Boston, 1988, Martinus Nijhoff Publishers.

154. Bashein G, Townes BD, Nessly ML, et al: A randomized study of carbon dioxide management during hypothermic cardiopulmonary bypass, Anesthesiology 72:7-15, 1990.

155. Gravlee GP, Roy RC, Stump DA, et al: Regional cerebrovascular reactivity to carbon dioxide during cardiopulmonary bypass in patients with cerebrovascular disease, J Thorac Cardiovasc Surg 99:1022-1029, 1990.

156. Prough DS, Stump DA, and Troost BT: Pa_{CO_2} management during cardiopulmonary bypass: intriguing physiologic rationale, convincing clinical data, evolving hypothesis? Anesthesiology 72:3-6, 1990.

157. Rebeyka IM, Coles JG, Wilson GJ, et al: The effect of low-flow cardiopulmonary bypass on cerebral function: an experimental and clinical study, Ann Thorac Surg 43:391-396, 1987.

158. Shevde K and DeBois WJ: Pro: Pulsatile flow is preferable to nonpulsatile flow during cardiopulmonary bypass, J Cardiothorac Anesth 1:165-168, 1987.

159. Finlayson DC: Con: Nonpulsatile flow is preferable to pulsatile flow during cardiopulmonary bypass, J Cardiothorac Anesth 1:169-170, 1987.

160. Hickey PR, Buckley MJ, and Philbin DM: Pulsatile and nonpulsatile bypass: review of a counterproductive controversy, Ann Thorac Surg 36:720-737, 1983.

161. Watanabe T, Orita H, Kobayashi M, et al: Brain tissue pH, oxygen tension, and carbon dioxide tension in profoundly hypothermic cardiopulmonary bypass: comparative study of circulatory arrest, nonpulsatile low-flow perfusion, and pulsatile low-flow perfusion, J Thorac Cardiovasc Surg 97:396-401, 1989.

162. Sanderson JM, Wright G, and Sims FW: Brain damage in dogs immediately following pulsatile and nonpulsatile blood flows in extracorporeal circulation, Thorax 27:275-285, 1972.

163. Anderson K, Waaben J, Husum B, et al: Nonpulsatile cardiopulmonary bypass disrupts the flow-metabolism couple in the brain, J Thorac Cardiovasc Surg 90:570-578, 1985.

164. Berryessa RG, and Tyndal CM: Perfusion techniques that may decrease brain injury during cardiopulmonary bypass. In Hilberman M, editor: Brain injury and protection during heart surgery, Boston, 1988, Martinus Nijhoff Publishers.

165. Sotaniemi KA, Mononen H, and Hokkanen TE: Long-term cerebral outcome after open-heart surgery, Stroke 17:410-416, 1986.

166. Kirklin JW and Barratt-Boyes: Hypothermia, circulatory arrest, and cardiopulmonary bypass. In Kirklin JW and Barratt-Boyes BG, editors: Cardiac surgery, New York, 1986, John Wiley & Sons.

167. Hickey PR and Anderson NP: Deep hypothermic circulatory arrest: a review of pathophysiology and clinical experience as a basis for anesthetic management, J Cardiothorac Anesth 1:137-155, 1987.

168. Muraoka R, Yokota M, Aoshima M, et al: Subclinical changes in brain morphology following cardiac operations as reflected by computed tomographic scans of the brain, J Thorac Cardiovasc Surg 81:364-369, 1981.

169. Kramer RS, Sanders AP, Lesage AM, et al: The effect of profound hypothermia on preservation of cerebral ATP content during circulatory arrest, J Thorac Cardiovasc Surg 56:699-709, 1968.

170. Fisk GC, Wright JS, Hicks RG, et al: The influence of duration of circulatory arrest at 20° C on cerebral changes, Anesth Intensive Care 4:126-134, 1976.

171. Treasure T, Naftel DC, Conger KA, et al: The effect of hypothermic circulatory arrest time on cerebral function, morphology, and biochemistry, J Thorac Cardiovasc Surg 86:761-770, 1983.

172. Haneda K, Thomas R, Sands MP, et al: Whole body protection during three hours of total circulatory arrest: an experimental study, Cryobiology 23:483-494, 1986.

173. Zingg W and Kantor S: Observations on the temperature in the brain during extracorporeal differential hypothermia, Surgical Forum 11:192-193, 1960.

174. Molina JE, Einzig S, Mastri AR, et al: Brain damage in profound hypothermia: perfusion versus circulatory arrest, J Thorac Cardiovasc Surg 87:596-604, 1984.

175. Barratt-Boyes BG, Neutze JM, Clarkson P, et al: Repair of ventricular septal defect in the first two years of life using profound hypothermic-circulatory arrest techniques, Ann Surg 184:376-390, 1976.

176. Ehyai A, Fenichel GM, and Bender HW: Incidence and prognosis of seizures in infants after cardiac surgery with profound hypothermia and circulatory arrest, JAMA 252:3165-3167, 1984.

177. Brunberg JA, Reilly EL, and Doty DB: Central nervous system consequences in infants of cardiac surgery using deep hypothermia and circulatory arrest, Circulation 50(suppl II):60-68, 1974.

178. Clarkson PM, MacArthur BA, Barratt-Boyes BG, et al: Developmental progress following cardiac surgery in infancy using profound hypothermia and circulatory arrest, Circulation 62:855-861, 1980.

179. Stewart RW, Blackstone EH, and Kirklin JW: Neurological dysfunction after cardiac surgery. In Parenzan L, Crupi G, and Graham G, editors: Congenital heart disease in the first three months of life: medical and surgical aspects, Bologna, Italy, 1981, Patron Editore.

180. Egerton N, Egerton WS, and Kay JH: Neurologic changes following profound hypothermia, Ann Surg 157:366-374, 1963.

181. Wright JS, Hicks RG, and Newman DC: Deep hypothermic arrest: observations on later development in children, J Thorac Cardiovasc Surg 77:466-468, 1979.

182. Wells FC, Coghill S, Caplan HL, et al: Duration of circulatory arrest does influence the psychological development of children after cardiac operation in early life, J Thorac Cardiovasc Surg 86:823-831, 1983.

183. Messmer BJ, Schallberger U, Gattiker R, et al: Psychomotor and intellectual development after deep hypothermia and circulatory arrest in early infancy, J Thorac Cardiovasc Surg 72:495-502, 1976.

184. Dickinson DF and Sambrooks JE: Intellectual performance in children after circulatory arrest with profound hypothermia in infancy, Arch Dis Child 54:1-6, 1979.

185. Haka-Ikse K, Blackwood MJA, and Steward DJ: Psychomotor development of infants and children after profound hypothermia during surgery for congenital

heart disease, Dev Med Child Neurol 20:62-70, 1978.

186. Ergin MA, O'Connor J, Guinto R, et al: Experience with profound hypothermia and circulatory arrest in the treatment of aneurysms of the aortic arch, J Thorac Cardiovasc Surg 84:649-655, 1982.

187. Lundar T, Froysaker T, and Nornes H: Cerebral damage following open-heart surgery in deep hypothermia and circulatory arrest, Scand J Thorac Cardiovasc Surg 17:237-242, 1983.

188. Luosto R, Maamies T, Peltola K, et al: Hypothermia and circulatory arrest in reconstruction of aortic arch: a report of nine cases, Scand J Thorac Cardiovasc Surg 21:113-117, 1987.

189. Sweeney MS, Cooley DA, Reul GJ, et al: Hypothermic circulatory arrest for cardiovascular lesions: technical considerations and results, Ann Thorac Surg 40:498-503, 1985.

190. Silverberg GD, Reitz BA, and Ream AK: Hypothermia and cardiac arrest in the treatment of giant aneurysms of the cerebral circulation and hemangioblastoma of the medulla, J Neurosurg 55:337-346, 1981.

191. Baumgartner WA, Silverberg GD, Ream AK, et al: Reappraisal of cardiopulmonary bypass with deep hypothermia and circulatory arrest for complex neurosurgical operations, Surgery 94:242-249, 1983.

192. O'Connor JV, Wilding T, Farmer P, et al: The protective effect of profound hypothermia on the canine central nervous system during one hour of circulatory arrest, Ann Thorac Surg 41:255-259, 1986.

193. Busija DW and Leffler CW: Hypothermia reduces cerebral metabolic rate and cerebral blood flow in newborn pigs, Am J Physiol 253:H869-H873, 1987.

194. Norwood WI, Norwood CR, and Castaneda AR: Cerebral anoxia: effect of deep hypothermia and pH, Surgery 86:203-209, 1979.

195. Harden A, Pampiglione G, and Waterston DJ: Circulatory arrest during hypothermia in cardiac surgery: an EEG study in children, Br Med J 2:1105-1108, 1966.

196. Weiss M, Weiss J, Cotton J, et al: A study of the electroencephalogram during surgery with deep hypothermia and circulatory arrest in infants, J Thorac Cardiovasc Surg 70:316-329, 1975.

197. Cohen ME, Olszowka JS, and Subramanian S: Electroencephalographic and neurological correlates of deep hypothermia and circulatory arrest in infants, Ann Thorac Surg 23:238-244, 1977.

198. Hicks RG and Poole JL: Electroencephalographic changes with hypothermia and cardiopulmonary bypass in children, J Thorac Cardiovasc Surg 81:781-786, 1981.

199. Coselli JS, Crawford ES, Beall AC, et al: Determination of brain temperatures for safe circulatory arrest during cardiovascular operation, Ann Thorac Surg 45:638-642, 1988.

200. Mizrahi EM, Patel VM, Crawford ES, et al: Hypothermic-induced electrocerebral silence, prolonged circulatory arrest, and cerebral protection during cardiovascular surgery, Electroencephalogr Clin Neurophysiol 72:81-85, 1989.

201. Tharion J, Johnson DC, Celermajer JM, et al: Profound hypothermia with circulatory arrest: nine years clinical experience, J Thorac Cardiovasc Surg 84:66-72, 1982.

202. Rossi R, Ekroth R, and Thompson RJ: No flow or low flow? A study of the ischemic marker creatine kinase BB after deep hypothermic procedures, J Thorac Cardiovasc Surg 98:193-199, 1989.

203. Greeley WJ, Ungerleider RM, Kern FH, et al: Effects of cardiopulmonary bypass on cerebral blood flow in neonates, infants, and children, Circulation 80(suppl I):I-210–215, 1989.

204. Steward DJ, Da Silva C, and Flegel T: Elevated blood glucose levels may increase the danger of neurological deficit following profoundly hypothermic cardiac arrest, Anesthesiology 68:653, 1988.

205. Zucker HA, Nicolson SC, Steven JM, et al: Blood glucose concentrations during anesthesia in children undergoing hypothermic circulatory arrest, Anesthesiology 69:A739, 1988.

206. Breuer AC, Furlan AJ, Hanson MR, et al: Neurologic complications of open heart surgery: computer-assisted analysis of 531 patients, Cleve Clin Q 48:205-206, 1980.

207. Hanson MR, Breuer AC, Furlan AJ, et al: Mechanism and frequency of brachial plexus injury in open-heart surgery: a prospective analysis, Ann Thorac Surg 36:675-679, 1983.

208. Seyfer AE, Grammer NY, Bogumill GP, et al: Upper extremity neuropathies after cardiac surgery, J Hand Surg 10:16-19, 1985.

209. Vander Salm TJ, Cutler BS, and Okike ON: Brachial plexus injury following median sternotomy: Part II, J Thorac Cardiovasc Surg 83:914-917, 1982.

210. Wey JM and Guinn GA: Ulnar nerve injury with open-heart surgery, Ann Thorac Surg 39:358-360, 1985.

211. Markand ON, Moorthy SS, Mahomed Y, et al: Postoperative phrenic nerve palsy in patients with open-heart surgery, Ann Thorac Surg 39:68-73, 1985.

212. Gray R et al: Low cardiac output states after open heart surgery, Chest 80:16, 1981.

213. McGee MG et al: Retrospective analyses of the need for mechanical circulatory support (intra-aortic balloon pump/abdominal left ventricular assist device or partial artificial heart) after cardiopulmonary bypass, Am J Cardiol 46:135, 1980.

214. DePaulis R et al: The total artificial heart: indications and preliminary results, J Cardiovasc Surg 2:275, 1987.

215. Larach DR: Anesthetic management during cardiopulmonary bypass. In Hensley FA and Martin DE, editors: The practice of cardiac anesthesia, Boston, 1990, Little, Brown & Co.

216. Watson BG: Unilateral cold neck: a new sign of misplacement of the aortic cannula during cardiopulmonary bypass, Anaesthesia 38:659-681, 1983.

217. Krous HF, Mansfield PB, and Sauvage LR: Carotid hyperperfusion during open heart surgery, J Thorac Cardiovasc Surg 66:118-121, 1973.

218. Ross WT, Lake CL, and Wellons HA: Cardiopulmonary bypass complicated by inadvertent carotid cannulation, Anesthesiology 54:85-86, 1981.

219. Chapin JW and Yarbrough JW: Facial paleness, Anesth Analg 61:475, 1982 (Letter).

220. Dalal FY and Patel KD: Another sign of inadvertent carotid cannulation Anesthesiology 55:487, 1981 (Letter).

221. McLesky CH and Cheney FW: A correctable complication of cardiopulmonary bypass Anesthesiology 56:214-216, 1982.

222. Jobes DR, Schwartz, Ellison N, et al: Monitoring heparin anticoagulation and its neutralization, Ann Thorac Surg 31:161-166, 1981.

223. Bull BS, Korpman RA, Huse WM, et al: Heparin therapy during extracorporeal circulation, I. J Thorac Cardiovasc Surg 69:674-684, 1975.

224. Young JA, Kisker CT, and Doty DB: Adequate anticoagulation during cardiopulmonary bypass determined by activated clotting time and the appearance of fibrin monomer, Ann Thorac Surg 26:231-240, 1978.

225. Cardoso PFG, Yamazake F, Keshavjee S, et al: A re-evaluation of heparin requirements for cardiopulmonary bypass, J Thorac Cardiovasc Surg 101:153-160, 1991.

226. Metz S and Keats AS: Low activated coagulation time during cardiopulmonary bypass does not increase postoperative bleeding, Ann Thorac Surg 49:440-444, 1990.

227. Gravlee GP, Haddon S, Rothberger HK, et al: Heparin dosing and monitoring for cardiopulmonary bypass: a comparison of techniques with measurement of subclinical plasma coagulation, J Thorac Cardiovasc Surg 99:518-527, 1990.

228. Lytle BW et al: Perioperative risk of bilateral internal mammary artery grafting: analysis of 500 cases from 1971-1984, Circulation 74(5 Pt 2):III-37, 1986.

229. McGregor CGA et al: Myocardial infarction related to valve replacement surgery, Br Heart J 51:612, 1984.

230. Akins CW: Early and late results following emergency isolated myocardial revascularization during hypothermic fibrillatory arrest, Ann Thorac Surg 43:131, 1987.

231. Loop FD et al: An 11-year evolution of coronary arterial surgery (1967-1978), Ann Surg 190:444, 1979.

232. Leung JM et al: Prognostic importance of postbypass regional wall-motion abnormalities in patients undergoing coronary artery bypass graft surgery, Anesthesiology 71:16-25, 1989.

233. Mangano DT: Perioperative cardiac morbidity, Anesthesiology 72:253-184, 1990 [Review].

234. Nussmeier NA, and Slogoff S: Verapamil treatment of intraoperative coronary artery spasm, Anesthesiology 62:539-541, 1985.

235. Kennedy JW et al: Clinical and angiographic predictors of operative mortality from the collaborative study in Coronary Artery Surgery (CASS), Circulation 63:793-802, 1981.

236. Braunwald E, and Rutherford JD: Reversible ischemic left ventricular dysfunction: evidence for the "hibernating myocardium," J Am Coll Cardiol 8:1467, 1986.

237. Ellis SG et al: Response of reperfusion-salvaged, stunned myocardium to inotropic stimulation, Am Heart J 107:13, 1984.

238. Oldham HN: Complications of cardiac surgery and trauma. In Greenfield LJ, editor: Complications in surgery and trauma, Philadelphia, 1990, JB Lippincott. Co.

239. Lichtenstein SV, Ashe KA, El Dalati H, et al: Warm heart surgery, J Thorac Cardiovasc Surg 101:269-274, 1991.

240. Bolli R et al: Attenuation of dysfunction in the postischemic "stunned" myocardium by dimethylthiourea, Circulation 76:458, 1987.

241. Buckberg GD: Strategies and logic of cardioplegic delivery to prevent, avoid, and reverse ischemic and reperfusion damage, J Thorac Cardiovasc Surg 93:127, 1987.

242. Daggett WM et al: The superiority of cold oxygenated dilute blood cardioplegia, Ann Thorac Surg 43:397, 1987.

243. Johnson DL et al: Free radical scavengers improve functional recovery of stunned myocardium in a model of surgical coronary revascularization, Surgery 102:334, 1987.

244. Otani H et al: Cardiac performance during reperfusion improved by pretreatment with oxygen free-radical scavengers, J Thorac Cardiovasc Surg 91:290, 1986.

245. Pasque MK and Wechsler AS: Metabolic intervention to affect myocardial recovery following ischemia, Ann Surg 200:1, 1984.

246. Stewart JR et al: Free radical scavengers and myocardial preservation during transplantation, Ann Thorac Surg 42:390, 1986.

247. Zumbro GL et al: Mechanical assistance for cardiogenic shock following cardiac surgery, myocardial infarction, and cardiac transplantation, Ann Thorac Surg 44:11, 1987.

248. Pace WE et al: Long-term results of ventricular assist pumping in postcardiogenic shock, J Thorac Cardiovasc Surg 93:434, 1987.

249. Conahan TJ: Complications of cardiac surgery. In Kaplan JA, editor: Cardiac anesthesia, ed 2, New York, 1987, Grune & Stratton, Inc.

250. Horrow JC: Protamine: a review of its toxicity, Anesth Analg 64:348-361, 1985.

251. Morel DR, Zapol WM, Thomas SJ, et al: C5a and thromboxane generation associated with pulmonary vaso- and broncho-constriction during protamine reversal of heparin, Anesthesiology 66:597-604, 1987.

252. Best N, Sinosich MJ, Teisner B, et al: Complement activation during cardiopulmonary bypass by heparin-protamine interaction, Br J Anaesth 56:339-343, 1984.

253. Colman RW: Humoral mediators of catastrophic reactions associated with protamine neutralization, Anesthesiology 66:595-596, 1987.

254. Cavarocchi NC, Schaff HV, Orszulak TA, et al: Evidence for complement activation by protamine-heparin interaction after cardiopulmonary bypass, Surgery 98:525-530, 1985.

255. Kirklin JK, Chenoweth DE, Naftel DC, et al: Effects of protamine administration after cardiopulmonary bypass on complement, blood elements, and the hemodynamic state, Ann Thorac Surg 41:193-199, 1986.

256. Lowenstein E, Johnston WE, Lappas DG, et al: Catastrophic pulmonary vasoconstriction associated with protamine reversal of heparin, Anesthesiology 59:470-473, 1983.

257. Levy JH, Schwieger IM, Zaidan JR, et al: Evaluation of patients at risk for protamine reactions, J Thorac Cardiovasc Surg 98:200-204, 1989.

258. Lake CL: Anesthesia and pericardial disease, Anesth Analg 62:431-443, 1983.

259. Gallagher JD, Moore RA, McNicholas KW, et al: Comparison of radial and femoral arterial blood pressure in children after cardiopulmonary bypass, J Clin Monitor 1:168-171, 1985.

260. Mohr R, Lavee J, and Goor DA: Inaccuracy of radial artery pressure measurement after cardiac operations, J Thorac Cardiovasc Surg 94:286-290, 1987.

261. Stern DH, Gerson JI, Allen FB, et al: Can we trust the direct radial artery pressure immediately following cardiopulmonary bypass? Anesthesiology 62:557-571, 1985.

262. Pauca AL, Hudspeth AS, Wallenhaupt SL, et al: Radial artery-to-aorta pressure difference after discontinuation of cardiopulmonary bypass, Anesthesiology 70:935-941, 1989.

263. Salerno TA, Henderson M, Keith FM, et al: Hypertension after coronary operation, J Thorac Cardiovasc Surg 81:396-399, 1981.

264. Estafanous FG, and Tarazi RC: Systemic arterial hypertension associated with cardiac surgery, Am J Cardiol 46:685-694, 1980.

265. Gray RJ: Postcardiac surgical hypertension, J Cardiothorac Anesth 2:678-682, 1988.

266. Reves JG: Adrenergic response to cardiopulmonary bypass, Mt Sinai J Med 52:511-515, 1985.

267. Engelman RM, Haag B, Lemeshaw S, et al: Mechanism of plasma catecholamine increases during coronary artery bypass and valve procedures, J Thorac Cardiovasc Surg 86:608-615, 1983.

268. Reves JG, Karp RB, Buttner EE, et al: Neuronal and adrenomedullary catecholamine release in response to cardiopulmonary bypass in man, Circulation 66:49-55, 1982.

269. Wallach R, Karp RB, Reves JG, et al: Pathogenesis of paroxysmal hypertension developing during and after coronary bypass surgery: a study of hemodynamic and humoral factors, Am J Cardiol 46:559, 1980.

270. Samuelson PN, Reves JG, Kirklin JK, et al: Comparison of sufentanil and enflurane–nitrous oxide anesthesia for myocardial revascularization, Anesth Analg 65:217-226, 1986.

271. Flezzani P, Croughwell N, McIntyre RW, et al: Isoflurane decreases the cortisol response to cardiopulmonary bypass, Anesth Analg 65:1117-1122, 1986.

272. Reves JG, and Flezzani P: Perioperative uses of esmolol, Am J Cardiol 56:57F-62F, 1985.

273. Gray RJ, Bateman TB, Czer LSC, et al: Comparison of esmolol and nitroprusside for acute post–cardiac surgical hypertension, Am J Cardiol 59:887-892, 1987.

274. Flaherty JT, Magee PA, Gardner TL, et al: Comparison of intravenous nitroglycerin and sodium nitroprusside for treatment of acute hypertension developing after coronary artery bypass surgery, Circulation 65:1072-1077, 1982.

275. Morel DR, Forster A, and Suter PM: IV labetalol in the treatment of hypertension following coronary artery surgery, Br J Anaesth 54:1191-1196, 1982.

276. Flacke JW, Bloor BC, Flacke WE, et al: Reduced narcotic requirement by clonidine with improved hemodynamic and adrenergic stability in patients undergoing coronary bypass surgery, Anesthesiology 67:11-19, 1987.

277. Morris JJ, Hamm DP, Pellom GL, et al: Right ventricular sensitivity to metabolic injury during cardiopulmonary bypass, Arch Surg 121:338-344, 1986.

278. Christakis GT, Weisel RD, Mickle DAG, et al: Right ventricular function and metabolism, Circulation 82(suppl IV):IV-332–IV-340, 1990.

279. Rich JB, Akins CW, and Daggett WM: Right ventricular failure following cardiopulmonary bypass: Inadequate myocardial protection or incomplete revascularization? Ann Thorac Surg 45:693-696, 1988.

280. D'Ambra MN, LaRaia PJ, Philbin DM, et al: Prostaglandin E: a new therapy for refractory right heart failure and pulmonary hypertension after mitral valve replacement, J Thorac Cardiovasc Surg 89:567-572, 1985.

281. Bertrand CA et al: Disturbances of cardiac rhythm during anesthesia and surgery, JAMA 216:1615-1617, 1971.

282. Karis JH: Atrioventricular block after coronary artery bypass grafting. In Reves JG and Hall KD, editors: Common problems in cardiac anesthesia, Chicago, 1987, Year Book Medical Publishers, Inc.

283. Michelson EL, Morganroth J, and MacVaugh H: Postoperative arrhythmias after coronary artery and cardiac valvular surgery detected by long term electrocardiographic monitoring, Am Heart J 97:442-448, 1979.

284. Ellis RJ, Mavroudis C, Gardner C, et al: Relationship between atrioventricular arrhythmias and the concentration of K^+ ion in cardioplegic solution, J Thorac Cardiovasc Surg 80:517-526, 1980.

285. Smith PK et al: Supraventricular conduction abnormalities following cardiac operations, J Thorac Cardiovasc Surg 85:105-115, 1983.

286. Hirayama T et al: Association between arrhythmias and reduced red cell deformability following cardiopulmonary bypass, Scand J Thorac Cardiovasc Surg 22:179-180, 1988.

287. Smith R et al: Arrhythmias following cardiac valve replacement, Circulation 45:1018-23, 1972.

288. Dewar ML et al: Perioperative Holter monitoring and computer analysis of dysrhythmias in cardiac surgery, Chest 87:593-597, 1985.

289. Leitch JW: The importance of age as a predictor of atrial fibrillation and flutter after coronary artery bypass grafting, J Thorac Cardiovasc Surg 100:338-342, 1990.

290. Hashimoto K, Ilstrup DM, and Schaff HV: Influence of clinical and hemodynamic variables on risk of supraventricular tachycardia after coronary artery bypass, J Thorac Cardiovasc Surg 101:56-65, 1991.

291. Hartzler GO et al: Hemodynamic benefits of atrioventricular sequential pacing after cardiac surgery, Am J Cardiol 40:232-236, 1977.

292. Bagdonas AA et al: Effects of ischemia and hypoxia on the specialized conducting system of the canine heart, Am Heart J 61:206-281, 1961.

293. Rosenfelt FL and Watson DA: II. Interference with local myocardial cooling by heat gain during aortic cross-clamping, Ann Thorac Surg 27:1:13-16, 1979.

294. Holley FO, Ponganis KV, and Stanski DR: Effect of cardiopulmonary bypass on the pharmacokinetics of drugs, Clin Pharm 7:234-251, 1982.

295. Shiroka A, Rah KH, and Keenan RL: Bronchospasm during cardiopulmonary bypass, Anesth Analg 61:538-540, 1982.

296. Kyösola K, Takkunen O, Maamies T, et al: Bronchospasm during cardiopulmonary bypass: a potentially fatal complication of open-heart surgery, Thorac Cardiovasc Surg 35:375-377, 1987.

297. Tuman KJ, and Ivankovish AD: Bronchospasm during cardiopulmonary bypass: etiology and management, Chest 90:635-637, 1986.

298. Casella ES, and Humphrey LS: Bronchospasm after cardiopulmonary bypass in a heart-lung transplant recipient, Anesthesiology 69:135-138, 1988.

299. Matthay MA, and Wiener-Kronish JP: Respiratory management after cardiac surgery, Chest 95:424-432, 1989.

300. Korsten HHM, Spierduk LJ, Beneken JEW, et al: Pulmonary shunting after cardiopulmonary bypass, Eur Heart J 10:17-21, 1989.

301. Bermudez J, and Lichtiger M: Increases in arterial to end-tidal CO_2 tension differences after cardiopulmonary bypass, Anesth Analg 66:690-692, 1987.

302. Kirklin JK: The postperfusion syndrome: inflammation and the damaging effects of cardiopulmonary bypass. In Tinker JH, editor: Cardiopulmonary bypass: current concepts and controversies, Philadelphia, 1989, WB Saunders Co.

303. Howard RJ, Crain C, Franzini DA, et al: Effects of cardiopulmonary bypass on pulmonary leukostasis and complement activation, Arch Surg 123:1496-1501, 1988.

304. Asada S, and Yamaguchi M: Fine structural change in the lung following cardiopulmonary bypass, Chest 59:478-483, 1971.

305. Knudsen F, and Anderson LW: Immunological aspects of cardiopulmonary bypass, J Cardiothorac Anesth 4:245-258, 1990.

306. Ratliff NB, Young WG, Hackel DB, et al: Pulmonary injury secondary to extracor   ' circulation, J Tho-

rac Cardiovasc Surg 65:425-432, 1973.

307. Flick MR, Perel A, and Staub NC: Leukocytes are required for increased lung microvascular permeability after microembolization in sheep, Circ Res 48:344, 1981.

308. Chenoweth DE, Cooper SW, Hugli TE, et al: Complement activation during cardiopulmonary bypass: evidence for generation of C3a and C5a anaphylatoxins, N Engl J Med 304:497-503, 1981.

309. van Oeveren W, Kazatchkine MD, Descamps-Latscha B, et al: Deleterious effects of cardiopulmonary bypass: a prospective study of bubble versus membrane oxygenation, J Thorac Cardiovasc Surg 89:888-899, 1985.

310. Royston D, Fleming JS, Desai JB, et al: Increased production of peroxidation products associated with cardiac operations, J Thorac Cardiovasc Surg 91:759-766, 1986.

311. Kharazmi A, Andersen LW, Baek L, et al: Endotoxemia and enhanced generation of oxygen radicals by neutrophils from patients undergoing cardiopulmonary bypass, J Thorac Cardiovasc Surg 98:381-385, 1989.

312. Bando K, Pillai R, Cameron DE, et al: Leukocyte depletion ameliorates free radical–mediated lung injury after cardiopulmonary bypass, J Thorac Cardiovasc Surg 99:873-877, 1990.

313. Edmunds LH, and Alexander JA: Effect of cardiopulmonary bypass on the lungs. In Fishman AP, editor: Pulmonary disease and disorders, New York, 1980, McGraw-Hill Book Co.

314. Kirklin JK, Westaby S, Blackstone EH, et al: Complement and the damaging effects of cardiopulmonary bypass, J Thorac Cardiovasc Surg 86:845-847, 1983.

315. Tennenberg SD, Clardy CW, Bailey WW, et al: Complement activation and lung permeability during cardiopulmonary bypass, Ann Thorac Surg 50:597-601, 1990.

316. Maggart M, and Stewart S: The mechanisms and management of noncardiogenic pulmonary edema following cardiopulmonary bypass, Ann Thorac Surg 43:231-236, 1987.

317. Hashim SW: Noncardiogenic pulmonary edema after cardiopulmonary bypass, Am J Surg 147:560-564, 1984.

318. Latson TW, Kickler TS, and Baumgartner WA: Pulmonary hypertension and noncardiogenic pulmonary edema following cardiopulmonary bypass associated with an antigranulocyte antibody, Anesthesiology 64:106-111, 1986.

319. Pilato MA, Fleming NW, Katz NM, et al: Treatment of non-cardiogenic pulmonary edema following cardiopulmonary bypass with veno-venous extracorporeal membrane oxygenation, Anesthesiology 69:609-614, 1988.

320. Hilberman M et al: Acute renal failure following cardiac surgery, J Thorac Cardiovasc Surg 77:880-888, 1979.

321. Bhat JG et al: Renal failure after open heart surgery, Ann Intern Med 84:677-682, 1976.

322. Abel RM et al: Etiology, incidence, and prognosis of renal failure following cardiac operations, J Thorac Cardiovasc Surg 71:323-333, 1976.

323. Gailiunas IP et al: Acute renal failure following cardiac operations, J Thorac Cardiovasc Surg 79:241-243, 1980.

324. Heikkinen L, Harjula A, and Merikallio E: Acute renal failure related to open-heart surgery, Ann Chir Gynaecol 74:203-209, 1985.

325. Porter GA et al: Renal complications associated with valve replacement surgery, J Thorac Cardiovasc Surg 53:145-152, 1967.

326. Lange HW, Aeppli DM, and Brown DC: Survival of patients with acute renal failure requiring dialysis after open heart surgery: early prognostic indicators, Am Heart J 113:1138-1143, 1987.

327. Porter GA et al.: Relationship between alterations in renal hemodynamics during cardiopulmonary bypass and postoperative renal function, Circulation 34:1005, 1966.

328. Senning A et al.: Renal function during extracorporeal circulation at high and low flow rates: experimental studies in dogs, Ann Surg 151:163, 1960.

329. Bove EL and Kirsh MM: Complications of extracorporeal circulation. In Greenfield LJ, editor: Complications in surgery and trauma, ed 2, Philadelphia, 1990, JB Lippincott & Co.

330. Engelman RM et al.: The effect of diuretics on renal hemodynamics during cardiopulmonary bypass, J Surg Res 16:268-275, 1974.

331. Lawhorne TW, Davis JL, and Smith GW: General surgical complications after cardiac surgery, Am J Surg 136:254-256, 1976.

332. Wallwork J and Davidson KG: The acute abdomen following cardiopulmonary bypass surgery, Br J Surg 67:410-412, 1980.

333. Lucas A and Max MH: Emergency laparotomy immediately after coronary bypass, JAMA 224:1829-1831, 1980.

334. Hanks JB et al: Gastrointestinal complications after cardiopulmonary bypass, Surgery 92:394-400, 1982.

335. Pinson CW and Alberty RE: General surgical complications after cardiopulmonary bypass surgery, Am J Surg 146:133-136, 1983.

336. Reath DB, Maull KI, and Wolfgang TC: General surgical complications following cardiac surgery, Am Surg 49:11-14, 1983.

337. Moneta GL, Misbach GA, and Ivey TD: Hypoperfusion as a possible factor in the development of gastrointestinal complications after cardiac surgery, AM J Surg 149:648-650, 1985.

338. Welling RE et al.: Gastrointestinal complications after cardiac surgery, Arch Surg 121:1178-1180, 1986.

339. Leitman MI et al: Intra-abdominal complications of cardiopulmonary bypass operations, Surg Gynecol Obstet 165:251-254, 1987.

340. Krasna MJ et al: Gastrointestinal complications after cardiac surgery, Surgery 104:773-780, 1988.

341. Stanley TH et al: Plasma catecholamine and cortisol responses to fentanyl-oxygen anesthesia for coronary artery operations, Anesthesiology 53:250-253, 1980.

342. Hoar PF et al: Hemodynamic and adrenergic responses to anesthesia and operation for myocardial revascularization, J Thorac Cardiovasc Surg 80:242-248, 1980.

343. Sutherland AD et al: The effect of preoperative oral fluid and ranitidine in gastric fluid volume and pH, Can J Anaesth 34:117-121, 1987.

344. Priebe HJ and Skillman JJ: Methods of prophylaxis in stress ulcer disease, World J Surg 5:223-333, 1981.

345. Zinner MJ, Zuidema GD, Smith PL, et al: The prevention of upper gastrointestinal tract bleeding in patients in an intensive care unit, Surg Gynecol Obstet 153:214-220, 1981.

346. Lehot JJ et al: Should we inhibit gastric acid secretion before cardiac surgery? Anesth Analg 70:185-190, 1990.

347. Kivilaakso E and Silen W: Pathogenesis of experimental gastric-mucosal injury, N Engl J Med 301:364-369, 1979.

348. Taylor PC, Loop FD, and Hermann RE: Management of acute stress ulcer after cardiac surgery, Ann Surg 178:1-5, 1973.

349. Shockett E et al: Gastroduodenal perforation after open heart surgery, Am J Surg 134:643-646, 1977.

350. Hairston P and Lee WH Jr: Management of infected prosthetic heart valves, Ann Thorac Surg 9:229, 1970.

351. Firor WB: Infection following open-heart surgery with special reference to the role of prophylactic antibiotics, J Thorac Cardiovasc Surg 53:371, 1967.

352. Subramanian VA, McLeod J, and Gans H: Effect of extracorporeal circulation on reticuloendothelial function: I. Experimental evidence for impaired reticuloendothelial function following cardiopulmonary bypass in rats, Surgery 64:775, 1968.

353. Silva J Jr, Hoeksema H, and Fekety FR Jr: Transient defects in phagocytic functions during cardiopulmonary bypass, J Thorac Cardiovasc Surg 67:175, 1974.

354. Hairston P et al.: Depression of immunologic surveillance by pump-oxygenator perfusion, J Surg Res 9:587, 1969.

355. Salo M: Effect of anaesthesia and open-heart surgery on lymphocyte responses to phytohaemagglutinin and concanavalin A, Acta Anaesthesiol Scand 24:471-479, 1978.

356. Pollock R et al.: Protracted severe immune dysregulation induced by cardiopulmonary bypass: a predisposing etiology factor in blood transfusion–related AIDS? J Clin Lab Immunol 22:1-5, 1987.

357. Kusserow B, Larrow R, and Nichols J: Perfusion and surface-induced injury in leukocytes, Fed Proc 30:1516-1520, 1971.

358. Austin TW et al: Cephalothin prophylaxis and valve replacement, Ann Thorac Surg 23:333, 1977.

359. Lee WH et al.: Denaturation of plasma proteins as a cause of morbidity and death after intracardiac operations, Surgery 50:29, 1961.

360. Vervloet AFC, Edwards MJ, and Edwards ML: Minimal apparent blood damage in Lande Edwards membrane oxygenator at physiologic gas tensions, J Thorac Cardiovasc Surg 60:774, 1970.

361. Geldof WCP and Brom AG: Infections through blood from heart-lung machine, Thorax 27:395, 1972.

362. Hehrlein FW, Herrman H, and Kraus J: Complications of median sternotomy in cardiovascular surgery, J Thorac Cardiovasc Surg 13:390, 1972.

363. Londe S and Sugg WL: The challenge of reoperation in cardiac surgery, Ann Thorac Surg 17:157, 1974.

364. Macmanus Q et al.: Surgical considerations in patients undergoing repeat median sternotomies, J Thorac Cardiovasc Surg 69:138, 1975.

365. Culliford AT et al.: Sternal and costochondral infections following open-heart surgery: a review of 2,594 cases, J Thorac Cardiovasc Surg 72:714, 1976.

366. Ibarra F and Alonso-Lej F: Médiastinite et déhiscence sternale comme complication de la sternotomie médiane, Ann Chir Thorac Cardiovasc 13:35, 1974.

367. Arnold M: The surgical anatomy of sternal blood supply, J Thorac Cardiovasc Surg 64:596, 1972.

368. Grmoljez PF, Barner HH, Willman VL, et al.: Major complications of median sternotomy, Am J Surg 130:679, 1975.

369. Stein PD, Harken DE, and Dexter L: The nature and prevention of prosthetic endocarditis, Am Heart J 71:393, 1966.

370. Slaughter L, Morris JE, and Starr A: Prosthetic valvular endocarditis, Circulation 47:1319, 1973.

371. Myerowitz PD et al.: Antibiotic prophylaxis for open-heart surgery, J Thorac Cardiovasc Surg 73:625, 1977.

372. Tamiya T, Yamasaki M, Maeo Y, et al: Complement activation in cardiopulmonary bypass, with special reference to anaphylatoxin production in membrane and bubble oxygenators. Ann Thorac Surg 46:47-57, 1988.

373. Westaby S: Organ dysfunction after cardiopulmonary bypass: a systemic inflammatory reaction initiated by the extracorporeal circuit, Intensive Care Med 13:89-95, 1987.

374. Moore FD, Warner KG, Assousa S, et al: The effects of complement activation during cardiopulmonary bypass: attenuation by hypothermia, heparin, and hemodilution, Ann Surg 208:95-103, 1988.

375. Cavarocchi NC, Pluth JR, Schaff HV, et al: Complement activation during cardiopulmonary bypass: comparison of bubble and membrane oxygenators, J Thorac Cardiovasc Surg 91:252-258, 1986.

376. Knudsen F, Pedersen JO, Juhl O, et al: Complement and leukocytes during cardiopulmonary bypass: effects on plasma C3d and C5a, leukocyte count, release of granulocyte elastase and granulocyte chemotaxis, J Cardiothorac Anesth 2:164-170, 1988.

377. Antonsen S, Brandslund I, Clemensen S, et al: Neutrophil lysosomal enzyme release and complement activation during cardiopulmonary bypass, Scand J Thor Cardiovasc Surg 21:47-52, 1987.

378. Hind CRK, Griffen JF, Pack S, et al: Effects of cardiopulmonary bypass on circulating concentrations of leukocyte elastase and free radical activity, Cardiovasc Res 22:37-41, 1988.

379. Riegel W, Spillner G, Schlosser V, et al: Plasma levels of main granulocyte components during cardiopulmonary bypass, J Thorac Cardiovasc Surg 95:1014-1019, 1988.

380. Tennenberg SD, Bailey WW, Cotta LA, et al: The effects of methylprednisolone on complement-mediated neutrophil activation during cardiopulmonary bypass, Surgery 100:134-142, 1986.

381. Andersen LW, Baek L, Thomsen BS, et al: Effect of methylprednisolone on endotoxemia and complement activation during cardiac surgery, J Cardiothorac Anesth 3:544-549, 1989.

382. Bonser RS, Dave JR, Davies ET, et al: Reduction of complement activation during bypass by prime manipulation, Ann Thorac Surg 49:279-283, 1990.

383. Hammerschmidt DE, Stroncek DF, Bowers TK, et al: Complement activation and neutropenia occurring during cardiopulmonary bypass, J Thorac Cardiovasc Surg 81:370-377, 1981.

384. Ryhänen P, Herva E, Hollmen A, et al: Changes in peripheral blood leucocyte counts, lymphocyte subpopulations, and in vitro transformation after heart valve replacement, J Thorac Cardiovasc Surg 77:259-266, 1979.

385. Tonnesen E, Brinklov MM, Christensen NJ, et al: Natural killer cell activity and lymphocyte function during and after coronary artery bypass grafting in relation to the endocrine stress response, Anesthesiology 67:526-533, 1987.

386. Ide H, Kakiuchi T, Furuta N, et al: The effect of cardiopulmonary bypass on T cells and their subpopulations, Ann Thorac Surg 44:277-282, 1987.

387. Ryhänen P, Huttunen K, and Ilonen J: Natural killer cell activity after open-heart surgery, Acta Anaesthesiol Scand 28:490-492, 1984.

388. van Velzen-Blad H, Dijkstra YJ, Schurink GA, et al: Cardiopulmonary bypass and host defense functions in human beings: I. Serum levels and role of immunoglobulins and complement in phagocytosis, Ann Thorac Surg 39:207-211, 1985.

389. Kress HG, Gehrsitz P, and Elert O: Predictive value of skin test in neutrophil migration and C-reactive protein for postoperative infections in cardiopulmo-

nary bypass patients, Acta Anaesthesiol Scand 31:397-404, 1987.

390. Campbell FW, Jobes DR, and Ellison N: Coagulation management during and after cardiopulmonary bypass. In Hensley FA and Martin DE, editors: The practice of cardiac anesthesia, Boston, 1990, Little, Brown & Co.

391. Ellison N, Jobes DR, and Schwartz AJ: Heparin therapy during cardiac surgery. In Ellison N and Jobes DR, editors: Effective hemostasis in cardiac surgery, Philadelphia, 1988, WB Saunders Co.

392. Kolff WJ, Effler DB, Groves LK, et al: Disposable membrane oxygenator (heart-lung machine) and its use in experimental surgery, Cleve Clin Q 23:69-75, 1956.

393. Ellison N, Beatty CP, Blake DR, et al: Heparin rebound, studies in patients and volunteers, J Thorac Cardiovasc Surg 67:723-729, 1974.

394. Pifarre R, Babka R, Sullivan HJ, et al: Management of postoperative heparin rebound following cardiopulmonary bypass, J Thorac Cardiovasc Surg 81:378-381, 1981.

395. McKenna R et al: The hemostatic mechanism after open heart surgery. II. Frequency of abnormal platelet functions during and after extracorporeal circulation, J Thorac Cardiovasc Surg 70:298-308, 1975.

396. Friedenbrug WR et al: Platelet dysfunction associated with cardiopulmonary bypass, Ann Thorac Surg 25:298-305, 1978.

397. Harker LA et al: Mechanism of abnormal bleeding in patients undergoing cardiopulmonary bypass: acquired transient platelet dysfunction associated with selective alpha granule release, Blood 56:824-834, 1980.

398. Harker LA: Bleeding after cardiopulmonary bypass, N Engl J Med 314:1446-1448, 1986.

399. Valeri CR et al: Hypothermia-induced reversible platelet dysfunction, Ann Surg 205:175-181, 1987.

400. Lambert CJ et al: The treatment of postperfusion bleeding using epsilon-aminocaproic acid, cryoprecipitate, fresh-frozen plasma, and protamine sulfate, Ann Thorac Surg 28:440-444, 1979.

401. Marengo-Rowe AJ and Leveson JE: Fibrinolysis: a frequent cause of bleeding. In Ellison N and Jobes DR, editors: Effective hemostasis in cardiac surgery, Philadelphia, 1988, WB Saunders Co.

402. Umlas J: Fibrinolysis and disseminated intravascular coagulation in open heart surgery, Transfusion 16:460-463, 1976.

403. Kalter RD et al: Cardiopulmonary bypass–associated hemostatic abnormalities, J Thorac Cardiovasc Surg 77:430, 1979.

404. Miller RD et al: Coagulation defects associated with massive blood transfusions, Ann Surg 174:794-801, 1971.

405. Mammen EF et al: Hemostasis changes during cardiopulmonary bypass surgery, Semin Thromb Hemost 11:281-292, 1985.

406. Mannucci PE et al: 1-Deamino-8-D-arginine vasopressin shortens the bleeding time in uremia, N Engl J Med 308:8-12, 1983.

407. Kobrinsky NL et al: Shortening of bleeding time by 1-deamino-8-D-arginine vasopressin in various bleeding disorders, Lancet 1:1145-1148, 1984.

408. Rocha E et al: Does desmopressin acetate reduce blood loss after surgery in patients on cardiopulmonary bypass? Circulation 77:1319-1323, 1988.

409. Czer L et al: Prospective trial of DDAVP in treatment of severe platelet dysfunction and hemorrhage after cardiopulmonary bypass, Circulation 72(suppl III):III-130, 1985.

410. Salzman EW et al: Treatment with desmopressin acetate to reduce blood loss after cardiac surgery: a double-blind randomized trial, N Engl J Med 314:1402-1406, 1986.

411. Lazenby WD, Russon I, Zadeh BJ, et al: Treatment with desmopressin acetate in routine coronary artery bypass surgery to improve postoperative hemostasis, Circulation 82(suppl IV):IV-413–IV-419, 1990.

412. Solen KA, Whiffen JD, and Lightfoot EN: The effect of shear, specific surface, and air interface on the development of blood emboli and hemolysis, J Biomed Mater Res 12:381-386, 1978.

413. Clark RE, Beauchamp RA, Magrath RA, et al: Comparison of bubble and membrane oxygenators in short and long perfusions, J Thorac Cardiovasc Surg 78:655-660, 1979.

414. Harris EA, Seelye ER, and Barratt-Boyes BG: Respiratory and metabolic acid-base changes during cardiopulmonary bypass in man, Br J Anaesth 42:912, 1970.

415. Pacifico AD, Digerness S, and Kirklin JW: Acute alternations of body composition after open intracardiac operations, Circulation 41:331, 1970.

416. Vitez TS: Pro: Calcium salts are contraindicated in the weaning of patients from cardiopulmonary bypass, J Cardiothorac Anesth 2:567-569, 1988.

417. Koski G: Con: Calcium salts are contraindicated in the weaning of patients from cardiopulmonary bypass after coronary artery surgery, J Cardiothorac Anesth 2:570-575, 1988.

418. Abbott TR: Changes in serum calcium fractions and citrate concentrations during massive blood transfusions and cardiopulmonary bypass, Br J Anaesth 55:753-759, 1983.

419. Hysing ES, Kofstad J, Lilleaasen P, et al: Ionized calcium in plasma during cardiopulmonary bypass, Scand J Clin Lab Invest 46:119-123, 1986.

420. Urban P, Scheidigger D, Buchmann B, et al: The hemodynamic effects of heparin and their relation to ionized calcium levels, J Thorac Cardiovasc Surg 91:303-306, 1986.

421. Kancir CB, Madsen T, Petersen PH, et al: Calcium, magnesium and phosphate during and after hypothermic cardiopulmonary bypass without temperature correction of acid-base status, Acta Anaesthesiol Scand 32:676-680, 1988.

422. Heining MPD, Linton RAF, and Band DM: Plasma ionized calcium during open heart surgery, Anaesthesia 40:237-241, 1985.

423. D'Hollander A, Primo G, Hennart D, et al: Compared efficacy of dobutamine and dopamine in association with calcium chloride on termination of cardiopulmonary bypass, J Thorac Cardiovasc Surg 83:264-271, 1982.

424. Shapira N, Schaff HV, White R, et al: Hemodynamic effects of calcium chloride injection following cardiopulmonary bypass: response to bolus injection and continuous infusion, Ann Thorac Surg 37:133-140, 1984.

425. Borgers M: The role of calcium in the toxicity of the myocardium, Histochem J 13:839-848, 1981.

426. Baker JE, Kemmenoe BH, Hearse DJ, et al: Calcium delivery and time: factors affecting the progression of cellular damage during the calcium paradox in the rat heart, Cardiovasc Res 18:361-370, 1984.

427. Chernow B, Smith J, Rainey TG, et al: Hypomagnesemia: implications for the critical care specialist, Crit Care Med 10:193-196, 1981.

428. Kuntschen FR, Galletti PM, Hahn C, et al: Alterations of insulin and glucose metabolism during car-

diopulmonary bypass under normothermia, J Thorac Cardiovasc Surg 89:97-106, 1985.

429. Kuntschen FR, Galletti PM, and Hahn C: Glucose-insulin interactions during cardiopulmonary bypass: hypothermia versus normothermia, J Thorac Cardiovasc Surg 91:451-459, 1986.

430. Kriauciunas KM, Grigorescu F, and Kahn R: Effects of heparin on insulin binding and biological activity, Diabetes 36:163-168, 1987.

431. Johnson CA, Amidon G, Reichert JE, et al: Adsorption of insulin to the surface of peritoneal dialysis solution containers, Am J Kidney Dis 3:224-228, 1983.

432. Watson BG, Elliott MJ, Pay DA, et al: Diabetes mellitus and open heart surgery, Anaesthesia 41:250-257, 1986.

433. Mori A, Tabata R, Matsuda M, et al: Carbohydrate metabolism during pulsatile cardiopulmonary bypass under profound hypothermia, Jpn Circ J 47:528-535, 1983.

434. Sladen RN: Temperature and ventilation after hypothermic cardiopulmonary bypass, Anesth Analg 64:816-820, 1985.

435. Wong KC: Physiology and pharmacology of hypothermia, West J Med 138:227-232, 1983.

436. Ralley FE, Wynands E, Ramsay JG, et al: The effects of shivering on oxygen consumption and carbon dioxide production in patients rewarming from hypothermic cardiopulmonary bypass, Can J Anaesth 35:332-337, 1988.

437. Guffin AV, Girard D, and Kaplan JA: Shivering following cardiac surgery: hemodynamic changes and reversal, J Cardiothorac Anesth 1:24-28, 1987.

438. Zwischenberger JB, Kirsh MM, Dechert RE, et al: Suppression of shivering decreases oxygen consumption and improves hemodynamic stability during postoperative rewarming, Ann Thorac Surg 43:428-431, 1987.

Chapter 13

Causes and Consequences of Hyperglycemia and Hypoglycemia

John D. Wasnick
Bart Chernow

I. Glucose Homeostasis
II. Hyperglycemia
III. Management of the Diabetic Patient in the Perioperative Period
IV. Hyperglycemia and Neuroanesthesia
V. Hypoglycemia
VI. Summary

Derangements in blood glucose concentration may account for clinically important perioperative morbidity. Altered glucose homeostasis may occur as a consequence of the hormonal responses to surgical stress.[1] Diabetic patients are equally subject to perioperative alterations in blood glucose concentration. Additionally, the diabetic patient's surgical course may be complicated by the systemic consequences of long-standing diabetes mellitus.[2] Both hypoglycemia and hyperglycemia may adversely effect anesthetic management and postoperative recovery. Well-planned glucose management may prevent perioperative morbidity.

I. GLUCOSE HOMEOSTASIS

Glucose is an essential nutrient of the cells within the central nervous system.[3] The brain is unable to synthesize glucose and requires a continuous supply of glucose via the circulation. Because prolonged hypoglycemia may produce irreversible neurologic injury, elaborate mechanisms have developed to ensure a sufficiently high concentration of blood glucose to provide for the energy needs of the central nervous system.

Plasma glucose concentration is normally maintained in the range of 60 to 120 mg/dl. Glucose is supplied to the body from dietary sources as well as through endogenous production. Glucose is formed in the liver by glycogenolysis and glucogenesis. Both exogenous and endogenous sources of glucose production are essential to provide the brain with glucose. Upwards of 50% of circulating glucose is used by the central nervous system as an energy source.

Blood glucose concentration is under tight hormonal control. Insulin is the dominant glucoregulatory hormone. Secreted by the beta cells of the pancreatic islets, insulin suppresses glycogenolysis and gluconeogenesis and promotes the tissue uptake of glucose. A deficiency in insulin results in hyperglycemia, whereas an excess of insulin causes hypoglycemia. Insulin is not the sole glucoregulatory hormone. Counterregulatory hormones include glucagon, epinephrine, norepinephrine, cortisol, and growth hormone.[3] The counterregulatory hormones increase the blood glucose concentration. Glucagon is secreted from the alpha cells of the pancreatic islets. Glucagon induces glycogenolysis and gluconeogenesis. Like glucagon, epinephrine also promotes glucose formation. Additionally, epinephrine decreases tissue glucose utilization. Cortisol and growth hormone similarly antagonize the actions of insulin.

Acute surgical stress may increase the concentrations of counterregulatory hormones such as cortisol.[4] Stress-induced increases in the counterregulatory hormones may account for unexpectedly high perioperative blood glucose values. Other sources of perioperative hyperglyce-

---

List 13-1. Sources of Perioperative Hyperglycemia

Poorly controlled diabetes mellitus
Excessive dextrose administration
Hyperalimentation
Hormonal response to surgical stress

---

mia are presented in List 13-1. No matter what factor initiates hyperglycemia, the concentration of insulin or the peripheral response to insulin is inadequate to maintain effective glucose homeostasis.

II. HYPERGLYCEMIA

Uncontrolled hyperglycemia leads to hyperosmolarity, and it may, in the type I or juvenile onset diabetic, lead to the development of diabetic ketoacidosis (DKA). DKA occurs when insufficient insulin is available to provide for glucose regulation. Frequently the stress of surgery with its associated increase in counterregulatory hormones leads to inadequate glucose control in the diabetic patient. Insulin deficiency in the setting of a relative excess of glucagon and other counterregulatory hormones permits unchecked glycogenolysis and gluconeogenesis. Progressive hyperglycemia follows because of increased glucose production and decreased glucose utilization.

Ketogenesis occurs as a response to the insulin deficiency. Acetoacetate and beta-hydroxybutyrate blood concentrations increase to provide an alternative central nervous system nutrient. Ketosis is a protective mechanism by which an alternative energy source is provided to the brain because of its inability to utilize glucose because of the insulin deficiency.

Patients with DKA present with symptoms of polyuria, polydipsia, abdominal pain, generalized malaise, and diminished mentation. Physical findings include tachycardia, tachypnea, and orthostatic hypotension. Deep inspirations (Kussmaul's respiration) are often seen and herald the presence of a metabolic acidemia. The signal laboratory finding in the patient with DKA is hyperglycemia (usually an average plasma glucose concentration of greater than 500 mg/dl).[5] Metabolic acidemia occurs because of the production of acetoacetate and beta-hydroxybutyrate. Hyponatremia is seen and results from the osmotic actions of glucose drawing water into the extracellular space. Hypertriglyceridemia may also account for decreased serum sodium concentrations.[5] Hyperkalemia or hypokalemia may be observed. Initially the potassium concentration is high secondary to the metabolic acidosis; however, potassium is lost with the glucosuria-induced osmotic diuresis.

Identification of diabetic ketoacidosis may be difficult in the patient under general anesthesia. Patients with a history of diabetes mellitus who undergo major surgery should be carefully monitored for the development of DKA. Unexpectedly high urine output or an unexplained metabolic acidemia may be the early signs of perioperative diabetic ketoacidosis.

Often patients become hyperglycemic without developing ketosis or acidemia. Hyperosmolarity produces many of the same signs and symptoms characteristic of DKA. Often the patient who develops a nonketotic hyperosmolar coma rather than DKA is elderly and has type II or adult onset diabetes mellitus. The patient who presents with DKA is generally younger with type I or juvenile onset diabetes mellitus.

The treatment of perioperative hyperglycemia is designed to replace insulin and to provide appropriate supportive care. Insulin counteracts the effects of glucagon and increases tissue glucose uptake. Regular insulin is administered intravenously by continuous infusion. Regular insulin is administered at an intravenous rate of 0.5 to 10 units/hour. The insulin infusion is frequently preceded by a regular insulin intravenous bolus of 5 to 20 units.[5] The infusion rate and the bolus insulin administration schedule are determined by frequent laboratory measurements of plasma glucose concentration, arterial pH, and serum potassium concentration. Additional therapy is directed toward correcting the underlying fluid deficit and the acid/base imbalance. The adult patient being treated for diabetic ketoacidosis is frequently several liters in negative fluid balance at the time of the initiation of therapy. Fluid replacement with saline is essential to restore the normal intravascular volume. Supplemental potassium is given to correct hypokalemia. Bicarbonate administration may be necessary when the pH falls below 7.0. This latter suggestion is controversial. We usually do not give bicarbonate for the DKA patient with an arterial pH of greater than 7.0 However, should the pH be less than 7.0, we administer one half to one ampule of bicarbonate.

Profound hyperglycemia and acidemia may lead to shock. Volume replacement and correction of the underlying metabolic acidemia usually restores hemodynamic stability. Rarely, cerebral edema presents after the initiation of therapy.[6] Cerebral edema is believed to occur as a result of an osmotic disequilibrium across the blood-brain barrier resulting from too rapid a decline in the plasma blood glucose. The decline in plasma glucose produces a decrease in the plasma osmolarity to a degree faster than the cerebral osmolarity. Fluid then crosses the blood-brain barrier following the concentration gradient.[7] Ideally, the plasma glucose concentration should not be decreased to less than 300 mg/dl during initial therapy.[7] If cerebral edema occurs, therapy is begun with mannitol and hyperventilation.

III. MANAGEMENT OF THE DIABETIC PATIENT IN THE PERIOPERATIVE PERIOD

By careful preoperative evaluation and management the majority of diabetic patients can safely undergo surgery and receive anesthesia without incident. Nevertheless, the diabetic patient presents many specific concerns to the anesthesiologist. Of paramount importance to the anesthesiologist is the realization that diabetes mellitus is a systemic disease affecting all organ systems. The cardiovascular status of the diabetic patient is often of foremost concern to the anesthetist. The diabetic frequently suffers from hypertension. Tight out-patient blood pressure control has been advocated to decrease the occurrence of diabetic nephropathy and atherosclerotic heart disease.[8,9]

On presentation to the operating room, the diabetic patient may be receiving several antihypertensive medications. Antihypertensive therapy should be continued throughout the operating room course and into the postoperative period. The patient with poorly treated hypertension may demonstrate increased hemodynamic lability throughout the anesthetic course.

Blood pressure regulation may be further aggravated by diabetic autonomic neuropathy. As a consequence of autonomic neuropathy, the diabetic patient may fail to exhibit tachycardia as a response to surgical stresses and volume loss. Indeed, diabetic patients demonstrate a greater need for vasopressor support during general anesthesia.[10]

The frequency of painless myocardial infarction or ischemia is increased in the diabetic population; however, this event has not been positively correlated with the presence of autonomic neuropathy.[11] The increased risk of atherosclerotic heart disease in the diabetic patient warrants a careful preoperative examination directed toward establishing the patient's cardiovascular reserve. Evaluation by a cardiologist is often helpful in the preoperative assessment of the diabetic patient.

Autonomic dysfunction may place the diabetic patient at increased risk for aspiration.[12] Diabetic gastroparesis must be considered an additional risk factor in the patient with autonomic neuropathy. Airway management may be further compromised by the diabetic "stiff joint syndrome."[13] Stiff joint syndrome comprises juvenile onset diabetes mellitus, short stature, and joint contractures. These changes may complicate endotracheal intubation. The diabetic patient should have a careful airway assessment before the induction of general anesthesia. Should difficulties be anticipated, fiberoptic intubation may be indicated when the patient is awake.

Diabetes mellitus, hypertension, and vascular disease may contribute to the diabetic person's developing chronic renal failure.[14] All diabetic patients should have preoperative laboratory determinations of creatinine and blood urea nitrogen concentrations before the induction of anesthesia. The patient with renal failure requires specific considerations, which are described in Chapter 19.

Lastly, the diabetic patient's blood glucose must be monitored during the operating room course to prevent hyperglycemia, hypoglycemia, or diabetic ketoacidosis. Several regimens have been advocated to provide perioperative glucose control.[15-18] Methods vary from institution to institution, but the goals are essentially the same. Ideally, perioperative glucose management should prevent hyperglycemia in the patient undergoing surgical stress but not create hypoglycemia in the patient who has been fasted.

The most frequently encountered approach to perioperative insulin coverage involves the administration of one half to one fourth of the patients daily morning intermediate-acting insulin on the day of surgery. A D5W infusion at a fixed infusion rate is started at the time of insulin administration. This approach fails to protect the patient against intraoperative increases in blood glucose resulting from surgical stress. Watts et al. showed in a study of 191 operative patients that both unacceptable hyperglycemia and hypoglycemia may occur with this regimen.[17] Others have advocated the use of a continuous infusion of insulin-glucose-potassium during the perioperative period.[18] In this setting, a regular insulin infusion is begun at the rate of 2 to 5 units/hour and is administered with supplemental potassium and glucose. Frequent blood samples must be obtained so that one can determine the plasma glucose and potassium concentrations. The insulin-glucose-potassium infusion is adjusted depending on the laboratory results. Thomas et al.[18] have reported that such infusions result in lower postoperative blood glucose and beta-hydroxybutyrate concentrations.

Watts et al.[17] have suggested that protocols for glucose and insulin administration be abandoned in the perioperative period. They advocate that frequent blood glucose and potassium monitoring be employed with intermittent intravenous injections of regular insulin with or without dextrose administration as guided by laboratory results. In this fashion, each patient's glucose, insulin, and potassium needs are addressed by the anesthesiologist on a moment-to-moment basis.

The practitioner must determine which approach in providing perioperative insulin administration is most suitable to his or her practice. We choose to administer a fraction of the patient's daily intermediate-acting insulin on the morning of surgery with a supplemental infusion of D5W. On the other hand, in brittle diabetics we often administer a continuous insulin infusion. We frequently monitor blood glucose concentration during the perioperative course. We provide supplemental, regular insulin intravenously if indicated by a blood glucose concentration greater than 200 mg/dl.

IV. HYPERGLYCEMIA AND NEUROANESTHESIA

We aim to maintain the blood glucose concentration between 150 and 200 mg/dl because recent work has focused attention on the role of hyperglycemia in exacerbating ischemic neurologic injury. In 1977, Myers and Yamaguchi[19] reported a study of 13 juvenile monkeys given brief periods of cardiac arrest. These investigators noted that those monkeys who received a dextrose infusion before asystole had a far worse outcome than fasted monkeys who had not received a glucose infusion. Other investigators have likewise shown that an infusion of glucose before a neurologic injury may worsen ischemic damage.[20-23] Hyperglycemia is believed to contribute paradoxically to ischemic neurologic injury by providing the brain cells with an increased supply of glucose. The augmented glucose stores are available to the ischemic brain to perform anerobic glycolysis during the period of hypoperfusion. As a result, the brain made ischemic during a period of glucose excess produces an increased amount of lactic acid. The intracellular accumulation of lactate is believed to be injurious to neural tissues.[20]

The majority of studies demonstrating the detrimental effects of hyperglycemia in ischemic neurologic injury have been performed in animal models. Pulsinelli et al.[23] have retrospectively examined outcome in patients admitted to the hospital with the diagnosis of ischemic stroke. Outcome was found to be significantly worse in the diabetic population when compared with the nondiabetic stroke population. These investigators concluded that hyperglycemia may accentuate ischemic brain injury in humans. Additionally, Pulsinelli et al.[23] advocate that blood glucose concentration should be maintained at near-normal concentration in the patient who has had a stroke.[23]

List 13-2. Sources of Perioperative Hypoglycemia

Insulin overdosage
Insulin-secreting tumor
Hepatic failure

The implications of these findings to the anesthesiologist are that blood glucose concentrations should probably be held near normal limits during the perioperative period. Glucose-containing solutions should be avoided in patients undergoing surgery likely to involve periods of cerebral ischemia such as carotid endarterectomy. We hasten to point out that controlled clinical trials in human subjects are lacking.

V. HYPOGLYCEMIA

In controlling the blood glucose concentration, care must be taken not to produce unintentional hypoglycemia. Hypoglycemia occurs frequently in the hospitalized patient as an iatrogenic event. It is a rare occurrence in the non–insulin dependent diabetic.[3] Sources of perioperative hypoglycemia are listed in List 13-2.

The diagnosis of hypoglycemia may be masked by the administration of general anesthesia. A plasma glucose concentration of less than 45 mg/dl after an overnight fast is considered to indicate hypoglycemia. Symptoms of hypoglycemia include those related to epinephrine release (such as anxiety, palpitations, tremulousness, and diaphoresis) in addition to those from cerebral dysfunction (such as somnolence, coma). Many of these signs and symptoms are not readily apparent in the anesthetized patient. Nevertheless, hypoglycemia should be suspected in any patient who has a delayed emergence from anesthesia. Therapy for hypoglycemia is with dextrose administration.

VI. SUMMARY

The perioperative period may mask both the signs and the symptoms of hyperglycemia and hypoglycemia. The anesthesiologist must be aware of the potential morbidity associated with both extremes in circulating glucose concentration. Perioperative glucose regulation is the responsibility of the anesthesiologist in his or her role as the intensivist of the operating room.

REFERENCES

1. Rossini A and Hare J: How to control the blood glucose level in the surgical diabetic patient, Arch Surg 111:945-949, 1976.

2. Alberti K and Thomas D: The management of diabetes during surgery, Br J Anaesth 51:693-710, 1979.
3. Cryer P and Gerich J: Glucose counterregulation, hypoglycemia, and intensive insulin therapy in diabetes mellitus, N Engl J Med 313:222-241, 1986.
4. Chernow B, Alexander R, Smallridge R, et al: Hormonal responses to graded surgical stress, Arch Intern Med 147:1273-1277, 1987.
5. Foster D and McGarry J: The metabolic derangements and treatment of diabetic ketoacidosis, N Engl J Med 309:159-169, 1983.
6. Rosenbloom A, Riley W, Weber F, et al: Cerebral edema complicating diabetic ketoacidosis in childhood, J Pediatr 96:357-361, 1980.
7. Arieff A and Kleeman C: Studies on mechanisms of cerebral edema in diabetic comas: effects of hyperglycemia and rapid lowering of plasma glucose in normal rabbits, J Clin Invest 52:571-583, 1973.
8. Peiris A and Gustafson A: Current therapeutic concepts in diabetic hypertension, Diabetes Care 9:409-414, 1986.
9. Ewing J and Clarke B: Diabetic autonomic neuropathy: present insights and future prospects, Diabetes Care 9:648-665, 1986.
10. Burgos L, Ebert T, Asiddao C, et al: Increased intraoperative cardiovascular morbidity in diabetics with autonomic neuropathy, Anesthesiology 70:591-597, 1989.
11. Hume L, Oakley GD, Boulton AJ et al: Asymptomatic myocardial ischemia in diabetes and its relationship to diabetic neuropathy: an exercise electrocardiography study in middle-aged diabetic men, Diabetes Care 9:384-388, 1986.
12. Mulhall BP and O'Fearghail M. Diabetic gastroparesis, Anaesthesia 39:468-469, 1984.
13. Salzarulo H and Taylor L: Diabetic "stiff joint syndrome" as a cause of difficult endotracheal intubation, Anesthesiology 64: 366-368, 1986.
14. Ciccarelli L, Ford C, and Tseuda K: Autonomic neuropathy in a diabetic patient with renal failure, Anesthesiology 64:283-287, 1986.
15. Palumbo P: Blood glucose control during surgery, Anesthesiology 55:94-95, 1981.
16. Bowen D, Nancekievill M, Proctor E, and Norman J: Peri-operative management of insulin dependent diabetic patients: use of a continuous intravenous infusions of insulin-glucose-potassium solutions, Anaesthesia 37:852-859, 1987.
17. Watts L, Miller J, Davidson M, and Brown J: Perioperative management of diabetes mellitus, Anesthesiology 55:104-109, 1981.
18. Thomas D, Platt H, and Alberti K: Insulin dependent diabetes during the peri-operative period, Anaesthesia 39:629-637, 1984.
19. Myers R and Yamaguchi S: Nervous system effects of cardiac arrest in monkeys, Arch Neurol 34:65-74, 1977.
20. Drummond CJ and Moore SS: The influence of dextrose administration on neurologic outcome after temporary spinal cord ischemia in the rabbit, Anesthesiology 70:64-70, 1989.
21. Siemkowicz E: The effect of glucose upon restitution after transient cerebral ischemia: a summary, Acta Neurol Scand 71:414-417, 1985.
22. Nedergaard M: Transient focal ischemia in hyperglycemic rats is associated with increased cerebral infarction, Brain Res 408:79-85, 1987.
23. Pulsinelli W, Levy D, Sigsbee B, et al: Increased damage after ischemic stroke in patients with hyperglycemia with or without established diabetes mellitus, 74:540-543, 1983.

Chapter 14

Causes and Consequences of Hypothermia and Hyperthermia

Henry Rosenberg
Jan Charles Horrow

I. HEAT BALANCE PHYSIOLOGY

A. Heat and temperature

Heat, which is energy in the form of molecular motion, differs from temperature, which is a measure of the concentration of heat energy. When a substance is divided into two equal parts, each half contains half as much heat as the original but the same temperature. Heat, like other forms of energy, follows conservation laws. Heat transfer, however, depends on the existence of a temperature gradient. By analogy, gas contents (mass) are conserved, whereas gas transfer occurs with differences in partial pressure.

Heat and temperature are related by the ability of a substance to contain heat, termed "specific heat." The specific heat of water and thus of body tissues defines the unit of heat energy, the calorie: the addition of 1 calorie to 1 gram of water results in a 1 Celsius degree increase in temperature.

B. Heat production

Basal metabolic energy appears as heat at the rate of 1 $kcal \cdot kg^{-1} \cdot hr^{-1}$, or 44 $watts \cdot m^{-2}$. Were all this heat retained, body temperature would increase at the rate of $1° C \cdot hr^{-1}$. The liver, heart, and skeletal muscle serve as major heat generators, whereas skin and respiratory muscosal surfaces provide opportunities for heat dissipation. Muscle tension alone, in the absence of shivering, generates additional heat. In hypothyroidism, a depressed basal metabolic rate results in decreased heat production. Likewise, impaired catecholamine excretion or inhibition of catecholamine peripheral action will decrease heat generation and may lead to symptoms and heat-conserving behaviors. Furthermore, thyroid hormone potentiates the calorigenic effects of epinephrine.[1]

C. Heat loss

Approximately 3000 kcal of heat are lost per day by the average adult male. Ninety-five percent of those 3000 kcal dissipate through the skin and respiratory mucosa. Warming of inspired air (3%) and elimination of urine and feces (2%) account for the remainder. The four mechanisms of heat loss are convection, evaporation, conduction, and radiation. Convective transfer, accounting for 15% of total heat loss, occurs by moving air. The loss increases with the square of air speed, up to 60 miles per hour.

Conductive heat loss occurs by direct contact with a cooler material, such as the cold mattress of a stretcher or by intravenous infusion of cold solution. (Strictly speaking, since the fluid becomes part of the body, the total heat content remains constant even though temperature decreases.) Normally there is little conductive heat loss.

Conversion of 1 ml of water from a liquid to a vapor state, that is, evaporation, from the skin or respiratory tract permits dissipation of 0.58 kcal of energy. Evaporation is facilitated by low ambient humidity and hindered in damp atmospheres. Nearly 1 ounce of water is lost each hour from the skin (two thirds) and lungs (one third) at room temperature, accounting for 17 kcal of energy.

Radiation of heat through the skin constitutes the major mechanism of heat loss, reaching 50% of the total, or about 50 $kcal \cdot hr^{-1}$,

when a person is naked. Radiant heat transfer occurs by infrared electromagnetic waves traveling from a hotter object to a cooler one. Radiant heat loss increases with the temperature differential and with the amount of exposed surface. By increasing skin temperature, vasodilatation promotes heat loss.

D. Thermoregulation

The hypothalamus manipulates multiple-organ systems in an effort to stabilize its own temperature. Hypothalamic thermal receptors respond to temperature on an absolute rather than a relative scale. Thermal receptors also exist outside the brain. Skin contains abundant warm and cold temperature sensors. Additional sensors reside in abdominal organs.

What role does the peripheral information play in themoregulation? Skin temperature modulates the hypothalamic output. It affects both the central temperature at which heat generation begins and the intensity of that response[2] (Fig. 14-1). Age, exercise, time of day, medications, hormonal milieu, and other factors determine the hypothalamic "set point" to which body temperature is compared. When temperature is below the set point, heat generation and conservation effector activity ensues; when the temperature is above it, the hypothalamus activates heat loss mechanisms. Pyrogens from leukocytes move the set point higher, resulting in fever, whereas aspirin restores the set point toward normal.

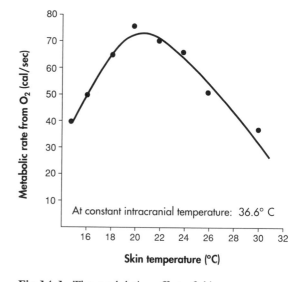

Fig.14-1. The modulating effect of skin temperature on hypothalamic effector activity. Notice that at the same cranial temperature higher skin temperature is associated with less heat production. (From Benzinger TH, Pratt AW, and Kitzinger C: Proc Natl Acad Sci 47:730, 1961.)

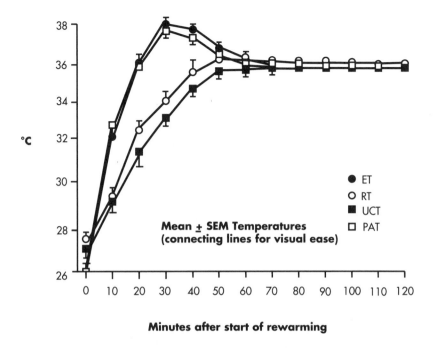

Fig. 14-2. Temperatures at four sites beginning with warming during extracorporeal circulation. *ET*, Esophageal; *RT*, rectal; *UCT*, urinary catheter; *PAT*, pulmonary arterial temperatures. Notice that ET and PAT behave similarly and rise more steeply than RT and UCT. (From Horrow JC and Rosenberg H: unpublished data, 1989, Philadelphia.)

Heat-balance effector sites include higher cortical centers, skeletal muscle, the vasculature, fat, adrenal medulla, and sweat glands. Higher cortical centers afford behaviors that converge or dissipate heat. Skeletal muscle provides heat by basal tone and shivering. With hypothermia, sympathetic nervous system activation initiates vasoconstriction of the vasculature, nonshivering thermogenesis of adipose tissue and other organs, notably liver and skeletal muscle, and catecholamine secretion from the adrenal gland. Diaphorsis, also sympathetically mediated, is increased greatly during hyperthermia.

E. Body temperature

Temperature measurements differ all over and within the living organism. The estimation of total body heat requires multiple surface and invasive temperature measurements.[3] The innermost core of the body, represented by the liver, contains the highest temperatures. Peripheral areas, such as the extremities, display the lowest temperatures, with transitional temperatures in intermediate zone areas such as rectum and bladder.[4] The interrelationship of temperatures in these areas is complex: for example, warming the skin will decrease central temperatures.[5]

With minimal thermal disequilibrium, the multiple measures of central (distal esophageal, nasopharyngeal, pulmonary arterial, tympanic

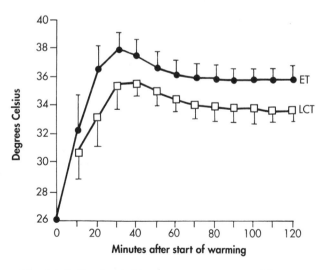

Fig. 14-3. Forehead skin temperature, measured by a liquid crystal device *(LCT)*, tracks the central temperature measured in the distal esophagus *(ET)*. Compared with RT and UCT (see Fig. 14-2), the LCT curve follows changes in ET, whereas UCT and RT continue to increase when ET is decreasing. (From Allen G, Horrow JC, and Rosenberg H: Can J Anaesth 37:659, 1990.)

membrane) and intermediate zone (rectal, urinary catheter) temperature agree. Large thermal gradients, such as occur during extracorporeal circulation warming, generate great discrepancies among the central and intermediate zone measures (Fig. 14-2).

Skin surface temperatures such as those of the axilla, great toe, or forehead are about to 3 to 4 Fahrenheit degrees cooler than central measures. Curiously, axillary skin temperature lags behind central measures in both absolute measure as well as time response, whereas forehead temperature displays only an absolute offset without time lag (Fig. 14-3). When patient temperature measurements determine clinical decisions, central measurements are indicated.

II. HYPERTHERMIA
A. Causes of hyperthermia

Body temperature depends on an intricate interplay between environmental temperature and mechanisms of heat gain and heat loss controlled by the central thermoregulatory centers. Hyperthermia may therefore be a result of an inadequate or inappropriate response to increased environmental temperature, an alteration of the internal "thermostat" located deep within the central nervous system, or overwhelming peripheral heat production.

Common environmental causes of hyperthermia include inability to vasodilate or perspire because of drugs or disease.[6] Examples include Parkinson's disease, anticholinergic medications, and unadapted persons exposed to high environmental temperatures, as may occur in vigorous exercise in the untrained athlete.[7] Centrally, hyperthermia may occur as a response to pyrogens, substances produced by bacteria or white blood cells that produce an increase in the set point for body temperature.[8]

1. Iatrogenic causes. The preceding generalizations about hyperthermia apply also to the anesthetized patient. Environmental temperature is controlled in the operating room theatre in general as well as in the microenvironment of the patient. During anesthesia, iatrogenic hyperthermia results from active warming of patients (particularly pediatric patients), as may occur during application of warming blankets or unintentional overuse of heated airway humidifiers.[9] Although hypothermia is far more common in the operating room, hyperthermia, usually mild, may occur during long procedures where the patient is covered with nonpermeable drapes and the operative area is small. Less common reasons have been reported. Application of tourniquets to either upper or lower extremities for prolonged periods of time will, es-

pecially in children, induce hyperthermia.[10] This is probably secondary to increased catecholamines. For reasons still poorly understood, the injection of arteriovenous malformations with sclerosing solution may increase body temperature.[11] Induced hyperthermia for patients undergoing treatment for malignancy is another iatrogenic cause of hyperthermia.[12] This modality of treatment of malignancy is no longer commonly used.

In days before temperature control of the operating room and air conditioning, heat stroke during anesthesia was a not uncommon problem.[13] The cause for such temperature elevation was believed to be high environmental temperature and humidity along with increased catecholamine release as occurs with the then commonly used agents ether and cyclopropane, especially in the face of hypercapnia.

Recent studies by Sessler et al. have shown that the normal vasoconstriction response to cold is depressed during anesthesia.[14] He also hypothesizes that vasodilatation normally occurring in response to increased body temperature is also altered during anesthesia, such that instead of occurring when body temperature exceeds 37.5° C central temperature, vasodilatation and sweating may not occur until the body temperature exceeds 38° or 39° C.[15] That is, during anesthesia the patient is poikilothermic over a wider range of body temperatures.

2. Hyperthermia Secondary to Diseases

a. Pheochromocytoma. As already indicated, catecholamine increase may cause hyperthermia. *Pheochromocytoma* results in the most profound increase in circulating catecholamines. Many cases of mild to significant hyperthermia have been reported during or in the absence of anesthesia in patients with a pheochromocytoma.[16]

b. Thyrotoxicosis and thyroid storm. Thyrotoxicosis and thyroid storm may also cause intraoperative hyperthermia.[17] Thyroid storm, an uncommon diagnosis in this era, presents with hypertension, hyperthermia, and tachycardia. Unlike with malignant hyperthermia, muscle rigidity does not occur and acidosis is unusual. Clinical observation indicates that thyroid gland surgery causes mild hyperthermia, perhaps because of release of thyroid hormone with manipulation of the gland. Alternatively, the increased temperature may be unrelated to thyroid surgery itself but related to inadequate heat dissipation from the small surgical site in a completely draped patient. The hypermetabolism of thyroid-induced hyperthermia is sodium-potassium ATPase mediated,[18] in contradistinction to that of malignant hyperthermia (MH), in which intracellular calcium is elevated.[19]

c. Riley-Day syndrome. Elevated body temperature also complicates the Riley-Day syndrome,[20] in which dopamine beta-hydroxylase is deficient. Persons having this syndrome exhibit pronounced instability of the autonomic nervous system with wide variation in blood pressure, heart rate, and temperature, apparently unrelated to external stimuli.

d. Osteogenesis imperfecta. Hyperthermia occurs during anesthesia in patients with osteogenesis imperfecta,[21] a metabolic bone disease characterized by easy and frequent bone fractures and blue scleras. Although a few episodes of true malignant hyperthermia have been reported with osteogenesis imperfecta, in many cases clinical and laboratory testing reveal that malignant hyperthermia was mistakenly diagnosed.

e. Central nervous system dysfunction. CNS dysfunction may induce hyperthermia.[22] Patients with status epilepticus develop fever, presumably secondary to the intense muscle activity. However, any major central nervous system catastrophe may also lead to hyperthermia: patients who experience hypoxic encephalopathy characteristically develop hyperthermia. After resuscitation from cardiac arrest, hyperthermia may accompany loss of consciousness, seizures, and increased muscle tone manifest by abnormal posturing. If cardiac arrest has occurred under anesthesia, the combination of autonomic imbalance associated with hypoxic encephalopathy, hyperthermia, and muscle rigidity render the distinction from malignant hyperthermia difficult.

f. Bacteremia and sepsis. Bacteremia and sepsis may lead to hyperthermia. Body temperature usually decreases when febrile patients are anesthetized. However, hyperthermia recurs after surgery, characterized by rigors and intense peripheral vasoconstriction. Sepsis, bacteremia, and hyperthermia may be induced by surgical manipulation, leading to postoperative hyperthermia. Appendectomy constitutes a common scenario for this occurrence, with fever engendered by release of pyrogens with handling of the septic organ. Fever may occur during surgery for head trauma, particularly with disruption of the oral cavity. In this case, the bountiful oral bacteria can readily enter the bloodstream.

3. Drug-induced hyperthermia

a. Malignant hyperthermia. The two most important pathophysiologic states causing hyperthermia from drug administration are malignant hyperthermia (MH)[23] and the neuroleptic malignant syndrome (NMS).[24] MH occurs in genetically predisposed persons anesthetized with certain potent inhalation agents or succi-nylcholine. The incidence of MH ranges from approximately from 1 in 15 to 1 in 200,000 anesthetics, with most authorities claiming an incidence of 1 in 50,000 anesthetics. The incidence depends on the gene pool for MH as well as the frequency of use of triggering anesthetic agents. Anesthesiologists who never use triggering agents will not see MH, whereas those who use such drugs regularly will see a higher frequency of MH. Also, elderly patients seem resistant to MH triggers; therefore anesthesiologists caring primarily for elderly patients will see MH infrequently.

The precise cause of MH remains elusive. However, increased intracellular calcium-ion concentration in skeletal muscle cells clearly constitutes one of the final pathophysiologic steps. Controversy exists as to whether animals or patients who are MH susceptible have increased intracellular calcium concentration before exposure to triggering anesthetics[25] and whether elevation of intracellular calcium-ion concentration occurs in cells other than skeletal muscle cells. In swine, intracellular calcium-ion concentration increases before the induction of MH and then rises dramatically during an MH episode. However, in vitro studies utilizing different measurement techniques document normal resting calcium levels in skeletal muscle that rise only upon exposure to MH trigger agents.

What leads to the increased intracellular calcium-ion levels? Perhaps an alteration in excitation contraction coupling in skeletal muscle of MH susceptible patients permits excessive release of calcium from sarcoplasmic reticulum upon exposure to triggering agents.[26] Perhaps mitochondrial oxidative phosphorylation and calcium uptake are altered.[27] Perhaps elevated intracellular calcium results from elevation of certain free fatty acids within the cell, which in turn leads to calcium-ion release from the sarcoplasmic reticulum.[28] The consequences of elevated intracellular calcium are clear: activation of ATPases with ensuing depletion of ATP, actin-myosin interaction causing muscle contraction or increased muscle tone, breakdown of glucose and glycogen, and generation of heat. With sufficient ATP depletion, compromise of membrane integrity occurs, leading to increased cellular permeability and release of intrcellular potassium, myoglobin, creatine kinase, and tissue thromboplastin. The clinical consequences include hyperkalemia, myoglobinemia, and disseminated intavascular coagulation.

The gene responsible for MH is located on chromosome 19 in humans and chromosome 6 in pigs.[29] Patients with Duchenne muscular dystrophy (DMD) may experience MH-like episodes on exposure to MH triggering drugs.[30] The X chromosome contains the gene for Duchenne dystrophy. Chronically increased intarcellular calcium produces progressive muscle destruction in DMD.[31] Since inhalation agents normally cause calcium release from the sarcoplasmic reticulum,[32] in DMD the normal response of intracellular calcium to inhalation agents against a background of intracellular hypercalcemia may lead to an MH-like syndrome. Whether the same process underlies MH occurring in the unusual myopathies (central core disease, myotonic dystrophy, King-Denborough syndrome) is largely speculative. Clinically, they all present and require the same treatment as MH.

MH occurrence requires both a susceptible patient and exposure to specific drugs. The "trigger" drugs are the potent inhalation agents, including halothane, insoflurane, enflurane, cyclopropane, ether, and methoxyflurane, and the depolarizing venromuscular relaxant succinylcholine. Whether the depolarizing relaxant decamethonium triggers MH remains unknown. Local anesthetics, both amides and esters, do *not* trigger MH,[33] nor do intravenous induction agents, including propofol, barbiturates, and benzodiazapines. Other drugs that do *not* trigger malignant hyperthermia include digitalis, calcium, parasympatholytics, anticholinesterases, and nondepolarizing muscle relaxants. Hyperkalemia, however, may trigger MH or may retrigger an episode of MH.[34] We believe that catecholamines do not trigger MH, though others state that they should not be employed during MH episodes. Cocaine toxicity, particularly in association with alcohol abuse, leads to hyperthermia, increased muscle tone, arrhythmias, and ventricular fibrillation.[35] This toxic effect of the drug is not related to MH.

Malignant hyperthermia may occur in pigs without drug intervention. Case reports indicate that MH-susceptible patients may be at increased risk to heat stroke;[36] likewise, in pigs high environmental temperatures and stress may induce an episode of MH. However, in humans there is no direct evidence that full-blown MH may occur without being induced by drugs. In some instances, drug exposure is insidious: one patient with hyperthermia, muscle aches, and malaise had been exposed to a hydrocarbon with a structure similar to halothane; symptoms resolved after removal of the compound from the environment.[37]

b. Neuroleptic malignant syndrome. Psychiatrists have noted a syndrome characterized by hyperthermia, muscle rigidity, rhabdomyolysis, arrhythmia, acidosis, and death. It is precipitated by haloperidol alone or with phenothiazines, or occasionally with antidepressant medications. This neuroleptic malignant syndrome (NMS) should not be confused with hyperthermia and arrhythmias induced by overdose of monoamine oxidase (MAO) inhibitors or by combination of MAO inhibitor and meperidine,[38] which originate from a different mechanism.

Despite the clinical similarity to MH, the cause of NMS is probably different from that of MH. Most believe that NMS results from blockade of dopamine receptors in the central nervous system. The dopamine agonist bromocriptine is one of the drugs effective in treating NMS. Treatment of NMS appears below.

The question, Is the patient also at risk for MH? arises when one is anesthetizing a patient who has experienced NMS. Studies yield conflicting results, with some diagnostic muscle biopsy studies indicating susceptibility and others not.[39,40] Succinylcholine, if preceded by barbiturate, as may occur for electroconvulsive therapy,[41] does not precipitate MH syndrome in the patient with NMS. There is little experience, however, with general anesthesia in patients who have experienced NMS.

B. Consequences of hyperthermia

Hyperthermia itself increases metabolic rate and oxygen consumption. Increased cardiac output, heart rate, and stroke volume ensue. Patients unable to increase their cardiac output may develop significant acidemia and myocardial ischemia. Hyperthermic patients may perspire during anesthesia but usually not until body temperature exceeds 38° or 39° C. Children may exhibit seizures. Coma and brain damage occur with pronounced hyperthermia. Seizures increase the metabolic demand for oxygen even further. Despite temperatures greater than 41° C, vigorous treatment of hyperthermia may reverse central nervous system dysfunction.[42] Although documentation is poor, case reports before air conditioning record death during anesthesia from hyperthermia, presumably because of acidosis.[13]

1. Clinical diagnosis of malignant hyperthermia. The signs and symptoms of MH may be classified as specific or nonspecific. Nonspecific responses in MH include tachycardia, tachypnea, and diaphoresis. In animals, increased levels of catecholamines lead to peripheral vasoconstriction, represented by mottled cyanosis in some cases of MH. Temperature elevation is a nonspecific, late sign of MH that follows the increase in oxygen consumption. More specific signs of MH include skeletal muscle rigidity, sometimes only involving the masseter muscles, muscle destruction with increase levels of creatine kinase (CK), myoglobinuria and myoglobinemia, hyperkalemia, and hypercalcemia. Respiratory and metabolic acidosis frequently accompany MH. Acidemia is mild when cardiac output and oxygen delivery to the periphery are maintained. In more dramatic cases, however, acidosis and hyperkalemia produce arrhythmias, myocardial depression, and cardiac arrest. Disseminated intravascular coagulation (DIC) occurs in severe MH; evidence of DIC should be sought in all MH cases.

Masseter muscle rigidity (MMR) presages MH.[43] Masseter muscle rigidity occurs in pediatric patients after halothane and succinylcholine induction as often as 1 in 100 cases.[44] Fifty percent of those patients when biopsied and tested with the halothane-caffeine contracture test demonstrate MH susceptibility. Clinically, however, a much smaller number of those experiencing MMR go on to develop MH. This discrepancy may arise from a high false-positive rate of diagnostic muscle biopsy, or because subclinical MH susceptibility occurs more frequently in the population than otherwise suspected.

2. Clinical diagnosis of neuroleptic malignant syndrome. Despite its presumed central nervous system cause (dopamine receptor alteration), NMS displays manifestations that imply direct involvement of skeletal muscle, such as rhabdomyolysis, rigidity, and release of CK. In contrast to MH, however, nondepolarizing muscle relaxants block the muscle rigidity of NMS. Fever, autonomic imbalance, and acidosis are a consequence of the hyperthermia.

C. Prevention of hyperthermia

A thorough history and familiarity with a patient's preoperative condition as well as careful attention to application of heating devices is essential in the prevention of intraoperative hyperthermia. It is important to know whether a patient has hypothyroidism or has a history suggestive of pheochromocytoma. Similarly, a preoperative history should seek evidence of myopathy. Osteogenesis imperfecta should be suspected in a patient with multiple fractures and blue scleras. A family or personal history of an adverse response to anesthesia should arouse suspicions of MH. MH is not the most common cause of intraoperative morbidity and mortality however. Therefore not all cases of unexplained death in the perioperative period should be ascribed to MH. Intraoperative monitoring plays a key role in the early diagnosis of

MH. Unexplained elevation in end-tidal CO_2 constitutes the earliest most sensitive sign of MH.[45] A doubling or tripling of end-tidal CO_2 may occur in less than 3 to 5 minutes. Hemoglobin oxygen saturation may or may not decrease during acute episodes of MH, depending on the degree of concomitant vasoconstriction and delivery of oxygen to the periphery. Routine monitoring of end-tidal CO_2 during general anesthesia is strongly advised.

More controversial is the role of routine temperature monitoring during anesthesia. We believe that temperature is a vital sign that should be recorded in all patients undergoing general anesthesia. Despite being a late sign of MH, temperature elevation may nevertheless be the determining clinical indicator of MH.

How best to monitor temperature intraoperatively has aroused controversy as well. Most authorities agree that central measures provide maximal accuracy and reliability. Less accurate monitors of central temperature include rectal and urinary catheter temperature.[46] The role of skin temperature monitors in anesthesia, particularly in relationship to MH, remains undetermined. No studies provide data on changes in skin temperature change. Theoretically vasoconstriction from catecholamine release during MH might render skin temperature monitoring inaccurate. However, if the heat load is sufficient, peripheral vasodilatation to transfer heat to the skin may occur during MH. Skin and central temperatures do not correlate during small thermal changes, such as those during routine anesthesia.[5] However, changes in skin temperature reflect larger thermal changes (central temperature 5 to 6 Celsius degrees) with accuracy.[47] Finally, skin temperature monitoring is better than no temperature monitoring. The American Society of Anesthesiologists standards indicate that temperature monitoring should be employed wherever temperature changes are anticipated. We contend that temperature changes should be anticipated with every general anesthetic.

Dantrolene, a hydantoin derivative, inhibits the release of calcium from sarcoplasmic reticulum and may enhance reuptake of calcium into the SR as well. Prophylaxis against MH is by dantrolene administration before surgery in a dose of 2 to 2.5 mg·kg^{-1} intravenously. The same blood levels may be achieved with 5 mg·kg^{-1} orally over 24 hours.[48] Dantrolene may exacerbate preexisting muscle weakness and elicit nausea and vomiting. Dantrolene prophylaxis may be omitted if regional anesthesia alone is employed and during general anesthetics employing end-tidal CO_2 monitoring where the diagnosis of MH has not been firmly made. Dantrolene should be available in all locations where general anesthesia is administered.

D. Treatment of hyperthermia

1. Nonspecific. The management of intraoperative hyperthermia *not* attributable to MH consists in removal of warming devices such as heating blankets, heated humidifiers, and coverings. Blowing cool air with a fan over the patient and cooling the room provide additional means of heat dissipation. In hyperthermia not related to MH, these simple surface-cooling maneuvers should prove sufficient to restore normothermia. With more pronounced hyperthermia ice packs should be placed along the superficial sites of major blood vessels such as the neck, groin, and axilla, and scalp.

Iced-solution lavage of the stomach, rectum, and wound provides internal cooling, as does infusion of iced intravenous fluid. Peritoneal lavage, in cases where the abdomen is not open, has also been reported to be effective.[49] In extreme cases cardiopulmonary bypass will rapidly cool patients. This highly invasive step is reserved for the most desperate situations. Only when heart rate exceeds 160 beats per minute with compromise of cardiac output or signs of myocardial ischemia should beta-blocker administration occur.

2. Specific for malignant hyperthermia. Upon diagnosing malignant hyperthermia, one should discontinue anesthetics and institute hyperventilation at twice the predicted minute ventilation. Hypotension or other cardiovascular compromise indicate use of sodium bicarbonate, 1 to 2 mg·kg^{-1} IV. However, rapid conversion of bicarbonate to CO_2 requires that minute ventilation be increased further.

Dantrolene, the specific drug treatment for MH, is prepared as a lyophilized solution of 20 mg per vial. Since it must be reconstituted with 60 ml of distilled water or 5% glucose solution, additional help should be sought to mix and solubilize the drug. Once mixed, 2.5 mg·kg^{-1} of the drug should be given intravenously, titrated to heart rate, body temperature, and muscle rigidity. Despite the recommended upper dosage limit of 10 mg·kg^{-1}, more may be administered if needed to establish control. This is rarely necessary. Once under control, dantrolene should be continued for at a least 48 hours, with use of an empiric dose of 2 mg·kg^{-1} IV every 4 to 6 hours. Total amounts of greater than 10 mg·kg^{-1} may be necessary with recrudescence or persistence of the syndrome. Dantrolene's half-life is approximately 12 hours.[50] Once the patient has responded to treatment and is awake, orally administered dantrolene is appropriate.

Upon diagnosing MH, one should measure arterial blood gases, activated partial thromboplastin time, platelet count, plasma fibrinogen, fibrinogen degradation products (if available), and calcium and phosphate ion concentrations. Base-line creative kinase (CK) as well as myoglobin levels in the blood and the urine should be obtained. Since CK peaks 24 hours after an MH episode, it should not be elevated initially. Myoglobinuria may occur at the time of first diagnosis of MH. Liver enzymes are also elevated in many patients.

Utilization of dantrolene, hyperventilation, and cooling measures usually prevent the occurrence of arrhythmias. Procainamide, not lidocaine, is recommended first should drug treatment for arrhythmia be necessary. Although amide local anesthetics do not trigger malignant hyperthermia, there is little information to indicate whether they might exacerbate an episode. We believe they do not, since amide local anesthetics do not exacerbate MH episodes in MH swine[51] and since lidocaine has allowed successful management of arrhythmias during MH.[52]

The use of calcium-channel blockers should be avoided. The combination of dantrolene, hyperkalemia, and hypotension complicate the use of calcium-channel blocking drugs in MH.[53] Similarly, coagulation abnormalities and DIC frequently revert with control of the underlying disorder. MH does not modify the customary treatment of acute DIC; many clinicians will wish to enlist the aid of a hematologist to treat DIC.

Once resuscitated, the patient should undergo observation in an intensive care unit for at least 24 hours. Recrudescence may occur within that period of time, and dantrolene should be administered for at least 48 hours. Serial CK levels serve to detect ongoing muscle destruction. Muscle weakness and myalgias are common after an episode of MH, since a massive amount of muscle destruction may occur.

The specific management of MMR is controversial.[54] We and others advocate that trismus is an indication to stop an anesthetic for elective surgery. Since it is not clear whether MH may supervene and since myoglobinuria is expected after MMR whether or not MH supervenes, others prefer converting to nontriggering anesthetics. Yet a third group contends that masseter muscle rigidity is an insignificant event; they would continue a triggering anesthetic. This approach is distinctly brazen. Serum CK should be measured at 6, 12, and 24 hours after muscle masseter rigidity. Myoglobinuria as well as hyperkalemia may occur. Since myoglobinuria carries particular renal morbidity, we recommend 1 to 2 mg·kg^{-1} dantrolene after an episode of masseter rigidity, even in the absence of other signs of MH.

After an episode of MH or MMR, patients should receive follow-up counseling for MH susceptibility through organizations such as the Malignant Hyperthermia Association of the United States, P.O. Box 191, Westport, Connecticut 06881-0191. Relatives of these patients should also consider being tested for MH.

At the present time, the only agreed upon diagnostic test for MH is the halothane-caffeine contracture test. Performed in over 40 centers worldwide, the test involves removal of 1 to 2 g muscle with testing for a contracture response to halothane and caffeine. Muscle from MH patients displays a contracture to halothane and "left-shifted" dose-response curve to caffeine. Although the sensitivity and specificity of the test are not clearly defined, no patient with a negative biopsy has subsequently developed MH, even when challenged.[55] A variety of other diagnostic tests have been found to be of no value, including the calcium uptake test, the calcium ATPase test, the platelet ATP depletion test, and a test of released calcium from lymphocytes. Serum CK levels are not an appropriate screening test for MH. Recent identification of the gene for MH on chromosome 19 holds prospect for a DNA-based test that could be performed on white cells.

Measurements of intracellular high-energy phosphates utilizing magnetic resonance imaging of arm muscles reveal a depletion of creatine kinase in MH-susceptible patients.[56] Since reduced levels of creatine kinase in muscle are also found in patients with a variety of other muscle disorders, this test may prove useful for screening family members once MH has been otherwise diagnosed.

3. Neuroleptic malignant syndrome. The management of NMS consists in discontinuing the offending psychotropic drug, administration of dantrolene and bromocriptine, and supportive treatment. We would also avoid triggering anesthetics. Dantrolene's effectiveness in NMS may be related to a nonspecific reduction of muscle tone and thus heat production or to blocking of a specific pathophysiologic process of heat production related to calcium release from the sarcoplasmic reticulum in muscle.

4. Other syndromes. The management of patients who have fevers unrelated to MH and NMS includes the administration of salicylates. Of course, specific treatment for pheochromo-

cytoma and hyperthyroidism should be instituted in those situations where these are the precipitating causes of hyperthermia.

III. HYPOTHERMIA
A. Effect of anesthetics on heat balance
Drugs can modify heat balance by altering one or more of the three components of the thermoregulatory system: the afferent pathway, the central control mechanism, or the efferent paths. Atropine, for example, may result in hyperthermia by blocking the efferent sympathetic diaphoresis response to warm environments. The effects of anesthetic agents on each segment of the thermoregulatory response are, for the most part, unknown. However, investigative studies of the effects of some drugs do explain the thermal behavior of anesthetized patients.

1. Sedatives. Direct cerebral application of barbiturates induces an increase in skin blood flow with resultant radiant heat loss to the environment.[57] Promethazine, a phenothiazine antihistamine, and chlorpromazine, a phenothiazine major tranquilizer, are two of the three components (the third is meperidine, see below) of the "cocktail" utilized in the past for intraoperative induced hypothermia. It is probable that central inhibition of normal thermoregulatory responses ensues from use of sedative-class drugs.

2. Opioids. Intracerebral morphine decreases body heat production.[58] All opioids in high doses cause hypothermia.[59] A nitrous oxide–fentanyl combination did not abolish the thermoregulatory response of cutaneous vasoconstriction to hypothermia in 6 of 10 patients during donor nephrectomy. Rather, the set point occurs at a lower temperature, that is, 34.2° C.[60] The other four patients, who did not respond with vasoconstriction, may not have become cool enough to demonstrate such a response. Meperidine can abolish postanesthetic tremor as well as depress the thermoregulatory response to hypothermia (see p. 353).

3. Inhaled anesthetics. Since inhaled anesthetics increase skin blood flow, they should augment radiant heat loss. Halothane resets the central thermoregulatory response to hypothermia: five patients receiving 1% end-tidal halothane did not demonstrate cutaneous vasoconstriction until central temperature decreased by 2.5 Celsius degrees.[61] Not surprisingly, increasing depth of anesthesia appears to create a graded central depression: abolition of cutaneous vasoconstriction in one patient required 0.94% halothane at 34.0° C but only 0.75% halothane at 34.2° C.[61]

4. Regional anesthesia. In contrast to general anesthetics, epidural or spinal anesthesia do not modify central thermoregulatory behavior. However, conduction anesthesia can decrease body temperature more than general anesthesia: sympatholysis causes vasodilatation, which augments radiant heat loss and prevents vasoconstriction below the level of the block. Motor blockade impairs the shivering response as well as decreasing heat production from muscle (see below). Reduction of circulating catecholamines reduces heat production. Cutaneous vasodilatation affords subjective warmth, despite loss of body heat.

5. Neuromuscular relaxants. Paralyzed patients cool more rapidly.[62] A dual mechanism may explain this effect: first, relaxants block the thermoregulatory shivering response; second, muscle relaxation decreases metabolic rate by impairing heat production in muscle.

B. Alterations of homeostasis with hypothermia

1. Cardiovascular. Hypothermia induces intense reflex sympathetic stimulation, resulting in increases in heart rate, stroke volume, cardiac output, and blood pressure. These effects accompany pronounced increases in total body oxygen consumption (see the discussion of shivering, p. 348). In the anesthetized patient, however, this reflex sympathetic response is blunted. Instead, the cardiovascular changes reflect decreased tissue needs for oxygen and substrate. Heart rate slows in proportion to decreased metabolism, and so it is halved at about 28° C. Stroke volume and contractility remain unchanged. Decreases in cardiac output reflect the bradycardia. Systemic vascular resistance and blood pressure increase.

Whether a patient is anesthetized or not, heart rate slows as temperature decreases to less than 33° C. This slowing results from prolongation of systole, unlike physiologic bradycardia in which diastole is prolonged.[63] Conduction velocity decreases throughout the hypothermic heart, yielding prolonged PR and QT intervals as well as a widening of the QRS complex on the electrocardiogram. Both J-point elevations, termed "Osborne waves," and T-wave flattening or inversions occur at hypothermia

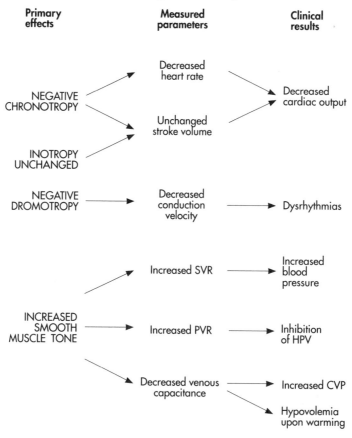

Fig. 14-4. The cardiovascular sequelae of hypothermia. *CPV,* Central venous pressure; *HPV,* hypoxic pulmonary vasoconstriction; *PVR,* pulmonary vascular resistance; *SVR,* systemic vascular resistance.

and should not be interpreted as signs of myocardial ischemia. Atrial fibrillation is common. It results from atrial stretching because of increased central blood volume. Between 28° and 30° C ventricular fibrillation develops. Hypothermia-induced ventricular fibrillation is refractory to pharmacologic therapy. Fig. 14-4 summarizes the cardiovascular sequelae of hypothermia.

2. Respiratory. Whole body carbon dioxide production decreases with hypothermia. The magnitude of this decrease reflects the behavior of most enzyme-controlled biologic phenomena, that is, a halving of activity with fall in temperature of 10° C. This halving is formally expressed as a Q_{10}, or quotient of measured activities at two temperatures 10 Celsius degrees apart, of approximately 2. Few patients undergo so radical a change in temperature. Thus the percentage change in CO_2 production per Celsius degree change in temperature would represent more useful information. Since arithmetic changes in temperature beget multiplicative changes in CO_2 production, this factor is not simply one tenth of 2 but rather the tenth root of 2, or 1.072. (By analogy, investments double in value after 10 years of 7.2% annual earnings when compounded.) Numerous experiments have verified that CO_2 production indeed changes by about 7% per Celsius degree.[64-66]

Initially, cooling increases respiratory rate by central stimulation; ventilatory depression supervenes. Decreases in both tidal volume and respiratory rate contribute to the decreased minute ventilation. Body CO_2 content remains constant at hypothermia. One might expect the magnitude of decrease in minute ventilation to parallel that of CO_2 production. However, ventilatory dead space enlarges at hypothermia, thus blunting the decrease in minute ventilation.[67]

As with other gases, CO_2 solubility increases with cooling. Since content is the product of solubility and partial pressure, preservation of CO_2 blood content in the face of increased solubility yields a decreased $Paco_2$ with hypothermia. Solubility changes are not enzymatically mediated and thus do not follow a "$Q_{10} = 2$" rule; $Paco_2$ changes only about 4.5% per Celsius degree. Fortunately, one may apply a convenient rule of thumb regarding the relationship of $Paco_2$ to temperature: normocapnia occurs when the temperature-corrected $Paco_2$ in mm Hg numerically equals the temperature measured in Celsius degrees. Thus a patient at 33° C should display a blood temperature-corrected $Paco_2$ of 33 mm Hg. Fig. 14-5 demonstrates that this approximation provides at most a 2 mm Hg error of predicted normocapnia in the range of 15° to 37° C. Blood pH increases by 0.015 units per Celsius degree, in parallel

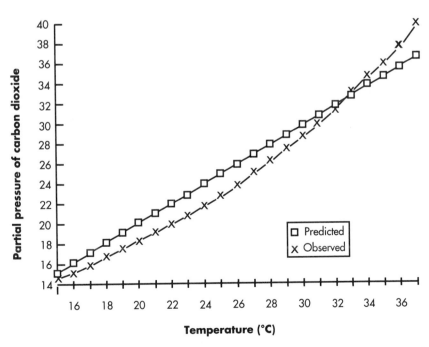

Fig. 14-5. Actual versus predicted values for $Paco_2$ using the rule of thumb that a patient's temperature-corrected $Paco_2$ is approximately equal to his temperature measured in Celsius degrees.

with the elevation of the pH of water with cold.

Hypothermia blunts the ventilatory response to CO_2. The slope of the CO_2 response curve decreases from 0.38 $L \cdot min^{-1} \cdot mm^{-1}$ Hg at 37° C to 0.10 $L \cdot min^{-1} \cdot mm^{-1}$ Hg at 28° C.[68]

The respiratory quotient, or ratio of CO_2 production to oxygen utilization, does not change with hypothermia. Thus oxygen utilization decreases at the same rate as CO_2 production. Like CO_2 content, oxygen content does not change. An increase of oxygen solubility in blood compounds an overall 7.5% per Celsius degree increase in oxygen affinity of hemoglobin. Thus Pa_{O_2} decreases with cooling. Even mild hypothermia induces pulmonary vasoconstriction, which thwarts hypoxic pulmonary vasconstriction.[69]

3. Central nervous system. The cerebral metabolic rates of oxygen and glucose decrease approximately 7% per Celsius degree, reflecting the "$Q_{10} = 2$" rule.[66,70] By reducing the need for oxygen and substrate, hypothermia protects the brain from hypoxic or ischemic insult. Cerebral blood flow reductions parallel those of metabolic rate. Although the brain can withstand complete ischemia of only 4 minutes at 38° C, it can tolerate 16 minutes of ischemia at 22° C. At hypothermia, temperature-adjusted (true) hypocapnia results in an exaggerated decrease in cerebral blood flow.

Hypothermia slows the electroencephalogram. Both power (amplitude) and peak power frequency decrease. Burst suppression may occur around 24° C. Electrical silence develops around 20° C. Brainstem auditory evoked potentials as well as cortical and spinal somatosensory evoked potentials display a progressive increase in latency with hypothermia. These alterations, like those of the electroencephalogram, resemble neuraxis ischemia. For the brain and spinal cord, as with the heart, hypothermia-induced electrical changes call for therapeutic restraint rather than intervention.

The minimum alveolar concentration of anesthetic gases (MAC) obeys the "$Q_{10} = 2$" principle: MAC changes about 7% per Celsius degree. Although the decreased cardiac output of hypothermia acts to increase the alveolar partial pressure of anesthetic, the increased solubility of anesthetic in blood blunts this rise in partial pressure, thus delaying delivery of drug to the brain. Speed of induction, a balance of these factors, remains unchanged. Cold alone obtunds cerebral function: memory is mildly impaired at 35° C; sedation occurs at 33° C and cold narcosis at 30° C.

4. Hematologic. Hypothermia increases blood viscosity by increasing plasma viscosity and by increasing hematocrit by fluid shifts from extracellular to intracellular spaces. The red blood cells in colder, more viscous blood tend to aggregate and form rouleaus more easily. Capillary flow suffers and ceases at profound hypothermia (below 15° C). Hypothermia induces splanchnic sequestration of platelets with resultant thrombocytopenia. Coagulation effects are discussed on p. 349.

5. Renal and hepatic. Mild hypothermia results in diuresis because of increases in central compartment volume, cardiac output, and blood pressure. Progressive hypothermia decreases renal blood flow and glomerular filtration rate. Tubular reabsorption ceases, impairing urinary concentrating and diluting ability. Urine output eventually slows. Renal blood flow reduction far exceeds that predicted by the "$Q_{10} = 2$" rule: at 20° C, flow decreases by twelvefold, rather than fourfold. Only skeletal muscle and the extremities experience greater reductions in blood flow with hypothermia. Perhaps this deviation reflects the kidney's minimal oxygen requirements. Drugs normally cleared by the kidney exhibit prolonged half-lives at hypothermia because of reduced delivery to the kidney, impaired tubular activity, or both (see p. 350).

Splanchnic blood flow and hepatic metabolism decrease with hypothermia. Drugs dependent on hepatic biotransformation, such as heparin, exhibit prolonged half-lives at hypothermia.

6. Neuromuscular. Cooling alone increases the strength of muscle contraction. However, neuromuscular transmission is impaired, possibly because of decreased acetylcholine release. Adductor pollicis twitch decreases as a patient's extremities cool during anesthesia.[71]

C. Consequences of hypothermia

1. Shivering. At emergence from anesthesia, the time comes to "pay the piper" for the many benefits of hypothermia during surgery, that is, cold narcosis, reduced minimum alveolar concentration, brain protection, and decreases in oxygen consumption, ventilatory requirement, and cardiac output. The impaired thermoregulatory response engendered by anesthetics becomes reengaged at emergence. In an attempt to warm to the set point, the hypothalamic control center activates the shivering response. Such muscle activity without mechanical purpose during emergence from anesthesia, termed "postanesthetic tremor," may result in trauma to teeth, wound, and surgical repair, as well as increases in oxygen demand and ventilatory requirement, with resultant hypoxemia. Oxygen consumption and CO_2 production may increase fourfold during intense shivering. Fig. 14-6 depicts the physiologic consequences of increased metabolism accompanying shivering. These changes have serious implications for patients with ischemic or other heart disease who cannot meet the cardiovascular demands. In some cases, patients with ischemic heart disease or impaired ventilatory reserve are best left anesthetized, intubated, and mechanically ventilated while warming proceeds, rather than risk the stressful sequelae of intact thermoregulation.

Postanesthetic tremor encompasses other phenomena besides shivering.[72-74] Fig. 14-7 displays the distinction between electromyographic activity of normal shivering, in which an underlying 8 Hz signal is modulated within an envelope of 4 to 8 cycles per minute, and that of postanesthetic tremor in a normothermic patient, in which the modulation is absent. The latter type of postanesthetic tremor may originate from a disequilibrium of spinal cord reflexes rather than the regain of central thermoregulatory control. Muscular activity after anesthesia in most patients probably represents a combination of true shivering and other neuraxis phenomena.

2. Bleeding. Four mechanisms contribute to impaired coagulation. First, activation of coagulation factors depends heavily on enzymatic cleavage; hypothermia retards enzymatic activity. Little more is known about this aspect, though it is likely that the "$Q_{10} = 2$" rule applies. Factor structure remains unaltered at cold temperature.

Second, hypothermia accentuates fibrinolysis.[75] Clot breakdown results in renewed bleeding and the formation of fibrin-degradation products, which impair subsequent fibrin polymerization. Warming restores fibrinolysis to normal. Frank disseminated intravascular coagulation may accompany accidental hypothermia but rarely complicates induced hypothermia.

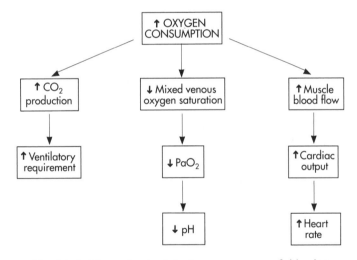

Fig. 14-6. The pathophysiologic consequences of shivering.

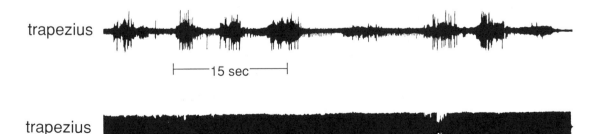

Fig. 14-7. Electromyogram of trapezius muscle from an unanesthetized shivering patient, **A,** and from a patient recovering from anesthesia, **B.** Muscle shivering activity is modulated within a 4 to 8 cycle/min envelope, whereas postanesthetic tremor is continuous. (Modified from Sessler DI, Israel D, Pozos RS, et al: Anesthesiology 68:843, 1988.)

Although hypothermia accompanying trauma surgery rarely causes concurrent disseminated intravascular coagulation, the release of tissue thromboplastin with trauma can trigger intravascular coagulation and fibrinolysis. Theoretically, however, cold-induced vascular endothelial cell injury alone can release thromboplastin in the absence of trauma.

Third, decreased body temperature is associated with doubling of activity of a specific heparin-like factor X_a inhibitor[76] that cannot be neutralized with protamine.[77] Fourth, platelet sequestration in the splanchnic circulation accompanies hypothermia.[78,79] Platelets undergo a shape change and increased adhesiveness at decreased temperature; ADP-induced aggregation is inhibited. The resultant thrombocytopenia reverses over an hour after warming. Transient platelet dysfunction may occur.[80] Both platelet thromboxane A_2 and endothelial cell prostacyclin synthesis are retarded with cold.[81]

The easy reversibility of cold-induced thrombocytopenia indicates that hypothermic patients should not receive platelet transfusions unless their coagulopathy requires immediate remedy. Likewise, trauma patients may require treatment of disseminated intravascular coagulation, including replacement of clotting factors and platelets and, in some cases, heparin administration.

3. Vasoconstriction. Increased tone characterizes the response of vascular smooth muscle to cold. Systemic vascular resistance increases progressively with immersion hypothermia, and so it is elevated by 147% at 30° C.[82] Pulmonary vascular resistance achieves a twofold increase at 30° C. At very cold temperatures, a cold-induced paralysis of smooth muscle results in seemingly paradoxical vasodilatation.[63] These events recur upon rewarming, explaining the biphasic blood pressure response during warming on cardiopulmonary bypass, that is, initial hypertension followed by hypotension. Systemic and pulmonary hypertension contribute to increased afterload of the left and right ventricles, thus acting to increase myocardial oxygen demand. Venous capacitance beds constrict, increasing central blood volume and cardiac preload, which also acts to increase myocardial oxygen demand.

More severe problems occur, however, after warming. With the return of normal venous tone, previously constricted capacitance vessels now dilate, pooling blood and decreasing venous return. Cardiac output and systemic blood pressure decrease in response to decreased preload. Warming patients may require several liters of fluid hourly to maintain adequate circu-

lating blood volume. This fluid replaces that lost during cold-induced diuresis. Fluid forced into interstitial spaces may remobilize slowly, causing increased lung water and decreased Pao_2. Rapid core warming, such as that accompanying cardiopulmonary bypass, establishes thermal gradients that require hours to equilibrate, thus establishing a prolonged and sometimes insidious continuing fluid requirement for the patient.

4. Altered drug clearance. Hypothermia potentially affects all aspects of drug pharmacokinetics. The volume of distribution may alter by closure of peripheral vascular channels in favor of central ones and by modified plasma protein binding. If the principles of alpha-stat pH management are followed,[83] ionization fractions of drugs should parallel those of water, to result in little change in drug activity for the weak acids and bases whose diffusion into cells is pH dependent.

Biotransformation of drugs generally utilizes enzymes, which, we have noted, follow a "$Q_{10} = 2$" rule. Nearly all drugs excreted via the liver undergo transformation, whether it be conjugation, oxidation, reduction, hydrolysis, or another process. Renal excretion involves filtration or active secretion, with or without intermediate tubular absorption. Most glomerular filtration depends on passive physical parameters such as perfusion pressure and filtration fraction. However, some drugs such as penicillin undergo active glomerular transport. Tubular secretion is an active, enzyme-mediated process.

The excretion of *d*-tubocurarine and pancuronium, which depend on renal clearance, is retarded during hypothermia, as is the hepatic clearance of vecuronium. Atracurium prolongation derives from the dependence of normal activity of both plasma cholinesterase and Hofmann elimination on normothermia. Mild hypothermia probably little affects the duration of action of neuromuscular blockers. Overall, the effects of hypothermia on clearance of various drugs is largely unknown. In general, one could assume that drug clearance is impaired at cold temperature and that the magnitude of the effect follows the "$Q_{10} = 2$" rule.

D. Prevention of hypothermia

1. Convective losses. Prevention of convective heat loss constitutes the most effective means of preserving temperature during surgery. Adequate ambient temperature of the operating room provides the most significant factor: intraoperative hypothermia does not occur in tropical operating rooms without air conditioning. Unfortunately, comfort of operating room personnel confounds efforts to maintain an environment compatible with patient normothermia. An operating room temperature at or above 24° C renders an esophageal temperature above 36° C.[84] The greatest loss of body heat occurs in the first hour after induction of anesthesia. Although one might expect that maintenance of room temperature above 24° C during skin preparation and until covering of exposed areas with surgical drapes would prevent much of this decrease, this outcome does not materialize.[85]

The frequency of room air exchanges affects convective heat loss much in the same manner as wind speed accentuates cooling, the so-called wind-chill factor. Operating rooms with more frequent ventilation turnover require higher temperatures to prevent patient cooling. Ideally, individual controls should permit rapid alteration of the ventilation rate, temperature, and humidity of each operating room.

Since convective losses are most significant, by corollary one should maximally cover exposed surfaces. It is prudent to minimize the room air exposure of open body cavities and of skin, both prepped and dry. The kinds of wraps available include paper, blankets, plastic, and reflective foil. A plastic scalp covering forms the simplest, cheapest, and most effective measure an anesthesiologist could employ. One study detected the greatest heat loss with uncovering of the patient during transfer to the recovery area.[86]

2. Evaporative losses. The evaporation of fluid from wet skin preparations decreases body temperature more than 1 Celsius degree in the first hour of surgery. Since the majority of the heat loss arises from the phase change from liquid to vapor and not from actual warming of the fluid, employment of heated skin preparation solutions contributes little to the prevention of hypothermia. Since heated solutions increases the risk of chemical burn from iodinated compounds, their use is discouraged.

Although heat loss through the skin exceeds respiratory heat loss, heating respiratory gases successfully attenuates hypothermia.[87-90] Dry gas flows of 5 liters·min^{-1} dissipate about 7 kcal of heat each hour. Heated humidified airway gases may even warm the patient slightly (≈ 0.5 Celsius degree) after the first hour of anesthesia.[85,88-90] Without concomitant humidification, however, heating of respiratory gases is futile and dangerous. The specific heat of dry gases is so low that heating the gas alone carries little heat to the patient compared with the heat lost by cooling of humid exhaled gas. The low

specific heat allows heated nonhumidified gas to attain high temperature and also produce a risk of tracheal burn.[91] Thus active gas heaters always employ humidifiers. Verification of proper humidifier function and measurement of delivered gas temperature are essential to safe airway gas heating. Gas temperature at the endotracheal tube should not exceed 41° C. Other potential pitfalls of heated gases include bacterial contamination of humidity sources and "rain-out" of humidity in airway tubing leading to impaired ventilation.

Heat and moisture exchange (HME) devices provide passive collection of exhaled water vapor in a hygroscopic material placed near the endotracheal tube. Subsequent inspired gases then become humidified upon passage through the device. After the first hour drop in central temperature in children, passive HME devices provide an additional 0.5 Celsius degree compared with no device but less than the 1.0 Celsius degree advantage afforded by active, heated humidified gases.[87]

One novel approach to achieve airway gas heating and humidification utilizes the carbon dioxide absorber, which creates both water vapor and heat:

$$CO_2 + Ca(OH)_2 \rightarrow CaCO_3 + H_2O + 13.7 \text{ kcal}$$

These modified carbon dioxide absorbers direct exhaled gases down the absorber to the inspiratory valve via a central outlet channel.[92] They have not enjoyed widespread use.

Employment of gas flows greater than those needed to ensure adequate removal of carbon dioxide from the anesthesia circuit exacerbates patient cooling by the airway. Truly low-flow or closed-system anesthesia allows maximal benefit of retained heat and humidity.

3. Radiation losses. Radiant warmers supply heat by infrared or incandescent lamps placed above the patient's surface. Because these devices strongly hinder the performance of surgery, they are useful only before incision, after operation, to the neonate after delivery, or during surgery on neonates. Feedback skin sensors should be employed to prevent skin burns.

4. Conductive loses. One liter of room-temperature clear fluid or two units (≈ 600 ml) of packed red cells from the refrigerator accept about 16 kcal of heat by conduction, which lowers body temperature about 0.5 Celsius degree. Fluid warmers permit rapid volume administration without the attendant hypothermia.

Warming blankets alone neither prevent nor ameliorate intraoperative hypothermia. In combination with other modalities, however, heating blankets contribute to heat savings.[85,90] Warming blankets placed ventrally on a supine patient are more effective than radiant heaters at increasing skin temperature.[5] Warming blankets carry the risk of skin burns in patients with poor circulation.

E. Treatment of hypothermic patients

1. Decrease losses. The first intervention in treatment of hypothermia should be to limit on-going heat loss. Fresh gas flows should be decreased and fluids warmed. One should heat and humidify airway gases by passive or preferably active means, apply warming blankets, and elevate ambient room temperature. All exposed surfaces should be covered with minimally porous material.

2. External heat. Radiant warmers, warming blankets, heated airway devices, and forced air warmers provide external sources of heat energy. Applied heat in any form should proceed with caution, since skin or mucosal burns can occur.

Victims of cold exposure respond to external heat application with peripheral vasodilatation. The resultant washout of peripheral acid, increased demand on a yet cold heart, and unmasking of hypovolemia lead to arrhythmias and hypotension.[93] Skin surface warming leads to a paradoxical decrease in central temperature.[5] Immersion in warm water complicates monitoring and other therapeutic interventions and is not recommended.[94] The contraindication for external rewarming applies to victims of chronic moderate (less than 32° C) hypothermia.

3. Internal heat. So-called core rewarming techniques include gastric, mediastinal, and peritoneal lavage and extracorporeal circulation. These modalities permit warming more rapidly than the $1\ °C \cdot hr^{-1}$ achieved by passive means alone. They also avoid initial peripheral vasodilatation.[93,94] The patient suffering from chronic, severe hypothermia from exposure benefits from these procedures. Although patients rendered hypothermic during operation should not require such heroic restorative measures, they are not specifically contraindicated.

4. Prevention of shivering. Appropriate insulating coverings or applied heat as discussed above will help the patient with postanesthetic

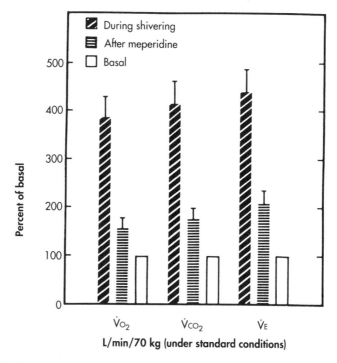

Fig. 14-8. Abolition of shivering with meperidine decreases oxygen consumption, carbon dioxide production, and minute ventilation. The decreases go far toward but do not achieve basal rates. (From Macintyre PE, Pavlin EG, and Dwersteg JF: Effect of meperidine on oxygen consumption, carbon dioxide production, and respiratory gas exchange in postanesthesia shivering, Anesth Analg 66:751, 1987.)

tremor or frank shivering. Several drugs may abolish shivering without supplying heat. Early reports recommended methylphenidate for this purpose.[95,96] More recent studies document the efficacy of the opioids morphine, meperidine, and fentanyl in this regard.[97] Meperidine, 25 mg IV, decreases oxygen consumption, carbon dioxide production, and minute ventilation.[98] Fig. 14-8 demonstrates that meperidine reduced these measurements from levels four times those of basal to roughly 150% of basal.

5. Prevention of arrhythmia. Bradyarrhythmias induced by moderate to severe hypothermia do not respond to atropine or pacing. Ventricular ectopic activity is notoriously resistant to pharmacologic therapy and countershock. In this setting, cardiopulmonary resuscitation may prove the only useful treatment of pulseless ventricular tachycardia or ventricular fibrillation. Repeat doses of antiarrhythmic medications in patients with mild hypothermia require adjustment for the associated impaired excretory mechanisms. Unfortunately, there is little available, aside from warming the patient, to treat cold-induced arrhythmias.

IV. SUMMARY

Our homeothermic physiology permits maintenance of function in hostile environments. However, compensatory mechanisms can be overwhelmed with the sudden, rapid heat production of malignant hyperthermia or with chronic exposure to cold. Furthermore these mechanisms may be obtunded by general anesthetics and the patient may be left later to pay the hypothermic consequences of inattentiveness. Good anesthetic care requires prevention of the causes and treatment of the consequences of altered body temperature.

REFERENCES

1. Ring GC: The importance of the thyroid in maintaining an adequate production of heat during exposure to cold, Am J Physiol 137:582-588, 1942.
2. Benzinger TH, Pratt AW, and Kitzinger C: The thermostatic control of human metabolic heat production, Proc Natl Acad Sci USA 47:730-739, 1961.
3. Colin J, Timbal J, Houdas Y, et al: Computation of mean body temperature from rectal and skin temperatures, J Appl Physiol 31:484-489, 1971.
4. Parbrook GD, Davis PD, and Parbrook EO: Basic physics and measurement in anesthesia, ed 2, Norwalk, Conn, 1986, Appleton-Century-Crofts, p 126.
5. Sessler DI and Maoyeri A: Skin-surface warming: heat flux and central temperature, Anesthesiology 73:218-224, 1990.
6. Clark WG and Lipton JM: Drug-related heatstroke, Pharmacol Ther 26:345-388, 1984.
7. Kim RC, Collins G, Cho C, et al: Heat stroke: report of three fatal cases with emphasis on findings in skeletal muscle, Arch Pathol Lab Med 104:345-349, 1980.
8. Bernheim HA, Block LH, and Atkins E: Fever: pathogenesis, pathophysiology, and purpose, Ann Intern Med 91:261-270, 1979.
9. Clark RE and Orkin LR: Body temperature studies in anesthetized man, JAMA 154:311-319, 1954.
10. Bloch EC: Hyperthermia resulting from tourniquet application in children, Ann R Coll Surg Engl 68:193-4, 1986.
11. Gomes AS, Busuttil RW, Baker JD, et al: Congenital arteriovenous malformations, Arch Surg 118:817-825, 1983.
12. Henderson MA and Pettigrew RT: Induction of controlled hyperthermia in the treatment of cancer, Lancet 1:1275-1277, 1971.
13. Moschcowitz AV: Post-operative heat stroke, Surg Gynecol Obstet 23:443-451, 1916.
14. Stoen R and Sessler DI: The thermoregulatory threshold is inversely proportional to isoflurane concentration, Anesthesiology 72:822-827, 1990.
15. Sessler DI: Perianesthetic thermal regulation, ASA Metropolitan Refresher Course Outline, 104, Park Ridge, Ill, March 1990, American Society of Anesthesiologists.
16. Crowley KJ et al: Phaeochromocytoma—a presentation mimicking malignant hyperthermia, Anaesthesia 43:1031-1032, 1988.
17. Bennett MH and Wainwright AP: Acute thyroid crisis on induction of anaesthesia, Anaesthesia 44:28-30, 1989.
18. Ismail-Beigi F and Edelman IS: The mechanism of the calorigenic action of thyroid hormone, J Gen Physiol 57:710, 1971.
19. Iaizzo PA, Klein W, and Lehmann Horn F: Fura-2 detected myoplasmic calcium and its correlation with contracture force in skeletal muscle from normal and malignant hyperthermia susceptible pigs, Pflugers Arch 411:648-653, 1988.
20. Axelrod FB et al: Anesthesia in familial dysautonomia, Anesthesiology 68:631-635, 1988.
21. Rampton AJ et al: Occurrence of malignant hyperpyrexia in a patient with osteogenesis imperfecta, Br J Anaesth 56:1443-1446, 1984.
22. Plum F, Posner JB, and Hain RF: Delayed neurological deterioration after anoxia, Arch Intern Med 110:18-25, 1962.
23. Rosenberg H and Seitman D: Pharmacogenetics. In Barash PG, Cullen BF, and Stoelting RK, editors: Clinical anesthesia, Philadelphia, 1989, JB Lippincott Co.
24. Lazarus A, Mann SC, and Caroff SN: The neuroleptic malignant syndrome and related conditions, Washington, DC, 1989, American Psychiatric Press, Inc., pp 1-56.
25. Lopez JR et al: [Ca^{2+}]$_i$ in muscles of malignant hyperthermia susceptible pigs determined in vivo with Ca^{2+} selective microelectrodes, Muscle Nerve 9:85-6, 1986 [Letter].
26. Mickelson JR, Gallant EM, Litterer LA, et al: Abnormal sarcoplasmic reticulum ryanodine receptor in malignant hyperthermia, J Biol Chem 263:9310-9315, 1988.
27. Cheah KS: Skeletal-muscle mitochondria and phospholipase A$_2$ in malignant hyperthermia, Biochem Soc Trans 12:358-360, 1984.
28. Fletcher JE et al: Triglycerides, not phospholipids, are the source of elevated free fatty acids in muscle from patients susceptible to malignant hyperthermia, Eur J Anaesthesiol 6(5):355-362, 1989.
29. McCarthy TV: Localization of the malignant hyperthermia susceptibility locus to human chromosome

19q12-13.2, Nature 343(6258):562-564, 1990.

30. Brownell AK et al: Malignant hyperthermia in Duchenne muscular dystrophy, Anesthesiology 58:180-182, 1983.

31. Bertorini TE, Bhattacharya SK, Palmieri GM, et al: Muscle calcium and magnesium content in Duchenne muscular dystrophy, Neurology 32:1088-1092, 1982.

32. Masayuki K: Volatile anesthetics decrease calcium content of isolated myocytes, Anesthesiology 70:954-960, 1989.

33. Paasuke RT and Brownell AK: Amide local anaesthetics and malignant hyperthermia Can Anaesth Soc J 33:126-129, 1986 [Editorial].

34. Gronert GA et al: Effect of CO_2, calcium, digoxin, and potassium on cardiac and skeletal muscle metabolism in malignant hyperthermia susceptible swine, Anesthesiology 64:24-28, 1986.

35. Loghmanee F and Tobak M: Fatal malignant hyperthermia associated with recreational cocaine and ethanol abuse, Am J Forensic Med Pathol 7:246-248, 1986.

36. Nagarajan K et al: Calcium uptake in frozen muscle biopsy sections compared with other predictors of malignant hyperthermia susceptibility, Anesthesiology 66:680-685, 1987.

37. Denborough MA, Hopkinson KC, and Banney DG: Firefighting and malignant hyperthermia, Br Med J Clin Res 296(6634):1442-1443, 1988.

38. Mirchandani H and Reich LE: Fatal malignant hyperthermia as a result of ingestion of tranylcypromine (Parnate) combined with white wine and cheese, J Forensic Sci 30:217-220, 1985.

39. Caroff SN et al: Malignant hyperthermia susceptibility in neuroleptic malignant syndrome, Anesthesiology 67:20-25, 1987.

40. Krivosic Horber R et al: Neuroleptic malignant syndrome and malignant hyperthermia: in vitro comparison with halothane and caffeine contracture tests, Br J Anaesth 59:1554-1556, 1987.

41. Geiduschek J et al: Repeated anesthesia for a patient with neuroleptic malignant syndrome, Anesthesiology 68:134-137, 1988.

42. Cabral R et al: Reversible profound depression of cerebral electrical activity in hyperthermia, Electroencephalogr Clin Neurophysiol 42:697-701, 1977.

43. Rosenberg H and Fletcher JE: Masseter muscle rigidity and malignant hyperthermia susceptibility, Anesth Analg 65:161-164, 1986.

44. Schwartz L, Rockoff MA, and Koka BV: Masseter spasm with anesthesia: incidence and implications, Anesthesiology, 61:772-775, 1984.

45. Baudendistel L et al: End-tidal CO_2 monitoring: its use in the diagnosis and management of malignant hyperthermia, Anaesthesia 39:1000-1003, 1984.

46. Horrow JC and Rosenberg, H: Does urinary catheter temperature reflect core temperature during cardiac surgery? Anesthesiology 69:986-989, 1988.

47. Lees DE, Bee WS, Bull, JM, et al: An evaluation of liquid-crystal thermometry as a screening device for intraoperative hyperthermia, Anesth Analg 57:669-674, 1978.

48. Allen GC et al: Plasma levels of dantrolene following oral administration in malignant hyperthermia-susceptible patients, Anesthesiology 69:900-904, 1988.

49. Horowitz BZ: The golden hour in heat stroke: use of iced peritoneal lavage, Am J Emerg Med 7:616-619, 1989.

50. Ward A, Chaffman MO, and Sorkin EM: Dantrolene: a review of its pharmacodynamic and pharmacokinetic properties and therapeutic use in malignant hyperthermia, the neuroleptic malignant syndrome and an update of its use in muscle spasticity, Drugs 32:130-168, 1986.

51. Rosenberg H and Fletcher JE: Failure of carbocaine to exacerbate malignant hyperthermia in swine. (In preparation.)

52. Katz D: Recurrent malignant hyperthermia during anesthesia, Anesth Analg 49:225-230, 1975.

53. Rubin AS and Zablocki AD: Hyperkalemia, verapamil, and dantrolene, Anesthesiology 66:246-249, 1987.

54. Rosenberg H: Trismus is not trivial, Anesthesiology 67:453-455, 1987 [Editorial].

55. Allen GC, Rosenberg H, and Fletcher JE: Safety of general anesthesia in patients previously tested negative for malignant hyperthermia susceptibility, Anesthesiology 72:619-622, 1990.

56. Olgin J et al: Non-invasive evaluation of malignant hyperthermia susceptibility with phosphorus nuclear magnetic resonance spectroscopy, Anesthesiology 68:507-513, 1988.

57. Lomax P: The hypothermic effect of pentobarbital in the rat: sites and mechanisms of action, Brain Res 1:296-302, 1966.

58. Lotti VJ, Lomax P, and George R: Heat production and heat loss in the rat following ntracerebral and systemic administration of morphine, Int J Neuropharmacol 5:75-83, 1966.

59. Rosow CE, Miller JM, Pelikan EW, et al: Opiates and thermoregulation in mice. I. Agonists, J Pharmacol Exp Ther 213:273-283, 1980.

60. Sessler DI, Olofsson CI, and Rubinstein EH: The thermoregulatory threshold in humans during nitrous oxide–fentanyl anesthesia, Anesthesiology 69:357-364, 1988.

61. Sessler DI, Olofsson CI, Rubinstein EH, et al.: The thermoregulatory threshold in humans during halothane anesthesia, Anesthesiology 68:836-842, 1988.

62. Goldberg MJ and Roe CF: Temperature changes during anesthesia and operations, Arch Surg 93:365-369, 1966.

63. Hervey GR: Hypothermia, Proc R Soc Med 66:1053-1057, 1973.

64. Bigelow WG, Lindsay WK, Harrison RC, et al.: Oxygen transport and utilization in dogs at low body temperatures, Am J Physiol 160:125-137, 1950.

65. Harper AM, Bain WH, Glass HI, et al: Temperature difference in organs and tissues with observations on total oxygen uptake in profound hypothermia, Surg Gynecol Obstet 112:519-525, 1961.

66. Michenfelder JD and Theye RA: Hypothermia: effects on canine brain and whole-body metabolism, Anesthesiology 29:1107-1112, 1968.

67. Severinghaus JW and Stupfel M: Respiratory dead space increase following atropine in man, and atropine, vagal or ganglionic blockade and hypothermia in dogs, J Appl Physiol 8:81-87, 1955.

68. Regan MJ and Eger EI: Ventilatory responses to hypercapnia and hypoxia at normothermia and moderate hypothermia during constant-depth halothane anesthesia, Anesthesiology 27:624-633, 1966.

69. Benumof JL and Wahrenbrock EA: Dependency of hypoxia pulmonary vasoconstriction on temperature, J Appl Physiol 42:56-58, 1977.

70. Hägerdal M, Harp J, and Siesjö BK: Effect of hypothermia upon organic phosphates, glycolytic metabolites, citric acid cycle intermediates and associated amino acids in rat cerebral cortex, J Neurochem 24:743-748, 1975.

71. Heier T, Caldwell JE, Sessler DI, et al.: The relationship between adductor pollicis twitch tension and core, skin, and muscle temperature during nitrous oxide–isoflurane anesthesia in humans, Anesthesiology 71:38-384, 1989.

72. Rosenberg H, Clofine F, and Bialik O: Neurologic changes during awakening fronanesthesia, Anesthesiology 54:125-130, 1981.

73. Sessler DI, Israel D, Pozos RS, et al: Spontaneous post-anesthetic tremor does not resemble thermoregulatory shivering, Anesthesiology 68:843-850, 1988.

74. Pozos RS, Israel D, McCutcheon R, et al.: Human studies concerning thermal-induced shivering, postoperative "shivering," and cold-induced vasodilation, Ann Emerg Med 16:1037-1041, 1987.

75. Yoshihara H, Yamamoto T, and Mihara H: Changes in coagulation and fibrinolysis occurring in dogs during hypothermia, Thrombosis Res 37:503-512, 1985.

76. Paul J, Cornillon B, Baguet J, et al.: In vivo release of a heparin-like factor in dogs during profound hypothermia, J Thorac Cardiovasc Surg 82:45-48, 1981.

77. Cornillon B, Mazzorana M, Dureau G, et al: Characterization of a heparin-like activity released in dogs during deep hypothermia, Eur J Clin Invest 18:460-464, 1988.

78. Villalobos TJ, Adelson E, and Barila TG: Hematologic changes in hypothermic dogs, Proc Soc Exp Biol Med 89:192-196, 1955.

79. Hessell EA, Schmer G, and Dillard DH: Platelet kinetics during deep hypothermia, J Surg Res 28:23-34, 1980.

80. Kattlove HE and Alexander B: The effect of cold on platelets. I. Cold-induced platelet aggregation, Blood 38:39-47, 1971.

81. Valeri CR, Feingold H, Cassidy G, et al.: Hypothermia-induced reversible platelet dysfunction, Ann Surg 205:175-181, 1987.

82. Bigelow WG, Mustard WT, and Evans JG: Some physiologic concepts of hypothermia and their applications to cardiac surgery, J Thorac Surg 28:463, 1954.

83. Rahn H: Introduction. In Rahn H and Prakash O, editors: Acid-base regulation and body temperature, Boston, 1985, Martinus Nijhoff Publishers, pp 1-12.

84. Morris RH: Influence of ambient temperature on patient temperature during intra-abdominal surgery, Ann Surg 173:230-233, 1971.

85. Roizen MF, Sohn YJ, L'Hommedieu CS, et al.: Operating room temperature prior to surgical draping: effect on patient temperature in recovery room, Anesth Analg 59:852-855, 1980.

86. Holdcroft A and Hall GM: Heat loss during anaesthesia, Br J Anaesth 50:157-164, 1978.

87. Bissonnette B and Sessler DI: Passive or active inspired gas humidification increases thermal steady-state temperatures in anesthetized infants, Anesth Analg 69:783-787, 1989.

88. Stone DR, Downs JB, Paul WL, et al.: Adult body temperature and heated humidification of anesthetic gases during general anesthesia, Anesth Analg 60:736-741, 1981.

89. Tausk HC, Miller R, and Roberts RB: Maintenance of body temperature by heated humidification, Anesth Analg 55:719-723, 1976.

90. Tølløfsrud SG, Gundersen Y, and Andersen R: Peroperative hypothermia, Acta Anaesthesiol Scand 28:511-515, 1984.

91. Klein EF Jr and Graves SA: "Hot pot" tracheitis, Chest 65:225-226, 1974.

92. Chalon J, Patel C, Ramanathan S, et al.: Humidification of the circle absorber system, Anesthesiology 48:142-146, 1978.

93. Lønning PE, Skulberg A, and Abyholm F: Accidental hypothermia, Acta Anaesthesiol Scand 30:601-613, 1986.

94. Reuler JB: Hypothermia: pathophysiology, clinical settings, and management, Ann Intern Med 89:519-527, 1978.

95. Brichard G and Johnstone M: The effect of methylphenidate (Ritalin) on post-halothane muscular spasticity, Br J Anaesth 42:718-722, 1970.

96. Liem ST and Aldrete JA: Control of post-anaesthetic shivering, Can Anaesth Soc J 21:506-510, 1974.

97. Pauca AL, Savage RT, Simpson S, et al.: Effect of pethidine, fentanyl and morphine on post-operative shivering in man, Acta Anaesthesiol Scand 28:138-143, 1984.

98. Macintyre PE, Pavlin EG, and Dwersteg JF: Effect of meperidine on oxygen consumption, carbon dioxide production, and respiratory gas exchange in postanesthesia shivering, Anesth Analg 66:751-755, 1987.

Chapter 15

Impaired Central Nervous System Function

Gregory Crosby

Central nervous system (CNS) dysfunction is a fundamental characteristic of the anesthetic state. In fact, general anesthesia would not occur without it. Hence, some degree of postoperative CNS impairment is a natural consequence of general anesthesia and is present in all patients in the immediate postanesthetic period. The degree of dysfunction is typically mild, short lived, and, despite present day pharmacologic advances, unavoidable. Only when the dysfunction is prolonged or bizarre does it becomes worrisome enough to be labeled as a complication. In addition, anesthesia complicates diagnosis of significant CNS events that do occur infrequently in anesthetized patients. On the other hand, because of the profound CNS effects of most anesthetics, the anesthesia provider is at least theoretically in a position to positively affect the incidence or severity of CNS injury inherent in certain surgical procedures.

Accordingly, this chapter focuses on perioperative CNS complications of anesthesia as well as those that are properly considered risks of particular surgical procedures. The first section is organized into four main topics: the "normal" cognitive and psychologic consequences of anesthesia; delirium, causes of new neurologic deficits in the perioperative period, and an approach to evaluation of delayed or abnormal emergence. The second section is concerned with neurologic risks inherent in a few surgical procedures. This chapter does not deal with the neurologic complications of spinal, epidural, or regional anesthesia, or with injury to the peripheral nervous system because these are covered in Chapters 3, 4, and 7 respectively.

The information presented here should be tempered with the realization that most data on CNS dysfunction in the perioperative period are epidemiologic in nature: the frequency of a particular event is associated with certain patient characteristics, medications, physiologic changes, procedures, and so on. Rarely have cause-and-effect relationships been established directly. Rarer still is reliable information that physiologic or anesthetic management influences neurologic outcome. Nevertheless, the information presented aims to help the clinician develop a rational and realistic approach to anticipating, avoiding, identifying, and managing CNS dysfunction in the perioperative period.

I. CNS DYSFUNCTION AFTER NON-CNS, NONCARDIAC SURGERY

A. "Normal" postanesthetic cognitive and psychomotor dysfunction

Clinicians and patients recognize that general anesthesia and surgery leave many people feeling lethargic, unable to concentrate or retain information, and with apparent deterioration of verbal and fine motor skills. In fact, it is not possible to administer a general anesthetic that does not produce postoperative CNS dysfunction because all agents used for premedication, induction, and maintenance have some lingering CNS effects. Intramuscular diazepam or meperidine, for example, impair reaction and coordination skills for as long as 5 to 12 hours in healthy volunteers.[1] Feelings of anxiety and restlessness may occur 24 to 36 hours postoperatively in nearly a fourth of outpatients receiving droperidol 1.25 mg intravenously for prophylaxis of vomiting.[2] Even drugs generally regarded to have a short duration of action may produce relatively long-lasting CNS dysfunction. Memory is impaired to the same extent 5 hours after sedative doses of midazolam or the longer-acting diazepam,[3] and although gross clinical recovery is faster after methohexital than after thiopental administration, residual effects of methohexital are evident on psychomotor testing 12 hours after a single dose.[4] Even propofol, with a very short elimination half-life, has lingering CNS effects. Compared with methohexital or thiopental for induction of enflurane anesthesia for brief procedures, propofol produces more rapid awakening and recovery of cognitive and psychomotor skills[5] such that little impairment is present 30 minutes after anesthesia. Inhalation anesthetics, of course, also have prolonged effects on mental function. In fact, psychomotor performance is worsened significantly for 5 hours after inhalation induction and maintenance of anesthesia for only 3½ minutes with halothane or enflurane in normal volunteers.[6] As the duration of anesthesia increases, so too does the duration of postanesthetic CNS impairment. In volunteers anesthetized with halothane or isoflurane (with or without nitrous oxide) for a mean of 6.6 to 7.2 hours, somatic and behavioral symptoms persisted for 6 to 8 days,[7] whereas perceptual-motor and intellectual function required 2 days to normalize after approximately 10 to 14 MAC-hours of halothane or enflurane anesthesia.[8]

In addition to producing transient neuropsychologic sequelae, some claim that, particularly in the elderly, general anesthesia produces prolonged or permanent changes in memory and cognitive ability.[9-12] Careful studies thus far yield no evidence to support that notion, however; neuropsychologic testing of elderly patients identifies no decrement in performance relative to preanesthesia scores 1 to several months after anesthesia.[13-16] Some of the psychologic and cognitive changes attributed to general anesthesia are not unique to it and may be related to the surgical experience (that is, anxiety, surgery, pain, hospitalization, and so on). Studies comparing the short- and long-term psychologic and cognitive effects of general anesthesia with those of regional anesthesia, for example, indicate that performance after regional anesthesia is essentially no better than after general anesthesia, particularly if intravenous sedation is used to supplement a regional technique.[14-17] Thus all general anesthetics produce subtle psychologic and intellectual changes that persist for hours or days.

Descriptions of CNS impairment after general anesthesia have seldom been complemented by investigation of the causes. The most obvious explanation for persistent neuropsychologic dysfunction after general anesthesia, and the reason for emphasis on agents with rapid and predictable redistribution and clearance in modern anesthesia practice, is that a small amount of anesthetic agent remains in the brain even when gross clinical recovery is complete.[18] Recent nuclear magnetic resonance (NMR) studies[19,20] show, for example, that 20% of the NMR signal for halothane is still detectable in rat brain 90 minutes after a 1-hour anesthetic with 1% halothane and 15% of the isoflurane signal remains 90 minutes after 1.5 hours of 1.5% isoflurane in rabbits. Another study [21] indicates that as much as 40% of the NMR signal of halothane or its metabolites is detectable in rabbit brain 7 hours after anesthesia though it is suggested that much of the signal that was originally believed to originate from brain actually represents anesthetic remaining in tissues outside of the brain.[20] In any event the lingering presence of small amounts of anesthetic in the brain would be of little significance were it not for the fact that complex brain functions are probably very sensitive to anesthetic drug effects. One indication of this is that at least in animals gross clinical recovery occurs at a time of significant cerebral metabolic depression; at emergence (defined by ability to withdraw from a pinch), the cerebral metabolic rate for oxygen of dogs anesthetized with either pentobarbital or halothane is still 20% below normal.[22] In humans, about the only nonbehavioral measure of persistent dysfunction that has been evaluated carefully is natural sleep. Electrophysiologic data indicate that natural patterns of rapid-eye-movement and slow-wave sleep in humans are disrupted for 24 hours after a brief anesthetic[23] and remain abnormal for several days after anesthesia and surgery.[24]

Part of the problem of postanesthetic CNS dysfunction, even with rapidly eliminated anesthetics, may be that anesthetic requirements are determined clinically by crude indices of anesthetic depth (such as blood pressure, heart rate) that may have little direct relationship to the state of higher brain function or consciousness. Whatever the reason, awakening and recovery from anesthesia is normally associated with cerebral metabolic, neurophysiologic, behavioral, and cognitive changes that persist for hours to days from the time of exposure. Almost by definition, however, these changes are considered side effects—the "cost of doing business"—rather than complications of anesthesia and, at the current level of sophistication, cannot be entirely prevented. These seemingly minor CNS side effects of anesthesia result in patient dissatisfaction and, on occasion, add to hospital expense (for example, if hospitalization of an outpatient is required) but are fundamentally benign and self-limited. The more worrisome types of postoperative CNS dysfunction begin with delirium and include permanent structural or functional damage to the nervous system.

B. Delirium

Delirium, which is not simply an exaggerated form of "normal" postoperative CNS dysfunction, is evidently a common clinical problem, but its exact incidence is unknown.[25-27] Postoperative delirium is frightening and disturbing to patients and staff, can be dangerous if an agitated, combative patient disconnects monitoring and intravenous tubing or life-support equipment such as endotracheal tubes and ventilators, and may result in lengthened hospitalization.[28]

The differential diagnosis is extensive[27,29,30] and of more than academic interest because postoperative delirium can be a warning of serious but treatable underlying disease. Many causes of postoperative delirium are not treatable however.[25-30] Preexisting organic brain disease, psychiatric disorders, the extremes of age, and the type of surgery (particularly cardiac,[31,32] ophthalmologic,[33] and hip repair[10,17]) all increase the risk of postoperative delirium. Delirium on emergence may also be a manifestation of awareness during anesthesia[34,35] and is presumably a response to stress. Of greatest clinical interest are the potentially treatable causes of postoperative delirium. In particular, conditions that unbalance the normally close relationship between cerebral oxygen supply and demand are the most ominous and important to recognize. Thus cerebral hypoxia,[10,26,27,36] whether caused by hypoventilation, pulmonary embolism, hypotension, severe anemia, or cerebral ischemia, must be considered immediately in any patient who is delirious in the perioperative period. Only after the possibility of cerebral hypoxia has been excluded

should one consider other treatable causes of delirium such as endocrine or ionic imbalances, postoperative pain, bowel or bladder distension, language difficulties, the porphyrias (acute intermittent and variegate), and drugs.[26,27,29,30]

A delirious patient's medication history is important. High-dose steroids may produce an acute psychotic reaction,[37] and delirium may occur during withdrawal from drugs of abuse such as alcohol, opioids, and hallucinogens. Certain anesthetic agents and adjuvants have also been implicated in postoperative confusional states. Ketamine, a derivative of phencyclidine (PCP), has hallucinogenic and convulsive properties that are primarily related to the negative stereoisomer in the racemic clinical preparation; emergence delirium as well as vivid unpleasant dreams, perceptual distortion, disorientation, agitation, and nightmares may occur.[38] The incidence of psychologic disturbances with ketamine can be reduced by administration of benzodiazepines intravenously before awakening,[38-40] and, for unknown reasons, in the elderly and young children troublesome CNS effects of ketamine are less common.[41] Anticholinergic medication such as atropine and scopolamine is another classic pharmacologic cause of postoperative confusion, particularly in the elderly.[36,42-44] Not only has a good correlation been demonstrated between increasing plasma anticholinergic concentrations and impairment of cognitive function,[43] but also, in elderly patients receiving either epidural or halothane anesthesia for hip fracture repair, the factor that best predicts development of postoperative confusion is use of anticholinergic medication.[36] Glycopyrrolate, however, has essentially no CNS effects because its quaternary ammonium structure prevents it from crossing the blood-brain barrier.[42] The psychotropic or neurologic effects of other anesthetic agents and adjuvants could be mistaken for a perioperative confusional state. Droperidol, a butyrophenone, has psychotropic effects characterized by dysphoria and ill-defined anxiety that are severe enough that some patients who receive droperidol premedication refuse surgery.[45] Droperidol may also produce extrapyramidal reactions[46] that respond well to treatment with diphenhydramine. Even propofol has been implicated in unusual perioperative behavior characterized by hallucinations,[47] muscular hypotonus,[48] abnormal posturing,[49] amorous behavior,[50] difficulty with eye opening,[51] and possibly seizures.[52,53] Since pharmacologic causes of postanesthetic delirium are fundamentally benign and self-limited, it is most important to be certain that delirium is not mistakenly attributed to a drug effect when cerebral hypoxia or some other correctable metabolic disturbance is actually the cause.

C. New neurologic impairment after routine surgery

In contrast to the ubiquitous but essentially benign consequences of general anesthesia just discussed, major neurologic complications such as stroke, seizures, or hypoxia after nonneurologic, noncardiac surgery are rare but potentially very devastating. In a recent prospective, randomized study[54] of outcome after anesthesia in 17,201 patients, only 7 patients (0.04%) had a stroke. A retrospective study[55] involving a 2-year period and 58,907 anesthetics reported only three patients with a new focal deficit upon emergence from anesthesia. The elderly [56] and those having peripheral vascular surgical procedures[57,58] are at higher risk for perioperative stroke, presumably because of coexisting cerebral or carotid vascular disease. Stroke is not the only cause of new postoperative neurologic morbidity, however. Seizures and hypoxic brain injury also occur but probably much less frequently than stroke does. For example, in a large retrospective review of insurance claims made on just over 1 million anesthetics administered to American Society of Anesthesiologists physical status 1 and 2 patients at nine teaching hospitals affiliated with a major university,[59] eight of the 11 claims were related to severe CNS injury attributed to hypoxia, usually attributable to catastrophes of airway management. From a clinical perspective, therefore, the central questions are what precipitates perioperative neurologic events, can they be prevented, and how does one distinguish between cerebral disease and "normal" CNS dysfunction in the patient recovering from anesthesia?

1. Perioperative stroke. Development of a new focal neurologic deficit during the perioperative period is uncommon and unpredictable but probably not random. One report,[60] for example, cites 12 strokes in a general surgical population when epidemiologic data concerning the yearly incidence of stroke in age-matched nonhospitalized people predicted only one such event. Another study[55] cites 3 cases of perioperative stroke when only 0.1 was predicted from epidemiologic data. Thus the risk of stroke is apparently increased perioperatively, but the conditions that predispose some surgical patients to stroke are not obvious. There is unanimity of opinion, for example, that an asymptomatic carotid bruit, usually considered a sign of cerebrovascular disease and present in about 14% of surgical patients 55 years or older and 20% of vascular surgical patients, is

not a risk factor for perioperative stroke.[61,66] Perhaps the reason is that a bruit is audible before critical narrowing of the vessel occurs[62] or because changes in flow characteristics such as anemia may create a bruit without vascular obstruction.

The relationship between symptomatic cerebrovascular disease and perioperative stroke is controversial however. A few studies[61,63] indicate that patients with transient ischemic attacks (TIAs) or amaurosis fugax have a significantly higher incidence of stroke in the perioperative period than asymptomatic individuals, but others refute any such relationship.[57,65,67] There is little guidance even in the extreme case of a person who has had a recent stroke. Although it is often recommended that surgery be delayed for 6 weeks after a stroke because of a period of vulnerability for reinfarction,[68] no careful investigation of the issue exists. Intraoperative hypotension is another time-honored explanation for perioperative stroke that is not entirely credible. The simple observation that intraoperative hypotension is frequent but stroke is rare raises questions about an association between the two, as does the fact that TIAs typically occur without meaningful changes in blood pressure.[69] Furthermore, studies indicate that many patients who suffer a postoperative stroke experienced and survived intraoperative hypotension without neurologic sequelae.[60,63,65] More direct evidence that challenges the role of hypotension as a cause of stroke comes from a study[70] of 37 patients with TIAs deliberately exposed to nearly a 60% decrease in systolic blood pressure. Such profound hypotension recreated a true TIA in only 1 person; some patients developed unrelated focal signs, but 17 had no focal findings at all. Similarly, an autopsy study[71] of the brains of 135 patients who survived at least 1 day after a cardiac arrest (and hence a hypotensive episode) found a relationship between the severity of cerebral atherosclerosis and brain infarction in only 7 patients. This is not to suggest that hypotension is benign but rather that it has probably been blamed for more neurologic events than is warranted.

What therefore does cause perioperative stroke? Thrombotic and embolic events, common causes of stroke in nonhospitalized patients with cerebrovascular disease,[72] are also responsible for most perioperative strokes. Cardiogenic embolism was considered the most common mechanism of cerebral infarction in a retrospective review[60] and accounted for 5 of 12 (42%) perioperative strokes; only 1 stroke was attributed to hypotension. Furthermore, nearly all (83%) of the strokes occurred postoperatively; 17% of the patients had an antecedent myocardial infarction, and 33% were in atrial fibrillation at the time of the stroke.[60] Similarly, among three recently reported cases of new focal neurologic deficits detected upon emergence from anesthesia, two were attributed to embolism (one cardiogenic, the other paradoxical embolization of CO_2) and one was caused by a cerebral hemorrhage.[55] In this context, it is noteworthy that arterial embolization is a rare consequence of venous air embolism even though a probe-patent foramen ovale is present in about 25% of autopsy specimens.[73] Because most perioperative strokes are embolic, a thorough cardiac examination should not be neglected when one is evaluating a patient afflicted with a new postoperative focal deficit.

2. *Perioperative seizures.* Perioperative seizures may be idiopathic or related to hypoxia, metabolic disorders such as hypocalcemia and hypoglycemia, fever, or occult concomitant CNS disease (such as cerebrovascular disease, brain tumor).[74] Anesthetic agents may also have a role in the genesis of perioperative seizures, however.[75,76] Several anesthetics produce intraoperative electroencephalographic (EEG) and clinical evidence of seizures, but evidence that these agents precipitate postoperative convulsions is comparatively weak. Enflurane, for example, produces epileptiform EEG activity that is influenced both by the depth of anesthesia and the Pa_{CO_2}. In healthy people at normal Pa_{CO_2}, EEG spiking is maximal at end-tidal concentrations of 2% to 3%, and grand mal seizure patterns occur at 3% to 6%.[77,78] At a given enflurane concentration, hyperventilation increases seizure activity and hypoventilation decreases it such that the minimum epileptogenic concentration is approximately 1% lower at a Pa_{CO_2} of 20 mm Hg and 1% higher at a Pa_{CO_2} of 60 mm Hg than it is at 40 mm Hg.[77,78] Even though seizures have been reported hours to days after enflurane anesthesia in nonepileptic patients,[79-84] EEG documentation of postoperative seizure activity is rare.[79,84,85] In volunteers followed for 6 to 30 days with surface EEG recordings after receiving 9.6 MAC-hours of enflurane, only nonepileptiform changes were observed even though one half the volunteers had clinical and EEG evidence of seizures during anesthesia.[86] It is also interesting that enflurane, like most anesthetics, has anticonvulsant properties; it reduces the frequency of seizure-like EEG activity relative to the awake or natural sleep EEG in patients with seizure disorders[87] and has been used successfully to stop status epilepticus in children.[87] Halothane,[88,89] isoflurane,[90-92] and nitrous oxide[88] have also been the subject of isolated case reports of seizure-like activity during exposure, but none are believed to cause postoperative seizures.

Seizure activity has also been associated with certain intravenous anesthetics. Etomidate produces involuntary myoclonic movements during induction of anesthesia that occasionally persist into the recovery period,[93-95] but this myoclonic activity is not associated with EEG spikes in nonepileptic patients.[93,96,97] On the other hand, seizure activity occurs in a large percentage of epileptic patients anesthetized with etomidate[87,98-100] and appeared in 20% of nonepileptic patients undergoing open-heart surgery under etomidate anesthesia.[98] There is no evidence that such intraoperative events increase the risk of postoperative seizures, however. Ketamine is another agent that activates epileptogenic foci and may increase seizure frequency in patients with a seizure disorder[101,102] but does not produce electroencephalographic seizures in nonepileptic patients.[76,103-106] As mentioned previously, propofol may activate preexisting seizure foci[52] but evidently does not precipitate epileptiform activity in patients without a seizure disorder.[53,107,108] In fact, propofol reduces seizure duration during electroconvulsive therapy[109,110] and has been used successfully to treat status epilepticus.[111] Methohexital, well-known to produce excitatory phenomena such as tremor and muscle movements, has never been demonstrated to precipitate clinical or EEG seizures in patients with generalized convulsive disorders but is epileptogenic in patients with psychomotor epilepsy.[112-114]

There has been some concern about the seizure potential of opioid analgesics as well. Meperidine, or more accurately, its metabolite normeperidine, may produce tremulousness, myoclonus, and seizures.[115,116] Since normeperidine has a long half-life (14 to 21 hours), this effect may persist into the postoperative period, particularly in patients with reduced clearance because of renal failure[117] or in those receiving very large doses of meperidine for chronic pain.[117,118] Morphine, on the other hand, has no seizure activity in humans.[76] The reports of grand mal seizure-like behavior after administration of fentanyl, sufentanil, and alfentanil[119-127] often lack EEG confirmation. Indeed, with the exception of two studies[128,129] that reported isolated sharp waves, abnormal EEG patterns have not been documented in patients treated with fentanyl or its analogs.[128-133]

Therefore, although selected inhalational and intravenous anesthetics may produce abnormal

EEG activity in normal persons and activate seizure foci in epileptics, it is uncertain whether these electrophysiologic events are neurologically meaningful, require treatment, or respond appropriately to it. Traditional seizure therapy with diazepam[79] or low-dose thiopental,[134] for example, may actually intensify enflurane-induced seizures. In any case, evidence that intraoperative seizure activity increases the risk of postoperative seizures, even in seizure-prone patients, is weak.

D. Clinical evaluation of CNS dysfunction upon emergence

Emergence from anesthesia may be neurologically unsatisfactory because of prolonged drowsiness, delirium, an obvious focal neurologic deficit, or even true coma (that is, unresponsiveness to painful stimuli). The most important diagnostic question in such a situation is whether the problem is attributable to exaggerated anesthetic-induced dysfunction or a neurologic event.

In practical terms, delayed emergence from anesthesia is defined by the clinician's expectation in a specific circumstance; the patient "should be awake by now" but isn't. Unfortunately, other than personal experience, there is little guidance as to what constitutes prolonged emergence under actual clinical circumstances. In a recent study[54] involving over 17,000 patients randomized to receive one of four anesthetic agents (enflurane, halothane, isoflurane, and fentanyl), 6% and 3% were scored as "not recovered" at respectively 60 and 90 minutes after anesthesia. Since the incidence of stroke and other major CNS events in this population was only 0.04 %, one can safely assume that non-CNS problems (such as protracted vomiting, pain, hemodynamic or respiratory instability) accounted for low recovery scores in most patients. Data specifically concerning neurologic recovery after anesthesia are surprisingly few. Outpatients who received about 1 hour of propofol or thiopental-isoflurane anesthesia responded to commands, opened their eyes, and were oriented within about 10 minutes of discontinuance of nitrous oxide.[135] However, a prospective study involving all surgical patients admitted to the recovery room during a single month reported that 41 out of 443 (9%) were unarousable for as long as 15 to 90 minutes after entering the recovery room even though none had a neurologic event. This illustrates two features of postanesthesia neurologic recovery: (1) most patients awaken promptly after anesthesia, but the variability is large; and (2) delayed arousal is much more commonly attributable to drug effects than to neurologic events.[136]

The first step in evaluating a patient whose emergence from anesthesia is abnormal or delayed is to perform a neurologic examination. However, very little neurologically acceptable investigation exists in patients recovering from anesthesia, and only gross evaluation of cognition, motor function, pupillary signs, and reflexes is practical. The possibility of a simple explanation for an alarming finding (such as dilated pupils caused by mydriatics or eye trauma) must always be considered, as must the possibility that intravenous tubing and catheters, monitoring devices, pain, and surgical appliances are interfering with the patient's ability to execute commands. Moreover, even neurologically normal patients awakening from anesthesia frequently have abnormal eye signs and "pathologic" reflexes.[137] For instance, 40% to 100% of neurologically normal patients have an absent pupillary response to light 20 minutes after anesthesia, and in 10% the pupillary and lid responses can be depressed for 40 minutes.[137] Biceps and quadriceps hyperreflexia, sustained and unsustained ankle clonus, and a plantar (Babinski) reflex occur in a large percentage of neurologically intact patients recovering from anesthesia, and in many cases abnormalities are present even when patients are fully awake.[137] The type of anesthesia influences the incidence of transient neurologic abnormalities; abnormal reflexes occur more commonly in patients recovering from enflurane or halothane than from nitrous oxide–opiate anesthesia.[137] A variety of other transient neurologic abnormalities have been reported during recovery from anesthesia; opisthotonus[49] and difficulty with eye opening [51] have been associated with propofol, extrapyramidal reactions with droperidol,[46] and seizures with several agents.[75,76] Certain findings on neurologic examination are inconsistent with a drug effect and point toward a primary neurologic event or intracranial process, however. Reflex changes associated with emergence from anesthesia are always bilateral,[137] unless of course reflex asymmetry (perhaps caused by a prior CNS or peripheral injury) existed preoperatively. Thus unilateral reflex changes are a worrisome finding. In addition, the snout, grasp, palmomental, and Hoffman reflexes cannot be attributed to medication[137] and ophthalmoplegia may signal thrombosis of the basilar artery.[138]

When recovery does not occur promptly, a neurologic examination may not be comprehensive. Since CNS dysfunction is produced deliberately every time induction of general anesthesia occurs, one should think first of an exaggerated drug effect as a cause of delayed emergence. Failure to awaken promptly and lucidly from anesthesia because of a drug effect, though clearly undesirable and anxiety provoking, is, however, not life threatening so long as the problem is recognized and supportive management (such as airway protection and ventilation) is appropriate. One could argue, in fact, that it is important to determine whether a prolonged or difficult emergence is caused by anesthesia only to the extent that it allows one to be sure that it is not attributable to a neurologic event.

Since an individual patient may have received several drugs capable of obtunding consciousness (an inhalational agent; sedatives such as barbiturates, benzodiazepines, and anticholinergics; opioids such as fentanyl and morphine; and muscle relaxants), identifying a pharmacologic cause may not be easy. A relative opioid overdosage might be suspected clinically in a patient with slow, deep inspirations and pinpoint pupils, whereas midposition pupils and rapid, shallow breathing may point toward lingering inhalation agent. The possibility of continuing neuromuscular blockade, which might limit patient cooperation but does not explain drowsiness or unconsciousness, can be evaluated by hand grasp strength, ability to sustain a head lift, or by train-of-four testing. More often than not, a combination of drugs, rather than a single agent, is the cause of delayed emergence, and determining whether anesthetics are responsible is further complicated by the fact that only a few anesthetic agents and adjuvants have pharmacologic antagonists. In this context, pharmacologic antagonists such as naloxone, physostigmine, and flumazenil should be viewed as diagnostic aids, not just therapy. Given the limited selection of antagonists and the multiplicity of drugs a patient may have received, one must be pragmatic; if in doubt, reverse what can be reversed. The goal of this approach is to permit a brief period of arousal during which clinical neurologic evaluation can be performed.[139,140]

Residual drug-induced paralysis is usually easily corrected with an anticholinesterase and antimuscarinic agent such as atropine or glycopyrrolate. If opioids have been administered, a very small dose of naloxone (40 to 80 μg intravenously) typically will reverse respiratory depression and awaken the patient transiently without intensifying incisional pain or producing nausea and vomiting.[139] Some caution should be exercised when one is using naloxone, however, since even small dosages rarely may produce severe hypertension and arrhythmias.[141,142] An attempt to reverse the CNS effects of an inhalational agent with a nonspecific analeptic such as physostigmine should be considered. Physostigmine (2 mg intravenously) produces transient EEG arousal and few side effects, but clinical arousal is unreliable and short lived. Physostigmine is the antagonist of choice for CNS depression or agitation caused by scopalamine or atropine[143] and may produce improvement in postoperative somnolence caused by benzodiazepines.[144] The benzodiazepine antagonist flumazenil will strengthen our diagnostic and therapeutic armamentarium substantially. Flumazenil produces prompt recovery from benzodiazepine sedation with minimal side effects and should prove useful in any postoperative patient whose emergence is believed to be delayed by lingering effects of diazepam or midazolam.[145,146] The underlying assumption of this approach is that if a patient is arousable (even if only transiently) by pharmacologic means and is neurologically intact, no further evaluation is necessary and recovery from anesthesia can proceed naturally. Judgments as to the need for continued support such as intubation and mechanical ventilation in such patients should be made according to the usual criteria, with recognition that the clinical effect of anesthetic antagonists is typically brief.

Failure to awaken sufficiently to perform even a crude neurologic examination despite passing of a reasonable period of time and attempts to reverse components of the anesthetic is worrisome and requires an active search for other causes of prolonged coma. A careful review of the history, particularly with respect to previous transient ischemic attacks, subarachnoid hemorrhage, seizures, or medical conditions that are associated with coma (such as diabetes,[147] porphyria[148]) is essential.[27] Hypothermia may delay awakening,[149,150] particularly in the elderly, but coma probably does not occur unless body temperature is 18° to 21° C.[67] Chronic medications, such as cimetidine,[151] may slow metabolism or elimination of anesthetic drugs and adjuvants. Severe hyperglycemia,[147] hyperosmolarity, and illicit drug usage should also be considered at this stage. An active seizure focus can depress consciousness, but in the absence of gross tonic-clonic movements the diagnosis requires EEG documentation. Finally, an unrecognized preexisting intracranial mass lesion such as a meningioma or new intracerebral hemorrhage may delay emergence from anesthesia.[152] The absence of focal findings on neurologic examination would be unusual with an intracranial mass lesion and the diagnosis would have to be confirmed by computerized tomography (CT) scan.

If a new and persistent focal neurologic deficit is identified, both additional diagnostic procedures and neurologic consulation are required. The history should be carefully reviewed for cardiac conditions such as arrhythmias, recent myocardial infarction, and intracardiac shunts that could predispose to emboli.[55,60] A thorough auscultatory examination of the heart should be performed with the same objective in mind. A CT scan is required to identify an intracranial mass lesion such as tumor or hemorrhage and, if contrast is used, may help identify a vascular anomaly (such as arteriovenous malformation) as well. A newly ischemic area will appear normal on CT scan for hours to days,[153] however, and so a negative CT scan in the immediate perioperative period does not exclude a diagnosis of stroke. In view of the high incidence of embolic causes of stroke,[55,60] an echocardiogram can be diagnostically helpful and is essential whenever the history or physical examination is suggestive of an intracardiac source for emboli. A precordial echocardiogram is not reliable for detecting a patent foramen ovale, however, and so a negative study does not eliminate the possibility of paradoxical embolism.[73] Arteriography may be appropriate at some stage of the evaluation if carotid or vertebrobasilar insufficiency is suspected or surgical evacuation of a hemorrhage or tumor is necessary. EEG, though useful to diagnose a seizure disorder, is not particularly helpful for determining the cause of delayed emergence or a focal deficit and therefore in general should not be one of the first studies obtained.

II. NEUROLOGIC DYSFUNCTION ASSOCIATED WITH SPECIFIC SURGICAL PROCEDURES

Carotid endarterectomy, open-heart surgery, and procedures on the thoracoabdominal aorta have inherent risks of perioperative CNS injury. The assumption and hope is that because these risks are predictable they can be minimized with meticulous intraoperative management, and the incidence of perioperative neurologic dysfunction is thereby reduced. Although this may be an unrealistic expectation in many situations, prevention, rather than postoperative recognition and management, of procedure-specific CNS complications is nevertheless the ideal objective in these cases.

A. Carotid endarterectomy

Although various neurologic complications have been attributed to carotid endarterectomy (CEA), the most common cause of neurologic dysfunction is stroke. Since CEA is the clinical prototype of transient focal cerebral ischemia with reperfusion, a 2% to 20% incidence of stroke associated with this procedure is not surprising.[154,155] Stroke in the perioperative period of CEA may be caused by hypoperfusion because of carotid cross-clamping, emboli occurring during shunt insertion or reperfusion of the carotid,[156] and perhaps reperfusion cerebral hyperemia.[157] Despite what one may imagine, many strokes during CEA are not related to cerebral hypoperfusion caused by carotid cross-clamping. In fact, studies of CEA performed under local anesthesia in awake patients[158-160] or with EEG monitoring in anesthetized patients[161] indicate that stroke is commonly embolic in origin because neurologic events often occur at the moment of clamping or reperfusion of the carotid. Some of these emboli may be related to surgical technique; in one study[162] the incidence of stroke was greater if a shunt was used than when it was not, presumably because of emboli released at the time of shunt insertion. Furthermore, strokes commonly occur postoperatively; a recent retrospective review of 561 CEAs identified 38 perioperative strokes (incidence 6.7%) and 60% of these occurred postoperatively.[163] Thus, since many strokes associated with CEA are related to surgical technique and occur postoperatively,[162-164] the degree to which it is possible to prevent neurologic complications during CEA by meticulous intraoperative management is probably limited.

Nevertheless, intraoperative physiologic and anesthetic management may be important in terms of reducing the risk of cerebral ischemic events. A goal of management therefore is to prevent ischemia by maintaining an acceptable balance between cerebral metabolic demand and blood supply or, alternatively, to minimize the consequences of cerebral ischemia once it occurs. Both strategies imply that one is capable of recognizing cerebral ischemia before it becomes severe enough to produce permanent CNS injury. In practice, this requires following neurologic status in an awake patient under local anesthesia or using an index of cerebral ischemia such as EEG in anesthetized patients, since stump pressure[165] or transconjunctival oxygen tension[166] measurements do not correlate well with regional cerebral blood flow. Routine shunting without EEG monitoring, selective shunting with EEG, and surgery under superficial cervical plexus block each has proponents, but whether one approach leads to improved neurologic outcome remains controversial. The rationale for EEG monitoring during CEA is based on the concept that characteristic EEG changes occur when cerebral blood flow (CBF) falls below a critical level,[167] which itself changes with the anesthetic state.[168] As CBF decreases, it reaches a level that is inadequate to support neuronal activity but is still sufficient to prevent neuronal death.[169] This hypothetical zone has been termed the "penumbra" and is characterized by electrically (and functionally) silent but viable neurons[169,170] and hence represents at least theoretically a situation of recoverable loss of function. EEG cannot distinguish between this level of hypoperfusion and a flow state so low that neuronal death occurs because neurons become electrically silent before their structural integrity is threatened.[169,170] Therefore EEG changes are not necessarily indicative of irreversible neuronal injury. Nevertheless, although direct comparison of EEG and neurologic examination during CEA performed under local anesthesia indicates that both false-positive and false-negative EEGs occur,[160] agreement between the two is usually good. In fact, so-called "false-positive" EEGs may reflect neurologically meaningful decreases in CBF that cannot be detected by the crude neurologic examination possible during surgery in a conscious patient under local anesthesia. However, whether EEG monitoring positively influences neurologic outcome remains a matter of speculation because no prospective, controlled studies have yet been performed. The possibility that intraoperative interventions to normalize the EEG are effective in preventing stroke is suggested indirectly by the fact that major, untreated, cross clamp–associated EEG changes are predictive of stroke in some patients.[161,171] Moreover, EEG monitoring permits selective shunting, which itself may reduce the incidence of major neurologic morbidity.[172]

Surgeons attempt to preserve adequate CBF during CEA by limiting cross-clamp time or inserting a shunt. Routine shunt insertion is controversial, however, because shunt insertion may cause cerebral emboli and increase neurologic morbidity;[162,172] hence many surgeons perform a shunt selectively. Chief among nonsurgical techniques for maintaining an adequate CBF are attention to blood pressure and arterial carbon dioxide (Pa_{CO_2}). The basis for concern about these physiologic parameters is that vessels in ischemic areas are maximally dilated because of tissue acidosis and are therefore incapable of autoregulating normally.[173,174] Thus a decrease in arterial pressure may reduce CBF in ischemic areas, whereas moderate induced hypertension may improve flow to marginal regions.[175,176] Accordingly, moderate induced hypertension is used occasionally during the pe-

riod of carotid cross-clamping in an attempt to improve CBF. Similar reasoning postulates that because cerebral vessels in ischemic areas are incapable of dilatation or constriction, one should avoid hypercapnia because blood may be shunted away from ischemic zones by dilatation of normal vessels (the so-called cerebral steal).[177] Hyperventilation, though theoretically capable of improving blood flow to ischemic regions by constriction of normal areas (the so-called Robin Hood phenomenon),[178] has not proved to be of benefit in acute ischemic stroke.[179] These theoretic considerations notwithstanding, hypocapnia or hypercapnia has not been shown to contribute to the risk of intraoperative stroke during CEA.[180] Thus, although normocapnia is usually recommended, it seems unlikely that either hypocapnia or hypercapnia has a significant impact on the likelihood of stroke during CEA.

Yet another physiologic consideration that may be important in patients at risk for cerebral ischemia is the plasma glucose concentration. Studies in animals[181-183] and humans[184,185] demonstrate that hyperglycemia worsens neurologic outcome from ischemic brain injury, at least in part because anaerobic metabolism of glucose to lactate during a critically low-flow state produces such severe tissue acidosis that irreversible neuronal injury ensues.[186] However, data[187] that hyperglycemia is deleterious during focal incomplete ischemia (the type that occurs during CEA, vascular neurosurgery, and probably cardiopulmonary bypass) are not as consistent as those for global complete ischemia (such as cardiac arrest), and the blood glucose threshold for increasing the risk of injury is not well defined. Therefore, extrapolating such information to the clinical setting of CEA is difficult, but one reasonable measure is to avoid administering glucose-containing solutions to nondiabetic patients or to maintain plasma glucose within broadly normal limits in diabetics. On the other hand, hypoglycemia has its own risks, and data do not yet warrant more aggressive intraoperative control of plasma glucose.

Another approach to preventing cerebral ischemia during carotid surgery relies on the potential of anesthetic agents, particularly the barbiturates and isoflurane, to improve the tolerance of the brain to low-flow states.[188] In a retrospective review of over 2000 patients who underwent CEA, intraoperative cerebral ischemia as determined by EEG criteria was significantly less common during isoflurane anesthesia (18%) than either enflurane (26%) or halothane (25%).[189] There was, however, no difference in neurologic outcome among the three groups, presumably because ischemic EEG changes, once detected, were treated effectively with insertion of a shunt.[189] These data agree with CBF measurements in CEA patients that show that the "critical" CBF (that is, the CBF below which ischemic EEG changes occur) is lower (approximately 10 ml/100 g/min) with isoflurane anesthesia than either halothane or enflurane (about 18 ml/100 g/min).[167,168] These data have been interpreted to indicate that isoflurane improves the brain's ability to tolerate ischemia, but recent studies[190,191] challenge this notion. Consequently, isoflurane's role in reducing the neurologic complications of CEA remains unsettled. Historically, barbiturates have been most closely associated with "brain protection." These agents have a beneficial effect in some laboratory models of focal cerebral ischemia[192-195] and have been used clinically during CEA,[175,196-198] but no controlled clinical trials of barbiturate therapy for CEA have been performed. Furthermore, issues related to timing, dose, and duration of therapy need to be addressed before such therapy can confidently be considered protective during CEA.

Despite meticulous intraoperative management, some patients will awaken from CEA with a neurologic deficit. In this situation, the first step is to rule out anesthetic-induced neurologic dysfunction in the manner described previously. Of particular note in these patients is the widely held view that an otherwise clinically mild focal neurologic deficit may be worsened transiently by anesthesia. Evidence for this concept is largely anecdotal,[138,199,200] but the possibility should be considered in the stroke-prone CEA population. The only surgically remediable cause of stroke after CEA is carotid occlusion.[156] Therefore the patient awakening from CEA with a dense hemiplegia or other major focal deficit should be evaluated promptly with carotid noninvasive studies or angiography once nonsurgical causes of the problem have been excluded.

If one assumes that no surgically correctable reason for stroke exists, the problem is what, other than supportive physiologic management, can be done to reverse or minimize the permanent consequences of the injury. Although discussion of the various treatment modalities is beyond the scope of this chapter, a few recent advances in stroke management are worth mentioning. Normovolemic hemodilution improves EEG activity and increases CBF in patients with acute stroke[201] and, if initiated early, may improve clinical outcome.[202] Other strategies to ameliorate ischemic neuronal injury are based upon improved understanding of the pathophysiology of cerebral ischemia, particularly with respect to the neurotoxic potential of calcium and excitatory amino acid neurotransmitters.[186,203] A prospective, randomized, placebo-controlled, double-blind study[204] indicates, for example, that nimodipine (30 mg every 6 hours begun within 24 hours) improves neurologic outcome and reduces mortality in patients suffering an acute ischemic stroke; curiously the benefits are confined to men. Excitatory amino acid antagonists such as MK-801 and ketamine also show promise in ameliorating ischemic brain injury,[203,205] but no controlled clinical trials have yet been performed. Finally, based on the assumption that deficits in the availability or activity of neuronotrophic factors contribute to ischemic neuronal death, the ganglioside G_{m1} has been tested in patients with acute stroke with encouraging results.[206] The role of these treatment modalities in the acute management of perioperative stroke is unclear, however, and must be determined in consultation with a neurologist.

B. Cardiac surgery and cardiopulmonary bypass (also see Chapter 12)

Despite numerous technical advances in the field, neurologic and neuropsychologic dysfunction continue to be significant and undeniable risks of cardiac surgery. For example, fatal cerebral damage occurs in as many as 2% of patients undergoing cardiac procedures,[207-210] and the reported incidence of gross neurologic deficits, depending on the rigor and thoroughness of evaluation, varies from 2% to 61%.[211,212] Such obvious neurologic injury, though certainly very important because of the emotional and economic costs,[213] is only one small subset of all CNS dysfunction associated with cardiac surgery; subtle deterioration of cognitive or neuropsychologic function is much more common. In one study,[212] careful testing revealed impaired neuropsyciatric function in 79% of 312 patients undergoing coronary artery bypass surgery (CABG), and in 24% the deterioration was judged to be moderate or severe. In contrast, none of a simultaneously studied control group of patients undergoing major peripheral vascular surgery had a moderate or severe neuropsychologic deficit. Other studies[210,212,214] in cardiac surgical patients confirm substantial decrements in performance on neuropsycholgic tests in the perioperative period and find cerebrospinal fluid evidence of subclinical brain injury in a high percentage of patients.[215] Some reports indicate that most of the deterioration in cognitive and neuropsychologic performance present immediately post-operatively in nearly all cardiac surgical patients resolves over a period of months or years,[210,216] but as many as 11% to 35% of patients may still be neuropsychologically impaired 12 months later.[210,217]

The potential causes of cerebral dysfunction during cardiac surgery fall into two general categories: cerebral hypoperfusion or embolic phenomena. Global cerebral hypoperfusion (or hypoxia) and massive embolism of air or debris can certainly cause catastrophic cerebral injury in cardiac surgical procedures complicated by cardiac arrest, equipment malfunction, or human error. However a few studies also claim that global hypoperfusion is a cause of CNS dysfunction during routine cardiopulmonary bypass (CPB).[218-220] In fact, studies of global CBF during CPB at a perfusion pressure of about 50 mm Hg provide evidence of so-called luxury perfusion (that is, a CBF: cerebral metabolic rate [$CMRO_2$] ratio higher than normal) rather than hypoperfusion,[221] preserved coupling of CBF and $CMRO_2$ at arterial pressures as low as 20 mm Hg,[222] and, provided that CO_2 is not added to the pump (so-called alpha-stat management), intact cerebral autoregulation.[221,223] Most recent studies[209,214,224-226] argue convincingly that perfusion pressure during normal cardiopulmonary bypass (CPB) is not a major determinant of CNS dysfunction and suggest instead that microemboli, consisting of air, fat, plastic, or aggregates of cellular elements,[227] are responsible for most neurologic and neuropsychologic deficits. Microemboli have been documented in the retina of patients undergoing CPB[228,229] and have been observed in the left ventricle by echocardiography.[230] The higher incidence of neurologic deficits in open-versus-closed cardiac procedures in some studies[208,209,231] and evidence that arterial filtration reduces the incidence of CNS dysfunction[232] provide additional support for the microemboli theory, as does the demonstration of diffuse microvascular obstruction at autopsy in patients that died after cardiac surgery.[233]

Although there are certain intrinsic neurologic risks of cardiac surgery and CPB, other factors may add to them. Procedures involving open cardiac chambers[208,209,215] or a longer duration of CPB[207-209,215,219,225,234] appear to increase the risk of CNS dysfunction, as do coexisting hemodynamically significant or symptomatic cerebrovascular disease[235,236] and advancing age.[209,210,237] These are not consistent findings in all studies, however. For example, the conclusion that open-cardiac procedures, such as valve replacement, are associated with a higher incidence of postoperative neurologic or neuropsychologic deficits than CABG surgery has not been confirmed in recent comparative studies,[210,214] and in some series involving only open procedures the incidence of gross neurologic deficits (4% to 8%) is comparable to that reported for CABG.[238,239] On the other hand, asymptomatic carotid artery disease does not increase the likelihood of stroke or neuropsychologic dysfunction in patients undergoing cardiac surgery,[57,58,240,241] which is consistent with data in non–cardiac surgical patients.[61]

Efforts to reduce the risk of CNS complications during cardiac surgery make the reasonable assumption that various technical or physiologic details of CPB are important determinants of neurologic outcome. Thus some suggest that membrane oxygenators are preferable to bubble oxygenators,[242] that arterial filtration is beneficial,[232] or that a higher perfusion pressure is critical.[220] What represents optimal CO_2 management during CPB has been a long and heated debate. On one side of the argument are those concerned that hypercapnia could increase CBF and thereby predispose to cerebral microembolism, whereas others fear that hypocapnia might result in cerebral hypoperfusion.[243] What complicates resolution of these theoretic concerns is a long-standing debate over what constitutes normocapnia in hypothermic individuals.[244,245] One approach, termed "alpha-stat management," aims for normal pH and $Paco_2$ values as measured in the blood-gas machine at 37° C, whereas the other strategy, so-called pH-stat management, corrects the measured values for body temperature and requires addition of CO_2 to the pump to maintain pH. In practical terms, the pH-stat method increases $Paco_2$ approximately 50% at a body temperature of 28° C and produces "luxury perfusion," uncoupling of CBF and metabolism, and impaired autoregulation during CPB.[222,223] On the other hand, alpha-stat management is associated with maintained CO_2 responsiveness, intact autoregulation, and, like pH-stat management, global CBF exceeding metabolic demand.[222,223,243] Despite what may seem to be meaningful differences in CBF physiology with these methods of CO_2 management, there has been no demonstration that one is associated with worse neurologic outcome. In fact, a recent prospective, randomized study[214] of neuropsychologic function in 86 patients undergoing CPB failed to identify differences in outcome based on the two CO_2 management strategies. The question of what $Paco_2$ is preferable during CPB remains open, however, partially because neuropsychologic function has not been correlated with actual CBF or $CMRO_2$ measurements.[243]

Brain "protection" is probably used more commonly in cardiac surgery than any place in the operating room. Hypothermia, widely regarded to protect the brain from anoxic or ischemic events,[224,246-248] is a mainstay of CPB protocol in many institutions. By decreasing neuronal activity and reducing the metabolic demands associated with maintenance of cellular integrity,[249,250] hypothermia narrows the discrepancy between supply and demand and improves neuronal tolerance for a low substrate delivery state. Hypothermia also has membrane-stabilizing and blood-brain barrier effects that may contribute to this protection.[251] However, data for hypothermic brain protection are best for global ischemia or anoxia, which occur only rarely during normal CPB. Moreover, microembolic CNS injury may occur when deep hypothermia is not practical such as during aortic cannulation[252] or when normal cardiac rhythm is restored. Indeed, the high incidence of post-CPB CNS dysfunction despite use of hypothermia is adequate justification to search for supplementary efforts to protect the brain during CPB. Thiopental may have potential benefit in this regard. In a prospective, controlled study[238] of patients undergoing open ventricle procedures during normothermic CPB that stands as the only valid demonstration of barbiturate protection in humans,[239] thiopental, administered as a bolus before aortic cannulation, was shown to reduce the frequency of persistent neuropsychiatric deficits. The disadvantages of high-dose thiopental treatment (such as longer period of postoperative intubation, more inotropic support)[238] as well as questions as to its applicability to other cardiac surgical centers have evidently discouraged its widespread use. There is, however, some recent evidence from an uncontrolled clinical trial[211] that thiopental, administered by continuous infusion before aortic cannulation or as a bolus before weaning the patient from CPB, is associated with a low incidence of gross neurologic deficits. Nevertheless, thiopental's role in protecting the brain during CPB continues to be controversial,[253] particularly since a recent study of patients undergoing CABG failed to show "protection" with barbiturates.[253a]

Treatment of a patient with a post-CPB neurologic deficit is primarily supportive with the aim of preventing a secondary neurologic insult because of hypoxia, hypoventilation, or hypoperfusion. However, one unique and rare cause of post-CPB CNS injury, that is, cerebral embolization of large amounts of air, lends itself to an unusual and specific form of treatment. Hyperbaric therapy capitalizes on the fact that a gas-filled space will decrease in size as pressure surrounding it increases.[254] Thus hyperbaric therapy is believed to reduce the size of cerebral air emboli and speed reabsorption. Comparatively few patients have been treated this way,[255-257] probably reflecting the limited number of such chambers and the practical difficulties encountered in caring for critically ill patients in such a device.[254] Results have nonetheless been encouraging, even when treatment is begun hours after the embolic event.

C. Thoracoabdominal aortic surgery

Paraplegia is not a complication unique to surgery on the thoracoabdominal aorta, but it is a prominent neurologic risk of such procedures. The incidence of paraplegia after thoracoab-

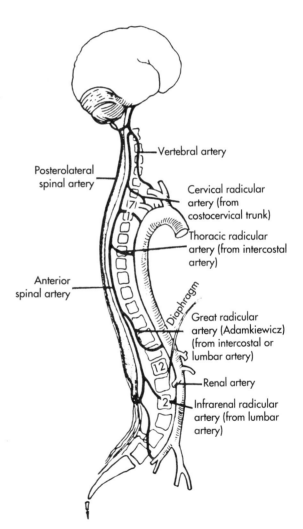

Fig. 15-1. A longitudinal view of the arterial blood supply to the spinal cord. In some people, portions of the anterior spinal artery are so narrow that supplemental blood flow from radicular (segmental) vessels is essential for normal spinal cord function. (From Szilagyi DE et al: Surgery 83:38, 1978.)

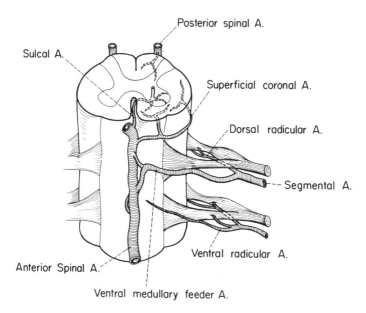

Fig. 15-2. Cross section of the spinal cord illustrating blood supply through the anterior and posterior spinal arteries. Notice that the flow through the anterior spinal artery is supplemented at various levels by segmental (radicular) arteries arising from the aorta. The anterior spinal artery provides flow to the ventral two thirds of the spinal cord, whereas the posterior spinal arteries supply the dorsal one third.

dominal surgery varies from 0.1% in coarctation repair to 24% for emergency resection of dissecting thoracic aneurysms[258,259] but is also affected by the adequacy of collateral flow, location and extent of the surgical lesion, and urgency of treatment.

To understand why aortic surgery poses a risk of ischemic spinal cord injury, one must understand possibly unfamiliar spinal vascular anatomy (Figs. 15-1 and 15-2). The spinal cord has essentially separate anterior and posterior circulations, with both arising from the vertebral arteries.[258] A single anterior spinal artery provides flow to the ventral two thirds of the spinal cord, including motor neurons in the anterior horn and the corticospinal tracts. Paired posterior spinal arteries from a plexus like arrangement on the dorsal surface of the cord and supply the dorsal third of the spinal cord parenchyma, including the posterior columns. The anterior spinal artery travels the entire length of the spinal cord but may be very narrow or even occluded in some areas,[258,260] thus rendering the spinal cord in some people heavily dependent on collateral flow from segmental vessels arising from the aorta. Of these segmental vessels, only six to eight of the 62 present at birth remain into adult life and 45% of the population has less than five;[261] they are unpaired and typically arise on the left from intercostal or

lumbar arteries.[258] One segmental vessel of note is the artery of Adamkiewicz (or great radicular artery), which arises from the aorta usually between the eighth thoracic and third lumbar nerve roots.[258,262] This vessel supplies 50% of the entire spinal cord in some people,[262] and its location relative to the site of aortic cross-clamping and resection can be a decisive factor insofar as risk of ischemic spinal injury is concerned. The clinical dilemma is that the extent to which the spinal cord depends on flow through aortic collaterals is quite variable among patients and it is often impossible to identify those at greatest risk for spinal ischemia preoperatively.

On the basis of these anatomic considerations, it is apparent that aortic surgery can interfere with spinal blood supply either by producing hypoperfusion through segmental vessels distal to the aortic cross-clamp or by sacrificing a critical segmental vessel during the aortic repair. Another less obvious possibility relates to the observation that aortic cross-clamping increases cerebrospinal fluid pressure (CSFP) in some patients. This phenomenon was initially described in animals,[263] but one subsequent report[264] of a patient who developed paraplegia after coarctation repair drew attention to the problem. In that particular person, aortic cross-clamping produced the dangerous combination of increased CSFP and distal aortic hypotension;calculated spinal cord perfusion pressure during the cross-clamp interval was negative 3 mm Hg.[264] The fact that CSFP increases in some neurologically normal patients during aortic cross-clamping has since been documented in other studies,[265,266] but the mechanism remains unclear. One theory attributes increased CSFP to breakthrough of cerebral autoregulation produced by arterial hypertension proximal to the aortic clamp, but since control of arterial blood pressure does not seem to reduce CSFP,[267-269] other mechanisms not yet identified must also be involved.

Tactics to reduce the incidence of spinal neurologic dysfunction during thoracoabdominal aortic surgery address the general problem of spinal cord hypoperfusion and range from efforts to identify patients at most risk to administration of putatively protective agents directly into the subarachnoid space. Preoperative angiography is rarely helpful in identifying critical radicular branches of the aorta that could be avoided or reattached during surgery,[270] and so intraoperative means of assessing the spinal cord have been explored. Experimental work suggests that somatosensory evoked potential (SEP) monitoring[271] and qualitative hydrogen clearance type of measurements of cord perfusion[272] may offer promise in this regard. Intraoperative SEP monitoring may be helpful in identifying patients with poor collateral flow or to assess adequacy of efforts to perfuse the distal aorta.[271,273-277] For example, animal work indicates that loss of the SEP correlates with a substantial decrease in spinal cord blood flow (SCBF)[278] but that the SEP may not recover fully during reperfusion despite spinal hyperemia. SEP studies also reveal a large incidence of reversible spinal ischemia (that is, recoverable loss of the SEP without permanent spinal cord dysfunction) during thoracoabdominal aortic surgery;[279] complete loss of the SEP occurs in 16% to 18% of patients undergoing coarctation repair[274,280] and in 48% to 77% of those having repair of descending thoracic or thoracoabdominal aneurysms.[275,277] Time to loss of the SEP after cross-clamping is extremely variable (5 to 40 min),[275,277,280] however, and probably reflects considerable patient-to-patient variability in collateral flow. The duration of SEP loss that can be tolerated without permanent neurologic injury also varies,[275,277,280] and therefore failure of SEP conduction cannot be used to predict how much longer a given patient could tolerate ongoing spinal cord ischemia. In addition, questions as to how distal hypotension affects conduction in the peripheral nerves from which SEPs are generated, whether the tolerance of motor tracts can reliably be determined from monitoring dorsal column function (the conduction pathway for SEPs) and whether SEP monitoring during this type of surgery improves neurologic outcome remain to be answered before this monitoring modality becomes widely accepted for this type of surgery.

One direct approach to reducing the incidence of neurologic complications during aortic surgery is to attempt to improve distal perfusion using bypass procedures or shunts. Some workeres[276,277,281] claim that maintaining distal aortic pressure above 60 mm Hg with some form of bypass or shunt if necessary is beneficial, whereas others assert that shunting or bypass are unnecessary,[282,283] harmful,[284] or ineffective.[285] Another way to improve spinal cord perfusion pressure and potentially positively influence neurologic outcome is to attenuate or prevent an increase in CSFP during aortic cross-clamping.[263,264] In fact, in animal models, reducing CSFP either with osmotic diuretics or withdrawal of CSF increases spinal cord blood flow and is effective in reducing the incidence of paraplegia associated with occlusion of the thoracic aorta.[263,266,286] Although CSF drainage is promising, a few reports dispute efficacyin animals,[262,268,287] and clinical studies are either too small to confirm a benefit[266] or lack an appropriate (that is, concurrent rather than historical)control group.[288] The mechanism for a beneficial effect of CSF drainage is also unclear; although it improves spinal cord blood flow during aortic cross-clamping, flow remains well below normal.[286] Inasmuch as CSF drainage prevents spinal hyperemia during reperfusion,[286] however, it may prevent reperfusion injury.[186]

Many pharmacologic and physiologic tactics employed to improve the ability of the brain to tolerate ischemic injury have also been tried for spinal cord "protection" in models of thoracic aortic occlusion, but only a few have been investigated thoroughly enough to warrant consideration. Systemic and regional hypothermia,[289-291] thiopental,[290,292] and magnesium[289,290] improve the tolerance of the spinal cord to ischemia in animals, as does anesthesia with halothane, fentanyl, or subarachnoid lidocaine.[293] Massive dosages of steroids, but not naloxone, have proved of value in a prospective, randomized study of spinal cord trauma in humans,[294] but whether such therapy would benefit patients at risk for ischemic cord injury is unknown.[295] Sodium nitroprusside, often used to control the hypertension that develops proximally to an aortic cross-clamp, may increase CSFP and compromise spinal cord blood flow[268] and hence is avoided by some practitioners. A potentially important physiologic consideration concerns the role of plasma glucose in exacerbation of ischemic spinal cord injury. Studies in animal models[296,297] show convincingly that as little as a 40 mg% increase in plasma glucose has an adverse effect on neurologic outcome, and one[298] even suggests that insulin-induced hypoglycemia is advantageous. Although hypoglycemia can be dangerous and should be avoided, these data indicate that it is prudent to avoid exogenous glucose in patients having surgery that places the spinal cord at risk for ischemia.

Finally and predictably, some workers have reasoned that a subarachnoid catheter placed for drainage of CSF could also be used to administer putatively protective agents intrathecally. Thus far, intrathecal papaverine, selected because it improves spinal cord blood flow in the thoracic cord of primates during aortic cross-clamping,[285] is about the only agent for which a small clinical experience exists. Although no adverse effects of intrathecal papaverine are reported,[285,299,300] and the incidence of paraparesis or paraplegia was reduced from 42% in patients treated with conventional methods (that is, no CSF drainage or papaverine) to 9% in those treated with CSF drainage and papaverine before aortic cross-clamping,[299,300] there were only 11 patients in the papaverine group. It is also curious, given the potential adverse effect of hyperglycemia in spinal ischemia,[296,297] that the papaverine was prepared and administered in a vehicle of 10% dextrose. Inasmuch as clinical experience with this technique is quite limited and thorough preclinical testing of intrathecal medication has been advocated before clinical trials,[301] protection of the spinal cord by direct intrathecal administration of drugs should still be regarded as experimental.

REFERENCES

1. Korttila K and Linnoila M: Psychomotor skills related to driving after intramuscular administration of diazepam and meperidine, Anesthesiology 42:685-691, 1975.
2. Melnick B, Sawyer R, Karambelkar D, et al: Delayed side effects of droperidol after ambulatory general anesthesia, Anesth Analg 69:748-751, 1989.
3. Skelly AM, Boscoe MJ, Dawling S, et al: A comparison of diazepam and midazolam as sedatives for minor oral surgery, Eur J Anaesthesiol 1:253, 1984.
4. Korttila K, Linnoila M, Ertama P, et al: Recovery and simulated driving after intravenous anesthesia with thiopental, methohexital, propanidid, or alphadione, Anesthesiology 43:291, 1975.
5. Mackensie N and Grant IS: Comparison of the new emulsion formulation of propofol with methohexitone and thiopentone for induction of anesthesia in day cases, Br J Anaesth 57:725, 1985.
6. Korttila K, Tammisto T, Ertama P, et al: Recovery, psychomotor skills, and simulated driving after brief inhalational anesthesia with halothane or enflurane combined with nitrous oxide and oxygen, Anesthesiology 46:20, 1977.
7. Davison LA, Steinhelber JC, Eger EI, and Stevens WC: Psychological effects of halothane and isoflurane anesthesia, Anesthesiology 43:313-324, 1975.
8. Storms LH, Stark AH, Calverley RK, et al: Psychological functioning after halothane or enflurane anesthesia, Anesth Analg 59:245, 1980.
9. Smith RJ, Roberts NM, Rodgers RJ, et al: Adverse effects of general anaesthesia in young and elderly patients, Int Clin Psychopharmacol 1:253-259, 1986.
10. Hole A, Terjesen T, and Breivik H: Epidural versus general anesthesia for total hip arthroplasty in elderly patients, Acta Anaesthesiol Scand 24:279-287, 1980.
11. Blundell E: A psychological study of the effects of surgery on eighty-six elderly patients, Br J Soc Psychol 6:297-303, 1967.
12. Bedford PD: Adverse effects of anaesthesia in the elderly, Lancet 2:259-263, 1955.
13. Chung F, Seyone C, Dyck B, et al: Age-related cognitive recovery after general anesthesia, Anesth Analg 71:217-224, 1990.
14. Chung FF, Chung A, Meier RH, et al: Comparison of perioperative mental function after general anaesthesia and spinal anaesthesia with intravenous sedation, Can J Anaesth 36:382-387, 1989.
15. Ghoneim MM, Hinrichs JV, O'Hara MW, et al: Comparison of psychologic and cognitive functions after general or regional anesthesia, Anesthesiology 69:507-515, 1988.
16. Riis J, Haxholdt O, Kehlet H, et al: Immediate and long-term mental recovery from general versus epidural anesthesia in elderly patients, Acta Anaesthesiol Scand 27:44-49, 1983.
17. Chung F, Meier R, Lautenschlaeger E, et al: General or spinal anesthesia: which is better in the elderly? Anesthesiology 67:422-427, 1987.
18. Bruce DI and Bach MJ: Effects of trace anesthetic gases on behavioral performance of volunteers, Br J Anaesth 48:871-876, 1976.
19. Litt L, González-Méndez R, James TL, et al: An in vivo study of halothane uptake and elimination in the rat brain with fluorine nuclear magnetic resonance spectroscopy, Anesthesiology 67:161-168, 1987.
20. Mills P, Sessler DI, Moseley M, et al: An in vivo 19F nuclear magnetic resonance study of isoflurane elimination from the rabbit brain, Anesthesiology 67:169-173, 1987.
21. Wyrwicz AM, Pszenny HM, Schofield JC, et al: Noninvasive observations of fluorinated anesthetics in rabbit brain by fluorine-19 nuclear magnetic resonance, Science 222:428-430, 1983.
22. Albrecht RF, Miletich DJ, Rosenberg R, and Zahed B: Cerebral blood flow and metabolic changes from induction to onset of anesthesia with halothane or pentobarbital, Anesthesiology 47:252-256, 1977.
23. Moote CA and Knill RL: Isoflurane anesthesia causes a transient alteration in nocturnal sleep, Anesthesiology 69:327-331, 1988.
24. Knill RL, Moote CA, Skinner MI, et al: Anesthesia with abdominal surgery leads to intense REM sleep during the first postoperative week, Anesthesiology 73:52-61, 1990.
25. Titchener JL, Zwerling I, Gottschalk I, et al: Psychosis in surgical patients, Surg Gynecol Obstet 102:59-65, 1956.

26. Eckenhoff JE, Kneale DH, and Dripps RD: The incidence and etiology of postanesthetic excitement, Anesthesiology 22:667-673, 1961.

27. Seibert CP: Recognition, management, and prevention of neuropsychological dysfunction after operation, Int Anesthesiol Clin 24:39-58, 1986.

28. Tune L and Folstein MF: Post-operative delirium. In Guggenheim FG, editor: Psychological aspects of surgery, Basel, 1986, S Karger AG.

29. Lipowski ZJ: Delirium in the elderly patient, N Engl J. Med 320:578-582, 1989.

30. Weinger MB, Swedlow NR, and Millar WL: Acute postoperative delirium and extrapyramidal signs in a previously healthy parturient, Anesth Analg 67:291-295, 1988.

31. Svensson IS: Postoperative psychosis after heart surgery, J Thorac Cardiovasc Surg 70:717, 1975.

32. Heller SS, Franj KA, Kornfeld DS, et al: Psychological outcome following openheart surgery, Arch Intern Med 134:908, 1974.

33. Summers WK and Riech TC: Delirium after cataract surgery: review and two cases Am J Psychiatry 136:386, 1979.

34. Hutchinson R: Awareness during surgery: a study of its incidence, Br J Anaesth 33:463, 1960.

35. McIntyre JWR: Awareness during general anesthesia: preliminary observations, Can Anaesth Soc J 13:495, 1966.

36. Berggren D, Gustafson Y, Eriksson B, et al: Postoperative confusion after anesthesia in elderly patients with femoral neck fractures, Anesth Analg 66:497-504, 1987.

37. Lewis DA and Smith RE: Steroid-induced psychiatric syndromes: a report of 14 cases and a review of the literature, J Affective Disord 5:319, 1983.

38. White PF, Way WL, and Trevor AJ: Ketamine—its pharmacology and therapeutic uses, Anesthesiology 56:119-136, 1982.

39. Kothary SP and Zsigmond EK: A double-blind study of the effective antihallucinatory doses of diazepam prior to ketamine anesthesia, Clin Pharmacol Ther 21:108-109, 1977.

40. Lilburn JK, Dundee JW, Nair SG, et al: Ketamine sequelae: evaluation of the ability of various premedicants to attenuate its psychic actions, Anesthesia 33:307-311, 1978.

41. Sussman DR: A comparative evaluation of ketamine anesthesia in children and adults, Anesthesiology 40:459-464, 1974.

42. Smith DS, Orkin FK, Gardner SM, et al: Prolonged sedation in the elderly after intraoperative atropine administration, Anesthesiology 51:348, 1979.

43. Tune LE, Holland A, Folstein MF, et al: Association of postoperative delirium with raised serum levels of anticholinergic drugs, Lancet 26:651, 1981.

44. Simpson KH, Smith RJ, and Davies LF: Comparison of the effects of atropine and glycopyrrolate on cognitive function following general anesthesia, Br J Anaesth 59:966-969, 1987.

45. Lee CM and Yeakel AE: Patient refusal of surgery following Innovar premedication, Anesth Analg 54:224-226, 1975.

46. Melnick BM: Extrapyramidal reactions to low-dose droperidol, Anesthesiology 69:424-426, 1988.

47. Nelson VM: Hallucinations after propofol, Anaesthesia 43:170, 1988.

48. Celleno D, Capogna G, Tomasetti M, et al: Neurobehavioral effects of propofol on the neonate following elective caesarean section, Br J Anaesth 62:649-654, 1989.

49. Laycock GJA: Opisthotonus and propofol: a possible association, Anaesthesia 43:257, 1988.

50. Hunter DN, Thornily A, and Whitburn R: Arousal from propofol. Anaesthesia 42:1128-1129, 1988.

51. Marsh SCU and Schaefer HG: Problems with eye opening after propofol anesthesia, Anesth Analg 70:127-128, 1990.

52. Hodkinson BP, Frith RW, and Mee EW: Propofol and the electroencephalogram, Lancet 2:1518, 1987.

53. Yate PM, Maynard DE, Major E, et al: Anaesthesia with ICI 35,868 monitored by the cerebral function analyzing monitor (CFAM), Eur J Anaesth 3:159-166, 1986.

54. Forrest JB, Cahalan MK, Rehder K, et al: Multicenter study of general anesthesia. II. Results, Anesthesiology 72:262-268, 1990.

55. Oliver SB, Cucchiara RF, Warner MA, et al: Unexpected focal neurologic deficit on emergence from anesthesia: a report of three cases, Anesthesiology 67:823-826, 1987.

56. Wilder AJ and Fishbein RH: Operative experience with patients over 80 years of age, Surg Gynecol Obstet 113:205-212, 1961.

57. Turnipseed WD, Berkoff HA, and Belzer FO: Postoperative stroke in cardiac and peripheral vascular disease, Ann Surg 192:365-367, 1980.

58. Barnes RW, Liebman PR, Marzalek PB, et al: The natural history of asymptomatic carotid disease in patients undergoing cardiovascular surgery, Surgery 90:1075-1081, 1981.

59. Eichhorn JH: Prevention of intraoperative anesthesia accidents and related severe injury through safety monitoring, Anesthesiology 70:572-577, 1989.

60. Hart R and Hindman B: Mechanisms of perioperative cerebral infarction, Stroke 13:766-773, 1982.

61. Ropper AH, Wechsler LR, and Wilson LS: Carotid bruit and risk of stroke in elective surgery, N Engl J Med 307:1388, 1982.

62. Hertzer NR, Beven EG, Young JR et al: Incidental asymptomatic bruits in patients scheduled for peripheral vascular reconstruction: results of cerebral and coronary angiography, Surgery 96:535, 1984.

63. Carney WI, Stewart WB, DePinto DJ, et al: Carotid bruit as a risk factor in aorto-iliac reconstruction, Surgery 81:567, 1977.

64. Evans WE and Cooperman M: The significance of asymptomatic unilateral carotid bruits in preoperative patients, Surgery 83:521, 1978.

65. Treiman RL, Foran RF, Cohen JL, et al: Carotid bruit: a follow-up report on its significance in patients undergoing an abdominal aortic operation, Arch Surg 114:1138, 1979.

66. Van Ruiswyk J, Noble H, and Sigmann P: The natural history of carotid bruits in elderly persons, Ann Intern Med 112:340-343, 1990.

67. Kartchner MM and McRae LP: Carotid occlusive disease as a risk factor in major cardiovascular surgery, Arch Surg 117:1086, 1982.

68. Knapp RB, Topkins MJ, and Artusio JF: The cerebrovascular accident and coronary occlusion in anesthesia, JAMA 182:332, 1962.

69. Millikan CH: The pathogenesis of transient focal cerebral ischemia, Circulation 32:438, 1965.

70. Kendell RE and Marshall J: Role of hypotension in the genesis of transient focal cerebral ischemic attacks, Br Med J 2:344-348, 1963.

71. Torvick A and Skullerud K: How often are brain infarcts caused by hypotensive episodes? Stroke 7:255-257, 1976.

72. Kistler JP, Ropper AH, and Heros RC: Therapy of ischemic cerebral vascular disease due to atherothrombosis, N Engl J Med 311:27, 1984.

73. Black SB, Muzzi DA, Nishimura RA, et al: Preopera-

tive and intraoperative echocardiography to detect right-to-left shunt in patients undergoing neurosurgical procedures in the sitting position, Anesthesiology 72:436-438, 1990.

74. Manner JM and Wills A: Post-operative convulsions: a review based on a case report, Anaesthesia 26:66-77, 1971.

75. Modica PA, Tempelhoff R, and White PF: Pro- and anticonvulsant effects of anesthetics (Part I), Anesth Analg 70:303-315, 1990.

76. Modica PA, Tempelhoff R, and White PF: Pro- and anticonvulsant effects of anesthetics (Part II), Anesth Analg 70:433-444, 1990.

77. Lebowitz MH, Blitt CD, and Dillon JB: Enflurane-induced central nervous system excitation and its relation to carbon dioxide tension, Anesth Analg 51:355-363, 1972.

78. Burchiel KJ, Stockard JJ, Myers RR, et al: Metabolic and electrophysiologic mechanisms in the initiation and termination of enflurane-induced seizures in man and cats, Electroencephalogr Clin Neurophysiol 38:55, 1975.

79. Kruczek M, Albin MS, Wolf S, and Bertoni JM: Post-operative seizure activity following enflurane anesthesia, Anesthesiology 53:175-176, 1980.

80. Allan NS: Convulsions after enflurane, Anesthesia 39:605-606, 1984.

81. Yazji NS and Seed RF: Convulsive reaction following enflurane anesthesia, Anesthesia 39:1249, 1984.

82. Nicoll JMV: Status epilepticus following enflurane anaesthesia, Anaesthesia 41:927-930, 1986.

83. Grant IS: Delayed convulsions following enflurane anaesthesia, Anaesthesia 41:1024-1025, 1986.

84. Ohm WW, Cullen BF, Amory DW, and Kennedy RD: Delayed seizure activity following enflurane anesthesia, Anesthesiology 42:367-368, 1975.

85. Fariello RG: Epileptogenic properties of enflurane and their clinical interpretation, Electroencephalogr Clin Neurophysiol 48:595-598, 1980.

86. Burchiel KJ, Stockard JJ, Calverly RK, and Smith NT: Relationship of pre- and postanesthetic EEG abnormalities to enflurane-induced seizure activity, Anesth Analg 56:509-514, 1977.

87. Opitz A, Marschall M, Degan R, and Koch D: General anesthesia in patients with epilepsy and status epilepticus. In Delgado-Escueta AV, Wasterlain CG, Treiman DM, and Porter RJ, editors: Status epilepticus: mechanisms of brain damage and treatment, New York, 1983, Raven Press.

88. Krenn J, Porges P, and Steinbereithner K: Case of anesthesia convulsions under nitrous oxide–halothane anesthesia, Anaesthesist 16:83-85, 1967.

89. Smith PA, McDonald TR, and Jones CS: Convulsions associated with halothane anaesthesia, Anaesthesia 21:229-233, 1966.

90. Hymes JA: Seizure activity during isoflurane anesthesia, Anesth Analg 64:367-368, 1985.

91. Harrison JL: Postoperative seizures after isoflurane anesthesia, Anesth Analg 65:1235-1236, 1986.

92. Poulton TJ and Ellingson RJ: Seizure associated with induction of anesthesia with isoflurane, Anesthesiology 61:471-476, 1984.

93. Meinck H, Molenhof O, and Kettler D: Neurophysiologic effects of etomidate, a new short acting hypnotic, Electroencephalogr Clin Neurophysiol 50:515-522, 1980.

94. Laughlin TP and Newberg LA: Prolonged myoclonus after etomidate anesthesia, Anesth Analg 64:80-82, 1985.

95. Grant IS and Hutchison G: Epileptiform seizures during prolonged etomidate sedation, Lancet 2:511-512, 1983 (Letter).

96. Ghoneim MM and Yamada T: Etomidate: a clinical and electroencephalographic comparison with thiopental, Anesth Analg 56:479-485, 1977.

97. Doenicke A, Loffler B, Kugler J, et al: Plasma concentration and EEG after various regimens of etomidate, Br J Anaesth 54:393-399, 1982.

98. Krieger W, Copperman J, and Laxer KD: Seizures with etomidate anesthesia, Anesth Analg 64:1226-1227, 1985 (Letter).

99. Gancher S, Laxer KD, and Krieger W: Activation of epileptogenic foci by etomidate, Anesthesiology 61:616-618, 1984.

100. Ebrahim ZY, DeBoer GE, Luders H, et al: Effect of etomidate on the electroencephalogram of patients with epilepsy, Anesth Analg 65:1004-1006, 1986.

101. Ferrer-Allado T, Brechner VL, Dymond A, et al: Ketamine-induced electroconvulsive phenomena in the human limbic and thalamic regions, Anesthesiology 38:333-344, 1973.

102. Bennett DR, Madsen JA, Jordan WS, and Wiser WC: Ketamine anesthesia in brain-damaged epileptics: electroencephalographic and clinical observations, Neurology 23:449-460, 1973.

103. Thompson CE: Ketamine-induced convulsions, Anesthesiology 37:662-663, 1972 (Letter).

104. Wyant GM: Intramuscular Ketalar (CI-581) in paediatric anesthesia, Can Anaesth Soc J 18:72-83, 1971.

105. Elliott E, Hanid TK, Arthur LJH, and Kay B: Ketamine anesthesia for medical procedures in children, Arch Dis Child 51:56-59, 1976.

106. Page P, Morgan M, and Loh L: Ketamine anesthesia in paediatric procedures, Acta Anaesthesiol Scand 16:155-160, 1972.

107. White PF: Propofol: pharmacokinetics and pharmacodynamics, Semin Anesth 7(suppl):4-20, 1988.

108. Stephan H, Sonntag H, Schenk HD, and Kohlhausen S: Effects of Disoprivan (propofol) on cerebral blood flow, cerebral oxygen consumption, and cerebral vascular reactivity, Anaesthesist 36:60-65, 1987.

109. Simpson KH, Halsall PJ, Carr CME, and Stewart KG: Propofol reduces seizure duration in patients having anaesthesia for electroconvulsive therapy, Br J Anaesth 61:343-344, 1988.

110. Rampton AJ, Griffin RM, Stuart CS, et al: Comparison of methohexital and propofol for electroconvulsive therapy: effects on hemodynamic responses and seizure duration, Anesthesiology 70:412-417, 1989.

111. Wood PR, Browne GPR, and Pugh S: Propofol infusion for the treatment of status epilepticus Lancet 1:480-481, 1988 (Letter).

112. Gumpert J and Paul R: Activation of the electroencephalogram with intravenous Brietal (methohexitone): the findings in 100 cases, J Neurol Neurosurg Psychiatry 34:646-648, 1971.

113. Musella L, Wilder BJ, and Schmidt RP: Electroencephalographic activation with intravenous methohexital in psychomotor epilepsy, Neurology 21:594-602, 1971.

114. Ryder W: Methohexitone and epilepsy, Br Dent J 126:343, 1969.

115. Goetting MG and Thirmam MJ: Neurotoxicity of meperidine, Ann Emerg Med 14:1007-1009, 1985.

116. Andrews HL: Cortical effects of Demerol, J Pharmacol Exp Ther 76:89-94, 1942.

117. Szeto HH, Inturrisi CE, Houde R, et al: Accumulation of normeperidine, an active metabolite of meperidine in patients with renal failure and cancer, Ann Intern Med 86:738-741, 1977.

118. Kaiko RF, Foley KM, and Grabinski PY: Central nervous system excitatory effects of meperidine in cancer patients, Ann Neurol 13:180-185, 1983.

119. Rao TLK, Mummaneni N, and El-Etr AA: Convulsions: an unusual response to intravenous fentanyl administration, Anesth Analg 61:1020-1021, 1982.

120. Safwat AM and Daniel D: Grand mal seizure after fentanyl administration, Anesthesiology 59:78, 1983 (Letter).

121. Hoien AO: Another case of grand mal seizure after fentanyl administration, Anesthesiology 60:387-388, 1984 (Letter).

122. Goroszeniuk T, Albin M, and Jones RM: Generalized grand mal seizure after recovery from uncomplicated fentanyl-etomidate anesthesia, Anesth Analg 65:979-981, 1986.

123. Rosenberg M and Lisman SR: Major seizure after fentanyl administration: two case reports, J Oral Maxillofac Surg 44:577-579, 1986.

124. Bailey PL, Wilbrink J, Zwanikken P, et al: Anesthetic induction with fentanyl, Anesth Analg 64:48-53, 1985.

125. Molbegott LP, Flashburg MH, Karasic L, and Karlin BL: Probable seizures after sufentanil, Anesth Analg 66:91-93, 1987.

126. Katz RI, Eide TR, Hartman A, and Poppers PJ: Two instances of seizure-like activity in the same patient associated with two different narcotics, Anesth Analg 67:289-290, 1988.

127. Strong WE and Matson M: Probable seizure after alfentanil, Anesth Analg 68:692-693, 1989.

128. Sebel PS, Bovill JG, Wauquier A, and Rog P: Effects of high-dose fentanyl anesthesia on the electroencephalogram, Anesthesiology 55:203-211, 1982.

129. Wauquier A, Bovill JG, and Sebel PS: Electroencephalographic effects of fentanyl-, sufentanil-, and alfentanil anesthesia in man, Neuropsychobiology 11:203-206, 1984.

130. Smith NT, Dec-Silver H, Sanford TJ, et al: EEGs during high dose fentanyl-, sufentanil-, or morphine-oxygen anesthesia, Anesth Analg 63:386-393, 1984.

131. Murkin JM, Moldenhauer CC, Hug CC Jr, and Epstein CM: Absence of seizures during induction of anesthesia with high-dose fentanyl, Anesth Analg 63:489-494, 1984.

132. Bovill JG, Sebel PS, Wauquier A, and Rog P: Electroencephalographic effects of sufentanil anesthesia in man, Br J Anaesth 54:45-52, 1982.

133. Bovill JG, Sebel PS, Wauquier A, et al: The influence of high-dose alfentanil anesthesia on the electroencephalogram: correlation with plasma levels, Br J Anaesth 55:1995-2005, 1983.

134. Furgang FA and Sohn JJ: The effect of thiopentone on enflurane-induced cortical seizures, Br J Anaesth 49:127-132, 1977.

135. Korttila K, Faure E, Apfelbaum J, et al: Recovery from propofol versus thiopental-isoflurane in patients undergoing outpatient anesthesia, Anesthesiology 69:A-564, 1988.

136. Zelcer J and Wells DG: Anaesthetic-related recovery room complications, Anaesth Intensive Care 15:168, 1987.

137. Rosenberg H, Clofine R, and Bialik O: Neurologic changes during awakening from anesthesia, Anesthesiology 54:125-130, 1981.

138. Ropper AH and Kennedy SK: Postoperative neurosurgical care. In Ropper AH and Kennedy SK, editors: Neurological and neurosurgical intensive care, Rockville, Md, 1988, Aspen Publishers.

139. Finck AD, Salcman M, and Balis E: Alleviation of prolonged postoperative central nervous system depression after treatment with naloxone, Anesthesiology 47:392, 1977.

140. Artru AA and Hui GS: Physostigmine reversal of general anesthesia for intraoperative neurological testing: associated EEG changes, Anesth Analg 65:1059-1062, 1986.

141. Azar I and Turndorf H: Severe hypertension and multiple atrial premature contractions following naloxone administration, Anesth Analg 58:524-525, 1979.

142. Prough DS, Roy R, Bumgarner J, et al: Acute pulmonary edema in healthy teenagers following conservative doses of naloxone, Anesthesiology 60:485-486, 1984.

143. Holzgrafe RE, Vondrell JJ, and Mintz SM: Reversal of postoperative reaction to scopolamine with physostigmine, Anesth Analg 52:921, 1973.

144. Bidwai AV, Stanley TH, Rogers C, et al: Reversal of diazepam-induced post-anesthetic somnolence with physostigmine, Anesthesiology 51:256, 1979.

145. Dodgson MS, Skeie B, Emhjellen S, et al: Antagonism of diazepam-induced sedative effects by Ro15-1788 in patients after surgery under lumbar epidural block, Acta Anaesthesiol Scand 31:629, 1987.

146. Darragh A, Lambe R, Brick I, et al: Reversal of benzodiazepine-induced sedation by intravenous Ro15-1788, Lancet 2:1042, 1981.

147. Toker P: Hyperosmolar hyperglycemic nonketotic coma, a cause of delayed recovery from anesthesia, Anesthesiology 41:284, 1974.

148. Mustajoki P and Heinonen J: General anesthesia in "inducible" porphyrias, Anesthesiology 53:15, 1980.

149. Johnston KR and Vaughan RS: Delayed recovery from general anaesthesia, Anaesthesia 43:1024, 1988.

150. Regan MJ and Eger EI II: Effect of hypothermia in dogs on anesthetizing and apneic doses of inhalational agent: determination of the anesthetic index (apnea/MAC), Anesthesiology 28:689, 1967.

151. Lam AM and Parkin JA: Cimetidine and prolonged postoperative somnolence, Can Anaesth Soc J 28:450, 1981.

152. Fraser AC and Goat VA: Unrecognized presentation of a meningioma: delayed recovery after general anesthesia presenting as a sign of intracranial pathology, Anaesthesia 38:128, 1983.

153. Davis O and Kobrine A: Computed tomography. In Youmans JR, editor: Neurological surgery, Philadelphia, 1982, WB Saunders Co.

154. Fode NC, Sundt TM Jr, Robertson JT, et al: Multicenter retrospective review of results and complications of carotid endarterectomy in 1981, Stroke 17:370-376, 1986.

155. Toronto Cerebrovascular Study Group: Risks of carotid endarterectomy, Stroke 17:848-852, 1986.

156. Warlow C: Carotid endarterectomy: does it work? Stroke 15:1068-1076, 1984.

157. Reigel MM, Hollier LH, Sundt TM Jr, et al: Cerebral hyperperfusion syndrome: a cause of neurologic dysfunction after carotid endarterectomy, J Vasc Surg 5:628, 1987.

158. Peitzman AB, Webster MW, Loubeau J-M, et al: Carotid endarterectomy under regional (conductive) anesthesia, Ann Surg 196:59, 1982.

159. Grundy BL, Webster MW, Richey ET, et al: EEG changes during carotid endarterectomy: drug effect and embolism, Br J Anaesth 57:445, 1985.

160. Evans WE, Hayes JP, Waltke EA, et al: Optimal cerebral monitoring during carotid endarterectomy: neurologic response under local anesthesia, J Vasc Surg 2:775, 1985.

161. Chiappa KH, Burke SR, and Young RR: Results of electroencephalographic monitoring during 367 carotid endarterectomies: use of a dedicated minicomputer, Stroke 10:381, 1979.

162. Prioleau WH Jr, Aiken AF, and Hairston P: Carotid endarterectomy: neurological complications as related to surgical techniques, Ann Surg 185:678-681, 1977.

163. Sieber FE, Toung TJ, Diringer NM, and Wang MD: Factors influencing stroke outcome following carotid endarterectomy, Anesth Analg 70:S-370, 1990.

164. Asiddao C, Donegan JH, Whitesell R, et al: Factors associated with perioperative complications during carotid endarterectomy, Anesth Analg 61:631, 1982.

165. McKay RD, Sundt TM Jr, Michenfelder JD, et al: Internal carotid artery stump pressure and cerebral blood flow during carotid endarterectomy: modification by halothane, enflurane, and Innovar, Anesthesiology 45:390, 1976.

166. Gibson BE, McMichan JG, and Cucchiara RF: Lack of correlation between transconjunctival O_2 and cerebral blood flow during carotid artery occlusion, Anesthesiology 64:277, 1986.

167. Sharbrough FW, Messick JM Jr, and Sundt TM: Correlation of continuous electroencephalograms with cerebral blood flow measurements during carotid endarterectomy, Stroke 4:674-683, 1973.

168. Messick JM, Casement B, Sharbrough FW, et al: Correlation of regional cerebral blood flow (rCBF) with EEG changes during isoflurane anesthesia for carotid endarterectomy: critical rCBF, Anesthesiology 66:344-349, 1987.

169. Astrup J, Siesjo BK, and Lymon L: Thresholds in cerebral ischemia: the ischemic penumbra, Stroke 12:723, 1981.

170. Heiss WD: Flow thresholds of functional and morphological damage of brain tissue, Stroke 14:329, 1983.

171. Blume WT, Ferguson GG, and McNeill DK: Significance of EEG changes at carotid endarterectomy, Stroke 17:891, 1986.

172. Cho I, Smullens SN, Streletz LJ, et al: The value of intraoperative EEG monitoring during carotid endarterectomy, Ann Neurol 20:508, 1986.

173. Harper AM: Autoregulation of cerebral blood flow: influence of arterial blood pressure on the blood flow through the cerebral cortex, J Neurol Neurosurg Psychiatry 29:398, 1966.

174. Hoedt-Rasmussen K, Skinhoj E, Paulson OB, et al: Regional cerebral blood flow in acute apoplexy: the "luxury perfusion syndrome" of brain tissue, Arch Neurol 17:271, 1967.

175. Gross CE, Adams HP Jr, Sokoll MD, et al: Use of anticoagulants, electroencephalographic monitoring, and barbiturate cerebral protection in carotid endarterectomy, Neurosurgery 9:1, 1981.

176. Drummond JC, Yong-Seok O, Cole DJ, et al: Phenylephrine-induced hypertension reduces ischemia following middle cerebral artery occlusion in rats, Stroke 20:1538, 1989.

177. Boysen G, Ladegaard-Petersen HJ, Henriksen H, et al: The effects of $Paco_2$ on regional cerebral blood flow and internal carotid arterial pressure during carotid clamping, Anesthesiology 35:286, 1971.

178. Mohr LL, Smith LL, and Hinshaw DB: Blood gas and carotid pressure: factors in stroke risk, Ann Surg 184:723, 1976.

179. Christensen MS, Paulson OB, Olesen J, et al: Cerebral apoplexy (stroke) treated with and without prolonged artificial hyperventilation: I. Cerebral circulation, clinical course, and cause of death, Stroke 4:568, 1973.

180. Baker WH, Rodman JA, Barnes RW, and Hoyt JL: An evaluation of hypocarbia and hypercarbia during carotid endarterectomy, Stroke 7:451-454, 1976.

181. Myers RE and Yamaguchi T: Nervous system effects of cardiac arrest in monkeys, Arch Neurol 34:65, 1974.

182. Pulsinelli WA, Waldman S, Rawlinson D, et al: Moderate hyperglycemia augments ischemic brain damage: a neuropathologic study in the rat, Neurology 32:1239, 1982.

183. Lanier WL, Strangland KJ, Scheithauer BW, et al: The effects of dextrose infusion and head position on neurologic outcome after complete cerebral ischemia in primates: examination of a model, Anesthesiology 66:39, 1987.

184. Pulsinelli WA, Levy DE, Sigsbee B, et al: Increased damage after ischemic stroke in patients with ischemic stroke in patients with hyperglycemia with or without established diabetes mellitus, Am J Med 74:540, 1986.

185. Candelize L, Landi G, Orazio EN, et al: Prognostic significance of hyperglycemia in stroke, Arch Neurol 42:661, 1985.

186. Raichle ME: The pathophysiology of brain ischemia, Ann Neurol 13:2, 1983.

187. Ginsberg MD, Prado R, Dietrich WD, et al: Hyperglycemia reduces the extent of cerebral infarction in rats, Stroke 18:570, 1987.

188. Messick JM, Newberg LA, Nugent M, and Faust RJ: Principles of neuroanesthesia for the nonneurosurgical patient with CNS pathophysiology, Anesth Analg 64:174, 1985.

189. Michenfelder JD, Sundt TM Jr, Fode N, and Sharbrough FW: Isoflurane when compared to enflurane and halothane decreases the frequency of cerebral ischemia during carotid endarterectomy, Anesthesiology 67:336-340, 1987.

190. Nehls DG, Todd MM, Spetzler RF, et al: A comparison of the cerebral protective effects of isoflurane and barbiturates during temporary focal ischemia in primates, Anesthesiology 66:453-464, 1987.

191. Gelb AW, Boisvert DP, Tang C, et al: Primate brain tolerance to temporary focal cerebral ischemia during isoflurane- or sodium nitroprusside–induced hypotension, Anesthesiology 70:678, 1989.

192. Shapiro HM: Barbiturates in brain ischemia, Br J Anaesth 57:82-95, 1985.

193. Michenfelder JD, Milde JH, and Sundt TM: Cerebral protection by barbiturate anesthesia: use of middle cerebral artery occlusion in Java monkeys, Arch Neurol 33:345, 1976.

194. Smith AL, Hoff JT, Nielsen SL, et al: Barbiturate protection in acute focal cerebral ischemia, Stroke 5:1-7, 1974.

195. Selman WR, Spetzler RF, Roessmann VR, et al: Barbiturate-induced coma therapy for focal cerebral ischemia: effect after temporary and permanent MCA occlusion, J Neurosurg 55:220-226, 1981.

196. Spetzler RF, Martin N, Hadley MN, et al: Microsurgical endarterectomy under barbiturate protection: a prospective study, J Neurosurg 65:63, 1986.

197. McMeniman WJ, Fletcher JP, and Little JM: Experience with barbiturate therapy for cerebral protection during carotid endarterectomy, Ann R Coll Surg Engl 66:361, 1984.

198. Gelb AW, Floyd R, Lok P, et al: A prophylactic bolus of thiopental does not protect against prolonged focal cerebral ischemia, Can Anaesth Soc J 33:173, 1986.

199. Miller RA, Crosby G, and Sundaram P: Exacerbated spinal neurologic deficit during sedation of a patient

with cervical spondylosis, Anesthesiology 67:844, 1987.

200. Benzel EC, Hadden TA, Nossaman BD, et al: Does sufentanil exacerbate marginal neurological dysfunction? J Neurosurg Anesthesiol 2:50, 1990.

201. Wood JH, Polyzoidis KS, Epstein CM, et al: Quantitative EEG alterations after isovolemic-hemodilutional augmentation of cerebral perfusion in stroke patients, Neurology 34:764-768, 1984.

202. Italian Acute Stroke Study Group: The Italian hemodilution trial in acute stroke, Stroke 18:670-676, 1987.

203. Rothman SM and Olney JW: Glutamate and the pathophysiology of hypoxicischemic brain damage, Ann Neurol 19:105, 1986.

204. Gelmers HJ, Gorter K, de Weerdt CJ, and Wiezer HJA: A controlled trial of nimodipine in acute ischemic stroke, N Engl J Med 318:203-207, 1988.

205. Olney JV, Price MT, Fuller TA, et al: The anti-excitotoxic effects of certain anesthetics, analgesics, and sedative-hypnotics, Neurosci Lett 68:28, 1986.

206. Argentino C, Sacchetti ML, Toni D, et al: G_{M1} ganglioside therapy in acute ischemic stroke, Stroke 20:1143-1149, 1989.

207. Branthwaite MA: Prevention of neurological damage during open heart surgery, Thorax 30:258, 1975.

208. Sotaniemi KA: Brain damage and neurological outcome after open heart surgery, J Neurol Neurosurg Psychiatry 43:127, 1980.

209. Slogoff S, Girgis KZ, and Keats AS: Etiologic factors in neuropsychiatric complication associated with cardiopulmonary bypass, Anesth Analg 61:903-911, 1982.

210. Townes BD, Bashien G, Hornbein TF, et al: Neurobehavioral outcomes in cardiac operations, J Thorac Cardiovasc Surg 98:744-782, 1989.

211. Metz S and Slogoff S: Thiopental sodium by single bolus dose compared to infusion for cerebral protection during cardiopulmonary bypass, J Clin Anesth 2:226-231, 1990.

212. Shaw PJ, Bates D, Cartlidge NEF, et al: Neurologic and neuropsychological morbidity following major surgery: comparison of coronary artery bypass and peripheral vascular surgery, Stroke 18:700-707, 1987.

213. Weintraub WS, Jones EL, Craver J, et al: Determinants of prolonged length of hospital stay after coronary bypass surgery, Circulation 80:276-284, 1989.

214. Bashein G, Townes BD, Nessly ML, et al: A randomized study of carbon dioxide management during hypothermic cardiopulmonary bypass, Anesthesiology 72:7-15, 1990.

215. Aberg T, Ronquist G, Tydén H, et al: Adverse effects on the brain in cardiac operations as assessed by biochemical, psychometric, and radiologic methods, J Thorac Cardiovasc Surg 87:99-105, 1984.

216. Klonoff H, Clark C, Kavanagh-Gray D, et al: Two-year follow-up study of coronary artery bypass surgery, J Thorac Cardiovasc Surg 97:78-85, 1989.

217. Venn G, Klinger L, Smith P, et al: Neuropsychologic sequelae of bypass twelve months after coronary artery surgery, Br Heart J 57:565, 1987.

218. Henriksen L: Evidence suggestive of diffuse brain damage following cardiac operations, Lancet 1:816, 1984.

219. Tufo HM, Ostfeld AM, and Shekelle R: Central nervous system dysfunction following open-heart surgery, JAMA 212:1333, 1970.

220. Stockard JJ, Bickford RG, and Schauble JF: Pressure dependent cerebral ischemia during cardiopulmonary bypass, Neurology 23:321-329, 1973.

221. Henriksen L: Brain luxury perfusion during cardiopulmonary bypass in humans: a study of the cerebral blood flow response to changes in CO_2, O_2, and blood pressure, J Cereb Blood Flow Metab 6:366-378, 1986.

222. Murkin JM, Farrar JK, Tweed WA, et al: Cerebral autoregulation and flow/metabolism coupling during cardiopulmonary bypass: the influence of P_{aCO_2}, Anesth Analg 66:825-832, 1987.

223. Roger AT, Stump DA, Gravlee GP, et al: Response of cerebral blood flow to phenylephrine infusion during hypothermic cardiopulmonary bypass: influence of P_{aCO_2} management, Anesthesiology 69:547-551, 1988.

224. Ellis RJ, Wisniewski A, Potts R, et al. Reduction of flow rate and arterial pressure at moderate hypothermia does not result in cerebral dysfunction, J Thorac Cardiovasc Surg 79:173-180, 1980.

225. Kolkka R and Hilberman M: Neurologic dysfunction following cardiac operation with low-flow, low-pressure cardiopulmonary bypass, J Thorac Cardiovasc Surg 79:432-437, 1980.

226. Fish KJ, Helms KN, Sarnquist FH, et al: A prospective, randomized study of the effects of prostacyclin on neuropsychologic dysfunction after coronary artery operation, J Thorac Cardiovasc Surg 93:609-615, 1987.

227. Solis RT, Noon GP, Beall AC, and DeBakey ME: Particulate microembolism during cardiac surgery, Ann Thorac Surg 17:332-344, 1974.

228. Williams IM: Retinal vascular occlusions in open heart surgery, Br J Ophthalmol 59:81, 1975.

229. Blauth CI, Arnold JV, Schulenberg WE, et al: Cerebral microembolism during cardiopulmonary bypass: retinal microvascular studies in vivo with fluorescein angiography, J Thorac Cardiovasc Surg 95:668-676, 1988.

230. Roigas PC, Meyer FJ, Haasler GB, et al: Intraoperative 2-dimensional echocardiography: ejection of microbubbles from the left ventricle after cardiac surgery, Am J Cardiol 50:1130-1132, 1982.

231. Aberg T and Kihlgren M: Effect of open-heart surgery on intellectual function, Scand J Thorac Cardiovasc Surg 15(suppl):1, 1974.

232. Aris A, Solanes H, Camara ML, et al: Arterial line filtration during cardiopulmonary bypass: neurologic, neuropsychologic, and hematologic studies, J Thorac Cardiovasc Surg 91:526-533, 1986.

233. Moody DM, Bell MA, and Challa VR: Focal encephalic microvascular alterations following cardiopulmonary bypass pump, Soc Neurosci Abs tr 15:27, 1989.

234. Smith PLC, Newman S, Treasure T, et al: Cerebral consequences of cardiopulmonary bypass, Lancet 1:823-824, 1986.

235. Kartchner MM and McRae LP: Carotid occlusive disease as a risk factor in major cardiovascular surgery, Arch Surg 117:1086, 1982.

236. Jones EL, Craver JM, Michalik RA, et al: Combined carotid and coronary operations: when are they necessary? J Thorac Cardiovasc Surg 87:7, 1984.

237. Gardner TJ, Horneffer PJ, Manolio TA, et al: Stroke following coronary artery bypass grafting: a ten-year study, Ann Thorac Surg 40:574-581, 1985.

238. Nussmeier NA, Arlund C, and Slogoff S: Neuropsychiatric complications after cardiopulmonary bypass: cerebral protection by a barbiturate, Anesthesiology 64:165-170, 1986.

239. Michenfelder JD: A valid demonstration of barbiturate-induced cerebral protection in man—at last, Anesthesiology 64:140-142, 1986.

240. Ivey TD, Strandness E, Williams DB, et al: Management of patients with carotid bruit undergoing cardiopulmonary bypass, J Thorac Cardiovasc Surg 87:183, 1984.
241. Harrison MJG, Schneidau, A, Ho R, et al: Cerebrovascular disease and functional outcome after coronary artery bypass surgery, Stroke 20:235-237, 1989.
242. Blauth CI, Smith PL, Arnold JV, et al: Influence of oxygenator type on the prevalence and extent of microembolic retinal ischemia during cardiopulmonary bypass: assessment by digital image analysis, J Thorac Cardiovasc Surg 99:61-69, 1990.
243. Prough DS, Stump DA, and Troost BT: $Paco_2$ management during cardiopulmonary bypass: intriguing physiologic rationale, convincing clinical data, evolving hypothesis? Anesthesiology 72:3-6, 1990.
244. Williams JJ and Marshall BE: A fresh look at an old question, Anesthesiology 56:1-2, 1982.
245. Swain JA: Hypothermia and blood pH: a review, Arch Intern Med 148:1643-1646, 1988.
246. Wolfe KB: Effect of hypothermia on cerebral damage resulting from cardiac arrest, Am J Cardiol 6:809, 1960.
247. Norwood WJ, Norwood CR, and Casteneda AR: Cerebral anoxia: effect of deep hypothermia and pH, Surgery 86:203, 1979.
248. Molina JE, Einzig S, Mastri AR, et al: Brain damage in profound hypothermia, J Thorac Cardiovasc Surg 87:596, 1984.
249. Michenfelder JD and Theye RA: Hypothermia: effect on canine brain and whole body metabolism, Anesthesiology 29:1107, 1968.
250. Steen PA, Newberg LA, Milde JH, et al: Hypothermia and barbiturates: individual and combined effects on canine cerebral oxygen consumption, Anesthesiology 58:527, 1983.
251. Busto R, Dietrich, WD, Globus MY-T, et al: Differences in intraischemic brain temperature critically determine the extent of ischemic neuronal injury, J Cereb Blood Flow Metab 7:729, 1987.
252. Barzilai B, Marshall WG Jr, Saffitz JE, and Kouchoukos N: Avoidance of embolic complications by ultrasonic characterization of the ascending aorta, Circulation 80: I275-I279, 1989.
253. Prough DS and Mills SA: Should thiopental sodium administration be a standard of care for open cardiac procedures? J Clin Anesth 2:221-223, 1990.
253a. Zaidan JR, Klochany A, Martin W, et al: Effect of thiopental on neurologic outcome following coronary artery bypass grafting, Anesthesiology 74:406-411, 1991 (plus editorial).
254. Moon RE and Camporesi EM: Clinical care in the hyperbaric environment. In Miller RE, editor: Anesthesia, New York, 1990, Churchill Livingstone.
255. Kindwall EP: Massive surgical air embolism treated with brief recompression to six atmospheres followed by hyperbaric oxygen, Aerospace Med 44:663, 1973.
256. Winter PM, Alvis HG, and Gage AA: Hyperbaric treatment of cerebral air embolism during cardiopulmonary bypass, JAMA 215:1786, 1971.
257. Bove AA, Clark JM, Simon AJ, and Lambertson CJ: Successful therapy of cerebral air embolism with hyperbaric oxygen at 2.8 ATA, Undersea Biomed Res 9:75, 1982.
258. Ross RT: Spinal cord infarction in disease and surgery of the aorta, Can J Neurol Sci 12:289-295, 1985.
259. Szilagyi DE, Hageman JH, Smith RF, and Elliott JP: Spinal cord damage in surgery of the abdominal aorta, Surgery 83:38-56, 1978.
260. Domisse GF: The blood supply of the spinal cord, J Bone Joint Surg 56B:225, 1974.

261. Adams HD and Van Geertruyden HH: Neurological complications of aortic surgery, Ann Surg 144:574, 1956.
262. Wadouh F, Lindemann EM Ardnt CF, et al: The arteria radicularis magna anterior as a decisive factor influencing spinal cord damage during aortic occlusion, J Thorac Cardiovasc Surg 88:1-10, 1984.
263. Blaisdell FW and Cooley DA: The mechanism of paraplegia after temporary thoracic aortic occlusion and its relationship to spinal fluid pressure, Surgery 51:351-355, 1962.
264. Berendes JN, Bredee JJ, Schipperheyn JJ, et al: Mechanisms of spinal cord injury after cross-clamping of the descending thoracic aorta, Circulation 66:I-112, 1982.
265. Hantler CB and Knight PR: Intracranial hypertension following cross-clamping of the thoracic aorta, Anesthesiology 56:146, 1982.
266. McCullough JL, Hollier LH, and Nugent M: Paraplegia after thoracic aortic occlusion: influence of cerebrospinal fluid drainage: experimental and early clinical results, J Vasc Surg 7:153-160, 1988.
267. D'Ambra MN, Dewhirst W, Jacobs M, et al: Cross-clamping the thoracic aorta: effect on intracranial pressure, Circulation 78:III-198, 1988.
268. Woloszyn TT, Marini CP, Coons MS, et al: Cerebrospinal fluid drainage does not counteract the negative effect of sodium nitroprusside on spinal cord perfusion pressure during aortic cross-clamping, Curr Surg 46:489, 1989.
269. Piano G and Gewertz BL: Mechanism of increased cerebrospinal fluid pressure with thoracic aortic occlusion, J Vasc Surg 11:695, 1990.
270. Crawford ES, Snyder DM, Cho GC, and Roehm JO Jr: Progress in treatment of thoracoabdominal and abdominal aortic aneurysms involving celiac, superior mesenteric, and renal arteries, Ann Surg 188:404-422, 1978.
271. Laschinger JC, Cunningham JN Jr, Baumann G, et al: Monitoring of somatosensory evoked potentials during surgical procedures on the thoracoabdominal aorta. III. Intraoperative identification of vessels critical to spinal cord blood supply, J Thorac Cardiovasc Surg 94:271-274, 1987.
272. Svensson LG, Patel V, Coselli JS, and Crawford ES: Preliminary report of localization of spinal blood supply by hydrogen during aortic operations, Ann Thorac Surg 49:528-535, 1990.
273. Mizrahi EM and Crawford ES: Somatosensory evoked potentials during reversible spinal cord ischemia in man, Electroencephalogr Clin Neurophysiol 58:120-126, 1984.
274. Dasmahapatra HK, Coles JG, Taylor MJ, et al: Identification of risk factors for spinal cord ischemia by use of monitoring of somatosensory evoked potentials during coarctation repair, Circulation 76(suppl III):14-18, 1987.
275. Laschinger JC, Cunningham JN, Cooper MW, et al: Monitoring of somatosensory evoked potentials during surgical procedures on the thoracoabdominal aorta. I. Relationship of aortic cross-clamp duration, changes in somatosensory evoked potentials, and incidence of neurologic dysfunction, J Thorac Cardiovasc Surg 94:260, 1987.
276. Laschinger JC, Cunningham JN, Baumann G, et al: Monitoring of somatosensory evoked potentials during surgical procedures on the thoracoabdominal aorta. II. Use of somatosensory evoked potentials to assess adequacy of distal aortic bypass and perfusion after thoracic aortic cross-clamping, J Thorac Cardiovasc Surg 94:266, 1987.

277. Cunningham JN Jr, Laschinger JC, and Spencer FC: Monitoring of somatosensory evoked potentials during surgical procedures on the thoracoabdominal aorta. IV. Clinical observations and results, J Thorac Cardiovasc Surg 94:275-285, 1987.

278. Kaplan BJ, Friedman WA, Gravenstein N, et al: Effects of aortic occlusion on regional spinal cord blood flow and somatosensory evoked potentials in sheep, Neurosurgery 21:668, 1987.

279. Laschinger JC, Cunningham J, Catinella FC, et al: Detection and prevention of intraoperative spinal cord ischemia after cross-clamping of the thoracic aorta: use of somatosensory evoked potentials, Surgery 92:1109, 1982.

280. Kaplan BJ, Friedman WA, Alexander JA, and Hampson SR: Somatosensory evoked potential monitoring of spinal cord ischemia during aortic operations, Neurosurgery 19:82-90, 1986.

281. Krieger KH and Spencer FC: Is paraplegia after repair of coarctation of the aorta due principally to distal hypotension during aortic cross-clamping? Surgery 97:2-6, 1985.

282. DeBakey ME, McCollum CH, Crawford ES, et al: Dissection and dissecting aneurysms of the aorta: twenty year follow-up of five hundred twenty-seven patients treated surgically, Surgery 92:1118-1134, 1982.

283. Livesay JJ, Cooley DA, Ventemiglia RA, et al: Surgical experience in descending thoracic aneurysmectomy with and without adjuncts to avoid ischemia, Ann Thorac Surg 39:37, 1985.

284. Crawford ES and Rubio PA: Reappraisal of adjuncts to avoid ischemia in the treatment of aneurysms of the descending thoracic aorta, J Thorac Cardiovasc Surg 66:693-704, 1973.

285. Svensson LG, Rickards E, Coull A, et al: Relationship of spinal cord blood flow to vascular anatomy during thoracic aortic cross-clamping and shunting, J Thorac Cardiovasc Surg 91:71-78, 1986.

286. Bower TC, Murray MJ, Gloviczki P, et al: Effects of thoracic aortic occlusion and cerebrospinal fluid drainage on regional spinal cord blood flow in dogs: correlation with neurologic outcome, J Vasc Surg 9:135-144, 1988.

287. Svensson LG, Von Ritter CM, Groeneveld HT, et al: Cross-clamping of the thoracic aorta: influence of aortic shunts, laminectomy, papaverine, calcium channel blocker, allopurinol, and superoxide dismutase on spinal cord blood flow and paraplegia in baboons, Ann Surg 204:38-47, 1986.

288. Wynn MM and Archer CW: Improved neurologic outcome using naloxone and spinal fluid drainage in surgery of the thoracoabdominal aorta, Anesthesiology 73:A64, 1990.

289. Vacanti FX and Ames A III: Mild hypothermia and Mg^{++} protect against irreversible damage during CNS ischemia, Stroke 15:695-698, 1984.

290. Robertson CS, Foltz R, Grossman RG, and Goodman JC: Protection against experimental ischemic spinal cord injury, J Neurosurg 64:633-642, 1986.

291. Colon R, Frazier OH, Cooley DA, and McAllister HA: Hypothermic regional perfusion for protection of the spinal cord during periods of ischemia, Ann Thorac Surg 43:639-643, 1987.

292. Oldfield EH, Plunkett RJ, Nylander WA Jr, et al: Barbiturate protection in acute experimental spinal cord ischemia, J Neurosurg 56:511-516, 1982.

293. Cole DJ, Shapiro HM, Drummond JC, et al: Halothane, fentanyl/nitrous oxide, and spinal lidocaine protect against spinal cord injury in the rat, Anesthesiology 70:967, 1989.

294. Bracken MB, Shepard MJ, Collins WF, et al: A randomized, controlled trial of methylprednisolone or naloxone in the treatment of acute spinal cord injury: results of the Second National Acute Spinal Cord Injury Study, N Engl J Med 322:1405, 1990.

295. Woloszyn TT, Marini CP, Coons MS, et al: Cerebrospinal fluid drainage and steroids provide better spinal cord protection during aortic cross-clamping than does either treatment alone, Ann Thorac Surg 49:78, 1990.

296. Drummond JC and Moore SS: The influence of dextrose administration on neurologic outcome after temporary spinal cord ischemia in the rabbit, Anesthesiology 70:64, 1989.

297. Lundy EF, Ball TD, Mandell MA, et al: Dextrose administration increases sensory/motor impairment and paraplegia after infrarenal aortic occlusion in the rabbit, Surgery 102:737-741, 1987.

298. Robertson CS and Grossman RG: Protection against spinal cord ischemia with insulin-induced hypoglycemia, J Neurosurg 67:739-744, 1987.

299. Svensson LG, Stewart RW, Cosgrove DM, et al: Intrathecal papaverine for the prevention of paraplegia after operation on the thoracic or thoracoabdominal aorta, J Thorac Cardiovasc Surg 96:823-829, 1988.

300. Svensson LG, Grum DF, Bednarski M, et al: Appraisal of cerebrospinal fluid alterations during aortic surgery with intrathecal papaverine administration and cerebrospinal fluid drainage, J Vasc Surg 11:423-429, 1990.

301. Yaksh TL: Effects of spinally administered agents on spinal cord blood flow: need for further studies, Anesthesiology 59:173, 1983.

Chapter 16

Immunologic Complications

Michael E. Weiss

Jerrold H. Levy

Among the many adverse events that can occur in the perioperative period, immunologic complications are important causes of morbidity and mortality. Anaphylaxis is the most severe of these complications and requires immediate intervention. Although the first reported case of anaphylaxis was recorded in hieroglyphics in 2600 B.C. after a fatal bee sting,[1] it wasn't until 1902 that Portier and Richet coined the word "anaphylaxis." They noted that a second sublethal injection of a sea anemone extract, which had produced minimal effects after first injection, caused dogs to die of profound shock. Thus the term was initially used to describe a phenomenon in which repeated exposure to a foreign protein produced an adverse reaction rather than the intended immunization or prophylaxis.

The profusion of terms used to describe immunologic mechanisms can be confusing. We presently consider that allergic reactions are untoward physiologic events triggered by immune processes. When we speak of an immunologic reaction, we mean the interaction of a foreign antigen with an immunospecific antibody or sensitized lymphocyte. When the antigen bridges cell surface IgE antibodies, the antibodies undergo conformational changes that may produce inflammation in the host. This inflammation produces pathophysiologic changes in the cardiopulmonary, vascular, cutaneous, and gastrointestinal systems.

Over 80 years after the original description, we now understand that anaphylaxis is a clinical syndrome produced by an IgE antibody–mediated reaction, resulting in immediate, severe alterations in the cutaneous (urticaria/angioedema), respiratory (asthma, laryngeal edema), gastrointestinal (nausea, vomiting, abdominal pain, diarrhea), or cardiovascular (hypotension, tachycardia, cardiovascular collapse) systems. The same clinical manifestations may occur consequent to non–IgE mediated reactions and have previously been termed "anaphylactoid reactions."

I. CLASSIFICATION OF ALLERGIC REACTIONS

Gell and Coombs classified four types of immunopathologic reactions[2] as follows:

A. Type I reactions: immediate hypersensitivity

Type I reactions result from the interaction of antigens with preformed antigen-specific IgE antibodies that are bound to tissue mast cells or circulating basophils by high-affinity IgE receptors. Cross-linking two or more IgE receptors, by antigen, liberates both preformed and newly generated mediators, producing urticaria, laryngeal edema, and bronchospasm with or without cardiovascular collapse.

B. Type II reactions: cytotoxic antibodies

Type II reactions result when IgG or IgM antibody reacts with a cell-bound antigen (that is, blood group antigens, penicillin determinants bound to red blood cells). The antigen-antibody interaction activates the complement system resulting in cell lysis. Type II reactions may also be complement independent. IgG or IgM antibody may bind to cell membrane–bound antigen. Neutrophils or macrophages may then attach to the antibody through their Fc receptors, and this opsonization can result in injury to the antigen-laden cell. Examples of type II reactions include ABO-incompatible transfusion reactions, drug-induced hemolytic anemia or thrombocytopenia, Rh disease of the newborn, and Goodpasture's syndrome.

C. Type III reactions: immune complexes (Arthus reaction)

Antigen-specific IgG or IgM antibodies form circulating complexes with antigens. The complexes lodge in tissue sites, fix complement, and attract polymorphonuclear leukocytes, which attempt to phagocytize the immune complexes. The release of proteolytic enzymes from the phagocytic cells results in tissue damage. Immune complex reactions typically appear 7 to 14 days after continual exposure to antigen. Examples include serum sickness and possibly drug fever.

D. Type IV reactions: cell-mediated hypersensitivity

Type IV reactions are not mediated by an antibody but rather by T-lymphocytes that are specifically sensitized to recognize a particular antigen. After being modified by antigen-processing cells (that is, macrophages, Langerhans cells), the modified antigen is presented, in association with major histocompatibility (MHC) class II molecules, to the T-lymphocyte. The sensitized T-lymphocyte recognizes the processed antigen through an antigen-specific T-cell receptor. This triggers the T-cell to release substances, known as "cytokines," that orchestrate the immune response by recruiting and stimulating proliferation of other lymphocytes and mononuclear cells, which ultimately cause tissue inflammation and injury. Examples of cell-mediated immune reactions are tuberculin skin testing, contact dermatitis (as from poison ivy), and graft-versus-host disease.

E. Idiopathic reactions

The immunologic pathogenesis of some reactions are unclear and are considered to be idiopathic in nature. Examples include eosinophilia, Stevens-Johnson syndrome, exfoliative dermatitis, and maculopapular eruptions.

II. MEDIATOR RELEASE

Anaphylaxis (involving mast cell or basophil mediator release) is the most important clinical example of an allergic reaction because of its potential for sudden onset with catastrophic outcome. Tissue mast cells or circulating basophils may be triggered to release their mediators by both IgE and non-IgE mechanisms. The various mechanisms inducing mediator release are considered next.

A. IgE-mediated anaphylaxis

Foreign molecules capable of stimulating IgE antibody production may cause IgE-mediated anaphylaxis on reexposure. Drugs and other small molecules (such as penicillin) that are too small to stimulate immune responses become complete antigens by binding to serum proteins to stimulate antibody production.[3] IgE antibodies, once produced, become fixed to tissue mast cells or circulating basophils, both of which contain high-affinity IgE receptors.[4] This attachment takes place at the Fc region of the IgE molecule, which allows the antigen binding (Fab) region of the IgE antibody to bind antigen. Reexposure to antigens or haptens that are functionally multivalent (have two or more antigenic sites) is required to cross-link IgE antibodies bound to mast cells or basophils. Cross-linking of IgE antibodies causes the direct bridging of IgE receptor molecules on mast cell and basophil cell membranes, which induces activation of membrane-associated enzymes, causing complex biochemical cascades that lead to an influx of extracellular calcium and a mobilization of intracellular calcium with subsequent release of preformed granule-associated mediators and the generation of new mediators from cell-membrane phospholipids[5,6] (Fig. 16-1). Examples of IgE antibody-mediated allergic reactions include those induced by insulin, chymopapain, muscle relaxants, and penicillin (hapten).

B. Complement-mediated reactions

Activation of the complement system results in generation of a membrane attack unit and the liberation of low-molecular-weight peptides C3a, C4a, and C5a, known as the "anaphylatoxins"[7] (Fig. 16-2). The anaphylatoxins are capable of causing mast-cell and basophil mediator release, directly increasing vascular permeability, contracting smooth muscles, aggregating platelets, and stimulating macrophages to produce thromboxane[7,8] (Fig. 16-1). The complement cascade may be activated either through the classical pathway or through the alternative pathway. Complement activation

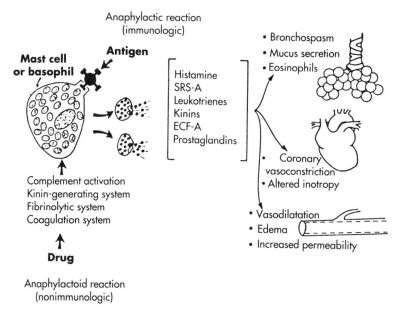

Fig. 16-1. Summary of the pathophysiologic changes producing anaphylactic and anaphylactoid reactions. *Upper left,* **Anaphylactic reactions:** The allergen enters the body and combines with allergen-specific IgE antibodies on the surface of mast cells and basophils. This interaction causes mast cell and basophil activation, releasing vasoactive mediators (histamine, leukotrienes, kinins, eosinophilic chemotactic factor–anaphaylaxis (ECF-A), prostaglandins, and others). The release of these substances may cause the signs and symptoms of anaphylaxis, that is, bronchospasm; pharyngeal, glottic, and plumonary edema; vasodilatation; hypotension; alterations in cardiac contractility and dysrhythmias; subcutaneous edema; and urticaria. *Lower left,* **Anaphylactoid reactions:** The offending agent enters the body and works by non-immunologically activating systems that cause degranulation of mast cells and basophils or activation of other humoral amplification systems. The systems that can be activated to cause release of mediators from basophils and mast cells include the complement system, the coagulation and fibrinolytic system, and the kinin-generating system. Activation of these systems can result in the release of the same mediators from basophils and mast cells and can result in a syndrome that is clinically indistinguishable from anaphylaxis. (From Levy JH, Roiven MF, and Morris JM: Spine 11:282-291, 1986.)

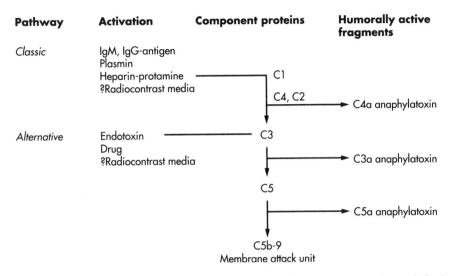

Fig. 16-2. Complement activation pathways, the involved component proteins and the humorally active fragments. (Modified from Levy JH: Anaphylactic reactions in anesthesia and intensive care, Boston, 1986, Butterworth & Co.)

through the classical pathway can be initiated through IgG or IgM antibody binding to antigens, as in hemolytic ABO-incompatible blood transfusion reactions. Heparin-protamine complexes have also been shown in vitro[9] and in vivo[10,11] to activate complement by the classical pathway. Injection of preformed immune complexes or IgG aggregates can activate complement and mimic clinical anaphylaxis.[12] Patients lacking IgA antibody may develop IgG anti-IgA antibodies after receiving multiple transfusions, which may result in complement activation and anaphylactic reactions.[13] Complement activation by the alternative pathway may be stimulated by cell membranes from gram-negative or gram-positive bacteria (endotoxin or exotoxin),[14] cell wall products from fungi (zymosan),[14] Althesin,[15] radiocontrast media,[16] and membranes used for cardiopulmonary bypass and dialysis.[17]

C. Pharmacologic (nonimmunologic) mast-cell activators

A variety of unrelated molecules can release histamine by a nonimmunologic mechanism (Fig. 16-1). The exact mechanism of nonimmunologic mediator release is poorly understood, but release is noncytotoxic. Drugs that induce nonimmunologic release include the opiates (morphine, meperidine, codeine)[18,19] and benzylisoquinoline-derived neuromuscular blocking agents (*d*-tubocurarine, metocurine, atracurium)[20] and vancomycin. Although less frequent, true allergic reactions to the neuromuscular blocking agents can also release mast-cell

mediators by means of IgE antibodies directed against quaternary or tertiary ammonium-ion epitopes.[21-23]

D. Mediators of anaphylactic reactions

Mast cell or basophil activation releases both preformed mediators that are stored in granules and those newly generated mediators that are stored in granules and those newly generated mediators after immunologic activation. The released mediators cause various pathophysiologic responses that may result in life-threatening clinical manifestations. The various preformed and newly generated mediators released by mast cells or basophils and their biologic actions and physiologic manifestations are shown in Table 16-1.

III. CLINICAL MANIFESTATIONS OF ANAPHYLAXIS

The time of onset and manifestations of anaphylaxis can vary. Usually signs and symptoms begin within minutes after parenteral injection of the causative agent but may be delayed for up to 1 or 2 hours after oral administration. The primary targets of anaphylaxis in humans are organs in the cutaneous, gastrointestinal, respiratory, and cardiovascular systems (Table 16-2). In a large study of numerous fatal anaphylactic reactions caused by bee stings, 70% of the deaths were ascribed to respiratory complications and 24% to cardiovascular complications.[24] However, cardiovascular collapse accounted for 80% of anaphylactic reactions to perioperative anesthetic agents.

Table 16-1. Biologic actions and clinical manifestations of mast cell/basophil mediators, both preformed *(A)* and newly synthesized *(B)*

Mediators	Biologic actions	Clinical Manifestations
A. *Preformed*		
Histamine	Smooth muscle relaxation	Vasodilatation, hypotension
	Smooth muscle contraction	Bronchospasm, coronary spasm, increased gastrointestinal motility
	Increases capillary permeability	Angioedema, urticaria, influx of inflammatory cells
	Positive inotropic	Increased contractility
	Positive chronotropic	Tachycardia
ECF-A (eosinophilic chemotactic factor of anaphylais)	Eosinophil chemotaxis	Inflammation
NCA (neutrophilic chemotactic factor	Neutrophil chemotaxis	Inflammation
Neutral proteases	Proteolysis	Inflammation
Heparin	Anticoagulant	Coagulopathy
B. *Newly synthesized*		
Prostaglandin D_2	Smooth muscle relaxation	Vasodilatation, hypotension
	Smooth muscle contraction	Bronchospasm, coronary spasm, increased gastrointestinal motility
	Stimulates mucus secretion	Bronchorrhea, rhinorrhea
	Enhances basophil mediator release	Potentiates reactions
	Inhibits platelet aggregation	
Leukotrienes (C_4, D_4, E_4)	Smooth muscle relaxation	Vasodilatation, hypotension
	Smooth muscle contraction	Bronchospasm, coronary spasm, increased gastrointestinal motility
	Increases capillary permeability	Angioedema, urticaria, influx of inflammatory cells
	Stimulates mucus secretion	Bronchorrhea, rhinorrhea
	Negative inotropic	Myocardial depression, hypotension
Platelet activating factor (PAF)	Smooth muscle relaxation	Vasodilatation, hypotension
	Smooth muscle contraction	Bronchospasm, coronary spasm, increased gastrointestinal motility
	Increases capillary permeability	Angioedema, urticaria, influx of inflammatory cells
	Neutrophil aggregation	Neutrophil activation
	Platelet aggregation	Platelet activation

Table 16-2. Recognition of anaphylaxis during regional and general anesthesia

Systems	Symptoms	Signs
Respiratory	Dyspnea Chest discomfort	Coughing, wheezing, sneezing, laryngeal edema, decreased pulmonary compliance, fulminant pulmonary edema, acute respiratory distress
Cardiovascular	Dizziness Malaise Retrosternal oppression	Disorientation, diaphoresis, loss of consciousness, hypotension, tachycardia, dysrhythmias, decreased systemic vascular resistance, cardiac arrest, pulmonary hypertension
Cutaneous	Itching Burning Tingling	Urticaria (hives), flushing, periorbital edema, perioral edema

From Levy JH: Allergic reactions and intraoperative use of foreign substances. In Barash P: Refresher Courses in Anesthesiology 13:129-141, 1985.

A. Cardiovascular manifestations

Cardiovascular complications include cardiovascular collapse, atrial and ventricular arrhythmias, and myocardial infarction. Symptoms include light-headedness, faintness, and a sense of impending doom.

B. Respiratory manifestations

Upper respiratory tract involvement may include laryngeal edema, which may progress to asphyxia. Early symptoms of laryngeal edema include hoarseness, dysphonia, or sensations of a "lump in the throat." Lower respiratory tract involvement is often indicated by chest tightness, shortness of breath, cough, or wheezing.

C. Cutaneous manifestations

Initial signs and symptoms may include erythema, flushing, and pruritus (especially of the palms, soles, and groin), which often progress to urticaria and angioedema. Angiodema refers to edema in serosal and other vascular-rich tissues that can produce edema in the glottis and larynx.

D. Gastrointestinal manifestations

Gastrointestinal findings include nausea, cramping abdominal pain, vomiting, and severe diarrhea, which may be bloody.

Other signs and symptoms reported in anaphylaxis include nasal, ocular, and palatal pruritus, sneezing, diaphoresis, disorientation, and incontinence. Some patients redevelop manifestations of anaphylaxis 8 to 24 hours after successful resuscitation.

E. Intraoperative and perioperative anaphylaxis

The diagnosis and treatment of patients who develop anaphylaxis in the operating room is difficult, even for the experienced physician. In the perioperative period, multiple medications are frequently given either simultaneously or in rapid succession, making temporal relationships more difficult to interpret. In addition, patients are frequently unconscious and draped, potentially masking early signs and symptoms of anaphylaxis.[25] Anesthetics themselves have been shown in vitro to alter mediator release, possibly delaying early recognition of the syndrome.[26] Often the only observable manifestation of anaphylaxis occurring during anesthesia is cardiovascular collapse,[27] a relatively late event in the syndrome. In suspected anaphylactic reactions in patients undergoing hemodynamic monitoring, cardiovascular changes were characterized by decreases in systolic, diastolic, and mean arterial pressure.[27] Systemic vascular resistance also decreased, while cardiac output and stroke volume increased.[27] Sudden decreases in pulmonary compliance and increases in airway resistance may be manifested by an increase in airway pressures during positive-pressure ventilation.

F. Differential diagnosis

In the awake patient, anaphylaxis is most easily confused with a vasovagal reaction, which may occur after an injection or the onset of intense pain. In vasovagal reactions, the patient looks pale and complains of nausea before syncope but does not become pruritic or cyanotic. Respiratory difficulty does not occur, and symptoms are almost immediately relieved once the patient is supine. The syndrome is usually accompanied by profuse diaphoresis and bradycardia, without flushing, urticaria, angioedema, pruritus, or wheezing. A differential diagnosis of sudden collapse perioperatively may also include dysrhythmia, myocardial infarction, and pulmonary or air embolism.

In the presence of laryngeal edema, especially

when accompanied by abdominal pain, the diagnosis of hereditary angioedema should be considered. When respiratory symptoms are present, globus hystericus and fictitious asthma are included in the differential diagnosis.

Other conditions that can mimic anaphylaxis include sedation from analgesics, overdose of vasodilators, or inadvertent discontinuation of vasopressors, cold urticaria (especially if generalized), idiopathic urticaria, carcinoid tumors, and systemic mastocytosis.

IV. TREATMENT OF ANAPHYLAXIS

Anaphylactic reactions must be recognized immediately because death may occur within minutes.[28] The longer initial therapy is delayed, the greater is the incidence of death.[24] Since anaphylactic reactions are primarily associated with compromised cardiovascular and respiratory function, close monitoring of vital signs, especially blood pressure and airway patency and ventilation, is most important in the assessment of the severity of the reaction and the response to therapy. Treatment of anaphylactic reactions can be divided into initial and secondary therapies and will be considered with suggested doses. Therapy must be titrated to clinical effect (see List 16-1).

A. Initial therapy

First, steps should be taken to interrupt further drug administration, when possible, and decrease absorption of the offending agent. Intravenous infusions of suspected allergens should be stopped immediately. If the antigen has been given subcutaneously (that is, insulin or immunotherapy), a venous tourniquet should be placed proximally to the site, and 0.01 ml/kg of aqueous epinephrine 1:1000 (maximal dose 0.3 to 0.5 ml) should be injected directly into the antigen source to reduce the local circulation and systemic absorption of antigen.

Second, maintain the airway and administer 100% oxygen; adequate oxygenization should be monitored using arterial blood gases. If the patient is not already intubated and there is any suggestion of airway compromise secondary to laryngeal edema, the patient should be intubated immediately. If laryngospasm or laryngeal edema is present, epinephrine, either aerosolized (3 inhalations of 0.16 to 0.20 mg of epinephrine per inhalation) or nebulized (8 to 15 drops of 2.25% epinephrine in 2 ml of normal saline) may be useful. If laryngospasm or laryngeal edema is refractory to these measures or is progressing too rapidly, a catheter cricothyrotomy or emergency surgical cricothyrotomy may be necessary.

Third, discontinue all anesthetic agents, since they have negative inotropic properties and may decrease systemic vascular resistance, interfering with the reflex compensatory response to hypotension. Halothane also sensitizes the heart to catecholamines, which may be required for resuscitation.

List 16-1. Management of Anaphylaxis

Initial therapy
1. STOP ADMINISTRATION OF ANTIGEN
2. MAINTAIN AIRWAY WITH 100% OXYGEN.
3. DISCONTINUE ALL ANESTHETIC AGENTS.
4. START INTRAVASCULAR VOLUME EXPANSION (2 to 4 liters of crystalloid with hypotension).
5. GIVE EPINEPHRINE (4 to 8 μg IV bolus with hypotension, titrate as needed; 0.1 to 0.5 mg IV with cardiovascular collapse).

Secondary treatment
1. ANTIHISTAMINES (0.5 to 1 mg/kg diphenhydramine).
2. CATECHOLAMINE INFUSIONS (starting doses: epinephrine 2 to 4 μg/min, norepinephrine 2 to 4 μg/min, *or* isoproterenol 0.5 to 1 μg/min as a drip, titrated to desired effects).
3. AMINOPHYLLINE (5 to 6 mg/kg over 20 minutes for persistent bronchospasm).
4. CORTICOSTEROIDS (0.25 to 1 g of hydrocortisone; alternatively 1 to 2 mg/kg methylprednisolone; methylprednisolone may be the drug of choice if one suspects that the reaction is mediated by complement).
5. SODIUM BICARBONATE (0.5 to 1 mEq/kg with persistent hypotension or acidosis).
6. AIRWAY EVALUATION (before extubation).

From Levy JH: Allergic reactions and intraoperative use of foreign substances. In Barash P: Refresher Courses in Anesthesiology 13:129-141, 1985.

Fourth, rapid intravenous volume administration of 25 to 50 ml/kg (2 to 4 liters in an adult) of isotonic crystalloid (lactated Ringer's or normal saline) or colloidal solutions is important in the initial therapy shock. Military antishock trousers (MAST suit) can be useful in patients suffering hypotension secondary to anaphylaxis.[29,30] The MAST suit provides perfusion to vital organs and may also be helpful in obtaining peripheral venous access in the upper extremities.[30]

Fifth, epinephrine is the mainstay of initial treatment and should be given intravenously. The exact dose depends on the clinical condition and common sense. In cases of severe hypotension, an initial dose of 0.05 to 0.1 ml of 1:10,000 epinephrine (100 μg/ml) should be given intravenously and increased until blood pressure improves. Depending on the patient's condition, the dosage may need to be higher, especially in the patient who is partially sympathectomized after spinal or epidural anesthesia.[31] If an intravenous line is not in place, 0.5 ml of 1:1000 epinephrine can be given intramuscularly or 10 ml of 1:10,000 epinephrine can be administered through the endotracheal tube. However, in a patient in shock, the absorption of intramuscular or subcutaneous epinephrine is unreliable.

B. Secondary treatment

Once a patient's condition has begun to stabilize, administration of other pharmacologic agents may be warranted.

First, an antihistamine, such as diphenhydramine (1 mg/kg, up to 50 mg), given either intravenously or intramuscularly, will be helpful for symptomatic relief of itching. Although there is no evidence demonstrating the effectiveness of H_2-receptor antagonists in the treatment of anaphylaxis, ranitidine (1 mg/kg IV) may be useful in combination with an H_1-receptor antagonist when hypotension is persistent, since peripheral vasodilatation may be exacerbated by the effects of histamine on endothelial H_2-receptors.

Second, for persistent hypotension, catacholamine infusions may be used. Epinephrine may be useful if both hypotension and bronchospasm persist. Suggested starting doses of epinephrine are 0.02 to 0.05 μg/kg/min (2 to 4 μg/min), which should be titrated to increase blood pressure. If greater than 8 to 10 μg/min is required, tachycardia may be a significant side effect, in which case norepinephrine may be a more effective alternative. Suggested starting dose for norepinephrine is 0.05 μg/kg/min (2 to 4 μg/min) titrated to maintain systemic perfusion pressure. If the patient has persistent

bronchospasm, pulmonary hypertension, or right ventricular failure, then isoproterenol should be considered, at a starting dose of 0.01 to 0.02 μg/kg/min (0.05 to 1 μg/min).

Third, if bronchospasm persists despite beta$_2$-catecholamine administration, aminophylline, 5 to 6 mg/kg administered over 20 minutes may be useful.

Fourth, glucocorticoids may be useful in preventing potential late-phase reactions but will have no immediate effect. Hydrocortisone, 5 mg/kg (up to a 200 mg initial dose) and then 2.5 mg/kg every 6 hours, or methylprednisolone, 1 mg/kg initially and every 6 hours for the first 24 hours, may be given. If the reaction is suspected of being complement mediated, higher doses of methylprednisolone may be given.

Fifth, if acidosis is suspected, sodium bicarbonate (0.5 to 1 mg/kg) should be administered initially. Acid-based status must be monitored by use of arterial blood gas levels to guide further therapeutic interventions.

Sixth, before extubation the airway should be evaluated for patency, especially if the patient has developed angioedema.

Despite all the above measures, some patients may be refractory to therapy. In one study where the efficacy of immunotherapy for insect-sting allergy was assessed by deliberate sting challenge, investigators found that even when they were totally prepared to treat anaphylaxis in an intensive care unit setting there occurred severe, persistent hypotension that was difficult to treat despite repeated doses of intravenously administered epinephrine.[32] During spinal or epidural anesthesia, patients may be partially sympathectomized and require larger doses of epinephrine. Treatment of anaphylaxis may also be complicated by the increased use of beta-adrenergic receptor blocking agents (such as propranolol).[33]

V. DETERMINING THE CAUSE OF ALLERGIC REACTIONS

Patients who have suffered anaphylactic reactions to drugs administered in the operating room require evaluation to identify the causal agents and to guide selection and use of future medications.

A. Detailed History

Evaluation should start with a detailed history including any concurrent illness or prior allergic or anesthetic encounters.[120] The patient's reaction should be carefully reviewed to determine the temporal relationship between the clinical manifestations of the reaction and the medications received, including indications, when initiated, dosage, and duration of therapy. Equally important information is previous exposure to the same or structurally related medications, effect of drug discontinuation, response to treatment, and any prior diagnostic testing or rechallenge. Medications should be considered with regard to their known propensity for causing anaphylaxis. The proximity of drug administration to the onset of acute reactions should also be documented. In general, agents that have been used for long, continuous periods of time before the onset of an acute reaction are less likely to be implicated than agents recently introduced or reintroduced. However, in the perioperative period, it is common for patients to receive many medications in temporal proximity, making a diagnosis more difficult by history alone.

B. Immunodiagnostic tests

1. Skin testing for immediate hypersensitivity reactions. Skin testing is a standardized procedure commonly used by allergists to diagnose immediate hypersensitivity to pollens and bee stings. However, evaluating anesthetic drug allergy is complicated by the unavailability of relevant drug metabolites or appropriate multivalent testing reagents. Intradermal skin tests are still the most readily available and generally useful diagnostic tests for drug allergy. Skin testing has an established role in the evaluation of IgE-mediated penicillin allergy,[34] and it is also useful in the evaluation of allergy to muscle relaxants,[23,35] barbiturates,[35,36] chymopapain,[37] streptokinase,[38] insulin,[39] and miscellaneous other drugs. Specific protocols for skin testing are well documented[40,41] but are not discussed in detail here.

For safety, a scratch or puncture (epicutaneous) test should be performed before the more definitive intradermal test.[41] When one is skin testing with drugs or reagents that have not been well validated previously, all positive skin-test responses should be confirmed by skin testing of five normal persons with the same drug concentration as an appropriate control for irritative, false-positive skin responses. Appropriate skin-testing concentrations of medications commonly used in anesthesia practice have been published.[23,42] It is prudent to discount negative skin-test results unless prior studies have established their reliability. Skin testing must be done in the absence of medications that will affect the skin-test response (especially H_1-antihistamines, trycyclic antidepressants, and sympathomimetic agents). Appropriate positive

(histamine or codeine) and negative (diluent) controls should be used.

2. In vitro tests

a. Total serum IgE concentrations. Although increased total serum IgE concentrations have been reported after allergic reactions,[43] the level of total IgE is rarely if ever helpful in establishing the diagnosis of an allergic drug reaction.

b. Assays to measure complement activation. Assays to measure complement activation include measuring decreases in complement components (that is, C4, C3, or total hemolytic complement [C_H50]) and assays to measure the generation of products of complement activation (C3a, C4a, C5a, and so forth). These assays may implicate, if positive, complement activation in specific reactions.

c. Release of histamine and other mediators by basophils and mast cells. Washed leukocytes containing basophils with IgE antibody on their cell surface release histamine and other mediators when incubated with relevant antigens.[44] In general, results appear to correlate with the results of the direct immediate skin test.[45,46] Although the in vitro basophil histamine release assay avoids exposing a patient to a drug, the assay is time consuming and requires whole blood drawn immediately before the test and its availability is limited. Leukocyte histamine release has been used to demonstrate sensitivity to thiopental,[47] muscle relaxants,[23,48] and penicillins.[49]

d. Measurements of mediators. During or shortly after allergic reactions, blood may be obtained and analyzed for the release of various mediators such as histamine, prostaglandin D_2 (PGD_2), or high-molecular-weight neutrophil chemotactic factor.[32,50] Urine may also be analyzed for metabolites of histamine or PGD_2. Plasma histamine and PGD_2 levels remain elevated only briefly, limiting their clinical utility. Bioassays to measure serum neutrophil chemotactic factor are cumbersome to perform and suffer from large interassay variability. Recently, assays to measure serum tryptase (a protease released specifically from mast cells) appears promising in the clinical assessment of mast cell–mediated allergic reactions.[51] Serum tryptase may remain elevated for hours after release from mast cells.

e. RAST testing. A solid-phase radioimmunoassay, termed the "radioallergosorbent test" (RAST), was first introduced in 1967. The RAST measures circulating allergen-specific IgE antibody, and its basic principle is quite simple. Allergen is attached to a solid phase (carbohydrate particle, paper disk, or the wall of a polystyrene test tubes or plastic microtiter wells) and incubated with serum under study, during which time specific antibody of all immunoglobulin classes is bound. The particles are then washed, and a second incubation is undertaken with a radiolabeled, highly specific, anti-IgE antibody. After washes, the bound radioactivity is directly related to the allergen-specific IgE antibody content in the original serum. When appropriately done, RAST correlates well with skin-test end-point titration, basophil histamine release, and provocation tests.[45,52-54] Results from the serum under study are compared to a positive reference serum and a negative control serum. Application of the RAST to the diagnosis of a drug hypersensitivity attributable to IgE antibody has been limited because of insufficient knowledge of the drug metabolite acting as antigen or hapten. In 1971, a RAST was developed to measure IgE antibody to the major determinant of penicillin,[55] and more recently RASTs have been developed to measure IgE antibody to insulin,[39] chymopapain,[37] muscle relaxants,[21,22] thiopental,[56] trimethoprim,[57] and protamine.[58] False-positive test results may occur because of large nonspecific binding, high total serum IgE levels, or poor technique.[59] False-negative results may occur because of interference of high levels of IgG "blocking antibodies" or inability to maximize assay sensitivity.[60]

In recent years, the commercialization of the RAST has led to abuses. Some commercial laboratories have offered RAST for testing numerous substances not known to cause IgE-mediated allergic disease (that is, local anesthetics and radiocontrast media). Relying upon misleading information from such inappropriate RASTs should be discouraged.

f. Measurement of specific IgG or IgM antibodies. Except for drug-induced thrombocytopenia, hemolytic anemia, and agranulocytosis, there often is little correlation between the presence of antigen-specific IgG and IgM antibodies and the occurrence of an allergic drug reaction. Recent evidence indicates that certain protamine reactions are mediated through protamine-specific IgG antibody.[58]

VI. MANAGEMENT OF THE ALLERGIC PATIENT

If a patient has a history of an allergic reaction to a specific medication but requires its use again, the physician must weigh the risks and benefits of using that medication. If an equally effective, non–cross reacting, alternative drug is available, it should be used. If alternative drugs are unavailable or induce unacceptable side effects or are clearly less effective, cautious administration of the offending drug, with use of a premedication regimen or a desensitization protocol, may be considered.

Premedication regimens have been tested, validated, and utilized mostly in patients who have had previous reactions to ionic radiocontrast agents and who again require procedures using radiocontrast.[16] There is little evidence supporting the use of premedication regimens to prevent IgE-mediated anaphylaxis, and premedication with antihistamines or steroids is not recommended for reactions mediated by IgE antibodies.[61,62] Desensitization protocols have been developed and utilized in patients with acute allergic reactions to penicillin,[63,64] insulin,[65] sulfonamides,[66] and heterologous antisera.[65] In general, desensitization protocols utilize the initial administration of low doses (usually 1:10,000 of a conventional dose) of the suspect drug. Oral or parenteral doses are usually doubled every 15 to 30 minutes, and full doses are usually achieved within 4 to 8 hours, though longer intervals are frequently needed for aspirin desensitization. Desensitization should be performed only by a physician appropriately trained and in an intensive care setting. However, desensitization is not usually practical for the anesthesiologist.

VII. SPECIFIC ALLERGIC REACTIONS SEEN BY THE ANESTHESIOLOGIST

Almost any drug may produce an anaphylactic reaction. However, some drugs have been implicated more often than others or have been investigated in greater detail. We will consider those drugs most often suspected of causing life-threatening anaphylactic reactions and discuss their pathophysiology. Blood products and related agents are considered in Chapter 21.

A. Antibiotics

1. Penicillin. Of all the medications capable of causing allergic drug reactions, penicillin antibiotics are the most frequent offenders. Various studies report an incidence of 0.7% to 0.8% of allergic reactions to penicillin.[67] Anaphylaxis occurs in 0.004% to 0.015% of penicillin treatment cases.[67] Fatality from penicillin anaphylaxis occurs about once in every 50,000 to 100,000 treatment cases,[67] causing approximately 400 to 800 deaths per year.[68] Penicillin can produce all four types of immunopathologic reaction described by Gell and Coombs, including anaphylaxis (type I), penicillin-induced hemolysis (type II), serum sickness (type III), and contact dermatitis (type IV).[2] Some reactions to penicillin have an obscure pathogenesis and have been labeled idiopathic. Among these are the common maculopapular rash, eosinophilia, Stevens-Johnson syndrome, exfoliative dermatitis, and toxic epidermal necrolysis. For reasons presently unknown, ampicillin induces rashes with much greater frequency than penicillin does.[34,69] Pseudoanaphylactic reactions have been observed after intramuscular or inadvertent intravenous injection of procaine penicillin, most likely because of a combination of toxic and embolic phenomena from the procaine.[70]

Penicillin has a low molecular weight (356 daltons) and must first covalently combine with tissue macromolecules (presumably serum albumin) to produce multivalent hapten-protein complexes, which are required for both sensitization, with production of immunospecific antibodies, and elicitation of an allergic reaction.[71] Levine and Parker showed that the beta-lactam ring in penicillins spontaneously opens under certain physiologic conditions, forming the penicilloyl group.[72] Recent evidence indicates that this reaction may be facilitated by low-molecular-weight molecules in serum.[73] The penicilloyl group has been designated the *major determinant* because about 95% of the penicillin molecules irreversibly combine with proteins from penicilloyl groups.[3] This reaction occurs with the prototype benzylpenicillin and with virtually all semisynthetic penicillins. Benzylpenicillin can also be degraded by other metabolic pathways to form additional antigenic determinants.[74] These derivatives are formed in small quantities and stimulate a variable immune response and thus have been termed the *minor determinants*. Therefore IgE antibodies can be produced against several haptenic derivatives of the major and minor determinants to penicillin and other beta-lactams. Anaphylactic reactions to penicillin are usually mediated by IgE antibodies directed against minor determinants, though some anaphylactic reactions have occurred in patients with only penicilloyl-specific IgE antibodies.[3,74,75,84] Accelerated and late urticarial reactions are generally mediated by penicilloyl-specific IgE antibody (major determinant).[3]

Parenteral administration of penicillin produces more allergic reactions than oral administration of penicillin does.[63] Recent evidence indicates that this may be more related to dose than to route of administration. When equivalent doses of penicillin are given orally, the incidence of allergic reactions is comparable to that of intramuscularly administered procaine penicillin.[76] Persons with a history of previous penicillin reactions have a fourfold to sixfold increased risk of subsequent reactions to penicillin compared to those without previous histories.[77] However, most serious and fatal allergic reactions to penicillin and beta-lactam antibiotics occur in persons who have never had a prior allergic reaction to these drugs. Sensitization of these persons may have occurred from a previous therapeutic course of penicillin.

Approximately 10% to 20% of hospitalized patients claim a history of penicillin allergy. However, studies have shown that many of these patients have been incorrectly labeled as allergic to penicillin or have lost their sensitivity to it. The most useful single piece of information in the assessment of a person's potential for an immediate IgE-mediated reaction is his skin-test response to major and minor penicillin determinants.[121] RASTs have been developed to detect IgE antibodies to the penicilloyl determinant.[55] At present, there is no in vitro RAST for minor determinant antibodies. Therefore RAST and other in vitro analogs have limited clinical utility.

2. Cephalosporins. Cephalosporins possess a beta-lactam ring like penicillins, but the five-membered thiazolidine ring of penicillin is replaced by the six-membered dihydrothiazine ring of cephalosporins. Shortly after the cephalosporins came into clinical use, allergic reactions, including anaphylaxis, were reported, and the question of cross-reactivity between cephalosporins and penicillins was raised.[78] Studies in both animals and man have clearly demonstrated cross-reactivity between penicillins and cephalosporins using immunoassays and bioassays to evaluate IgG, IgM, and IgE antibodies.[79-81] Primary cephalosporin allergy in non–penicillin allergic patients has been reported, but the exact incidence is not clear.[82,83] Studies have been limited because the haptenic determinants involved in cephalosporin allergy are unknown. The exact incidence of clinically relevant cross-reactivity between the penicillins and the cephalosporins is unknown and probably small, but anaphylactic cross-reactivity has occurred.[84]

3. Vancomycin. Hypotension is the most serious adverse effect associated with intravenous vancomycin. Non–immunologically mediated histamine release[20,88] has been reported recently as the mechanism of vancomycin-induced hypotension. Hypotension occurs when the drug is rapidly infused or when it is administered in a concentrated solution.[20,87] Vancomycin can produce the "red-neck syndrome," alternatively called the "red-man's syndrome," which is characterized by an intense erythematous discoloration of the upper trunk, arms, and neck, and pruritus. To minimize the risk of histamine release, vancomycin should be infused over a period of at least 60 minutes and in a dilute solution (500 mg/dl). Hypotension should be treated by discontinuance of the vancomycin infusion and by volume and vasopressor administration.

B. Muscle relaxants

The benzylisoquinoline-derived muscle relaxants, such as *d*-tubocurarine, metocurine, atracurium, doxacurium, and mivacurium, produce nonimmunologic histamine release.[27] However, Vervloet et al. and Baldo et al.[21-23,48] have also demonstrated IgE-mediated anaphylactic reactions to muscle relaxants. Evidence supporting an IgE-mediated mechanism includes positive passive transfer tests, basophil histamine release studies, inhibition of basophil histamine release after desensitization to anti-IgE, and the demonstration of drug-specific IgE antibodies in sera from patients who have had adverse reactions to muscle relaxants.[21-23,48] It appears that IgE antibodies are directed against the quaternary or tertiary ammonium ions present in muscle relaxants.[21] Extensive in vitro cross-reactivity has been reported between the muscle relaxants and other compounds that contain quaternary and tertiary ammonium ions.[21] These compounds occur widely in many drugs, foods, cosmetics, disinfectants, and industrial materials. The clinical significance of this in vitro cross-reactivity is unclear, though it has been postulated that patients may become sensitized through environmental contact with these various compounds.[21] Since the muscle relaxants contain two ammonium ions, they appear to be functionally divalent, capable of cross-linking cell-surface IgE and initiating mediator release from mast cells and basophils without haptenizing to carrier molecules.[48] Molecules with ammonium ions at or less than 0.4 nm apart appear incapable of inducing histamine release, whereas the optimal length for cross-linking cell-surface IgE appears to be at or greater than 0.6 nm.[89] Muscle relaxants with a rigid backbone between the two ammonium ions (such as pancuronium and vecuronium) appear to be less likely than flexible molecules in initiating mediator release.[89]

Atopy does not appear to be a risk factor for the occurrence of anaphylactic reactions to muscle relaxants.[90] It is of interest that 90% to 95% of anaphylactic reactions to muscle relaxants occur in females.[91] The reason for this is unclear. However, sensitization to ammonium-ion epitopes in cosmetics has been postulated

to explain the predominance of reactions in women.[21]

Skin testing and RAST can be used to evaluate the presence of IgE antibody directed against muscle relaxants.[21,35,66] However, more studies are needed to determine the predictive value of these tests.

C. Barbiturates

Anaphylaxis has been reported after thiobarbiturate administration, most often associated with thiopental.[27] Proposed mechanisms for thiobarbiturate reactions include non–immunologically induced mediator release and IgE-mediated reactions.[27] Positive skin tests to thiopental have been reported in patients who have had anaphylactic reactions after induction of general anesthesia.[35,92] Recently a thiopental RAST has been reported,[56] but the value of skin testing and RAST in predicting reactions to thiopental is uncertain at present.

D. Local anesthetics

Despite the fact that patients commonly report adverse reactions to local anesthetics and are advised that they are "allergic" to these agents, true allergic reactions to injected local anesthetics are rare. Reactions to local anesthetics are often the result of vasovagal changes, toxic reactions (probably because of inadvertent intravenous injection), side effects from epinephrine, or psychomotor responses, including hyperventilation. Toxic symptoms often involve the central nervous and cardiovascular systems and may produce slurred speech, euphoria, dizziness, excitement, nausea, emesis, disorientation, or convulsions.[93] Vasovagal reactions are usually associated with bradycardia, sweating, pallor, and rapid improvement in symptoms when the patient is supine. Sympathetic stimulation, either from epinephrine or anxiety, may result in tremor, diaphoresis, tachycardia, or hypertension. Rarely, symptoms of reaction to local anesthetics are consistent with IgE-mediated reactions, such as urticaria, bronchospasm, and anaphylactic shock. However, acceptable documentation of IgE-mediated reactivity against local anesthetics in such patients is almost totally lacking.[94] IgE-mediated sensitivity has also been reported, though rarely, for methylparaben, which is a preservative used in local anesthetics.[95] Local anesthetics are divided into two chemical groups: group I comprises chemicals containing benzoate esters, which may cross-react with each other but not with group II drugs; group II agents include mostly amides, which do not substantially cross-react with each other.

Evaluation of a patient with a history of adverse reaction to local anesthetics should include a complete history of the episode and skin testing, along with incremental drug challenge.[93,94] The local anesthetic tested should be one that is appropriate for the proposed procedure and that would not be expected to cross-react with the drug implicated in the previous reaction. If the previous drug is unknown, a group II anesthetic (probably lidocaine) should be chosen. In a patient with a history suggestive of methylparaben sensitivity, preparations without paraben should be used for testing, challenge, and treatment. Preparations without epinephrine should be used for skin testing because epinephrine may mask a positive skin test[96] and may induce toxic effects.

E. Opioids

Morphine, meperidine, and codeine cause non–immunologically mediated histamine release from cutaneous mast cells.[18] In vitro studies indicate that the cutaneous mast cell is uniquely sensitive to opioids and that neither the gastrointestinal nor the lung mast cell nor the circulating basophil releases histamine when exposed to these agents.[97] Most opiate-induced reactions are self-limiting cutaneous reactions, restricted to hives and pruritus or mild hypotension treated by fluid administration. However, anaphylaxis induced by meperidine, fentanyl, and morphine has been documented.[98-100] Recent evidence indicates that IgE antibodies may be induced, which bind epitopes contained in opiates.[98-100]

F. Radiocontrast media

The incidence of reactions induced by radiocontrast media (RCM) injections is between 5% and 8%.[16] Vasomotor reactions (nausea, vomiting, flushing, or warmth) occur in 5% to 8% of patients.[16] Anaphylactoid reactions (urticaria, angioedema, wheezing, dyspnea, hypotension, or death) occur in 2% to 3% of patients receiving intravenous or interarterial infusions.[65] Fatal reactions occurring after radiocontrast media administration occur in about 1:50,000 intravenous procedures,[65] and it has been estimated that as many as 500 deaths per year are attributable to reactions to radiocontrast media. Most reactions begin 1 to 3 minutes after intravascular administration. Patients with a previous anaphylactoid reaction to RCM have approximately a 33% (range 17% to 60%) chance of a repeat reaction upon reexposure.[65] The cause or causes of adverse reactions to RCM are unknown at present. Histamine liberation appears to be a feature of some reactions,[16] though elevations in plasma histamine have occurred without hemodynamic changes or anaphylactic reactions.[16] Activation of serum complement occurs after the intravascular injection of RCM[16] and may occur by the classical or alternative pathway. Therefore it has been suggested that production of anaphylatoxins with subsequent mast cell and basophil mediator release is the cause of RCM reactions. Yet, RCM is capable of inducing nonimmunologic histamine release from mast cells and basophils in the absence of complement activation.[16] It has been suggested that the hypertonicity of RCM results in nonimmunologic mediator release from mast cells and basophils.[16] Although it appears clear that the vasomotor reactions (pain, nausea, vomiting, and warmth) as well as histamine release in vitro are caused by hyperosmolarity, it is unclear if hyperosmolarity is the cause of all RCM reactions in man. There is no evidence that IgE-mediated mechanisms play a role in radiocontrast media reactions.

A patient who requires radiocontrast media administration and who has had a previous reaction to it has an increased (35% to 60%) risk for a reaction on reexposure.[16] Pretreatment of these high-risk patients with prednisone (50 mg) 13 hours, 7 hours, and 1 hour before RCM administration, along with diphenhydramine (50 mg) 1 hour before RCM administration, reduces the risk of reactions to 9%.[101] Almost all reactions in pretreated patients are so mild as to be of no clinical importance (that is, mild urticaria).[16] The addition of ephedrine (25 mg) 1 hour before RCM administration (in patients without angina, arrhythmia, or other contraindications for ephedrine) resulted in a reaction rate of 3.1%.[16] It might be expected that the addition of an H_2-receptor antagonist, such as cimetidine or ranitidine, would further decrease the incidence of RCM reactions, but up to now, no study has shown a benefit from the addition of H_2-receptor antagonists to RCM pretreatment regimens. A recent study showed that steroid pretreatment before the administration of hyperosmolar RCM is as effective as and much less expensive than the use of recent nonhyperosmolar RCM.[102]

G. Protamine

Protamine sulfate is a polycationic, strongly basic small protein with a molecular weight of 4300. Protamine is extracted from salmon milt in a protein-purification process and is used medicinally to reverse heparin anticoagulation and to retard the absorption of certain insulins, namely, neutral protamine Hagedorn (NPH) and protamine zinc insulin (PZI). The use of intravenous protamine has increased in the last decade with the advent of cardiopulmonary bypass technology, cardiac catherization, and hemodialysis. This increase in intravenous protamine use has resulted in more frequent reports of adverse reactions.

Adverse reactions to intravenous protamine administration include rash, urticaria, bronchospasm, pulmonary vasoconstriction, and systemic hypotension leading at times to cardiovascular collapse and death.[103-105]

Diabetic patients receiving daily subcutaneous injections of insulins containing protamine have a thirtyfold to fiftyfold increased risk for life-threatening reactions when given protamine intravenously.[103-105] The actual risk for anaphylactic reactions in NPH insulin–dependent diabetics is 0.6% to 2%.[104,105] Another group putatively at increased risk for protamine reactions are men who have undergone vasectomies. With disruption of the blood-testis barrier, studies have shown that 20% to 33% of such men develop hemagglutinating autoantibodies against protamine-like compounds.[106] It has been postulated that these autoantibodies may cross-react with medicinal protamine, causing adverse reactions.[107] Although protamine reactions in vasectomized men have been reported,[108] Levy et al. did not observe any clinical reactions in a prospective evaluation of 16 vasectomized patients undergoing cardiac surgery with protamine reversal of heparin.[105] Fish-allergic persons also represent a group at theoretic risk for protamine reactions. Since protamine is produced from the matured testis of salmon or a related species of fish belonging to the family Salmonidae or Clupeidae, it has been suggested that persons allergic to fish may have serum antibodies directed against protamine. On the other hand, commercial protamine preparations may be contaminated with fish proteins that fish-allergic patients may react to. Up to now, evidence supporting the increased risk for protamine reactions in fish-allergic patients is lacking and is limited to case reports.[108] Levy et al. did not observe any clinical reactions to protamine in six patients with a history of fish allergy after cardiac surgery.[105]

Finally, previous exposure to intravenous protamine given for reversal of heparin anticoagulation may increase the risk of a reaction on subsequent protamine administration.[116]

The exact mechanisms by which acute protamine reactions occur are incompletely understood. Animal studies initially indicated that protamine may be able to cause direct, nonimmunologic release of histamine in hamster and rat peritoneal mast cells in vitro.[122] However, studies using human basophils and human mast cells have been unable to demonstrate significant histamine release from protamine at concentrations up to 100 μg/ml.[123] Some protamine reactions may be associated with complement activation, either through protamine-heparin complexes[9-11,111] or through protamine and complement fixing, and antiprotamine IgG antibody interaction.[112] These reactions may lead to pulmonary artery pressure elevation and have been associated with the generation of thromboxane, a pulmonary vasoconstrictor.[113,114] Recent evidence indicates that protamine may inhibit the action of plasma carboxypeptidase N, which cleaves the C-terminal arginine residue from the anaphylatoxins and bradykinin, converting them to their less active *des arg* metabolites.[115]

Lakin et al.[112] provided evidence that protamine-specific IgG antibodies could cause protamine reactions by activating complement, whereas others[116,117] have also reported the presence of protamine-specific IgG antibodies in small numbers of protamine reactors. Weiss et al., in a case-control study, showed that in diabetic patients who had received previous protamine-insulin injections the presence of antiprotamine IgE antibody was a significant risk factor for acute protamine reactions (relevant risk = 95), as was the presence of antiprotamine IgG (relative risk = 38).[58] In patients without prior exposure to protamine-insulin injections, antiprotamine IgG antibody was also a risk factor for protamine reactions (relative risk = 25).[58] It appears that in protamine-insulin–dependent diabetic patients antibody-mediated mechanisms are the likely cause for the increased risk of protamine reactions seen in this group. Prescreening high-risk patients (protamine-insulin–dependent diabetics) for the presence of antiprotamine antibodies before elective procedures that would involve the administration of intravenous protamine might be worthwhile. If such antibodies are present, special precautions could be taken, or alternative heparin antagonists, such as hexadimethrine, could be substituted.[118]

Skin testing with protamine does not appear to be useful in discriminating between subjects with significant serum antiprotamine IgE antibody and control subjects.[124, 125] It has been suggested that protamine may be an incomplete or univalent antigen that first must combine with a tissue macromolecule, or possibly heparin, to become a complete, multivalent antigen capable of eliciting mediator release. Thus it appears likely that more than one mechanism may be responsible for the adverse reactions associated with protamine.[126]

H. Chymopapain

Chymopapain is injected intradiskally for chemonucleolysis of herniated lumbar intervertebral disks. The incidence of anaphylaxis to chymopapain is about 1%, whereas the incidence of fatal anaphylaxis appears to be about 0.14%.[37] Women appear to be three times more likely to develop anaphylaxis than men.[106] Chymopapain is obtained from a crude fraction, called "papain," that is extracted from the papaya tree and may be found in meat tenderizers, cosmetics, beer, and soft contact lenses.[17] Evidence indicates that chymopapain reactions may be IgE mediated.[37,65] Both in vivo skin tests and in vitro immunoassays have been used to detect antichymopapain IgE antibody,[37] but more studies are required to determine the predictive value of these tests.

I. Mannitol

The administration of mannitol or other hyperosmotic agents may cause direct, nonimmunologic histamine release from circulating basophils and mast cells.[27] There is no evidence that mannitol causes immunologically mediated reactions. It is believed that slow infusion helps to avoid this problem.

J. Methylmethacrylate

Methylmethacrylate (bone cement) is used during orthopedic surgery to attach a prosthetic joint to raw bone. Cardiopulmonary complications from the use of methylmethacrylate include hypotension, hypoxemia, noncardiogenic pulmonary edema, and cardiac arrest. Many reasons have been postulated for these physiologic manifestations, none of which implicate mechanisms that are allergic in nature.[27]

VIII. EFFECTS OF ANESTHESIA ON IMMUNE RESPONSES

Patients undergoing both anesthesia and surgery develop depressions of both T-cell mediated and B-cell mediated lymphocyte responsiveness as well as depression of nonspecific host resistance mechanisms including phagocytosis.[119] A spectrum of anesthetic drugs have been shown in vitro to decrease immune responses; however the effects are short lived and may be modified by multiple other factors such as increases in stress responses that occur perioperatively.[119] Immune competence during surgery can be affected by direct and hormonal effects of anesthetic drugs, immunologic consequences of other drugs used, type of surgery,

and coincidence infections. Although multiple studies demonstrate in vitro alterations of immune function, no studies have ever demonstrated the actual clinical significance or actual importance.[119] Furthermore, they are likely to be of minor importance when compared with the general systemic hormonal aspects of stress responses and their abilities to depress immune function transiently.

REFERENCES

1. Ovary Z: The history of immediate hypersensitivity, Hosp Pract Feb.:99-109, 1989.
2. Gell PGH and Coombs RRA: Classification of allergic reactions responsible for clinical hypersensitivity and disease. In Gell PGH, Coombs RRA, and Hachmann PJ, editors: Clinical aspects of immunology, Oxford, Engl, 1975, Blackwell Scientific Publications.
3. Levine BB: Immunologic mechanisms of penicillin allergy: a haptenic model system for the study of allergic diseases of man, N Engl J Med 275:1115-1125, 1966.
4. Metzger H, Alcaraz G, Hohman R, et al: The receptor with high affinity for immunoglobulin E, Ann Rev Immunol 4:419-470, 1986.
5. Ishizaka T: Mechanisms of IgE-mediated hypersensitivity. In Middleton E Jr, Reed CE, Ellis EF, et al, editors: Allergy: principles and practice, ed 3, St. Louis, 1988, The CV Mosby Co.
6. Siraganian RP: Histamine secretion from mast cells and basophils, Trends Pharmacol Sci 4:432-437, 1983.
7. Ghebrehiwet B: The complement system: mechanisms of activation, regulation, and biological functions. In Kaplan AP, editor: Allergy, New York, 1985, Churchill Livingstone.
8. Yancey KB, Hammer CH, Harvath L, et al: Studies of human C5a as a mediator of inflammation in normal human skin, J Clin Invest 75:486-495, 1985.
9. Rent R, Ertel N, Eisenstein R, and Gewurz H: Complement activation by interaction of polyanions and polycations. I. Heparin-protamine induced consumption of complement, J Immunol 114:120-124, 1975.
10. Kirklin JK, Chenoweth DE, Naftel DC, et al: Effects of protamine administration after cardiopulmonary bypass on complement, blood elements, and the hemodynamic state, Ann Thorac Surg 41:193-199, 1986.
11. Best N, Sinosich MJ, Teisner B, et al: Complement activation during cardiopulmonary bypass by heparin-protamine interaction, Br J Anaesth 56:339, 1984.
12. Wasserman SI and Marquardt DL: Anaphylaxis. In Middleton E Jr, Reed CE, Ellis EF, et al, editors: Allergy: principles and practice, ed 3, St. Louis, 1988, The CV Mosby Co.
13. Vyas GN, Perkins HA, and Fundenberg HH: Anaphylactoid transfusion reactions associated with anti-IgA, Lancet 2:312, 1968.
14. Frank MM: Complement: a brief review, J Allergy Clin Immunol 84:411-420, 1988.
15. Watkins J, Clark A, Appleyard TN, Padfield: Immune mediated reactions to althesin (alphaxalone). Br J Anaesth 55:231, 1976.
16. Greenberger PA: Contrast media reactions, J Allergy Clin Immunol 74:600-605, 1984.
17. Craddock PR, Fehr J, Brigham KL, et al: Complement and leukocyte-mediated pulmonary dysfunction

in hemodialysis, N Engl J Med 296:769-774, 1977.

18. Levy JH, Brister NW, Shearin A, et al: Wheal and flare responses to opioids in humans, Anesthesiology 70:756-760, 1989.

19. North FC, Kettelkamp N, and Hirshman CA: Comparison of cutaneous and in vitro histamine release by muscle relaxants, Anesthesiology 66:543-546, 1987.

20. Levy JH, Kettelkamp N, Goertz P, et al: Histamine release by vancomycin: a mechanism for hypotension in man, Anesthesiology 67:122-125, 1987.

21. Baldo BA and Fisher MM: Substituted ammonium ions as allergenic determinants in drug allergy, Nature 306:262-264, 1983.

22. Harle DG, Baldo BA, and Fisher MM: Detection of IgE antibodies to suxamethonium after anaphylactoid reactions during anaesthesia, Lancet 1:930-932, 1984.

23. Vervloet D, Nizankowska E, Arnaud A, et al: Adverse reactions to suxamethonium and other muscle relaxants under general anesthesia, J Allergy Clin Immunol 71:552-559, 1983.

24. Barnard JH: Studies of 400 Hymenoptera sting deaths in the United States, J Allergy Clin Immunol 52:259, 1973.

25. Laxenaire MC, Moneret-Vautrin DA, Boileau S, and Moeller R: Adverse reactions to intravenous agents in anaesthesia in France, Klin Wochenschr 60:1006-1009, 1982.

26. Kettelkamp NS, Austin DR, Cheek DBC, et al: Inhibition of d-tubocurarine–induced histamine release by halothane, Anesthesiology 66:666-669, 1987.

27. Levy JH: Anaphylactic reactions in anesthesia and intensive care, Boston, 1986, Butterworth & Co.

28. James LP and Austen KF: Fatal systemic anaphylaxis in man, N Engl J Med 270:597, 1964.

29. Bickell WH and Dice WH: Military antishock trousers in a patient with adrenergic-resistant anaphylaxis, Ann Emerg Med 13:189, 1984.

30. Loehr MM: Suit up against anaphylaxis, Emerg Med April:127-128, 1985.

31. Levy JH: Cardiovascular changes during anaphylactic/anaphylactoid reactions in man, J Clin Anesth 1:426-430, 1989.

32. Smith PL, Kagey-Sobotka A, Bleecker ER, et al: Physiologic manifestations of human anaphylaxis , J Clin Invest 66:1072-1080, 1980.

33. Jacobs RL, Geoffrey WR Jr, Fournier DC, et al: Potentiated anaphylaxis in patients with drug-induced beta-adrenergic blockade, J Allergy Clin Immunol 68:125-127, 1981.

34. Weiss ME and Adkinson NF Jr: Immediate hypersensitivity reactions to penicillin and related antibiotics, Clin Allergy 18:515-540, 1988.

35. Fisher MM: Intradermal testing in the diagnosis of acute anaphylaxis during anaesthesia: results of five years' experience, Anaesth Intensive Care 7:58-61, 1979.

36. Moscicki RA, Sockin SM, Corsello BF, et al: Anaphylaxis during induction of general anesthesia: subsequent evaluation and management, J Allergy Clin Immunol 86:325-332, 1990.

37. Grammer LC and Patterson R: Proteins: chymopapain and insulin, J Allergy Clin Immunol 74:635-640, 1984.

38. Dykewicz MS, McGrath KG, Davison R, et al: Identification of patients at risk for anaphylaxis due to streptokinase, Arch Intern Med 146:305-307, 1986.

39. Hamilton RG, Rendell M, and Adkinson NF Jr: Serological analysis of human IgG and IgE anti-insulin antibodies by solid-phase radioimmunoassays, J Lab Clin Med 96:1022-1036, 1980.

40. Norman PS: Skin testing. In Rose NR, Friedman H, and Fahey JL, editors: Manual of clinical laboratory immunology, ed 3, Washington, DC, 1986, American Society for Microbiology.

41. Adkinson NF Jr: Tests for immunological drug reactions. In Rose NF, Friedman H, and Fahey JL, editors: Manual of clinical immunology, ed 3, Washington, DC, 1986, American Society for Microbiology.

42. Fisher M: Intradermal testing after anaphylactoid reaction to anaesthetic drugs: practical aspects of performance and interpretation, Anaesth Intensive care 12:115-120, 1984.

43. Etter MS, Helrich M, and Mackenzie CF: Immunoglobulin E fluctuation in thiopental anaphylaxis, Anesthesiology 52:181-183, 1980.

44. Lichtenstein LM and Osler AG: Studies on the mechanisms of hypersensitivity phenomena. IX. Histamine release from leukocytes by ragweed pollen antigen, J Exp Med 120:507-530, 1964.

45. Norman PS, Lichtenstein LM, and Ishizaka K: Diagnostic tests in ragweed hay fever: a comparison of direct skin tests, IgE antibody measurements, and basophil histamine release, J Allergy Clin Immunol 52:210-224, 1973.

46. Bruce CA, Rosenthal RR, Lichtenstein LM, and Norman PS: Diagnostic tests in ragweed-allergic asthma: a comparison of direct skin tests, leukocyte histamine release, and quantitative bronchial challenge, J Allergy Clin Immunol 53:230-239, 1974.

47. Hirshman CA, Peters J, and Cartwright-Lee I: Leukocyte histamine release to thiopental, Anesthesiol 56:64-67, 1982.

48. Vervloet D, Arnaud A, Senft M, et al: Leukocyte histamine release to suxamethonium in patients with adverse reactions to muscle relaxants, J Allergy Clin Immunol 75:338-342, 1985.

49. Pienkowski MM, Kazmier WJ, and Adkinson NF Jr: Basophil histamine release remains unaffected by clinical desensitization to penicillin, J Allergy Clin Immunol 82:171-178, 1988.

50. Atkins PC, Norman M, Weiner H, and Zweiman B: Release of neutrophil chemotactic activity during immediate hypersensitivity reactions in humans, Ann Intern Med 86:415-418, 1977.

51. Schwartz LB, Metcalfe DD, Miller JS, et al: Tryptase levels as an indicator of mast-cell activation in systemic anaphylaxis and mastocytosis, N Engl J Med 316:1622-1626, 1987.

52. Council on Scientific Affairs: In vitro testing for allergy. Report II of the Allergy Panel, JAMA 258:1639, 1987.

53. Plaut M, Lichtenstein LM, and Henney CS: Properties of a subpopulation of T cells bearing histamine receptors, J Clin Invest 55:856-874, 1975.

54. Santrach PJ, Parker JL, Jones RT, and Yuninger JW: Diagnostic and therapeutic applications of a modified radioallergosorbent test and comparison with the conventional radioallergosorbent test, J Allergy Clin Immunol 67:97-105, 1981.

55. Wide L and Juhlin L: Detection of penicillin allergy of the immediate type by radioimmunoassay of reagins (IgE) to penicilloyl conjugates, Clin Allergy 1:171-177, 1971.

56. Harle DG, Baldo BA, Smal MA, et al: Detection of thiopentone-reactive IgE antibodies following anaphylactoid reactions during anaesthesia, Clin Allergy 16:493-498, 1986.

57. Harle DG, Baldo BA, Smal SA, and Van Nunen SA: An immunoassay for the detection of IgE antibodies to trimethoprim in the sera of allergic patients, Clin Allergy 17:209-216, 1987.

58. Weiss ME, Nyhan D, Zhikang P, et al: Association of protamine IgE and IgG antibodies with life-threatening reactions to intravenous protamine, N Engl J Med 320:886-892, 1989.

59. Hamilton RG and Adkinson NF Jr: Serological methods in the diagnosis and management of human allergic disease, CRC Crit Rev Clin Lab Sci 21:1-18, 1984.

60. Zeiss CR, Grammer LC, and Levitz D: Comparison of the radioallergosorbent test and a quantitative solid-phase radioimmunoassay for the detection of ragweed-specific immunoglobulin E antibody in patients undergoing immunotherapy, J Allergy Clin Immunol 67:105-110, 1981.

61. Mathews KP, Hemphill FM, Lovell RG, et al: A controlled study on the use of parenteral and oral antihistamines in preventing penicillin reactions, J Allergy 27:1-15, 1956.

62. Sciple GW, Knox JM, and Montgomery CH: Incidence of penicillin reactions after an antihistaminic simultaneously administered parenterally, N Engl J Med 261:1123-1125, 1959.

63. Sullivan TJ, Yecies LD, Shatz GS, et al: Desensitization of patients allergic to penicillin using orally administered beta-lactam antibiotics, J Allergy Clin Immunol 69:275-282, 1982.

64. Adkinson NF Jr: Penicillin allergy. In Lichtenstein LM and Fauci A, editors: Current therapy in allergy, immunology and rheumatology, Burlington, Ontario, 1983, BC Decker.

65. Patterson R, DeSwarte RD, Greenberger PA, and Grammer LC: Drug allergy and protocols for management of drug allergies, N Engl Reg Allergy Proc 4:325-342, 1986.

66. Smith RM, Iwamoto GK, Richerson HB, and Flaherty JP: Trimethoprim-sulfamethoxazole desensitization in the acquired immunodeficiency syndrome, Ann Intern Med 106:335, 1987.

67. Idsoe O, Guthe T, Willcox RR, and De Weck AL: Nature and extent of penicillin side-reactions, with particular reference to fatalities from anaphylactic shock, Bull WHO 38:159-188, 1968.

68. Sheffer AL: Anaphylaxis, J Allergy Clin Immunol 75:227-233, 1985.

69. Shapiro S, Siskind V, Slone D, et al: Drug rash with ampicillin and other penicillins, Lancet 2:969-972, 1969.

70. Galpin JE, Chow AW, Yoshikawa TT, and Guze LB: "Pseudoanaphylactic" reactions from inadvertent infusion of procaine penicillin G, Ann Intern Med 81:358, 1974.

71. Eisen HN: Hypersensitivity to simple chemicals. In Lawrence HS, editor: Cellular and humoral aspects of the hypersensitive states, New York, 1959, PB Hoeber.

72. Levine BB: Immunochemical mechanisms involved in penicillin hypersensitivity in experimental animals and in human beings, Fed Proc 24:45-50, 1965.

73. Sullivan TJ: Facilitated haptenation of human proteins by penicillin, J Allergy Clin Immunol 83:255, 1989 (Abstract).

74. Levine BB and Redmond AP: Minor haptenic determinant-specific reagins of penicillin hypersensitivity in man, Int Arch Allergy 35:445-455, 1969.

75. Levine BB, Redmond AP, Fellner MJ, et al: Penicillin allergy and the heterogeneous immune responses of man to benzylpenicillin, J Clin Invest 45:1895-1906, 1966.

76. Adkinson NF Jr and Wheeler B: Risk factors for IgE-dependent reactions to penicillin. In Kerr JW and Ganderton MA, editors: XI International Congress of Allergology and Clinical Immunology, London, 1983, MacMillan Press Ltd., pp 55-59.

77. Sogn DD: Prevention of allergic reactions to penicillin, J Allergy Clin Immunol 78:1051-1052, 1987.

78. Grieco MH: Cross-allergenicity of the penicillins and the cephalosporins, Arch Intern Med 119:141-146, 1967.

79. Petz L: Immunologic cross-reactivity between penicillins and cephalosporins: a review, J Infect Dis 137:S74-S79, 1978.

80. Shibata K, Atsumi T, Horiuchi Y, and Mashimo K: Immunological cross-reactivities of cephalothin and its related compounds with benzylpenicillin (penicillin G), Nature 212:419-420, 1966.

81. Abraham GN, Petz LD, and Fudenberg HH: Immunohaematological cross-allergenicity between penicillin and cephalothin in humans, Clin Exp Immunol 3:343-357, 1968.

82. Abraham GN, Petz LD, and Fudenberg HH: Cephalothin hypersensitivity associated with anti-cephalothin antibodies, Int Arch Allergy 34:65-74, 1968.

83. Ong R and Sullivan T: Detection and characterization of human IgE to cephalosporin determinants, J Allergy Clin Immunol 81:222, 1988.

84. Saxon A, Beall GN, Rohr AS, and Adelman DC: Immediate hypersensitivity reactions to beta-lactam antibiotics, Ann Intern Med 107:204-215, 1987.

85. Adkinson NF Jr, Swabb EA, and Sugerman AA: Immunology of the monobactam aztreonam, Antimicrob Agents Chemother 25:93-97, 1984. [Not in text.]

86. Adkinson NF Jr, Wheeler B, and Swabb EA: Clinical tolerance of the monobactam aztreonam in penicillin allergic subjects. Abstract (WS-26-4) presented at the 14th International Congress of Chemotherapy, June 23-28, Kyoto, Japan, 1984. [Not in text.]

87. Southorn PA, Plevak DJ, Wright AJ, and Wilson WR: Adverse effects of vancomycin administered in the perioperative period, Mayo Clin Proc 61:721-724, 1986.

88. Verburg KM, Bowsher RR, Israel KS, et al: Histamine release by vancomycin in humans, Fed Proc 44:1247, 1985.

89. Didier A, Cador D, Bongrand P, et al: Role of the quaternary ammonium ion determinants in allergy to muscle relaxants, J Allergy Clin Immunol 79:578-584, 1987.

90. Charpin D, Benzarti M, Hemon Y, et al: Atopy and anaphylactic reactions to suxamethonium, J Allergy Clin Immunol 82:356-360, 1988.

91. Youngman PR, Taylor KM, and Wilson JD: Anaphylactoid reactions to neuromuscular blocking agents, Lancet 2:597-599, 1983.

92. Dolovich J, Evans S, Rosenbloom D, et al: Anaphylaxis due to thiopental sodium anesthesia, Can Med Assoc J 123:292-294, 1980.

93. Schatz M: Skin testing and incremental challenge in the evaluation of adverse reactions to local anesthetics, J Allergy Clin Immunol 606:616-1984, 1989.

94. deShazo RD and Nelson HS: An approach to the patient with a history of local anesthetic hypersensitivity: experience with 90 patients, J Allergy Clin Immunol 63:387-394, 1989.

95. Nagel JE, Fuscaldo JT, and Fireman PL: Paraben allergy, JAMA 237:1594, 1977.

96. DeSwarte RD: Drug allergy. In Patterson R, editor: Allergic diseases: diagnosis and management, ed 3, Philadelphia, 1989, JB Lippincott Co.

97. Lawrence ID, Warner JA, Cohan VL, et al: Purification and characterization of human skin mast cells: evidence for human mast cell heterogeneity, J Immunol 139:3062-3069, 1987.

98. Harle DG, Baldo BA, Coroneos NJ, and Fisher MM: Anaphylaxis following administration of papaveretum. case report: implication of IgE antibodies that react with morphine and codeine, and identification of an allergenic determinant, Anesthesiology 71:489-494, 1989.

99. Zucker-Pinchoff B and Ramanathan S: Anaphylactic reaction to epidural fentanyl, Anesthesiology 71:599-601, 1989.

100. Levy JH and Rockoff MR: Anaphylaxis to meperidine, Anesth Analg 61:301-303, 1982.

101. Kelly JF, Patterson R, Lieberman P, et al: Radiographic contrast media studies in high risk patients, J Allergy Clin Immunol 62:181-184, 1978.

102. Lasser EC, Berry CC, Talner LB, et al: Pretreatment with corticosteroids to alleviate reactions to intravenous contrast material, N Engl J Med 317:845-849, 1987.

103. Sharath MD, Metzger WJ, Richerson HB, et al: Protamine-induced fatal anaphylaxis, J Thorac Cardiovasc Surg 90:86-90, 1985.

104. Levy JH, Zaidan JR, and Faraj BA: Prospective evaluation of risk of protamine reactions in NPH insulin–dependent diabetics, Anesth Analg 65:739-742, 1986.

105. Levy JH, Schwieger IM, Zaidan JR, et al: Evaluation of patients at risk for protamine reactions, J Thorac Cardiovasc Surg 98:200-204, 1989.

106. Samuel T: Antibodies reacting with salmon in human protamines in sera from infertile men and from vasectomized men and monkeys, Clin Exp Immunol 30:181, 1977.

107. Watson RA, Ansbacher R, Barry M, et al: Allergic reaction to protamine: a late complication of elective vasectomy? Urology 22:493, 1983.

108. Knape JTA, Schuller JL, De Haan P, et al: An anaphylactic reaction to protamine in a patient allergic to fish, Anesthesiology 55:324-325, 1981.

109. Keller R: Interrelations between different types of cells, Int Arch Allergy 34:139-144, 1968.

110. Levy JH, Faraj BA, Zaidan JR, and Camp VM: Effects of protamine on histamine release from human lung, Agents Actions 28:70-72, 1989.

111. Cavarocchi NG, Schaff HV, Orszulak TA, et al: Evidence for complement activation by protamine-heparin interaction after cardiopulmonary bypass, Surgery 98:525, 1985.

112. Lakin JD, Blocker TJ, Strong DM, and Yocum MW: Anaphylaxis to protamine sulfate mediated by a complement-dependent IgG antibody, J Allergy Clin Immunol 61:102-107, 1977.

113. Degges RD, Foster ME, Dang AQ, and Read RC: Pulmonary hypertensive effect of heparin and protamine interaction: evidence for thromboxane B_2 release from the lung, Am J Surg 154:696-699, 1987.

114. Morel DR, Zapol WM, Thomas SJ, et al: C5a and thromboxane generation associated with pulmonary vaso- and broncho-constriction during protamine reversal of heparin, Anesthesiology 66:597-604, 1987.

115. Skidgel RA, Tan F, Jackman H, et al: Protamine inhibits plasma carboxypeptidase N (CPN), the inactivator of anaphylatoxins and kinins, Fed Proc 2:A1382, 1988 (Abstract).

116. Grant JA, Cooper JR, Albyn KC, et al: Anaphylactic reactions to protamine in insulin-dependent diabetics after cardiovascular procedures, J Allergy Clin Immunol 73:180, 1984 (Abstract).

117. Gottschlich GM and Georgitis JW: Protamine-specific antibodies in protamine anaphylaxis, Ann Allergy 60:249, 1988 (Abstract).

118. Doolan L, McKenzie I, Krafchek J, et al: Protamine sulphate hypersensitivity, Anaesth Intensive Care 9:147, 1981.

119. Stevenson GW, Hall SC, Rodnick S, et al: The effect of anesthetic agents on the human immune response, Anesthesiology 72:542-552, 1990.

120. Weiss ME, Adkinson NF Jr, and Hirshman CA: Evaluation of allergic drug reactions in the perioperative period, Anesthesiology 71:483-486, 1989.

121. Weiss ME and Adkinson NF Jr: Immediate hypersensitivity reactions to penicillin and related antibiotics, Clin Allergy 18:515-540, 1988.

122. Keller R: Interrelations between different types of cells, Int Arch Allergy 34:139-144, 1968.

123. Foreman JC and Lichtenstein LM: Induction of histamine secretion by polycations, Biochim Biophys Acta 629:587-603, 1980.

124. Weiler JM, Gelhaus MA, Carter JG, et al: A prospective study of the risk of an immediate adverse reaction to protamine sulfate during cardiopulmonary bypass surgery, J Allergy Clin Immunol 85:713-719, 1990.

125. Weiss ME, Chatham F, Kagey-Sobotka A, and Adkinson NF Jr: Serial immunological investigations in a patient who had a life-threatening reaction to intravenous protamine, Clin Exp Allergy 20:713-721, 1990.

126. Weiss ME and Adkinson NF Jr: Allergy to protamine. In Vervloet, editor: Clinical reviews in allergy: anesthesiology and allergy, New York, 1991, Elsevier Pub Co, Inc.

Chapter 17

Nausea and Vomiting

Janice M. Bitetti
Herbert D. Weintraub

Nausea and vomiting have been the bane of anesthesia for more than a century. The earliest accounts of diethyl ether and nitrous oxide administration include tales of patients retching and vomiting. The medical literature of that era is replete with proposed remedies and etiologies. In the days of ether and cyclopropane, almost 80% of patients experienced nausea and vomiting and therapies were often limited to what today seem like voodoo: meat-free diets, mustard leaves to the epigastrium, black coffee, and iced water.[1,2]

Fortunately, there has been some progress over the past 100 years in reducing the incidence of postoperative nausea and vomiting (PNV). Fluorinated inhalation agents and new intravenous anesthetics have lowered the current incidence of PNV to between 20% and 50%. However, even today, there is up to an 80% incidence of PNV in select groups such as young women undergoing laparoscopy and children having eye muscle surgery.[3,4] And now that death is no longer a common sequela of anesthesia, PNV has emerged as one of the more important and annoying complications. This is particularly true in the outpatient setting, where PNV can significantly delay discharge, thereby increasing costs. PNV's impact on anesthesia costs can only grow if, as predicted, over 50% of all surgery performed in the United States is on an outpatient basis within the next 5 years. In recent times, great efforts have been made to evaluate patient and surgical risk factors for PNV, to analyze the effects of different anesthetic agents on this complication, and to develop better prophylaxis and treatment. In this chapter, we review the physiology of nausea and vomiting, the preoperative risk factors, and predisposing conditions. In addition, we discuss the impact of anesthetic agents and surgery on PNV and will conclude with a description of treatment options, both prophylactic and therapeutic.

I. PHYSIOLOGY OF NAUSEA AND VOMITING

Nausea and vomiting conjure up unpleasant images and are undoubtedly adverse aspects of anesthesia. Nevertheless, they derive from centrally mediated reflexes and pathways that are extremely advantageous to the human organism. Survival strategies of many higher organisms include the ability to discriminate between desirable and undesirable material for ingestion. Even many lower animal forms demonstrate this ability through well-developed senses of sight, taste, and smell. Vomiting—the expulsion of something toxic that has been swallowed despite these senses—thus serves as a safety mechanism. Interestingly the vomiting reflex, a finely coordinated maneuver, exists in lower animal forms like the frog and the bird but is not uniformly present in mammals.[5] Cats, dogs, and ferrets, like humans, have a well-developed vomiting reflex, and vomiting in these animals is often studied to approximate human vomiting.

The central nervous system (CNS) serves as the control center for nausea and vomiting. The CNS receives input from peripheral sensors and the cerebral cortex, and after integrating this information, it activates the autonomic system and the motor fibers of the thorax and gastrointestinal tract to initiate vomiting.

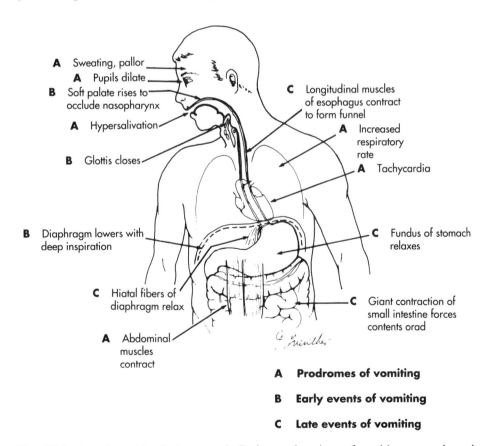

A Sweating, pallor
A Pupils dilate
B Soft palate rises to occlude nasopharynx
A Hypersalivation
B Glottis closes
B Diaphragm lowers with deep inspiration
C Hiatal fibers of diaphragm relax
A Abdominal muscles contract

C Longitudinal muscles of esophagus contract to form funnel
A Increased respiratory rate
A Tachycardia
C Fundus of stomach relaxes
C Giant contraction of small intestine forces contents orad

A **Prodromes of vomiting**

B **Early events of vomiting**

C **Late events of vomiting**

Fig. 17-1. Act of vomiting in humans. A, Early warning signs of vomiting occur through activation of autonomic nuclei near the vomiting center. B, Act of vomiting itself begins with closure of the glottis, elevation of the soft palate, and lowering of the diaphragm. C, Contractions of the intestines and abdominal muscles then force food into the relaxed stomach, and the esophageal muscles contract to form a funnel through which food can exit.

A. The vomiting reflex

The act of vomiting is a complex, almost convulsive, reflex maneuver involving both visceral and striated muscle (Fig. 17-1). Vomiting begins with a deep inspiration, elevation of the soft palate to occlude the nasopharynx, and glottic closure. Then the proximal area of the stomach relaxes and a giant contraction of the small intestine forces previously ingested contents orad into the relaxed stomach, diluting and buffering the gastric acid. Finally, contracture of the esophageal muscles pulls the stomach into the thorax, forming an esophageal funnel, and food is forced out of the stomach by contraction of the abdominal muscles against the lowered diaphragm. If the glottis is closed, only retching results; if the pharynx is relaxed, the contents exit through the mouth.[6,7]

In humans, vomiting is often preceded by nausea, a difficult to describe feeling of impending vomiting. Several autonomic signs accompany nausea and are probably attributable to the proximity of the autonomic nuclei to the center for vomiting. These warning signs (which should cause an alert observer to quickly proffer a basin) include excessive salivation, dilated pupils, tachypnea, swallowing, pallor, sweating, and tachycardia. If the nausea proceeds to retching, bradycardia may replace tachycardia. Unlike the intense gastrointestinal activity associated with vomiting, there are no known gastrointestinal correlates of nausea.[5,6,7]

B. Anatomic control of vomiting: the chemoreceptor trigger zone

There are two anatomic sites for CNS control of vomiting: the chemoreceptor trigger zone (CTZ) and the vomiting center (Fig. 17-2). The CTZ is located in the area postrema (AP), a spongiform vascular body protruding into the fourth ventricle. Early in this century researchers observed that the area postrema, unlike most brain tissue, had a peculiar uptake of blood-borne dyes. However, little was understood about the significance of the CTZ until the 1950s, when Borison and Wang identified it as the major chemosensory area for inducing vomiting.[8] Blood vessels supplying the area

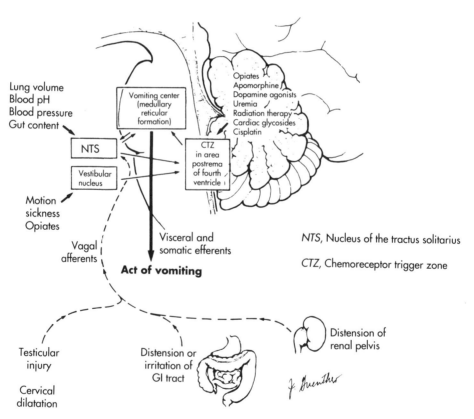

Fig. 17-2. Central control of vomiting. The act of vomiting is mediated by the vomiting center in the medullary reticular formation. Input to the vomiting center comes from the chemoreceptor trigger zone (CTZ), the nucleus of the tractus solitarius (NTS), and the cerebral cortex. Both the NTS and the vestibular nucleus can induce vomiting through effects on the CTZ.

postrema leak injected dye into the underlying tissue; the area postrema also exchanges solutes directly with the cerebrospinal fluid. These properties could represent a countercurrent mechanism for concentrating blood-borne toxins, bypassing the blood-brain barrier.[5,9]

The CTZ is rich in enkephalins, opiate receptors, and dopamine receptors. Stimulation of the CTZ by injection of apomorphine, L-dopa, and numerous other substances leads to vomiting. The CTZ is believed to be responsible for the vomiting associated with opiates, cardiac glycosides, and the dopaminergic agonists. Ablation of the CTZ prevents the vomiting associated with uremia, motion sickness, and radiation therapy. There is afferent input to the area postrema from the vagal and glossopharyngeal nerves, which can provide information on blood pressure, arterial gas composition, lung volume, and gut content.

C. Anatomic control of vomiting: the vomiting center

The CTZ acts only as a sensor; it induces vomiting by signaling the vomiting center, located deep in the medulla in the lateral reticular formation. Electrical stimulation of the vomiting center leads to emesis through both visceral and somatic efferents. These include the fifth, seventh, ninth, tenth, and twelfth cranial nerves as well as spinal nerves that innervate the diaphragm and abdominal muscles. Nearby nuclei associated with vasomotor and bulbar activity, respiration, and salivation are often activated in concert with the vomiting center and lead to the autonomic prodromes of vomiting. Input to the vomiting center comes from the CTZ, the cerebral cortex, the vestibular nucleus, and the nucleus of the tractus solitarius (NTS).

D. The nucleus of the tractus solitarius

The NTS is the terminus in the lower medulla for all general and special visceral afferent fibers of the cranial nerves. Although vagal fibers predominate, fibers from the seventh, ninth, and possibly spinal nerves end there as well.[5] The NTS could therefore serve as the pathway whereby pharyngeal stimulation, gut irritation or distension, distension of the renal pelvis, testicular injury, or cervical dilatation leads to nausea and vomiting.

E. The vestibular nucleus

The vestibular nucleus is the relay station for spatial and motion input, and through its action on the CTZ it can mediate the nausea and vomiting of "motion sickness" or "seasickness." Bursts of acceleration or deceleration set the endolymph in the inner ear into motion and generate impulses that are conducted centrally via the eight cranial nerve. Cortical activity can sometimes override and destruction of the CTZ can eliminate the vomiting response to motion.

F. The cerebral cortex

The role of the cerebral cortex in nausea and vomiting is not well described; however, it is clear that the sensation of nausea involves conscious perception. Nausea often precedes or accompanies vomiting, but it is not a necessary concomitant. For example, the vomiting seen with intracranial hypertension is rarely associated with nausea. Psychologic factors are well known to modulate the nausea and vomiting associated with chemotherapy and cancer; perception of pain is believed to play a role in PNV. Temporary staying of the vomiting reflex can occur through voluntary effort, though a strong enough stimulus cannot be voluntarily overridden.

G. Hormonal influences

The NTS, vestibular cortex, and cerebral cortex are well established as furnishing important input to the vomiting center or CTZ. A large number of hormones are also suspected of having such an impact. The prominent emetic effects of the sympathomimetic anesthetics, ether and cyclopropane, have led to the investigation of catecholamines as causes of PNV. In cats, even when blood pressure is controlled, intraventricular injection of alpha-adrenergic receptor agents leads to vomiting and the emesis is blocked by alpha-blockers but not beta-blockers. Beta-adrenergic receptor stimulation is associated with deactivation of the vomiting response.[10] Numerous other peptide hormones, listed in List 17-1, have been implicated in causing nausea and vomiting, but the search for a circulating "emetic" substance continues. A recently discovered hormone, peptide YY, has been isolated from animal ileum and is a very potent emetic in dogs and ferrets. However, most evidence indicates that nausea and vomiting in humans is influenced by numerous pathways, hormonal action being only one of them.[11]

H. The antiemetic center

Work in the cat has led to postulation of an antiemetic center. It has been noted that opiates at low doses may have antiemetic effects but at higher doses stimulate the CTZ. An antiemetic center with different types of opiate receptors from those of the CTZ could explain some of these bimodal results.[9,12]

List 17-1. Peptides Implicated in Causing Nausea and Vomiting

---

Norepinephrine
ACTH
Vasopressin
Human chorionic gonadotropin
Angiotensin II
Leu-enkephalin
Met-enkephalin
Cholecystokinin
Insulin
Gastrin
Oxytocin
Bombesin
Thyrotropin-releasing hormone
Peptide YY
Neurotensin
Vasoactive intestinal peptide

I. Physiologic complications of nausea and vomiting

There are several physiologic complications of nausea and vomiting that are of concern to the anesthetist. Significant complications include possible acid aspiration, visceral or wound dehiscence from the steep rise in intrathoracic and intra-abdominal pressure, and electrolyte disorders from prolonged vomiting.

1. Aspiration pneumonitis. In an unanesthetized patient, laryngeal reflexes accompany the vomiting reflex, preventing aspiration of gastric contents. If laryngeal reflexes are blunted, however, vomiting can result in regurgitated gastric contents entering the trachea with the attendant risk of aspiration pneumonitis.

2. Visceral and wound dehiscence. The act of vomiting causes a considerable increase in both intrathoracic and intra-abdominal pressure. If the pharyngeal sphincter is incompletely relaxed at this time, esophageal rupture can occur. Severe retching or vomiting also can lead to small esophageal tears, known as "Mallory-Weiss tears." In the postsurgical setting, the rise in intra-abdominal pressure can stress visceral

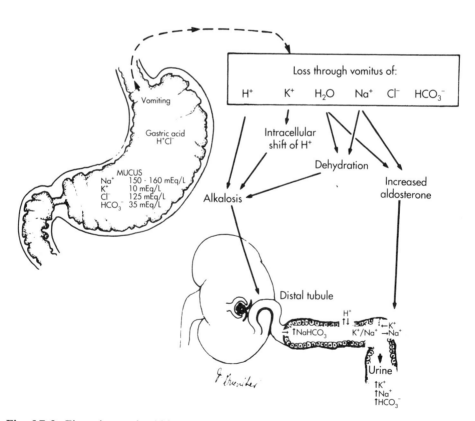

Fig. 17-3. Electrolyte and acid-base consequences of vomiting. Metabolic consequences of vomiting include loss of acid and water from the stomach, a contraction alkalosis and elevated aldosterone from dehydration, and a loss of potassium and bicarbonate through the kidneys in response to alkalosis and dehydration.

anastomoses as well as dehisce wound closures. There may also be an initiation of postsurgical bleeding secondary to raised intravascular pressures.

3. Electrolyte disorders. Severe, prolonged vomiting, such as that seen in children with pyloric stenosis, causes electrolyte depletion, dehydration, and gastric acid loss. The predominant resulting disorder is metabolic alkalosis (Fig. 17-3). Hypokalemia and hyponatremia can occur as well and are exacerbated by renal excretion of K^+ and Na^+ in an effort to conserve H^+.[6,13]

II. PREOPERATIVE STATES PREDISPOSING TO NAUSEA AND VOMITING

Hormonal or neural imbalances, central nervous system diseases, and gastrointestinal disturbances can lead to nausea and vomiting. These disorders, when present in the preoperative period, increase the likelihood of PNV. Specific conditions that make PNV more likely include diabetes mellitus, uremia, intracranial hypertension, pregnancy, motion sickness, and abdominal disorders. In addition, perioperative pain, certain medications, or even anxiety can increase the incidence of PNV. Factors such as female sex, young age, emergency operation, and obesity seem to predispose to PNV as well. In prepubital children, there is no difference in the incidence of PNV according to gender.[2,14]

A. Diabetes mellitus

Impaired gastric motility without anatomic obstruction can lead to nausea and vomiting. This commonly occurs in diabetics who have an autonomic neuropathy involving visceral as well as cardiac fibers. The visceral neuropathy can lead to delayed gastric emptying, early satiety, and nausea and vomiting, and it can predispose diabetic patients to aspiration after induction of anesthesia. Patients with diabetes mellitus respond well to administration of metoclopramide.

B. Uremia

No one completely understands how uremia causes nausea and vomiting, but it appears to act through the CTZ because ablation of this area eliminates uremic vomiting. Some have suggested that the inciting agent is the elevated level of vasopressin seen in uremic patients. Intravenous infusion of vasopressin in humans causes nausea and vomiting and increases the firing of neurons in the area postrema. Several other disorders of fluid balance, such as water intoxication, intracranial hypertension, and

acute severe hyponatremia, also elevate vasopressin levels. This may explain the high incidence of nausea and vomiting observed in these disorders.[11,15] Whether delayed gastric emptying occurs in uremia is controversial;[13,16] if present, it too could contribute to nausea.

C. Intracranial hypertension

The vomiting associated with raised intracranial pressure typically occurs in the morning, without preceding nausea, and can be projectile. It presumably results from direct pressure on the vomiting center but also may be related to high levels of vasopressin. One treats it by relieving the intracranial hypertension.

D. Pregnancy

Vomiting commonly occurs in the first 14 to 16 weeks of pregnancy; nausea occurs in 50% to 90% of pregnancies and vomiting in 25% to 55%.[13] Nausea and vomiting are more frequent in primigravidas, younger women, nonsmokers, the obese, and those with a prior history of nausea and vomiting. Nausea and vomiting have no known adverse effects on the fetus and, in fact, a lower rate of spontaneous abortion has been noted among women with nausea. Severe vomiting, known as "hyperemesis gravidarum," occurs in 3.5 of 1000 pregnancies and results in significant fluid and electrolyte losses requiring hospitalization. Some suspect a hormonal cause for the nausea of pregnancy and human chorionic gonadotropin (hCG) is often implicated. hCG is elevated not only in pregnancy, but also in the third to fourth week of the menstrual cycle, when a higher incidence of PNV has been observed.[17] Molar pregnancy and multiple gestations are also associated with nausea and elevated hCG. The low levels of hCG in patients over 70 years of age would be consistent with the minimal PNV observed in this age group. However, studies using radioimmunoassay techniques have failed to show any relationship between nausea and vomiting and hCG, LH, FSH, TSH, prolactin, and numerous other hormones.[11] The treatment of pregnancy-related nausea is usually supportive; however, metoclopramide (Reglan) and prochlorperazine have been used with success in severe cases.[18]

E. Abdominal disorders

Irritation or distension of viscera can lead to emesis; this is seen in multiple abdominal disorders including peritonitis, bowel or gastric outlet obstruction, and viral gastroenteritis. Distension of the ureter by renal calculi, testicular pain, or cervical dilatation will also induce nausea and vomiting. These stimuli are carried by splanchnic and vagal afferents to the area postrema and the vomiting center. Vagotomy eliminates vomiting caused by these stimuli; ablation of the area postrema does not.

F. Motion sickness

Motion sickness is caused by excitation of vestibular afferents by movement and is eliminated by destruction of the vestibular apparatus or the CTZ.[6] In humans, motion sickness causes a pronounced antidiuresis and the magnitude of vasopressin secretion is closely related to the degree of nausea and vomiting. However, emesis also occurs in patients with diabetes insipidus, making the significance of vasopressin questionable.[11] Opiates predispose humans to PNV by sensitizing the vestibular apparatus to movement. A history of motion sickness increases the likelihood of PNV, and the high incidence of motion sickness in children may contribute to their propensity for PNV. The timing of PNV indicates that the vestibular component may be significant; a great proportion occurs during transport out of the recovery room. PNV in ambulatory patients most often occurs on arising from the stretcher or during the ride home. Anticholinergics have been successful in treating motion sickness. Sensorial cells for motion are not cholinergic; therefore the anticholinergics must act at the level of the vestibular nucleus or the area postrema, which both contain cholinergic neurons. Histamine blockers are also useful in treating motion sickness through their effect on sensorial cells.[18]

G. Perioperative pain

Clinical studies show that pain is a stimulus to nausea and vomiting and that pain relief, regardless of analgesic used, can decrease nausea and vomiting. In a study of 104 postoperative patients, complete cessation of pain relieved nausea in 80% of episodes and only 10% of patients experienced nausea without pain.[19] Naloxone itself does not cause nausea, but nausea often accompanies the pain occurring after a naloxone overdose. Whether activation of the sympathetic nervous system plays a role in the nausea of pain is not known.

H. Medications

There are numerous pathways whereby medications may affect nausea and vomiting. List 17-2 lists medications commonly associated with nausea and vomiting. Two of the most notorious classes of medications encountered in preoperative patients are the opiates and the chemotherapeutic agents.

List 17-2. Some of the Drugs Causing Nausea and Vomiting

L-Dopa
Bromocryptine
Opiates
Chemotherapeutic agents
Cardiac glycosides
Alcohol
Nonsteroidal anti-inflammatory drugs
Antibiotics

I. Opioids

Many patients take opioids before surgery. Opioids can cause nausea and vomiting by stimulating the CTZ, by sensitizing the vestibular system, and by delaying gastric emptying. The CTZ has a high concentration of enkephalins and opiate receptors, and the opioids probably induce vomiting through stimulation of these receptors. This differs from the action of apomorphine, which acts through dopaminergic receptors in the CTZ. Pain relief and possible stimulation of an antiemetic center may moderate the nausea and vomiting response to opioids.

Opioid effects on the vestibular system are prominent in patients with PNV. In a study of 411 patients given morphine, the ambulatory group experienced significantly more nausea than the bedridden patients did. In almost every instance, one could relieve the nausea by lying down.[20] Other studies have corroborated the relationship of movement to opiate-induced nausea and vomiting; increasing dose is an additional risk factor.[21]

J. Chemotherapeutic agents

The most potent emetics encountered in the preoperative setting are chemotherapeutic agents, particularly cisplatin. Others are listed in Table 17-1. The frequency and severity of vomiting after chemotherapy have led to numerous trials of antiemetics, and the resulting data have been useful in designing treatments for PNV. Animal studies have shown that cisplatin produces vomiting through stimulation of the CTZ. Since ablation of the area postrema does not entirely eliminate drug-induced emesis, there also may be peripheral drug effects. Metabolic intermediates having indirect as well as direct effects on the CTZ and vomiting center could explain the delayed emetic response seen with some cytotoxic agents.

Table 17-1. Chemotherapeutic agents causing nausea and vomiting

Highly emetogenic	Moderately emetogenic
Cisplatin	L-Asparaginase
Dacarbazine	5-Azacytidine
Nitrogen mustard	Daunorubicin
Streptozotocin	Doxorubicin
Nitrosoureas	5-Fluorouracil
Actinomycin D	Hexamethylamine
Cyclophosphamide	Mitomycin C
Mithramycin	
Mitotane	
Procarbazine	

The incidence and severity of vomiting after chemotherapy are related to the particular agent used, the dose, and the rapidity of administration.[22] Additional risk factors are a propensity to develop motion sickness, female sex, and youth.

A well-described aspect of chemotherapy-induced emesis is "anticipatory nausea and vomiting," which can occur in up to 57% of patients.[23] It occurs more frequently with highly emetic agents, with unusual taste sensations during infusions, and with severe vomiting after initial therapy. Younger patients and those with a history of motion sickness are more susceptible. Psychologic studies cannot demonstrate a clear-cut relationship between anticipatory nausea and vomiting and the degree of anxiety; it is postulated to be a physiologic "pavlovian" response. Support for this hypothesis comes from evidence that reducing the severity of the initial nausea and vomiting, or reducing the perception of it, reduces anticipatory nausea. Benzodiazepines and behavioral therapy have some therapeutic effect on anticipatory nausea and vomiting; antiemetics have very little efficacy except in reducing the severity of the initial event.

Treatment of chemotherapy-induced emesis often requires much higher doses of antiemetics than those given for PNV. Dopamine receptor antagonists and 5-hydroxytryptamine-3 antagonists work well, but antihistamines are relatively unsuccessful.[22,24] It is possible that the high-dose antiemetic combination regimens used for chemotherapy might be helpful in the recovery room as well. The obvious disadvantage in the PNV context is that sedation may delay recovery and discharge. Further discussion on treatment is covered in the section on therapy for PNV.

K. Miscellaneous risk factors

Female sex, youth, obesity, type of surgery, and history of previous postanesthetic nausea and vomiting are risk factors for PNV. The highest incidence of PNV is in the newborn to 19-year-old age group, and it decreases with increasing age.[2,12,14,17,25,26] The reason for the predisposition in children is not readily explained but may be related to differences in vagal tone or vestibular afferents. In the general population there are people who will vomit at the slightest exposure to provocative stimuli. Although this may be psychosomatic, it is also possible that the vomiting reflex is variably developed. For example, dentists have observed significant differences among patients in their response to stimuli that can provoke a gag reflex. Even the skill of the anesthesiologist has been known to influence the incidence of vomiting.

III. ANESTHESIA AND ITS EFFECTS ON NAUSEA AND VOMITING
A. Premedication

Current anesthetic agents and techniques have helped eliminate the need for routine premedication. In addition, the high frequency of outpatient surgery has reduced opportunities for premedication. However, the goal of a relaxed but not overly sedated preoperative patient is still desirable. A wide variety of medications can be used toward this goal, but there remains a need for an informed preoperative discussion to alleviate patient anxiety. The prevention of acid aspiration is a new goal in premedication and is made possible by the wide availability of histamine-2 (H_2) receptor blockers and gastrokinetic agents. The effects of these drugs on the incidence of PNV is difficult to ascertain since few controlled studies are available.[12,27]

1. Barbiturates. Barbiturates have long been used as premedicants. The most commonly used, secobarbital and pentobarbital, are generally considered to have very little effect on PNV.

2. Tranquilizers. Proponents of tranquilizers as premedicants cite their sedative, antiemetic, and antihistaminic properties. Phenothiazine derivatives such as promethazine are considered to be good for sedation in addition to having antiemetic and antihistaminic capabilities. Hydroxyzine is considered to be an excellent anxiolytic and has antiemetic, bronchodilatory, anticholinergic, and antihistaminic effects. Droperidol, a butyrophenone, was commonly used as a premedicant when administered in a fixed combination with fentanyl as the drug Innovar. Although droperidol is an effective antiemetic, in larger dosages it is long acting, may produce dysphoria and extrapyramidal symptoms, and is a weak alpha-adrenergic receptor blocking agent.[2,17,21,28]

Diazepam, lorazepam, and midazolam, the commonly used benzodiazepines, have been very popular as premedicants because of their overall anxiolytic, sedative, and amnestic properties. They produce minimal cardovascular depression, have anticonvulsant activity, and do not contribute to PNV. Lorazepam is long acting, whereas midazolam has a rapid onset and quick recovery.

3. Opioids. The routine use of opioids as premedicants, despite the absence of preoperative pain, is based largely on tradition. Opioids are associated with a high incidence of nausea and vomiting. Other undesirable properties associated with opioid premedication include orthostatic hypotension, spasm of the sphincter of Oddi, bronchoconstriction, delayed gastric emptying, constipation, urinary retention, and respiratory depression. To minimize these, narcotics are often combined with other drugs such as scopolamine or droperidol.

4. Anticholinergics. Previously used anesthetics like diethyl ether provoked the production of copious secretions. Anticholinergics were used as premedicants to obviate this serious airway problem. With the newer anesthetic agents, secretion production is minimal. It was also believed that the anticholinergics were needed to suppress vagal reflexes related to the stimulation of the airway during instrumentation before endotracheal intubation. They are no longer used for this purpose, and at present they are primarily administered intravenously to prevent the oculocardiac reflex or before a second dose of succinylcholine in children. Hyoscine and atropine are believed to have antiemetic actions. Although these drugs may decrease gastric secretions and increase gastric pH, they may also produce unpleasant CNS effects such as hallucinations, restlessness, and delirium. Today the desirable gastrointestinal effect of scopolamine and atropine are better achieved with other agents. Glycopyrrolate is the preferred agent for drying of secretions, and because it is a quaternary ammonium, it does not cross the blood-brain barrier and has no CNS effects.

Pneumonitis aspiration of acidic particulate matter remains a concern in the perioperative period. Current practice is to minimize this risk by preoperative administration of antacids, H$_2$-receptor blockers, and drugs affecting gastric motility.[29]

5. Antacids. Particulate antacids, if aspirated, can cause pneumonitis. Most clinicians advocate the use of nonparticulate sodium citrate when the risk of aspiration is high and there is insufficient time for H$_2$-receptor blockers to take effect.

6. H$_2$-receptor blockers. It is common practice to use H$_2$-receptor antagonists (such as ranitidine or cimetidine) preoperatively when time permits and there is a risk of acid aspiration. These drugs may be used in combination with gastrokinetic agents or antacids. The H$_2$-receptor antagonists increase gastric pH by decreasing nocturnal and basal acid production, and they decrease gastric volume as well. Cimetidine has been shown to reduce gastric volume by two thirds of the control if given 1 hour before induction of anesthesia. Its side effects include confusion, restlessness, and hallucinations. It also prolongs the elimination half-life of diazepam, lidocaine, and propranolol. Ranitidine has a longer duration and fewer side effects than cimetidine. Patients treated with H$_2$-receptor antagonists have been found to have a greater variety of gastric bacteria because of the increase in gastric pH.[6,30,31]

7. Metoclopramide. Metoclopramide is a dopamine antagonist that increases the tone of the lower esophageal sphincter, improves gastric motility, and depresses the vomiting center. It has recently been shown to produce a dose-dependent, potent, noncompetitive inhibition of human plasma cholinesterase and acetylcholinesterase activities. Therefore patients receiving metoclopramide and succinylcholine should be "monitored carefully."[32]

Anticholinergics have been shown to reduce both volume and acidity of gastric contents. One study reported a 50% decrease in gastric residual with glycopyrrolate, but other studies have reached conflicting conclusions.[30]

B. General anesthesia

1. Nitrous oxide. The literature concerning the emetic effects of nitrous oxide (N$_2$O) contains controversial findings. Several properties of N$_2$O could contribute to PNV: sympathetic stimulation, opioid-like effects, and closed-space expansion.

Alpha-adrenergic receptor agonism has been shown to cause nausea and vomiting in animals, and the sympathomimetic effects of N$_2$O have been postulated to do the same. In a study of volunteers given N$_2$O at 1.5 atmospheres, all subjects developed signs of sympathetic stimulation and vomited.[33]

Changes in middle ear pressure and bowel gas volume can also cause nausea and vomiting. Studies by Eger have shown that 75% N$_2$O can increase the volume of bowel gas by 80% to

100% after 2 hours.[34] Since intestinal distension is a known stimulus to vomiting, this can contribute to PNV after long surgical procedures. Even 30 minutes of 80% N_2O can raise middle ear pressures to a range that causes emesis. On the other hand, during the recovery period from N_2O inhalation, middle ear pressures can reach negative values if the eustachian tube is not functioning. This irritates the vestibular system by producing traction on the round window and could lead to nausea and vomiting.[35,36]

There is evidence that N_2O reacts at the receptor level with the endogenous opioid system and that some of the analgesic effects of N_2O can be reversed by naloxone.[37] Such opioid properties could have emetic effects.

Clinical trials to ascertain the degree of emetic properties of N_2O have produced conflicting results. Some of the major trials that found N_2O to be an emetic were by Lonie and Harper, Melnick, and Alexander[38,39,40] Lonie and Harper compared the emetic effects of enflurane/O_2/N_2O and enflurane/O_2/air as anesthetics for laparoscopy. All patients received fentanyl as well. The incidence of nausea was similar between groups, but vomiting occurred 49% of the time in patients receiving N_2O versus only 17% of the time in those not given N_2O. Alexander did a similar study of anesthesia for laparoscopy comparing N_2O/O_2/fentanyl, isoflurane/O_2/fentanyl, and isoflurane/O_2. Alexander found that PNV occurred 61% of the time with N_2O and only 30% and 25% of time in the other groups respectively. Melnick compared isoflurane/O_2 with isoflurane/N_2O/O_2 for minor gynecologic procedures and did not use narcotics or neuromuscular reversal agents. PNV occurred in 25% of the N_2O group but in only 3.6% of the group with isoflurane alone. The recovery stay was noted to be longer in those patients with nausea and vomiting.

Several other studies, however, have found no evidence that N_2O contributes significantly to PNV.[3,41-43] Sengupta looked at enflurane/O_2/N_2O and enflurane/O_2 as anesthetics for laparoscopy. All patients received fentanyl and were mask ventilated. Sengupta noted a trend for greater emesis with N_2O but found no significant difference in PNV between groups or any difference in time to discharge or resumption of normal activity. Korttila compared isoflurane/O_2/N_2O and isoflurane/O_2/air as anesthetics for gynecologic operations. All patients received preoperative and intraoperative narcotics. PNV occurred in 62% to 67% of patients in both groups. Risk factors for nausea were

previous nausea with anesthesia or a history of motion sickness. Muir studied 780 patients and compared enflurane/O_2/N_2O, enflurane/O_2/air, isoflurane/O_2/N_2O, and isoflurane/O_2/air. All patients were given narcotics at the end of the operations, which did not include procedures known to predispose to PNV. There was no difference in PNV among groups either in the recovery room or at 24 hours postoperatively. Interestingly, there was a pronounced increase in PNV in all groups after the time of recovery room discharge, corroborating previous work that correlated PNV with movement. Hovorka also found no difference when comparing isoflurane/O_2/N_2O, enflurane/O_2/N_2O, and isoflurane/O_2/air for outpatient laparoscopy.

These conflicting results probably reflect differences in operation, patient selection, and concomitant intravenous anesthetics. It is therefore impossible to draw conclusions about the contribution of N_2O to PNV. However, the high incidence of PNV after gynecologic procedures like laparoscopy confirms the persistent inadequacy of current methods for controlling PNV.

2. Potent inhalation anesthetics. Historically the potent inhalation agents were notorious for prolonged emetic action. Beecher and Knapp in the 1950s reported a 78% incidence of PNV with ether anesthesia whereas contemporaneous reports noted a 40% incidence of PNV with nonether anesthesia. Chloroform and cyclopropane were similar to ether in producing vomiting.[1,14] The advent of halothane, enflurane, and isoflurane has reversed the notoriety of the potent agents, and, in fact, animal work indicates that halothane may have an antiemetic effect.[44] Most studies comparing the three newer agents have shown no difference between them in inducing PNV[42,43,45] and they seem to cause less PNV than anesthesia involving narcotics.[46,51]

3. Intravenous anesthetics. Intravenous anesthetic agents have variable emetic effects. PNV does not commonly occur after administration of ultrashort-acting barbiturates when used for induction or maintenance of anesthesia for brief, painless procedures. Of methohexital, thiamylal, and thiopental, the last is probably the most commonly used and least associated with PNV. Etomidate, another intravenous hypnotic agent, has been associated with PNV. In a comparison of etomidate/N_2O/O_2 with methohexital/N_2O/O_2 for anesthesia in unpremedicated women undergoing minor gynecologic procedures, etomidate was noted to cause more PNV in the first 6 postoperative hours. Ketamine may cause PNV more frequently than other intravenous anesthetic agents, though not to the extent that would require the routine preoperative administration of antiemetics.[52] When intravenous narcotics are used in large doses as the sole or major anesthetic agents, it is the clinical impression that postoperative emetic problems are very uncommon. It has been postulated that large doses of narcotics directly depress the vomiting center in the brain. Propofol, a new intravenous anesthetic, has been shown to have few emetic sequelae. It has been shown to reduce the emetic effect of opiate premedication in healthy patients undergoing minor gynecologic procedures.[53] One of the characteristics of neuroleptanalgesia, which combines an intravenously administered sedative with an analgesic, is a lower incidence of PNV.[54]

There is significant relationship between PNV and the antagonism of muscle relaxants by neostigmine and atropine. The incidence of vomiting was 47% in those patients in whom muscle relaxation was reversed versus only 11% in those in whom the neuromuscular block was allowed to wear off. All patients had joint replacement procedures, and determinations were made 24 hours postoperatively. It was concluded that the neostigmine, through an increase in gastrointestinal peristalsis and spasm, could contribute to PNV.[55] The addition of atropine or glycopyrrolate to neostigmine failed to reduce the incidence of PNV after administration of anesthesia using halothane and pancuronium.[56]

C. Regional anesthesia

1. Spinal anesthesia. The quoted incidence of emesis under spinal anesthesia ranges from 11% to 21%.[12] The postulated causes include an effect on the vomiting center through a reduction in cerebral blood flow or an increase in gastrointestinal peristalsis from preganglionic sympathetic blockade. Numerous studies have shown that hypotension is frequently the inciting episode for nausea.[12,57,58] Blood pressure may be maintained by preoperative infusion of 1 to 1.5 liters of crystalloid,[12,57,59] by ephedrine injection preoperatively, or by ephedrine infusion.[58]

Maintenance of blood pressure during conduction blockade does not assure eradication of PNV, and numerous medications have been tried as well. In women having spinal anesthesia for cesarean delivery, 2.5 mg of IV droperidol after the umbilical cord clamping decreased the incidence of nausea from 40% to 12%.[59] In contrast, neither 10 mg of IV metoclopramide nor 10 mg of IV domperidone lowered the in-

cidence of PNV compared to placebo when given before spinal anesthesia for orthopedic surgery.[60]

2. Epidural anesthesia. Nausea and vomiting associated with epidural anesthesia, like spinal anesthesia, seems to be related to hypotension and can be ameliorated by fluid and vasopressor infusion. In a study of patients undergoing lithotripsy, both spinal anesthesia and epidural anesthesia led to significantly less PNV than general anesthesia did (21% versus 27% versus 50%).[61]

Several recent studies have evaluated therapies for lowering the incidence of nausea and vomiting after administration of epidural narcotics.[62,63] Bromage reported a 60% incidence of nausea and a 50% incidence of vomiting after 10 mg of epidural morphine.[64] Stenseth studied 1085 patients receiving epidural morphine for postoperative pain relief, and PNV occurred in 34%. PNV was more frequent in women than in men; in men it occurred more often in those who had pain; and it often responded to treatment with metoclopramide or perphenazine. Naloxone relieved 90% of the pruritus associated with morphine but did not relieve the nausea and vomiting.[65] The ability of naloxone to reverse pruritus but not nausea and vomiting has also been noted with intrathecal narcotics.[62] In women receiving epidural morphine after umbilical cord clamping during cesarean delivery, Chestnut found that 0.15 mg/kg IV metoclopramide reduced both intraoperative and postoperative vomiting. Its efficacy was greatest in the 30-minute immediate postoperative period.[66] In a later study, Chestnut also noted that 0.5 mg of droperidol after umbilical cord clamping was as effective as 15 mg of metoclopramide in relieving PNV after epidural morphine and that both were more effective against vomiting than nausea.[67] In similar patients, transdermal scopolamine (TDS) reduced the incidence of PNV when compared with placebo.[63]

IV. TREATMENT OF NAUSEA AND VOMITING

Evaluating the literature on the treatment of PNV presents many difficulties. Reporting of PNV can be by oneself or by an observer; assessment scales of severity can be yes or no or can contain gradations of all kinds; duration may or may not be evaluated; retching may be scored as nausea, vomiting, or not at all. In addition, the definitions of indirect measures such as time to eating, to resumption of normal activities, or to recovery room discharge vary tremendously. The chemotherapeutic literature suggests that nausea and vomiting should be considered separately, that frequency, severity, and duration are separable phenomena, and that indirect measures of relief are very helpful.[68] The study of PNV presents additional problems in trial design; the multitude of factors contributing to PNV detracts from the significance of small trials. With these issues in mind, we review some of the general measures for treating or preventing PNV and then discuss in detail the antiemetics in common use.

A. General management of postoperative nausea and vomiting

Prevention of PNV is obviously desirable. Some have suggested that opioids be avoided as premedicants, but many believe that the beneficial effects of opioids outweigh any increase in PNV. Improved gastric emptying by metoclopramide may be useful in preventing PNV in the "full-stomach" patient, and minimizing positive pressure mask ventilation should diminish the likelihood of PNV from gastric distension. Avoidance of pharyngeal irritation during emergence from anesthesia, minimizing movement in the recovery period, and relieving postoperative pain should also lower the incidence of PNV. Whether routine prophylaxis with antiemetics is warranted depends on the risk of PNV for each specific individual and operation and on the efficacy, sedative properties, and other side effects of the antiemetic chosen. The routine suctioning of the stomach before extubation is advocated as a practical method of reducing emetic events in the postoperative period.

The antiemetic medications fall into several broad categories: anticholinergics, phenothi-

Table 17-2. Antiemetics for prevention and treatment of postoperative nausea and vomiting (PNV)

Drug		Initial average adult dose
ANTICHOLINERGICS	Atropine	0.4-0.6 mg IM
	Scopolamine	0.3-0.6 mg IM
		2.0 mg PO or transdermal patch
PHENOTHIAZINES	Chlorpromazine	25-50 mg IM
		10-50 mg PO
	Promethazine	12.5-50 mg IM/IV
(Piperazine ring at position 10:)	Perphenazine	2.5-5 mg IM
		2-4 mg PO
	Prochlorperazine	5-20 mg IM/PO
ANTIHISTAMINES	Promethazine	12.5-50 mg IM/IV
Piperazines	Cyclizine	25-50 mg IM/IV/PO
Ethanolamines	Diphenhydramine	25-50 mg IM/IV/PO
	Diphenhydrinate	25-50 mg IM/IV/PO
BUTYROPHENONES	Haloperidol	0.5-4 mg IM/IV
	Droperidol	0.005-0.175 mg/kg IV
		0.25-7.5 mg IV/IM
DOPAMINE ANTAGONISTS	Metoclopramide	10-20 mg PO/IV
		0.15-3 mg/kg PO/IV*
	Domperidone	4-15 mg IV/IM
DRUGS FOR ACID PROPHYLAXIS		
H$_2$-receptor blockers	Cimetidine	300-800 mg PO
		300 mg IV
	Ranitidine	150-300 mg PO
		50 mg IV
	Famotidine	20-40 mg PO
Nonparticulate antacids	Sodium citrate	30-60 cc PO

IM, Intramuscular; *IV,* intravenous; *PO,* per ōs, by mouth.
*High doses used for chemotherapy emesis.

azines, antihistamines, butyrophenones, dopamine antagonists, cannabinoids, and serotonin antagonists. The drugs in these categories and their commonly employed doses are listed in Table 17-2.

B. Anticholinergics

Seasickness of service personnel during World War II was the major impetus for the development of anticholinergic agents for treating and preventing emesis from this cause. For centuries, anticholinergics had been used in the form of crude extracts of hyoscyamus and belladonna. Their CNS rather than antivagal actions appear to be essential in preventing emesis. The two drugs used today are atropine (hyoscyamine) and scopolamine HBr (hyoscine HBr); glycopyrrolate has no antiemetic effect. Hyoscine is reportedly a more effective antiemetic and has more sedative properties than atropine. The anticholinergics are most efficacious in treating motion sickness; they are also used as premedicants in combination with narcotics to reduce PNV.[21] Several recent studies have evaluated the efficacy of scopolamine in preventing PNV. In one, 190 patients for minor surgery had less PNV with transdermal scopolamine (TDS) than with placebo; 31% of patients were nevertheless nauseated despite TDS.[69] A study of gynecologic patients given prophylactic TDS revealed it to be better than placebo in preventing PNV, despite a 68% incidence of PNV with the drug.[70] A comparison of TDS versus 1.25 mg of droperidol versus placebo showed both drugs to be only slightly more effective than placebo and droperidol caused more sedation than TDS.[71] A similar comparison of droperidol 7.5 mg and TDS in cholecystectomy patients revealed vomiting in 25% of the droperidol group and in 50% of the TDS group.[72] In a study of 283 female surgical patients, no advantage was seen with TDS[73] but it has been shown to reduce PNV after epidural narcotics.[63]

C. Phenothiazines

The phenothiazines are predominantly dopamine antagonists with some antihistaminergic and anticholinergic properties. They are used as major tranquilizers and sedatives and are particularly effective against drugs acting on the CTZ such as opioids. Phenothiazines in larger doses may suppress the vomiting center; they are not first-line agents for motion sickness. Substitution of a piperazine ring at position 10 on the tricyclic nucleus results in compounds that produce less sedation and have greater antiemetic activity. The two most commonly used piperazines are prochlorperazine (Compazine) and perphenazine (Fentazin); they are equally effective against vomiting, but perphenazine causes more sedation. A dose of 10 mg IM of prochlorperazine has an onset time of 30 to 60 minutes and lasts 4 hours. Administration of 2.5 to 5 mg IM or 2 to 4 mg PO of perphenazine is effective against emesis but can cause restlessness.[6] All the phenothiazine-related compounds, particularly the piperazine-substituted ones, can cause restlessness, dystonia, pseudoparkinsonism, and tardive dyskinesia. These symptoms, curiously enough, can usually be eliminated by promethazine, another phenothiazine, in a dose of 12.5 mg IV.

D. Antihistamines

The main action of the antihistamines is on the vomiting center and vestibular pathways, and these drugs are therefore useful in treating motion sickness. Except for promethazine, antihistamines have very little activity on the CTZ. The piperazines and the ethanolamines have antihistaminic properties. The ethanolamines include diphenhydramine (Benadryl) and dimenhydrinate (Dramamine); they are less effective than scopolamine in relieving motion sickness. The most effective of the piperazines is cyclizine, used for motion sickness and with opiates to prevent PNV. In a dose of 50 mg IM it was found to be more effective than 2.5 mg IM of perphenazine in reducing PNV.[74] It frequently causes sedation and dryness of the mouth but extrapyramidal effects are rare.

E. Butyrophenones

The butyrophenones are potent antiemetics and have alpha-blocking activity, extrapyramidal side effects, and sedative properties as well. The two drugs commonly used are haloperidol (Haldol) and droperidol. They are very similar; droperidol lasts longer when given intramuscularly though its half-life is shorter. Haloperidol causes less restlessness and sedation than prochlorperazine and, in doses of 0.15 to 4 mg IM preoperatively, is an effective antiemetic without noticeable effects on emergence.[27] It is also useful in treating established PNV.[75] Most of the clinical anesthesia studies involve droperidol because of its efficacy and long duration of action. Numerous trials have shown it to be superior to placebo in preventing PNV.[4,76-82] A recent study by Melnick, however, showed no advantage to 1.25 mg of droperidol in reducing PNV in ambulatory patients and found that its side effects were troublesome to patients after discharge.[28]

Many studies have sought to determine the

optimal dosing of droperidol for reducing PNV while minimizing droperidol's adverse side effects. In a study of dental outpatients, 0.25 mg of droperidol was more effective than 1.25 mg in reducing nausea and led to faster recovery times.[79] Another study found no difference in PNV using 2.5 mg of IM droperidol preoperatively versus 1.25 mg of IV droperidol postoperatively.[77] Outpatients having voluntary interruption of pregnancy had a similar incidence of PNV with 0.25 versus 0.5 mg of droperidol;[81] but for patients undergoing laparoscopy, 0.01 mg/kg was more effective than 0.005 mg/kg.[83] Dosing in children is somewhat different, and higher doses may be required for efficacy. In one trial of a group of children having strabismus surgery, m 0.05 mg/kg of droperidol did not decrease the high incidence of PNV.[84] Yet in similar patients a higher dose of 0.075 mg/kg was effetive in reducing PNV from 85% to 43%.[4]

Comparisons of droperidol and other antiemetics in perioperative patients have, in the limited studies available, found it to be as efficacious as or better than other agents. A dose of 0.5 mg of droperidol was equivalent to 15 mg of metoclopramide in reducing PNV in cesarean delivery patients.[67] A dose of 7.5 mg of droperidol was superior to TDS in preventing PNV in cholecystectomy patients.[72] In female orthopedic patients, 1.25 mg of IV droperidol lowered the incidence of PNV when compared with metoclopramide 20 mg IV.[76] Likewise, droperidol 2.5 mg was superior to both domperidone 20 mg and metoclopramide 10 mg in reducing PNV in gynecologic patients.[85]

The combination of droperidol with metoclopramide has been shown to be more efficacious than droperidol alone in outpatients, and the lower incidence of PNV greatly decreased recovery times.[86]

F. Dopamine antagonists

Metoclopramide, a procainamide derivative selective for dopamine-2 (D_2) receptors, and domperidone, a benzimidazole derivative with similar peripheral actions, are both effective antiemetics. Metoclopramide inhibits both the CTZ and the vomiting center through its antagonism of central D_2 receptors, and in higher doses it has antiserotoninergic activity. It inhibits the vestibular nucleus and may have an antivertigo action. Its peripheral actions are cholinomimetic effects on the gastrointestinal tract, mediated by blockade of inhibitory dopaminergic neurons. This results in increased tone of the lower esophageal sphincter, improved gastric emptying, and heightened intestinal peristalsis. Domperidone has similar actions peripherally but does not cross the blood-brain barrier. This does not exclude an action on the CTZ that is outside this barrier. Neither metoclopramide nor domperidone has antihistamine activity, and their sedative properties are not prominent. Metoclopramide can cause restlessness and occasional extrapyramidal reactions. The dystonic-dyskinetic reactions are most common in younger female patients and can be treated with benztropine, diphenhydramine, or diazepam. Older patients are more likely to develop parkinsonian side effects.[18]

Studies on the prophylactic efficacy of metoclopramide have shown mixed results. In female outpatients, premedication with oral metoclopramide reduced PNV,[87] and in orthopedic patients 20 mg IV was better than placebo but inferior to droperidol in reducing PNV.[76] Other studies have shown no reduction in PNV when metoclopramide was given as a premedicant.[88] In children having strabismus surgery, 0.15 mg/kg of metoclopramide reduced PNV, improved time to recovery, and produced no adverse side effects.[89]

In treating the emesis from cancer chemotherapy, doses of 1 to 3 mg/kg metoclopramide have been very effective, particularly in the treatment of cisplatin vomiting.[90] Treatment is more effective if initiated before nausea and vomiting begin, and side effects are ameliorated by the routine use of diphenhydramine prophylactically.[24,91,92] Combinations of metoclopramide with steroids or droperidol, or both, have been more effective than single-drug therapy.[90]

Studies using domperidone for PNV prophylaxis have shown mixed results; it appears to be better as treatment than as prevention. For established vomiting, a dose of 4 to 10 mg IV is effective and lasts for 2 to 4 hours.

G. Cannabinoids

Reports of reduced nausea and vomiting in young cancer patients smoking marijuana at the Sidney Farber Institute led to studies on the antiemetic efficacy of the cannabinoids. They do not inhibit dopamine, histamine, or cholinergic receptors and may act on opioid receptors in the forebrain or medullary reticular formation to inhibit the vomiting center.[9] The high incidence of dysphoric side effects limits widespread cannabinoid use.

H. Steroids

High-dose steroids, especially with metoclopramide, have been useful in treating the emesis associated with cancer chemotherapy. There is no experience, with their use in the perioperative setting.

I. Acupuncture

The application of low-frequency (10 Hz) electrical current for 5 minutes to an acupuncture point, P6 *(neiguan),* was found to be as effective as manual needling in the reduction of emetic sequelae in minor gynecologic operations. Both acupuncture techniques were slightly better, though not statistically, than the antiemetic effects of 50 mg of cyclizine.[93]

J. Serotonin antagonists

Our understanding of the emetic response has been broadened by the knowledge of the presence of serotonin receptors in the gastrointestinal tract and the area postrema. These receptors may be the principal mediators in an emetic reflex. Serotonin antagonists have recently been shown to be effective in the treatment of chemotherapy-induced vomiting.[94] Studies comparing the 5-hydroxytryptamine-3 antagonist ondansetron (GR 38032F) with high-dose metoclopramide in the control of cisplatin-induced vomiting have shown ondansetron to be more effective. This indicates that serotonin may be an important mediator of emesis related to cisplatin treatment.[95] It is postulated that high doses of metoclopramide may prevent emesis by blocking serotonin receptors. Published clinical trials to date have been limited to chemotherapy-induced nausea, and the effect of serotonin blockade on PNV has yet to be shown.[9]

V. SUMMARY

For physicians, anesthesia and surgery present numerous difficulties and require extensive expertise and vigilance. However, for patients these demands go unperceived, and PNV may be the most negative aspect of anesthesia. Despite greater understanding of the physiology of nausea and vomiting and despite the plethora of antiemetic medications, certain operations and risk factors are associated with an unacceptably high incidence of PNV. Therefore work must still be done in many areas to eliminate this major perioperative problem.

ACKNOWLEDGMENT

The authors wish to acknowledge Ms. Sandy Fricker for her help in the preparation of this chapter. No request was denied, and deadlines were always met with enthusiasm and professionalism. Thank you.

REFERENCES

1. Knapp MR and Beecher HK: Post-anesthetic nausea, vomiting and retching, JAMA 160(5):376-385, 1956.
2. Burtles R and Peckett BW: Postoperative vomiting, Br J Anaesth 29:114-123, 1957.
3. Sengupta P and Plantevin OM: Nitrous oxide and day-case laparoscopy: effects on nausea, vomiting and return to normal activity, Br J Anaesth 60:570-573, 1988.
4. Abramowitz MB et al: The antiemetic effect of droperidol following outpatient strabismus surgery in children, Anesthesiology 59(6):579-583, 1983.
5. Borison HL, Borison R, and McCarthy LE: Phylogenic and neurologic aspects of the vomiting process, J Clin Pharmacol 21:23S-29S, 1981.
6. Clarke RSJ: Nausea and vomiting, Br J Anaesth 56:19-27, 1984.
7. Lang, IM: Digestive tract motor correlates of vomiting and nausea, Can J Physiol Pharmacol 68:242-253, 1990.
8. Borison HL and Wang SC: Physiology and pharmacology of vomiting, Pharmacol Rev 5:193-230, 1953.
9. Edwards CM: Chemotherapy induced emesis—mechanisms and treatment: a review, J R Soc Med 81:658-662, 1988.
10. Jenkins LC and Lahay D: Central mechanisms of vomiting related to catecholamine response: anaesthetic implication, Can Anaesth Soc J 18(4):434-441, 1971.
11. Kucharczyk J and Harding RK: Regulatory peptides and the onset of nausea and vomiting, Can J Physiol Pharmacol 68:289-293, 1990.
12. Palazzo MGA and Strunin L: Anaesthesia and emesis. I: Etiology, Can Anaesth Soc J 31(2):178-187, 1984.
13. Feldman M: Nausea and vomiting. In Sleisinger MH and Ford JS, editors: Gastrointestinal disease, ed 4, Philadelphia, 1989, WB Saunders, vol 1, pp 222-237.
14. Purkis IE: Factors that influence postoperative vomiting, Can Anaesth Soc J 11(4):335-353, 1964.
15. Arieff AI: Effects of water, electrolyte and acid-base disorders on the central nervous system. In Arieff AI and DeFronzo RA, editors: Fluid, electrolyte and acid-base disorders, New York & London, 1985, Churchill Livingstone.
16. McCallum RW: What is the role of gastric emptying tests in a patient with nausea and vomiting? Am J Gastroenterol 83(8):803-805, 1988.
17. Bellville JW et al: Postoperative nausea and vomiting. IV: Factors related to postoperative nausea and vomiting, Anesthesiology 21(2):186-193, 1960.
18. Marin J, Ibañez MC, and Arribas S: Therapeutic management of nausea and vomiting, Gen Pharmacol 21(1):1-10, 1990.
19. Andersen R and Krohg K: Pain as a major cause of postoperative nausea, Can Anaesth Soc J 23(4):366-369, 1976.
20. Comroe JH and Dripps RD: Reactions to morphine in ambulatory and bed patients, Surg Gynecol Obstet 87:221-224, 1948.
21. Riding JE: Post-operative vomiting, Proc R Soc Med 53:671-675, 1960.
22. Stewart DJ: Cancer therapy, vomiting, and antiemetics, Can J Physiol Pharmacol 68:304-313, 1990.
23. Jacobsen PB and Redd WH: The development and management of chemotherapy related anticipatory nausea and vomiting, Cancer Invest 6(3):329-336, 1988.
24. Sanger GJ: New antiemetic drugs, Can J Physiol Pharmacol 68:314-324, 1990.
25. McKenzie SA and Halavan J: An investigation into post-anesthesia nausea and vomiting in a community hospital–based anesthesiology practice, J Am Assoc Nurse Anesthetists 55(5):427-433, Park Ridge, Ill, 1987.
26. Cote CJ: NPO after midnight for children—a reappraisal, Anesthesiology 72:589-592, 1990.

27. Palazzo MGA and Strunin L: Anaesthesia and emesis. II: Prevention and management, Can Anaesth Soc J 31(4):407-415, 1984.

28. Melnick B et al: Delayed side effects of droperidol after ambulatory general anesthesia, Anesth Analg 69:748-751, 1989.

29. Olsson GL, Hallen B, and Hambraeus-Jonzon K: Aspiration during anaesthesia: a computer-aided study of 185,358 anaesthetics, Acta Anaesthesiol Scand 30:84-92, 1986.

30. Laws H et al: Effects of preoperative medication on gastric pH, volume, and flora, Ann Surg 203(6):614-619, 1986.

31. Alpert CC, Baker JD, et al: A rational approach to anesthetic premedication, Drugs 37:219-228, 1989.

32. Kao YJ, Tellez J, and Turner DR: Dose-dependent effect of metoclopramide on cholinesterases and suxamethonium metabolism, Br J Anaesth 65:220-224, 1990.

33. Hornbein TF et al: The minimum alveolar concentration of nitrous oxide in man, Anesth Analg 61:553-556, 1982.

34. Eger EI and Saidman LJ: Hazards of nitrous oxide anesthesia in bowel obstruction and pneumothorax, Anesthesiology 26(1):61-66, 1965.

35. Perreault L et al: Middle ear pressure variations during nitrous oxide and oxygen anaesthesia, Can Anaesth Soc J 29(5):428-434, 1982.

36. Thomsen KA, Terkildsen K, and Arnfred, I: Middle ear pressure variations during anesthesia, Arch Otolaryngol 82:609-611, 1965.

37. Yang JC, Clark WC, and Ngai SH: Antagonism of nitrous oxide analgesia by naloxone in man, Anesthesiology 52:414-417, 1980.

38. Lonie DS and Harper JN: Nitrous oxide anaesthesia and vomiting, Anaesth 41:703-7, 1986.

39. Melnick BM, Johnson LS: Effects of eliminating nitrous oxide in outpatient anesthesia, Anesthesiology 67:982-4, 1987.

40. Alexander GD, Shupski JN, and Brown EM: The role of nitrous oxide in postoperative nausea and vomiting, Anesth Analg 63:175, 1985.

41. Korttila K, Hovorka J, and Erkola O: Nitrous oxide does not increase the incidence of nausea and vomiting after isoflurane anaesthesia, Anesth Analg 66:761-765, 1987.

42. Muir JJ et al: Role of nitrous oxide and other factors in postoperative nausea and vomiting: a randomized and blinded prospective study, Anesthesiology 66:513-518, 1987.

43. Hovorka J, Korttila K, and Erkola, O: Nitrous oxide does not increase nausea and vomiting following gynaecological laparoscopy, Can J Anaesth 36(2):145-148, 1989.

44. Zunini GS, Roth SH, and Lucier GE: The inhibitory effect of halothane on the emetic response in the ferret, Physiol Pharmacol 68(3):374-378, 1990.

45. Fisher DM et al: Comparison of enflurane, halothane, and isoflurane for diagnostic and therapeutic procedures in children with malignancies, Anesthesiology 63(6):647-650, 1985.

46. Rising S, Dodgson MS, and Steen PA: Isoflurane vs fentanyl for outpatient laparoscopy, Acta Anaesthesiol Scand 29(3):251-255, 1985.

47. Guggenberger H et al: Complaints in the postoperative phase related to anesthetics, Anaesthesist 37(12):746-751, 1988.

48. Zuurmond WW and VanLeeuwen L: Recovery from sufentanil anaesthesia for outpatient arthroscopy: a comparison with isoflurane, Acta Anaesthesiol Scand 31(2):154-156, 1987.

49. Zuurmond WW and Van Leeuwen L: Alfentanil v.

50. isoflurane for outpatient arthroscopy, Acta Anaesthesiol Scand 30(4):329-331, 1986.

50. Collins KM et al: Outpatient termination of pregnancy: halothane or alfentanil-supplemented anaesthesia, Br J Anaesth 57(12):1226-1231, 1985.

51. Metter SE et al: Nausea and vomiting after outpatient laparoscopy: incidence, impact on recovery room stay and cost, Anesth Analg 66:S116, 1987.

52. Dundee JW: Intravenous anaesthetic agents. Vol. 1. Current topics in anaesthesia, London, 1979, Edward Arnold (Publishers) Ltd.

53. Mulligan KR, McCollum JSC, and Dundee JW: An investigation into the antiemetic effect of propofol, Br J Clin Pharmacol 23:608-609, 1987.

54. Holderness MC, Chase PE, and Dripps RD: A narcotic analgesic and a butyrophenone with nitrous oxide for general anesthesia, Anesthesiology 24(3):336-340, 1963.

55. King MJ et al: Influence of neostigmine on postoperative vomiting, Br J Anaesth 61:403-406, 1988.

56. Takkunen O, Salmenpera M, and Heinonen J: Atropine vs. glycopyrrolate during reversal of pancuronium block in patients anaesthetized with halothane, Acta Anaesthesiol Scand 28:377-380, 1984.

57. Wollman SB and Marx GF: Acute hydration for prevention of hypotension of spinal anesthesia in parturients, Anesthesiology 29(2):374-380, 1968.

58. Kang YG, Abouleish E, and Cartis S: Prophylactic intravenous ephedrine infusion during spinal anesthesia for cesarean section, Anesth Analg 61(10):839-842, 1982.

59. Santos A and Datta S: Prophylactic use of droperidol for control of nausea and vomiting during spinal anesthesia for cesarean section, Anesth Analg 63a:85-87, 1984.

60. Spelina KR, Gerber HR, and Pagels IL: Nausea and vomiting during spinal anesthesia, Anaesthesia 39:132-137, 1984.

61. Rickford JK et al: Comparative evaluation of general, epidural, and spinal anaesthesia for extracorporeal shockwave lithotripsy, Ann R Coll Surg Engl 70(2):69-73, 1988.

62. Dailey PA et al: The effects of naloxone associated with the intrathecal use of morphine in labor, Anesth Analg 64:658-666, 1985.

63. Kotelko DM et al: Transdermal scopolamine decreases nausea and vomiting following cesarean section in patients receiving epidural morphine, Anesthesiology 71:675-678, 1989.

64. Bromage PR et al: Nonrespiratory side effects with epidural morphine, Anesth Analg 61:490-495, 1982.

65. Stenseth R, Sellevold O, and Breivik H: Epidural morphine for postoperative pain: experience with 1085 patients, Acta Anaesthesiol Scand 29:148-156, 1985.

66. Chestnut DH et al: Administration of metoclopramide for prevention of nausea and vomiting during epidural anesthesia for elective cesarean section, Anesthesiology 66(4):563-566, 1987.

67. Chestnut DH et al: Metoclopramide versus droperidol for prevention of nausea and vomiting during epidural anesthesia for cesarean section, South Med J 82(10):1224-1227, 1989.

68. Morrow GR: The assessment of nausea and vomiting, Cancer Suppl 53(10):2267-2278, 1984.

69. Wilkinson AR et al: Preoperative transdermal hyoscine for the prevention of postoperative nausea and vomiting, Anaesth Intensive Care 17(3):285-289, 1989.

70. Uppington J, Dunnet J, and Blogg CE: Transdermal hyoscine and postoperative nausea and vomiting, Anaesthesia 41:16-20, 1986.

71. Tigerstedt I, Salmela L, and Aromaa U: Double blind

comparison of transdermal scopolamine, droperidol and placebo against postoperative nausea and vomiting, Acta Anaesthesiol Scand 32:454-457, 1988.

72. Schuh R, Tolksdorf W, and Hucke H: Transdermal scopolamine or droperidol for prevention of postoperative nausea and vomiting in cholecystectomy patients, Anästh Intensivther Notfallmed 22(6):261-266, 1987.

73. Koski EM et al: Double blind comparison of transdermal hyoscine and placebo for the prevention of postoperative nausea, Br J Anaesth 64(1):16-20, 1990.

74. Chestnutt WN and Dundee JW: The influence of cyclizine and perphenazine on the emetic effect of meptazinol, Eur J Anaesthesiol 3(1):27-32, 1986.

75. Barton MD, Libonati M, and Cohen PJ: The use of haloperidol for treatment of postoperative nausea and vomiting: a double blind placebo-controlled trial, Anesthesiology 42(4):508-512, 1975.

76. Kauste A et al: Droperidol, alizapride and metoclopramide in the prevention and treatment of post-operative emetic sequelae, Eur J Anaesthesiol 3(1):1-9, 1986.

77. Korttila K et al: Droperidol prevents and treats nausea and vomiting after enflurane anaesthesia, Eur J Anaesthesiol 2(4):379-385, 1985.

78. Valanne J and Korttila K: Effect of a small dose of droperidol on nausea, vomiting and recovery after outpatient enflurane anaesthesia, Acta Anaesthesiol Scand 29(4):359-362, 1985.

79. O'Donovan N and Shaw J: Nausea and vomiting in day-case dental anaesthesia: the use of low-dose droperidol, Anaesthesia 39(12):1172-1176, 1984.

80. Winning TJ, Brock-Utne JG, and Downing JW: Nausea and vomiting after anesthesia and minor surgery, Anesth Analg 56:674-677, 1977.

81. Millar JM and Hall PJ: Nausea and vomiting after prostaglandins in day-case termination of pregnancy: the efficacy of low-dose droperidol, Anaesthesia 42(6):613-618, 1987.

82. Trapp LD: An evaluation of droperidol for preventing nausea and vomiting after deep intravenous sedation for ambulatory dental surgery, Anesth Prog 36(1):9-12, 1989.

83. Tripple GE, Holland MS, and Hassanein K: Comparison of droperidol 0.01 mg/kg and 0.005 mg/kg as a premedication in the prevention of nausea and vomiting in the outpatient for laparoscopy, J Am Assoc Nurse Anesthesiologists 57(5):413-416, Park Ridge, Ill, 1989.

84. Hardy JF et al: Nausea and vomiting after strabismus surgery in preschool children, Can Anaesth Soc J 33(1):57-62, 1986.

85. Madej TH and Simpson KH: Comparison of the use of domperidone, droperidol and metoclopramide in the prevention of nausea and vomiting following gynaecological surgery in day cases, Br J Anaesth 58(8):879-883, 1986.

86. Doze VA, Shafer A, and White PF: Nausea and vomiting after outpatient anesthesia: effectiveness of droperidol alone and in combination with metoclopramide, Anesth Analg 66:S41, 1987.

87. Miller CD and Anderson WG: Silent regurgitation in day case gynaecological patients, Anaesthesia 43(4):321-323, 1988.

88. Pandit SK et al: Premedication with cimetidine and metoclopramide, Anaesthesia 41:486-492, 1986.

89. Broadman LM et al: Metoclopramide reduces the incidence of vomiting following strabismus surgery in children, Anesthesiology 72:245-248, 1990.

90. Gralla RJ et al: The management of chemotherapy induced nausea and vomiting, Med Clin North Am 71(2):289-301, 1987.

91. Triozzi PL and Laszlo J: Optimum management of nausea and vomiting in cancer chemotherapy, Drugs 34:136-149, 1987.

92. Jacobsen PB and Redd WH: The development and management of chemotherapy related anticipatory nausea and vomiting, Cancer Invest 6(3):329-336, 1988.

93. Ghaly RG, Fitzpatrick KTJ, and Dundee JW: Antiemetic studies with traditional Chinese acupuncture, Anaesthesia 42:1108-1110, 1987.

94. Grunberg SM: Making chemotherapy easier, N Engl J Med 322:846-848, 1990.

95. Marty M, Pouillart P, Scholl S, et al: Comparison of the 5-hydroxytryptamine$_3$ (serotonin) antagonist ondansetron (GR 38032F) with high-dose metoclopramide in the control of cisplatin-induced emesis, N Engl J Med 322(12):816-821, comment 846-846, 1990.

Chapter 18

Liver Complications After Anesthesia

James D. Pearson
Simon Gelman

The differential diagnosis of postoperative hepatic dysfunction can be very difficult. The cause may become evident only after meticulous attention to small, sometimes seemingly unimportant details related to medical history, physical examination, laboratory tests, and environmental exposure. The surgical procedure itself as well as the stress of operation can affect hepatic function often to a greater extent than any one anesthetic technique or intraoperative event. When a patient develops postoperative hepatic dysfunction, the process may have begun before the patient ever presented for care but does not manifest itself until after the operation. It is important therefore to know and understand the many causes of postoperative hepatic dysfunction, criteria for diagnosis, prognosis, and how to distinguish preoperatively those patients at risk for such complication. The proper anesthetic can then be administered to minimize the impact of perioperative events on hepatic function.

I. INHALATIONAL ANESTHETICS
A. Halothane—mild injury

Anesthetic-induced hepatotoxicity is caused by either direct drug injury (chloroform, maybe halothane), an allergic response (halothane), or tissue hypoxia (all anesthetics). Life-threatening halothane-induced hepatotoxicity is rare, and the incidence of complete, sometimes lethal, halothane-induced hepatic necrosis is approximately 1 in 30,000 anesthetics.[1] More commonly, halothane causes mild postoperative changes in liver function.

Twenty-five percent of patients exposed to halothane may have a mild, postoperative increase in serum aminotransferase concentration.[2] These abnormalities of liver function may persist for as long as 2 weeks after anesthesia.[3-6] Although a change in serum aminotransferase activity is regarded as a sensitive measure of acute hepatic damage, an increased aminotransferase concentration is not specific to the liver because these enzymes are released from other tissues and plasma changes correlate poorly with hepatic histologic features.[7] Another liver enzyme, glutathione S-transferase (GST), has been measured after halothane or isoflurane anesthesia for urologic procedures.[8] Postoperative GST concentrations, which are a more sensitive measure of acute hepatic damage than aminotransferase activity, were abnormal 3 to 6 hours after surgery in one third of patients who received halothane in a mixture of 30% oxygen and 70% nitrous oxide and one fourth of the patients who received halothane in 100% oxygen. Patients who received isoflurane in a mixture of 30% oxygen and 70% nitrous oxide showed no significant increase in GST. No patients exhibited signs of hepatic dysfunction postoperatively, and there were no significant increases in aspartate aminotransferase (AST, SGOT), alanine aminotransferase (ALT, SGPT), alkaline phosphatase, or bilirubin concentrations. GST concentrations not only increased within 3 hours after operation, but also had another increase at 24 hours. The first increase is probably best explained by hepatic hypoxia attributable to the direct effect of halothane on hepatic blood flow, whereas the second increase possibly is a result of the production of toxic metabolites from halothane. In contrast to the periportal location of the aminotransferase enzymes, GST is primarily located in the centrilobular hepatocytes. Halothane hepatitis and other types of severe hepatic damage are morphologically associated with centrilobular necrosis; therefore the measurement of serum GST concentrations may be a more sensitive and specific test for anesthetic-induced hepatic dysfunction. This study implies that even a single halothane anesthetic for relatively minor surgery can produce hepatic damage, though transient.

Halothane causes minor changes in hepatic function in 25% of patients , though the majority of patients, even those with preexisting liver disease, may undergo repeated halothane anesthetics with little derangement in hepatic function. Twenty-five children who were anesthetized at least 10 times in 1 year with halothane were prospectively examined for postoperative changes in liver function, specifically aspartate aminotransferase (AST), alanine aminotransferase (ALT), gamma-glutamyl transferase (GGT), and alkaline phosphatase (AP). Postoperatively, serum AST concentrations were increased in 10.6% of patients and ALT concentrations in 4.7% of patients. Of children who received a repeat halothane anesthetic at intervals of less than 28 days, 2.7% had increases in postoperative GGT concentrations.

Preoperative liver enzyme induction with phenobarbital does influence the effect of halothane on postoperative liver function. Japanese investigators demonstrated a higher incidence of halothane-induced liver injury (7 of 100 versus 1 of 179, $p < 0.01$) in neurosurgical patients taking phenobarbital preoperatively than in those who required no phenobarbital treatment.[9] A subgroup of patients who had never before received halothane were also examined, and again the incidence of liver dysfunction was significantly higher in phenobarbital-treated than in the nontreated patients (4 of 71 versus 1 of 168, $p < 0.05$). In the laboratory, the same investigators demonstrated decreasing degrees of halothane hepatoxicity in rats with the following order: phenobarbital > controls = phenytoin > valproic acid. Although phenobarbital has been shown to induce both reductive and oxidative metabolism of halothane,[10] Nomura et al. [9] found it difficult to conclude whether the postoperative hepatic dysfunction in humans was caused by the metabolites of halothane (metabolic theory) or relative hepatic hypoxia created by enzyme induction with increase in oxygen demand in combination with altered hepatic oxygen delivery caused by halothane.

Are reversible, mild forms of halothane toxicity related to the more severe form of halothane hepatitis? The answer is unknown; however, a direct relationship seems unlikely. Unfortunately, animal models of hepatotoxicity consistently produce massive hepatic necrosis, not mild hepatic injury when halothane is administered.[11] The degree of liver damage in the rat directly correlates with serum inorganic fluoride concentration, implicating reductive metabolism of halothane as the cause of liver injury in this model. Enzyme induction and hypoxia are also required for hepatic damage in the rat, thus making it difficult to exclude hepatic ischemia as a contributing factor.

Reductive metabolism of halothane seems to play an important role in animal hepatoxicity. Animal studies demonstrate covalent binding of reductive halothane metabolites to proteins and phospholipids in the liver,[12] and this binding is increased by enzyme inducers (phenobarbital and polychlorinated biphenyls) in the rat in vitro and in vivo. Dehalogenation of halothane by hepatic cytochrome P-450 occurs both aerobically (oxidative) and anaerobically (reductive), with the former a detoxifying reaction and the latter a toxifying reaction (Fig. 18-1). More simply stated, reductive metabolism of halothane produces molecules toxic to hepatocytes, just as reductive metabolism of oxygen generates a molecule with an unpaired electron that has tremendous affinity for certain cellular components such as phospholipids, DNA, and mitochondrial structures. This is clearly the mechanism for the direct hepatotoxicity of carbon tetrachloride (CCl_4), which undergoes biotransformation by the hepatic microsomal cytochrome P-450 system. Biotransformation of CCl_4 generates a trichloromethyl radical that initiates a series of lipid peroxidation events resulting in subcellular membrane damage and cellular necrosis of the hepatocytes. Centrilobular necrosis is produced by the metabolism of CCl_4 possibly because the centrilobular hepatocytes contain the highest concentration of cytochrome P-450.[13] The final metabolites of reductive halothane metabolism do not cause hepatic damage; therefore it is likely that the reductive metabolism of halothane generates reactive intermediates that cause hepatocellular damage.

Liver damage may not be attributable to biotransformation of halothane, but rather hepatocellular hypoxia as a result of induced hypermetabolism in the centrilobular cells combined with anesthetic-induced depression of ventilation and particularly a reduction in splanchnic blood flow.[14] The guinea pig model of halothane-induced liver damage may offer pertinent data relating to injury observed in humans.[15] Hepatic necrosis was observed in nonpretreated, nonhypoxic guinea pigs after halothane but not after isoflurane anesthesia. Inorganic fluoride excretion was increased only after halothane anesthesia with hypoxia, whereas hepatic injury occurs with and without hypoxia. The authors using the guinea pig model speculated that hepatic oxygen supply during halothane and isoflurane anesthesia was similar because of similar changes in heart rate, blood pressure, and respiration. There are data however to show that equipotent doses of isoflurane and halothane are associated with very different patterns of hepatic circulatory disorders, resulting in a much better hepatic oxygen supply during isoflurane than during halothane anesthesia.[16,17] The study therefore only confirms that reductive metabolism of halothane is enhanced during hypoxia in the guinea pig. If hepatic damage were related to reductive halothane metabolism, the severity of liver injury should have been associated with an increase in metabolites produced during the reductive biotransformation of halothane; however, it was not observed.[18]

Other problems with the metabolic (biotransformation) theory have been highlighted:[19] (1) enflurane and isoflurane administered with hypoxia to rats pretreated with phenobarbital also produce hepatotoxicity, despite their minimal metabolism; (2) neither enflurane nor isoflurane are reductively metabolized; (3) fasting enhances the hepatotoxicity produced by the volatile anesthetics but has no effect on metabolism of the anesthetics; (4) the metabolites produced by the reductive metabolism of halothane have been isolated and identified (Fig. 18-2) but do not produce hepatotoxicity by themselves; (5) the guinea pig, which does

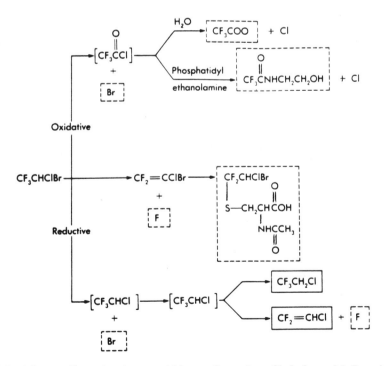

Fig. 18-1. Schema of hepatic microsomal biotransformation of halothane. [ ], Reactive intermediate; ----, excreted in urine. (From Smuckler EA: Patterns of reaction of the liver to injury. In Zakim D and Boyer TD, editors: Hepatology: a textbook of liver disease, Philadelphia, 1982, WB Saunders Co.)

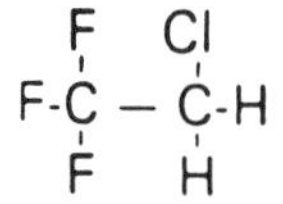

1,1,1-trifluoro-2-chloroethane

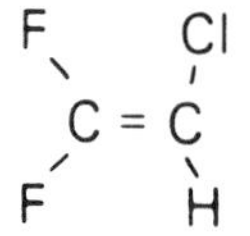

1,1-difluoro-2-chloroethylene

Fig. 18-2. Chemical structure of reductive metabolites of halothane. (From Brown BR, editor: Anesthesia in hepatic and biliary tract disease, Philadelphia, 1988, FA Davis Co.)

not metabolize halothane well without phenobarbital induction, develops hepatotoxicity without phenobarbital pretreatment or hypoxia; (6) higher doses with brief exposures to halothane are associated with more pronounced hepatic damage than lower concentrations with longer exposures; (7) triiodothyronine pretreatment of rats exposed to halothane without hypoxia or barbiturate pretreatment leads to hepatic necrosis despite the fact that T_3 treatment reduces cytochrome P-450 content, reducing the metabolism of halothane.

There is substantial evidence showing that halothane anesthesia causes mild, transient changes in liver enzymes. Evidence implicates biotransformation of the molecule, but reductive biotransformation requires cellular conditions that are hepatotoxic, that is, hypoxia. The first part of the discussion on halothane toxicity has been directed at attempts to explain the first type of adverse reaction to halothane, that is, mild toxicity. This type of reaction is rather common and involves quantitative enhancement of the reductive biotransformation by a variety of factors such as obesity, decreased hepatic blood flow as a result of the anesthetic, retractors, packs, genetic amplification of the reductive pathway and the influence of various hepatic enzyme-inducing drugs. The onset of noticeable liver damage is rapid but remains mild and does not progress to hepatic necrosis.[20]

B. Halothane—fatal hepatotoxicity

1. Fulminant halothane hepatitis. Halothane has also been linked to a probably entirely different and much more severe form of

liver necrosis. The basic event is most likely halothane biotransformation, which leads to conjugation of an intermediate with liver macromolecules, producing a hapten. Six to 10 days may elapse before hepatic dysfunction becomes apparent and may progress to fulminant halothane hepatitis. This is a rare clinical event that may be immunologically mediated and represents an entity completely different from other forms of perioperative liver injury.[21]

2. National halothane study. Several years after the introduction of halothane in 1955, cases of unexplained hepatitis after halothane anesthesia implicated this drug as a potential hepatotoxin. The Committee on Anesthesia of the National Academy of Sciences—National Research Council formed a group to study clinical aspects of halothane; the result was one of the largest epidemiologic studies ever completed. The National Halothane Study was a retrospective review by 35 institutions of anesthetics performed over a 4-year period from 1959 to 1962, with the aim of determining the incidence of massive hepatic necrosis after anesthesia. A total of 856,600 surgical anesthetics were reviewed and the following conclusions were drawn: (1) fatal, postoperative massive hepatic necrosis was very rare and was usually explainable on a nonanesthetic basis, and (2) halothane, compared with other anesthetics, was associated with an overall lower anesthetic mortality.

There are some problems with the study, however, that may not allow such reassuring conclusions. First, this retrospective study initially involved 54 centers of which 38 were able to comply with the limitations of the protocol and only 35 contributed data. Second, among these 35 institutions there were considerable differences in patterns of anesthetic use (halothane use varied from 6.2% to 62.7%), as well as considerable variation in the overall anesthesia death rate (0.27% to 6.41%). Third, the study was designed to look at only massive hepatic necrosis terminating in death and did not address the incidence of lesser degrees of hepatic involvement. Fourth, only cases in which necropsy was performed could be considered in the data analysis. Of the 15,722 deaths, the autopsy rate was 65%. Fifth, of the 946 cases believed to represent massive necrosis, 724 were excluded largely because of postmortem autolysis, making it impossible to assess hepatic morphology. Of the 222 cases believed to represent hepatic necrosis, all but 82 were eliminated by the reviewing pathologists as demonstrating less than "massive" necrosis, neglecting the fact that submassive necrosis might be fatal. Of the remaining 82 cases, only 9 were attributed to anesthetic toxicity and only 7 of those received halothane. In short, the true incidence of halothane hepatitis cannot be ascertained from the study,[22] which was reported as 1 of 35,000 anesthetics. Other more recent studies report the incidence as 1:6,000 to 1:20,000.[23,24]

There are two other factors that make the clinical diagnosis of halothane hepatitis even more difficult. First, Schemel has shown that the incidence of asymptomatic hepatitis in otherwise healthy, ASA physical status I patients is 1:700 and the incidence of clinical jaundice is 1:2540.[25] To obtain these data, 7620 elective surgical admissions were screened for abnormal elevations in routine liver functions over a 1-year period. Increased liver enzyme concentrations were attributable to infectious mononucleosis, viral hepatitis, cirrhosis, or alcoholic hepatitis. Although not clinically jaundiced at the time of the initial examination, 3 out of 11 patients later developed clinical jaundice that could have been easily attributed to halothane if the patient had received a halothane anesthetic. A similar incidence of unsuspected preoperative hepatic dysfunction has been documented by another investigation.[26]

It is also exceedingly difficult to differentiate halothane hepatitis from viral hepatitis on a morphologic basis.[27] Both cause centrilobular necrosis as evidence of direct cytotoxicity, not cholestatic liver injury. It is possible that the stress of anesthesia and surgery unmasks incubating or subclinical hepatitis and results in a fulminant course. Such a clinical course has been described after laparotomy in a patient with jaundice and suspected extrahepatic biliary obstruction in whom viral hepatitis was eventually found to be the etiologic factor.[28] A similar clinical picture developed after an enflurane anesthetic, but herpesvirus was eventually isolated as the cause of liver failure.[29] Serologic markers for hepatitis A, B, and non-A, non-B (hepatitis C) may be useful to document infection, but if the patient has recently been exposed to the virus, antigen titers may be very low and antibody titers nonexistent, an implication of other causes (that is, halothane) for postoperative hepatic dysfunction. Of note, the median age of the patient with fulminant viral hepatitis is much lower (30 versus 57) than that of the patient with halothane-associated fulminant hepatic failure[30] (Fig. 18-3).

3. Risk factors. There are certain factors that seem to enhance a person's susceptibility to halothane hepatitis (List 18-1). Multiple or prior exposures to halothane are common[31] (Table 18-1), and several cases of halothane hepatitis

in very young children have been documented after multiple exposures.[32] It is postulated that transplacental exposure to halothane may sensitize a person who then may react on a second exposure. Neuberger et al. state that the severe, idiosyncratic reaction to halothane is characteristically found after multiple anesthetics up to 10 times more frequently than that after a single exposure.[33] The shorter the interval between the two most recent exposures, the more rapid is the onset of jaundice ($r = 0.48$, p

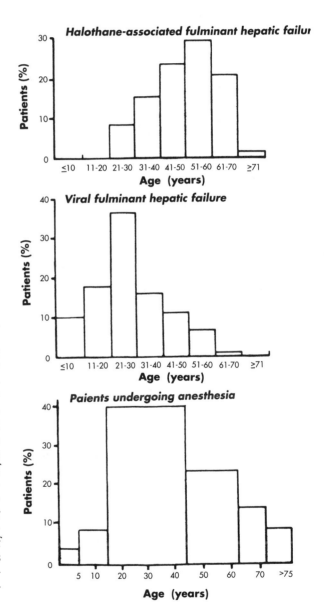

Fig. 18-3. Age distributions of patients admitted to liver failure unit with unexplained hepatic failure after halothane anesthesia or hepatic failure from viral hepatitis. (From Neuberger J and Williams R: Br Med J 289:1136, 1984.)

Table 18-1. Importance of multiple exposures in halothane jaundice in representative series

Series cases	Total exposures	% patients with multiple exposures
Moult and Sherlock (1975)	26	92
Klion et al. (1969)	42	71
Bottiger et al. (1976)	94	82
Walton et al. (1976)	76	95
Inman and Mushin (1974)	114	82
Peters et al. (1969)	41	80
TOTAL	393	MEAN 84

From Touloukian J and Kaplowitz N: Semin Liver Dis 1(2):134-142, 1981.

List 18-1. Features Stated to Increase the Risk of Hepatotoxicity of Halothane

Frequent or multiple exposures
Middle age (40 to 65 years)
Obesity
Female sex
Hispanic ethnicity

From Brown BR editor: Anesthesia in hepatic and biliary tract disease, Philadelphia, 1988, FA Davis Co.

Table 18-2. Clinical features of halothane jaundice

Latent period	Days
1. Single exposure	
To first symptom	6
To jaundice	11
2. Multiple exposure	
To first symptom	3
To jaundice	6
Systemic complaints	**% of cases**
Fever	75
Chills	30
Rash	10
Myalgia	20
Anorexia, nausea	50

From Touloukian J and Kaplowitz N: Semin Liver Dis 1(2):134-142, 1981.

List 18-2. Factors Associated with Poor Prognosis in Halothane Jaundice

Short latent period
Age >40 years
Obesity
Prothrombin time, >20 sec (associated with 100% mortality)
Bilirubin, >10 mg/dl (associated with 60% mortality)

From Touloukian J and Kaplowitz N: Semin Liver Dis 1(2):134-142, 1981.

=0.05). Women who develop the disease outnumber men 1.8 to 1, but men have a higher mortality from fulminant failure. Obese women[34,35] seem to be more likely to develop halothane hepatitis, possibly because of increased metabolism of halothane or prolonged exposure to halothane and its metabolites secondary to release from the adipose tissue long after the anesthetic has ended. Surgery is often minor, lasting less than 30 minutes. An allergic history may also be linked to the development of this sometimes fatal disease. Clinical features of the disease are outlined in Table 18-2. Evidence also indicates some ethnic groups (Mexican-American) as high risk,[36] and the disease may be linked genetically[37] because Japanese investigators have documented chromosomal differences between normal patients and patients who have recovered from halothane hepatitis.[38] Preexisting liver disease, such as hepatitis or cirrhosis, does not enhance the susceptibility of the liver to injury by halothane.[39,40] Once hepatic dysfunction develops, mortality may be as high as 40%, and several factors have been associated with poor prognosis (List 18-2).

4. Mechanisms of halothane hepatitis. What is the mechanism for fulminant hepatic failure after halothane anesthesia? Is there a single, as yet unexplained, mechanism responsible, or are

several mechanisms involved? Cousins et al. believe that reported cases of halothane hepatitis do not form a homogeneous group, and it would be too simplistic to expect a single mechanism to explain all the different types of hepatic toxicity from halothane.[41] Current hypotheses propose three distinct causes: (1) direct toxicity from the intermediates of halothane metabolism (biotransformation); (2)

Table 18-3. Evidence pertaining to the different mechanisms of halothane-induced liver disease

Direct toxicity	Hypersensitivity

1. Centrilobular necrosis
2. Short interval between exposures
3. 10% to 20% incidence of anicteric hepatitis with multiple exposures
4. Animal model
   a. Reductive hypoxic
      Inducible hepatic
      Biotransformation
   b. Covalent binding
   c. Centrilobular necrosis
   (a) to (c) require some form of hepatic hypoxia
    for hepatocellular damage.
	5. Low incidence
	6. Multiple exposures
	7. Autoantibodies (occurring in a minority of cases)
	8. Rash and eosinophilia (occurring in a minority of cases)
	9. Antibody to plasma membrane of halothane-exposed hepatocytes

From Touloukian J and Kaplowitz N: Semin Liver Dis 1(2):134-142, 1981.

hepatic oxygen deprivation either from the operation itself or from altered hepatic circulation from halothane, or both; and (3) immunologically mediated hepatic necrosis (Table 18-3).

5. Biotransformation. Animal models (hypoxic, phenobarbital-pretreated rats; nonhypoxic, triiodothyronine-pretreated rats; nonhypoxic, nonpretreated guinea pigs[42]) of halothane hepatotoxicity are set up under the assumption that enhanced metabolism of halothane by the cytochrome P-450 pathway generates toxic intermediates that cause liver damage. The intermediates are assumed to be responsible for toxicity because the final metabolites have never been shown to be hepatotoxic. These models consistently produce hepatic necrosis, but these data may not be applicable to the human disease. In animals, these models rely upon enhanced metabolism (that is, increased oxygen consumption) by means of the cytochrome P-450 system for toxicity and demonstrate decreased toxicity if the cytochromes are inhibited (that is, decreased oxygen consumption) by cimetidine.[43] The role of reductive metabolism of halothane in halothane hepatitis in humans is still questionable.

6. Ischemia. Almost all animal models of halothane hepatotoxicity require enhancement of hepatic metabolism, which increases oxygen demand. Certainly this is true for all rat models, but some strains of guinea pigs develop liver dysfunction after anesthesia even with normoxia and no phenobarbital pretreatment. Apparently, hepatic arterial blood flow in the guinea pig is very low, contributing only 2% to 3% of total hepatic arterial blood flow compared to other species where hepatic arterial blood flow represents 20% to 35% of the total hepatic blood flow. It is not surprising that this

may be responsible for the unusual sensitivity of the liver to any hypoxic-ischemia insult in the guinea pig. Liver injury can be induced by surgical stress and hemorrhage and even enflurane, isoflurane, and nitrous oxide. These observations can be explained only by the hypoxic hypothesis. Anesthesia, especially when superimposed with surgery, leads to different degrees of respiratory and circulatory depression, resulting in a reduction of hepatic oxygen supply and consequently a decrease in the hepatic oxygen supply-to-demand ratio. Halothane appears to cause the most severe liver dysfunction of all the anesthetics in the guinea pig model secondary to respiratory and circulatory depression, with pronounced hepatic oxygen deprivation.

There is an inverse correlation between hepatic injury and hepatic oxygen supply, regardless of the insult that is used to vary hepatic oxygen supply: halothane, isoflurane, or hemorrhage.[44] Experimental conditions that reduce hepatic oxygen consumption such as hypothermia, cimetidine, or metyrapone administration protect against hepatic injury in animal models.[45] It is interesting to note that ischemic hepatitis morphologically mimics halothane hepatitis. Van Dyke and Mason have demonstrated that halothane, enflurane, and isoflurane inhibit oxidative phosphorylation at the step of nicotinamide adenine dinucleotide (NAD) formation (Fig. 18-4). The results of this observation indicate that all three inhalational anesthetics, even at low concentrations, may increase intracellular calcium concentrations, which may contribute to hepatocellular injury.[46] Hepatic ischemia has been clearly documented to cause liver injury, but its contribution to fatal halothane hepatitis is not clear. The clinical characteristics of ischemic hepatitis are discussed in a later section.

7. Immune mechanisms. Although animal data support direct toxicity of halothane as the mechanism for hepatic necrosis, human data reflect an idiosyncratic reaction or more likely an immune response to halothane as the probable cause of halothane hepatitis. Most of the evidence is circumstantial. Hepatitis occurs most commonly after multiple exposures, not a single exposure (could this reflect cumulative toxicity in some patients?). The response is often delayed for several days, a further implication that the immune system is the cause of hepatotoxicity. The disease seems to be common in patients with an allergic history but uncommon in children. Other features of hypersensitivity include peripheral eosinophilia,[47] circulating immune complexes, and the appearance of organ nonspecific autoantibodies.[48] Lymphocytes from patients with halothane hepatitis are di-

rectly cytotoxic to halothane-pretreated hepatocytes.[49]

A case report describes a woman with a previous history of halothane hepatitis who received a nonhalothane anesthetic but still developed "halothane hepatitis" postoperatively. The authors speculate that halothane dissolved in the rubber in the machine resulted in an inadvertent reexposure in this already sensitized patient.[50] Klatskin and Kimberg[51] administered subanesthetic concentrations of halothane to an anesthesiologist who was known to have liver disease possibly from occupational exposure to halothane. Shortly after exposure, the anesthesiologist developed increased concentrations of hepatic enzymes, possibly indicating a response to the halothane challenge. Unfortunately, although somewhat convincing, these case reports are anecdotal, but it is not possible to prove the absence of toxicity.[52] However, patients who die from halothane hepatitis most

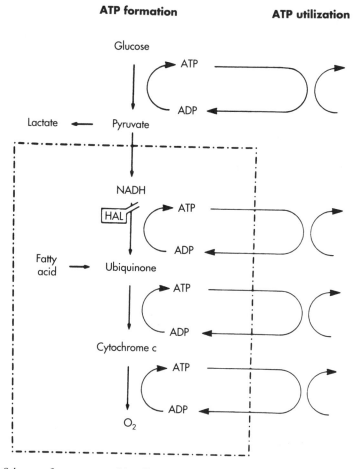

Fig. 18-4. Schema of sequence and localization of various reactions important to energy metabolism within a liver cell. *Rectangle,* Mitochondrial membrane. Other intracellular organelles are not shown. Notice where halothane interrupts NADH metabolism and therefore cellular oxygen metabolism. (From Becker GL: Anesth Analg 70:22, 1990.)

often develop an allergic picture, and laboratory data are surfacing to support this theory.

Strong evidence exists from not only human but also animal studies[53-57] that trifluoroacetic acid (TFA), an oxidative metabolite of halothane, binds covalently to hepatocytes thus allowing this hapten (TFA) combined with hepatocellular components to act as an antigen. The humoral immune system identifies this neoantigen as nonself and mounts the appropriate response to obliterate this foreign protein. The hepatocyte is then destroyed by the immune system. Other evidence supporting this theory includes the almost absolute requirement for a recent and sometimes a remote halothane exposure before the immune response can cause significant hepatic necrosis. Morphologically, centrilobular necrosis is the hallmark of halothane hepatitis, which is the zone of the liver with the highest concentration of cytochrome P-450, the enzyme responsible for oxidative metabolism of halothane. The antibody generated by patients with halothane hepatitis is also of the IgG class, an indication that the immune response is highly specific. The role of the cellular immune system in this response is not clear.[58]

Early immunoreactive techniques for the detection of the "halothane antibody" were technically suspect,[59] but development of the enzyme-linked immunosorbent assay (ELISA) has eliminated some of the technical problems associated with detection of the antibody in patients who have recovered from halothane hepatitis. The technique still lacks sensitivity and specificity evidenced by a 75% positive and 12% false-positive rate of antibody identification. Still, this test may be useful in identifying patients at risk for the development of halothane hepatitis. Some investigators still challenge the TFA hapten theory, believing instead that the antigen-antibody response is a result of hepatic injury, not its cause. Of particular interest, covalent binding of halothane metabolites to hepatocytes is increased with low oxygen concentrations in vitro again an implication that hepatic oxygen deprivation is playing a role in the hepatic damage.

8. Recommendations. Recommendations by Stock and Strunin[60] have been made regarding the use of halothane. First, halothane has very low potential for liver damage in children, even with repeated exposures. Second, preexisting, compensated liver disease is not a contraindication to the use of halothane; the outcome is correlated with the degree of liver disease and type of surgery rather than with the anesthetic itself. Third, severe liver damage is uncommon after a single exposure to halothane. Fourth, repeated exposure to adults, especially obese, middle-aged women over a short period of time (less than 6 weeks) might result in liver damage, though rarely. Fifth, if a repeated halothane anesthetic is planned within a short period of time, the use of halothane should be justified. Sixth, the mechanism of halothane hepatitis is complex but probably involves the immune system. Seventh, there is no reliable test for the detection of patients susceptible to halothane liver damage. I (J.D.P) believe that halothane has a very limited place in modern anesthesia practice considering other factors associated with halothane anesthesia such as decrease in cardiac output and overall tissue perfusion, substantial decrease in hepatic blood flow and often occurring mild temporary liver injury, availability of other effective but less dangerous volatile anesthetics, and possible legal implications.

C. Enflurane

Enflurane is probably not hepatotoxic, but it is always difficult to disprove toxicity. Lewis et al.[61] examined reports of liver damage that had occurred since the introduction of enflurane in 1972. He concluded enflurane had caused liver damage in some patients because they had signs, symptoms, and histories reminiscent of halothane-induced hepatitis. The morphologic lesion often was the same as that produced by halothane, that is, centrilobular necrosis.

Eger et al.[62] disagreed with Lewis et al. and reanalyzed the same data. Eger created a "syndrome score" for all patients with probable postanesthetic enflurane hepatitis. Patients were analyzed for 12 different points, including presence of fever, chills, nausea, rash, eosinophilia, death, and hepatic morphology. Syndrome scores from patients who had postoperative hepatitis from other causes (such as sepsis, shock) were compared to patients who were identified as having enflurane hepatitis. "Syndrome scores" were the same between these two groups of patients with postoperative hepatitis. Eger et al. believed that no conclusion could therefore be made concerning the incidence or even the existence of enflurane hepatitis based on these case-control studies.

Enflurane has been deemed hepatotoxic by association with halothane, but there are several characteristics of enflurane that clearly differentiate it from halothane. The current theories of halothane hepatotoxicity assume liver injury results from the metabolites of halothane. Whereas 20% of halothane is metabolized by the body, only 2.4% of enflurane is metabolized.[63] Enflurane does not undergo reductive metabolism, and experimental conditions that produce reductive metabolites of halothane produce no such metabolites of enflurane.[63] One key requirement for the development of halothane hepatitis is a prior exposure to the drug. This has been shown to be important with halothane because the number of cases of halothane hepatitis has increased with the number of years since the introduction of the drug (Fig. 18-5). This increase does not appear to be true with enflurane.

Enflurane metabolites in the rat have been shown to react with serum from patients who have recovered from halothane hepatitis.[64] Even though the acyl haptens produced by oxidative metabolism of enflurane (difluoromethoxydifluoroacetyl halide) and halothane (trifluoroacetyl halide) are chemically distinct, the liver protein adducts containing these haptens are similar enough to be recognized by serum antibodies from patients with halothane hepatitis. Proposed pathways for the formation of acylating intermediates from the oxidative metabolism of several inhalational agents are shown in Fig. 18-6. It is yet unclear if there is true immune crossover sensitivity between halothane and enflurane. Although laboratory evidence seems to indicate the possibility, there are no human data in this regard. If only the possi-

ble (that is, unexplained) cases of enflurane hepatitis are considered as enflurane-induced, the incidence of hepatitis is 0.36 cases per million(!), which is 200 times less than that observed with halothane.

D. Isoflurane

Isoflurane is an inhalational anesthetic that undergoes minimal biodegradation,[65] preserves hepatic oxygen supply even during laparotomy,[66] and does not undergo reductive metabolism. It has also been shown to protect the liver from carbon tetrachloride toxicity by inhibiting the cytochrome P-450 metabolism of CCl_4 and possibly dismutating haloperoxyl radicals.[67] Isoflurane does not influence hepatic function in rats with CCl_4-induced cirrhosis,[68] but, under certain experimental conditions, isoflurane can cause centrilobular necrosis.[69]

Clinical reports of isoflurane hepatitis have been published,[70] and they prompted an investigation of this drug as a potential hepatotoxin. A subcommittee of four members of the Anesthetic and Life Support Advisory Committee of the Federal Drug Administration evaluated these adverse drug reports to determine if a causal association existed between administration of isoflurane and subsequent hepatic dysfunction. The committee concluded that "cur-

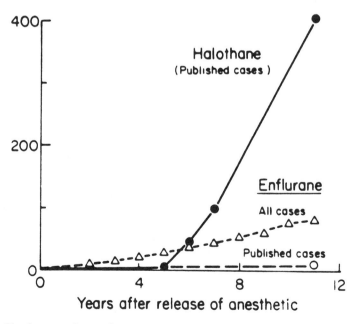

Fig. 18-5. Total reported cases from release of halothane or enflurane to date of liver injury or jaundice. The number of published reports of hepatic injury after halothane anesthesia dramatically increased about 5 years after the introduction of halothane (●) into clinical practice. No such upturn appeared in the 11-year period after the release of enflurane (---○). (From Eger EI, Smuckler EA, and Ferrell LD: Anesth Analg 65:21, 1986.)

rent evidence does not indicate a reasonable likelihood of an association between the use of isoflurane and the occurrence of postoperative hepatic dysfunction."[71] The committee members were in most cases able to implicate another cause for hepatic dysfunction such as sepsis, hypoxia, biliary obstruction, nutritional deficiency, circulatory shock, viral hepatitis (including herpesvirus), and antibiotic therapy (erythromycin estolate). There were two reports of postoperative hepatic injury in pregnant patients treated with a beta$_2$-receptor agonist and undergoing cholecystectomy. The stress of upper abdominal surgery and chronic administration of a drug that may decrease hepatic blood flow may have been enough to cause hepatic dysfunction. Table 18-4 is a comparison of halothane, enflurane, and isoflurane on issues relevant to hepatotoxicity of these inhalational agents.

E. Desflurane

Desflurane, though in the initial stages of human investigation, has not exhibited hepatotoxicity in enzyme-induced, hypoxic rats.[72] Theoretically, the incidence of hepatic dysfunction after desflurane anesthesia would probably be similar to that quoted for enflurane or isoflurane anesthesia. In other words, desflurane should possess no intrinsic toxicity because it is not metabolized, but patients might develop hepatic dysfunction after administration of the drug because of unidentifiable causes.

F. Nitrous oxide

Nitrous oxide administered by itself has little effect on hepatic function[73] but may enhance the hepatotoxicity of halothane in hypoxic rats.[74] Fifty-percent nitrous oxide inhibits the enzyme methionine synthetase resulting in de-

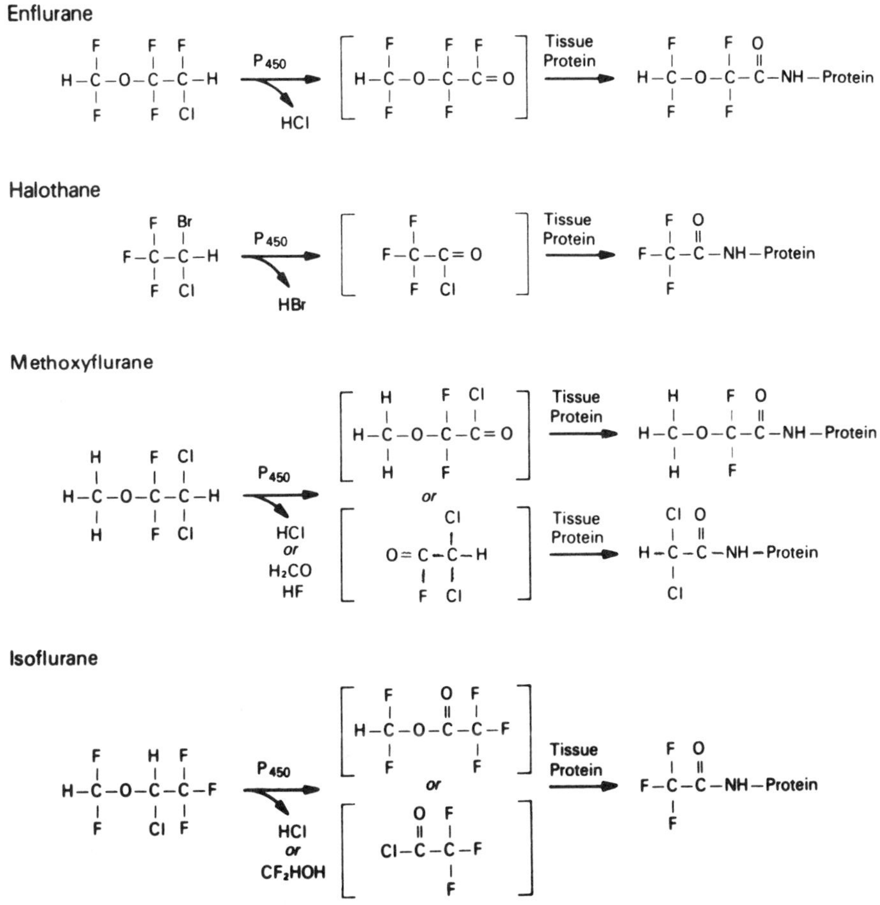

Fig. 18-6. Possible pathways for the formation of acylating intermediates from the oxidative metabolism of enflurane, halothane, methoxyflurane, or isoflurane. (From Christ DD, Kenna JG, and Kammerer W: Anesthesiology 69:833, 1988.)

Table 18-4. Differences between halothane, enflurane, and isoflurane relevant to considerations of hepatotoxicity

	Halothane	Enflurane	Isoflurane
Stable in sunlight	No	Yes	Yes
Toxic breakdown products	Yes	—	No
Stable in soda lime	No	Yes	Yes
Extent of metabolism	15% to 20%	2.4%	0.2%
Reductive metabolism	Yes	No	No
Metabolism to free radicals	Yes	No	No
Tissue binding of metabolites	Yes	No	—
Hepatic oxygen delivery	Decreased	Slightly decreased	Unchanged

From Eger EI: Anesthetic-induced hepatitis, International Anesthesia Research Society Refresher Course Lectures, Cleveland, Ohio, 1986, pp 116-120.

rangement of folate and methionine metabolism.[75] Nitrous oxide causes a 1.7 times higher incidence of liver disease in dentists who are chronically exposed to the drug compared to other professionals not chronically exposed to N_2O.[76] However, patients with mild alcoholic hepatitis show no significant changes in postoperative liver function when a nitrous oxide–opioid anesthetic is used for peripheral surgery. Other studies support these conclusions.[77]

II. INTRAVENOUS ANESTHETICS

Thiopental may depress liver function if administered in large doses (greater than 750 mg) but in clinically used doses causes little alteration in liver function.[78,79]

Ketamine has been shown to affect postoperative liver function probably depending on the total dose.[80] Fourteen of 34 patients anesthetized with ketamine and oxygen for intermediate procedures developed significant elevations in postoperative hepatic enzyme levels compared to 7 of 34 who received a "control" anesthetic. The authors state that postoperative changes in liver function could be attributed to a hepatotoxic effect, enzyme induction, or changes in liver metabolism. Altered hepatic blood flow could be implicated because ketamine increases serum catecholamine levels, which certainly influence oxygen delivery.

Etomidate, midazolam, propofol, and althesin have not been shown to significantly alter hepatic function in patients undergoing minor surgery.[81] However, if major surgery is performed with these drugs, significant increases in plasma concentrations of liver enzymes are observed.[82] Sear states that "it appears that single infusions of all the intravenous hypnotic agents (with the possible exceptions of thiopental and ketamine) cause only minimal alterations in plasma concentrations of the routinely measured liver function tests."[83]

Opioids can cause spasm of the sphincter of Oddi with subsequent severe abdominal pain from the increase in intrabiliary pressure. Equipotent doses of fentanyl and morphine cause the largest increases in biliary pressure, whereas meperidine and pentazocine are associated with modest increases.[84] Nalbuphine does not cause biliary spasm.

Opioids have been shown in mice to cause fatty infiltration in the liver and up to a tenfold increase in AST concentrations after single intraperitoneal injections. These changes are blocked by naloxone, reserpine, or propranolol administration thus implicating a sympathetic response with subsequent decrease in hepatic blood flow as the cause of this liver dysfunction. It is difficult to relate these data to humans undergoing major surgery but may have some importance when taking care of opioid addicts with liver failure.[85]

III. MISCELLANEOUS CAUSES OF HEPATIC DYSFUNCTION RELATED TO ANESTHESIA
A. Ischemic hepatitis

Extreme liver injury has been reported in patients with prolonged shock or sepsis where there may be total infarction of a lobe or the entire liver with no evidence of portal or hepatic arterial occlusion.[86] However, with lesser degrees of hypotension, a hepatitis-like illness may occur. Morphologically, ischemic hepatitis is characterized by centrilobular necrosis with little or no inflammatory response[87] and may present as clinically apparent liver disease with pronounced elevation of serum transaminases, jaundice, and even systemic symptoms. In contrast, hepatic congestion alone causes only minor damage to the liver. Hepatic dysfunction after period of documented ischemia is usually mild, and prognosis depends on the underlying cardiac or systemic illness. Abnormal liver function tests secondary to ischemia usually persist for 3 to 11 days. Ischemic hepatitis can be differentiated from viral hepatitis on clinical and biochemical criteria alone, a characteristic that is fortunate because liver biopsy specimens in both cases show centrilobular necrosis. Clinically, ischemic hepatitis occurs in patients with a probable history of inadequate systemic perfusion. Biochemically the increase in liver enzyme concentrations is usually greater with ischemic hepatitis than viral hepatitis. The role of oxygen-free radicals in postischemic hepatitis has yet to be elucidated but has clearly been implicated because hepatocytes contain some of the highest concentrations of xanthine oxidase in the body.

B. Anesthesia, surgery, and hepatic function

Inhalational anesthetics affect hepatic oxygen supply and demand in various ways and to different degrees. Halothane decreases hepatic blood flow and oxygen supply to a much greater extent than isoflurane does.[88] However, in comparison to the negative effects of exploratory laparotomy on hepatic oxygen supply, the inhalational anesthetics have only mild though potentiating effects.

Certain responses to surgical stress such as an increase in circulating catecholamines, cortisol, growth hormone, antidiuretic hormone, aldosterone, and activation of the renin-angiotensin system are well known. Specific effects of stress on hepatic function have been studied to a lesser degree. Available data strongly indicate that laparotomy by itself may reduce blood flow through the intestine and the liver.[89] Laparotomy is associated with pronounced mesenteric vasoconstriction and a decrease in gastrointestinal blood flow, which can be abolished by hypophysectomy.[90] Phenobarbital-pretreated (liver enzyme-induced) rats anesthetized with halothane develop liver necrosis after laparotomy alone or after laparotomy with ligation of the hepatic artery.[91] Under similar conditions, halothane anesthesia without laparotomy is not associated with hepatic necrosis. This indicates that laparotomy may be accompanied by a reduction in the liver oxygen supply severe enough to cause hepatic necrosis in these particular experimental conditions. It has been shown that major surgery is associated with a substantial increase in the concentration of enzymes supposedly released from the liver. The degree of such an increase depends more on the type of surgery than on a particular anesthetic technique; such increases are rarely observed after minor surgery.[92,93]

Thus surgery, particularly laparotomy, affects liver function but usually without serious consequences. However, in patients with advanced hepatic disease, laparotomy is often accompanied by extremely high postoperative morbidity and mortality.[94,95] Patient with marginal hepatic function are probably not able to tolerate the significant changes in hepatic oxygen supply induced by surgical stress. Patients with marginal hepatic function may undergo a peripheral procedure, even with halothane, without postoperative hepatic complications.

IV. NONANESTHETIC CAUSES OF POSTOPERATIVE LIVER DYSFUNCTION

A. Preoperative unsuspected liver disease

In patients with preexisting liver disease, surgery and anesthetic-induced decrease in hepatic oxygen supply is more likely to result in overt liver dysfunction or even hepatic failure than in patients without liver failure. Large surveys have confirmed that the risk of a postoperative hepatic complication is greatly increased in patients with preexisting liver disease, especially with emergency operations.[96] Chronic alcoholism is notoriously difficult to determine by a quick patient history and may not be evident unless the patient exhibits end-stage disease. Laboratory values can be misleading (Table 18-5), and chronic alcohol abuse can create a spectrum of liver disease from fatty liver to cirrhosis. Patients may be remarkably well compensated even with extensive disease, with a poor correlation between the clinical presentation and histologic extent of damage.[97] Although elective surgery is not contraindicated in patients with fatty livers, the mortality from acute alcoholic hepatitis, even without surgery, is significant. Animals pretreated with alcohol are more likely than controls to develop centrilobu-

Table 18-5. Preoperative characteristics in 30 patients with mild alcoholic hepatitis

Variable	Mean ± SD
Age (years)	43± 11
Hemoglobin (g/dl)	12.4±2.1
White blood cells (1000/mm^3)	8.2±2.2
Blood urea nitrogen (mg/dl)	10± 5
Prothrombin time (sec)	10.9±1.1
Serum albumin (g/dl)	3±0.7

From Zinn SE, Fairley HB and Glenn JD: Anesth Analg 64:487-490, 1985.

lar necrosis after exposure to halothane because alcohol is believed to enhance hepatic hypoxia. Therefore a complete patient history in regard to long-term and recent alcohol use may offer evidence warranting further examination of liver function.

Clearly, surgical risk is increased in patients with cirrhosis and is greater for abdominal surgery than for nonabdominal surgery. Operative mortality correlates with Child's class of hepatic dysfunction (A, 10%; B, 31%; C, 76%).[98] Child's classification also correlates with the incidence of postoperative complications, which include liver failure, bleeding, infection, sepsis, renal failure, pulmonary failure, and ascites.[99] Fortunately it is relatively easy to detect this disease by thorough history and laboratory data. Postoperative hepatic dysfunction should raise the question of preoperative alcohol excess.

Whereas chronic ethanolism can be relatively easy to detect, postoperative hepatic dysfunction secondary to viral hepatitis can be an elusive diagnosis. There are a variety of hepatotrophic agents that may cause hepatic dysfunction including hepatitis A virus (HAV, infectious hepatitis), hepatitis B virus (HBV, serum hepatitis), hepatitis D virus (delta), and non-A, non-B virus. Acute hepatitis may rarely be caused by cytomegalovirus (CMV), Epstein-Barr virus (EBV), herpesvirus, measles virus, and coxsackievirus. CMV hepatitis is more common in the immunosuppressed patient but may occur in the routine postsurgical patient. The disease is often benign with only minor changes in hepatic function. The diagnosis can be made on the basis of the pathognomonic cytoplasmic inclusions in the hepatocytes. Whereas other DNA viruses, such as herpes simplex virus[100] and varicella-zoster virus, produce intranuclear inclusions, they do not produce cytoplasmic inclusions.[101] Hepatitis secondary to EBV also affects the lymphoreticular tissue, resulting in prominent lymphadenopathy. Many of these lesser known causes of hepatitis are anicteric thus escaping detection by the surgical and anesthesia teams, but in unusual cases they may lead to complete hepatic failure and death. Therefore these causes must be considered if liver failure occurs after an anesthetic.

HAV, HBV, and NANB viral infections can cause clinically evident disease; serologic diagnosis is therefore necessary to identify or exclude them as the cause of hepatic dysfunction. An antibody of the IgM class to the HAV capsid is used to document a HAV infection. Either the HBsAg or antibody of the IgM class to the HBV core identifies an HBV infection. However, hepatitis B viral DNA has been identified in patients with chronic liver disease with concurrent negative tests for hepatitis B surface antigen.[102] Hepatitis delta virus (HDV) may be identified by an antibody to the HDV core, but HBsAg is also detected because HDV requires the HBV for viral replication. If serologic markers are all negative, NANB hepatitis is the diagnosis by exclusion in 90% of cases.

Older clinical studies report significant postoperative mortality in patients operated on with active hepatitis. In the past, laparotomy was usually performed in patients with liver failure to obtain a diagnosis; the detrimental effects of laparotomy on hepatic oxygen supply probably resulted in complete hepatic failure. Today, improved serologic tests, transhepatic cholangiography, and endoscopic retrograde cholangiography as well as percutaneous needle biopsy have all combined to obviate the need for exploratory laparotomy.

The patient with incubating hepatitis may still undergo an anesthetic and operation and may not manifest the disease until well into the recovery period (6 to 8 days), which is exactly the course of anesthetic-induced hepatitis. An incidence of unsuspected liver disease in a healthy surgical population is 1 out of 700, and 1 out of 3 of these patients develops jaundice.[103,104] Clinical features of HAV infection are an incubation period of 3 to 4 weeks, no connection to blood transfusion, and a very limited viremia. There are no chronic carriers of HAV, and chronic liver disease is not usually associated with HAV infection. The incubation period for transfusion-associated hepatitis (HBV) is approximately 11.8 weeks, but even screening tests for HBsAg cannot detect the virus at levels below 10E8 to 10E9 particles/ml. Posttransfusion hepatitis B occurs in no greater than 0.4% of patients transfused with HBsAg-negative blood obtained from volunteers.[105] Since all available evidence discounts HAV and HBV as the culprits of posttransfusion hepatitis, NANB hepatitis seems more likely. Although there are no satisfactory methods to identify persons who are susceptible to, are immune to, or are carriers of NANB hepatitis, epidemiologic information indicates that it is spread by all routes. The incubation period is 7.8 weeks, which closely mimics the 7-week incubation period recorded in the 1960s for all cases of transfusion-associated hepatitis, an indication that, even before HBsAg screening of donor blood, most posttransfusion hepatitis might have been of the NANB type. NANB hepatitis, unfortunately, more frequently progresses to chronic liver disease than other less common viral hepatitis infections do. A serologic test for non-A, non-B hepatitis has been developed and may soon be released for blood donor screening.

Gilbert's syndrome (familial unconjugated hyperbilirubinemia) is the most common cause of jaundice in the United States. It is exacerbated by stress, fasting, fever, or infection and is associated with jaundice without dark urine. These patients may not exhibit impairment of hepatic function and may not know they have the disease until the second decade of life. These patients have decreased hepatic bilirubin uptake and a partial deficiency of bilirubin glucuronyl transferase. Crigler-Najjar syndrome (type II) may also cause unconjugated hyperbilirubinemia; surgical and anesthetic-related problems are apparently minimal. Dubin-Johnson syndrome can be exacerbated after surgery.

B. Drug-induced hepatic dysfunction

Patients who undergo major surgery often receive a myriad of drugs. Drug interactions are commonly described where one drug may increase or decrease the metabolism of another leading to altered effect or toxicity. Drug toxicity can be either dose related, as with acetominophen, or idiosyncratic, as with halothane. Induction of hepatic microsomal drug-metabolizing systems often play a role because increased drug metabolism (and the formation of reactive intermediates) may lead to increased liver damage from an otherwise nontoxic substance.

Acetaminophen, isoniazid, furosemide, and methyldopa can cause centrilobular necrosis in the liver. Other cytotoxic drugs include ox-yphenisatin, rifampin, papaverine, and phenytoin.[106] Cholestatic reactions are caused by chlorpromazine, phenylbutazone, and androgenic and anabolic steroids. Erythromycin (ethylsuccinate form) has caused hepatic failure that was first attributed to halothane administration. The combination of trimethoprim-sulfamethoxazole is nearly five times more frequently associated with hepatotoxicity than the administration of sulfamethizole alone. Paracetamol overdose is the most common cause of fulminant hepatic failure in the United Kingdom.[107] Phenobarbital administration enhances halothane liver injury,[108] and other drugs that may affect postoperative hepatic function include chemotherapeutic agents (methotrexate) and antibiotics (tetracycline).[109] Dantrolene may cause hepatic failure if administered for more than 60 days for muscle spasms. Indomethacin, monoamine oxidase inhibitors, and amitriptyline have also been implicated.[110] A partial list of drugs that can cause hepatic dysfunction is provided in Table 18-6.

C. Other causes of postoperative hepatic dysfunction

Jaundice after surgery and anesthesia can be caused by overproduction or overload of bilirubin, impaired excretion secondary to hepatocellular injury or congenital defect in bilirubin metabolism, or cholestasis secondary to biliary tract obstruction. Transfusion of 500 ml of blood results in a bilirubin load of approximately 250 mg, which is easily handled by the normal liver. Excessive transfusion results in an even greater bilirubin load, which can lead to unconjugated hyperbilirubinemia until the liver

Table 18-6. Partial listing of drugs proved or suspected of producing liver dysfunction

Drugs that cause hepatic necrosis	Drugs that cause cholestatic reaction	Drugs that cause direct hepatotoxicity
Alpha-methyldopa	Amitriptyline	Actinomycin
Chlordiazepoxide	Carbamazepine	Chloroform
Chlortetracycline	Chlorpromazine	Mithramycin
Ergot alkaloids	Chlorpropamide	Tetracyclines
Halothane	Chlorthiazide	
Idomethacin	Estrogens	
Isoniazid	Erythromycin estolate	
Papaverum	Methimazole	
Phenelzine	Prochlorperazine	
Phenylbutazone	Promazine	
Sulfamethoxypyridine	Thioridazine	
Tranylcypromine	Thiouracil	
Verapamil	Tolbutamide	

From Brown BR, editor: Anesthesia in hepatic and biliary tract disease, Philadelphia, 1988, FA Davis Co.

is able to excrete the excess bilirubin. At least 10% of transfused red blood cells die during the first 24 hours after transfusion. Other sources of excess bilirubin include hemolysis from sickle cell anemia crisis, prosthetic heart valves, and glucose-6-phosphate dehydrogenase deficiency (G-6-PD). Hemolysis may be induced in patients with G-6-PD deficiency by drugs such as sulfonamides, chloramphenicol, nitrofurantoin, and aspirin. Reabsorption of large surgical hematomas might also lead to jaundice without evidence of hepatocellular dysfunction.

Hepatocellular injury not only causes jaundice but also is accompanied by increased liver enzymes, decreased production of all liver-produced moieties, and sometimes encephalopathy. Incubating viral hepatitis can present as postoperative hepatic failure. Stress of surgery, especially an upper abdominal operation, can lead to hepatocellular dysfunction secondary to derangements in hepatic oxygen supply-and-demand relationships. Although cardiac and central nervous systems have tremendous intrinsic autoregulatory mechanisms compensating for decreased oxygen delivery, autoregulation of hepatic oxygen supply is grossly affected by anesthetics, surgical manipulation, positive-pressure ventilation, hypercapnia, and acidosis.[111] Therefore, although no obvious cardiac or central nervous system damage is seen occurring after a difficult anesthetic, hepatocellular function may not have been preserved. The liver, fortunately, has remarkable regenerative capacity and, given optimal hemodynamics and oxygenation, usually recovers without sequelae. Pregnancy-induced hypertension may affect hepatic function, presumably on the basis of marginal hepatic perfusion secondary to profound peripheral vasoconstriction accompanied by hypovolemia and starvation.[112]

Cholestasis may also cause postoperative jaundice. Extrahepatic biliary obstruction can be caused by stones in the duct, iatrogenic stricture, or pancreatitis. Benign postoperative intrahepatic cholestasis refers to a syndrome that often follows severe shock, hypoxemia, major surgical procedures, and blood transfusion. Bilirubin concentrations may exceed 40 mg/dl, but hepatocellular function is well preserved. Mortality is uncommon unless concurrent disease, such as sepsis, cardiac failure, or renal failure, is severe.[113]

Cardiac failure itself does not usually lead to significant hepatic dysfunction, but jaundice and hepatocellular necrosis may occur in patients who experience severe hypotension.[114] Cardiopulmonary bypass with low-flow states and nonpulsatile perfusion can probably aggravate preexisting hepatic dysfunction. If catecholamine administration is necessary for cardiac performance, either before or after bypass, hepatic oxygen delivery may be compromised. Hypothermia during cardiopulmonary bypass probably limits the hepatic damage created by the abnormal hemodynamics, thus limiting the development of liver damage.

V. PREVENTION AND TREATMENT OF HEPATIC INJURY

Thorough preoperative evaluation including history of fever after prior anesthetics, alcohol intake, hepatitis, illicit and prescribed drug use, transfusion, and occupational exposure to hepatic enzyme–inducing substances may be helpful in excluding the patients most at risk for the development of postoperative hepatic dysfunction. Halothane hepatitis is most commonly seen in patients with a history of fever or jaundice after a prior anesthetic. The history is usually there, just ignored. If the history is highly suggestive of halothane hepatitis, an anesthesia machine that has never been equipped with a halothane vaporizer should be used to prevent inadvertent exposure of the patient to trace concentrations of the gas.[115] Patients addicted to alcohol may deceive the anesthesiologist because they look normal and may have normal laboratory tests but have pronounced impairment of hepatic function and even alcoholic hepatitis. Although not a contraindication to anesthesia and surgery, this information would certainly be useful if postoperative hepatic dysfunction should develop. Drug addicts may have impairment of hepatic function as a result of chronic exposure to cocaine (increased catecholamine concentrations) or shared needles (chronic active hepatitis). Prescribed drugs may also impinge on hepatic function, and the anesthesiologist should be familiar with the most common ones (that is, cimetidine, ranitidine, indomethacin, phenytoin, phenobarbital, rifampin, isoniazid, tetracycline, estrogen, and erythromycin, to name a few). Some cause hepatocellular damage, whereas others lead to cholestatic disease. Recent blood transfusion may lead to non-A, non-B hepatitis with an incubation period of about 8 weeks. Hepatic microsomal enzymes responsible for detoxifying almost all anesthetic drugs can probably be induced by certain environmental chemicals (phenols, polycylic compounds) that might increase metabolism of certain drugs such as halothane.

There is probably no one anesthetic technique that is best for the liver. An anesthetic that maximizes hepatic oxygen delivery while minimizing pertubations in cardiopulmonary function is desirable. Although this may not be so important for peripheral and minor surgery, when the impact of operation on splanchnic blood flow is minimal, anesthetic choice may be crucial for hepatic function if major portal triad surgery is planned. Isoflurane, fentanyl, or sufentanil can be recommended for anesthetic management because they seem to preserve cardiac output and hepatic oxygen supply-and-demand relationships and adequate oxygenation and ventilation. In patients with preexisting hepatic disease, general anesthesia, either balanced or inhalation, as well as spinal anesthesia have all been used with some degree of success. Aggressive monitoring of the circulation should be planned if a major operation is scheduled, and the anesthesiologist should be ready for rapid treatment of acute hypovolemia. A patient with normal hepatic function may tolerate hepatic hypoperfusion without deleterious effects, but the chronic alcoholic or a patient recovering from infectious hepatitis may not tolerate periods of hepatic hypoperfusion as liver blood flow and autoregulation may already be compromised.

Treatment of hepatic injury is usually symptomatic as it would be for any patient with hepatic dysfunction. A thorough search must be made for any reversible cause of hepatic injury. Percutaneous liver biopsy may identify the pathogen or at least document the type of liver injury. Sources of sepsis should be sought and treated. All drugs must be examined for hepatotoxic potential and withdrawn if suspect. If possible, delineation of hepatocellular from cholestatic dysfunction may be useful not only to determine the cause, but also the prognosis. If halothane hepatitis is suspect, corticosteroid therapy may be useful,[116] but others have used corticosteroids, plasmapheresis, and cyclophosphamide with no obvious beneficial effect.[117]

VI. SUMMARY

The incidence of postoperative liver dysfunction varies as a function of diverse patient populations and differing criteria for the diagnosis of hepatic injury and dysfunction. Mild changes in liver function tests occur after almost all major operations. Approximately 20% of patients who receive a halothane anesthetic develop minor changes in liver function. Jaundice after major operations is common secondary to blood transfusion and reabsorption of surgical hematomas. Although current surgical mortality may approach 2%, the risk of halothane hepatitis does not exceed 1 in 10,000 anesthetic instillations (0.01%), and the incidence may be

Table 18-7. Clinical details and results of biochemical tests in seven children with halothane hepatitis

Case number	Age (years)	Sex	Last operation	Number of halothane exposures	Bilirubin (mg%) (normal <15)	Serum aspartate transaminase (IU/L) (normal <40)	Halothane antibody	Outcome
1	13	F	Ureterocele	3	37.2	3755	+	Alive
2	1½	F	Scar removal	3	Not assessed	>1500	+	Alive
3	1	M	Fistula repair	6	21.4	5080	+	Alive
4	14	F	Orthopedic repair	3	30.0	4000	+	Alive
5	15	F	Orthopedic manipulation	2	21.5	1005	+	Alive
6	3½	M	Hypospadias	3	86.1	960	+	Died
7	4	M	Orthopedic repair	2	9.3	3120	−	Alive

From Kenna JG, Neuberger J, Mieli-Vergani G, et al: Br Med J 294:1210, 1987.

even lower. The incidence of postoperative jaundice from a preoperatively acquired viral infection is probably 1 of 2500. Therefore the diagnosis of anesthetic-induced postoperative hepatic dysfunction can be a diagnosis of exclusion because no reliable tests are currently available to document halothane hepatitis.

There seem to be several risk factors that predispose certain patients to the development of the fatal form of halothane hepatitis. Middle-aged, obese females seem to be at higher risk for the development of this very uncommon syndrome. Interestingly enough, halothane hepatitis has been most commonly seen after short anesthetics with only brief halothane exposure. If one definitive risk factor were to be identified, it would probably be a recent (within 28 days) exposure to halothane, which has been recorded in 80% of patients by Inman and Mushin.[118] Fever or unexplained jaundice after a previous halothane anesthetic is probably a contraindication to another halothane anesthetic. Children have long been considered to be immune from halothane hepatitis, but several cases that are highly suspect because no other risk factors were identified have been reported. Table 18-7 characterizes seven children who developed halothane hepatitis. Still, the inherent safety of halothane for pediatric anesthesia outweighs the risks of using the drug. Should a child receive halothane within a month of receiving a prior halothane anesthetic? A difficult question, but the answer might be yes, if one considers the other significant benefits of halothane when anesthetizing children. Family history of liver dysfunction after a prior halothane anesthetic may identify at-risk children.

Should halothane be avoided because of medicolegal problems associated with use of the drug? If one malpractice claim resulted in a $500,000 loss after a halothane anesthetic and one anesthetic with isoflurane costs $5 per hour, the wise financial decision would be to use only isoflurane because it would cost approximately $15 per anesthetic to pay for the loss in consideration of a maximum incidence of 1 of 30,000 cases.[119]

Enflurane, isoflurane, and N_2O have been accused of causing hepatitis but only by association. All current evidence seems to indicate that these agents are completely free of hepatotoxicity. All three of these drugs are minimally biotransformed, are relatively insoluble, and do not undergo reductive metabolism. The oxidative metabolites are also benign, though there is suspicion that halothane metabolite antibodies recognize enflurane metabolite antigens. Definite conclusions are not available at present. It is important to keep in mind that although the incidence of halothane hepatitis increased yearly after introduction of the drug (possibly because of an ever-enlarging pool of sensitized patients), such an increase has not occurred with enflurane.

The immune theory of halothane hepatitis appears to offer an explanation for many of the cases of halothane hepatitis, but liver dysfunction occurs not only after halothane anesthesia, but also after other types of anesthetics. Although halothane probably causes the most profound derangement of hepatic circulation and oxygen-demand ratios of all the anesthetic drugs, its influence is probably only a modifying one when compared to the effects of surgical stress, especially during laparotomy. All anesthetics decrease portal blood flow as cardiac output decreases, and although hepatic arterial flow may increase, the net result is usually decreased total hepatic blood flow during anesthesia. Whether this decrease in total hepatic blood flow plays a role in postoperative hepatic dysfunction, 20% of patients exposed to halothane develop abnormal liver function tests postoperatively. Animal models consistently develop postanesthetic liver dysfunction when liver metabolism is artificially enhanced and hypoxic gas mixtures are used. Some animals develop liver dysfunction without enzyme induction or hypoxia, but experimental conditions often allow spontaneous ventilation while nothing is done to ensure adequate systemic perfusion, thus leading to the possibility of inadequate hepatic perfusion.

REFERENCES

1. Eger EI: Anesthetic-induced hepatitis, International Anesthesia Research Society Review Course Lectures, Cleveland, Ohio, 1986, p 116.
2. Neuberger J and Williams R: Halothane anaesthesia anesthesia and liver damage, Br Med J 289:1136-1139, 1984.
3. Neuberger J: Halothane hepatitis. Institute for Scientific Information Atlas of science: Pharmacology 309-313, 1988, and Halothane hepatitis, Dig Dis 6:52-64, 1988.
4. Trowell J, Peto R, and Campton-Smith A: Controlled trial of repeated halothane hepatitis in patients of the uterine cervix treated with radium, Lancet 1:824-827, 1975.
5. Wright R et al: A controlled prospective study of the effect on liver function of multiple exposures to halothane, Lancet 1:824-827, 1975.
6. Fee JPH et al: A prospective study of liver enzyme and other changes following repeat administration of halothane and enflurane, Br J Anaesth 51:1133-1141, 1979.
7. Sherman M et al: Radioimmunoassay of human ligandin, Hepatology 3:162-169, 1983.
8. Allan LG et al: Hepatic glutathione S-transferase re-

lease after halothane anaesthesia: open randomized comparison with isoflurane, Lancet 1:771, 1987.

9. Nomura F et al: Effects of anticonvulsant agents on halothane-induced liver injury in human subjects and experimental animals, Hepatology 6:952-956, 1986.

10. Van Dyke RA: Metabolism of volatile anesthetics. III. Induction of microsomal dechlorinating and ether-cleaving enzymes, J Pharmacol Exp Ther 154:364-369, 1966.

11. Neuberger J and Williams R: Halothane anaesthesia and liver damage, Br Med J 289:1136, 1984.

12. Touloukian J and Kaplowitz N: Halothane-induced hepatic disease, Semin Liver Dis 1(2):134-142, 1981.

13. Brown BR and Gandolfi AJ: Adverse effects of volatile anaesthetics, Br J Anaesth 59:14-23, 1987.

14. Carmichael FJ: Mechanism of liver necrosis in hyperthyroid rats, Anesthesiology 59:591, 1983.

15. Lunam CA, Cousins MJ, and Hall P de la M: Guinea-pig model of halothane-associated hepatotoxicity in the absence of enzyme induction and hypoxia, J Pharmacol Exp Ther 232:802-809, 1985.

16. Gelman S, Fowler KC, and Smith LR: Liver circulation and function during isoflurane and halothane anesthesia, Anesthesiology 61:726-730, 1984.

17. See ref. 16.

18. Gelman S: Halothane hepatoxicity—again? Anesth Analg 65:831-834, 1986.

19. Gelman S and Van Dyke R: Mechanism of halothane-induced hepatotoxicity: another step on a long path, Anesthesiology 68:479-482, 1988.

20. Brown BR and Gandolfi AJ: Adverse effects of volatile anesthetics, Br J Anaesth 59:20, 1987.

21. Gelman S: Halothane hepatotoxicity—again? Anesth Analg 65:831-834, 1986.

22. Touloukian J and Kaplowitz N: Halothane-induced hepatitis, Semin Liver Dis 1(2):134, 1981.

23. Inman WHW and Mushin WW: Jaundice after repeated exposure to halothane: an analysis of reports to the Committee on Safety of Medicines, Br Med J 21:5, 1974.

24. Bottinger LE, Dalen E, and Hallen B: Halothane-induced liver damage: an analysis of the material reported to the Swedish Adverse Drug Reaction Committee 1966-1973, Acta Anaesthesiol Scand 20:40, 1976.

25. Schemel WH: Unexpected hepatic dysfunction found by multiple laboratory screening, Anesth Analg 55:810, 1976.

26. Wataneeyawech M and Kelly KA: Hepatic diseases—unsuspected before surgery, NY State J Med 75:1278-1281, 1975.

27. Summary of the National Halothane Study, JAMA 197:775, 1966.

28. Morley TJ: Halothane hepatitis, JAMA 225:1659, 1973.

29. Douglas HJ et al: Halothane hepatic necrosis associated with viral infection after enflurane anesthesia, N Engl J Med 296:553, 1977.

30. Neuberger J and Williams R: Halothane anaesthesia and liver damage, Br Med J 289:1136, 1984.

31. Halothane-associated liver damage, Lancet 1:1251-1252, 1986 (Editorial).

32. Kenna JG et al: Halothane hepatitis in children, Br Med J 294:1209-1210, 1987.

33. Neuberger J and Williams R: Halothane anaesthesia and liver damage, Br Med J 289: 1136-1139, 1984.

34. Mushin WW, Rosen M, and Jones EB: Post-halothane jaundice in relation to previous administration of halothane, Br Med J 3:18, 1971.

35. Biermann JS et al: Metabolism of halothane in obese Fischer 344 rats, Anesthesiology 71:431-437, 1989.

36. Brown BR Jr and Gandolfi AJ: Adverse effects of volatile anaesthetics, Br J Anaesth 59:14, 1987.

37. Hoft RH et al: Halothane hepatitis in three pairs of closely related women, N Engl J Med 304:1023-1024, 1981.

38. Otsuka S et al: HLA antigens in patients with unexplained hepatitis following halothane anesthesia, Acta Anaesthesiol Scand 29:497-501, 1985.

39. Brown BR Jr: General anesthetics and hepatic toxicity, Ariz Med 34:5, 1977.

40. Nomura F et al: Halothane hepatotoxicity and reductive metabolism of halothane in acute experimental liver injury in rats, Anesth Analg 67:448-452, 1988.

41. Cousins MJ, Plummer JLW, and Hall PM: Toxicity of volatile anaesthetic agents, Can Anaesth Soc J 32:S52-S55, 1985.

42. Gelman S: Halothane hepatotoxicity—again? Anesth Analg 65:831-834, 1986.

43. Stock JGL and Strunin L: Unexplained hepatitis following halothane, Anesthesiology 63:424-439, 1985.

44. Gelman S: General anesthesia and hepatic circulation, Can J Physiol Pharmacol 65:1762-1779, 1987.

45. Gelman S and Van Dyke R: Mechanism of halothane-induced hepatotoxicity: another step on a long path, Anesthesiology 68:479, 1988.

46. Van Dyke RA and Madson TH: Stimulation of phosphorylase activity by volatile anesthetics in isolated rat hepatocytes, Fed Proc 45:699, 1986.

47. Fujiwara M et al: Clinical significance of eosinophilia in the diagnosis of halothane-induced liver injury, Acta Med Okayama 38:35-40, 1984.

48. Hubbard AK et al: Halothane hepatitis patients generate an antibody response toward a covalently bound metabolite of halothane, Anesthesiology 68:791-796, 1988.

49. Neuberger J: Halothane and the liver—the present situation, J Clin Pharm Therap 12:269-271, 1987.

50. Varma RR, Whitesell RC, and Iskandarani MM: Halothane hepatitis without halothane: role of inapparent circuit contamination and its prevention, Hepatology 5:1159-1162, 1985.

51. Klatskin G and Kimberg KV: Recurrent hepatitis attributable to halothane sensitization in an anesthetist, N Engl J Med 280:515, 1969.

52. Eger EI et al: Is enflurane hepatotoxic? Anesth Analg 65:21-30, 1986.

53. Callis AH, Gandolfi AJ, Roth TP, et al: Circulating anti-halothane antibodies in patients with unexplained hepatitis following halothane exposure, Anesthesiology 65:A235, 1986.

54. Hals J et al: Halothane-associated liver damage and renal failure in a young child, Acta Anaesthesiol Scand 30:651-655, 1986.

55. Martin JL, Kenna JG, and Pohl LR: Antibody assays for the detection of patients sensitized to halothane, Anesth Analg 70:154-159, 1990.

56. Neuberger J et al: Specific serological markers in the diagnosis of fulminant hepatic failure associated with halothane anaesthesia, Br J Anaesth 55:15-18, 1983.

57. Kenna JG, Neuberger J, and Williams R: Specific antibodies to halothane-induced liver antigens in halothane-associated hepatitis, Br J Anaesth 59:1286-1290, 1987.

58. Hubbard AK, Roth TP, and Gandolfi AJ: Elicitation of a cell-mediated immune response to a reactive intermediate of halothane, Toxicologist 8:12, 1988.

59. Martin JL, Kenna JG, and Pohl LR: Antibody assays for the detection of patients sensitized to halothane, Anesth Analg 70:154-159, 1990.

60. Stock JGL and Stunin L: Unexplained hepatitis following halothane, Anesthesiology 63:424, 1985.

61. Lewis JH et al: Enflurane hepatotoxicity: a clinico-pathologic study of 24 cases, Ann Intern Med 98:984-992, 1983.

62. Eger EI et al: Is enflurane hepatotoxic? Anesth Analg 65:21-30, 1986.

63. Chase RE, Holaday DA, Fiserova-Bergerova V, et al: The biotransformation of ethrane in man, Anesthesiology 35:262-267, 1972.

64. Christ DD et al: Enflurane metabolism produces covalently bound liver adducts recognized by antibodies from patients with halothane hepatitis, Anesthesiology 69:833-838, 1988.

65. Holaday DA et al: Resistance of isoflurane to biotransformation in man, Anesthesiology 43:325, 1975.

66. Gelman S, Dillard E, and Bradley DL: Hepatic circulation during surgical stress and anesthesia with halothane, isoflurane, or fentanyl, Anesthesiology 66:936-943, 1987.

67. Gil F, Fiserova-Bergerova V, and Altman N: Hepatic protection from chemical injury by isoflurane, Anesth Analg 67:860-867, 1988.

68. Baden J: Hepatotoxicity and metabolism of isoflurane in rats with cirrhosis, Anesth Analg 68:214-218, 1989.

69. Van Dyke RA: Hepatic centrilobular necrosis in rats after exposure to halothane, enflurane or isoflurane, Anesth Analg 61:812-819, 1982.

70. Carrigan TW and Straughen WJ: A report of hepatic necrosis and death following isoflurane anesthesia, Anesthesiology 67:581-583, 1987.

71. Stoelting RK et al: Hepatic dysfunction after isoflurane anesthesia, Anesth Analg 66:147-153, 1987.

72. Eger EI et al: Studies of the toxicity of I-653, halothane, and isoflurane in enzyme-induced, hypoxic rats, Anesth Analg 66:1227-1229, 1987.

73. Zinn SE, Fairley B, and Glenn JD: Liver function in patients with mild alcoholic hepatitis after enflurane, nitrous oxide–narcotic, and spinal anesthesia, Anesth Analg 64:487-490, 1985.

74. Ross JA, Monk SA, and Duffy SW: Nitrous oxide increases halothane hepatotoxicity in the hypoxic rat model, Br J Anaesth 55:1162P, 1983.

75. Lumb N et al: The effect of nitrous oxide inactivation of vitamin B_{12} on rat hepatic folate: implications for the methylfolate-trap hypothesis, Biochem J 186:933-936, 1980.

76. Cohen EN et al: Occupational disease in dentistry and chronic exposure to trace anesthetic gases, J Am Dent Assoc 101:21-31, 1980.

77. Clarke RSJ, Doggart JR, and Lavery T: Changes in liver function after different types of surgery, Br J Anaesth 48:119-128, 1976.

78. Clarke RSJ et al: Clinical studies of induction agents. XIII: Liver function after propanidid and thiopentone anaesthesia, Br J Anaesth 37:415-421, 1965.

79. Dundee JW: Thiopentone as a factor in the production of liver dysfunction, Br J Anaesth 27:14, 1955.

80. Dundee JW et al: Changes in serum enzyme levels following ketamine infusions, Anaesthesia 35:12-16, 1980.

81. Gelman S: Anesthesia and the liver. In Barash PG, Cullen BF, and Stoelting RK, editors: Clinical anesthesia, Philadelphia, 1989, JB Lippincott Co.

82. Sear JW, Prys-Roberts C, and Dye A: Hepatic function after anaesthesia for major vascular reconstructive surgery: a comparison of four anaesthetic techniques, Br J Anaesth 55:606, 1983.

83. Sear JW: Toxicity of i.v. anaesthetics, Br J Anaesth 59:24, 1987.

84. Arguelles JE et al: Intrabiliary pressure changes produced by narcotic drugs and inhalation anesthetics in guinea pigs, Anesth Analg 58:120, 1979.

85. Needham WP et al: Liver damage from narcotics in mice, Toxicol Appl Pharmacol 58:157-170, 1981.

86. Bynum TE, Boitnott JK, and Maddrey WC: Ischemic hepatitis, Dig Dis Sci 24:129-135, 1979.

87. Gibson PR and Dudley FJ: Ischemic hepatitis: clinical features, diagnosis and prognosis, Aust N Z J Med 14:822-825, 1984.

88. Gelman S, Fowler K, and Smith LR: Liver circulation and function during isoflurane and halothane anesthesia, Anesthesiology 61:726-730, 1984.

89. Gelman S: Effects of anesthetics on splanchnic circulation. In Altura BM and Halevy S, editors: Cardiovascular action of anesthetics and drugs used in anesthesia, Basel, 1986, S. Karger AG.

90. McNeill JR and Pang CC: Effect of pentobarbital anesthesia and surgery on the control of arterial pressure and mesenteric resistance in cats: role of vasopressin and angiotensin, Can J Physiol Pharmacol 60:363, 1982.

91. Harper MH et al: Postanesthetic hepatic injury in rats: influence of alterations in hepatic blood flow, surgery, and anesthesia time, Anesth Analg 61:79, 1982.

92. Clarke RSJ, Doggar JR, and Lavery T: Changes in liver function after different types of surgery, Br J Anaesth 48:119, 1976.

93. Viegas O and Stoelting RK: LDH_5 changes after cholecystectomy or hysterectomy in patients receiving halothane, enflurane, or fentanyl, Anesthesiology 51:556, 1979.

94. Aranha GV and Greenlee HB: Intra-abdominal surgery in patients with advanced cirrhosis, Arch Surg 121:275, 1986.

95. Powell-Jackson P, Greenway B, and Williams R: Adverse effects of exploratory laparotomy in patients with unsuspected liver disease, Br J Surg 69:449-451, 1982.

96. Friedman LS and Maddrey WC: Surgery in the patient with liver disease, Med Clin North Am 71:454, 1987.

97. Maddrey WC: Alcoholic hepatitis. In Williams R and Maddrey WC, editors: Liver, London, 1984, Butterworth & Co.

98. Bloch RS, Allaben RD, and Walt AJ: Cholecystectomy in patients with cirrhosis: a surgical challenge, Arch Surg 120:669-672, 1985.

99. Brown MW and Burk RF: Development of intractable ascites following upper abdominal surgery in patients with cirrhosis, Am J Med 80:879-883, 1986.

100. Douglas HJ et al: Hepatic necrosis associated with viral infection after enflurane anesthesia, N Engl J Med 296:553-555, 1977.

101. Scully RE et al: Case records of the Massachusetts General Hospital, N Engl J Med 322:318-325, 1990.

102. Brechot C et al: Hepatitis B virus DNA in patients with chronic liver disease and negative tests for hepatitis B surface antigen, N Engl J Med 312:270-276, 1985.

103. Schemel WH: Unexpected hepatic dysfunction found by multiple laboratory screening, Anesth Analg 55:810-812, 1976.

104. Wataneeyawech M and Kelly KA: Hepatic diseases unsuspected before surgery, NY State J Med 75:1278-1281, 1975.

105. Dienstag JL: Non-A,non-B hepatitis. I. Recognition, epidemiology, and clinical features, Gastroenterology 85:439-462, 1985.

106. Dossing M and Andreasen PB: Drug-induced liver disease in Denmark, Scand J Gastroenterology 17:205-211, 1982.

107. Neuberger J: Halothane and the liver—the present situation, J Clin Pharm Therap 12:269-271, 1987.
108. Nomura F et al: Effects of anticonvulsant agents on halothane-induced liver injury in human subjects and experimental animals, Hepatology 6:952-956, 1986.
109. Gilman AG et al: The pharmacological basis of therapeutics, ed 7, New York, 1985, MacMillan Publishing Co.
110. Brown BR: Anesthesia in hepatic and biliary tract disease, Philadelphia, 1988, FA Davis Co.
111. Gelman S: Carbon dioxide and hepatic circulation, Anesth Analg 69:149-151, 1989.
112. James FM, Wheeler AS, and Dewan DM: Obstetric anesthesia: the complicated patient, Philadelphia, 1988, FA Davis Co.
113. Schmid M, Hefti ML, Gattiker R, et al: A benign postoperative intrahepatic cholestasis, N Engl J Med 272:545, 1965.
114. Maze M and Baden JM: Anesthesia for patients with liver disease. In Miller R, editor: Anesthesia, New York, 1986, Churchill Livingstone.
115. Varma RR, Whitesell RC, and Iskandarani MM: Halothane hepatitis without halothane: role of inapparent circuit contamination and its prevention, Hepatology 5:1159-1162, 1985.
116. Moore DH and Benson GD: Prolonged halothane hepatitis—prompt resolution of severe lesion with corticosteroid therapy, Dig Dis Sci 31:1269-1272, 1986.
117. Neuberger J and Williams R: Halothane hepatitis, Dig Dis Sci 6:52-64, 1988.
118. Inman WHW and Mushin WW: Jaundice after repeated exposure to halothane: an analysis of reports to the Committee on Safety on Medicines, Br Med J 1:5-10, 1974.
119. Taylor MS and Lack JA: Letter to the editor, Br Med J 293:335, 1986.

Chapter 19

Hypovolemia and Renal Dysfunction

Donald S. Prough
Gary Zaloga

ABBREVIATIONS

ADH	Antidiuretic hormone
ANH	Atrial natriuretic hormone
ARF	Acute renal failure
BUN	Blood urea nitrogen
Cao$_2$	Systemic oxygen transport
CAVH	Continuous arteriovenous hemofiltration

CAVHD	Continuous arteriovenous hemodialysis
C$_B$	Concentration of solute in blood
CCr	Creatinine clearance
C$_D$	Concentration of solute in dialysate
CO	Cardiac output
CVP	Central venous pressure
D	Diffusion coefficient of the membrane
D5W	5% dextrose in water

ECF	Extracellular fluid	P_{BC}	Bowman's capsule hydraulic pressure
ECV	Extracellular volume	PEEP	Positive end-expiratory pressure
FENa	Fractional excretion of sodium	P_{GC}	Glomerular capillary hydraulic pressure
FF	Filtration fraction	π_{GC}	Bowman's capsule plasma oncotic
Fio_2	Fractional inspired concentration of		pressure
	oxygen	PGE_2	Prostaglandin E_2
GFR	Glomerular filtration rate	PGI_2	Prostacyclin
ICU	Intensive care unit	Pio_2	Inspiratory pressure of oxygen
ICV	Intracellular volume	P_{onc}	Plasma oncotic pressure
IF	Interstitial fluid	P_{tm}	Transmembrane hydrostatic pressure
J_s	Solute flux		gradient
K	Filtration characteristics of membrane	PV	Plasma volume
K_f	Glomerular filtration coefficient	Q_f	Flow of filtrate
LRS	Lactated Ringer's solution	RBF	Renal blood flow
NOARF	Nonoliguric acute renal failure	RE	Respiratory excretion
NSAIDs	Nonsteroidal anti-inflammatory drugs	SCr	Serum clearance
Pao_2	Arterial oxygen tension	TBW	Total body water
P_{AO_2}	Alveolar oxygen tension	Tx	Thromboxane
PAOP	Pulmonary artery occlusion pressure	UNa	Urinary sodium concentration

I. INCIDENCE OF PERIOPERATIVE RENAL FAILURE

Acute renal failure (ARF) represents an abrupt reduction of renal function, with or without oliguria, resulting in retention of nitrogenous waste products. Perioperative ARF, which accounts for one half of all patients who require acute dialysis,[1] is associated with a mortality exceeding 50%.[2-4] Although the incidence of perioperative ARF has gradually declined, the mortality has remained similar for 30 years.[2,3,5-8] Even intensive dialytic therapy, once believed to improve outcome in comparison to less aggressive dialysis,[9] appears to produce no significant benefit in patients with ARF.[6]

Acute elevation of blood urea nitrogen (BUN) and creatinine occurs in approximately 5% of all general hospital admissions and in up to 20% of intensive care unit (ICU) patients. After nonemergent surgery, 23% of patients demonstrate an increase in serum creatinine of 20% or greater.[10] Eleven percent experience at least 11% decrease in creatinine clearance measured 4 to 5 days postoperatively.[10] In traumatized patients, the risk of ARF increases as the severity and number of injuries increase. Cardiovascular surgery (that is, cardiac valve replacement, myocardial revascularization, and aortic aneurysm repair) is now the primary cause of ARF.[11] Vascular surgical procedures threaten renal perfusion in several ways. First, vascular procedures often involve extensive tissue manipulation, substantial loss of plasma volume into the interstitium, and variable, sometimes massive, hemorrhage. Aortic and renal vascular procedures also produce frank renal

ischemia or disturbed renal hemodynamics[12,13] because of suprarenal or infrarenal aortic cross-clamping or temporary occlusion of the renal arteries.

In patients who undergo thoracic aortic cross-clamping, the incidence of ARF is 2.7% to 13.8%.[14-16] The incidence of less severe renal dysfunction is 50%.[15] In patients undergoing infrarenal aortic cross-clamping, 15% of patients develop an increase in serum creatinine of 0.5 mg·dl^{-1} or more.[17] In a series of 47 patients who developed ARF as a consequence of aortic aneurysm surgery, 79% died and only 15% regained renal function; the remainder required chronic hemodialysis.[11] Aggressive medical management of patients with ARF after repair of a ruptured abdominal aortic aneurysm has been associated with improved survival in some small series.[18] However, larger series report poor survival,[19] most commonly as a consequence of infection related to prolonged ventilatory, nutritional, and cardiovascular support.

ARF also occurs frequently in patients undergoing certain gastrointestinal procedures,[7,20] in patients with hepatic insufficiency,[21] and in patients with sepsis or volume depletion. McMurray et al.[19] reported that gastrointestinal surgery was responsible for 32% of postoperative ARF. Postoperative ARF developed in 6.8% of 103 jaundiced patients compared with 0.1% of 2353 emergency gastric surgeries, despite equal or greater degrees of hypotension.[21] Overall, volume depletion may account for at least 17% of cases of hospital-acquired ARF in surgical and medical patients.[21] Ten percent to 50% of intensive care unit patients suffering from respiratory failure, sepsis, or hepatic failure will develop ARF; the majority of those affected will succumb.

Postoperative, hemodynamically mediated ARF can be divided into three distinct patterns.[22,23] In some patients, glomerular filtration abruptly declines at the time of surgery and then promptly recovers (Fig. 19-1, *A*). In such patients, the peak increase in serum creatinine may be reached as the glomerular filtration rate (GFR) is already returning toward normal. Dialysis is rarely required. The second pattern of ARF is associated with prolonged hemodynamic insufficiency (Fig. 19-1, *B*). As hemodynamic function recovers, GFR will increase and serum creatinine will decline. The third category of ARF is highly lethal, usually developing in association with delayed septic complications, recurrent episodes of hypotension, and failure of other organ systems (Fig. 19-1, *C*). Recurrent episodes of renal ischemia may induce new renal lesions and prevent healing of existing lesions, resulting in permanent loss of renal function. Renal replacement therapy then becomes part of an escalating series of therapeutic interventions in progressively worsening, often terminal illness.

To reduce the incidence, morbidity, and mortality of ARF, the surgical team must recognize threatened renal ischemia, attempt to prevent ARF and, for patients who develop ARF, provide adequate renal replacement therapy.

II. RENAL PHYSIOLOGY
A. Physiology and pharmacology of urine formation

The kidneys perform three major functions: filtration, reabsorption, and secretion. Acute oliguria results from physiologic or pathologic alterations in renal blood flow (RBF), glomerular filtration, or tubular reabsorption. RBF equals 20% to 25% of total cardiac output (approximately 1000 to 1250 ml·min^{-1}), 10% of which is normally filtered. Therefore normal GFR is ≤125 ml·min^{-1}, equivalent to a total filtration volume ≤180 L per day (Fig. 19-2). Blood enters the glomeruli via the afferent arterioles, which arise from the renal arteries, and leaves the glomeruli via the efferent arterioles. The amount of filtrate produced depends on RBF, vascular resistance in the afferent arterioles, the resistance of the efferent arteriole (which is the primary determinant of glomerular hydrostatic pressure), glomerular capillary integrity, intratubular pressure, and oncotic pressure. Reducing glomerular filtrate to a final urinary volume of 1 to 2 L per day necessitates reabsorption of 99% of the filtered solute as it

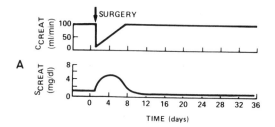

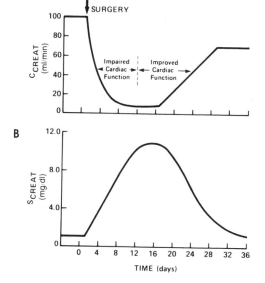

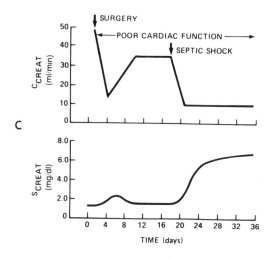

Fig. 19-1. Three patterns of hemodynamically mediated acute renal failure (ARF) occur after major trauma or surgery. **A** (Abbreviated ARF), acute reduction in creatinine clearance (C$_{Creat}$) with prompt recovery. Serum creatinine (S$_{Creat}$) may be increasing even as C$_{Creat}$ recovers. **B** (Overt ARF), concurrent, mirror-image decreases in C$_{Creat}$ and increases in S$_{Creat}$, usually in association with compromised cardiac function followed by recovery. **C** (Protracted ARF), development as a consequence of prolonged hemodynamic compromise, often complicated by systemic sepsis. (From Myers BD and Moran SM: N Engl J Med 314:97-105, 1986.)

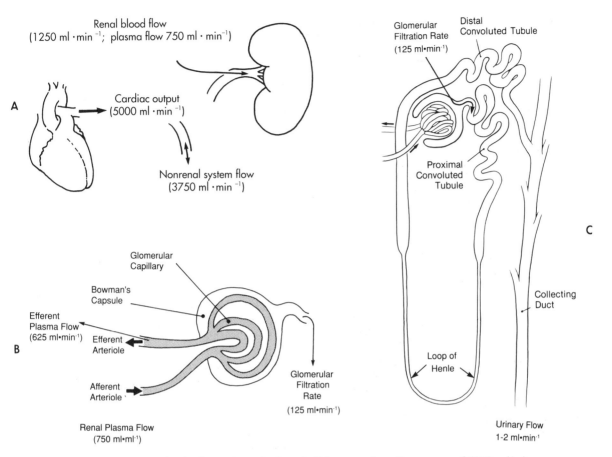

Fig. 19-2. Stages in the formation of urine. **A,** Of a normal cardiac output of 5000 ml/min, approximately 3750 ml/min is distributed to nonrenal tissue and 1250 ml/min to the kidneys. **B,** Of the total renal plasma flow of 750 ml/min, approximately 125 ml/min is filtered in the glomeruli; the remainder of renal plasma flow leaves through the efferent arterioles, together with an unchanged volume of red blood cells. **C,** After leaving Bowman's capsule, the glomerular filtrate is progressively altered by the processes of reabsorption and secretion to produce a final urinary flow of 1 to 2 ml/min.

passes through the renal tubules and collecting ducts.

B. Sodium filtration and reabsorption

The concentration of sodium in glomerular filtrate is similar to that in plasma. Roughly 65% of filtered sodium and water are reabsorbed in the proximal renal tubule. Because equal percentages are reabsorbed, the concentration of sodium remains similar throughout the proximal tubule. An increased percentage is reabsorbed during hypovolemic states. An additional 25% of filtered sodium is reabsorbed by a primary active process as the filtrate passes through the ascending limb of Henle's loop. The remaining 10% of sodium undergoes continued reabsorption in the distal tubules and collecting ducts by means of both aldosterone-dependent and aldosterone-independent processes. Only 1% of the sodium originally filtered by the glomeruli is ultimately excreted in the urine.

C. Water filtration and reabsorption

As noted above, 65% of filtered water is reabsorbed in the proximal tubule. In Henle's loop, proportionately less water than sodium is reabsorbed. Although fluid leaving the loop is isosmotic, about half of the total osmolar content consists of urea rather than sodium and chloride. The countercurrent multiplier system in Henle's loop is a critical component of renal sodium and water conservation. The vasa recta, medullary vessels arising from the efferent renal arterioles, preserve the hypertonicity of medullary interstitium. Either increases or decreases in flow within the vasa recta may diminish the gradient, as will sodium depletion and malnutrition. In addition, an increased filtrate flow rate through Henle's loop reduces renal concentrating ability; a greatly accelerated flow rate, such as that produced by the infusion of mannitol, may "wash out" the concentrating gradient. Water is reabsorbed to a variable extent in the

Table 19-1. Sodium, water, and osmolar excretion*

	Flow rate (ml·min^{-1})	[Na$^+$] (mEq·L^{-1})	Urea (mg·dl^{-1})	Osmolality (mOsm·kg^{-1})
Plasma	750	140	10	290
Filtrate	125	140	10	290
Proximal tubule	44	140	50	290
Henle's loop	25	70	50	150
Distal tubule	20	10	50	100
Final urine	2	100	250	100

Modified from Prough, DS: Perioperative management of acute renal failure. In Stoelting RK, Barash PG, and Gallagher TJ, editors: Advances in Anesthesia, 5:129-172, Chicago, 1988, Mosby–Year Book, Inc.
* All numbers refer to expected values in euvolemic, normally hydrated persons.

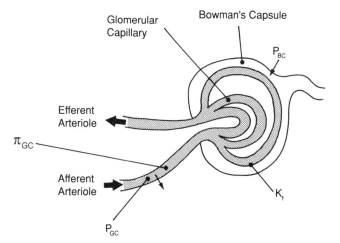

Fig. 19-3. The afferent arteriole enters the glomerular capillary tuft; the efferent arteriole carries blood away from the glomerular capillary tuft. Filtration through the glomerulus is a function of the glomerular filtration coefficient (K_f), the hydrostatic pressure within the glomerular capillaries (P_{GC}), the opposing hydrostatic pressure within Bowman's capsule (P_{BC}), and the oncotic pressure within the glomerular capillary (π_{GC}). Constriction of the afferent arteriole will reduce P_{GC}; constriction of the efferent arteriole will tend to increase P_{GC} by restricting exiting flow. An increase in π_{GC} will oppose filtration; a decrease in π_{GC} will enhance filtration.

distal tubules, cortical collecting tubules, and medullary collecting ducts. This reabsorption depends primarily on the presence of antidiuretic hormone (ADH). A summary of the stages of urine formation and sodium excretion is presented in Table 19-1.

D. Physiologic control of glomerular filtration and solute reabsorption

The physiologic factors that determine GFR include the glomerular filtration coefficient (K_f), which is the product of glomerular membrane permeability and surface area, the glomerular capillary hydraulic pressure (P_{GC}), the hydraulic pressure in Bowman's capsule (P_{BC}), and the plasma oncotic pressure (π_{GC}), according to the equation:[24]

$$GFR = K_f \times (P_{GC} - P_{BC} - \pi_{GC})$$

P_{GC} is subject to the greatest physiologic variation. P_{GC} and RBF are determined by inflow resistance and outflow resistance. The P_{GC} will decline if the resistance in the afferent arterioles (the arterioles leading to the glomerulus) increases *or* if resistance in the efferent arterioles decreases (Fig. 19-3). Conversely, a decrease in afferent arteriolar resistance or an increase in efferent arteriolar resistance will increase P_{GC}. The renin-angiotensin and prostaglandin systems alter afferent and efferent resistance to maintain RBF at similar levels over a range of renal perfusion pressure of 80 to 160 mm Hg.[25] Sympathetic nervous system activation and high levels of circulating catecholamines can induce afferent arteriolar constriction that overrides autoregulatory mechanisms and decreases cortical perfusion and GFR.[25] However, afferent arteriolar constriction reduces GFR less than RBF because efferent arteriolar vasoconstriction supports P_{GC} and enhances the filtration fraction (FF), according to the equations:

$$GFR = \text{Afferent arteriolar plasma flow} - \\ \text{Efferent arteriolar plasma flow}$$

$$FF = \frac{\text{Afferent arteriolar plasma flow} - \text{Efferent arteriolar plasma flow}}{\text{Afferent arteriolar plasma flow}} \times 100$$

III. REGULATION OF EXTRACELLULAR FLUID VOLUME

Alterations in extracellular fluid (ECF) volume result in parallel changes in plasma volume. Thus the primary monitors of ECF volume are located within the vascular system. The body protects ECF volume by controlling the secretion of sodium and water.

A. Afferent limb of ECF volume control

Low-pressure intrathoracic volume receptors are located within the cardiac atria, great veins, cardiac ventricles, and pulmonary capillaries.[26] Since 85% of circulating blood volume resides within the high-compliance venous system, these receptors are of primary importance for detecting decreases in intravascular and ECF volume. Stimulation of atrial stretch receptors by volume expansion results in the release of atrial natriuretic hormone (ANH) and natriuresis. High-pressure arterial receptors are found within the carotid sinuses, aortic arch, and intrarenal arterioles. These receptors, relatively insensitive to small changes in intravascular volume, act to preserve perfusion when blood pressure is already decreased. Stimulation of these high-pressure arterial receptors by volume overload induces natriuresis. Intrarenal baroreceptors cause renin release in response to decreased renal perfusion pressure. Renin increases the production of angiotensin and aldosterone. These hormones increase blood pressure, increase afferent glomerular arteriolar tone (decreasing renal blood flow), and stimulate sodium reabsorption. The renal baroreceptors also stimulate natriuresis in response to increased perfusion pressure.

B. Efferent limb of ECF volume control

Adequate circulating blood volume is essential for maintenance of organ perfusion and survival. Afferent signals are converted to efferent signals, which serve to maintain ECF volume and vital organ perfusion.[26] Activation of the sympathetic nervous system, renin-angiotensin-aldosterone axis, ADH secretion, and suppression of ANH release serve to increase systemic vascular resistance and conserve sodium and water during volume depletion. Thirst and salt craving are activated in an attempt to increase intake. Aldosterone also decreases salt loss in sweat. Insufficiency of these systems or the use of pharmacologic antagonists may aggravate hypovolemic states.

C. Renal response to ECF volume depletion

Under normal conditions, RBF remains constant (that is, autoregulates) over a wide range of perfusion pressure. However, RBF decreases when perfusion pressure decreases below the autoregulatory range. In addition, autoregulation may be diminished or lost during acute hypovolemia.[26-28] An increase in renal vascular resistance during acute hypovolemia may result from secretion of alpha-adrenergic catecholamines[29] and angiotensin II and from renal sympathetic stimulation. RBF during acute hypovolemia is determined by a balance among opposing factors: intrinsic renal autoregulatory capacity, the vasodilatory capacity of prostaglandins to maintain RBF, and the ability of the renal sympathetic nerves, angiotensin II, and catecholamines to decrease RBF.[30] In addition to changes in total RBF, hypovolemia also changes the intrarenal distribution of perfusion. There is a redistribution of blood from outer cortical nephrons to inner cortical nephrons,[26] which have longer loops of Henle and tend to conserve more sodium and thus protect circulating blood volume.

GFR may be either maintained or decreased in the setting of volume depletion. As noted above, GFR depends on glomerular plasma flow, P_{GC}, π_{GC}, and glomerular capillary ultrafiltration. During hypovolemia, plasma flow decreases but filtration pressure tends to increase secondary to increase efferent arteriolar resistance, thereby serving to increase the FF.

The kidney responds to ECF volume depletion by retaining water and salt. Reabsorption of filtered water and sodium is heavily influenced by the hormonal factors ADH, ANH, and the renal prostaglandins (Fig. 19-4). Diminished water excretion is accomplished by ADH-dependent and ADH-independent mechanisms. ADH secretion from the posterior pituitary responds both to changing osmolarity and to changing intravascular volume. ADH is released in response to stimulation of the hypothalamic osmoreceptors by increased blood osmolarity. A 1% to 2% change in osmolality significantly alters ADH secretion. ADH release is stimulated by decreased stretch of the atrial baroreceptors. However, the ADH response to volume depletion is less sensitive than the response to changes in osmolality. A 10% to 20% decrease in blood volume is necessary to stimulate ADH secretion. ADH acts primarily on the medullary collecting ducts and to a lesser extent on the cortical collecting tubules, to increase water permeability, resulting in greater water reabsorption and the excretion of smaller volumes of more highly concentrated urine. Urinary volume may vary a hundredfold, depending on ADH concentration (Table 19-2). Water excretion is further reduced in volume-depleted patients by impaired delivery of tubular fluid to distal nephron sites and by ADH-inde-

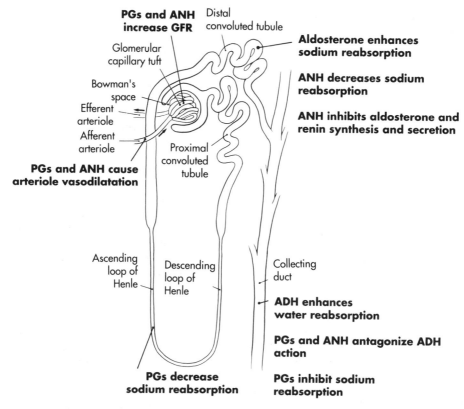

Fig. 19-4. Important neuroendocrine modifiers of glomerular and tubular function include aldosterone, antidiuretic hormone (ADH), atrial natriuretic hormone (ANH), and the renal prostaglandins (PGs). The primary sites of action include the afferent and efferent arterioles, glomerular filtration, loop of Henle, the distal convoluted tubule, and the collecting ducts (ADH). GFR, Glomerular filtration rate.

Table 19-2. Renal effects of antidiuretic hormone (ADH)

	Urinary flow rate (ml·min^{-1})	[Na$^+$] (mEq·L^{-1})	Urea (mg·dl^{-1})	Osmolality (mOsm·kg^{-1})
Euvolemic, young adult	2.0	100	250	300
Maximal ADH secretion	0.2	300	1000	1200
Minimal ADH secretion	20	10	50	50

pendent water reabsorption by the collecting ducts.

In volume-depleted states, sodium conservation results both from decreased filtration of sodium (decreased GFR) and from increased tubular reabsorption of sodium. The major effectors of sodium reabsorption are activation of the renin-angiotensin-aldosterone axis and suppression of ANH secretion. However, increased peritubular capillary oncotic pressure and autonomic nervous system activation also contribute to increased tubular sodium reabsorption.

Aldosterone, the most important humoral regulator of sodium reabsorption, is produced by the renal cortex as the final product of a series of endocrine events: (1) renin is released from the granular cells of the juxtaglomerular apparatus in response to activation of the sympathetic nervous system, stimulation of intrarenal baroreceptors, or reduced delivery of so-

Table 19-3. Renal effects of aldosterone secretion

	Urinary flow rate $(ml \cdot min^{-1})$	$[Na^+]$ $(mEq \cdot L^{-1})$	Urea $(mg \cdot dl^{-1})$	Osmolality $(mOsm \cdot kg^{-1})$
Euvolemic, young adult	2.0	100.0	250	300
Maximal aldosterone secretion	2.0	1.0	250	300

dium chloride to the macula densa;[31-33] (2) renin then catalyzes the release of angiotensin I from angiotensinogen (synthesized in the liver); (3) angiotensin-converting enzyme converts angiotensin I to angiotensin II; and (4) angiotensin II stimulates adrenocortical cells to synthesize and release aldosterone. Acting primarily in the distal tubules, high concentrations of aldosterone may reduce urinary concentration of sodium nearly to zero, whereas low levels of aldosterone permit excretion of urine high in sodium (Table 19-3). Table 19-3 illustrates the effects on urine composition of maximal aldosterone stimulation.

ANH is released from the cardiac atria in response to increased atrial stretch. Although its complete physiologic role has yet to be defined, ANH exerts vasodilatory effects and increases the renal excretion of sodium and water.[34-42] Many of the physiologic effects of ANH appear to be mediated by hemodynamic effects that increase GFR and thus result in diuresis. Acute sodium loading significantly increases ANH secretion; in contrast, chronic sodium loading does not significantly affect ANH levels.[35] ANH secretion is decreased during volume depletion.

The kidney also contains large quantities of prostaglandin metabolites, including PGE_2 and thromboxane A_2. These products appear to modulate the renal effects of other hormones.[43,44] For instance, the vasodilator PGE_2 decreases the contraction of glomerular mesangial cells produced by angiotensin II.[45] Vasodilatory prostaglandins are important for maintaining RBF during states of ECF volume depletion. Thromboxane A_2, in contrast, produces mesangial contraction.[45]

The kidney has a remarkable ability to perform its homeostatic functions despite substantial reductions in ECF volume. Renal adaptation to decreases in ECF volume (and cardiac output) occurs through three primary mechanisms: RBF, glomerular filtration, and tubular reabsorption.[46] Initially RBF is maintained as perfusion pressure decreases (that is, by autoregulation) by reductions in renal vascular resistance (primarily at the level of the afferent arteriole). Prostaglandins may play a crucial role in

protecting the kidney from the effects of systemic vasoconstrictor hormones and for maintaining RBF during hypovolemia. The protective effect of endogenous renal prostaglandins is emphasized by the numerous reports of ARF in patients in whom circulatory compromise was superimposed upon treatment with nonsteroidal anti-inflammatory drugs.[46] Further decreases in cardiac output may decrease the fraction of cardiac output delivered to the kidneys. Increases in renal vascular resistance shunt blood away from the kidneys in an attempt to preserve central circulating volume. This response may result in renal ischemia and the development of ARF.

The FF normally increases as ECF volume decreases. As RBF decreases, the efferent arterioles constrict, primarily in response to angiotensin II and norepinephrine. The net result is that GFR tends to be preserved despite reduced ECF volume. However, stimulation of the sympathetic nervous system and release of ADH and aldosterone increase sodium and water reabsorption.

There is a limit to the ability of these mechanisms to compensate without producing excessive vasoconstriction, decreased RBF, and renal ischemia. Postischemic ARF is usually multifactorial, and both vascular (that is, renal vasoconstriction, altered glomerular function) and tubular factors (that is, intraluminal obstruction, backleak) combine to reduce GFR. Factors that appear to enhance the risk of ARF include volume depletion, sepsis, liver failure, nephrotoxic antibiotics and other drugs, and myoglobinuria. It is also important to remember that loop diuretics (such as furosemide) may impair autoregulatory vasodilatation and sodium reabsorption during decreases in ECF volume and thus predispose to further renal ischemia.[47]

IV. PERIOPERATIVE HYPOVOLEMIA
A. Distribution of body fluid compartments

Accurate replacement of fluid deficits necessitates an understanding of the distribution spaces of water, sodium, and colloid (Fig. 19-5). Total body water (TBW), the distribution volume of sodium-free water, approximates

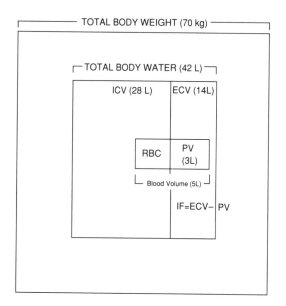

Fig. 19-5. The distribution volume of water is approximately 60% of total body weight and includes both the extracellular (ECV) and intracellular volume (ICV). Sodium is distributed primarily in the extracellular volume (ECV). If capillary integrity is preserved, the concentration of colloid is higher in the plasma volume (PV) than in interstitial fluid (IF).

60% of total body weight, or 42 L in a 70 kg person. TBW consists of intracellular volume (ICV), which constitutes 40% of total body weight (28 L in a 70 kg person), and extracellular volume (ECV), which constitutes 20% of body weight (14 L). Plasma volume (PV) equals approximately 3 L, or about one fifth of ECV. The remainder of ECV is interstitial fluid (IF). Red blood cell volume, approximately 2 L, is part of ICV.

The distribution volumes of infused fluid can be illustrated best when one considers a specific example. Assume that a 70 kg patient has suffered an acute blood loss of 2000 ml, approximately 40% of the predicted 5 L blood volume. Further assume that 5% dextrose in water (D5W), lactated Ringer's solution (LRS), 5% human serum albumin, or 25% human serum albumin, could be chosen to replace that volume. The formula describing the effects of fluid infusion on PV is as follows:

$$\text{PV increment} = \frac{\text{Volume infused} \times \text{PV}}{\text{Distribution volume}}$$

To achieve restoration of blood volume using D5W (which distributes throughout TBW), it would be necessary to administer 28 L.

$$2 \text{ L} = \frac{28 \text{ L} \times 3 \text{ L}}{42 \text{ L}}$$

where 2 L is the desired PV increment, 3 L is the normal estimated plasma volume, and 42 L = TBW in a 70 kg person.

If LRS were chosen (which distributes throughout ECV), a 2.0 L PV increment would require infusion of approximately 9.3 L.

$$2 \text{ L} = \frac{9.3 \text{ L} \times 3 \text{ L}}{14 \text{ L}}$$

where 14 L = ECV in a 70 kg person.

If 5% human serum albumin were chosen (which distributes initially only in PV), nearly all the infused volume would remain in the vascular tree, perhaps osmotically drawing additional interstitial fluid into the vascular space. If 25% human serum albumin were infused, each 100 ml would initially expand the PV by approximately 400 ml, reflecting the additional 300 ml increment in PV because of translocation of interstitial fluid.

B. Traumatic sequestration of interstitial fluid

However, replacement of acute intravascular losses also necessitates compensation for the sequestration of IF that accompanies trauma, hemorrhage, and tissue manipulation. This sequestration of fluid secondary to surgery, often called "third-space" loss,[48,49] is surprisingly extensive. Healthy subjects undergoing gastric or gallbladder surgery demonstrated a decline in ECV of approximately 1.9 L and an acute 13% decline in GFR when they received no intraoperative sodium.[48] In contrast, patients who received LRS maintained ECV and increased GFR by 10%. These data indicate that upper abdominal surgery, not involving major hemorrhage, may be associated with a 15% decline in functional ECV, the reservoir available for physiologic compensation for hypovolemia. In more extensive surgical procedures, the decline is presumably much greater. Failure to recognize and replace sequestered fluid may result in hypovolemia and hypoperfusion.

Based upon estimates of the magnitude of sequestration of fluid associated with extensive tissue manipulation, guidelines have been developed for replacement of third-space losses during high-risk surgical procedures.[50] The simplest formula provides, in addition to maintenance fluids and replacement of estimated blood loss, 4 ml·kg^{-1}·hr^{-1} for procedures involving minimal trauma, 6 ml·kg^{-1}·hr^{-1} for those involving moderate trauma, and 8 ml·kg^{-1}·hr^{-1} for those involving extreme trauma.[50]

An important corollary of third-space sequestration of fluid is the delayed mobilization and

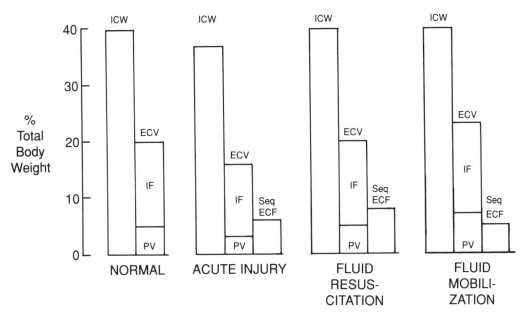

Fig. 19-6. Fluid distribution after injury. In the presence of surgical trauma, the functional extracellular volume (ECV) is diminished by sequestration of sodium and water that is unavailable to the systemic circulation. During recovery, the sequestered sodium and water is returned to the plasma volume (PV), at which time it must be excreted by the kidneys. If the cardiovascular system and kidneys cannot adequately manage the mobilized fluid, pulmonary edema may result. ECF, Extracellular fluid.

return of accumulated fluid to the ECV and the PV (Fig. 19-6). In most patients, mobilization occurs on approximately the third postoperative day, though it may occur sooner or later, depending on patient characteristics and the circumstances of the initial insult. If the cardiovascular system and kidneys can effectively transport and excrete mobilized fluid, no important physiologic consequences follow. However, should the cardiovascular system be unable to accommodate the increase in intravascular volume or the kidneys be unable to increase urinary volume (that is, because of renal insufficiency or stress-induced secretion of ADH), hypervolemia and pulmonary edema may occur.

C. Implications of perioperative administration of crystalloid and colloid fluids

As is evident from the earlier calculations, fluids containing colloids, such as albumin or hydroxyethyl starch, preferentially expand PV rather than IF. Sufficiently concentrated colloid-containing solutions translocate some IF into the PV. Intuitively, PV expansion without IF expansion offers apparent advantages: lower fluid requirements, less peripheral and pulmonary edema accumulation, and reduced concern

about delayed fluid mobilization. However, exhaustive research has failed to establish the superiority of either colloid-containing or crystalloid-containing fluids. The most commonly cited advantages of colloid solutions include a smaller initial infused volume, a more prolonged increase in PV, limited peripheral edema, and less tendency to increase intracranial pressure (Table 19-4). Crystalloid, on the other hand, is less expensive, tends to enhance GFR, and more effectively replaces third-space losses. However, each type of fluid also has disadvantages (Table 19-4). Crystalloid fluids exert more transient hemodynamic effects and, when used for massive resuscitation, inevitably produce peripheral edema. Crystalloid solutions are also associated with pulmonary edema, usually as a consequence of an increase in left atrial pressure or perhaps of a reduction of the gradient between plasma oncotic pressure and pulmonary capillary pressure.[51] The disadvantages of colloid-containing fluids include expense, possible coagulopathy (especially with dextran), a reduction in ionized calcium (with albumin), impaired crossmatching (dextran), a reduction in GFR, and osmotic diuresis. Colloid solutions have also been associated with pulmonary edema, especially in disease states associated

Table 19-4. Colloid versus crystalloid: reported advantages and disadvantages

Solution	Advantages	Disadvantages
Colloid	Smaller volume required	Expensive
	Sustained plasma volume increase	Coagulopathy (dextran > hydroxyethyl-starch)
		Pulmonary edema in capillary leak states
	Less peripheral edema	Decreased Ca^{++} (albumin)
	Lower intracranial pressure (with conflicting data)	Decreased glomerular filtration rate
		Osmotic diuresis
		Impaired cross-match (dextran)
Crystalloid	Inexpensive	Transient hemodynamic effects
	Promotes urinary flow	Peripheral edema
	Restores third-space losses	Pulmonary edema (with conflicting data)

Table 19-5. Possible end points for comparison of resuscitation fluids

End point	Advantages	Disadvantages
Equal fluid volume	Simple calculation	Different acute effects
		Different time course
Equal preload (that is, central venous pressure, pulmonary artery occlusion pressure)	Simple, continuous measurement	Determined by multiple, simultaneously changing variables
Equal cardiac output	Simple measurement, can be repeated	Misleading if fluids differentially affect hemoglobin concentration
Equal oxygen delivery	Logical, physiologically sound end point	Difficult calculation to make frequently; calculated from two simultaneously changing variables

with increased alveolar capillary permeability (that is, sepsis or adult respiratory distress syndrome).

One reason for the failure to resolve the controversy regarding the superiority of crystalloid or colloid solutions is the inability to clearly define comparable experimental end points (Table 19-5). Colloid-induced PV expansion persists longer than that produced by crystalloid. Therefore any valid comparison should take into account the necessity for additional administration of crystalloid to maintain comparable systemic hemodynamics. Even if the experimental design adjusts for the differing temporal effects, the two types of solutions exert effects on more than one variable. For instance, if sufficient LRS or 5% albumin is administered to achieve similar degrees of hemodilution, the latter solution will be associated with depression of ionized calcium, reduction of GFR, and an increase in viscosity and vascular resistance in comparison to LRS. Depending on the extent to which the multivariate changes produced by crystalloid and colloid are considered in the ex-

perimental design, studies may demonstrate apparent rather than real differences between the solutions.

D. Diagnosis of hypovolemia and tissue hypoperfusion

This section contrasts two methods of assessing the adequacy of intravascular volume. The first, conventional clinical assessment, is appropriate for most patients; the second, goal-directed therapy, may be superior for high-risk surgical patients.

1. Conventional clinical assessment of intravascular volume. The clinical ability to estimate the adequacy of intravascular volume and ECV is a critical skill. Unfortunately, although estimation of expected distribution volumes is straightforward, actual quantification of intravascular volume and ECV is difficult. Accurate quantification begins with a recognition of clinical settings in which deficits are likely. Such situations include protracted gastrointestinal losses, bowel obstruction, bowel perforation, preoperative bowel preparation, chronic hypertension, chronic diuretic use, sepsis, burns, pancreatitis, and trauma.

The physical signs of ECV depletion are relatively insensitive and nonspecific. However, suggestive evidence includes oliguria, supine hypotension, and a positive "tilt test." Supine hypotension implies a blood volume deficit exceeding 30%. However, arterial blood pressure within the normal range could represent relative hypotension in an elderly or chronically hypertensive patient. Substantial depletion of ECF volume and organ hypoperfusion may occur in patients with a normal blood pressure and heart rate.

One of the traditional methods of assessing intravascular volume depletion is the tilt test, in which a positive response is defined as an increase in heart rate exceeding 20 beats per minute and a decline in systolic blood pressure exceeding 20 mm Hg upon assumption of the upright position. However, a high incidence of false-positive and false-negative findings limits the value of the test. Of the few data that objectively examine postural changes in blood pressure, most were accumulated four or five decades ago. Shenkin et al., in 1944, subjected 18 young, healthy volunteers to an acute blood loss of 500 ml and 17 to an acute blood loss of 1000 ml.[52] In the 18 subjects bled 500 ml, the heart rate increased variably upon assumption of the upright position while blood pressure changed little. In those bled 1000 ml, the heart rate increased prominently; in most subjects, systolic blood pressure declined 10 to 30 mm Hg after 1 to 2 minutes in the upright position. In a single subject bled 1000 ml and reinfused after 24 hours, as much as 3 to 11 minutes were tolerated on repeated occasions before systolic blood pressure declined and signs of cerebral hypoperfusion developed. Therefore young, healthy subjects can withstand hemorrhage equaling 20% of blood volume while demonstrating only orthostatic tachycardia and variable orthostatic hypotension. Similar studies have not been performed in elderly persons, those with autonomic dysfunction, those on chronic hypertensive therapy, and those who have reduced cardiovascular reserve. Twenty percent to 30% of elderly subjects may demonstrate orthostatic changes in blood pressure despite normal blood volume.[53]

Recent data indicate that orthostatic changes in filling pressure, coupled with assessment of the response to fluid infusion, may represent a more sensitive test of the adequacy of circulating blood volume. Amoroso et al. recently examined changes in central venous pressure (CVP) as a function of position in a group of patients with chronic renal failure.[54] Base-line CVP, averaging 0.1 cm H_2O, declined precipitously to a mean value of -9.7 cm H_2O upon assuming a 45-degree sitting posture. Infusion of fluid resulted in a small increase in CVP to 2.3 cm H_2O but eliminated the pronounced orthostatic decline in CVP. Other signs suggestive of underlying volume depletion include improvement in urinary output, a decrease in circulating lactate levels, or an improvement in mixed venous oxygen saturation after volume infusion.

During anesthesia and surgery, a variety of readily available data permit inferential assessment of the adequacy of fluid resuscitation. Maintenance of adequate blood pressure during anesthesia with potent inhalational agents indicates that fluid administration is sufficient. However, normalization of blood pressure and heart rate following resuscitation after trauma in nonanesthetized patients may still be associated with significant organ hypoperfusion. If direct arterial pressure monitoring is employed, a prominent reduction in pulse pressure associated with positive-pressure ventilation indicates that intravascular volume may be inadequate to compensate for small changes in the resistance to venous return produced by transient increases in intrathoracic pressure.

Excluding anesthetic overdosage, profound hypotension is a specific indicator of inadequate cardiac output and therefore of inadequate fluid replacement in patients with normal left ventricular contractile function. Tachycardia, though not diagnostic of inadequate fluid replacement, is highly suggestive. However, changes in heart rate are insufficiently sensitive and specific to reflect the adequacy of volume resuscitation in most patients. Urinary output is a useful surveillance monitor of the adequacy of systemic circulation, despite limited sensitivity and specificity. Urinary output may be unreliable as a result of the use of diuretics (osmotically active substances, such as mannitol, radiocontrast dye, and glucose) and in patients with renal tubular disease. Postural changes in blood pressure and heart rate cannot be assessed easily in the operating room. In patients who have developed sufficient hypovolemia that metabolic acidosis occurs, resolution of the metabolic acidosis implies that perfusion has been substantially improved.

2. Management of perioperative perfusion using goal-directed therapy. No intraoperative monitor is sufficiently sensitive or specific to detect hypoperfusion in all patients. Moreover, certain postoperative surgical complications, such as renal failure, hepatic failure, and sepsis, may result from unrecognized, subclinical tissue hypoperfusion during the immediate perioperative period. Several important studies suggest that possibility.[55-57] Average cardiac output (CO) and systemic oxygen transport (CO × CaO_2) are greater in high-risk surgical patients who survive than in those who succumb to critical illness.[55,56] Therefore Shoemaker et al. adjusted hemodynamic therapy to achieve the higher values for CO and systemic oxygen delivery previously associated with improved survival in postsurgical patients.[57] In the first of two studies they compared conventional management of a control surgical group to a protocol that utilized hemodynamic values of previous survivors as goals for therapy. In the protocol group, in which CO and oxygen delivery were elevated above control values as guided by pulmonary artery catheterization, survival was improved and complications were reduced.[57] The control group received conventional monitors, including a central venous pressure catheter. In a second study, combined with the first study for publication, an additional control group received conventional monitoring, supplemented by pulmonary artery catheterization without specific management guidelines. As in the first series, the protocol group demonstrated improved mortality and reduced complications. The control group that underwent pulmonary artery catheterization and treatment without specific hemodynamic goals had a mortality and complication rate equal to the group managed without a pulmonary artery catheter.[57] These data indicate that aggressive, goal-directed hemodynamic support avoids clinically inapparent hypoperfusion and as a consequence limits the incidence of mortality and morbidity secondary to that process. Confirmation, however, is essential before this concept can be applied routinely.

V. SYSTEMIC AND RENAL RESPONSES TO TRAUMA, ANESTHESIA, AND HYPOVOLEMIA

The physiologic stress of trauma and surgery is associated with reduced urinary excretion of sodium and water, which occurs in response to changes in intravascular and extracellular volume and to secondary neuroendocrine effects, especially the release of ADH, catecholamines, and aldosterone.[58,59] Although anesthetics may not directly stimulate release of ADH and aldosterone, anesthetic-related changes in hemodynamic function may trigger those neuroendocrine responses. Table 19-6 summarizes the average and maximal effects of surgical stress on urinary flow, urinary sodium, and water excretion.

Anesthetic drugs may alter renal blood flow, glomerular filtration, or tubular function. Anesthetics may directly alter renal function or exert indirect effects, secondary to changes in cardiovascular function or neuroendocrine activity. Anesthetic drugs and techniques exert diverse effects on myocardial contractility, intravascular volume, regional blood flow, autonomic reflexes, coronary blood flow, vascular tone, and the response to catecholamines.[60] In high concentrations, potent inhalational anesthetics decrease myocardial contractility and reduce cardiac output. Spinal or epidural anesthesia may reduce cardiac output through sympathectomy-induced venodilatation. Either an increase or a decrease in peripheral vascular resistance may indirectly reduce RBF.

Because anesthesia interferes with compensatory hemodynamic responses, physiologic insults such as hemorrhage may produce exaggerated hemodynamic effects in comparison to the conscious state.[60] After moderate hemorrhage in anesthetized animals, there is intense peripheral vasoconstriction of renal, muscular, and mesenteric vascular beds. In conscious animals, renal vasodilatation occurs despite vasoconstriction in mesenteric and limb circulations.[60] The coronary vascular response to norepinephrine and dopamine is diminished in anesthetized animals. In addition, the inotropic response to dobutamine and dopamine is increased in anesthetized animals.[60]

Other perioperative interventions also directly and indirectly modify renal function. Mechanical ventilation and positive end-expiratory pressure (PEEP) are associated with reduced urinary output,[61] which improves in response to volume expansion.[62] Ventilation with PEEP reduces both urinary sodium excretion and plasma levels of ANH, an indication of a role of that hormone in the renal response to increased intrathoracic pressure.[63] In contrast, ADH release appears to exert little effect on renal function during ventilation with PEEP.[64]

A. Effects of inhaled anesthetics

1. Methoxyflurane. Now rarely used, methoxyflurane produces dose-dependent renal toxicity, including hyposmotic diuresis, azotemia, hypernatremia, and hyperosmolality,[65] which is mediated by inorganic fluoride ion, a methoxyflurane metabolite.[66] Clinical toxicity occurs consistently at serum inorganic fluoride levels exceeding 50 $\mu mol \cdot ml^{-1}$.[67]

2. Enflurane and isoflurane. Enflurane decreases GFR and urinary output.[68] Although

Table 19-6. Renal responses to surgery or trauma

	Urinary flow rate (ml·min^{-1})	[Na$^+$] (mEq·L^{-1})	Urea (mg·dl^{-1})	Osmolality (mOsm·kg^{-1})
Euvolemic, young adult	2.0	100.0	250	300
"Average" perioperative patient	0.5	20.0	500	800
Maximal antidiuretic hormone and aldosterone	0.2	1.0	1000	1200

isoflurane does not reduce RBF, it does reduce GFR and urinary output.[69,70] Enflurane, unlike halothane or isoflurane, releases significant amounts of fluoride ion.[68] After prolonged (about 9 hours of) enflurane anesthesia, fluoride concentrations of 30 to 40 μmol·ml^{-1}, sufficient to decrease urinary concentrating ability, have been reported.[71] Potentially harmful concentrations of fluoride ion (greater than 50 μmol·ml^{-1}) accumulate in obese patients after prolonged exposure to enflurane and in patients who have received isoniazid.[72]

3. Halothane. Clinical doses of halothane decrease renal vascular resistance but have little effect on RBF.[73] Halothane-induced hypotension does not reduce RBF until mean arterial pressure is ≤60 mm Hg.[74] When added to halothane, nitrous oxide reduces urine flow.[75] Even during acute hemorrhagic hypovolemia in halothane-anesthetized animals, autoregulation remains intact and decreased renal vascular resistance maintains RBF at normal levels.[76]

B. Effects of intravenous induction agents

1. Thiopental. Low doses of thiopental produce little change in systemic blood pressure, renal vascular resistance, or RBF.[77] Higher doses produce venodilatation and decrease cardiac preload and myocardial contractility.[78] RBF is preserved during thiopental administration by reduced renal vascular resistance.[78]

2. Opioids. Morphine, even when given in doses that lower blood pressure, does not reduce RBF.[79] Fentanyl decreases urine flow and GFR; the effects of fentanyl on RBF are less defined.[80,81]

C. Effects of regional anesthesia

The renal and systemic hemodynamic responses to spinal and epidural anesthesia are strongly influenced by preanesthetic intravascular volume. Spinal anesthesia (T1 level) only slightly decreases GFR and RBF.[82] Epidural block per-

formed with epinephrine-free solutions generates little change in systemic hemodynamics and only a small decrease in GFR and RBF.[83] Thoracic levels of epidural block, using epinephrine-containing local anesthetics, moderately reduce RBF and GFR in parallel with the decrease in mean arterial pressure.[84]

In summary, virtually all anesthetic agents and techniques have been associated with a decrease in GFR and urinary output under certain conditions. Nevertheless, few agents or techniques generate direct renal toxicity. Few data describe interactions among the many drugs commonly combined in clinical anesthesia. Specific responses vary with respect to the characteristics of the subjects studied, the control of confounding variables, and the choice of measurement techniques. Surprisingly little is known about the integrity of RBF autoregulation during the administration of various individual anesthetic drugs and combinations of anesthetic drugs and adjuvants.

VI. ACUTE RENAL DYSFUNCTION

Acute renal dysfunction is conventionally divided into three categories: postrenal, prerenal, and renal.[85] Although acute renal dysfunction may be heralded by oliguria, renal dysfunction frequently is nonoliguric. Because both prerenal and postrenal dysfunction may progress to ARF, rapid treatment may restore urinary flow and prevent the development of ARF.

A. Postrenal dysfunction

Postrenal (obstructive) oliguria presents variably as anuria, oliguria, erratically fluctuating urinary output, or nonoliguric renal failure. Treatment necessitates identification of the site of obstruction, including evaluation of the patency of existing urinary catheters. Abdominal ultrasonography, computerized tomography, cystoscopy, and retrograde pyelography occasionally may be necessary for accurate diagnosis.

B. Prerenal dysfunction

Prerenal dysfunction, often evidenced by oliguria (urinary output <0.5 ml·kg^{-1}·hr^{-1}), is initiated by decreased renal perfusion. In response to circulatory compromise, renin, angiotensin II, aldosterone, and ADH avidly conserve sodium and water. The renal vasodilating prostaglandins, especially PGE$_2$, act to preserve RBF and GFR. Autonomic nervous system activation helps to maintain blood pressure and RBF.

In response to decreased afferent arteriolar pressure,[86] to catecholamine secretion, and to increasing tubular concentrations of sodium and chloride delivered to the macula densa,[87] renin is released from the juxtaglomerular apparatus. Angiotensin II is generated and constricts both afferent and efferent arterioles, thereby reducing GFR, and releases aldosterone, which leads to increased sodium reabsorption in the distal tubule. Renal hypoperfusion also is associated with reduction of factors that facilitate sodium excretion. Circulating levels of ANH are reduced during hypotensive hemorrhage,[88] and the response to exogenous ANH is reduced.[89] Moderate hypovolemia reduces the stimulation of atrial stretch receptors, thereby initiating ADH release and increasing reabsorption of water from urine in the collecting ducts. Frank hypotension stimulates the vagally innervated aortic arch and carotid sinus baroreceptors, leading to further ADH secretion. Although maximal ADH stimulation can increase urinary osmolality to nearly 1200 mOsm·L^{-1}, surgical patients typically cannot achieve maximal urinary concentration. To excrete the normal dietary solute load of 400 to 600 mOsm per day, the kidneys must excrete 300 to 500 ml per day of urine. Excretion of increased catabolic waste, a necessity in hypermetabolic patients, may require even greater urinary flow. Failure to excrete these waste products indicates prerenal failure.

The renal response to hypovolemia and hypotension depends on the severity of the insult. Severely reduced renal perfusion depletes high-energy phosphates and initiates a series of biochemical insults that may lead to progressive renal injury.[90] Such responses are particularly likely if mean arterial pressure declines below the level necessary to preserve renal autoregulation.[91] In experimental models, GFR declines more profoundly if acute hypotension is superimposed on preexisting renal hypoperfusion, produced by acute water deprivation or congestive heart failure.[92]

Although the kidneys are capable of substantial compensation in response to declining per-

Table 19-7. Mechanisms contributing to the initiation and maintenance of acute renal failure

Initiation	Maintenance
Renal hypoperfusion Nephrotoxins	Decreased renal blood flow Decreased glomerular filtration Tubular obstruction Tubular dysfunction

fusion, at some point decompensation ensues.[93] When renal hypoperfusion precipitates prerenal oliguria, the primary treatment is to improve renal perfusion. Prompt restoration of RBF may increase urinary flow, diminish hormonal responses to circulatory depression, and prevent ARF. Failure to restore RBF may lead to postischemic ARF. Thus there is a continuum between prerenal azotemia and postischemic ARF.

C. Acute renal failure

Established ARF cannot be corrected by improving prerenal or postrenal factors.[94] Contributing mechanisms to hemodynamically mediated ARF include both factors that initiate and processes that maintain ARF (Table 19-7).[23,95,96] After initiation by renal hypoperfusion or nephrotoxins (that is, causes of renal ischemia or direct toxic injury), ARF is maintained by one or more of the following mechanisms:

Reduced renal blood flow. When total RBF declines because of ECF volume depletion or compensatory vasoconstriction, blood flow is redistributed from cortical to juxtamedullary nephrons.[97] Although improvements in RBF improve GFR in prerenal states, increases in RBF do not increase GFR in established ARF. The exact cause or mediator of this persistent vasoconstriction is unknown. Cortical vasoconstriction is augmented by intrarenal renin, released by increased delivery to the macula densa of sodium and chloride, which are no longer adequately absorbed by ischemic tubular epithelium. In ARF, the kidneys lose the ability to autoregulate and are more dependent on renal artery pressure for perfusion than normal kidneys are.[98,99] Such kidneys are susceptible to repeated ischemic insults.

In the renal cortex, one potent mechanism resisting the development of ARF involves the vasodilating prostaglandins PGE$_2$ and PGI$_2$ (prostacyclin), which modulate renin release and reduce renal vascular resistance.[100,101] Nonsteroidal anti-inflammatory drugs (NSAIDs), by inhibiting the production of vasodilating prostaglandins, potentially increase the risk of ARF.[46,101] Exogenous vasodilator prostaglandins protect against development of ischemic renal failure.[102,103]

Decreased glomerular filtration. In postischemic ARF, glomerular filtration declines, although the glomeruli appear structurally normal. GFR also remains depressed despite near-normalization of RBF. This finding indicates that reduced glomerular permeability may contribute to the ARF.

Tubular obstruction. Obstruction of tubular flow by intratubular debris, produced by ischemic desquamation of brush-border microvilli[104] or by pigmented casts, can result in back pressure that opposes glomerular filtration.[105] Tubular obstruction may maintain but rarely initiates ARF (except that caused by pigmenturia or crystalluria). Mannitol, by increasing tubular flow and relieving tubular obstruction during prerenal insults, ameliorates some experimental models of ARF.[106]

Tubular dysfunction. Disruption of the integrity of tubular epithelium permits pathologic reabsorption, called "backleak," of filtered waste products from the tubular lumen into the peritubular interstitium and peritubular capillaries. Backleak, aggravated by tubular obstruction from intraluminal debris, may prevent excretion of nearly 50% of total filtrate, leading to azotemia and sodium and water retention.[23,107,108]

1. Nephrotoxic acute renal dysfunction

a. Aminoglycoside nephrotoxicity. Aminoglycoside nephrotoxicity, occurring in 10% to 26% of patients,[109-111] is characterized by enzymuria, reduced glomerular permeability, decreased concentrating ability, and progressively declining GFR.[109-111] Neomycin, the most toxic aminoglycoside, may be absorbed from surgical irrigation fluid. In a prospective, controlled trial[112] 8% to 10% of patients receiving gentamicin developed nephrotoxicity in contrast to 18% of those receiving tobramycin. The risk of aminoglycoside nephrotoxicity is increased by sustained high blood levels, advanced age, volume depletion, cephalosporin antibiotics, potent diuretics, acidemia, endotoxemia, and a history of recent exposure to aminoglycosides and nonsteroidal anti-inflammatory drugs.

b. Myoglobin-induced ARF. Myoglobin, if released in sufficient quantities from injured or ischemic skeletal muscle, causes ARF. Several clinical situations associated with myoglobin-induced ARF include (1) embolic arterial ischemia and rhabdomyolysis; (2) the crush syndrome, which combines muscle injury and hypovolemia; (3) nontraumatic myonecrosis; (4) severe hypokalemia, especially if combined with exercise,[113,114] and (5) severe hypophosphatemia.

Myoglobin toxicity is enhanced by dehydration and by acidic urine (pH <5.6). Urinary alkalinization prevents conversion of myoglobin to ferrihematin, decreases tubular obstruction, and reduces tubular toxicity.[115] Myoglobinemia is associated with a precipitous fall in GFR, probably related both to swelling of glomerular epithelial cells and mesangial cells and to tubular obstruction. Mannitol in doses of 25 to 50 g induces diuresis and prevents tubular obstruction by decreasing glomerular edema and maintaining tubular flow. In experimental models, furosemide aggravates myoglobinuria-induced ARF.

C. Contrast medium–induced ARF. Nearly all patients undergoing elective or emergent major vascular surgery and many of those requiring surgery after trauma will have undergone radiographic procedures that require contrast media. The risk of contrast medium–induced ARF is increased by multiple risk factors, most importantly preexisting renal insufficiency (List 19-1). If serum creatinine is less than 1.5 mg%, the risk of contrast medium–induced ARF is 0.6%, increasing to 3% if serum creatinine is 1.5 to 4.5 mg%.[116] Other risk factors include diabetes mellitus, dehydration, congestive heart failure, multiple myeloma, liver disease, and vascular disease. The combination of diabetes mellitus and renal insufficiency is associated with an incidence of contrast-induced ARF of nearly 9%.[117] After radiographic contrast studies, renal injury produces evidence of azotemia beginning 24 to 48 hours after exposure; serum creatinine rapidly increases 3 to 5 days after in-

---

List 19-1.   Risk Factors Contributing to the Development of Contrast-Induced Acute Renal Failure

---

Definite risk factor
  Preexisting renal insufficiency
Probable risk factors
  Diabetes mellitus
  Dehydration
  Large dose of contrast medium
  Prior contrast medium–induced acute renal failure
  Congestive heart failure
  Multiple myeloma

---

jury and then typically becomes normal within 2 weeks.

Agents that alter the agglutination of red cells (dextran and volume expansion) protect against ARF induced by contrast media. Mannitol attenuates experimental contrast-induced ARF.[118,119] Volume expansion effectively reduces the risk of contrast-induced ARF by minimizing proteinaceous tubular obstruction.[120,121] Minimizing the total dose of contrast media used also helps to limit injury. The newer radiocontrast agents are minimally toxic in the absence of risk factors.[122]

2. Atheroembolic renal disease. Atheromatous material can be dislodged by thoracic or abdominal trauma, by cardiac or aortic surgery, or by intra-aortic catheters. The clinical diagnosis, often difficult, requires a high index of suspicion and the recognition of peripheral embolization (such as ischemic injury to fingers and toes). No specific findings or laboratory values are diagnostic; the only clinical manifestation may be oliguria with increasing hypertension. Livedo reticularis, an irregular skin mottling at sites of small vessel occlusion, is strongly suggestive of atheroembolic disease. There is no specific therapy.

3. Nonoliguric acute renal failure (NOARF). NOARF, once uncommon, now represents the most frequently observed form of ARF.[5,122-125] The changing proportion of nonoliguric ARF has been attributed to increasing use of aminoglycosides, improved detection because of routine chemistry panels, improved fluid resuscitation,[126] and frequent use of potent loop diuretics[127] and dopamine. Improved intraoperative fluid and hemodynamic management appears to favor the development of NOARF rather than oliguric ARF after severe trauma.[126,128]

In most patients, NOARF represents a milder form of oliguric ARF. NOARF often follows brief intervals of total renal ischemia.[94] Glomerular filtration and tubular function are better maintained than in oliguric ARF.[123] In a heterogeneous population of patients with NOARF, the complications, duration, and mortality are reduced in comparison to oliguric ARF.[123] Severely traumatized patients with NOARF also demonstrate reduced mortality and morbidity in comparison to oliguric ARF.[126] However, conversion of established, oliguric ARF to NOARF using high doses of loop diuretics and dopamine does not improve outcome.[129]

D. Prevention of acute renal failure

Because of the high mortality associated with the progression from prerenal insults to ARF,

renal ischemia must be prevented or limited in duration. Efforts to prevent or attenuate renal ischemia should be particularly emphasized in patients who are at greater risk for ARF, including those who are elderly or have underlying renal disease, hepatic disease, sepsis, and cardiac disease. The fundamental strategy for the prevention of ARF is to limit the magnitude and duration of renal ischemia. ARF usually results from inadequate renal perfusion as a consequence of systemic hypoperfusion. Preoperative and intraoperative restoration and maintenance of intravascular volume are essential, especially in patients who are hypovolemic because of angiography, bowel preparation, or prolonged fasting.[130] Data indicate that optimal volume loading, using information derived from Swan-Ganz catheterization, can reduce renal injury associated with vascular surgery.[130,131] In the previously described study by Shoemaker and colleagues, goal-directed hemodynamic therapy was associated with a negligible incidence of ARF in high-risk surgical patients.[57]

Most clinical approaches to the reduction of perioperative ARF are based upon inferences from animal models that consist in complete renal ischemia.[132] Mannitol, dopamine, and furosemide promote urinary flow and reduce the renal damage produced by experimental renal ischemia.[132-142] Mannitol improves renal cortical blood flow and may exert cellular protective effects.[133-135] However, mannitol does not reverse the profound reduction in GFR and RBF induced by suprarenal aortic cross-clamping for 60 minutes in dogs.[137] Dopamine, a selective renal vasodilator, increases renal cortical blood flow with minimal systemic effects at doses of 1 to 3 $\mu g \cdot kg^{-1} \cdot min^{-1}$.[138] Dopamine induces natriuresis, increases GFR, and improves urinary flow.[138,139] Like mannitol, dopamine is ineffective in reversing the renal injury produced by thoracic aortic crossclamping.[137] There is no evidence that use of low-dose dopamine alters the course of established ARF. Furosemide improves renal perfusion and GFR in experimental models of complete renal ischemia,[134,135] though less effectively than mannitol. In established oliguric ARF, furosemide does not improve outcome or reduce the frequency at which dialysis is required.[129,140] The greatest risk associated with the administration of diuretics in patients at risk for ARF is that chemically induced diuresis, in the absence of adequate volume expansion, may delay effective therapy and further deplete intravascular volume.

Recently, fenoldopam, a novel dopamine₁ adrenergic receptor agonist, has been investigated. The drug substantially enhances urinary flow, sodium excretion, and creatinine clearance while reducing systemic vascular resistance.[143-146] Although fenoldopam will likely become a valuable perioperative adjunct, its precise role in the management of renal functions remains to be demonstrated.

In addition to the commonly discussed renal protective effects of volume expansion, mannitol, dopamine, and furosemide, a variety of agents demonstrate efficacy in experimental models of ARF. The intense investigative activity in this field indicates that improved pharmacologic renal protective therapy will be available within the decade. Numerous reviews address recent research that may lead to therapeutic progress.[147-153] Some of the more promising approaches are summarized below.

Renal hypoperfusion reduces the concentration of high-energy phosphates.[154] The thick ascending limb of Henle's loop may be particularly vulnerable to ischemic injury.[155-158] Infusion of adenine nucleotides in combination with magnesium chloride preserves postischemic renal function.[159,160] Inhibition of 5'-nucleotidase similarly enhances metabolic and functional recovery after renal ischemia.[161] Infusion of fructose-1,6-diphosphate, a high-energy metabolite, also enhances the ability of the kidney to withstand ischemic injury.[162] Presumably the renal protective effects of hypothermia are also dependent on preservation of high-energy phosphates.[163]

In the kidney, as in other organs, ischemia causes an increase in intracellular free calcium. Pretreatment with calcium-channel blockers limits renal injury produced by experimental complete renal ischemia,[164-166] though additional clinical evidence is necessary before calcium-channel blockers can be added to management of patients who must undergo complete renal ischemia.[167] In partial renal ischemia, calcium-channel blockers may produce salutary or deleterious effects, depending on the magnitude of drug-induced blood pressure decline and the cause of the renal hypoperfusion.[168-170]

Oxygen free radicals, arachidonate metabolites, leukotrienes, and neutrophils have also been implicated in ischemic renal damage. Oxygen free radicals probably are produced in large quantities during and after renal ischemia,[171] an observation that may explain why superoxide dismutase or allopurinol reduce experimental renal ischemic injury when administered before ischemia.[172] Evidence indicates that the balance between the synthesis of the vasodilator prostaglandin PGI_2 and the vasoconstrictor thromboxane (Tx) A_2 regulates renal vascular tone. Inhibition of TxA_2 synthesis protects against tubular necrosis after experimental ischemia in the rat[173] and improves renal function in patients with lupus nephritis.[174] Scavengers of oxygen free radicals also inhibit synthesis of TxA_2 and improve renal outcome in experimental models.[175]

Just as inhibition of the production of vasoconstrictive arachidonate metabolites attenuates experimental renal injury, so too does therapeu-

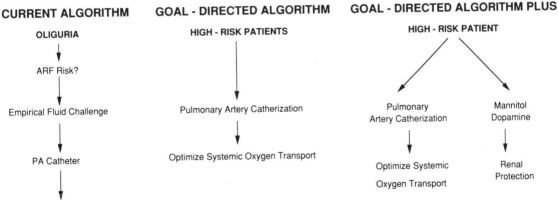

Fig. 19-7. Three possible approaches to prevention of acute renal failure, ARF. The left-hand algorithm is derived from the approach used by many clinicians. Once oliguria is recognized, the diagnostic and therapeutic approach consists in empirical volume expansion, supplemented if necessary by pulmonary artery (PA) catheterization, with subsequent data-directed therapy consisting in fluid, dopamine, inotropic support, mannitol, or furosemide. In contrast, the goal-directed algorithm is based upon identification of high-risk patients. Such patients would undergo pulmonary artery catheterization with subsequent support of systemic oxygen transport (cardiac output × arterial oxygen content) at levels associated with improved survival in high-risk surgical patients.[57] The right-hand figure combines goal-oriented therapy with early pharmacologic support.

tic administration of vasodilator prostaglandins such as $PGE_2,^{174,176}$ $PGE_1,^{103,177}$ and prostacyclin $(PGI_2).^{178}$ Leukotrienes, presumably derived from neutrophils, appear to partially mediate ischemic renal injury; neutrophil depletion improves postischemic renal function.[179]

Although a variety of agents appear promising, clinical application requires cumbersome testing. Clinical ARF is more heterogeneous than experimental ARF, frequently involving elderly patients with reduced renal reserve and highly variable degrees of renal ischemia. Two experimental studies particularly emphasize the extent to which small differences in preischemic status could affect the subsequent course of ARF. In rats, protein intake in the weeks before renal ischemia profoundly affects renal function and survival.[180] Rats maintained before ischemia on no- or low-protein diets survive, whereas those maintained on normal- or high-protein diets have a higher mortality.[181] *Post*ischemic protein ingestion does not affect recovery. Seguro and colleagues have demonstrated that preischemic potassium depletion greatly accentuated renal injury secondary to ischemia.[181]

Fig. 19-7 summarizes three possible approaches to the prevention of ARF. The left-hand algorithm, similar to that used by many clinicians, emphasizes the essential role of volume expansion, supplemented by hemodynamic data and pharmacologic therapy in patients who fail to respond to volume expansion. The middle algorithm, based on extrapolations from the data of Shoemaker and colleagues,[57] depends on identification of high-risk patients rather than recognition of oliguria and emphasizes support of systemic oxygen transport in those patients at an optimal level. The right-hand algorithm combines aggressive hemodynamic support with preventive pharmacotherapy.

VII. MONITORING AND EVALUATION OF HYPOVOLEMIA AND RENAL FUNCTION

Challenging diagnostic and therapeutic problems confront physicians in clinical situations in which ARF constitutes a potential threat (Fig. 19-8). Because the only readily available monitor of renal function is oliguria (<30 ml·hr^{-1} in perioperative patients), only a fraction of renal ischemia will be clinically evident. Urinary output will exceed 30 ml·hr^{-1} in the remainder of patients. To further complicate matters, even adequate renal perfusion may be associated with oliguria,[182] though the majority of pa-

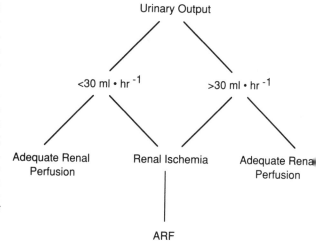

Fig. 19-8. Prevention of acute renal failure (ARF) is complicated by the difficulty of recognizing inadequate renal perfusion. Oliguria, less than 30 ml/hr, the most easily recognized sign of acute renal ischemia, can be associated with adequate renal perfusion, especially under circumstances in which salt and water conservation is maximum. On the other hand, urinary output exceeding 30 ml·hr^{-1} (or 0.5 ml·kg^{-1}·hr^{-1} may accompany either adequate renal perfusion or renal ischemia. Thus ARF may follow oliguria or occur unexpectedly without sentinel oliguria. Satisfactory renal function may follow either acceptable urinary output or oliguria.

List 19-2. Criteria for Effective Renal Monitoring

Must relate renal ischemia to acute renal failure
Must be a quantitative indicator of renal ischemia
The monitoring device should be continuous and based on the quantitative indicator
Direction of therapy facilitated by monitor-derived data
Outcome is improved by being based on monitor-based intervention

---

tients with adequate renal perfusion will have adequate urinary output. Of the patients with renal ischemia, some are oliguric and some are not; only some of the patients with oliguria will proceed to ARF, as will some patients without a clearly defined antecedent oliguric episode. Consequently, controlled clinical trials of promising interventions are essential.

An effective renal monitor must fulfill several criteria (List 19-2). First, the monitor must relate to an underlying pathophysiologic process, that is, renal ischemia, that can produce ARF. Second, a quantifiable indicator of renal isch-

---

List 19-3. Operational Characteristics of Monitors

Sensitivity
Specificity
Speed
Utility

---

emia must be identified. Third, a functional monitor, using frequent (ideally continuous) analysis of the indicator, must be developed. Fourth, data derived from the monitor must facilitate alteration of therapy. Finally, the use of the monitor to manage therapy should result in an objective improvement in outcome.

Current and potential monitors of renal function also must satisfy several practical, operational criteria (List 19-3). An ideal monitor should be sensitive, specific, and fast and should be useful in titrating therapeutic support. *Sensitivity* refers to whether the monitor identifies all patients who could ultimately go on to develop organ injury. *Specificity* refers to whether the monitor incorrectly identifies patients who would not progress to injury. A monitor with poor sensitivity (many false negatives) will be associated with the development of unexpected injury. In contrast, a nonspecific monitor that generates many false-positive results may prompt unnecessary concern and treatment. The concept of *speed* in a monitor incorporates both the rate at which information can be produced and the rate at which the marker changes after a critical event. For instance, serum creatinine can be analyzed in less than 1 hour but increases at a rate of only 1 to 3 $mg \cdot dl^{-1}$ per day even if glomerular filtration ceases. The final operational characteristic of a worthwhile monitor, *utility,* refers to the ability of monitor-derived information to facilitate the clinical reasoning process, alter therapy, and ultimately improve outcome.

A. Laboratory evaluation of renal function

1. Blood and urine tests. Renal function tests are influenced by base-line renal function, by the renal capacity to reabsorb indicators, by intravascular and extracellular volume, by cardiovascular function, and by neuroendocrine factors such as ADH and aldosterone. Therefore no simple, inexpensive test adequately quantifies renal function. The readily available tests of renal function, including urinalysis, BUN, serum creatinine (SCr), and creatinine clearance (CCr), are most inaccurate in elderly, malnourished, and dehydrated patients (Table 19-8).

The urinalysis provides qualitative information that must be interpreted with caution. Pyuria (more than four white blood cells per high-power field) occurs in patients with urinary tract inflammation. It has a low specificity

Table 19-8. Diagnostic evaluation of renal function

Test	Normal range	Limitations
BUN	8-20 $mg \cdot dl^{-1}$	Dehydration Variable protein intake Gastrointestinal bleeding Catabolism Recent major trauma or surgery
Serum creatinine (SCr)	0.5-1.2 $mg \cdot dl^{-1}$	Advanced age Muscle mass Rhabdomyolysis Catabolic state Recent major trauma or surgery
Creatinine clearance (CCr) Estimated*	120 $ml \cdot min^{-1}$	Similar to serum creatinine Weight dependency Recent major trauma or surgery
Measured	120 $ml \cdot min^{-1}$	Inaccurate urine volume measurement Unsteady state Varying hydration

*Using the formula: $CCr = \dfrac{(140 - Age)\, Wt}{72 \times SCr}$

for urinary tract infection.[183] Although urine may normally contain hyaline and granular casts, cellular casts (either red cell or white cell) represent a pathologic finding.[183]

Both BUN and SCr offer rapid but inexact estimates of CCr. The actual measurement of CCr constitutes the best routinely available indicator of GFR. However, all three measurements require careful interpretation. BUN, a product of protein metabolism, is increased by high protein intake, gastrointestinal bleeding, or accelerated catabolism (such as traumatized or septic patients, glucocorticoid administration). Hepatic dysfunction decreases the synthesis of urea and reduces BUN. Freely filtered at the glomerulus, urea is reabsorbed to a large and variable extent. The reabsorption of urea increases (approximately 60% of the filtered load) when urinary flow is low. Creatinine, a product of the catabolism of skeletal muscle, is produced at a lower rate in the elderly than in young adults and in females than in males. In debilitated or malnourished patients, creatinine production may be reduced. Consequently, in many patients SCr may fail to increase in proportion to nephron loss. In contrast, in muscular or acutely catabolic patients, SCr may exceed the normal range because of more rapid muscle breakdown. Combining the evaluation of BUN and SCr provides more information than the evaluation of either alone. If the BUN:SCr ratio exceeds the normal range of 10 to 20, one should suspect dehydration or one of the individual factors that alter the serum concentration of the two metabolites.

CCr may be estimated from the following equation:

$$GFR = \frac{(140 - Age)\, Wt}{72 \times SCr}$$

where *Wt* is weight in kilograms and *GFR* and *CCr* are assumed to be equal. The calculated value is multiplied by 0.8 in females.

However, precise measurements of CCr require collection of timed urine samples, using the following formula:

$$GFR = \frac{UV}{P}$$

where *U* is urinary concentration of creatinine (mg·dl^{-1}), *V* is volume of urine (in ml·min^{-1}), and *P* is plasma concentration of creatinine (in mg·dl^{-1}).

Although 24-hour specimens are usually used, a 2-hour sample, collected through a urinary catheter, provides an acceptable estimate of 24-hour values.[184] GFR may also be determined by serial measurement of the clearance

rates of insulin or radiolabeled tracers. However, these tests are not yet clinically applicable to early diagnosis of ARF.

Short-term analysis of CCr in the perioperative period necessitates certain considerations. First, CCr can be reduced despite normal urinary output, normal BUN, and normal SCr.[185] Second, CCr estimates require hemodynamic stability at least for the duration of the CCr determination. Third, variations in urinary output and the state of hydration may adversely affect the validity of the measurements.[186-188]

2. Use of tests in patients with acute renal dysfunction

a. Oliguria. A decrease in urinary output (that is, oliguria) to less than 0.5 ml·kg^{-1}·hr^{-1} is suggestive of the possibility of renal hypoperfusion. However, this monitor of renal function may be unreliable (Fig. 19-8). Zaloga and Hughes[182] reported a subset of postoperative patients in whom oliguria appeared to be secondary to excess ADH secretion without evidence of sodium conservation. In addition, although prerenal azotemia is usually associated with oliguria, Miller et al.[189] reported 9 patients with polyuric, prerenal failure in which a urinary concentration defect was present (that is, as a result of malnutrition, protein deficiency, urea depletion, or salt depletion). These patients have a form of nephrogenic diabetes insipidus. Oliguria may also be absent in patients with nonoliguric acute renal failure and in patients with renal failure who receive diuretics.

b. Serum creatinine. An acute increase in SCr exceeding 0.5 mg·dl^{-1} is suggestive of ARF, though SCr determinations may be artificially elevated by noncreatinine chromogens and ketone bodies. Artifactual increases in SCr result in underestimation of CCr. SCr may also be elevated somewhat because of dehydration.

c. Urinary sodium and urinary concentration. Oliguria, urinary sodium conservation, and retained concentrating ability are strongly suggestive of an intense prerenal physiologic state (Table 19-9). In prerenal oliguria, tubular function is intact and sodium reabsorption in the distal tubule usually reduces urinary sodium to ≤20 mEq·L^{-1}. These patients retain the ability to concentrate urine (that is, osmolality greater than 500; urine/plasma creatinine ratio greater than 40:1). However, the specificity and sensitivity of urinary sodium measurements are inadequate in most acute situations.

Concentrating ability ideally is assessed by use of urinary osmolality. In prerenal oliguria, urinary osmolality should exceed 500 mOsm· kg^{-1} (1.3 × serum osmolality); in ARF, the

Table 19-9. Urinary diagnostic tests in acute oliguria

	Prerenal	Renal (acute renal failure)
Urine sodium ($mEq \cdot L^{-1}$)	<20	>40
Urine osmolality ($mOsm \cdot kg^{-1}$)	>500	<350
Urine/plasma osmolality	>1.3:1	<1.1:1
Urine/plasma urea	>8:1	<3:1
Urine/plasma creatinine	>40:1	<20:1
Fractional excretion of sodium (FENa) (%)	<1	>2

Table 19-10. Characteristics of urinary diagnostic tests in oliguric postoperative patients

	Avid water conservation; without sodium conservation (normovolemic)	Avid water and sodium conservation (hypovolemic)
Number	11	7
Urinary output ($ml \cdot hr^{-1}$)	13 ± 2	17 ± 2
Urinary osmolality ($mOsm \cdot kg^{-1}$ of H_2O)	522 ± 36	525 ± 34
Urinary Na^+ ($mEq \cdot L^{-1}$)	83 ± 12*	11 ± 2
Fractional excretion of sodium (FENa)	1.15 ± 0.2*	0.15 ± 0.03

From Zaloga GP and Hughes SS: Anesthesiology 72:598-602, 1990.
*p <0.05 compared to hypovolemic group.

loss of concentrating ability results in isosthenuria (approximately 285 to 300 $mOsm \cdot kg^{-1}$).

d. Fractional excretion of sodium (FENa). One calculates FENa by dividing the urine-plasma sodium ratio by the urine−to−plasma creatinine ratio and then multiplying by 100.[190-192] Values less than 1% are suggestive of prerenal azotemia; increased values are suggestive of ARF (Table 19-9). Despite early enthusiasm, the diagnostic and prognostic utility of the FENa calculation is limited in acute oliguria.[193,194] Postoperative patients commonly demonstrate oliguria and high urinary osmolality despite normal or high urinary sodium concentration and normal FENa[182] (Table 19-10). This combination, consistent with increased levels of ADH in association with normal levels of aldosterone, is suggestive of normovolemia. In sodium-avid patients (those with liver failure, nephrotic syndrome, cirrhosis, and glomerulonephritis), FENa may remain low despite inexorably progressive renal failure.[195,196] Thus some patients with ARF retain enough tubular integrity to respond to salt-retaining stimuli, and a low FENa is not a reliable predictor of hypoperfusion that is reversible with volume expansion. Overaggressive volume expansion may lead to pulmonary edema in these patients. On the other hand, occasional patients with prerenal (hypoperfusion) oliguria may have a FENa greater than 1%. Inability to concentrate urine despite considerable volume depletion may occur in patients with hypertensive and diabetic nephrosclerosis and other chronic parenchymal renal diseases. Most importantly, high values of FENa may be suggestive of established parenchymal injury at a time when hemodynamically mediated prerenal factors could be reversed, thereby delaying or halting appropriate efforts to improve renal perfusion.

e. Pulmonary artery catheterization. Intravascular volume cannot be accurately estimated in critically ill patients. Although pulmonary artery catheterization provides no specific information about renal status, it provides data that may facilitate fluid management of patients at risk for renal failure. When empiric fluid administration seems unduly hazardous, pulmonary artery catheterization permits optimal volume expansion while reducing the risk of pulmonary edema.

3. Monitoring perioperative renal function. Rapid changes in hemodynamics and extracellular volume during anesthesia and surgery, coupled with the transient effects of anesthetic drugs and noxious stimulation, virtually preclude precise assessment of renal function. The problems involved in monitoring renal function

Table 19-11. Perioperative renal monitoring

	Sensitivity	Specificity	Speed	Utility
Urinary output	2+	2+	4+	3+
BUN, SCr	1+	1+	1+	1+
CCr	4+	3+	2+	2+
UNa	1+	2+	3+	1+
Urinary osmolality	1+	2+	3+	1+
FENa	1+	3+	3+	1+
Pulmonary artery catheterization	1+	1+	4+	4+

BUN, Blood urea nitrogen; *CCr,* creatinine clearance; *FENa,* fractional excretion of sodium; *SCr,* serum creatinine; *UNa,* urinary sodium concentration; a range of 1+, poor, to 4+, good.

in critically ill patients have recently been reviewed.[197] Table 19-11 lists available tests of renal function, including Swan-Ganz catheterization, an indirect measure of circulatory adequacy, and estimates on a scale of 1+ (poor) to 4+ (good) the value of those tests or techniques for renal monitoring in the perioperative period. Each of the current and potential monitors of renal function can be analyzed in terms of how well they meet several operational criteria (Table 19-11).

VIII. RENAL REPLACEMENT THERAPY

In patients who develop perioperative ARF, excess water and sodium and metabolic wastes can be eliminated by hemodialysis, peritoneal dialysis, continuous arteriovenous hemofiltration (CAVH), continuous arteriovenous hemodialysis (CAVHD), and venovenous hemofiltration. Several principles are the basis for all forms of renal replacement therapy; nevertheless, the physiologic effects and complications differ among the various forms of therapy.[198-205]

A. Principles of renal replacement therapy

Ultrafiltration and dialysis are the two essential components of renal replacement therapy. Ultrafiltration is the movement of serum and solutes through pores in membranes at rates that depend on hydrostatic pressure, molecular weight, and pore size. If molecules are sufficiently small to pass freely through the pores in the membrane, filtration will vary directly with the magnitude of hydrostatic pressure. Dialysis describes diffusive transport of solute down an osmotic gradient across a semipermeable membrane. Accumulated waste solutes such as urea and potassium move from high concentrations in blood into a chemically prescribed dialysate.

Substances such as bicarbonate move from higher concentrations in the dialysate into blood.

B. Hemodialysis

Transport of substances from blood into dialysate across the semipermeable dialysis membrane is governed by a relationship expressed mathematically as

$$J_s = DA(C_B - C_D)$$

where J_s is solute flux, D is the diffusion coefficient of the membrane for the solute, A is the area of membrane, C_B is the concentration of the solute in blood, and C_D is the concentration of the solute in the dialysate. In the hollow-fiber type of dialyzer the membrane area available for solute exchange is 0.8 to 2.0 m^2.[206]

The diffusive transport of substances across a dialyzer membrane differs both quantitatively and qualitatively from the convective transport of substances across the renal glomerular membrane. The glomerulus quantitatively filters molecules, independent of size, up to a molecular weight of 7000 to 10,000 daltons, beyond which glomerular filtration rapidly declines until the upper limit of filtration size (around 100,000 daltons) is attained. In contrast, clearance of solutes by dialysis is inversely proportional to molecular weight across the entire range of 0 to 100,000 daltons. Small molecules, such as urea, are cleared readily by dialysis, their clearance being dependent primarily on blood flow through the dialyzer.

Hemodialysis efficiently removes small molecules. Hemodialyzers are also capable of convective transport, or ultrafiltration, the magnitude of which is directly proportional to the transmembrane hydrostatic pressure. Ultrafiltration clears solutes inefficiently because only the solute present in the filtrate is removed. Although the human kidney also initiates urine formation by ultrafiltration, high clearances result from the high rate of filtration and subsequent tubular modification of filtrate. Normal adult kidneys filter approximately 20% of renal plasma flow, or approximately 7 L per hour. Therapeutic ultrafiltration filters far less volume per hour and does not modify the filtrate.

The plastic surface of the dialyzer activates the coagulation cascade; therefore systemic or regional anticoagulation must be provided. Regional heparinization is used to limit the risk of systemic heparinization. Heparin is added to the blood in the arterial line and is neutralized with protamine before returning to the patient through the venous line. Careful monitoring of anticoagulation is required during either systemic or regional heparinzation.

Hemodialysis, CAVH, CAVHD, and venovenous ultrafiltration necessitate high-capacity vascular access. Double-lumen catheters[207,208] permit simultaneous withdrawal and return through a single percutaneous access site, usually the subclavian vein. Emergent perioperative hemodialysis is less often performed through a percutaneously inserted Shaldon catheter. Blood is returned through a peripheral vein or, when necessary, through a second Shaldon catheter inserted in the same or a contralateral femoral vein. Chronic hemodialysis is usually performed through a surgically constructed arteriovenous fistula.

C. Peritoneal dialysis

Peritoneal dialysis takes advantage of the natural semipermeable membrane consisting of the tissue layers that separate peritoneal capillary blood from intraperitoneal dialysate. The extensive peritoneal capillary network provides contact between blood and dialysate. Peritoneal dialysis clears small molecules such as urea more slowly than hemodialysis but clears larger molecules such as inulin more rapidly.[209]

Clearance of solute during peritoneal dialysis depends on the rate of blood flow in the peritoneal capillaries, the permeability and area of the tissue interface, the volume and composition of the dialysate, and the circulation of the fluid film in the peritoneal cavity. The rate of ultrafiltration of water and solute out of the capillary bed may be increased by increasing the concentration of dextrose in the dialysate, that is, by increasing the osmotic pressure in the peritoneal cavity. The osmotic pressure gradient across the peritoneal membrane governs ultrafiltration as the hydraulic gradient does across the hemodialysis membrane.

Peritoneal dialysis is performed through an indwelling peritoneal catheter.[210] Short-term peritoneal access may be obtained with a percutaneously inserted catheter,[211] but there is risk of bowel perforation or catheter loss.[212,213]

D. Continuous arteriovenous hemofiltration

CAVH removes fluid and solute using only convective forces.[214,215] The hydraulic driving pressure is provided by systemic arterial pressure or by the addition of a blood pump to increase pressure in the circuit. The apparatus consists of an arterial withdrawal cannula, a filter, and a venous return cannula. The rate of ultrafiltration with these devices is described by the equation

$$Q_f = KA(P_{tm} - P_{onc})$$

where Q_f is flow of filtrate, K is the filtration characteristic of the membrane, A is membrane area, P_{tm} is transmembrane hydrostatic pressure gradient, and P_{onc} is plasma oncotic pressure. Like the human glomerulus, CAVH eliminates solutes in a manner independent of molecular weight up to 10,000 daltons. Urea clearance equals the filtration rate, which rarely exceeds 35 to 40 ml·min^{-1} and usually is less than 10 ml·min^{-1}. In contrast, hemodialysis may clear urea from 150 ml of plasma in 1 minute.

The rate of ultrafiltration is directly proportional to mean arterial pressure and to blood flow through the filter and is inversely proportional to the plasma oncotic pressure. Either the addition of a pump on the arterial side or the application of negative pressure to the ultrafiltrate line will increase the rate of ultrafiltration by increasing P_{tm}.[216] CAVH removes large quantities of protein-free fluid containing solute in roughly the same concentrations as serum. The solute concentration remaining in serum is then reduced by dilution according to the concentration in intravenous fluid. CAVH removes sufficient salt and water to permit full-calorie, high-protein nutritional support of critically ill patients.[19] CAVHD is a modification of CAVH, in which dialysate resembling peritoneal dialysate is passed through the CAVHD device, thereby adding the clearance capabilities of diffusive transport to that achieved by convection alone.

The relative indications for and limitations of hemodialysis, peritoneal dialysis, and CAVH are listed in Table 19-12.

E. Physiologic effects and complications of renal replacement therapy

Although renal replacement therapy limits the complications of ARF, the therapy itself generates other complications.[217,218] The most im-

Table 19-12. Selection of renal replacement therapy

Therapy	Indications	Limitations
Hemodialysis	Rapid catabolism Severe volume, electrolyte, or acid-base disorders	Hypotension Anticoagulation risk Need for vascular access
Peritoneal dialysis	Lower cost Anticoagulation risk Difficult vascular access Hypotension Infants and small children	Rapid catabolism Diaphragmatic defects Severe volume, electrolyte, or acid-base disorders
Continuous arteriovenous hemofiltration (CAVH)	Hemodynamic instability Inexpensive equipment	Rapid catabolism Severe volume, electrolyte, or acid-base disorders Anticoagulation

portant physiologic effects and complications of renal replacement therapy involve the central nervous system, the cardiovascular system, and the respiratory system.

1. Central nervous system effects. The disequilibrium syndrome is an uncommon, potentially severe complication of acute hemodialysis.[219,220] Usually mild, the syndrome may progress to stupor, coma, and seizures. Predisposing factors include a predialysis BUN >150 mg·dl^{-1}, hypernatremia, profound acidemia, and preexisting brain disease. The mechanism is not established; however, most data implicate a transient increase in brain-tissue osmolality relative to serum osmolality.[221] Management of the disequilibrium syndrome is primarily preventive; that is, greatly elevated levels of BUN and serum sodium should be reduced gradually.

2. Cardiovascular effects. Symptomatic hypotension complicates 25% of chronic hemodialysis treatments.[222] The cause of hemodialysis-induced hypotension is multifactorial. Although intravascular volume is reduced, patients undergoing hemodialysis often fail to vasoconstrict in response to reductions in plasma volume and cardiac output. Uremic patients appear to have defective carotid and aortic body reflex arcs.[223,224] Peripheral resistance declines during hemodialysis despite hypotension and decreased cardiac filling pressures.[225]

The failure of compensatory vasoconstriction may be attributable to acetate, added to dialysate to replace bicarbonate expended in buffering accumulated acid wastes. Acetate, a vasodilator that interferes with reflex vasoconstriction,[226,227] is metabolized in the liver to bicarbonate. Removal of fluid and solute by dialysis against a bicarbonate bath may produce less hemodynamic instability than removal of similar quantities of fluid with acetate-containing dialysate.[226-229]

Recent studies indicate that an increase in plasma ionized calcium may be an important factor in the preservation of left ventricular contractility during dialysis.[230] An increase in the calcium concentration of dialysate from 5.5 to 7.5 mg·dl^{-1} produces substantially higher intradialytic blood pressure.[231]

Hemodialysis-induced hypotension is less severe if plasma volume is reduced slowly. Leg elevation, intravenous fluid administration, and occasionally vasoconstrictors can be used for the short-term management of hypotension. Myers and Moran hypothesize that norepinephrine may be the drug of choice for blood pressure elevation during hemodialysis in patients with ARF[22] because of the blunted renal response to vasoconstrictors in such patients.[232]

Hypotension occurs less commonly during peritoneal dialysis and CAVH. Hypotension during peritoneal dialysis, usually caused by excessively rapid removal of water and solute, may require substitution of dialysate containing a lower dextrose concentration. CAVH is associated with a low incidence of hypotension.[214] Since P_{tm} determines the rate of ultrafiltration, a decrease in systemic blood pressure will decrease the rate of ultrafiltration, thereby limiting further rapid fluid removal. However, if a blood pump is included in the arterial circuit, intravascular volume can be depleted rapidly.[215,216] Appropriate intravenous replacement of fluid will prevent excessive depletion of intravascular volume. Because CAVH does not interfere with sympathetic reflex responsiveness, even critically ill septic patients tolerate the modality well.[215]

3. Respiratory system effects. Two mechanisms contribute to the frequent occurrence of hypoxemia during hemodialysis: ventilation-perfusion mismatch and hypoventilation.[233,234] Patients may hypoventilate during hemodialysis without becoming hypercapnic,[235] perhaps the only situation in which hypoventilation and hypercapnia are not synonymous. The decline in Pa_{O_2} during hemodialysis may be explained partially by loss of carbon dioxide across the dialyzer membrane, as can be understood by use of the alveolar gas equation:

$$P_{A}O_2 = Pi_{O_2} - \frac{Pa_{CO_2}}{RE}$$

where $P_{A}O_2$ is alveolar oxygen tension, Pi_{O_2} is $Fi_{O_2} \times$ (barometric pressure $- 47$), Fi_{O_2} is the fractional inspired concentration of oxygen, and RE (respiratory excretion) is CO_2 excretion by the lung $\div$ by oxygen consumption. During dialysis against acetate, CO_2 is both excreted by the lungs and lost through the dialyzer membrane. The decline in CO_2 excretion by the lungs decreases RE. Thus, if the $P(A-a)_{O_2}$ remains the same, Pa_{O_2} must fall. If the decrease in Pa_{O_2} exceeds the decrease in $P_{A}O_2$, ventilation-perfusion mismatch also must be increased.[236] De Backer et al.[237] examined the relative contributions of changes in ventilation-perfusion relationships and of acetate-associated hypoventilation. Cuprophan membranes were associated consistently with ventilation-perfusion disturbances, whereas polyacrylonitryl membranes were not. Acetate dialysate was related to a decrease in Pa_{O_2}, whereas bicarbonate dialysate was not. Substitution of bicarbonate for acetate in the dialysate limits CO_2 loss through the dialyzer.[236] Hypoxemia during hemodialysis responds to an increase in Fi_{O_2}.

During peritoneal dialysis, hypoxemia may occur if upward displacement of the diaphragm impairs ventilation or if fluid traverses the diaphragm. Hypoxemia seldom occurs during CAVH.

IX. SUMMARY

Hypovolemia is common in critically ill patients and may result in renal dysfunction. The body has developed multiple mechanisms (that is, renal and hormonal) for coping with volume depletion. Renal adaptation to decreases in circulating volume involves alterations in renal blood flow, glomerular filtration, and tubular reabsorption. However, there is a limit to the ability of the kidneys to compensate for hypovolemia. If volume depletion persists, renal ischemia may occur and result in acute renal failure. Concomitant sepsis, organ failure, and nephrotoxic drugs increase the risk of acute re-

nal failure in volume-depleted patients. The development of acute renal failure in critically ill patients substantially increases mortality. Better understanding of basic renal physiology, the regulation of extracellular fluid volume, causes of hypovolemia, the diagnosis of hypovolemia and tissue hypoperfusion, and the management of volume status should help reduce the incidence of renal dysfunction.

REFERENCES

1. Kasiske BL and Kjellstrand CM: Perioperative management of patients with chronic renal failure and postoperative acute renal failure, Urol Clin North Am 10:35-50, 1983 (Review).
2. Abreo K, Moorthy AV, and Osborne M: Changing patterns and outcome of acute renal failure requiring hemodialysis, Arch Intern Med 146:1338-1341, 1986.
3. Lordon RE and Burton JR: Post-traumatic renal failure in military personnel in Southeast Asia: experience at Clark USAF Hospital, Republic of the Philippines, Am J Med 53:137-147, 1972.
4. Hou SH, Bushinsky DA, Wish JB, et al: Hospital-acquired renal insufficiency: a prospective study, Am J Med 74:243-248, 1983.
5. Gillum DM, Dixon BS, Yanover MJ, et al: The role of intensive dialysis in acute renal failure, Clin Nephrol 25:249-255, 1986.
6. Bullock ML, Umen AJ, Finkelstein M, et al: The assessment of risk factors in 462 patients with acute renal failure, Am J Kidney Dis 5:97-103, 1985.
7. Cameron JS: Acute renal failure in the intensive care unit today, Intensive Care Med 12:64-70, 1986 (Review).
8. Corwin HL and Bonventre JV: Acute renal failure in the intensive care unit. Part 1. Intensive Care Med 14:10-16, 1988, (Review).
9. Conger JD: A controlled evaluation of prophylactic dialysis in post-traumatic acute renal failure, J Trauma 15:1056-1063, 1975.
10. Charlson ME, MacKenzie CR, Gold JP, and Shires GT: Postoperative changes in serum creatinine, when do they occur and how much is important? Ann Surg 209:328-333, 1989.
11. Gornick CC Jr and Kjellstrand CM: Acute renal failure complicating aortic aneurysm surgery, Nephron 35:145-157, 1983.
12. Gamulin Z, Forster A, Morel D, et al: Effects of infrarenal aortic cross-clamping on renal hemodynamics in humans, Anesthesiology 61:394-399, 1984.
13. Gamulin Z, Forster A, Simonet F, et al: Effects of renal sympathetic blockade on renal hemodynamics in patients undergoing major aortic abdominal surgery, Anesthesiology 65:688-692, 1986.
14. Crawford E, Walker H, Salch S, et al: Graft replacement of aneurysm in descending thoracic aorta: results without bypass or shunting, Surgery 89:73-85, 1981.
15. Carlson DE, Karp RB, and Kouchoukos NT: Surgical treatment of aneurysms of the descending thoracic aorta: an analysis of 85 patients, Ann Thorac Surg 35:58-69, 1983.
16. Najafi H, Javid H, Hunter J, et al: Descending aortic aneurysmectomy without adjuncts to avoid ischemia, Ann Thorac Surg 30:326-335, 1980.
17. Alpert RA, Roizen MF, Hamilton WK, et al: Intra-

operative urinary output does not predict postoperative renal function in patients undergoing abdominal aortic revascularization, Surgery 95:707-711, 1984.

18. Sinicrope RA, Serra RM, Engle JE, et al: Mortality of acute renal failure after rupture of abdominal aortic aneurysms, Am J Surg 141:240-242, 1981.

19. McMurray SD, Luft FC, Maxwell DR, et al: Prevailing patterns and predictor variables in patients with acute tubular necrosis, Arch Intern Med 138:950-955, 1978.

20. Dawson JL: The incidence of postoperative renal failure in obstructive jaundice, Br J Surg 52:663-665, 1965.

21. Bushinsky DA, Wish JB, Hou SH, et al: Hospital acquired renal insufficiency, Kidney Int 16:875, 1979, (Abstract).

22. Myers BD and Moran SM: Hemodynamically mediated acute renal failure, N Engl J Med 314:97-105, 1986 (Review).

23. Vander AJ: Renal physiology, ed 3 New York, 1985, McGraw-Hill Book Co, pp 70-74.

24. Arendshorst WS, Finn WF, and Gottschalk CW: Autoregulation of renal blood flow in the rat kidney, Am J Physiol 228:127-133, 1975.

25. Kelleher SP and Berl T: Acute renal failure associated with hypovolemia. In Brenner BM and Lazarus JM, editors: Acute renal failure, Philadelphia, 1983, WB Saunders Co.

26. Stone AM and Stahl WM: Renal effects of hemorrhage in normal man, Ann Surg 172:825-836, 1970.

27. Aukland K, Kirkebo A, Loyning E, and Tyssebotn I: Effect of hemorrhagic hypotension on the distribution of renal cortical blood flow in anesthetized dogs, Acta Physiol Scand 87:514-525, 1973.

28. Henrich WL, Pettinger WA, and Cronin RE: The influence of circulating catecholamines and prostaglandins on canine renal hemodynamics during hemorrhage, Circ Res 218:424-429, 1981.

29. Henrich WL, Anderson RJ, Berns AS, et al: The role of renal nerves and prostaglandins in control of renal hemodynamics and plasma renin activity during hypotensive hemorrhage in the dog, J Clin Invest 61:744-750, 1978.

30. Badr KF and Ichikawa I: Prerenal failure: a deleterious shift from renal compensation to decompensation, N Engl J Med 319:623-629, 1988.

31. Laragh JH: The endocrine control of blood volume, blood pressure and sodium balance: atrial hormone and renin system interactions, J Hypertens 4:S143-S156, 1986.

32. Barajas L and Powers K: The structure of the juxtaglomerular apparatus (JGA) and the control of renin secretion: an update, J Hypertens 2:3-12, 1984.

33. Briggs JP and Schnermann J: Macula densa control of renin secretion and glomerular vascular tone: evidence for common cellular mechanisms, Renal Physiol 9:193-203, 1986 (Review).

34. Huang CL, Lewicki J, Johnson LK, et al: Renal mechanism of action of rat atrial natriuretic factor, J Clin Invest 75:769-773, 1985.

35. Salazar FJ, Romero JC, Burnett JC Jr, et al: Atrial natriuretic peptide levels during acute and chronic saline loading in conscious dogs, Am J Physiol 251:R499-R503, 1986.

36. Needleman P and Greenwald JE: Atriopeptin: a cardiac hormone intimately involved in fluid, electrolyte, and blood-pressure homeostasis, N Engl J Med 314:828-834, 1986 (Review).

37. Genest J: The atrial natriuretic factor, Br Heart J 56:302-316, 1986 (Review).

38. Roy LF, Ogilvie RI, Larochelle P, et al: Cardiac and vascular effects of atrial natriuretic factor and sodium nitroprusside in healthy men, Circulation 79:383-392, 1989.

39. Anand-Srivastava MB, Vinay P, and Genest J: Effect of atrial natriuretic factor on adenylate cyclase in various nephron segments, Am J Physiol 251:F417-F423, 1986.

40. Cernacek P, Maher E, and Crawhall JC: Renal dose response and pharmacokinetics of atrial natriuretic factor in dogs, Am J Physiol 255:R929-R935, 1988.

41. Shenker Y: Atrial natriuretic hormone effect on renal function and aldosterone secretion in sodium depletion, Am J Physiol 255:R867-R873, 1988.

42. Atlas SA, Volpe M, Sosa RE, et al: Effects of atrial natriuretic factor on blood pressure and the renin-angiotensin-aldosterone system, Fed Proc 45:2115-2121, 1986 (Review).

43. Makhoul RG and Gewertz BL: Renal prostaglandins, J Surg Res 40:181-192, 1986 (Review).

44. Raymond KH and Lifschitz MD: Effect of prostaglandins on renal salt and water excretion, Am J Med 80:22-33, 1986 (Review).

45. Scharschmidt LA, Lianos E, and Dunn MJ: Arachidonate metabolites and the control of glomerular function, Fed Proc 42:3058-3063, 1983.

46. Murray MD and Brater DC: Adverse effects of nonsteroidal anti-inflammatory drugs on renal function, Ann Intern Med 112:559-560, 1990 (Editorial).

47. Duchin KL, Peterson LN, and Burke TJ: Effect of furosemide on renal autoregulation, Kidney Int 12:379-386, 1977.

48. Roberts JP, Roberts JD, Skinner C, et al: Extracellular fluid deficit following operation and its correction with Ringer's lactate: a reassessment, Ann Surg 202:1-8, 1985.

49. Carrico CJ, Coln CD, Lightfoot SA, et al: Extracellular fluid volume replacement in hemorrhagic shock, Surg Forum 14:10-12, 1963.

50. Giesecke AH and Egbert LD: Perioperative fluid therapy crystalloids. In Miller R, editor: Anesthesia, New York, 1986, Churchill Livingstone.

51. Rackow EC, Falk JL, Fein IA, et al: Fluid resuscitation in circulatory shock: a comparison of the cardiorespiratory effects of albumin, hetastarch, and saline solutions in patients with hypovolemic and septic shock, Crit Care Med 11:839-850, 1983.

52. Shenkin HA, Cheney RH, Govons SR, et al: On the diagnosis of hemorrhage in man: a study of volunteers bled large amounts, Am J Med Sci 208:421-436, 1944.

53. Lipsitz LA: Orthostatic hypotension in the elderly, N Engl J Med 321:952-957, 1989 (Review).

54. Amoroso P and Greenwood RN: Posture and central venous pressure measurement in circulatory volume depletion, Lancet 2:258-260, 1989.

55. Bland RD, Shoemaker WC, Abraham E, et al: Hemodynamic and oxygen transport patterns in surviving and nonsurviving postoperative patients, Crit Care Med 13:85-90, 1985.

56. Bland RD and Shoemaker WC: Probability of survival as a prognostic and severity illness scorer in critically ill surgical patients, Crit Care Med 13:91-95, 1985.

57. Shoemaker WC, Appel PL, Kram HB, et al: Prospective trial of supranormal values of survivors as therapeutic goals in high-risk surgical patients, Chest 94:1176-1186, 1988.

58. Sladen RN: Effect of anesthesia and surgery on renal function, Crit Care Clin 3:373-393, 1987 (Review).

59. Philbin D and Coggins CH: Plasma antidiuretic hor-

mone levels in cardiac surgical patients during morphine and halothane anesthesia, Anesthesiology 49:95-98, 1978.

60. Vatner SF and Braunwald E: Cardiovascular control mechanisms in the conscious state, N Engl J Med 293:970-976, 1975.

61. Marquez JM, Douglas ME, Downs JB, et al: Renal function and cardiovascular responses during positive airway pressure, Anesthesiology 50:393-398, 1979.

62. Priebe H-J, Heimann JC and Hedley-Whyte J: Mechanisms of renal dysfunction during positive end-expiratory pressure ventilation, J Appl Physiol 50:643-649, 1981.

63. Andrivet P, Adnot S, Brun-Buisson C, et al: Involvement of ANF in the acute antidiuresis during PEEP ventilation, J Appl Physiol 65:1967-1974, 1988.

64. Payen DM, Farge D, Beloucif S, et al: No involvement of antidiuretic hormone in acute antidiuresis during PEEP ventilation in humans, Anesthesiology 66:17-23, 1987.

65. Crandell WB, Pappas SG, and Macdonald A: Nephrotoxicity associated with methoxyflurane anesthesia, Anesthesiology 27:591-607, 1966.

66. Mazze RI, Trudell JR, and Cousins MJ: Methoxyflurane metabolism and renal dysfunction: clinical correlation in man, Anesthesiology 35:247-252, 1971.

67. Cousins MJ and Mazze RI: Methoxyflurane nephrotoxicity: a study of dose response in man, JAMA 225:1611-1616, 1973.

68. Cousins MJ, Greenstein LR, Hitt BA, et al: Metabolism and renal effects of enflurane in man, Anesthesiology 44:44-53, 1976.

69. Lundeen G, Manohar M, and Parks C: Systemic distribution of blood flow in swine while awake and during 1.0 and 1.5 MAC isoflurane anesthesia with or without 50% nitrous oxide, Anesth Analg 62:499-512, 1983.

70. Gelman S, Fowler KC, and Smith LR: Regional blood flow during isoflurane and halothane anesthesia, Anesth Analg 63:557-565, 1984.

71. Mazze RI, Calverley RK, and Smith NT: Inorganic fluoride nephrotoxicity: prolonged enflurane and halothane anesthesia in volunteers, Anesthesiology 46:265-271, 1977.

72. Mazze RI, Woodruff RE, and Heerdt ME: Isoniazid-induced enflurane defluorination in humans, Anesthesiology 57:5-8, 1982.

73. Theye RA and Maher FT: The effects of halothane on canine renal function and oxygen consumption, Anesthesiology 35:54-60, 1971.

74. Ohmura A, Wong KC, Pace NL, et al: Effects of halothane and sodium nitroprusside on renal function and autoregulation, Br J Anaesth 54:103-108, 1982.

75. Hill GE, Lunn JK, Hodges MR, et al: N$_2$O modification of halothane-altered renal function in the dog, Anesth Analg 56:690-695, 1977.

76. Priano LL: Effect of halothane on renal hemodynamics during normovolemia and acute hemorrhagic hypovolemia, Anesthesiology 63:357-363, 1985.

77. Lebowitz PW, Cote ME, Daniels AL, et al: Comparative renal effects of midazolam and thiopental in humans, Anesthesiology 59:381-384, 1983.

78. Priano LL: Alteration of renal hemodynamics by thiopental, diazepam, and ketamine in conscious dogs, Anesth Analg 61:853-862, 1982.

79. Bidwai AV, Stanley TH, Bloomer HA, et al: Effects of anesthetic doses of morphine on renal function in the dog, Anesth Analg 54:357-360, 1975.

80. Hunter JM, Jones RS, and Utting JE: Effect of anaesthesia with nitrous oxide in oxygen and fentanyl on renal function in the artificially ventilated dog, Br J Anaesth 52:343-348, 1980.

81. Priano LL: Effects of high-dose fentanyl on renal hemodynamics in conscious dogs, Can Anaesth Soc J 30:10-18, 1983.

82. Kennedy WF Jr, Sawyer TK, Gerbershagen HY, et al: Simultaneous systemic cardiovascular and renal hemodynamic measurements during high spinal anaesthesia in normal man, Acta Anaesthesiol Scand Suppl 37:163, 1969.

83. Sivarajan M, Amory DW, and Lindbloom LE: Systemic and regional blood flow during epidural anesthesia without epinephrine in the rhesus monkey, Anesthesiology 45:300-310, 1976.

84. Kennedy WF Jr, Sawyer TK, Gerbershagen HY, et al: Systemic cardiovascular and renal hemodynamic alterations during peridural anesthesia in normal man, Anesthesiology 31:414-421, 1969.

85. Harrington JT and Cohen JJ: Acute oliguria, N Engl J Med 292:89-91, 1975 (Review).

86. Vander AJ: Control of renin release, Physiol Rev 47:359-382, 1967 (Review).

87. Thurau K, Schnermann J, Naggel W, et al: Composition of tubular fluid in the macula densa segment as a factor regulating the function of the juxtaglomerular apparatus, Circ Res 21(suppl 2):79-90, 1967.

88. Edwards BS, Zimmerman RS, Schwab TR, et al: Role of atrial peptide system in renal and endocrine adaptation to hypotensive hemorrhage, Am J Physiol 254:R56-R60, 1988.

89. Habib BR, Hanet C, van Mechelen H, et al: Effects of atriopeptin III on renal function, regional blood flows and left ventricular function in conscious dogs in presence or absence of hypovolaemia, Eur J Clin Invest 16:461-467, 1986.

90. Burke TJ, Burnier M, Langberg H, et al: Renal response to shock, Ann Emerg Med 15:1397-1400, 1986.

91. Hamaji M, Nakamura M, Izukura M, et al: Autoregulation and regional blood flow of the dog during hemorrhagic shock, Circ Shock 19:245-255, 1986.

92. Yoshioka T, Yared A, Kon V, et al: Impaired preservation of GFR during hypotension in preexistent renal hypoperfusion, Am J Physiol 256:F314-F320, 1989.

93. Badr KF and Ichikawa I: Prerenal failure: a deleterious shift from renal compensation to decompensation, N Engl J Med 319:623-629, 1988 (Review).

94. Schrier RW: Acute renal failure, JAMA 247:2518-2524, 1982.

95. Flamenbaum W: Pathophysiology of acute renal failure, Arch Intern Med 131:911-928, 1973 (Review).

96. Olsen S and Solez K: Acute renal failure in man: pathogenesis in light of new morphological data, Clin Nephrol 27:271-277, 1987.

97. Hollenberg NK, Adams DF, Oken DE, et al: Acute renal failure due to nephrotoxins, N Engl J Med 282:1329-1334, 1970.

98. Williams RJ, Thomas CE, Navor LG, and Evan AP: Hemodynamic and single nephron function during the maintenance phase of ischemic acute renal failure in the dog, Kidney Int 19:503-515, 1981.

99. Conger JD and Robinette JB: Loss of blood flow autoregulation in acute renal failure (ARF), Kidney Int 16:850, 1979 (Abstract).

100. Whelton A, Stout RL, Spilman PS, et al: Renal effects of ibuprofen, piroxicam, and sulindac in patients with asymptomatic renal failure: a prospective, randomized crossover comparison, Ann Intern Med 112:568-576, 1990.

101. Walshe JJ and Venuto RC: Acute oliguric renal failure induced by indomethacin: possible mechanism, Ann Intern Med 91:47-49, 1979.

102. Mauk RH, Patak RV, Fadem SZ, et al: Effect of prostaglandin E administration in a nephrotoxic and a vasoconstrictor model of acute renal failure, Kidney Int 12:122-130, 1977.

103. Tobimatsu M, Konomi K, Saito S, et al: Protective effect of prostaglandin E₁ on ischemia-induced acute renal failure in dogs, Surgery 98:45-53, 1985.

104. Donohoe JF, Venkatachalam MA, Bernard DB, et al: Tubular leakage and obstruction after renal ischemia: structural functional correlations, Kidney Int 13:208-222, 1978.

105. Thurau K: Pathophysiology of the acutely failing kidney, Clin Exp Dial Apheresis 7:9-24, 1983.

106. Oken DE, Arce ML, and Wilson DR: Glycerol-induced hemoglobinuric acute renal failure in the rat: I. Micropuncture study of the development of oliguria, J Clin Invest 45:724-735, 1966.

107. Myers BD, Carrie BJ, Yee RR, et al: Pathophysiology of hemodynamically mediated acute renal failure in man, Kidney Int 18:495-504, 1980.

108. Moran SM and Myers BD: Pathophysiology of protracted acute renal failure in man, J Clin Invest 76:1440-1448, 1985.

109. Porter GA and Bennett WM: Nephrotoxic acute renal failure due to common drugs, Am J Physiol 241:F1-F8, 1981 (Review).

110. Moore RD, Smith CR, Lipsky JJ, et al: Risk factors for nephrotoxicity in patients treated with aminoglycosides, Ann Intern Med 100:352-357, 1984.

111. Kaloyanides GJ and Pastoriza-Munoz E: Aminoglycoside nephrotoxicity, Kidney Int 18:571-582, 1980.

112. Matzke GR, Lucarotti RL, and Shapiro HS: Controlled comparison of gentamicin and tobramycin nephrotoxicity, Am J Nephrol 3:11-17, 1983.

113. Knochel JP and Schlein EM: On the mechanism of rhabdomyolysis in potassium depletion, J Clin Invest 51:1750-1758, 1972.

114. Dubrow A and Flamenbaum W: Acute renal failure associated with myoglobinuria and hemoglobinuria. In Brenner BM and Lazarus JM, editors: Acute renal failure, ed 2, New York, 1988, Churchill Livingstone.

115. Ron D, Taitelman U, Michaelson MD, et al: Prevention of acute renal failure in traumatic rhabdomyolysis, Arch Intern Med 144:277-280, 1984.

116. VanZee BE, Hoy WE, Talley TE, et al: Renal injury associated with intravenous pyelography in nondiabetic and diabetic patients, Ann Intern Med 89:51-54, 1978.

117. Parfrey PS, Griffiths SM, Barrett BJ, et al: Contrast material–induced renal failure in patients with diabetes mellitus, renal insufficiency, or both: a prospective controlled study, N Engl J Med 320:143-149, 1989.

118. Snyder HE, Killen DA, and Foster JH: The influence of mannitol on toxic reactions to contrast angiography, Surgery 64:640-642, 1968.

119. Anto HR, Chou SY, Porush JG, et al: Mannitol prevention of acute renal failure (ARF) associated with infusion intravenous pyelography (IIVP), Clin Res 27:407A, 1979.

120. Talner LB: Does hydration prevent contrast material renal injury? AJR 136:1021-1022, 1981 (Editorial).

121. Eisenberg RL, Bank WO, and Hedgcock MW: Renal failure after major angiography can be avoided with hydration, AJR 136:859-861, 1981.

122. Rasmussen HH and Ibels LS: Acute renal failure: multivariate analysis of causes and risk factors, Am J Med 73:211-218, 1982.

123. Anderson RJ, Linas SL, Berns AS, et al: Nonoliguric acute renal failure, N Engl J Med 296:1134-1138, 1977.

124. Diamond JR and Yoburn DC: Nonoliguric acute re-

nal failure, Arch Intern Med 142:1882-1884, 1982 (Review).

125. Dixon BS and Anderson RJ: Nonoliguric acute renal failure, Am J Kidney Dis 6:71-80, 1985 (Review).

126. Shin B, Mackenzie CF, McAslan TC, et al: Postoperative renal failure in trauma patients, Anesthesiology 51:218-221, 1979.

127. Myers BD, Hilberman M, Spencer RJ, et al: Glomerular and tubular function in non-oliguric acute renal failure, Am J Med 72:642-649, 1982.

128. Myers BD, Miller DC, Mehigan JT, et al: Nature of the renal injury following total renal ischemia in man, J Clin Invest 73:329-341, 1984.

129. Brown CB, Ogg CS, and Cameron JS: High dose frusemide in acute renal failure: a controlled trial, Clin Nephrol 15:90-96, 1981.

130. Hesdorffer CS, Milne JF, Meyers AM, et al: The value of Swan-Ganz catheterization and volume loading in preventing renal failure in patients undergoing abdominal aneurysmectomy, Clin Nephrol 28:272-276, 1987.

131. Bush HL Jr, Huse JB, Johnson WC, et al: Prevention of renal insufficiency after abdominal aortic aneurysm resection by optimal volume loading, Arch Surg 116:1517-1524, 1981.

132. Cronin RE, Erickson AM, de Torrente A, et al: Norepinephrine-induced acute renal failure: a reversible ischemic model of acute renal failure, Kidney Int 14:187-190, 1978.

133. Burke TJ, Cronin RE, Duchin KL, et al: Ischemia and tubule obstruction during acute renal failure in dogs: mannitol in protection, Am J Physiol 238:F305-F314, 1980.

134. Patak RV, Fadem SZ, Lifschitz MD, et al: Study of factors which modify the development of norepinephrine-induced acute renal failure in the dog, Kidney Int 15:227-237, 1979.

135. Hanley MJ and Davidson K: Prior mannitol and furosemide infusion in a model of ischemic acute renal failure, Am J Physiol 241:F556-F564, 1981.

136. Sinsteden TD, O'Neil TJ, Hill S, et al: The role of high-energy phosphate in norepinephrine-induced acute renal failure in the dog, Circ Res 59:93-104, 1986.

137. Pass LJ, Eberhart RC, Brown JC, et al: The effect of mannitol and dopamine on the renal response to thoracic aortic cross-clamping, J Thorac Cardiovasc Surg 95:608-612, 1988.

138. Henderson IS, Beattie TJ, and Kennedy AC: Dopamine hydrochloride in oliguric states, Lancet 2:827-828, 1980.

139. Schwartz LB and Gewertz BL: The renal response to low dose dopamine, J Surg Res 45:574-588, 1988 (Review).

140. Kleinknecht D, Ganeval D, Gonzales-Duque LA, et al: Furosemide in acute oliguric renal failure: a controlled trial, Nephron 17:51-58, 1976.

141. Lindner A, Cutler RE, and Goodman WG: Synergism of dopamine plus furosemide in preventing acute renal failure in the dog, Kidney Int 16:158-166, 1979.

142. Lindner A: Synergism of dopamine and furosemide in diuretic-resistant, oliguric acute renal failure, Nephron 33:121-126, 1983.

143. Elliott WJ, Weber RR, Nelson KS, et al: Renal and hemodynamic effects of intravenous fenoldopam versus nitroprusside in severe hypertension, Circulation 81:970-977, 1990.

144. Allison NL, Dubbs JW, Ziemniak JA, et al: The effect of fenoldopam, a dopaminergic agonist, on renal he-

modynamics, Clin Pharmacol Ther 41:282-288, 1987.

145. Murphy MB, McCoy CE, Weber RR, et al: Augmentation of renal blood flow and sodium excretion in hypertensive patients during blood pressure reduction by intravenous administration of the dopamine-1 agonist, fenoldopam, Circulation 76:1312-1318, 1987.

146. Hughes JM, Ragsdale NV, Felder RA, et al: Diuresis and natriuresis during continuous dopamine-1 receptor stimulation, Hypertension 11:I69-I74, 1988.

147. Bonventre JV: Mediators of ischemic renal injury, Annu Rev Med 39:531-544, 1988 (Review).

148. Corwin HL and Bonventre JV: Acute renal failure, Med Clin North Am 70:1037-1054, 1986.

149. Cronin RE: Drug therapy in the management of acute renal failure, Am J Med Sci 292:112-119, 1986.

150. Corwin HL and Bonventre JV: Acute renal failure in the intensive care unit. Part 2. Intensive Care Med 14:86-96, 1988.

151. Fildes RD, Springate JE, and Feld LG: Acute renal failure. II. Management of suspected and established disease, J Pediatr 109:567-571, 1986.

152. Epstein FH and Brown RS: Acute renal failure: a collection of paradoxes, Hosp Pract 23:171-175,179-183, 1988 (Review).

153. Mandal AK, Lightfoot BO, and Treat RC: Mechanisms of protection in acute renal failure, Circ Shock 11:245-253, 1983 (Review).

154. Ratcliffe PJ, Moonen CT, Holloway PA, et al: Acute renal failure in hemorrhagic hypotension: cellular energetics and renal function, Kidney Int 30:355-360, 1986.

155. Brezis M, Rosen S, Silva P, et al: Renal ischemia: a new perspective, Kidney Int 26:375-383, 1984 (Review).

156. Vetterlein F, Petho A, and Schmidt G: Distribution of capillary blood flow in rat kidney during postischemic renal failure, Am J Physiol 251:H510-H519, 1986.

157. Ratcliffe PJ, Endre ZH, Tange JD, et al: Ischaemic acute renal failure: why does it occur? Nephron 52:1-5, 1989 (Review).

158. Mason J, Torhorst J, and Welsch J: Role of the medullary perfusion defect in the pathogenesis of ischemic renal failure, Kidney Int 26:283-293, 1984.

159. Hirasawa H, Odaka M, Soeda K, et al: Experimental and clinical study on ATP-MgCl$_2$ administration for postischemic acute renal failure, Clin Exp Dial Apheresis 7:37-47, 1983.

160. Siegel NJ, Glazier WB, Chaudrey IH, et al: Enhanced recovery from acute renal failure by the postischemic infusion of adenine nucleotides and magnesium chloride in rats, Kidney Int 17:338-349, 1980.

161. van Waarde A, Stromski ME, Thulin G, et al: Protection of the kidney against ischemic injury by inhibition of 5'-nucleotidase, Am J Physiol 256:F298-F305, 1989.

162. Didlake R, Kirchner KA, Lewin J, et al: Protection from ischemic renal injury by fructose-1,6-diphosphate infusion in the rat, Circ Shock 16:205-212, 1985.

163. Zager RA, Gmur DJ, Bredl CR, et al: Degree and time sequence of hypothermic protection against experimental ischemic acute renal failure, Circ Res 65:1263-1269, 1989.

164. Wait RB, White G, and Davis JH: Beneficial effects of verapamil on postischemic renal failure, Surgery 94:276-282, 1983.

165. Goldfarb D, Iaina A, Serban I, et al: Beneficial effect

of verapamil in ischemic acute renal failure in the rat, Proc Soc Exp Biol Med 172:389-392, 1983.

166. Silverman M, Rose H, and Puschett JB: Modifications in proximal tubular function induced by nitrendipine in a rat model of acute ischemic renal failure, J Cardiovasc Pharmacol 14:799-802, 1989.

167. Russell JD and Churchill DN: Calcium antagonists and acute renal failure, Am J Med 87:306-315, 1989 (Review).

168. Leahy AL, Galla J, Fitzpatrick JM, et al: The canine kidney in haemorrhagic shock: effect of verapamil, Eur Urol 13:401-406, 1987.

169. Loutzenhiser RD and Epstein M: Renal hemodynamic effects of calcium antagonists, Am J Med 82:23-28, 1987 (Review).

170. Diamond JR, Cheung JY, and Fang LS: Nifedipine-induced renal dysfunction: alterations in renal hemodynamics, Am J Med 77:905-909, 1984.

171. Canavese C, Stratta P, and Vercellone A: The case for oxygen free radicals in the pathogenesis of ischemic acute renal failure, Nephron 49:9-15, 1988 (Review).

172. Ratych RE and Bulkley GB: Free-radical–mediated postischemic reperfusion injury in the kidney, J Free Radic Biol Med 2:311-319, 1986 (Review).

173. Lelcuk S, Alexander F, Kobzik L, et al: Prostacyclin and thromboxane A$_2$ moderate postischemic renal failure, Surgery 98:207-212, 1985.

174. Pierucci A, Simonetti BM, Pecci G, et al: Improvement of renal function with selective thromboxane antagonism in lupus nephritis, N Engl J Med 320:421-425, 1989.

175. Kaufman RP Jr, Klausner JM, Anner H, et al: Inhibition of thromboxane (Tx) synthesis by free radical scavengers, J Trauma 28:458-464, 1988.

176. Mandal AK and Miller J: Protection against ischemic acute renal failure by prostaglandin infusion, Prostaglandins Leukot Med 8:361-373, 1982.

177. Torsello G, Schror K, Szabo Z, et al: Effects of prostaglandin E$_1$ (PGE$_1$) on experimental renal ischaemia, Eur J Vasc Surg 3:5-13, 1989.

178. Lifschitz MD and Barnes JL: Prostaglandin I$_2$ attenuates ischemic acute renal failure in the rat, Am J Physiol 247:F714-F717, 1984.

179. Klausner JM, Paterson IS, Goldman G, et al: Postischemic renal injury is mediated by neutrophils and leukotrienes, Am J Physiol 256:F794-F802, 1989.

180. Andrews PM and Bates SB: Dietary protein prior to renal ischemia dramatically affects postischemic kidney function, Kidney Int 30:299-303, 1986.

181. Seguro AC, Shimizu MH, Monteiro JL, et al: Effect of potassium depletion on ischemic renal failure, Nephron 51:350-354, 1989.

182. Zaloga GP and Hughes SS: Oliguria in patients with normal renal function, Anesthesiology 72:598-602, 1990.

183. Zaloga GP and Hill T: Advances in diagnostic testing for urinary tract infection, Infections in Urology 2:117-125, 1989.

184. Sladen RN, Endo E, and Harrison T: Two-hour versus 22-hour creatinine clearance in critically ill patients, Anesthesiology 67:1013-1016, 1987.

185. Wilson RF, Soullier G, and Antonenko D: Creatinine clearance in critically ill surgical patients, Arch Surg 114:461-467, 1979.

186. Wilson RF and Soullier G: The validity of two-hour creatinine clearance studies in critically ill patients, Crit Care Med 8:281-284, 1980.

187. Preece MJ and Richardson JA: The effect of mild dehydration on one-hour creatinine clearance rates, Nephron 9:106-112, 1972.

188. Richardson JA and Philbin PE: The one-hour creati-

nine clearance rate in healthy men, JAMA 216:987-990, 1971.

189. Miller PD, Krebs RA, Neal BJ, et al: Polyuric prerenal failure, Arch Intern Med 140:907-909, 1980.

190. Espinel CH and Gregory AW: Differential diagnosis of acute renal failure, Clin Nephrol 13:73-77, 1980.

191. Mathew A and Berl T: Fractional excretion of sodium: use early to assess renal failure, J Crit Illness 4:45-52, 1988.

192. Miller TR, Anderson RJ, Linas SL, et al: Urinary diagnostic indices in acute renal failure: a prospective study, Ann Intern Med 89:47-50, 1978.

193. Oken DE: On the differential diagnosis of acute renal failure, Am J Med 71:916-920, 1981.

194. Pru C and Kjellstrand CM: The FE_{Na} test is of no prognostic value in acute renal failure, Nephron 36:20-23, 1984.

195. Diamond JR and Yoburn DC: Nonoliguric acute renal failure associated with a low fractional excretion of sodium, Ann Intern Med 96:597-600, 1982.

196. Zarich S, Fang LS, and Diamond JR: Fractional excretion of sodium: exceptions to its diagnostic value, Arch Intern Med 145:108-112, 1985.

197. Prough DS and Zaloga GP: Monitoring renal function, Crit Care Clin 4:573-589, 1988.

198. Prough DS and Adams PL: Physiologic effects of dialysis and ultrafiltration. In Barash PG, editor: ASA Refresher Courses in Anesthesiology, Philadelphia, 1987, JB Lippincott Co.

199. Beck CH Jr: Etiologies of acute renal failure: the dialytic treatment of acute renal failure. In Critical care: state of the art, vol 5, pp 1-27, Fullerton, Calif, 1984, Society of Critical Care Medicine.

200. Levey AS and Harrington JT: Continuous peritoneal dialysis for chronic renal failure, Medicine 61:330-339, 1982.

201. Nolph KD: Continuous ambulatory peritoneal dialysis, Am J Nephrol 1:1-10, 1981 (Review).

202. Kliger AS: Complications of dialysis: hemodialysis, peritoneal dialysis, CAPD. In Arieff AI and DeFronzo RA, editors: Fluid, electrolyte, and acid-base disorders, vol 2, New York, 1985, Churchill Livingstone.

203. Cogan MG and Garovoy MR, editors: Introduction to dialysis, New York, 1985, Churchill Livingstone.

204. Drukker W, Parsons FM, and Maher JF, editors: Replacement of renal function by dialysis: a textbook of dialysis, ed 2, Boston, 1983, Martinus Nijhoff Publishers.

205. Alfred HJ and Cohen AJ: Use of dialytic procedures in the intensive care unit. In Rippe JM, Irwin RS, Alpert JS, et al, editors: Intensive care medicine, Boston, 1985, Little, Brown & Co.

206. Gotch FA and Keen ML: Dialyzers and delivery systems. In Cogan MG and Garovoy MR, editors: Introduction to dialysis, New York, 1985, Churchill Livingstone.

207. Uldall PR, Joy C, and Merchant N: Further experience with a double-lumen subclavian cannula for hemodialysis, Trans Am Soc Artif Intern Organs 28:71-75, 1982.

208. Lewinstein C, Silberman H, Goren C, et al: Experience with a coaxial dialysis cannula for temporary vascular access, Trans Am Soc Artif Intern Organs 29:357-359, 1983.

209. Maher JF: Characteristics of peritoneal transport: physiological and clinical implications, Miner Electrolyte Metab 5:201-211, 1981.

210. Tenckhoff H and Schechter H: A bacteriologically safe peritoneal access device, Trans Am Soc Artif Intern Organs 14:181-187, 1968.

211. Weston RE and Roberts M: Clinical use of stylet-catheter for peritoneal dialysis, Arch Intern Med 115:659-662, 1965.

212. Simkin EP and Wright FK: Perforating injuries of the bowel complicating peritoneal catheter insertion, Lancet 1:64-66, 1968.

213. Cope C and Kramer MS: Laparoscopic retrieval of dialysis catheter, Ann Intern Med 81:121, 1974.

214. Synhaivsky A, Kurtz SB, Wochos DN, et al: Acute renal failure treated by slow continuous ultrafiltration: preliminary report, Mayo Clin Proc 58:729-733, 1983.

215. Lauer A, Saccaggi A, Ronco C, et al: Continuous arteriovenous hemofiltration in the critically ill patient: clinical use and operational characteristics, Ann Intern Med 99:455-460, 1983.

216. Kaplan AA, Longnecker RE, and Folkert VW: Continuous arteriovenous hemofiltration: a report of 6 months' experience, Ann Intern Med 100:358-367, 1984.

217. Freeman RB: Treatment of chronic renal failure: an update, N Engl J Med 312:577-579, 1985 (Editorial).

218. Twardowski ZJ and Nolph KD: Blood purification in acute renal failure, Ann Intern Med 100:447-449, 1984.

219. Mahoney CA and Arieff AI: Uremic encephalopathies: clinical, biochemical, and experimental features, Am J Kidney Dis 2:324-336, 1982 (Review).

220. Fraser Cl and Arieff AI: Nervous system complications in uremia, Ann Intern Med 109:143-153, 1988 (Review).

221. Arieff AI, Guisado R, Massry SG, et al: Central nervous system pH in uremia and the effects of hemodialysis, J Clin Invest 58:306-311, 1976.

222. Henderson LW: Symptomatic hypotension during hemodialysis, Kidney Int 17:571-576, 1980 (Review).

223. Lazarus JM, Hampers CL, Lowrie EG, et al: Baroreceptor activity in normotensive and hypertensive uremic patients, Circulation 47:1015-1021, 1973.

224. Lilley JJ, Golden J, and Stone RA: Adrenergic regulation of blood pressure in chronic renal failure, J Clin Invest 57:1190-1200, 1976.

225. Endou K, Kamijima J, Kakubari Y, et al: Hemodynamic changes during hemodialysis, Cardiology 63:175-187, 1978.

226. Graefe U, Milutinovich J, Follette WC, et al: Less dialysis-induced morbidity and vascular instability with bicarbonate in dialysate, Ann Intern Med 88:332-336, 1978.

227. Kirkendol PL, Devia CJ, Bower JD, et al: A comparison of the cardiovascular effects of sodium acetate, sodium bicarbonate and other potential sources of fixed base in hemodialysate solutions, Trans Am Soc Artif Intern Organs 23:399-405, 1977.

228. Raja R, Kramer M, Rosenbaum JL, et al: Prevention of hypotension during iso-osmolar hemodialysis with bicarbonate dialysate, Trans Am Soc Artif Intern Organs 26:375-377, 1980.

229. Fournier G and Man NK: Prevention of hemodialysis-induced hypoxemia by use of bicarbonate-containing dialysate, abstracted, Kidney Int 17:701-702, 1980 (Abstract).

230. Hung J, Harris PJ, Uren RF, et al: Uremic cardiomyopathy: effect of hemodialysis on left ventricular function in end-stage renal failure, N Engl J Med 302:547-551, 1980.

231. Maynard JC, Cruz C, Kleerkoper M, et al: Blood pressure response to changes in serum ionized cal-

cium during hemodialysis, Ann Intern Med 104:358-361, 1986.

232. Kelleher SP, Robinette JB, and Conger JD: Sympathetic nervous system in the loss of autoregulation in acute renal failure, Am J Physiol 246:F379-F386, 1984.

233. Craddock PR, Fehr J, Brigham KL, et al: Complement and leukocyte-mediated pulmonary dysfunction in hemodialysis, N Engl J Med 296:769-774, 1977.

234. Francos GC, Besarab A, Burke JF Jr, et al: Dialysis-induced hypoxemia: membrane dependent and membrane independent causes, Am J Kidney Dis 5:191-198, 1985.

235. Aurigemma NM, Feldman NT, Gottlieb M, et al: Arterial oxygenation during hemodialysis, N Engl J Med 297:871-873, 1977.

236. Romaldini H, Rodriquez-Roisin R, Lopez FA, et al: The mechanisms of arterial hypoxemia during hemodialysis, Am Rev Respir Dis 129:780-784, 1984.

237. De Backer WA, Verpooten GA, Borgonjon DJ, et al: Hypoxemia during hemodialysis: effects of different membranes and dialysate compositions, Kidney Int 23:738-743, 1983.

Chapter 20

Perioperative Electrolyte Disorders

Albert T. Cheung
Bart Chernow

I. **Sodium and Water**
   A. Physiologic Properties of Sodium and Water
   B. Regulation of Sodium and Water Metabolism
   C. Hyponatremia
      1. Causes of hyponatremia
         a. Hyponatremia without plasma hyposmolality
         b. Hyponatremia with plasma hyposmolality
      2. Clinical manifestations of hyponatremia
      3. Diagnostic strategy for hyponatremia
      4. Treatment of hyponatremia
   D. Hypernatremia
      1. Causes of hypernatremia
      2. Treatment of hypernatremia
      3. Evaluation of polyuria and diabetes insipidus
         a. Treatment of diabetes insipidus
II. **Potassium**
   A. Potassium Homeostasis
   B. The Regulation of Serum Potassium Concentration
      1. Regulation of internal potassium balance
      2. Regulation of external potassium balance
   C. Hypokalemia
      1. Causes of hypokalemia
         a. Dietary potassium deficiency
         b. Hypokalemia secondary to cellular uptake of potassium
         c. Hypokalemia secondary to renal and extrarenal potassium losses
      2. Clinical manifestations of hypokalemia
      3. Diagnostic evaluation of hypokalemia
      4. Treatment of hypokalemia
   D. Hyperkalemia

   1. Causes of hyperkalemia
      a. Pseudohyperkalemia
      b. Hyperkalemia secondary to cellular release of potassium
      c. Hyperkalemia secondary to excessive potassium administration
      d. Hyperkalemia secondary to impaired potassium excretion
   2. Clinical manifestations of hyperkalemia
   3. Treatment of hyperkalemia
III. **Calcium**
   A. Calcium Homeostasis
   B. Measurement of Circulating Calcium Concentrations
   C. Physiologic Regulation of Calcium Metabolism
   D. Physiologic Actions of Calcium
   E. Hypocalcemia
      1. Causes of hypocalcemia
      2. Clinical manifestations of hypocalcemia
      3. Treatment of hypocalcemia
   F. Hypercalcemia
      1. Causes of hypercalcemia
      2. Clinical manifestations of hypercalcemia
      3. Treatment of hypercalcemia
IV. **Magnesium**
   A. Magnesium Homeostasis
   B. Physiologic Actions of Magnesium
   C. Hypomagnesemia
      1. Causes of hypomagnesemia
      2. Clinical manifestations of hypomagnesemia
      3. Treatment of hypomagnesemia
   D. Hypermagnesemia
      1. Causes of hypermagnesemia
      2. Clinical manifestations of hypermagnesemia
      3. Treatment of hypermagnesemia

Laboratory measurements of circulating electrolyte concentrations are a routine part of the preoperative evaluation of virtually all surgical patients. This practice is based upon the presumed rationale that (1) electrolyte disturbances are common, (2) the measurement of electrolytes provides clues to the presence of coexisting conditions that may influence anesthetic and surgical management, and (3) prophylactic management or the immediate institution of therapy for preoperative electrolyte disturbances has a positive impact on anesthetic and surgical outcome.

The clinical management of perioperative electrolyte disorders in the surgical patient is a challenging problem. The majority of acute perioperative electrolyte disorders can be diagnosed accurately and corrected with appropriate therapy. Proper and timely therapy usually is followed by clinical improvement in the patient's condition.

I. SODIUM AND WATER

The evaluation and correction of common preoperative sodium (Na^+) and water disorders are an important part of anesthetic care. This care is especially important for patients who have suffered major fluid and electrolyte shifts because of gastrointestinal diseases, trauma, or febrile illnesses. Perioperative fluid management can alleviate the prexisting problem or compound it. Furthermore, some clinical disorders of Na^+ and water metabolism are unique to the perioperative period. A few examples of these problems include hyponatremia during transurethral resection of the prostate, hyponatremia from the nonosmotic release of antidiuretic hormone during surgery, hypernatremia from postoperative diuresis, and hypernatremia and polyuria from diabetes insipidus after craniotomy. The diagnosis and therapy for disorders of Na^+ and water balance can be based on physiologic principles.

A. Physiologic properties of sodium and water

Sodium is the predominant extracellular electrolyte. Along with its accompanying anions, Na^+ accounts for virtually all the osmotically active solute in the extracellular fluid. Consequently, the concentration of Na^+ in the extracellular fluid is the principle factor governing the osmolality of the extracellular fluid. Because all cell membranes are permeable to water, the extracellular and intracellular fluid must exist in osmotic equilibrium. The osmolality and the Na^+ concentration of the extracellular fluid therefore have a profound impact on cellular volume and cellular water content. Increasing the extracellular fluid osmolality causes the net movement of water out of cells and results in shrinkage of cells. In contrast, decreasing the extracellular fluid osmolality causes the net movement of water into cells and results in cellular swelling. Brain cells within the confines of the cranial vault are particularly sensitive to small changes in cellular volume and water content as illustrated by the clinical sequelae of severe hyponatremia and hypernatremia. By necessity, extracellular Na^+ and osmolality are closely regulated by the body.

Serum or plasma Na^+ concentration is normally maintained between 135 and 145 mEq/L. The serum Na^+ concentration is representative of the entire extracellular fluid compartment because of the rapid equilibration of Na^+ and water throughout this space. The intracellular concentration of Na^+ is only 5 mEq/L. Membrane-bound Na^+-K^+-adenosine triphosphatase (Na^+-K^+-ATPase) serves to maintain this transmembrane gradient through the expenditure of energy. Since the concentration of a substance is always in proportion to the quantity of solution, changes in the serum Na^+ concentrations are analyzed always in terms of changes in the amount of free water in the extracellular compartment. For example, hyponatremia can be caused either by loss of Na^+ in excess of free water or by gain in free water in excess of Na^+. The net Na^+ content of the body largely determines the volume of the extracellular space, and so disorders of serum concentration are analyzed also in relation to the body's volume status.

Plasma osmolality is expressed as the quantity in millimoles of nonionizable particles in solution per kilogram of water (mOsm/kg) and normally is maintained between 275 and 290 mOsm/kg. Normally, Na^+ and its accompanying anions contributes to greater than 90% of the total osmolality of the plasma and interstitial fluids. The plasma Na^+ concentration therefore reflects both extracellular and intracellular osmolality.

It is estimated that as a proportion of total body mass 55% to 60% of the average adult male consists of water. Lean body mass has a proportionally greater water content than adipose tissue. Because of differences in body composition, the total body water (TBW) of a newborn can be as high as 72% of his or her body weight, whereas the TBW of women and elderly persons averages between 45% and 50% of their body weight. The approximately 40 liters of TBW in the 70 kg adult male is distributed between the intracellular and extracellular fluid compartments of the body. Approximately 45% of TBW (18 liters) is extracellular and 55% of TBW (22 liters) is intracellular.[1,2] Extracellular water is further subdivided into plasma water (7.5% TBW), interstitial water (27.5% TBW), inaccessible bone water (7.5% TBW), and transcellular water (2.5%). Transcellular water refers to water present in the respiratory tracts, lumen of the gastrointestinal tract, urinary system, cerebrospinal fluid, and aqueous humor of the eye. With the exception of inaccessible bone water and transcellular water, water within the body moves freely and equilibrates rapidly between the intracellular, interstitial, and plasma fluid compartments to maintain osmotic equilibrium across cell membranes.

Sodium also has an important role in the electrophysiologic properties of excitable cells. The action potentials of nerve impulses, myocardial cells, and the motor end plates of skeletal muscles are all initiated through cellular influx of Na^+ through specialized Na^+ channels in the cell membrane. Because the extracellular Na^+ concentration is so much higher than the intracellular Na^+ concentration, clinical changes in the extracellular Na^+ concentration do not alter appreciably the transmembrane Na^+ gradient and therefore have only a minimal effect on the electrical properties of cells.

B. Regulation of sodium and water metabolism

The serum Na^+ concentration and plasma osmolality are regulated when the amount of solute-free fluids ingested through the triggering of thirst is varied and the volume and osmolality of the urine excreted by the kidneys are varied through the release of antidiuretic hormone. The physiologic control of intravascular volume status through the sympathetic nervous system, the renin-angiotensin-aldosterone system, and the secretion of atrial natriuretic peptide are intimately linked to these regulatory mechanisms.

Arginine vasopressin (AVP), the antidiuretic hormone in man, is a nonapeptide synthesized by neurons in the supraoptic and paraventricular nuclei of the hypothalamus.[3] It is transported down the neurohypophysis along with its neurophysin and released into the systemic circulation from the posterior pituitary gland. Circulating AVP causes the kidneys to decrease free water excretion and causes vascular smooth muscle to contract. These two separate actions of AVP operate through independent cell receptor systems. The primary site of action of AVP within the kidney is at the cortical and medullary collecting duct where it increases cellular permeability to water. Under the influence of AVP, water is permitted to be reabsorbed into the hypertonic medullary interstitium resulting in the excretion of a concentrated urine. Through this mechanism, the osmolality of the urine can be varied from 100 mOsm/kg in the absence of AVP to as great as 1200 mOsm/kg when maximally stimulated by AVP. Optimal

functioning of this mechanism is dependent on normal renal function and an adequate circulating blood volume.

The combined input of afferent signals from stress, osmoreceptors, and baroreceptors control the release of AVP. Plasma osmolality is sensed by osmoreceptors located in the anterior hypothalamus. Although the precise set point may vary, plasma osmolality greater than 280 mOsm/kg generally stimulates osmoreceptor-mediated release of AVP (Fig. 20-1). Normally, maximum antidiuresis and osmoreceptor-mediated release of AVP occur when the plasma osmolality exceeds 295 mOsm/kg. Sodium appears to be the most potent osmotically active solute that stimulates osmoreceptor-mediated AVP secretion. Baroreceptor-mediated AVP secretion occurs when a 5% decrease in arterial pressure is sensed by high-pressure baroreceptors in the carotid bodies and aortic arch or when a 10% decrease in intravascular volume is sensed through low-pressure baroreceptors located in the left atrium and large intrathoracic veins. The preservation of intravascular volume takes priority over the control of plasma osmolality. Baroreceptor-mediated AVP secretion occurs in the presence of normal or low plasma osmolality. Activation of the sympathetic nervous system, angiotensin II, hypoglycemia, nausea, vomiting, pain, and surgical stress all appear to enhance the nonosmotic secretion of AVP.

Thirst stimulates free water intake. It is a cortical process and is modulated by osmoreceptors, circulating hormones, and sensory input.[4] Osmoreceptors that specifically activate thirst are located within the hypothalamus. The osmotic threshold for thirst is a plasma osmolality of approximately 295 mOsm/kg, which is greater than the osmotic threshold for AVP release (Fig. 20-1). Increased circulating concentrations of angiotensin II, hypovolemia, and low cardiac output also provoke thirst. The effectiveness of thirst is disabled when access to water is restricted, when gastrointestinal absorption of fluids is impaired, or when the patient is under general anesthesia.

The renin-angiotensin-aldosterone system functions primarily in the control of net Na^+ balance and only indirectly influences serum Na^+ concentration and plasma osmolality. Plasma renin concentration and renin-stimulated release of angiotensin II and aldosterone vary inversely with net Na^+ balance. Angiotensin II and aldosterone promote renal Na^+ conservation by respectively decreasing glomerular filtration and increasing the tubular reabsorption of Na^+. This system is important for the

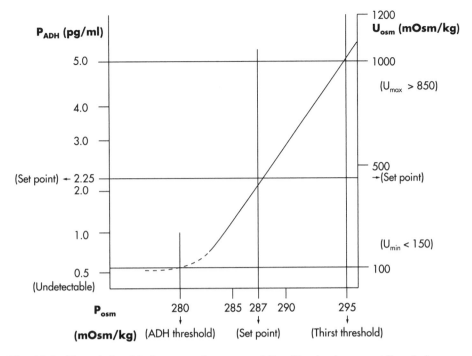

Fig. 20-1. The relationship between plasma osmolality (P_{osm}), plasma antidiuretic hormone concentration (P_{ADH}), and urine osmolality (U_{osm}). In humans, plasma osmolality greater than 280 mOsm/kg stimulates osmoreceptor-mediated antidiuretic hormone secretion. Antidiuretic hormone acts on the kidneys to promote the excretion of a concentrated urine. Thirst is activated when plasma osmolality exceeds 295 mOsm/kg. Plasma osmolality is normally maintained between 275 and 290 mOsm/kg. (From Morrison G and Singer I: Hyperosmolal states. In Maxwell MH, Kleeman CR, and Narins RG, editors: Clinical disorders of fluid and electrolyte metabolism, New York, 1980, Macmillan Publishing Co., Inc.)

maintenance of intravascular volume. Changes in intravascular volume influence serum Na^+ concentration and plasma osmolality through the nonosmotic secretion of AVP.

Atrial natriuretic peptide or atriopeptin[5,6] is a hormone secreted primarily from atrial cardiocytes in response to atrial distension. This hormone causes diuresis, natriuresis, arterial vasodilatation, and the translocation of plasma fluid into the interstitial space and also inhibits the release of aldosterone. Although its role in intravascular volume regulation is apparent, its role in regulating Na^+ and water metabolism is still being studied.

C. Hyponatremia

Hyponatremia is defined as a serum Na^+ concentration less than 135 mEq/L. Overall, hyponatremia is a serious clinical problem with reported mortality as high as 50%.[7] The prevalence of hyponatremia among all hospitalized patients has been reported to be 2.5%.[8] The frequency of postoperative hyponatremia has been reported to range from 4.4% to 40% de-

pending on the surgical procedure.[9] Recognition of this problem and appropriate fluid management potentially can decrease the frequency of this condition.

1. Causes of hyponatremia. Hyponatremia is clinically important only when it is associated with a reduction in plasma tonicity. The clinical manifestations of hyponatremia are the consequence of cellular edema secondary to reductions in extracellular fluid osmolality. For diagnostic and therapeutic purposes it is therefore useful to separate the clinical syndromes of hyponatremia into two major groups based on the plasma tonicity: (1) hyponatremia without plasma hyposmolality and (2) hyponatremia with plasma hyposmolality (List 20-1). The latter group of disorders is subdivided further according to the volume status of the patient (List 20-1).

a. Hyponatremia without plasma hyposmolality. The introduction of osmotically active solutes other than Na^+ into the extracellular fluid space causes the movement of free water out of cells in order to maintain transmembrane osmotic

---

List 20-1. Diagnostic Classification of
Hyponatremia

Hyponatremia without plasma hyposmolality
  Hyperglycemia
  Hypertonic mannitol administration
  Systemic absorption of glycine- or sorbitol-
    containing irrigants
  Hyperlipidemia
  Hyperproteinemia
Hyponatremia with plasma hyposmolality (classified
  according to volume status)
  Hypovolemic hyposmotic hyponatremia
    Diuretics
    Adrenal insufficiency
    Chronic renal failure
    Diarrhea
    Vomiting
    Burn injuries
    "Third-spacing"
  Isovolemic hyposmotic hyponatremia
    Hypotonic fluid administration
    Postoperative hyponatremia
    Oxytocin administration
    Pituitary insufficiency
    Syndrome of inappropriate antidiuretic hor-
      mone secretion (SIADH)
  Hypervolemic hyposmotic hyponatremia
    Congestive heart failure
    Cirrhosis
    Nephrotic syndrome
    Renal failure
    Mechanical ventilation with positive end-
      expiratory pressure (PEEP)

---

equilibrium. This free water entering the extracellular compartment decreases the serum Na^+ concentration. Changes in plasma osmolality are secondary and depend on the tonicity of the administered solute-containing solution and the degree of subsequent solute-induced diuresis. The most common examples of osmotically active solutes that lower the serum Na^+ concentration when they are introduced into the circulation are glucose, mannitol, sorbitol, and glycine. Increases in serum glucose can be measured directly. The presence of the other osmotically active solutes can be detected indirectly by comparison of the actual measured plasma osmolality with the plasma osmolality calculated from the serum Na^+, glucose, and urea concentrations. The difference in these two values is referred to as the "osmolar gap." An osmolar gap greater than 10 mOsm/kg indicates the presence of an unmeasured solute.

Calculated plasma osmolality:
osm (mOsm/kg) = 2[Na^+] (mEq/L) +
    [Glucose] (mg/dl)/18 + [BUN] (mg/dl)/2.8

Ethanol, methanol, or propylene glycol in the circulation are also osmotically active solutes that account for an increased osmolar gap. However, these substances do not cause hyponatremia because they readily cross cell membranes and do not cause the translocation of water into the extracellular space.

Hyperglycemia can be a cause for hyponatremia in conditions of insulin deficiency or insulin resistance. Diabetic ketoacidosis and nonketotic hyperosmolar states are extreme examples. Perioperative hyperglycemia can also be caused by surgical stress, perioperative glucocorticoid therapy, or the intravenous administration of dextrose-containing solutions.

Hypertonic mannitol solutions frequently are administered during neurosurgical procedures and for the acute treatment of increased intracranial pressure. This therapeutic use of mannitol can cause hyponatremia. A 20% solution of mannitol has an osmolality of 1098 mOsm/kg. When this solution of mannitol is administered intravenously at doses ranging from 0.25 to 2.0 g/kg, serum osmolality increases to approximately 300 mOsm/kg and serum Na^+ correspondingly decreases below 135 mEq/L.[10]

The systemic absorption of glycine- or sorbitol-containing bladder irrigants during transurethral prostate operations can be a cause of hyponatremia. Plasma osmolality in this condition of hyponatremia is usually normal or only slightly reduced, since isosmotic or nearly isosmotic irrigants are now used for this procedure. Cardiovascular instability and clinical symptoms of visual changes, hallucinations, nausea, and vomiting can sometimes accompany this form of hyponatremia. These symptoms are similar to those seen with hypotonic hyponatremia and are related to the degree of hyponatremia, but they are not related to changes in plasma osmolality.[11-13] Instead, the clinical manifestations that occur in this hyponatremic condition may be attributed to hypervolemia, the direct toxic effects of glycine, or encephalopathy produced by the biotransformation of glycine into ammonia.[12,13] The degree of hyponatremia reflects the quantity of bladder irrigant absorbed and the extent of hemodilution. Hyponatremia is unlikely to be directly responsible for clinical manifestations seen in this syndrome if the plasma osmolality is close to normal.

Hyponatremia as a laboratory artifact can be observed in patients with hyperlipidemia or hyperproteinemia. Abnormal increases in plasma lipid or protein content expand plasma volume and decrease the total plasma Na^+ concentration without changing the Na^+ concentration in the water fraction of plasma. Plasma osmolality remains normal in these conditions. This phenomenon is termed "pseudohyponatremia" and is most often observed in patients with diabetes mellitus, diabetic ketoacidosis, hyperlipidemia, or multiple myeloma. Patients receiving parenteral nutritional therapy with lipid emulsions also can have pseudohyponatremia. Pseudohyponatremia is observed even when the serum Na^+ concentration is measured by use of automated systems employing ion-selective electrodes, since approximately half these instruments (those utilizing indirect-reading ion-selective electrodes) perform the Na^+ measurements on diluted samples.[14]

b. Hyponatremia with plasma hyposmolality. Hyponatremic disorders associated with plasma hyposmolality are considered in terms of total body volume status. Measurement of plasma osmolality and estimation of the patient's volume status using clinical signs or invasive monitoring usually can lead to the correct diagnosis.

Hypovolemic hyposmolal hyponatremia is produced by renal or extrarenal loss of Na^+-containing fluid in combination with hypotonic fluid replacement. Hypovolemia stimulates the nonosmotic release of AVP and promotes water retention, thereby contributing to the development of hyponatremia. Causes of inappropriate renal loss of Na^+ and water include diuretic use, adrenal insufficiency, and chronic renal disease. A urine Na^+ concentration greater than 20 mEq/L in the presence of hypovolemia indicates renal Na^+ wasting. Diarrhea, vomiting, and burn injuries are some clinical conditions that cause extrarenal loss of Na^+ and water. Patients who have undergone extensive abdominal operations or patients with pancreatitis, peritonitis, or pseudomembranous colitis can lose large amounts of fluid internally. This phenomenon is often referred to as "third-spacing."

Isovolemic hyposmolal hyponatremia refers to disorders caused by antidiuretic hormone activity in excess of that dictated by the plasma osmolality. The retention of free water characterizes these conditions of isovolemic hyposmolal hyponatremia, but volume expansion and edema are not clinically evident. Free water retained by the body distributes evenly throughout the extracellular and intracellular compartments, and physiologic mechanisms controlling intravascular volume status remain intact. Conceivably, the excessive intake of large quantities of free water can cause isovolemic hyposmolal hyponatremia without abnormal antidiuretic hormone activity. However, the normal kidney has a capacity to excrete up to 1200 ml of free water per hour. Cases of pure psychogenic water intoxication requires water intake in excess of 20 liters per day and are extremely unusual.

Several factors contribute to the nonosmotic release of AVP in the perioperative period (Fig. 20-2). Administration of hypotonic fluids to surgical patients with elevated levels of AVP is

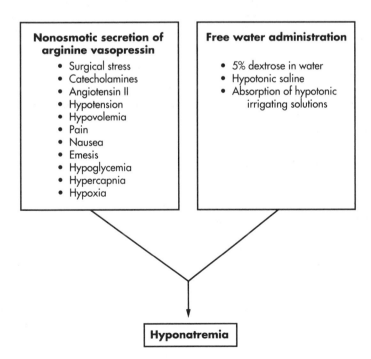

Fig. 20-2. Factors contributing to postoperative hyponatremia.

the most common cause of postoperative hyponatremia.[8,9,15] In the majority of cases, postoperative hyponatremia from this cause is mild and resolves with appropriate fluid management. However, severe cases of postoperative hyponatremia and even death from cerebral edema and transtentorial herniation have been reported in the literature.[15,16] Perioperative factors that provoke the nonosmotic secretion of AVP include surgical stress,[15,17,18] pain,[17] nausea and vomiting,[19] hypoxia,[20] hypercapnia,[21] hypoglycemia,[22] catecholamines,[23] and volume depletion. Attention to avoiding stimuli that cause the nonosmotic secretion of AVP together with appropriate fluid management and the avoidance of excessive hypotonic fluid therapy potentially can reduce the frequency of postoperative hyponatremia.

Oxytocin has direct antidiuretic actions. Oxytocin, used during the induction of labor or for therapeutic abortions, can cause hyponatremia when administered together with hypotonic fluids.[24]

The tonic inhibition of AVP release is among one of the actions of glucocorticoids. Hyponatremia associated with the inappropriate secretion of AVP has been reported among patients with hypopituitarism.[25] Hyponatremia in this group of patients can be provoked by surgical stress, infections, or fluid administration[26] and responds to treatment with hydrocortisone.[25]

The syndrome of inappropriate antidiuretic hormone secretion (SIADH) is a diagnosis often applied to conditions in which AVP secretion is sustained despite normal or low plasma osmolality. For clinical purposes, SIADH is a diagnosis of exclusion, which means that patients with this syndrome must satisfy the following clinical criteria: (1) hyponatremia in combination with reduced plasma osmolality, (2) urine osmolality less than maximally dilute when compared to the plasma osmolality, (3) absence of hypovolemia, hypotension, or edema-forming states, and (4) normal renal, thyroid, and adrenal function.[27] These exclusion criteria are necessary, since the nonosmotic release of AVP may be physiologically appropriate in certain conditions despite low plasma osmolality. SIADH is associated with a wide range of clinical conditions including central nervous system disorders, malignancies, lung diseases, and certain drugs (List 20-2). Autonomous production of bioactive and immunoreactive AVP by tumor has been demonstrated most commonly in patients with bronchogenic carcinoma of the lung.[28,29] Drug-induced release of AVP can occur with chlorpropamide,

---

List 20-2.   Causes of SIADH

Malignancy
  Bronchogenic carinoma of lung
  Pancreatic carcinoma
  Carinoma of duodenum
  Thymoma
  Lymphoma
  Prostatic carcinoma
Pulmonary disorders
  Pneumonia
  Lung abscess
  Empyema
  Tuberculosis
Central nervous system disorders
  Head trauma
  Brain tumors
  Intracranial hemorrhage
  Stroke
  Craniotomy
  Transsphenoidal hypophysectomy
  Encephalitis
  Meningitis
Drugs
  Chlorpropamide
  Vincristine
  Vinblastine
  Cyclophosphamide
  Carbamazepine

---

carbamazepine, clofibrate, vincristine, vinblastine, thiazides, monoamine oxidase inhibitors, and phenothiazines. Inappropriate release of AVP from the neurohypophysis can be caused by infections, vascular lesions, or direct injury to the pituitary gland.

A subset of patients with SIADH have as their underlying defect a primary disorder of osmoregulation.[30] In some of these patients the osmotic threshhold for AVP release is lower than normal ("reset osmostat" or "sick-cell syndrome"). In others, SIADH is caused by erratic release of AVP, nonsuppressible basal release of AVP, or abnormal end-organ sensitivity to the actions of AVP.

Hypervolemic hyposmolal hyponatremia occurs in patients with congestive heart failure, positive pressure ventilation with positive end-expiratory pressure (PEEP), cirrhosis, nephrotic syndrome, and advanced renal failure. In these conditions, total body water and Na^+ content are increased but the increase in total body water is proportionally greater than the increase in total body Na^+. The presence of edema is an indicator of extracellular volume excess in these conditions. Except for renal failure, the pathophysiologic mechanism underlying this set of disorders is the body's sensing of a low circulating blood volume. These signals initiate a sequence of events, which includes the nonosmotic secretion of AVP, that lead to avid Na^+ and water retention by the kidneys.[31] In patients with advanced renal failure, the impaired excretion of ingested water and Na^+ loads leads to the development of this form of hyponatremia.

2. Clinical manifestations of hyponatremia. The clinical manifestations of hyponatremia depend on the cause of the underlying condition. In hyponatremia caused by systemic absorption of glycine-containing bladder irrigants, hyperglycinemia and volume overload may explain the majority of symptoms and can be treated by termination of the surgical procedure and administration of a diuretic to assist in restoring normal intravascular volume status. In hyponatremia with hypovolemia, the majority of symptoms may be attributed to volume contraction and are resolved with intravascular volume expansion.

In conditions of hyponatremia with plasma hyposmolality, the clinical manifestations are the result of cellular swelling, cerebral edema, and in the extreme case herniation of the brain.[32] Depending on the severity of the condition, symptoms can range from lethargy, apathy, anorexia, and nausea to disorientation, psychosis, agitation, seizures, and coma. Signs include the detection of abnormal sensorium, diminished deep tendon reflexes, the elicitation of pathologic reflexes, Cheyne-Stokes respirations, cranial nerve palsy, and seizures. Acute changes in serum Na^+ and plasma osmolality are associated with the abrupt onset of symptoms followed soon thereafter by seizures and coma. In general, a serum Na^+ concentration of less than 120 mEq/L is associated with clinical symptoms and adverse outcome.[32] Patients with chronic hyponatremia are often asymptomatic or present with the insidious onset of nonspecific symptoms. Brain cells appear to adapt to chronic hyponatremia and plasma hyposmolality by losing intracellular solutes.

3. Diagnostic strategy for hyponatremia. The evaluation of the patient with hyponatremia needs to be performed in a systematic manner by (1) measurement of plasma osmolality, (2) exclusion of pseudohyponatremia caused by hyperlipidemia or hyperproteinemia, (3) measurement of serum glucose concentration, (4) calculation of the osmolar gap when the presence of other osmotically active solutes are suspected, (5) determination of intravascular volume status, (6) examination of the patient for signs of edema, and (6) evaluation of renal function.

The result of this initial evaluation usually leads to the correct diagnosis or assists in the decision to conduct specialized tests to establish the specific diagnosis.

4. Treatment of hyponatremia. Therapy for hyponatremia should first aim to resolve the underlying disorder. Postoperative hyponatremia from the inappropriate administration of hypotonic fluid corrects itself after fluid restriction. Hyponatremia from Na^+ wasting responds to volume expansion with Na^+-containing fluids. Hyponatremia with hyperglycemia in diabetic ketoacidosis resolves with the control of blood glucose. Drug-induced SIADH resolves with the discontinuation of the offending drug. Hyponatremia from mineralocorticoid or glucocorticoid deficiency responds to hormone replacement therapy. If it is not possible to treat the underlying disorder or neuropsychiatric manifestations of hyponatremia are present, symptomatic improvement can be accomplished with therapy directed at increasing plasma osmolality. In mild cases of SIADH, limiting water intake to 1000 ml/day is usually sufficient. In severe hyposmolal hyponatremia, plasma osmolality can be increased by the administration of hypertonic saline. An alternative method is to induce diuresis with a potent loop diuretic, such as furosemide, and replace the volume deficit by intravenous administration of isotonic or hypertonic saline.

Although the optimal rate and end point for the emergency correction of hyposmotic hyponatremia has not been established, it generally appears to be safe to increase serum Na^+ concentration at a rate of 1 to 2 mEq/L/hour.[33-35] Once a serum Na^+ concentration of 120 to 130 mEq/L is reached, the restoration of serum Na^+ concentration to normal can proceed in a more gradual manner. The major reported complication of therapy is central pontine myelinolysis, or osmotic demyelination syndrome.[36,37] This disastrous neurologic sequelae generally can be prevented by avoidance of overcorrection of serum Na^+ concentration in all patients and by avoidance of rapid correction in patients with chronic hyponatremia. Frequent measurements of serum Na^+ concentration are important for monitoring progress during therapy.

The correction of hyponatremia can be based on a calculation of the the amount of excess free water:

$$\text{Excess free water} = \text{TBW}\left(1 - \frac{\text{Measured serum }[Na^+]}{\text{Desired serum }[Na^+]}\right)$$

where

$$\text{TBW (liters)} = \text{Body weight (kg)} \times 0.6 \text{ (L/kg)}$$

One can eliminate the excess free water by administering a loop diuretic such as furosemide and by replacing urinary volume losses with isotonic saline. The urinary Na^+ concentration with diuretic administration is typically equivalent to 0.45% saline (77 mEq/L).

Example 1. To correct serum Na^+ concentration from 110 to 120 mEq/L in a 70 kg male by diuretic administration and replacement with isotonic saline, first calculate the excess free water:

$$\text{Excess free water} = 70 \text{ kg} \times 0.6 \text{ L/kg} \times \left(1 - \frac{110 \text{ mEq/L}}{120 \text{ mEq/L}}\right)$$
$$= 42 \text{ L} \times 0.083$$
$$= 3.5 \text{ L}$$

A urinary output of 7 liters over 5 to 10 hours accompanied by the intravenous administration of 3.5 liters of normal saline over the same time should increase the serum Na^+ concentration at a rate of 1 to 2 mEq/L per hour.

Alternatively, the administration of hypertonic saline can be used to increase the Na^+ concentration without changing net water balance.

Volume of hypertonic saline (in liters) necessary to restore serum Na^+ to desired concentration = Excess free water (L) × (Desired serum $[Na^+]$)/{($[Na^+]$ in the hypertonic saline solution)−(Desired serum $[Na^+]$)}

Example 2. To correct serum Na^+ concentration from 110 to 120 mEq/L in a 70 kg male with a 3% solution of hypertonic saline that has a Na^+ concentration of 513 mEq/L requires the following calculations:

$$\text{Excess free water} = 70 \text{ kg} \times 0.6 \text{ L/kg} \times \left(1 - \frac{110 \text{ mEq/L}}{120 \text{ mEq/L}}\right)$$
$$= 42 \text{ L} \times 0.083$$
$$= 3.5 \text{ L}$$

$$\text{Volume of 3\% saline} = 3.5 \text{ L} \times (120 \text{ mEq/L})/$$
$$(513 \text{ mEq/L} - 120 \text{ mEq/L})$$
$$= 1.07 \text{ L}$$

The 1.07 liter of 3% saline can be administered over 5 to 10 hours to correct the serum Na^+ concentration at a rate of 1 to 2 mEq/L per hour. Although these formulas may be helpful, the clinician is advised to serially monitor therapy by performing frequent serum Na^+ determinations.

D. Hypernatremia

Hypernatremia is defined as a serum Na^+ concentration greater than 145 mEq/L. A total body deficit of free water characterizes the disorders of hypernatremia. Plasma hyperosmolality is invariably present in conditions associated with hypernatremia. Normally, activation of thirst and subsequent drinking of water protects against the development of hypernatremia. Impaired thirst or conditions that limit the patient's ability to obtain and ingest water are essential for the pathogenesis of hypernatremic syndromes. Disorders of thirst and inadequate water intake are the most common causes of hypernatremia in mentally obtunded, mentally handicapped, or debilitated patients. Access to water is often denied to patients during the perioperative period or while they are in the intensive care unit. Neonates and small infants do not have the ability to obtain or drink water on their own. Anesthetized patients completely lack the ability to control water balance through thirst. In a study conducted to examine the frequency of hypernatremia in hospitalized patients over 60 years of age, hypernatremia was encountered most frequently among surgical patients in the postoperative period and was associated with a 51% mortality.[38]

1. Causes of hypernatremia. Hypernatremia can develop as a consequence of excessive hypotonic fluid losses combined with the inadequate intake of Na^+-free fluids. The insensible loss of hypotonic fluid from the skin and respiratory tract averages 500 to 1000 ml/day for the average adult in a controlled environment. Living in hot environments, breathing dry nonhumidifed gases, suffering febrile illnesses, and losing skin integrity from open wounds, burn injuries, or exfoliative skin diseases can increase drastically hypotonic fluid losses. The gastrointestinal tract can also be an extrarenal source of hypotonic fluid loss in vomiting and diarrheal illnesses, during abdominal operations, and with nasogastric suctioning. When thirst is rendered ineffective and free water intake is inadequate, failure to replace the free water deficit in these conditions eventually leads to the development of hypernatremia. Replacement of hypotonic fluid deficits with the sustained infusion of normal (154 mmol) also can cause hypernatremia and has been reported to be a common cause of hypernatremia among postoperative surgical patients.[38]

Hypernatremia caused by excessive renal loss of hypotonic urine occurs with polyuria from diabetes insipidus or with diuresis. Osmotic diuretics, such as mannitol or glucose, and loop diuretics, such as furosemide, impair renal concentrating mechanisms and result in the formation of hypotonic urine. Osmotic diuresis caused by hyperglycemia may contribute to the development of hypernatremia observed in patients receiving enternal or parenteral nutritional support.[38] In addition, solute diuresis can occur during the excretion of large quantities of urea after the relief of urinary tract obstruction or in patients being fed a high protein diet. Hypernatremia can also develop in surgical patients who have been volume loaded intraoperatively with isotonic saline and then subjected to postoperative diuretic therapy.

Diabetes insipidus (DI) is a disorder characterized by polydipsia, polyuria, and the inability to concentrate urine in response to increases in plasma tonicity. Patients with DI are dependent on an intact thirst mechanism and the ingestion of substantial quantities of water to protect themselves from developing hypernatremia. Two forms of DI have been recognized: (1) absent or diminished release of AVP in response to increases in plasma osmolality is the underlying defect in central or hypothalamic DI, and (2) renal unresponsiveness to the antidiuretic actions of AVP is the underlying defect in nephrogenic DI.

Neurosurgery and head trauma are the most common cause for acquired central DI. Central DI is a frequent complication after surgical resection of the pituitary gland or hypothalamic lesions. Patients undergoing transsphenoidal hypophysectomy for pituitary adenomas and frontal craniotomy for craniopharyngiomas, pituitary adenomas, and metastatic brain tumors appear to be at greatest risk for developing central DI postoperatively.[39,40] Injury to or destruction of hypothalamic osmoreceptors or the hypothalamic neurons synthesizing AVP is necessary to produce central DI. Injury to or resection of the posterior lobe of the pituitary gland in many instances does not cause permanent DI, since hypothalamic neurons can directly release AVP into the systemic circulation. Additional causes of central DI include central nervous system infections, granulomatous diseases, vascular lesions, familial DI, and idiopathic DI.

Nephrogenic DI can be caused by any number of conditions impairing renal concentrating mechanisms. A rare famial form of nephrogenic DI involves a primary defect in the cellular response to circulating AVP. Hypercalcemia and hypokalemia are two metabolic disorders that are associated with renal resistance to the actions of AVP. Lithium carbonate, demeclocycline, and inorganic fluoride (from the biotransformation of methoxyflurane) are examples of compounds that can induce nephrogenic DI. Practically any form of acute or chronic renal disease that affects the kidney's ability to concentrate urine has the potential for causing nephrogenic DI.

Finally, hypernatremia can also be caused iatrogenically by the administration of hypertonic solutions of Na^+ without net gain or loss of total body water. Sodium bicarbonate solutions used for resuscitation or for the emergency correction of metabolic acidosis typically contain 50 mEq of bicarbonate in a volume of 50 ml and has a Na^+ concentration of 1000 mEq/L. Excessive administration of hypertonic saline for volume expansion or correction of hyponatremia can cause hypernatremia. Hypertonic formulas used during enteral or parenteral nutritional therapy are another cause of iatrogenic hypernatremia.

2. Treatment of hypernatremia. Hypernatremia is associated with high mortality either as a direct consequence of the condition or as an indicator of severe underlying disease.[38,41] The therapeutic approach to the patient with hypernatremia is aimed at the restoration of the deficit in body water and solute, continued replacement of ongoing fluid losses, treatment of associated medical conditions, and finally identification and treatment of the underlying disorder responsible for the metabolic derangement.

Intravascular volume expansion with isotonic saline is effective for the initial treatment of hypernatremia associated with cardiovascular signs and symptoms of hypovolemia. The restoration of an effective circulating blood volume and the preservation of renal function takes priority over the replacement of the free water deficit. The determination of intravascular volume status is therefore an important step in the initial evaluation of the patient with hypernatremia.

Aside from hypovolemia, the clinical manifestations of hypernatremia are caused by the excessive tonicity of the extracellular fluid. Cellular dehydration occurs as water moves out of cells in accordance to the osmotic gradient. Shrinkage of brain cells results in progressive neurologic deterioration depending on the degree of hyperosmolality. Signs and symptoms are nonspecific and can include increased thirst, weakness, confusion, neuromuscular irritability, seizures, stupor, and coma. Acute hypernatremia and rapid changes in brain volume can cause the rupture of blood vessels, intracranial hemorrhages, and thrombosis of venous sinuses. The clinical manifestations of chronic hypernatremia are usually less dramatic. Brain cells adapt to gradual increases in extracellular tonicity by accumulating intracellular solutes and thus keeping cell volume constant. Rapid correction of chronic hypertonic states can paradoxically cause cerebral edema.

Once the intravascular volume deficit has been restored by isotonic volume expansion, ongoing fluid losses and the free water deficit can be replaced. The patient is allowed to drink or hypotonic solutions such as 5% dextrose in water or 5% dextrose in 0.45% saline is administered by intravenous infusion. It is unusual for pure water deficits to be associated with significant alterations in intravascular volume because water is proportionately lost from all body compartments and the corresponding decrease in blood volume is relatively minor in relation to the degree of hypernatremia. The free water deficit can be estimated with the following formula, which may be used as a guide for therapy:

$$\text{Free water deficit} = 0.6 \text{ L/kg} \times \text{Body weight (kg)} \times \left(1 - \frac{140 \text{ mEq/L}}{\text{Serum } [Na^+] \text{ mEq/L}}\right)$$

The optimal rate at which the serum Na^+ concentration should be corrected has not been established. Rapid correction, as mentioned earlier, can cause cerebral edema and neurologic sequelae. A general guideline that appears to be safe is replacement of half the water deficit within the first 12 to 24 hours and the remainder of the deficit over the next 24 to 48 hours. Alternatively, correcting the serum Na^+ concentration at a rate of 0.5 mEq/L per hour also appears to be safe. Close observation for changes in neurologic status and frequent measurement of serum Na^+ concentrations are important for monitoring the progress of therapy.

3. Evaluation of polyuria and diabetes insipidus.

Polyuria is defined as urine output greater than 2 ml/kg/hour. Hyperglycemia, hyperuricemia, diuretics, and renal failure cause polyuria and can be easily excluded in the initial diagnostic workup (Fig. 20-3). The diagnosis of DI should be suspected in all patients with polyuria, especially among neurosurgical patients or patients with head injuries. The presence of hypernatremia in combination with polyuria almost always is suggestive of the diagnosis of DI; however, hypernatremia does not usually occur in patients with DI unless they are deprived of water. Polyuria in the absence of diuretics and a urine osmolality less than 300 mOsm/kg, a plasma osmolality greater than 300 mOsm/kg, and a serum Na^+ concentration greater than 143 mEq/L in combination is also diagnostic of DI.[40] The water deprivation test[42] can be hazardous in critically ill patients and usually is not necessary for the clinical evaluation of perioperative polyuria in the surgical patient.

Postoperative central DI after neurosurgery can be either temporary or permanent. Infrequently, the onset of postoperative central DI is characterized by a "triphasic" pattern.[39,40] In the first phase, transient polyuria occurs within 24 hours of the operation and is caused by the

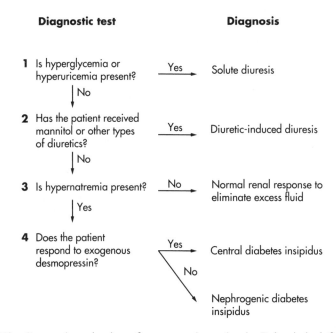

Diagnostic test   **Diagnosis**

1 Is hyperglycemia or hyperuricemia present? — Yes → Solute diuresis

| No

2 Has the patient received mannitol or other types of diuretics? — Yes → Diuretic-induced diuresis

| No

3 Is hypernatremia present? — No → Normal renal response to eliminate excess fluid

| Yes

4 Does the patient respond to exogenous desmopressin? — Yes → Central diabetes insipidus

No → Nephrogenic diabetes insipidus

Fig. 20-3. The diagnostic evaluation of postoperative polyuria. Polyuria is defined as a urine output exceeding 2 ml/kg/hr. Hypernatremia is defined as a serum sodium concentration greater than 145 mEq/L. Plasma hyperosmolality (plasma osmolality greater than 300 mOsm/kg) in the presence of an inappropriately dilute urine (urine osmolality less than 300 mOsm/kg) is highly suggestive of diabetes insipidus. A normal response to exogenous desmopressin is defined as an increase in urine osmolality above 300 mOsm/kg.

functional impairment of AVP release. This phase is then followed by remission or inappropriate antidiuresis (SIADH), which can last for 4 to 8 days. This second phase is believed to be caused by the release of AVP from damaged neurons. The final phase heralds the onset of permanent DI and is characterized by polyuria and polydipsia.

a. Treatment of diabetes insipidus. The treatment of central DI consists in restoring the water deficit, replacing ongoing losses, and administering antidiuretic hormone replacement therapy. Desmopressin (1-desamino-8-D-arginine vasopressin, or DDAVP) is a synthetic analog of AVP, which has minimal vasoactive effects and approximately twice the antidiuretic activity of the native hormone. The required dose of desmopressin for the treatment of central DI varies considerably between patients and must be adjusted for each individual. Desmopressin can be administered transmucosally (5 to 20 μg bid), subcutaneously (2 to 4 μg bid), intramuscularly (2 to 4 μg bid), or intravenously. (0.1 to 0.3 μg/kg). The plasma half-life of intravenous desmopressin is 1 to 2 hours. In longstanding untreated central DI, the renal medullary hypertonic gradient and corresponding ability to concentrate urine may take several days to develop after the initiation of desmopressin therapy.

Polyuria in a patient (who has not received diuretics) that does not respond to desmopressin is suggestive of the diagnosis of nephrogenic DI. Sometimes an underlying metabolic disturbance, such as hypercalcemia or hypokalemia, is responsible for the nephrogenic DI. In this situation, the DI improves or resolves after treatment of the underlying disorder. More frequently the treatment of nephrogenic DI is supportive, though thiazide diuretics may be effective in some patients.[43]

II. POTASSIUM

Disorders of potassium (K^+) homeostasis are a constant concern for the anesthesiologist in the perioperative management of surgical patients. It is well recognized that hypokalemia is particularly frequent among surgical patients with cardiovascular diseases, receiving diuretic therapy, or receiving intravenous fluid therapy. The frequency of hypokalemia among patients receiving diuretic therapy has been estimated to be as high as 50%.[44] A 43% frequency of hypokalemia has been found among a select group of patients undergoing elective cardiac or major vascular procedures.[45] A large survey reported that 21% of hospitalized patients had laboratory criteria for hypokalemia and this group of patients had a higher hospital mortality.[46] Hyperkalemia appears to be encountered much less frequently than hypokalemia and has been reported to be present in only 1% to 2% of hospitalized patients.[47] A less recent study, however, reported that hyperkalemia was a postoperative complication in 11% of patients undergoing cardiac operations in 1965.[48] Ironically, hyperkalemia has emerged as an important clinical problem because of the frequency of hypokalemia; iatrogenic hyperkalemia from K^+) supplementation is a major cause of fatality among hospitalized patients.[49] Although considerable controversy surrounds the perioperative management of patients with hypokalemia, there is unanimous agreement that clinically important hyperkalemia (such as serum $K^+ > 6.0$ mEq/L) should be treated as a medical emergency. The avoidance, prompt recognition, and treatment of hyperkalemia are essential to avoid catastrophy.

A. Potassium homeostasis

Potassium is predominantly an intracellular ion. The plasma K^+ concentration, which is representative of the K^+ concentration in the extracellular fluid, is normally 3.5 to 5.0 mEq/L. The serum K^+ concentration is usually 0.4 mEq/L higher than the plasma concentration because of the release of K^+ into the serum during clot formation. In comparison, the intracellular fluid has a K^+ concentration of 150 mEq/L. Although only about 2% of the body's total K^+ is present in the extracellular fluid compartment, this extracellular K^+ is critical for neuromuscular activity. The ratio of the extracellular to the intracellular K^+ concentration is the primary determinant of the transmembrane voltage potential in electrically excitable cells. The generation of membrane action potentials and the depolarization of neuronal, skeletal muscle, and cardiac cells are dependent on this transmembrane K^+ concentration gradient.

B. Regulation of serum potassium concentration

The net amount of K^+ in the extracellular fluid compartment is regulated closely. The addition or removal of a relatively small amount of K^+ to this extracellular compartment results in a large change in the K^+ concentration of the extracellular fluid. A large change in the extracellular K^+ concentration produces a proportionately large change in the ratio of intracellular to extracellular K^+ concentration, which has a pronounced effect on the electrical activity of cells. For example, a typical 70 kg adult male has an extracellular fluid volume of 15 liters, a

K^+ concentration of 4 mEq/L in his extracellular fluid, and a K^+ concentration of 150 mEq/L in his intracellular fluid. He thus has a total of 60 mEq of K^+ in the extracellular fluid compartment and an intracellular to extracellular K^+ concentration ratio of 37.5. The ingestion of 60 mEq of K^+ in a typical daily diet potentially can double his extracellular K^+ concentration, decrease his transmembrane K^+ concentration ratio to 18.8, and cause life-threatening hyperkalemia if the physiologic processes that normally control his extracellular K^+ balance are inactivated.

One can change the extracellular K^+) concentration by (1) shifting K^+ into or out of cells or (2) altering the net dietary intake or renal excretion of K^+ by the body (Fig. 20-4). The internal redistribution of K^+ between the intracellular and extracellular compartments changes the extracellular K^+ concentration without changing the total body K^+ content. Internal K^+ balance is regulated by catecholamines and endocrine hormones. Internal K^+ balance also is influenced by alterations in cell membrane integrity, blood pH, and extracellular fluid tonicity. Net external changes in total body K^+ content eventually lead to changes in the extracellular K^+ concentration. For example, continuous unreplaced losses of K^+ in the urine cause a decrease in the extracellular K^+ concentration, which is partially compensated by the transfer of K^+ out of cells. Eventually, intracellular K^+ stores become depleted; this depletion is manifested as severe extracellular hypokalemia. External K^+ balance is regulated almost exclusively by the renal excretion of K^+ under the influence of aldosterone.

1. Regulation of internal potassium balance.
The internal distribution of K^+ within the body is regulated by factors that influence the net movement of K^+ across cell membranes. The underlying transmembrane K^+ concentration gradient is maintained by the action of Na^+-K^+-ATPase. Na^+-K^+-ATPase is a membrane bound enzyme that uses energy to extrude Na^+ out of cells in exchange for K^+. Insulin, epinephrine, and alkalosis are factors that promote the net entry of K^+ into cells and cause a decrease in the extracellular K^+ concentration.[50] Acidosis, exercise, and extracellular fluid hypertonicity promote the exit of K^+ out of cells and increases the extracellular K^+ concentration.[50] The internal redistribution of K^+ between the intracellular and extracellular fluid compartments appears to be an important physiologic mechanism for attenuating changes in extracellular K^+ concentration in situations of acute K^+ loading.

Clinical and experimental evidence indicate that epinephrine may decrease serum K^+ concentration specifically through the stimulation of beta$_2$-adrenergic receptors.[51] In contrast to its beta-adrenergic actions, epinephrine's action as an alpha-adrenergic agonist can impair the cellular uptake of K^+.[52] This alpha-adrenergic action of epinephrine on internal K^+ balance explains the transient increase (1 to 3 minutes) in serum K^+ concentration observed immediately after the administration of epinephrine.[53] The importance of these physiologic effects are not certain, but they may have a role in modulating extracellular K^+ concentrations during exercise or stress.

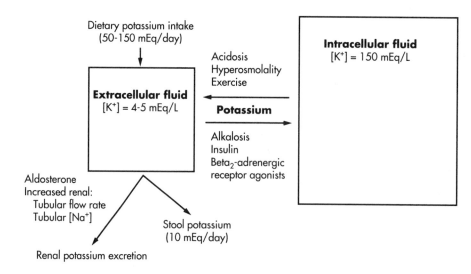

Fig. 20-4. Factors influencing internal and external potassium balance.

The effects of pH on serum K^+ concentrations are well recognized. Acidosis shifts K^+ out of cells, thereby increasing serum K^+ concentration, whereas alkalosis has an opposite effect. This effect of pH on internal K^+ balance traditionally has been explained by increases in intracellular hydrogen-ion concentrations, which cause the displacement of K^+ out of cells in order to maintain electrochemical neutrality. The general rule that serum K^+ concentration changes 0.6 mEq/L for each 0.1 unit change in pH has been advocated to predict the influence of pH on serum K^+ concentrations,[54] but clinical and experimental observations indicate that this rule is an oversimplification of what actually happens.[55] The magnitude of the alterations in serum K^+ concentration caused by acid-base disturbances depends on the acuteness of the condition and on the nature of the acid-base disorder. In general, the respective incremental changes in serum K^+ concentrations are greater with acidosis, acute pH changes, and metabolic acidosis than with alkalosis, chronic pH changes, and respiratory acidosis.

Insulin directly stimulates the cellular uptake of K^+. Experimental evidence indicates insulin may exert this effect by stimulating membrane bound Na^+-K^+-ATPase activity.[56] The intracellular uptake of K^+ induced by insulin is independent of its effect on glucose uptake. Pancreatic insulin secretion appears to be under the influence of plasma K^+ concentrations. Hyperkalemia stimulates insulin release, whereas normokalemia or hypokalemia inhibits insulin release. The K^+-lowering effect of insulin may be important in attentuating postprandial increases in the extracellular K^+ concentration.

Hyperosmolar states can alter internal K^+ balance,[50] Increasing the tonicity of the extracellular fluid induces the shift of K^+ out of cells. One explanation for this phenomenon is that solvent drag causes K^+ to accompany the movement of water out of cells in hyperosmotic conditions. Cellular dehydration and the resulting increase in the intracellular fluid K^+ concentration also may favor the movement of K^+ out of cells. In contrast, plasma hypotonicity has little or no effect on internal K^+ balance.

Exercise is associated with the release of K^+ from skeletal muscle cells. The exercise-induced increase in serum K^+ concentration is proportional to the grade of physical exertion.[50,57]

2. Regulation of external potassium balance.
A normal dietary intake of K^+ ranges from 50 to 100 mEq per day. This amount is nearly equal to or exceeds the entire K^+ content in the extracellular space. The uptake of K^+ into cells temporarily protects the body against hyperkalemia, but the long-term maintenance of external K^+ balance is dependent on renal excretion of this daily K^+ load. The gastrointestinal tract has a passive role in the normal regulation of external K^+ balance. Virtually all dietary K^+ is absorbed systemically from the gastrointestinal tract. Potassium loss in the stool is normally less than 10% of the dietary intake. Regulation of external K^+ balance is accomplished almost exclusively by renal K^+ excretion. Increases in K^+ intake are matched within hours by increases in the urinary excretion of K^+. Renal adaptation to hypokalemia takes days to weeks, eventually decreasing urinary K^+ excretion to an obligatory loss of 10 mEq per day. The renal excretion of K^+ is primarily under the influence of aldosterone but also is affected by changes in the ionic composition of the urine.

Renal K^+ excretion is dependent on the tubular secretion of K^+ into the urine because 90% of filtered K^+ automatically is reabsorbed by the proximal nephron. Potassium excretion into the urine occurs mainly in the late distal tubule and collecting duct. Specialized cells in these parts of the nephron actively transport K^+ into the tubule lumen. This active transport mechanism has functional similarities to Na^+-K^+-ATPase, since the tubular secretion of K^+ is coupled with the reabsorption of Na^+. Potassium secretion by these cells is greatly facilitated by aldosterone. In addition to aldosterone, several other conditions influence the renal handling of K^+.[57] Increases in plasma K^+ concentration, distal tubular flow rate, Na^+ delivery to the distal nephron, and luminal electronegativity (the urinary secretion of poorly permeant anions, such as sulfate, or anionic drugs, such as carbenicillin) promote the excretion of K^+ into the urine. Acute acidosis inhibits and acute alkalosis stimulates distal tubular K^+ secretion. Any condition resulting in chloride depletion is associated with enhanced renal K^+ excretion.

Aldosterone directly stimulates cells of the distal tubule and cortical collecting duct to secrete K^+ into the urine and reabsorb Na^+ into the circulation. Aldosterone secretion from the adrenal cortex is influenced directly by the plasma K^+ concentration and the intravascular volume status[58] (Fig. 20-5). Small increases in the extracellular K^+ concentration directly stimulate aldosterone secretion, whereas small decreases in the extracellular K^+ concentration directly inhibit aldosterone secretion. Hypotension, low cardiac output, decreased renal perfusion pressure, and Na^+-avid states stimulate aldosterone synthesis and release by activating the renin-angiotensin-aldosterone pathway. Sympathetic nervous system activation and de-

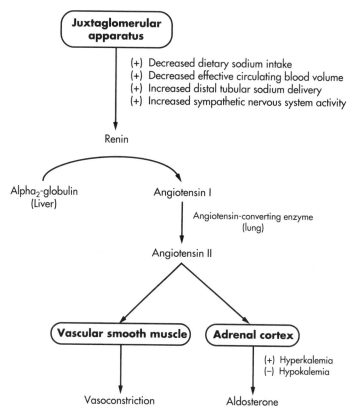

Fig. 20-5. Factors regulating the secretion of aldosterone.

creased Na^+ delivery to the distal nephron stimulate the juxtaglomerular apparatus to secrete renin. Circulating renin catalyzes the conversion of alpha$_2$-globulin, which is synthesized by the liver, to angiotensin I. Angiotensin I subsequently undergoes biotransformation in the lung to angiotensin II through the action of angiotensin-converting enzyme. Angiotensin II directly stimulates aldosterone secretion from the adrenal cortex and thereby promotes kaliuresis.

In renal failure, extrarenal excretion of K^+ by the colon becomes an important mechanism for K^+ disposal. In this condition, the active transport of K^+ into the lumen of the gastrointestinal tract may be facilitated by aldosterone. Renal failure also stimulates remaining functional nephrons to adapt and increase their relative ability to excrete K^+.

C. Hypokalemia

1. Causes of hypokalemia. Hypokalemia is defined as a serum K^+ concentration less than 3.5 mEq/L. Hypokalemia can be caused by dietary deficiency of K^+, cellular uptake of K^+, or excessive loss of K^+ through the urinary and gastrointestinal tracts (Fig. 20-6). Total body K^+ content is unchanged in conditions of hypokalemia caused by the internal redistribution of K^+. Hypokalemia from dietary deficiency, renal K^+ losses, or extrarenal K^+ losses are associated with a total body K^+ deficit.

a. Dietary potassium deficiency. Hypokalemia from dietary K^+ deficiency alone is rare, since the kidney normally can decrease K^+ secretion to as low as 10 mEq per day. Clay ingestion, which has been reported to occur among inhabitants of the southeastern United States, can cause dietary K^+ deficiency by binding K^+ and preventing it from being systemically absorbed.[59]

b. Hypokalemia secondary to cellular uptake of potassium. Internal redistribution of K^+ from the extracellular compartment into the intracellular compartment can cause hypokalemia without net changes in total body K^+ content. As mentioned earlier, factors that promote the cellular uptake of K^+ include alkalosis, insulin, and beta$_2$-adrenergic agonists.

Hypokalemia from the pharmacologic action of beta$_2$-adrenergic agonists can be of clinical importance in a variety of situations. Beta-adrenergic agonists (such as epinephrine, terbutaline, metaproterenol, or salbutamol) used for

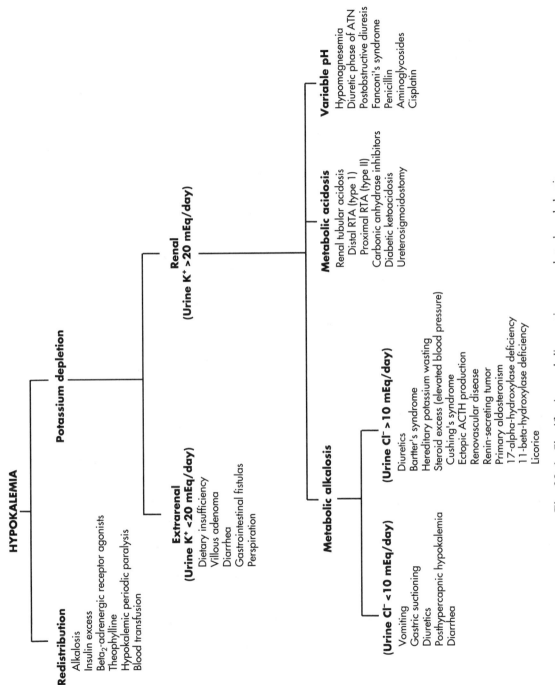

HYPOKALEMIA

Redistribution
Alkalosis
Insulin excess
Beta$_2$-adrenergic receptor agonists
Theophylline
Hypokalemic periodic paralysis
Blood transfusion

Potassium depletion

Extrarenal
(Urine K$^+$ <20 mEq/day)
Dietary insufficiency
Villous adenoma
Diarrhea
Gastrointestinal fistulas
Perspiration

Renal
(Urine K$^+$ >20 mEq/day)

Metabolic alkalosis

(Urine Cl$^-$ <10 mEq/day)
Vomiting
Gastric suctioning
Diuretics
Posthypercapnic hypokalemia
Diarrhea

(Urine Cl$^-$ >10 mEq/day)
Diuretics
Bartter's syndrome
Hereditary potassium wasting
Steroid excess (elevated blood pressure)
Cushing's syndrome
Ectopic ACTH production
Renovascular disease
Renin-secreting tumor
Primary aldosteronism
17-alpha-hydroxylase deficiency
11-beta-hydroxylase deficiency
Licorice

Metabolic acidosis
Renal tubular acidosis
Distal RTA (type 1)
Proximal RTA (type II)
Carbonic anhydrase inhibitors
Diabetic ketoacidosis
Ureterosigmoidostomy

Variable pH
Hypomagnesemia
Diuretic phase of ATN
Postobstructive diuresis
Fanconi's syndrome
Penicillin
Aminoglycosides
Cisplatin

Fig. 20-6. Classification and diagnostic approach to hypokalemia.

the treatment of bronchospasm, asthma, or heart failure can cause acute decreases in serum K^+ concentrations. In contrast, patients receiving beta-adrenergic antagonists (such as propranolol) or alpha-adrenergic agonists (such as phenylephrine) may have an impaired tolerance to conditions that produce increases in serum K^+. Theophylline decreases serum K^+ concentration by directly increasing intracellular cyclic-AMP, the intracellular second messenger coupled to beta-adrenergic receptor stimulation. The endogenous release of epinephrine induced by emotional, surgical, or anesthetic stress partially may explain the frequently observed decreases in perioperative serum K^+ concentrations.[60] Increases in circulating catecholamine concentrations also may provide an explanation for hypokalemia associated with hypothermia in postoperative surgical patients.[61]

Alkalosis causes hypokalemia by promoting the cellular uptake of K^+. The most common cause for alkalosis in the perioperative period is hyperventilation during anesthesia.[62] Acute respiratory alkalosis causes a 0.13 to 0.42 mEq/L decrease in serum K^+ concentration for a 0.1 unit increase in plasma pH.[55] A relationship of the same magnitude also applies to acute metabolic alkalosis from bicarbonate administration.[55]

Increases in circulating insulin concentrations can also cause hypokalemia by promoting the cellular uptake of K^+. The endogenous release of insulin is stimulated by hyperglycemia. Perioperative hyperglycemia can be caused by surgical stress or by the administration of dextrose-containing solutions. Exogenous administration of insulin, used in the treatment of diabetes mellitus, diabetic ketoacidosis, or nonketotic hyperosmolar states, can cause precipitous decreases in the serum K^+ concentration as cells reuptake extracellular K^+.

The uptake of extracellular K^+ by rapidly dividing cells can lead to hypokalemia. The acute anabolic state that occurs with vitamin B_{12} therapy for severe pernicious anemia is an example of this condition.[50] Transfusion of stored red blood cells can lead to hypokalemia. As the transfused cells enter the circulation, their metabolic activity is restored and K^+ is taken up by the cells.[63]

Hypokalemic periodic paralysis is a rare familial disorder of internal K^+ balance. It is characterized by spells of severe muscle weakness or paralysis that are associated with sudden shifts of K^+ into cells. These attacks often are precipitated by stress, infection, exercise, exposure to cold environments, or any circumstance that decreases extracellular K^+ concentration.

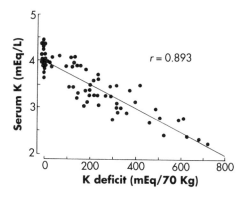

Fig. 20-7. The relationship between serum potassium concentration (K) and the total body potassium deficit in human subjects with uncomplicated potassium depletion. A 0.27 mEq/L reduction in the serum potassium concentration is equivalent to a 100 mEq total body potassium deficit. (From Sterns RH, Cox M, Feig PU, and Singer I: Medicine 60:339, 1981.)

In the unusual event that such a patient requires surgery, therapeutic agents and metabolic conditions that promote intracellular shifts in K^+ should be avoided to prevent triggering of an attack.[64]

c. Hypokalemia secondary to renal and extrarenal potassium losses. Hypokalemia from renal or extrarenal K^+ loss is associated with a net deficit in total body K^+. In these conditions, K^+ lost from the extracellular fluid compartment is accompanied by depletion of intracellular K^+. Metabolic studies indicate that the decrease in the extracellular K^+ concentration proportionately exceeds the decrease in the intracellular K^+ concentration; as a result, the extracellular to intracellular K^+ concentration gradient is reduced.[50] Depending on the presence of coexisting conditions that influence the internal distribution of K^+, a 1 mEq/L decrease in the serum K^+ concentration is associated with an approximately 300 to 400 mEq total body K^+ deficit[50] (Fig. 20-7).

The gastrointestinal tract is the major source of extrarenal K^+ losses. The K^+ concentrations of both upper and lower gastrointestinal secretions average 10 mEq/L. Gastrointestinal fluid losses from diarrhea, ureterosigmoidostomy, continuous nasogastric suctioning, vomiting, or pyloric stenosis alone can cause substantial K^+ deficits (such as nasogastric output of 2 liters per day equates to 20 mEq K^+ loss per day). Hypokalemia caused by these conditions is compounded by secondary renal K^+ loss. In these settings, renal K^+ losses can be as high as 100 to 200 mEq per day. The hypochloremic metabolic alkalosis that accompanies the loss of upper gastrointestinal secretions promotes kaliuresis through several mechanisms. Alkalosis and hypochloremia stimulate renal tubular secretion of K^+. Intravascular volume contraction stimulates the secretion of aldosterone, which further augments the secretion of K^+ into the urine. Hypokalemia predictably occurs within 4 to 5 days in postoperative surgical patients on continuous nasogastric suctioning if K^+ supplements are not provided.[65] Hypokalemia is an especially prominent clinical feature in patients with villous adenomas of the colon or rectum. The villous adenoma can secrete a large quantity of K^+-rich fluid in the stool. In this disorder, stool K^+ concentrations can range from 10 to 107 mEq/L.[66]

Renal K^+ wasting from diuretic therapy is perhaps the most common cause of hypokalemia in both medical and surgical patients. The frequency of hypokalemia in patients treated with diuretics can range from 20% to 50%.[44] Diuretic therapy is associated with hypokalemia for several reasons. All diuretics increase renal tubular flow rates, alkalinize the urine, cause chloride depletion, and increase the filtered load of Na^+ delivered to the distal nephron. Except for the K^+-sparing agents (amiloride, triamterene, and spironolactone), these actions of diuretics cause renal K^+ wasting. Furthermore, many clinical conditions in which diuretics are used are associated with hyperaldosteronism. Hyperaldosteronism potentiates diuretic-induced kaliuresis by directly stimulating K^+ secretion in the distal nephron. A decreased circulating blood volume provides the stimulus for aldosterone secretion in patients with congestive heart failure or cirrhosis who are being treated with diuretics. On the other hand, hyperreninemia stimulates aldosterone secretion in patients with renovascular hypertension who are being treated with diuretics. Finally, hypovolemia as a direct result of diuretic therapy stimulates the secretion of aldosterone.

Renal K^+ wasting is also a feature of clinical conditions associated with excess aldosterone or other mineralocorticoids. These syndromes are characterized by metabolic alkalosis, hypertension, and renal wasting of K^+ and chloride. Some clinical examples of conditions with mineralocorticoid excess that can cause hypokalemia are primary hyperaldosteronism from adenoma or glandular hyperplasia, Cushing's syndrome, adrenocorticotropic hormone (ACTH)– secreting tumors, and the syndromes of congenital adrenal hyperplasia (17-alpha-hydroxylase and 11-beta-hydroxylase deficiency). Liddle's syndrome is a renal disorder with clinical features identical to the syndromes of mineralocorticoid excess, but the primary defect is believed to be abnormal end-organ sensitivity to aldosterone.[67] Clinical examples of hyperreninemic states leading to hyperaldosteronism include renovascular hypertension, renin-secreting tumors, and Bartter's syndrome.[68] Finally the administration of mineralocorticoids or the ingestion of exogenous substances with mineralocorticoid activity, such as glycyrrhizinic acid (which is present in licorice), can cause hypokalemia from excessive urinary excretion of the electrolyte.

Hypokalemia can be caused by a variety of other renal diseases and metabolic conditions that are associated with excessive renal K^+ losses. Distal (type I) and proximal (type II) renal tubular acidosis are characterized by the excretion of an alkaline urine, renal K^+ wasting, and metabolic acidosis. Magnesium deficiency is associated with both renal K^+ wasting and intracellular K^+ depletion. Hypokalemia from Mg^{++} deficiency is often unresponsive to K^+ replacement therapy until the underlying hypomagnesemia is corrected.[69] Aminoglycoside antibiotics, amphotericin B, and cisplatin can cause nephrotoxicity, which is characterized by selective wasting of K^+ and Mg^{++} before the development of end-stage renal failure. Antibiotic therapy with penicillin G, carbenicillin, or its derivatives cause urinary K^+ wasting because these drugs are excreted in the urine as nonreabsorbable anions. The presence of these anions in the tubular fluid promotes the passive diffusion of K^+ into the tubular fluid. Renal K^+ wasting is a clinical feature of the diuretic phase of acute tubular necrosis as well as during the diuresis that occurs after the relief of urinary tract obstruction. Chronic hypercapnia induces renal bicarbonate retention and chloride depletion. The acute correction of chronic hypercapnia by hyperventilation results in a metabolic state characterized by hypochloremic alkalosis and hypokalemia.[70]

2. Clinical manifestations of hypokalemia. Neuromuscular dysfunction is the most prominent clinical manifestation of hypokalemia. The increased intracellular to extracellular K^+ concentration gradient hyperpolarizes cell membranes and increases the depolarization threshold for the action potential. Although individual variability exists, mild symptoms generally begin to appear when serum K^+ concentrations reach 2.5 to 3 mEq/L. The early symptoms often are nonspecific and can include complaints of weakness, fatigue, and malaise. Diminished deep tendon reflexes, weakness of the lower extremities, trunk, and arms become evident at serum K^+ concentrations of less than 2.5 mEq/L. Skeletal muscle weakness can be severe enough to cause respiratory failure and paralysis. Patients with this degree of hypokalemia have an increased sensitivity to nondepolarizing muscle relaxants.[71] Neostigmine may be less effective in antagonizing the nondepolarizing neuromuscular block in hypokalemic patients. At serum K^+ concentrations of less than 2 mEq/L, patients are at risk for rhabdomyolysis and skeletal muscle necrosis. The mechanism of hypokalemia-induced rhabdomyolysis and muscle necrosis is incompletely understood, but these conditions appear to be worsened by physical exercise or exertion.[72]

The effects of hypokalemia on the electrical activity of the heart can be manifested by changes on the surface ECG. The progressive changes of the ECG caused by hypokalemia are nonspecific and often do not correlate with the presence of other clinical signs and symptoms. A typical ECG pattern of hypokalemia is ST-segment depression followed by a reduction in the amplitude of the T wave, T-wave inversion, and finally the appearance of a U wave. A prolongation of the QT or QT_c interval actually may reflect the presence of a U wave rather than a genuine delay in repolarization.

The clinically important aspect of hypokalemia on the heart concerns the potential for cardiac dysrhythmias. Hypokalemia may predispose patients to cardiac dysrhythmias by shortening the effective refractory period of Purkinje cells, shortening the coupling intervals for ventricular premature contractions (VPCs), and increasing the frequency and complexity of VPCs.[73,74] These effects of hypokalemia can sensitize the heart to catecholamine-induced dysrhythmias. An association between hypokalemia and the risk of ventricular tachycardia and ventricular fibrillation has been reported among patients suffering acute myocardial infarctions.[75] The arrhythmogenic potential of hypokalemia is especially important among patients taking digitalis glycosides. Hypokalemia potentiates both digitalis-induced dysrhythmias and digitalis toxicity. This effect of hypokalemia is supported by clinical and experimental evidence. Hypokalemia exposes the myocardium to a higher concentration of digoxin by increasing the number of ouabain-binding sites on Na^+-K^+-ATPase in myocardial cells. Hypokalemic patients on digoxin therapy are susceptible to almost any type of cardiac rhythm disturbance. Digoxin toxicity is manifested in patients with hypokalemia at lower plasma digoxin concentrations than in patients without hypokalemia.[76]

Whether the arrhythmogenic effects of hypokalemia pose an actual risk to patients undergoing anesthesia is an important clinical question. Hypokalemia is one of the most frequently encountered preoperative electrolyte disturbances and is especially common in diuretic-treated patients with cardiovascular diseases. Based on the belief that hypokalemia predisposes the patient to life-threatening cardiac dysrhythmias during anesthesia, the traditional practice has been to treat hypokalemia preoperatively. This approach is often impractical, since it can prolong hospitalization, increase hospital costs, delay scheduled operations, and occasionally cause iatrogenic complications. Several recent studies have attempted to address this problem and determine if this traditional approach is warranted. A study conducted by Vitez et al.[77] found that intraoperative rhythm disturbances were not more frequent or more severe in 62 surgical patients with preoperative serum K^+ concentrations less than 3.5 mEq/L as compared to 88 normokalemic surgical patients. An editorial accompanying the study questioned whether the conclusion can be applied to all patients because the study population consisted only of patients at low risk for cardiac dysrhythmias.[78] This additional question was addressed by a recent study conducted by Hirsh et al. In this study, 447 patients undergoing cardiac and vascular operations were examined.[45] This study of "high-risk" patients also found that the frequency and severity of intraoperative dysrhythmias did not correlate with the degree of preoperative hypokalemia. Patients on long-term digoxin therapy and patients with congestive heart disease were at greatest risk of intraoperative arrhythmias regardless of their preoperative serum K^+ concentration. These reports suggest that preoperative K^+ replacement is often unnecessary in the patient with asymptomatic hypokalemia. Thus the traditional practice of preoperative K^+ replacement for all patients with hypokalemia probably needs to be reevaluated. We speculate that the more severe the hypokalemia, the more it is that replacement therapy is indicated.

3. Diagnostic evaluation of hypokalemia. Definitive therapy for hypokalemia requires the diagnosis and treatment of the underlying disorder. The underlying conditions responsible for hypokalemia usually can be elucidated from the patient's medical history and their therapeutic drug regimen. Hypokalemia caused by internal redistribution needs to be recognized, since K^+ supplementation is not indicated in this condition. Laboratory measurements of blood pH, serum glucose, and plasma osmolality are useful for determining whether internal redistribution is contributing to the low serum K^+ concentration. Vomiting, diarrhea, and nasogastric suctioning indicate sources of extrarenal K^+ loss. Alternatively, hypokalemia in combination with a urine K^+ concentration of greater than 20 mEq/L indicates renal K^+ wasting.

Measuring the blood pH, arterial carbon dioxide tension (P_{CO_2}), the urinary chloride concentration, and the patient's blood pressure is useful for distinguishing between the various disorders of renal K^+ wasting[79,57] (Fig. 20-6). Metabolic alkalosis with a urine chloride concentration less than 10 mEq/L indicates that renal K^+ wasting is secondary to upper gastrointestinal fluid losses or to rapid correction of chronic hypercapnia. Metabolic acidosis with a urine chloride concentration of greater than 10 mEq/L in association with hypertension indicates conditions of mineralocorticoid excess. The detection of metabolic acidosis indicates renal tubular acidosis, ureterosigmoidostomy, use of carbonic anhydrase inhibitors, or diabetic ketoacidosis.

All patients with hypokalemia should be evaluated for evidence of hypovolemia, since volume depletion is a potent stimulus for aldosterone secretion. Hypovolemia can be readily treated by intravascular volume expansion. In addition, the serum Mg^{++} concentration probably should be measured in all patients with hypokalemia. Hypomagnesemia frequently is associated with hypokalemia and can be a cause of renal K^+ wasting. Hypokalemia sometimes can be refractory to treatment in patients with underlying hypomagnesemia until the Mg^{++} deficit is restored.

4. Treatment of hypokalemia. Although more information is needed to establish strict guidelines for K^+-replacement therapy, the following scheme is applicable in most clinical situations. If a laboratory determination establishes the serum K^+ concentration to be less than 3 mEq/L, therapy for hypokalemia should be instituted even if clinical signs and symptoms of hypokalemia are absent. If the measured serum K^+ concentration is between 3 and 3.5 mEq/L and the patient has unequivocal signs and symptoms of hypokalemia in combination with ECG evidence of hypokalemia, treatment probably also should be initiated. Patients receiving digitalis glycosides pose a special clinical problem, and their serum K^+ concentrations should probably be maintained between 3.5 and 4.5 mEq/L. A patient with an acute metabolic acidosis with a serum K^+ concentration less than 3.5 mEq/L should be treated. An alkalotic patient with a serum K^+ concentration less than 3.5 mEq/L may be monitored without therapy.

Potassium chloride can be used to replace deficits in most clinical situations. This statement is especially true in patients with hypokalemia associated with hypochloremic alkalosis. Potassium phosphate sometimes is substituted for part of the K^+ replacement dose in patients with diabetic ketoacidosis because hypophosphatemia often accompanies this condition. Potassium chloride can be administered either orally or intravenously. Potassium administered orally is usually 90% absorbed except with extended release or enteric-coated formulations, which can have variable patterns of absorption. The usual dose for oral K^+ supplementation is 50 to 100 mEq per day.

Potassium chloride can be administered intravenously when oral administration is unfeasible or when it is desirable to rapidly restore the serum K^+ concentration to within the normal range. Intravenous administration of K^+ carries the risk of life-threatening cardiac toxicity from inadvertent overdose when it is administered too quickly. It is useful to remember that the extracellular fluid space contains only a total of 50 to 70 mEq of K^+ in the average adult and that K^+ administered into the intravascular space does not distribute instantaneously throughout the extracellular space. In addition, K^+ administered through a peripheral vein at concentrations greater than 40 mEq/L can cause pain. For the above reasons, intravenous potassium chloride should not be administered at rates greater than 40 mEq per hour except in life-threatening situations. When a concentrated solution of K^+ is used, it is preferable to infuse it through a central venous line or into a large vein. The risk of iatrogenic hyperkalemia can be reduced by continuous monitoring of the ECG for evidence of hyperkalemia, frequent measurement of the serum K^+ concentration during therapy, and placement of no more than 20 mEq of K^+ at a time into the intravenous administration apparatus. Furthermore, emergency drugs and the means to treat hyperkalemia must be immediately available.

As stated earlier, the serum K^+ concentration provides only an indirect indication of total body K^+ content. Although intravenous K^+ administration can quickly restore the serum K^+ concentration to within the normal range, continued K^+ administration for several days is usually necessary to replace the intracellular deficit.

D. Hyperkalemia

1. Cause of hyperkalemia. Hyperkalemia is defined as a serum K^+ concentration greater than 5.0 mEq/L. Hyperkalemia can be caused by internal redistribution of K^+ or by net

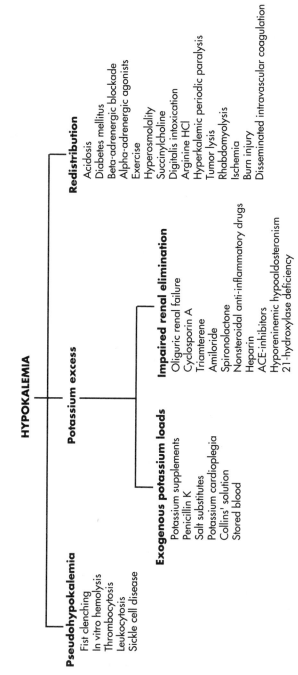

Fig. 20-8. Classification and diagnostic approach to hyperkalemia.

changes in external K^+ balance (Fig. 20-8). The release of K^+ from cells into the extracellular fluid and the impaired uptake of K^+ into cells cause hyperkalemia without net changes in the total body K^+ content. Excessive administration of K^+ and impaired ability to excrete K^+ cause hyperkalemia with increased net total body K^+ content.

a. Pseudohyperkalemia. The in vitro hemolysis of blood samples before electrolyte determination provides a falsely increased laboratory estimation of the actual serum K^+ concentration. Blood samples obtained by venipuncture in an arm after prolonged application of a tourniquet and repeated clenching of the fist can also result in falsely elevated laboratory determinations of serum K^+ concentrations.[80] Blood samples from patients with sickle cell disease, leukocytosis, and thrombocytosis are particularly prone to in vitro hemolysis. These laboratory artifacts commonly are referred to as "pseudohyperkalemia." When pseudohyperkalemia is suspected, the patient's ECG should be inspected for evidence of true hyperkalemia before one ignores the results or requests that the test be repeated.

b. Hyperkalemia secondary to cellular release of potassium. Because greater than 90% of the body's total K^+ store is intracellular, any process that causes the release of K^+ from cells into the extracellular fluid compartment can produce hyperkalemia. Tumor lysis, rhabdomyolysis, hemolytic transfusion reactions, disseminated intravascular coagulation, acidosis, exercise, burns, and severe tissue trauma are clinical conditions associated with hyperkalemia because intracellular K^+ is released into the circulation. Hyperkalemia also can occur after sudden reperfusion of a large mass of ischemic tissue. This circumstance occurs regularly during major vascular procedures involving the aorta or lower extremities. A lethal overdose of digitalis glycosides causes hyperkalemia by inhibiting membrane-bound Na^+-K^+-ATPase.[81] The therapeutic administration of hypertonic glucose, mannitol, or saline solutions to acutely increase plasma osmolality can increase the serum K^+ concentration by causing osmotically induced K^+ efflux from cells. Arginine hydrochloride, a cationic amino acid sometimes used for the treatment of metabolic alkalosis, also can cause hyperkalemia by inducing the shift of K^+ out of cells.[82]

Hyperkalemia is a well-recognized complication of succinylcholine administration.[83,84] In normal persons the administration of a paralyzing dose of succinylcholine is accompanied by a transient 0.5 mEq/L increase in serum K^+ concentration. This increase in serum K^+ is caused by the release of K^+ from skeletal muscle cells upon depolarization. In the process of depolarization, succinylcholine directly increases membrane permeability to K^+ within the neuromuscular junction by the sustained activation of nicotinic acetylcholine receptors. In the majority of patients, this drug-induced increase in serum K^+ is of minor clinical importance. However, an exaggerated response to succinylcholine resulting in acute hyperkalemia and cardiac arrest has been reported in certain groups of patients. Patients with denervation injuries, spinal cord transection, upper motor neuron injuries, severe muscle trauma, and burn injuries appear to be susceptible. Experimental studies indicate that the affected skeletal muscle in these susceptible patients are exquisitely sensitive to the actions of succinylcholine.[83] Injury or denervation causes both the sensitization and the proliferation of junctional and extrajunctional nicotinic acetylcholine receptors on muscle cells. The mass of skeletal muscle affected and the timing of succinylcholine administration after the acute injury determine the magnitude of the hyperkalemic response. It takes 5 to 10 days after injury for the affected muscle cells to develop sensitivity to succinylcholine. After 60 days, the K^+ content and mass of denervated muscle is reduced sufficiently so that hyperkalemia is unlikely. The risk of succinylcholine-induced hyperkalemia may extend indefinitely in patients with ongoing injuries, persistent infections, or upper motor neuron injuries. Tetanus, prolonged nerve block with local anesthetics, disuse muscle atrophy, intracranial lesions, and severe abdominal infections are other conditions that may cause a predisposition to succinylcholine-induced hyperkalemia. Fortunately the anticipation of this complication in susceptible patients and the alternative use of nondepolarizing muscle relaxants have made this problem exceedingly rare.

Hyperkalemia can result from clinical conditions that impair the ability of cells to take up K^+. The internalization of K^+ by cells is a normal physiologic mechanism to protect against hyperkalemia during acute K^+ loading. Experimental and clinical evidence demonstrate that patients with diabetes mellitus have a limited ability to dispose of acute K^+ loads.[85] Insulin deficiency or insulin unresponsiveness in these patients with diabetes mellitus impairs insulin-mediated K^+ uptake as well as glucose metabolism. Patients receiving beta-adrenergic antagonists and alpha-adrenergic agonists theoretically can develop hyperkalemia from acute K^+ loads. Propranolol, a nonselective beta-adrenergic blocker, is more effective than beta$_1$-selective drugs (such as atenolol, metoprolol, or nadolol) at inhibiting K^+ uptake by cells. Propranolol consistently produces minor increases in serum K^+ concentrations, but it is not clear whether these effects are clinically important.[82] Beta-adrenergic receptor blockade does not appear to cause an exaggerated hyperkalemic response to succinylcholine administration during anesthesia in humans.[86-88]

Familial hyperkalemic periodic paralysis is a rare disorder of episodic hyperkalemia caused by an underlying abnormality in the regulation of internal K^+ balance. In contrast to hypokalemic periodic paralysis, patients with the hyperkalemic varient are usually younger and suffer more frequent attacks of shorter duration. Infusing dextrose-containing solutions preoperatively, refraining from the use of succinylcholine during anesthesia, and avoiding conditions that increase extracellular K^+ concentrations have been advocated to prevent attacks in the perioperative period.[89]

c. Hyperkalemia secondary to excessive potassium administration. Potassium supplements, whether administered orally or intravenously can cause hyperkalemia in susceptible patients. A study that involved examination of 6199 hospitalized patients found 27 cases of fatal drug reactions.[49] Hyperkalemia from K^+ supplementation caused 19% (5 patients) of those deaths. In a separate study that involved examination of 4921 patients receiving potassium chloride supplementation, it was found that hyperkalemia is a complication in 3.6% of patients.[50] In 15% of those patients with hyperkalemia, it was life threatening or fatal. Elderly patients, patients with uremia, patients on diuretic therapy, and patients receiving both oral and parenteral potassium chloride are at greatest risk for developing hyperkalemia.

Potassium also may be administered unintentionally in various ways. Salt substitutes contain 10 to 13 mEq of K^+ per gram; penicillin K contains 1.7 mEq of elemental K^+ per million units of the drug; K^+ cardioplegic solutions typically contain 30 mEq/L of K^+; stored blood has a K^+ concentration that can range from 15 to 50 mEq/L depending on length of storage.[91] The excessive ingestion of salt substitutes, high-dose antibiotic therapy with penicillin K, intraoperative K^+ cardioplegia, and the rapid transfusion of large volumes of stored blood can cause hyperkalemia. Pediatric patients and patients who are hypothermic, acidotic, and actively hemorrhaging are particularly prone to hyperkalemia from blood transfusions.[92,93] Collins' solution used for organ preservation in transplantation operations contains 141 mEq/L of K^+. Cardiac arrest from hyperkalemia with rapid organ reperfusion has been reported during kidney and liver transplantation.[94,95] Intraoperative hyperkalemia can be prevented during organ transplantation by preoperative treatment of preexisting hyperkalemia and also by gradually reperfusing the new graft.

d. Hyperkalemia secondary to impaired potassium excretion. The kidneys are primarily responsible for the daily disposal of K^+. Renal failure of any cause can produce hyperkalemia. In chronic renal failure the capacity of the kidneys to excrete K^+ usually is preserved until the glomerular filtration rate (GFR) is reduced below 5 ml/min.[57] At this GFR, approximately 35 mEq per day of K^+ is excreted in the urine. The gastrointestinal system adapts during chronic renal failure and can excrete an additional 10 to 20 mEq of K^+ per day. Acute oliguric renal failure can cause the rapid clinical onset of hyperkalemia, especially in surgical patients with extensive tissue injuries, rhabdomyolysis, or a high catabolic rate.

Drugs can impair the renal excretion of K^+ by (1) causing direct renal toxicity, (2) changing the composition of urine to promote K^+ secretion, or (3) inhibiting the secretion or action of aldosterone. Aminoglycoside antibiotics and cyclosporin A are two examples of drugs used commonly in the perioperative period that can cause direct renal toxicity and impair urinary K^+ excretion. Severe reduction of the GFR usually is necessary for hyperkalemia to develop from aminoglycoside-induced nephrotoxicity. In contrast, hyperkalemia and metabolic acidosis are prominent clinical features of cyclosporin A−induced renal toxicity.[82] The K^+-sparing diuretics triamterene and amiloride block Na^+ reabsorption at the distal tubule. Potassium secretion into the urine is impaired by these drugs because Na^+-K^+ exchange by active transport mechanisms is inhibited. These two K^+-sparing diuretics also decrease the passive diffusion of K^+ into the urine by lowering the electronegativity of the tubular fluid, which is a consequence of the abnormally high tubular Na^+ concentration.

Disorders that affect any of the steps in the pathway that lead to aldosterone secretion or that inhibit aldosterone at its cellular site of action can produce hyperkalemia because aldosterone is important for promoting renal K^+ excretion. Heparin, even at doses used for the prophylaxis of deep vein thrombosis, impairs aldosterone synthesis by the adrenal cortex.[82] Primary adrenal insufficiency and congenital

21-hydroxylase deficiency are other examples of clinical disorders of aldosterone synthesis. Nonsteroidal anti-inflammatory drugs (NSAIDs), such as indomethacin, inhibit the renal synthesis of prostacyclin (PGI_2) and prostaglandin E_2 (PGE_2). PGI_2 and PGE_2 are vasodilating eicosanoids that act within the kidney to stimulate renin secretion and natriuresis. These actions of PGI_2 and PGE_2 promote aldosterone secretion and the tubular secretion of K^+. NSAID-induced nephropathy can cause the clinical syndrome of hyporeninemic hypoaldosteronism, which is characterized by hyperkalemia and metabolic acidosis in the presence of an adequate GFR. Cyclosporin A toxicity, diabetic glomerulosclerosis, and a variety of other diseases affecting the kidney can also cause the syndrome of hyporeninemic hypoaldosteronism.[96] The angiotensin-converting enzyme (ACE) inhibitors captopril and enalapril reduce angiotensin II–mediated aldosterone secretion but do not affect the direct stimulation of aldosterone release by K^+. The direct stimulation of aldosterone release by K^+ limits the ability of ACE inhibitors to cause hyperkalemia.[97] Finally the K^+-sparing diuretic spironolactone inhibits the tubular secretion of K^+ by competitively inhibiting the cytoplasmic aldosterone receptor within renal tubular cells.

2. Clinical manifestations of hyperkalemia. Hyperkalemia is a medical emergency. The potential for cardiac arrest from hyperkalemia is the most serious concern in this condition. Cardiac toxicity from hyperkalemia is a consequence of altered transmembrane electrical potential on the electrically excitable cells of the heart. Initial increases in the extracellular K^+ concentration lower the resting membrane potential, enhance depolarization, and shorten the duration of the action potential of myocardial cells, but further increases in the extracellular K^+ concentration ultimately suppress depolarization and conduction velocity.

Hyperkalemia causes characteristic changes on the surface ECG.[98]. At serum K^+ concentrations of 6 to 7 mEq/L, tall or "tented" T waves appear, the P-R interval lengthens, and the amplitude of P waves decreases. At serum K^+ concentrations of 8 to 10 mEq/L, P waves often are undiscernible, the QRS complex widens, the S wave becomes broad and deep, and the R-R interval becomes irregular. The morphology of the QRS complex on the ECG at serum K^+ concentrations of 9 to 10 mEq/L is often said to assume a sine-wave pattern. Serum K^+ concentrations greater than 10 mEq/L cause asystole or ventricular fibrillation. In animal experiments, lethal hyperkalemia causes asystole. True ventricular tachycardia or ventricular fibrillation is observed rarely in experimental hyperkalemia. During cardiac operations, the controlled administration of K^+ cardioplegic solutions into the heart also causes asystole. From this experience one can state that it is likely that in humans asystole is more common than ventricular fibrillation as a consequence of lethal hyperkalemia. In patients dependent on artificial cardiac pacemakers, the first sign of hyperkalemia may be failure to pace. At serum K^+ concentrations approaching 8 mEq/L, the energy threshold for pacing increases. Hyperkalemia affects the pacing threshold of the atria to a greater extent than that of the ventricles. Ventricular pacing is therefore more efficacious than atrial pacing for asystole caused by hyperkalemia.[98,99]

3. Treatment of hyperkalemia. Treatment of hyperkalemia is the same regardless of the underlying cause. All K^+-containing intravenous solutions should be immediately discontinued. Therapy is aimed at antagonizing the membrane effects of hyperkalemia, decreasing the extracellular K^+ concentration by promoting intracellular transfer of the electrolyte, and eliminating the excess K^+ burden from the body. As mentioned above, temporary ventricular pacing of the heart is indicated when cardiovascular arrest is caused by asystole, bradycardia, or atrioventricular dissociation.

Intravenous Ca^{++} chloride or calcium gluconate is the first drug of choice for the emergency treatment of hyperkalemia. Both calcium chloride 15 to 50 mg/kg and calcium gluconate 50 to 100 mg/kg can be administered by intravenous bolus injection and effectively antagonize the hyperkalemia-induced depolarization blockade. These Ca^{++} salts have an immediate onset of action, and their effects last between 30 and 60 minutes. Increasing the extracellular Na^+ concentration also antagonizes the membrane effects of hyperkalemia and partially may explain the efficacy of sodium bicarbonate therapy for hyperkalemia. Endogenous extracellular Na^+ and Ca^{++} can have similar pharmacologic actions. Patients with hyponatremia and hypocalcemia are more susceptible to hyperkalemia. Hyponatremic or hypocalcemic patients manifest clinical signs of hyperkalemia at lower serum K^+ concentrations than patients with normal serum Na^+ and Ca^{++} concentrations. Patients on hemodialysis undergoing parathyroidectomy for renal hyperparathyroidism are at increased risk of developing symptomatic hyperkalemia postoperatively. Postoperative hypocalcemia from transient parathyroid insufficiency is a possible explanation for this finding.[100]

Alkalinizing the blood promotes K^+ entry into cells and can be accomplished rapidly by administration of sodium bicarbonate at a dose of 1 to 2 mEq/kg intravenously. In addition, hyperventilating the patient is also an effective therapeutic measure for increasing the blood pH. The sodium bicarbonate should not be mixed together with Ca^{++}, since calcium carbonate precipitates out of solution. A 0.1 unit increase in the blood pH causes an approximately 0.13 mEq/L decrease in the serum K^+ concentration. Alkalinization lowers serum K^+ concentrations within 15 to 30 minutes.

Insulin promotes intracellular uptake of K^+. Regular insulin at a dose of 0.1 units/kg intravenously every 15 to 30 minutes decreases the serum K^+ concentration within 15 to 30 minutes. Insulin therapy usually is combined with glucose 250 to 500 mg/kg/hour IV to prevent hypoglycemia.

Potassium can be removed from the gastrointestinal tract by using the K^+-binding resin sodium polystyrene sulfonate (Kayexalate). Sodium polystyrene sulfonate can be administered at an oral dose of 0.5 to 1 g/kg every 2 to 4 hours. It is usually suspended in 70% sorbital to prevent constipation. Alternatively, sodium polystyrene sulfonate can be given as a retention enema at a dose of 0.5 to 1.0 g/kg every 2 to 4 hours. Each gram of sodium polystyrene sulfonate binds an average of 0.5 mEq of K^+ and causes a decrease in serum K^+ concentration within 60 minutes when given as an enema or within 4 to 6 hours when given orally. If renal function is normal, K^+ can be eliminated from the body by induction of kaliuresis with loop diuretics such as furosemide. When renal function is severely impaired, hemodialysis or peritoneal dialysis is necessary to eliminate K^+ from the body if sodium polystyrene sulfonate cannot be used. Peritoneal dialysis removes K^+ at a rate of 10 to 15 mEq per hour, and hemodialysis can remove K^+ at a rate of 25 to 50 mEq per hour. Several hours may be required to prepare a patient for hemodialysis or peritoneal dialysis.

Continuous monitoring of the ECG and frequent measurements of the serum K^+ concentration should be used for evaluation of the effectiveness of therapy at lowering the serum K^+ concentration. Furthermore, therapy appropriate for the severity of the clinical situation should be instituted with the first signs of hyperkalemia because delaying treatment can result in irreversible clinical deterioration.

The definitive treatment of hyperkalemia depends on the underlying cause. Dietary K^+ restriction and dialysis may be the only therapeutic options in the patient with oliguric renal failure. Hyperkalemia as a complication of K^+ supplementation resolves with discontinuation or readjustment of the dose of K^+ being administered. Drug-induced hyperkalemia resolves with discontinuation of the offending drug. The patient should be evaluated for coexisting hypocalcemia and hyponatremia because these two electrolyte disorders potentiate the toxic effects of hyperkalemia. Finally the patient should be evaluated for the presence of disorders causing aldosterone deficiency.

III. CALCIUM

Calcium (Ca^{++}) has a vital role in a diverse range of physiologic processes.[101-103] Free or ionized Ca^{++} is the second messenger system responsible for stimulus-excitation coupling and transmembrane signal transduction in a wide variety of cells. Calcium mediates the contraction of cardiac, vascular smooth muscle, and nonvascular smooth muscle cells. Calcium is required for the secretion of hormones, the release of neurotransmitters, and the initiation of blood coagulation. Calcium has a major influence on the electrical properties of neuronal cells and is essential for the generation of electrical impulses in cells of the cardiac conduction system. It is therefore not surprising that disorders of Ca^{++} homeostasis have broad clinical implications. Cardiovascular, neurologic, and neuromuscular functions are grossly affected by alterations in the extracellular Ca^{++} concentration. Other physiologic processes may also be variably affected by hypercalcemia or hypocalcemia and may explain, in part, the increase in morbidity and mortality among critically ill patients with abnormal serum Ca^{++} levels.[104-106]

A. Calcium homeostasis

Approximately 1% of the body's total Ca^{++} content exists within cells and their surrounding medium.[103] Only this small fraction of Ca^{++} can actively participate in physiologic processes. The remaining 99% of the body's total Ca^{++} is part of the mineral lattice of bone and serves as a structural support for the body. This large pool of Ca^{++} is potentially exchangeable with the much smaller pool of extracellular and intracellular Ca^{++} under the influence of hormonal systems that regulate Ca^{++} metabolism.

The normal serum Ca^{++} concentration ranges between 2.1 and 2.6 mmol/L. Approximately 40% of circulating Ca^{++} is bound to al-

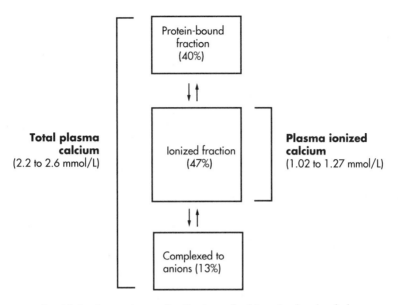

Fig. 20-9. Approximate distribution of calcium in the circulation.

bumin and other plasma proteins, whereas another 13% is complexed to bicarbonate, phosphate, lactate, and other anions present in the plasma. The remaining 47% of Ca^{++} present in the plasma exists as a free ionized form in solution (Fig. 20-9). This ionized fraction of plasma Ca^{++} diffuses freely throughout the extracellular space. This ionized fraction is responsible for the physiologic actions attributed to Ca^{++}; its concentration determines the activity of hormonal systems that control internal Ca^{++} homeostasis.

The intracellular concentration of ionized Ca^{++} ranges between 100 and 200 nmol or approximately 10,000 times less than the concentration of extracellular ionized Ca^{++}. This transcellular Ca^{++} gradient is maintained by electrogenic and energy-dependent membrane pumps that actively transport Ca^{++} out of cells. The majority of intracellular Ca^{++} is sequestered within mitochondria and specialized cell organelles, such as the sarcoplasmic reticulum and the transverse tubule system.

B. Measurement of circulating calcium concentrations

For clinical purposes, only the circulating Ca^{++} concentration is accessible for measurement. Since a large portion of circulating Ca^{++} is protein bound, measurement of the total serum Ca^{++} concentration often fails to provide an accurate indication of the ionized Ca^{++} concentration that is of physiologic importance. Changes in serum protein concentration alter the total serum Ca^{++} concentration without af-

fecting the ionized Ca^{++} concentration. Furthermore, factors that affect the binding of Ca^{++} to plasma proteins change the ionized Ca^{++} concentration without affecting the total serum Ca^{++} concentration. For example, alkalosis increases the plasma fraction of protein-bound Ca^{++} and thus decreases the ionized Ca^{++} concentration without changing the total serum Ca^{++} concentration. In contrast, acidosis decreases the plasma fraction of protein-bound Ca^{++} and thus increases the ionized Ca^{++} concentration without altering the total serum Ca^{++} concentration. Formulas that correct for differences in blood pH and the plasma albumin concentration have been devised to estimate the ionized Ca^{++} concentration from the total serum Ca^{++} concentration, but they have been shown to correlate poorly with direct measurements of the ionized Ca^{++} concentration.[107,108]

The development of automated instruments employing ion-selective electrodes has enabled the routine measurement of ionized Ca^{++} concentrations in most "acute-care" laboratories. The normal plasma ionized Ca^{++} concentration ranges between 1.02 to 1.27 mmol/L. Direct measurement of blood ionized Ca^{++} concentrations has replaced largely, and is always preferred over, the indirect estimation of ionized Ca^{++} concentration. Measurement of ionized Ca^{++} concentrations can be performed rapidly on heparinized blood samples and is clinically useful in the perioperative care of surgical patients when blood pH changes frequently, plasma albumin concentrations vary, and anions, which chelate Ca^{++}, are introduced into the bloodstream.

C. Physiologic regulation of calcium metabolism

The blood ionized Ca^{++} concentration is regulated within a narrow range by the combined actions of parathyroid hormone, calcitonin, and vitamin D[103,109] (Fig. 20-10). These hormones control the gastrointestinal absorption, renal conservation, and internal redistribution of Ca^{++}. A decrease in the blood ionized Ca^{++} concentration elicits the synthesis and release of parathyroid hormone from the parathyroid gland. Conversely, increases in blood ionized Ca^{++} concentrations suppress the synthesis and release of parathyroid hormone. Parathyroid hormone increases the ionized Ca^{++} concentration by promoting tubular reabsorption of Ca^{++} by the kidneys, enhancing the renal conversion of 25-hydroxyvitamin D (calcidiol) to 1,25-dihydroxyvitamin D (calcitriol), and activating osteoclast-mediated resorption of bone. 1,25-Dihydroxyvitamin D, the active form of vitamin D, increases blood ionized Ca^{++} concentrations by facilitating the dietary absorption of Ca^{++} in the small intestine, the mobilization of Ca^{++} from bone, and to a lesser extent the renal conservation of Ca^{++}. The body produces 1,25-dihydroxyvitamin D through a series of steps beginning with cholecalciferol (vitamin D), a fat-soluble vitamin that is consumed in the diet or synthesized by the skin during exposure to ultraviolet radiation. Cholecalciferol undergoes 25-hydroxylation in the liver to form 25-hydroxyvitamin D. 25-Hydroxyvitamin D is the substrate for 1-alpha-hydroxylase, an enzyme in the kidney that catalyzes the biotransformation of 25-hydroxyvitamin D to 1,25-dihydroxyvitamin D. 1,25-Dihydroxyvitamin D synthesis appears to be regulated by renal 1-alpha-hydroxylase activity. Increases in circulating parathyroid hormone stimulated by hypocalcemia promotes the enzymatic conversion of 25-hydroxyvitamin D to 1,25-dihydroxyvitamin D. Hypophosphatemia augments the renal synthesis of 1,25-dihydroxyvitamin D.

Counterregulation of blood ionized Ca^{++} concentration is mediated by calcitonin and negative feedback. Increases in 1,25-dihydroxyvitamin D or hyperphosphatemia inhibit renal 1-alpha-hydroxylase activity. Increases in blood ionized Ca^{++} concentrations stimulate the synthesis and release of calcitonin from parafollicular "C cells" located in the thyroid gland. Calcitonin decreases the blood ionized Ca^{++} con-

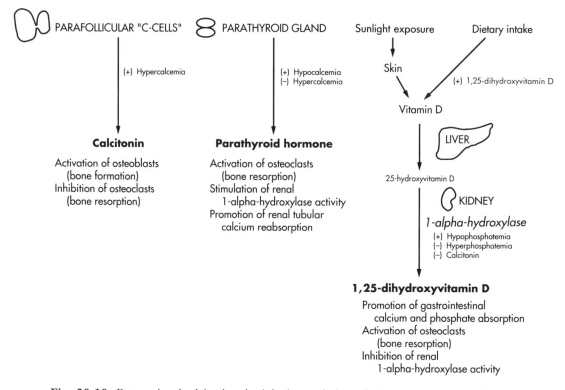

Fig. 20-10. Factors involved in the physiologic regulation of the plasma ionized calcium concentration.

centration by enhancing bone formation by osteoblasts and inhibiting bone resorption by osteoclasts. Through these physiologic actions, calcitonin functionally acts as a parathyroid hormone antagonist.

D. Physiologic actions of calcium

Ionized Ca^{++} has an important role in transmembrane signal transduction in many cell types. Cell activation initiates the transmembrane influx of Ca^{++}, which then triggers the secondary release of Ca^{++} from intracellular stores. Free cytosolic Ca^{++} then binds to specific effector proteins, such as calmodulin, troponin C, or protein kinase C, which trigger intracellular processes that lead to the final cellular response. The contraction of skeletal, cardiac, and smooth muscles is mediated through this mechanism. In addition, the replication of immune cells, the secretion of hormones by endocrine cells, the aggregation of platelets, the degranulation of leukocytes, and the release of neurotransmitters are initiated through Ca^{++}-dependent mechanisms.

Calcium has an additional physiologic role in electrically excitable cells. Calcium influx through specialized Ca^{++} channels located on the cell membrane is required for the formation and propagation of the electrical impulse in cardiac pacemaker cells, the specialized cells of the cardiac conduction system, and the plateau phase of the action potential in myocardial cells. The extracellular Ca^{++} concentration can influence electrical transmission in nerve and muscle cells by modifying the membrane permeability to Na^+ and K^+. Hypercalcemia increases the depolarization threshold for the action potential, whereas hypocalcemia decreases the depolarization threshold for the action potential.

The extracellular concentration of ionized Ca^{++} affects Ca^{++}-dependent cellular processes in varying degrees. Relatively small changes in blood ionized Ca^{++} affect nerve and muscle excitation by altering the electrical activity of cells. Intermediate changes in the ionized Ca^{++} concentration may affect Ca^{++}-mediated signal transduction. An extreme degree of hypocalemia must be reached before blood coagulation is impaired.

E. Hypocalcemia

1. Causes of hypocalcemia. Ionized hypocalcemia can be caused by disorders of vitamin D metabolism, parathyroid insufficiency, the chelation of free Ca^{++} by anions, or conditions that increase the protein-bound fraction of plasma Ca^{++} (List 20-3). In the clinical setting,

List 20-3. Causes of Ionized Hypocalcemia

Disorders of parathyroid hormone secretion or action
  Surgical ablation of parathyroid glands during neck operations
  Subtotal parathyroidectomy
  Idiopathic primary hypoparathyroidism
  Pseudohypoparathyroidism
  Late-neonatal hypocalcemia
  Hypomagnesemia
  Hypermagnesemia
Vitamin D deficiency and disorders of vitamin D metabolism
  Intestinal malabsorption
  Malnutrition
  Renal failure
  Hyperphosphatemia
Chelation of free calcium by anions
  Citrate intoxication during transfusion of stored blood products
  Hyperphosphatemia
Increased protein-bound calcium
  Albumin administration
  Alkalosis
  Increased plasma free fatty acids
Miscellaneous and multifactorial
  "Hungry-bone" syndrome
  Malignancy
  Cardiac operations employing cardiopulmonary bypass
  Pancreatitis
  Sepsis
  Chronic renal failure

more than one factor often plays a role in the pathogenesis of hypocalcemia.

Factors that increase Ca^{++} binding to plasma proteins cause ionized hypocalcemia without changing the total serum Ca^{++} concentration. An increase in blood pH from respiratory or metabolic alkalosis decreases the ionized Ca^{++} concentration by increasing the fraction of protein-bound Ca^{++} in the plasma. The decrease is usually small but can be clinically important in susceptible patients. Increases in plasma free fatty acids also increase the binding of Ca^{++} to plasma proteins.[110] Circulating free fatty acid concentrations often are increased in patients with severe illnesses, such as pancreatitis or sepsis. Administration of heparin, epinephrine, and intravenous lipids also increase free fatty acid levels.

Tumor lysis and rhabdomyolysis cause hypocalcemia by increasing the plasma concentration of anions that chelate free Ca^{++}.[111] Phosphate released from cells into the circulation in these two conditions complexes with plasma ionized Ca^{++} and lower the ionized Ca^{++} concentration. Citrate, used in the storage of blood products, prevents blood coagulation by chelating free Ca^{++}. The rapid transfusion of blood products can result in elevated plasma levels of citrate and ionized hypocalcemia. The severity of ionized hypocalcemia varies depending on the transfusion rate, but the duration of hypocalcemia is usually less than 10 to 15 minutes, or the time it takes for the body to metabolize the citrate load.[112,113] The transient ionized hypocalcemia potentially can cause hemodynamic instability. Extreme hypocalcemia induced by citrate has been reported in patients undergoing orthotopic liver transplantation who require large amounts of citrated blood products.[114] In these patients, impaired metabolism of citrate during the anhepatic stage of the transplantation operation results in plasma ionized Ca^{++} concentrations as low as 0.56 mmol/L and is associated with depressed cardiovascular function. Upon return of hepatic function, the citrate is metabolized and the ionized Ca^{++} concentration returns to normal.

Parathyroid insufficiency is a common cause of hypocalcemia among surgical patients. Hypocalcemia can develop in the postoperative period after subtotal parathyroidectomy, subtotal thyroidectomy, or extensive neck surgery for cancer if the parathyroid glands are injured or inadvertently removed. Postoperative hypocalcemia can be expected in patients undergoing subtotal parathyroidectomy even when an attempt is made to spare at least one functioning gland. Hypocalcemia is usually transient and lasts less than 5 days during the recovery of glandular function.

Other causes of parathyroid insufficiency include idiopathic primary hypoparathyroidism and pseudohypoparathyroidism.[115] Pseudohypoparathyroidism is a familial disorder characterized by end-organ resistance to the actions of parathyroid hormone. Rarely, acquired parathyroid insufficiency is caused by glandular destruction as a complication of hemochromatosis or metastatic invasion. Late-neonatal hypocalcemia can occur in children of mothers suffering from hyperparathyroidism.[116] Hypocalcemia in these infants appear within 2 weeks of age and can last up to 1 year. This condition is caused by the intrauterine transfer of maternal hypercalcemia, which suppresses the fetal parathyroid gland.

Vitamin D deficiency from intestinal malabsorption, malnutrition, or insufficient sunlight exposure can cause hypocalcemia. Vitamin D deficiency with hypocalcemia is especially common in surgical patients after subtotal gastrectomy or gastrojejunostomy.[117] Impaired renal conversion of 25-hydroxyvitamin D to 1,25-dihydroxyvitamin D contributes to hypocalcemia in patients with chronic renal failure. Inhibition of vitamin D synthesis can also be caused by hyperphosphatemia, which suppresses renal 1-alpha-hydroxylase activity.

Disorders of Mg^{++} metabolism often are associated with and are possibly a causative factor in hypocalcemia. Hypomagnesemia can cause parathyroid hormone resistance, whereas both hypomagnesemia[118] and hypermagnesemia[119] can inhibit the secretion of parathyroid hormone. Magnesium is a competitive inhibitor of Ca^{++}-mediated processes, and hypermagnesemia can potentially exacerbate the clinical consequences of hypocalcemia.[120]

Miscellaneous causes of hypocalcemia include the "hungry-bone syndrome," which manifests after thyroidectomy for hyperthyroidism, parathyroidectomy for hyperparathyroidism, or vitamin D therapy for rickets. In this syndrome, the rate of Ca^{++} deposition in bone exceeds Ca^{++} intake and causes extracellular hypocalcemia. Osteoblastic metastasis in cancer of the prostate, lung, or breast cause hypocalcemia by increased bone formation. The cause of hypocalcemia in association with cardiac operations, pancreatitis, sepsis, and chronic renal failure is probably multifactorial.[121]

2. Clinical manifestations of hypocalcemia. The classic clinical features of ionized hypocalcemia are characterized by enhanced neuromuscular excitability. Patients may complain of numbness or tingling in the fingertips or around the lips. Tetanic spasms from hypocalcemia may range in severity from carpopedal spasm (involuntary flexion of the wrist accompanied by adduction of the thumb, and extension of the fingers) to laryngospasm, seizures, and tetany of the extremities and trunk. In hypocalcemic patients without symptoms, one can elicit signs of neuromuscular irritability by tapping on the facial nerve and observing the contraction of the corresponding facial muscles (Chvostek's sign) or by inflating a blood pressure cuff applied to the arm and observing carpopedal spasms (Trousseau's sign).

Depression of cardiovascular function from hypocalcemia can be clinically important in patients during anesthesia, in intensive care, or with underlying heart disease.[122-124] Prolongation of the QT interval on the ECG correlates well with progressive ionized hypocalcemia but is a nonspecific sign. Ionized hypocalcemia can manifest itself as hypotension, cardiac failure, and arrhythmias that do not respond to vasoactive agents or volume expansion. Routine measurement of the plasma ionized Ca^{++} concentrations is important in the care of these critically ill patients.

3. Treatment of hypocalcemia. Hypocalcemia in patients with cardiovascular instability or clinical symptoms warrants immediate therapy. Administration of Ca^{++} often causes dramatic clinical improvement. Calcium chloride and calcium gluconate are two Ca^{++} salts available for parenteral therapy. The immediate bioavailability of Ca^{++} in either of these two preparations is the same when they are administered in equimolar quantities.[125] A 10% solution of calcium chloride contains 27 mg/ml (1.36 mEq of Ca^{++}/ml) of elemental Ca^{++} or approximately three times the amount of elemental Ca^{++} in an equal volume of a 10% solution of calcium gluconate. A 10% solution of calcium gluconate contains 9 mg/ml (0.45 mEq of Ca^{++}/ml) of elemental Ca^{++}. Doses in the range of 15 to 30 mg/kg of elemental Ca^{++} (calcium chloride 50 to 100 mg/kg or calcium gluconate 150 to 300 mg/kg) administered as an intravenous bolus injection over 5 to 10 minutes is usually effective for the initial treatment of hypocalcemia.

The administration of either calcium chloride or calcium gluconate causes an immediate increase in the plasma ionized Ca^{++} concentration. The increase in plasma ionized Ca^{++} concentration is usually transient; thus repeated bolus administration of calcium or the intravenous infusion of 1 to 2 mg/kg/hour of elemental Ca^{++} is necessary to keep the plasma ionized Ca^{++} concentration at a therapeutic level. Although overcorrection of ionized hypocalcemia is not recommended, transient hypercalcemia during therapy is usually well tolerated. Calcium should be administered cautiously to patients with hyperphosphatemia, since calcium phosphate has a low solubility coefficient and soft-tissue calcification is a complication of therapy. Calcium chloride is irritating to veins and can cause tissue injury with extravasation. For these reasons, calcium gluconate is usually preferred for use in pediatric patients or when Ca^{++} is administered through a peripheral venous line.

Vitamin D therapy is useful in the long-term treatment of patients with hypocalcemia caused by vitamin D deficiency or hypoparathyroidism. Calcitriol (1,25-dihydroxyvitamin D) is available for patients with renal disease whose ability to biotransform vitamin D to its active metabolite is impaired.

Definitive therapy for hypocalcemia requires the diagnosis and treatment of the primary disorder. Patients with underlying Mg^{++} disorders often respond poorly to intravenous Ca^{++} therapy until serum Mg^{++} concentrations are normalized. Measurement of serum Mg^{++} concentration probably should be performed in all patients with hypocalcemia. Other useful laboratory tests include measuring the serum alkaline phosphatase activity, creatinine concentration, and phosphate concentration. An elevated alkaline phosphatase activity can be an indication of osteomalacia or osteoblastic metastasis. Hyperphosphatemia can be suggestive of cell lysis or hypoparathyroidism. An increase in the serum creatinine concentration indicates renal disease.

F. Hypercalcemia

1. Causes of hypercalcemia. Although there are many causes for hypercalcemia, the majority of surgical patients with hypercalcemia have underlying primary hyperparathyroidism or humoral hypercalcemia of malignancy (List 20-4).

Primary hyperparathyroidism is characterized by the hypersecretion of parathyroid hormone innappropriate to the circulating Ca^{++} concentration. Primary hyperparathyroidism is most commonly caused by adenoma or glandular hyperplasia. Rarely, it can be caused by carcinoma of the parathyroid gland. Primary hyperparathyroidism sometimes is associated with other endocrine disorders in the same patient and occurs in a familial pattern. In multiple endocrine neoplasia (MEN) type I syndrome, hyperparathyroidism is associated with pituitary, pancreatic, adrenal, and thyroid tumors. In MEN type II syndrome, hyperparathyroidism is associated with pheochromocytoma and medullary thyroid tumors.

Abnormally high levels of circulating parathyroid hormone in patients with primary hyperparathyroidism cause hypercalcemia by increasing bone resorption, promoting the tubular reabsorption of Ca^{++} by the kidneys, and stimulating the renal synthesis of 1,25-dihydroxyvitamin D. Patients with primary hyperparathyroidism generally have laboratory findings of hypophosphatemia in association with hypercalcemia.

Cancer is one of the most common causes of hypercalcemia among hospitalized patients.[126] Squamous cell carcinomas of the lung and cancer of the breast are the two malignancies most often associated with hypercalcemia. The ectopic production of a substance with parathyroid hormone activity has long been suspected in some of these patients. Recently, a parathyroid hormone–related protein has been isolated from tumors and has been shown to possess biologic activity similar to that of the native hormone.[127] Researchers have found that patients with squamous cell tumors of the lung and also

---

List 20-4. Causes of Ionized Hypercalcemia

Hyperparathyroidism
  Adenoma of the parathyroid gland
  Hyperplasia of the parathyroid gland
  Carcinoma of the parathyroid gland
  MEN I (hyperparathyroidism associated with pituitary, pancreatic, adrenal, and thyroid tumors)
  MEN II (hypoparathyroidism, pheochromocytoma, medullary thyroid tumor)
Malignancy
  Squamous cell carcinoma of the lung
  Breast cancer
  Renal tumors
  Urothelial tumors
  Adenoma
  Multiple myeloma
  Lymphoma
Disorders of vitamin D excess
  Vitamin D toxicity
  Sarcoidosis
  Granulomatous diseases
  Post−renal transplantation condition
  Recovery from acute renal failure
Miscellaneous
  Calcium administration
  Milk-alkali syndrome
  Familial hypocalciuric hypercalcemia
  Immobilization
  Hyperthyroidism
  Thiazide diuretics

---

patients with renal, urothelial, and breast carcinomas, adenomas, multiple myeloma, and lymphoma have increased circulating levels of this parathyroid hormone−related protein in association with hypercalcemia.[128] Other possible causes for hypercalcemia in association with malignancies are the neoplastic production of 1,25-dihydroxyvitamin D[129] and osteoclast-activating factors.[130]

Any condition that increases the circulating concentrations of vitamin D can cause hypercalcemia. Excessive self-medication or treatment with any vitamin D compounds can cause hypercalcemia. In these cases, hypercalcemia is associated with hyperphosphatemia and secondary hypoparathyroidism. There is evidence that hypercalcemia in patients with sarcoidosis or granulomatous diseases may be caused by increased sensitivity to or the ectopic synthesis of 1,25-dihydroxyvitamin D.[109] Hypercalcemia developing after successful renal transplantation or with the recovery from acute renal failure may be mediated in part by the restoration of 1,25-dihydroxyvitamin D synthesis.[131,132]

Other causes for hypercalcemia include excessive administration of Ca^{++} salts, the milk-alkali syndrome, familial hypocalciuric hypercalcemia, immobilization, and hyperthyroidism.[103,133] Hypercalcemia can also be present in a small proportion of patients taking thiazide diuretics. Hypercalcemia in these patients usually is not clinically important unless it is associated with Ca^{++} administration or other disorders causing hypercalcemia.

2. Clinical manifestations of hypercalcemia. The clinical features of hypercalcemia can vary extensively between patients. Patients with hyperparathyroidism often have clinical features consistent with chronic hypercalcemia and present with bone disease, renal calculi, band keratopathy, hypertension, or cardiomyopathy. Patients with acute hypercalcemia from cancer experience symptoms at relatively lower plasma Ca^{++} concentrations and may present with anorexia, confusion, or acute neurologic deterioration.

The manifestations of hypercalcemia on the nervous system are attributed to the depressant effect of increased extracellular Ca^{++} concentrations on neuronal activity. Symptoms are usually nonspecific. Patients may complain of personality changes, depression, anorexia, or memory impairment. Severe hypercalcemia can cause psychosis, obtundation, and coma. The peripheral manifestations of hypercalcemia are muscular weakness, easy fatigability, diminished deep tendon reflexes, and muscular atropy.

Hypercalcemia causes both acute and chronic alterations in renal function. Acute hypercalcemia is associated with a reduction in renal blood flow and a reduction in the glomerular filtration rate. Renal concentrating ability is impaired. Extracellular volume contraction and dehydration as a consequence of renal Na^+ wasting compounds the clinical condition. The increased filtered load of Ca^{++} entering the urine can cause nephrolithiasis. Chronic interstitial nephritis and nephrocalcinosis as a consequence of glomerular and vascular deposition of Ca^{++} are long-term complications of hypercalcemia. Renal failure, nephrogenic diabetes insipidus, distal renal tubular acidosis (type I), and salt-losing nephritis are all potential renal complications of hypercalcemia.

The gastrointestinal symptoms of hypercalcemia typically are nausea, vomiting, and constipation. The direct depressant effects of hypercalcemia on nerve conduction and intestinal smooth muscle motility may partially explain these symptoms. Poor oral intake contributes to dehydration that usually accompanies states of hypercalcemia. Peptic ulcer disease and pancreatitis are more frequent among patients with hypercalcemia, but a direct pathophysiologic link between hypercalcemia and either of these two disorders is lacking.

Although Ca^{++} administration acutely increases the blood pressure and myocardial contractility in hypocalcemic patients, chronic hypercalcemia has adverse effects on the cardiovascular system. Chronic hypercalcemia can lead to the deposition of Ca^{++} within the myocardium, on the heart valves, and within the coronary and systemic vasculature. Hypercalcemia affects cardiac conduction, as manifested by shortening of the QT interval on the surface ECG, but is a rare cause of cardiac dysrhythmias. Hypertension is associated with hypercalcemia often in patients with hyperparathyroidism.[134] Sometimes hypertension resolves after parathyroidectomy upon normalization of the plasma ionized Ca^{++} concentrations. The role of hypercalcemia in the pathogenesis of hypertension in this subgroup of patients remains to be investigated further.

Osteopenia and osteoporosis are the most common skeletal manifestations of hyperparathyroidism and represent excessive bone resorption and turnover. Bone and skeletal pain in patients with hypercalcemia can also indicate bone metastasis from malignancy.

3. Treatment of hypercalcemia. The decision to initiate therapy for hypercalcemia depends on the severity of symptoms and the presence of reversible end-organ dysfunction. Patients presenting with asymptomatic hypercalcemia and mild skeletal involvement and who are scheduled for elective parathyroidectomy often require no special care, but patients with severe hypercalcemia, obtundation, and progressive renal insufficiency require emergent therapy. Before definitive therapy for the underlying disorder, acute therapy for decreasing the plasma ionized Ca^{++} concentration can reverse the early stages of renal dysfunction and improve the neurologic condition of patients with symptomatic hypercalcemia.

Intravascular volume expansion with isotonic saline is the first line of therapy. The majority of patients with hypercalcemia are volume depleted because of vomiting, poor oral intake, and renal dysfunction. Although restoration of intravascular volume decreases the plasma ionized Ca^{++} concentration by dilution alone, it also promotes the net loss of Ca^{++} in the urine by increasing the glomerular filtration rate. The diuresis induced by isotonic saline administration decreases the fractional reabsorption of Ca^{++} from the proximal tubule and thus enhances renal Ca^{++} excretion. Loop diuretics, such as furosemide or ethacrynic acid, inhibit the reabsorption of urinary Ca^{++} from the thick ascending limb of Henle's loop and help to potentiate the hypocalcemic effects of isotonic saline–induced diuresis.[135] A typical therapeutic regimen begins with the acute administration of 1 to 2 liters of normal saline intravenously. After the first 1 to 2 liters, normal saline at a rate of 300 to 500 ml/hour should be administered. The addition of furosemide 20 to 60 mg intravenously every 4 to 6 hours is administered to sustain the diuresis. This regimen usually causes an appreciable decrease in the plasma Ca^{++} concentration within 4 hours. One can augment the regimen by increasing the volume and rate of intravenous saline administration in combination with increasing the dose and frequency of furosemide for cases of severe hypercalcemia.

The patient's volume status should be monitored carefully to avoid dehydration from excessive diuresis or pulmonary edema from overhydration. In addition to measuring the plasma ionized Ca^{++} concentration, serum Na^+, K^+, and Mg^{++} concentrations should be checked frequently and corrected appropriately. Hemodialysis or peritoneal dialysis may be necessary for the treatment of symptomatic hypercalcemia in the patient with oliguric renal failure.

Alternatively, plasma Ca^{++} concentrations can be lowered acutely with agents that chelate free Ca^{++}. Intravenous administration of phosphate 15 mmol IV over 8 to 12 hours or ethylenediaminetetraacetic acid (EDTA) 10 to 50 mg IV over 4 hours works through this mechanism.[103] The use of these two agents usually is reserved for patients with life-threatening hypercalcemia refractory to saline diuresis. Severe hypocalcemia, soft-tissue calcifications, and nephrotoxicity are serious complications from this form of therapy.

Both mithramycin and calcitonin lower plasma Ca^{++} concentrations by inhibiting bone resorption; they are most effective in treating hypercalcemia from hyperparathyroidism or malignancy.[103] Mithramycin is an antineoplastic agent that is particularly effective against osteoclastic activity. A dose of mithramycin 25 μg IV over 4 hours usually causes a decrease in plasma Ca^{++} concentration within 24 hours. Its effects last for several days and can be readministered every 2 to 7 days. Nephrotoxicity, hepatotoxicity, and thrombocytopenia are reported side effects of mithramycin but usually occur only with high doses. Although calcitonin has fewer reported side effects and a faster onset of action than mithramycin, it is usually less effective at lowering plasma Ca^{++} concentrations. The therapeutic dose for calcitonin is 4

MRC (Medical Research Council) units/kg subcutaneously every 12 hours.

Glucocorticoids are effective hypocalcemic agents for hypercalcemia caused by hematologic malignancies, vitamin D toxicity, sarcoidosis, and granulomatous disease. The hypocalcemic action of glucocorticoids appears to operate by antagonizing vitamin D–facilitated intestinal absorption of Ca^{++}.[136] Prednisone 40 to 100 mg/day IV in divided doses lowers the plasma Ca^{++} concentration over 4 to 6 days in the above conditions.

IV. MAGNESIUM

Abnormalities of serum magnesium (Mg^{++}) concentrations may rank as the most common electrolyte disturbance among hospitalized patients. Disorders of Mg^{++} balance appear to be especially common among patients in intensive care. Laboratory evidence of hypomagnesemia was present in 61% of surgical patients being admitted for postoperative intensive care in a study conducted at our institution.[137] This frequency of hypomagnesemia was similar to the figure of 65% reported by Ryzen et al.[138] among patients in medical intensive care units. A study measuring serum Mg^{++} concentrations in all blood samples being submitted for electrolyte determinations detected hypomagnesemia in 47% of the samples and hypermagnesemia in 14% of the samples according to standard laboratory criteria.[139] The frequency of hypomagnesemia (19%) has also been found to be twice as common as the frequency of hy-

pokalemia (9%) among hospitalized patients receiving digitalis.[140] These reported frequencies of Mg^{++} disorders are not surprising when one considers the frequency of conditions that predispose hospitalized patients to abnormal Mg^{++} homeostasis.

A. Magnesium homeostasis

The distribution of Mg^{++} in the body resembles the distribution of Ca^{++} in many ways.[103] Approximately 60% to 70% of total body Mg^{++} exists within the mineral structure of bone and 30% to 40% exists within cells. Magnesium in the extracellular fluid accounts for only 1% of the body's total Mg^{++} content. Intracellular Mg^{++} is unevenly distributed. The majority of intracellular Mg^{++} is complexed to organophosphates, enzymes, proteins, phospholipids, and nucleic acids. The cytosolic concentration of free Mg^{++} is approximately 2 mEq/L and exchanges with the bound intracellular pool. The total Mg^{++} concentration in the serum normally ranges from 1.4 to 2.0 mEq/L (Fig. 20-11). Only 55% of the total serum Mg^{++} is in the physiologically active or ionized form. Of the remaining serum Mg^{++}, approximately 30% is protein bound and 15% is complexed to plasma anions. The total serum Mg^{++} concentration therefore reflects changes in the total serum protein concentration but not necessarily reflects the physiologically important concentration of Mg^{++}. Furthermore, the total serum Mg^{++} concentration is only an indirect measure of the intracellular Mg^{++} con-

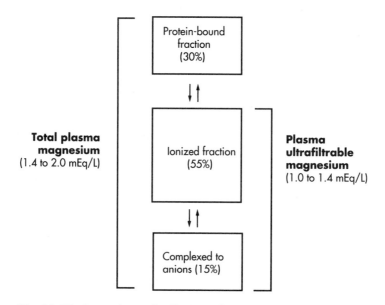

Fig. 20-11. Approximate distribution of magnesium in the circulation.

tent. Presently, only the total serum Mg^{++} concentration can be routinely measured in the clinical laboratory.

Total body Mg^{++} balance is largely determined by dietary intake and renal excretion of the electrolyte. The average dietary intake of Mg^{++} is 18 to 33 mEq per day. Dietary Mg^{++} is primarily absorbed by the small intestine. The proportion of dietary Mg^{++} absorbed ranges between 25% and 75%. The gastrointestinal absorption of Mg^{++} is more efficient when dietary intake is low. Magnesium entering the kidneys in the glomerular filtrate is reabsorbed in the proximal tubule and thick ascending limb of Henle's loop. In Mg^{++}-deficient states, the renal excretion of Mg^{++} can decrease to as little as 1 mEq per day. The renal threshold (T_m) for Mg^{++} excretion occurs at a serum Mg^{++} concentration of 1.3 to 1.7 mEq/L. This value for the T_m is very close to the normal range of serum Mg^{++} concentrations.[141] Acute increases in the serum Mg^{++} concentration above this T_m result in the rapid elimination of Mg^{++} by the kidneys. Restoring total Mg^{++} deficits by parenteral Mg^{++} administration therefore must proceed in a gradual manner and requires several days.

B. Physiologic actions of magnesium

Magnesium has diverse physiologic actions. Magnesium is an essential cofactor in over 300 intracellular and membrane-associated enzymatic reactions.[142] All cellular reactions that involve the transfer, storage, and utilization of energy in the form of nucleotide triphosphates require Mg^{++}. The active transport of ions across plasma membranes by Na^{++}-K^{++}-ATPase and $Ca^{++}Mg^{++}$-ATPase require Mg^{++} as a substrate. Magnesium is also important for the polymerization of nucleic acids, the reversible binding of messenger RNA to ribosomes, and the processing of DNA.

Although it is well established that Mg^{++} is necessary for many essential cellular processes, it is unclear to what extent each of these processes is affected at clinical levels of Mg^{++} deficiency or excess. Indirect evidence indicates that clinical hypomagnesemia can impair the normal functioning of Mg^{++}-dependent enzymes. Hypokalemia is associated frequently with Mg^{++}-deficient states and correction of underlying hypomagnesemia is a prerequisite for the restoration of normal serum K^+.[69] In this clinical condition, hypomagnesemia may impair the performance of Mg^{++}-dependent Na^+-K^+-ATPase, which is required for the tubular reabsorption of K^+. Hypocalcemia is another clinical condition associated with Mg^{++} deficiency

and may be caused by impairment of Mg^{++}-dependent adenylate cyclase. Activation of adenylate cyclase and subsequent generation of cyclic-AMP is necessary for both the secretion of and the end-organ responsiveness to parathyroid hormone.[118] Finally, clinical hypomagnesemia may render patients particularly sensitive to the cardiac glycosides, which act by inhibiting Mg^{++}-dependent Na^+-K^+-ATPase. This phenomenon may explain in part the predisposition of hypomagnesemic patients to digitalis toxicity.[143]

As a divalent cation, Mg^{++} resembles Ca^{++} in certain physiologic processes. The clinical signs and symptoms of hypomagnesemia parallel those seen in hypocalcemia. Furthermore, these signs and symptoms are more pronounced when hypocalcemia is associated with hypomagnesemia.[144] The membrane-stabilizing effects of Mg^{++} on electrically excitable cells of the central nervous system and the heart may be the result of Mg^{++}'s Ca^{++}-like action. In an analogous manner, Mg^{++} may also antagonize Ca^{++}-mediated cellular processes by acting as a nonspecific Ca^{++}-channel antagonist.[120] Magnesium interferes with Ca^{++}-mediated contractile process in vascular smooth muscle. Extracellular hypomagnesemia increases vascular smooth muscle reactivity, whereas hypermagnesemia decreases vascular tone.[145]

C. Hypomagnesemia

1. Causes of hypomagnesemia. Magnesium-deficient diets, intestinal malabsorption, internal redistribution of extracellular Mg^{++}, and excessive renal excretion of Mg^{++} are the major causes of clinical hypomagnesemia (List 20-5).

Cellular uptake of Mg^{++}, increases in the protein-bound fraction of serum Mg^{++}, or chelation of ionized Mg^{++} by anions cause extracellular hypomagnesemia by internal redistribution. Internal redistribution changes the extracellular Mg^{++} concentration without a net change in total body Mg^{++}. Uptake of Mg^{++} into newly formed tissue during anabolic states is an example of internal redistribution as a cause for hypomagnesemia. Additional clinical examples of redistribution are hypomagnesemia occurring after insulin therapy in patients with diabetic ketoacidosis and hypomagnesemia occurring after the restoration of normal mineral metabolism after parathyroidectomy in patients with hyperparathyroidism. Saponification and sequestration of Mg^{++} into injured tissues can be factors contributing to hypomagnesemia in patients with pancreatitis. Citrate, used in the storage of blood products, chelates Mg^{++} as well as Ca^{++} and potentially can cause transient

---

List 20-5. Causes of Hypomagnesemia

Dietary insufficiency
  Malnutrition
  Parenteral nutrition
  Alcoholism
Gastrointestinal losses
  Diarrhea
  Gastric suctioning
  Steatorrhea
Renal losses
  Saline diuresis
  Solute diuresis
  Diuretic therapy
  Aminoglycoside antibiotics
  Cisplatin
  Cyclosporin A
  Amphotericin B
  Ethanol
Internal redistribution
  Pancreatitis
  Diabetic ketoacidosis
  "Hungry-bone" syndrome
  Anabolic states
  Citrate

---

ionized hypomagnesemia during transfusion therapy.[146]

Gastrointestinal diseases cause hypomagnesemia by decreased dietary intake of Mg^{++}, intestinal malabsorption of dietary Mg^{++}, and loss of Mg^{++} in gastrointestinal fluids. Short bowel syndrome, extensive bowel resection, inflammatory bowel disease, sprue, and familial hypomagnesemia are clinical conditions in which gastrointestinal absorption of Mg^{++} is impaired.[147,148] The Mg^{++} content in gastrointestinal fluids can be substantial. Lower gastrointestinal tract secretions have a Mg^{++} concentration of 10 to 14 mEq/L, whereas the Mg^{++} concentration of gastric fluid is 1 to 2 mEq/L. Gastrointestinal fluid losses from prolonged nasogastric suctioning, diarrhea, intestinal or biliary fistulas, and the practice of preoperative intestinal antisepsis can cause clinical hypomagnesemia. The Mg^{++} content of stool in patients with steatorrhea can be even greater because Mg^{++} binds with insoluble intestinal soaps. Steatorrhea contributes to hypomagnesemia in patients with malabsorption syndromes and in patients with pancreatic insufficiency. Dietary restriction of Mg^{++} alone can be a cause of hypomagnesemia.[144] Alcoholism, malnutrition, protracted therapy with intravenous fluids, and total parenteral nutrition are conditions predisposing to dietary insufficiency of Mg^{++}.

Renal Mg^{++} excretion is increased by Na^+ loading, diuretics, and nephrotoxic drugs. The high frequency of hypomagnesemia noticed among patients on digoxin therapy, patients with hypertension, and patients with congestive heart failure may, in part, be caused by diuretic use. Loop diuretics such as furosemide, ethacrynic acid, and bumetanide cause the greatest degree of renal Mg^{++} wasting. However, thiazide diuretics and osmotic diuretics also impair renal Mg^{++} conservation. Osmotic diuresis from hyperglycemia probably plays a role in the development of hypomagnesemia in patients with diabetes.[149] Intravascular volume expansion with saline solutions, mannitol administration, diuretic use, and hemodilution may be factors contributing to the development of postoperative hypomagnesemia in patients undergoing cardiac operations.[150] Aminoglycosides,[151] cisplatin,[152] amphotericin B,[153] and cyclosporin A[154] have been associated with renal Mg^{++} wasting. Alcohol ingestion alone also increases renal magnesium excretion.[155]

The cause of hypomagnesemia in the majority of surgical patients cannot usually be explained by a single cause. Alcoholism, diuretic therapy, cardiac disease, cardiac surgical procedures, aminoglycoside antibiotic therapy, mannitol, and parenteral nutrition all appear to be risk factors for the development of hypomagnesemia through several possible mechanisms. Patients with hypomagnesemia should be evaluated for insufficient enteral or parenteral Mg^{++} intake, disorders that cause renal Mg^{++} wasting, and gastrointestinal diseases. The patient should also be evaluated for the presence of hypokalemia and hypocalcemia because these two electrolyte disorders are commonly associated with hypomagnesemia and can exacerbate the clinical symptoms of hypomagnesemia. Appropriate Mg^{++} supplementation and correction of associated electrolyte disorders usually can restore the Mg^{++} deficit and improve the symptoms caused by hypomagnesemia.

2. Clinical manifestations of hypomagnesemia. The signs and symptoms of hypomagnesemia are nonspecific and depend on the coexistence of hypocalcemia, hypokalemia, and other diseases.[144] Symptoms include apathy, weakness, anorexia, nausea, and vomiting. These symptoms usually precede the neuromuscular signs of hypomagnesemia. The clinical signs of hypomagnesemia are strikingly similar to those seen in patients with hypocalcemia and are characterized by neuronal excitability and tetany. Trousseau's sign, Chvostek's sign, muscle fasciculations, muscle spasticity, hyperreflexia, and seizures occur with progressive hypomagnesemia. Hypomagnesemia can cause subclinical respiratory muscle weakness in patients that improves after Mg^{++} supplementation.[156] Both hypomagnesemia and hypocalcemia prolong the QT interval on the ECG.

3. Treatment of hypomagnesemia. Magnesium salts administered parenterally are used for the acute treatment of hypomagnesemia. A typical dose for an adult is 64 to 96 mEq of elemental Mg^{++} given intravenously over 24 hours followed by 32 to 40 mEq daily for 3 to 4 days. A standard 2 ml ampule of 50% magnesium sulfate in solution contains 1 g of magnesium sulfate, which is equal to 8 mEq (98 mg) of elemental Mg^{++}. One gram of magnesium chloride is equal to 9 mEq (118 mg) of elemental Mg^{++}. The Mg^{++} salt can be diluted in dextrose- or saline-containing intravenous solutions and administered slowly. Concentrated solutions of Mg^{++} can be irritating to veins. Restoration of intracellular Mg^{++} deficits takes time because of the low renal threshold for Mg^{++} excretion. Therapy should be guided by periodic measurements of serum Mg^{++} concentration and by examination of the patient. The appearance of clinical signs suggestive of hypermagnesemia (Table 20-1) indicates that the dose of Mg^{++} needs to be reduced. Patients with renal insufficiency may develop hypermagnesemia from excessive therapy.

Several therapeutic regimens have been described for the use of Mg^{++} in the acute treatment of intractable ventricular arrhythmias. The administration of elemental Mg^{++} 9 mEq IV over 20 minutes repeated every 6 hours effectively increases and maintains the serum Mg^{++} concentration in a therapeutic range.[103] Alternatively, 16 mEq of elemental Mg^{++} can be administered intravenously over 1 minute followed by 80 mEq over the next 5 hours.[157] In a study conducted by Rasmussen et al.[158] prophylactic administration of an intravenous dose of magnesium chloride 60 mEq IV over 6

hours followed by 40 mEq IV over the next 18 hours was effective in reducing both the mortality and frequency of cardiac arrhythmias in patients suffering from acute myocardial infarctions. A preliminary study indicates that prophylactic Mg^{++} therapy to keep the serum Mg^{++} concentration greater than 2 mEq/L may effectively reduce the incidence of postoperative cardiac dysrhythmias in patients undergoing cardiac operations.[159]

In the absence of intestinal malabsorption syndromes, gradual Mg^{++} replacement can be instituted by supplementation of the diet with Mg^{++}-rich foods (seafoods, green vegetables, meat, dairy products, and cereals) or magnesium gluconate tablets.

D. Hypermagnesemia

1. Causes of hypermagnesemia. Iatrogenic hypermagnesemia and renal failure are the only recognized causes of clinical hypermagnesemia. The kidneys normally are extremely efficient at eliminating Mg^{++}. The low renal threshold for Mg^{++} excretion normally prevents even minor increases in the serum Mg^{++} concentration. Patients with a reduced GFR from acute or chronic renal failure are predisposed to develop hypermagnesemia, especially when Mg^{++} administration is not controlled. Often unrecognized sources of Mg^{++} include Mg^{++}-containing antacids, cathartics, intravenous solutions, and parenteral nutrition.

The therapeutic uses of Mg^{++} salts are expanding. Magnesium is used routinely for the treatment of hypertension and seizures associated with preeclampsia and eclampsia of pregnancy. Magnesium therapy in these mothers can potentially cause neonatal hypermagnesemia, since the ion readily crosses the placenta. Neonatal hypermagnesemia is manifested by flaccidity, hyporeflexia, and respiratory insufficiency. Intraoperatively, Mg^{++} salts are used in cardioplegic solutions, for spinal cord protection during ischemia,[160] and even for attenuation of the cardiovascular responses to tracheal intubation.[161] Magnesium has been advocated and used for the treatment of seizures,[162] asthma,[163] and cardiac arrhythmias.[143,157-159]

Parenteral administration of large doses of magnesium chloride or magnesium sulfate increases the serum Mg^{++} concentration by overwhelming the capacity of the kidneys to excrete the electrolyte. Extreme care is necessary if Mg^{++} is to be administered to patients with impaired renal function.

2. Clinical manifestations of hypermagnesemia. The signs and symptoms of hypermagnesemia correlate well with increases in serum

Table 20-1. Clinical manifestations of hypermagnesemia

Serum magnesium concentration (mEq/L)	Signs and symptoms
3-5	Nausea and vomiting
4-7	Muscle weakness Hyporeflexia
5-10	Hypotension Bradycardia
10-15	Coma Paralysis

Mg^{++} concentrations (Table 20-1). Signs and symptoms range from nausea and vomiting at serum Mg^{++} concentrations of 3 to 5 mEq/L to cardiac arrest at serum Mg^{++} concentrations of greater than 15 mEq/L. Muscle weakness and hyporeflexia manifests at serum Mg^{++} concentrations of 4 to 7 mEq/L, hypotension and bradycardia at 5 to 10 mEq/L, and coma and paralysis at 10 to 15 mEq/L. The diminution of deep tendon reflexes is a reliable clinical sign of hypermagnesemia and is useful for the clinical assessment of patients on Mg^{++} therapy.

Hypermagnesemic patients have an increased sensitivity to neuromuscular blocking agents. Increased serum Mg^{++} concentrations directly depress skeletal muscle contraction, inhibit the release of acetylcholine at the motor end plate, decrease the sensitivity of the postjunctional membrane to the depolarizing action of acetylcholine, and decrease the amplitude of the motor end-plate potential.[164] These pharmacologic properties of Mg^{++} potentiate and prolong the action of both depolarizing and nondepolarizing muscle relaxants.[165] Calcium and acetylcholinesterase inhibitors (neostigmine) do not completely antagonize the inhibitory effects of Mg^{++} on neuromuscular transmission.

The cardiovascular manifestations of hypermagnesemia are hypotension and conduction abnormalities. Serum Mg^{++} concentrations of 10 to 15 mEq/L are associated with the lengthening of the PR and QRS intervals on the surface ECG. Hypotension is a consequence of decreased vascular smooth muscle tone and decreased vascular smooth muscle reactivity to endogenous vasoconstrictors. General anesthesia or sympathetic blockade by regional anesthesia potentially can unmask the cardiovascular depressant effects of Mg^{++} in surgical patients with hypermagnesemia.

3. Treatment of hypermagnesemia. Discontinuing the administration of Mg^{++} is the first step in the treatment of hypermagnesemia. If the patient has evidence of respiratory failure from muscle weakness, tracheal intubation and ventilatory support may be necessary until renal excretion of Mg^{++} reduces the serum Mg^{++} concentration to nontoxic levels. In emergency situations, intravenous calcium chloride or calcium gluconate partially antagonizes the toxic effects of Mg^{++}, but the duration of action is limited. Hemodialysis or peritoneal dialysis may be necessary to treat symptomatic hypermagnesemia in the patient with renal failure.

REFERENCES

1. Fanestil DD: Compartmentalization of body water. In Maxwell MH, Kleeman CR, and Narins RG, editors: Clinical disorders of fluid and electrolyte metabolism, New York, 1987, McGraw-Hill Book Co.
2. Mudge GH: Water, salts, and ions. In Gilman AG, Goodman LS, and Gilman A, editors: Goodman and Gilman's The pharmacological basis of therapeutics, New York, 1980, Macmillan Publishing Co.
3. Bayliss PH: Vasopressin and its neurophysin. In DeGroot LJ, editor: Endocrinology, Philadelphia, 1989, WB Saunders Co.
4. Anderson B and Rundgren M: Thirst and its disorders, Annu Rev Med 33:321-329, 1982.
5. Cantin M and Genest J: The heart and atrial natriuretic factor, Endocrine Rev 6:107-127, 1985.
6. Goetz KL: Physiology and pathophysiology of atrial peptides, Am J Physiol 254:E1-15, 1988.
7. Arieff AI, Llach F, and Massry SG: Neurological manifestations and morbidity of hyponatremia: correlation with brain water and electrolytes, Medicine 55:121-129, 1976.
8. Anderson RJ, Chung HM, Kluge R, et al: Hyponatremia: a prospective analysis of its epidemiology and the pathogenic role of vasopressin, Ann Intern Med 102:164-168, 1985.
9. Chung HM, Kluge R, Schrier RW, and Anderson RJ: Postoperative hyponatremia: a prospective study, Arch Intern Med 146:333-336, 1986.
10. Cottrell JE, Robustelli A, Post K, and Turndorf H: Furosemide- and mannitol-induced changes in intracranial pressure and serum osmolality and electrolytes, Anesthesiology 47:28-30, 1977.
11. Desmond J: Serum osmolality and plasma electrolytes in patients who develop dilutional hyponatremia during transurethral resection, Can J Surg 13:116-121, 1970.
12. Rothenberg DM, Berns AS, and Ikanovich AD: Isotonic hyponatremia following transurethral prostate resection, J Clin Anesth 2:48-53, 1990.
13. Wang JM, Creel DJ, and Wong KC: Transurethral resection of the prostate, serum glycine levels, and ocular evoked potentials, Anesthesiology 70:36-41, 1989.
14. Weisberg LS: Pseudohyponatremia: a reappraisal, Am J Med 86:315-318, 1989.
15. Deutsch S, Goldberg M, and Dripps RD: Postoperative hyponatremia with the inappropriate release of antidiuretic hormone, Anesthesiology 27:250-256, 1966.
16. Arieff AI: Hyponatremia, convulsions, respiratory arrest, and permanent brain damage after elective surgery in healthy women, N Engl J Med 314:1529-1535, 1986.
17. Philbin DM and Coggins CH: Plasma antidiuretic hormone levels in cardiac surgical patients during morphine and halothane anesthesia, Anesthesiology 49:95-98, 1978.
18. Cochrane JP, Forsling ML, Gow NM, et al: Arginine vasopressin release following surgical operations, Br J Surg 68:209-213, 1981.
19. Rowe JW, Shelton RL, Helderman JH, et al: Influence of emetic reflex on vasopressin release in man, Kidney Int 16:729-735, 1979.
20. Anderson RJ, Pluss RG, Berus AS, et al: Mechanism of effect of hypoxia on renal water excretion in the dog, J Clin Invest 62:769-777, 1978.
21. Berns AS, Anderson RJ, and McDonald KM: Effect of hypercapnic acidosis on renal water excretion in the dog, Kidney Int 15:116-125, 1979.
22. Bayliss PH, Zerbe RL, and Robertson GL: Arginine

vasopressin response to insulin-induced hypoglycaemia in man, J Clin Endocrinol Metab 53:935-940, 1981.

23. Berl T, Cadnapaphornchai P, Harbottle JA, and Schrier RW: Mechanism of stimulation of vasopressin release during beta-adrenergic stimulation with isoproterenol, J Clin Invest 53:857-867, 1974.
24. Morgan DB, Kirwan NA, Hancock KW, et al: Water intoxication and oxytocin infusion, Br J Obstet Gynaecol 84:6-12, 1977.
25. Oelekers W: Hyponatremia and inappropriate secretion of vasopressin (antidiuretic hormone) in patients with hypopituitarism, N Engl J Med 321:492-496, 1989.
26. Bethune JE and Nelson DH: Hyponatremia in hypopituitarism, N Engl J Med 272:771-776, 1965.
27. Schwartz WB, Bennett W, Curelop S, and Bartter FC: A syndrome of renal sodium loss and hyponatremia probably resulting from inappropriate secretion of antidiuretic hormone, Am J Med 23:529-542, 1957.
28. Bower BF, Mason DM, and Forsham PH: Bronchogenic carcinoma with inappropriate antidiuretic activity in plasma and tumor, N Engl J Med 271:934-938, 1964.
29. Morton JJ, Kelly P, and Padfield PL: Antidiuretic hormone in bronchogenic carcinoma, Clin Endocrinol 9:357-370, 1978.
30. Zerbe R, Stropes L, and Robertson G: Vasopressin function in the syndrome of inappropriate antidiuresis, Annu Rev Med 31:315-327, 1980.
31. Schrier RW: Pathogenesis of Na$^+$ and water retention in high-output and low-output cardiac failure, nephrotic syndrome, cirrhosis, and pregnancy, N Engl J Med 319:1065-1072, 1127-1134, 1988.
32. Arieff AI, Llach F, and Massry SG: Neurological manifestations and morbidity in hyponatremia, Medicine 55:121-129, 1976.
33. Narins RG: Therapy for hyponatremia: Does haste make waste? N Engl J Med 314:1573-1575, 1986.
34. Berl T: Treating hyponatremia: Damned if we do and damned if we don't, Kidney Int 37:1006-1018, 1990.
35. Berl T: Treating hyponatremia: What is all the controversy about? Ann Intern Med 113:417-419, 1990.
36. Sterns RH, Riggs JE, and Schochet SS: Osmotic demyelination syndrome following correction of hyponatremia, N Engl J Med 314:1535-1542, 1986.
37. Papadakis MA, Fraser CL, and Arieff AI: Hyponatraemia in patients with cirrhosis, Q J Med 76:675-688, 1990.
38. Snyder NA, Feigal DW, and Arieff AI: Hypernatremia in elderly patients, Ann Intern Med 107:309-319, 1987.
39. Balestrieri FJ, Chernow B, and Rainey TG: Postcraniotomy diabetes insipidus: who's at risk? Crit Care Med 10:108-110, 1982.
40. Seckl J: Postoperative diabetes insipidus, BMJ 298:2-3, 1989.
41. Leaf A: Dehydration in the elderly, N Engl J Med 311:791-792, 1984.
42. Dashe AM, Cramm RE, Crist CA, et al: A water deprivation test for the differential diagnosis of diabetes insipidus, JAMA 185:699-703, 1963.
43. Alon U and Chan JC: Hydrochlorothiazide-amiloride in the treatment of congenital nephrogenic diabetes insipidus, Am J Nephrol 5:9-13, 1985.
44. Morgan DB and Davison C: Hypokalaemia and diuretics: an analysis of publications, BMJ 280:905-908, 1980.
45. Hirsch IA, Tomlinson DL, Slogoff S, and Keats AS: The overstated risk of preoperative hypokalemia, Anesth Analg 67:131-136, 1988.

46. Paice BJ, Paterson KR, Onyanga-Omara F, et al: Record linkage study of hypokalemia in hospitalized patients, Postgrad Med J 62:187-191, 1986.
47. Paice B, Gray JM, McBride D, et al: Hyperkalaemia in patients in hospital, BMJ 286:1189-1192, 1983.
48. Williams JF, Morrow AG, and Braunwald E: The incidence and management of "medical" complications following cardiac operations, Circulation 32:608-619, 1965.
49. Shapiro S, Slone D, Lewis GP, and Jick H: Fatal drug reactions among medical inpatients, JAMA 216:467-472, 1971.
50. Sterns RH, Cox M, Feig PU, and Singer I: Internal potassium balance and the control of plasma potassium concentration, Medicine 60:339-354, 1981.
51. Brown MJ and Murphy MB: Hypokalemia from beta$_2$-receptor stimulation by circulating epinephrine, N Engl J Med 309:1414-1419, 1983.
52. Williams ME, Rosa RM, Silva P, et al: Impairment of extrarenal potassium disposal by alpha-adrenergic stimulation, N Engl J Med 311:145-149, 1984.
53. Todd EP and Vick RL: Kalemotropic effect of epinephrine: analysis with adrenergic agonists and antagonists, Am J Physiol 220:1964-1969, 1971.
54. Burnell JM, Villamil MF, Uyeno BT, et al: The effect in humans of extracellular pH change on the relationship between serum potassium concentration and intracellular potassium, J Clin Invest 35:935-939, 1965.
55. Adrogue HJ and Madias NE: Changes in plasma potassium concentration during acute acid-base disturbances, Am J Med 71:456-467, 1981.
56. Clausen T, and Kohn PG: The effect of insulin on the transport of sodium and potassium on the rat soleus muscle, J Physiol (Lond) 265:19-42, 1977.
57. Tannen RL: Potassium disorders. In Kokko JP and Tannen RL, editors: Fluids and electrolytes, Philadelphia, 1990, WB Saunders Co.
58. Erhlich EN: Adrenocortical regulation of electrolyte and water metabolism. In DeGroot LJ, editor: Endocrinology, Philadelphia, 1989, WB Saunders Co.
59. Gonzales JJ, Owens W, Ungaro PC, et al: Clay ingestion: a rare cause of hypokalemia, Ann Intern Med 97:65-66, 1982.
60. Ossey K: Stress and hypokalemia, Anesthesiology 66:443-444, 1987.
61. Boelhouwer RU, Bruining HA, and Ong GL: Correlations of serum potassium fluctuations with body temperature after major surgery, Crit Care Med 15:310-312, 1987.
62. Edwards R, Winnie AP, and Ramamurthy S: Acute hypocapnic hypokalemia: an iatrogenic anesthetic complication, Anesth Analg 56:786-792, 1977.
63. Rao TL, Mathru M, Salem MR, and Adel AE: Serum potassium level following transfusion of frozen erythrocytes, Anesthesiology 52:170-172, 1980.
64. Horton B: Anesthetic experiences in a family with hypokalemic familial periodic paralysis, Anesthesiology 47:308-310, 1977.
65. Kassirer JP and Schwartz WB: Potassium deficiency in surgical patients: its recognition and management, Ann Surg 40:10-18, 1966.
66. Da Cruz GM, Gardner JD, and Peskin GW: Mechanism of diarrhea in villous adenomas of the rectum and sigmoid colon with severe electrolyte depletion, Ann Surg 155:806-816, 1962.
67. Liddle GW, Bledsoe T, and Coppage WS: A familial renal disorder simulating primary aldosteronism but with negligible aldosterone secretion, Trans Assoc Am Physicians 76:199-213, 1963.
68. Bartter FC, Pronove P, Gill JR, and MacCardle RC:

Hyperplasia of the juxtaglomerular complex with hyperaldosteronism and hypokalemic alkalosis: a new syndrome, Am J Med 33:811-828, 1962.

69. Whang R, Flink EB, Dyckner T, et al: Magnesium depletion as a cause of refractory potassium repletion, Arch Intern Med 145:1686-1689, 1985.

70. Polak A, Haynie GD, Hayes RM, et al: Effects of chronic hypercapnia on electrolyte and acid-base equilibrium, J Clin Invest 40:1223-1237, 1961.

71. Miller RD and Savarese JJ: Pharmacology of muscle relaxants and their antagonists. In Miller RD, editor: Anesthesia, New York, 1986, Churchill Livingstone.

72. Knockel JP: Neuromuscular manifestations of electrolyte disorders, Am J Med 72:521-535, 1982.

73. Fisch C: Relation of electrolyte disturbances to cardiac arrhythmias, Circulation 47:408-419, 1973.

74. Holland OB, Nixon JV, and Kuhnert L: Diuretic-induced ventricular ectopic activity, Am J Med 70:762-768, 1981.

75. Nordrehaug JE, Johannessen KA, and Lippe G: Serum potassium concentration as a risk factor for ventricular arrhythmias early in acute myocardial infarction, Circulation 71:645-649, 1985.

76. Smith TW, Antman EM, Freidman PL, et al: Digitalis glycosides: mechanisms and manifestations of toxicity, Prog Cardiovasc Dis 27:21-56, 1985.

77. Vitez TS, Soper LE, Wong KC, and Soper P: Chronic hypokalemia and intraoperative dysrhythmias, Anesthesiology 63:130-133, 1985.

78. McGovern B: Hypokalemia and cardiac arrhythmias, Anesthesiology 63:127-129, 1985.

79. Narins RG, Jones ER, Stom MC, et al: Diagnostic strategies in disorders of fluid, electrolyte, and acid-base homeostasis, Am J Med 72:496-520, 1982.

80. Don BL, Sebastian A, Cheitlin M, et al: Pseudohyperkalemia caused by fist clenching during phlebotomy, N Engl J Med 322:1290-1292, 1990.

81. Reza MJ, Kovick RB, Shine KI, and Pearce ML: Massive intravenous digoxin overdosage, N Engl J Med 291:777-778, 1974.

82. Ponce SP, Jennings AE, Madias NE, and Harrington JT: Drug-induced hyperkalemia, Medicine 64:357-370, 1985.

83. Gronert GA and Theye RA: Pathophysiology of hyperkalemia induced by succinylcholine, Anesthesiology 43:89-99, 1975.

84. Azar I: The response of patients with neuromuscular disorders to muscle relaxants: a review, Anesthesiology 61:173-187, 1984.

85. DeFonzo, RA, Lee R, Jones A, et al: Effect of insulinopenia and adrenal hormone deficiency on acute potassium tolerance, Kidney Int 17:586-594, 1980.

86. Maryniak JK, Henderson AM, Woodall NM, et al: Beta-adrenoreceptor blockade and suxamethonium-induced rise in plasma potassium, Anaesthesia 42:71-74, 1987.

87. From RP and Metha MP: Effects of beta-adrenergic blockade on serum potassium following succinylcholine, Anesth Analg 67:S63, 1988.

88. Halevy JD, Ornstein E, and Matteo RS: Esmolol is not associated with an exaggerated succinylcholine mediated hyperkalemic response, Anesthesiology 69:A424, 1988.

89. Aarons JJ, Moon RE, and Camporesi EM: General anesthesia and hyperkalemic periodic paralysis, Anesthesiology 71:303-304, 1989.

90. Lawson DH: Adverse reactions to potassium chloride, Q J Med 43:433-440, 1974.

91. Conroy JM, Baker JD, and Cooke JE: Supernatant potassium levels in stored blood, Anesth Analg 67:S38, 1988.

92. Brown KA, Bissonnette B, and McIntyre BG: Hyperkalemia during cardiac arrest in the pediatric patient, Anesthesiology 71:A1014, 1989.

93. Linko K and Saxelin I: Electrolyte and acid-base disturbances caused by blood transfusions, Acta Anesthesiol Scand 30:139-144, 1986.

94. Paulsen AW, Valek TR, Blessing DD, et al: Hemodynamics during liver transplantation with venovenous bypass, Transplant Proc 11:2417-2419, 1987.

95. Soulillou JP, Fillaudeau F, Keribin JP, and Guenel J: Acute hyperkalemia risks in recipients of kidney graft cooled with Collins' solution, Nephron 19:301-304, 1977.

96. Knochel JP: The syndrome of hyporeninemic hypoaldosteronism, Annu Rev Med 30:145-153, 1979.

97. Marks ES: Diuretics and other medications used in renal failure. In Chernow B, editor: The pharmacologic approach to the critically ill patient, Baltimore, 1988, Williams & Wilkins Co.

98. Ettinger PO, Regan TJ, and Oldewurtel HA: Hyperkalemia, cardiac conduction, and the electrocardiogram: a review, Am Heart J 88:360-371, 1974.

99. Barold SS, Kalkoff MD, Ong LS, et al: Hyperkalemia-induced failure of atrial capture during dual-chamber cardiac pacing, J Am Coll Cardiol 10:467-469, 1987.

100. Hayes JF, Gross GF, and Schuman ES: Surgical management of renal hyperparathyroidism, Am J Surg 143:569-571, 1982.

101. Rasmussen H: The calcium messenger system, N Engl J Med 314:1094-1101, 1164-1170, 1986.

102. Landers DF, Becker GL, and Wong KC: Calcium, calmodulin, and anesthesiology, Anesth Analg 69:100-112, 1989.

103. Zaloga GP and Chernow B: Divalent ions: calcium, magnesium, and phosphorus. In Chernow B, editor: The pharmacological approach to the critically ill patient, Baltimore, 1988, Williams & Wilkins Co.

104. Chernow B, Zaloga G, McFadden E, et al: Hypocalcemia in critically ill patients, Crit Care Med 10:848-851, 1982.

105. Zaloga GP and Chernow B: The multifactorial basis for hypocalcemia during sepsis, Ann Intern Med 107:36-41, 1987.

106. Forster J, Querusio L, Burchard KW, and Gann DS: Hypercalcemia in critically ill surgical patients, Ann Surg 202:512-518, 1985.

107. Zaloga GP, Chernow B, Cook D, et al: Assessment of calcium homeostasis in the critically ill surgical patient: the diagnostic pitfalls of the McLean-Hastings nomogram, Ann Surg 202:587, 1985.

108. Ladensen JH, Lewis JW, and Boyd JC: Failure of total serum calcium corrected for protein, albumin, and pH to correctly assess free calcium status, J Clin Endocrinol Metab 46:986-993, 1978.

109. Reichel H, Koeffler P, and Norman AW: The role of vitamin D endocrine system in health and disease, N Engl J Med 320:980-991, 1989.

110. Zaloga GP, Willey S, Tomasic P, and Chernow B: Free fatty acids alter calcium binding: a cause for misinterpretation of serum calcium values and hypocalcemia of critical illness, J Clin Endocrinol Metab 64:1010-1014, 1987.

111. Gabow PA, Kaehny WD, and Kelleher SP: The spectrum of rhabdomyolysis, Medicine 61:141-152, 1982.

112. Cote CJ, Drop LJ, Hoaglin DC, et al: Ionized hypocalcemia after fresh frozen plasma administration to thermally injured children, Anesth Analg 67:152-160, 1988.

113. Denlinger JK, Nahrwold ML, Gibbs PS, et al: Hypocalcemia during rapid blood transfusion in an anaesthetized man, Br J Anaesth 48:995-999, 1976.
114. Marquez J, Martin D, Virji MA, et al: Cardiovascular depression secondary to ionic hypocalcemia during hepatic transplantation in humans, Anesthesiology 65:457-461, 1986.
115. Bronsky D, Kushner DS, Dubin A, et al: Idiopathic hypoparathyroidism and pseudohypoparathyroidism: case reports and review of the literature, Medicine 37:317-352, 1958.
116. Delmonico FL, Neer RM, Cosimi AB, et al: Hyperparathyroidism during pregnancy, Am J Surg 131:328-337, 1976.
117. Morgan DB, Hunt G, and Paterson CR: The osteomalacia syndrome after stomach operations, Q J Med 39:395-410, 1970.
118. Anast CA, Winnacker JL, Forte LR, and Burns TW: Impaired release of parathyroid hormone in magnesium deficiency, J Clin Endocrinol Metab 42:707-717, 1976.
119. Cholst IN, Steinberg SF, Tropper PJ, et al: The influence of hypermagnesemia on serum calcium and parathyroid hormone levels in human subjects, N Engl J Med 310:1221-1225, 1984.
120. Iseri LT and French JH: Magnesium: nature's physiologic calcium blocker, Am Heart J 108:188-193, 1984.
121. Zaloga GP and Chernow B: Hypocalcemia in critical illness, JAMA 256:1924-1929, 1986.
122. Drop LJ and Laver MB: Low plasma ionized calcium and response to calcium therapy in critically ill man, Anesthesiology 43:300-306, 1975.
123. Connor TB, Rosen BL, Blaustein MP, et al: Hypocalcemia precipitating heart failure, N Engl J Med 307:869-872, 1982.
124. Koski G: Con: Calcium salts are contraindicated in weaning of patients from cardiopulmonary bypass after coronary artery surgery, J Cardiothorac Anesth 2:570-575, 1988.
125. Cote CJ, Drop LJ, Daniels AL, and Hoaglin DC: Calcium chloride versus calcium gluconate: comparison of ionization and cardiovascular effects in children and dogs, Anesthesiology 66:465-470, 1987.
126. Mundy GR, Ibbotson KJ, D'Souza SM, et al: The hypercalcemia of cancer, N Engl J Med 310:1718-1727, 1984.
127. Martin TJ: Properties of parathyroid hormone—related protein and its role in malignant hypercalcemia, Q J Med 76:771-786, 1990.
128. Burtis WJ, Brady TG, Orloff JJ, et al: Immunochemical characterization of circulating parathyroid hormone—related protein in patients with humoral hypercalcemia of cancer, N Engl J Med 322:1106-1112, 1990.
129. Rosenthal N, Insogna K, Godsall JW, et al: Elevations in 1,25-dihydroxyvitamin D in three patients with lymphoma-associated hypercalcemia, J Clin Endocrinol Metab 60:29-33, 1985.
130. Mundy GR, Rick ME, Turcotte R, et al: Pathogenesis of hypercalcemia in lymphosarcoma cell leukemia, Am J Med 65:600-606, 1978.
131. Schwartz GH, David DS, Riggio RR, et al: Hypercalcemia after renal transplantation, Am J Med 49:42-51, 1970.
132. Segal AJ, Miller M, and Moses A: Hypercalcemia during the diuretic phase of acute renal failure, Ann Intern Med 68:1066-1071, 1968.
133. Pak CY: Calcium disorders: hypercalcemia and hypocalcemia. In Kokko JP and Tannen RL, editors: Fluids and electrolytes, Philadelphia, 1990, WB Saunders Co.
134. Rosenthal FD and Roy S: Hypertension and hyperparathyroidism, BMJ 4:396-397, 1972.
135. Suki WN, Yium JJ, Von Minden M, et al: Acute treatment of hypercalcemia, N Engl J Med 283:836-840, 1979.
136. Frame B and Parfitt AM: Corticosteroid-responsive hypercalcemia with elevated serum 1-alpha,25-dihydroxyvitamin D, Ann Intern Med 93:449-451, 1980.
137. Chernow B, Bamberger S, Stoiko M, et al: Hypomagnesemia in postoperative intensive care, Chest 95:391-397, 1989.
138. Ryzen E, Wagers PW, Singer FR, and Rude RK: Magnesium deficiency in a medical ICU population, Crit Care Med 13:19-21, 1985.
139. Whang R and Ryder KW: Frequency of hypomagnesemia and hypermagnesemia, JAMA 263:3063-3064, 1990.
140. Whang R, Oei TO, and Watanabe A: Frequency of hypomagnesemia in hospitalized patients receiving digitalis, Arch Intern Med 145:655-656, 1985.
141. Quamme GA and Dirks JH: Magnesium metabolism. In Maxwell M, Kleeman CR, and Narins RG, editors: Clinical disorders of fluid and electrolyte metabolism, New York, 1987, McGraw Hill Book Co.
142. Wacker WE and Paresi AF: Magnesium metabolism, N Engl J Med 278:658-662, 712-717, 772-776, 1968.
143. Iseri LT, Freed J, and Bures A: Magnesium deficiency and cardiac disorders, Am J Med 58:837-846, 1975.
144. Shils ME: Experimental human magnesium depletion, Medicine 48:61-85, 1969.
145. Altura BM and Altura BT: Magnesium ions and the contraction of vascular smooth muscle: relationship to some vascular diseases, Fed Proc 40:2672-2679, 1981.
146. Killen DA, Grogen EL, Gower RE, et al: Response of canine plasma ionized calcium and magnesium to the rapid infusion of acid-citrate-dextrose (ACD) solution, Surgery 70:736-743, 1971.
147. Booth CC, Babouris N, Hanna S, et al: Incidence of hypomagnesemia in intestinal malabsorption, BMJ 2:141-144, 1963.
148. Paunier L, Radde IC, Kooh SW, et al: Primary hypomagnesemia with secondary hypocalcemia, J Pediatr 67:945, 1965.
149. Fort P and Lifshitz F: Magnesium status in children with insulin-dependent diabetes mellitus, J Am Coll Nutr 5:69-78, 1986.
150. Aglio LS, Stanford GG, Maddi R, et al: Hypomagnesemia is a common and important problem following cardiopulmonary bypass, Crit Care Med 17:S40, 1989.
151. Zaloga GP, Chernow B, Pock A, et al: Hypomagnesemia is a common complication of aminoglycoside therapy, Surg Gynecol Obstet 158:561-565, 1984.
152. Lam M and Adelstein DJ: Hypomagnesemia and renal magnesium wasting in patients treated with cisplatin, Am J Kidney Dis 8:164-169, 1986.
153. Masur H: Antimicrobials. In Chernow B, editor: The pharamacological approach to the critically ill patient, Baltimore, 1988, Williams & Wilkins Co.
154. Barton CH, Vaziri ND, Martin DC, et al: Hypomagnesemia and renal magnesium wasting in renal transplant recipients receiving cyclosporin, Am J Med 83:693-699, 1987.
155. Kalbfleisch JM, Linderman RD, Ginn HE, et al: Effects of ethanol administration on urinary excretion of magnesium and other electrolytes in alcoholics and normal subjects, J Clin Invest 42:1471-1475, 1963.
156. Dhing S, Solven F, Wilson A, and McCarthy DS:

Hypomagnesemia and respiratory muscle power, Am Rev Respir Dis 129:497-498, 1984.

157. Iseri LT, Chung P, and Tobis J: Magnesium therapy for intractable ventricular arrhythmias in normomagnesemic patients, Western J Med 138:823-828, 1983.

158. Rasmussen HS, Norregard P, Lindeneg O, et al: Intravenous magnesium in acute myocardial infarction, Lancet 1:234-235, 1986.

159. Schwieger I, Kopel ME, and Finlayson DC: Magnesium reduces incidence of postoperative dysrhythmias in patients after cardiac surgery, Anesthesiology 71:A1163, 1989.

160. Vacanti FX and Ames A: Mild hypothermia and magnesium protect against irreversible damage during CNS ischemia, Stroke 15:695-698, 1984.

161. James MF, Beer RE, and Esser JD: Intravenous magnesium sulfate inhibits catecholamine release associated with tracheal intubation, Anesth Analg 68:772-776, 1989.

162. Goldman RS and Finkbeiner SM: Therapeutic use of magnesium sulfate in cerebral ischemia and seizure, N Engl J Med 319:1224-1225, 1988.

163. Skobeloff EM, Spivey WH, McNamara RM, and Greenspon L: Intravenous magnesium sulfate for the treatment of acute asthma in the emergency department, JAMA 262:1210-1213, 1989.

164. Hubbard JI: Microphysiology of vertebrate neuromuscular transmission, Physiol Rev 53:674-723, 1973.

165. Ghonheim MM and Long JP: The interaction between magnesium and other neuromuscular blocking agents, Anesthesiology 32:23-27, 1970.

Chapter 21

Complications of Blood Transfusion

Norig Ellison
Ronald J. Faust

Since November 1975 reporting of all deaths associated with blood collection, transfusion, or plasmapheresis to the United States Food and Drug Administration has been required. In the first 10 years of reporting, 355 deaths (Table 21-1) from 14 causes (Table 21-2) in recipients and 12 deaths in donors (Table 21-3) have been reported.[1] An accompanying editorial points out that "a major fraction of the thirty million people who received transfusion during this period were kept alive by the blood they received."[2] Obviously these deaths are merely the worst cases and do not reflect the significant morbidity associated, for example, with chronic active hepatitis after transfusion or acute lung injury.

A "Circular of Information for the Use of Human Blood and Blood Components," prepared jointly by the American Association of Blood Banks, American Red Cross, and Council of Community Blood Centers and approved by the Center for Biologics Evaluation and Research of the Food and Drug Administration (FDA), is the equivalent of the package insert provided by pharmaceutical manufacturers with each drug.[3] Because of space limitations on blood and component container labels, the circular is necessary to supply the information required by applicable federal statutes and regulations of the FDA. Unlike drug package inserts, the circular is not routinely provided to physicians when blood is issued from the blood bank. This 30-page circular succinctly lists, among other things, the complications that may accompany the administration of a blood product (List 21-1). When one considers the large number of potential complications presented in

Table 21-1. Number of reports of transfusion-associated deaths per year, 1976-1985

Year	Number of reports
1976	12
1977	22
1978	36
1979	44
1980	46
1981	36
1982	32
1983	52
1984	37
1985	38
Total	355

From Sazama K: Transfusion 30:583-590, 1990.

the circular, why do physicians administer homologous blood? When the alternative is death from exsanguination, a lifesaving increase in oxygen transport capability or restoration of effective hemostasis clearly defines the reason homologous blood transfusion is judged a necessary risk in many cases.

Well over 50% of the homologous blood and virtually all the autologous blood transfused in America is administered to surgical patients in

Table 21-2. Cause of transfusion-associated deaths in order of reported frequency, 1976-1985

Number	Cause
158	Acute hemolysis
42	Non-A, non-B hepatitis
31	Acute pulmonary edema
26	Hepatitis B
26	Bacterial contamination
26	Delayed hemolysis
15	Not associated
12	Donation of blood product
8	Anaphylaxis
5	External hemolysis
3	AIDS*
1	Red blood cells not deglycerolized
1	Graft-versus-host disease†
1	Records unavailable

From Sazama K: Transfusion 30:583-590, 1990.
*Acquired immunodeficiency syndrome; 2 persons transfused in 1982, 1 in 1983.
†Immunocompromised recipient; nonirradiated product.

List 21-1. Potential Side Effects and Hazards of the Administration of Blood or Blood Components.

1. Hemolytic transfusion reaction, immediate or delayed
2. Disease transmission
   a. Viral hepatitis
   b. Cytomegalovirus (CMV)
   c. Other infections
3. Recipient alloimmunization
4. Graft-versus-host disease (GVHD)
5. Febrile reactions
6. Allergic reactions
   a. Angioedematous
   b. Anaphylactoid
7. Circulatory overload reactions
8. Bacterial contamination
9. Iron overload
10. Depletion of procoagulants and platelets
11. Microaggregates
12. Metabolic complications
    a. Hypothermia
    b. Citrate toxicity
    c. Acidosis
    d. Hypokalemia or hyperkalemia

From Circular of information for the use of human blood and blood components, Washington, DC, 1987, jointly by American Association of Blood Banks, American Red Cross, and Council of Community Blood Centers.

Table 21-3. Deaths of blood or plasma donors, 1976-1985

Year	Age	Gender	Product	Cause
1978	31	F	Plasma	Unknown
	33	M	Plasma*	Convulsion, myocardial infarction (?)
1979	?	M	White cells	Ruptured cerebral vascular aneurysm
	?	M	Plasma	Digoxin toxicity
1980	?	?	Plasma	Convulsion, myocardial infarction (?)
	48	F	Blood	Pheochromocytoma
1981†				
1982	?	?	Plasma	ABO error, group O donor received group A red blood cells
	47	M	Plasma	Acute myocardial infarction
1983	44	M	Blood*	Acute myocardial infarction (18 hours after phlebotomy)
	37	F	Blood	Acute myocardial infarction concurrent
1984	?	M	Plasma	Staphylococcal sepsis, endocarditis
	47	M	Plasma	Stroke (3 hours after donation)
1985‡				

From Sazama K: Transfusion 30:583-590, 1990.
*First-time donor.
†None reported.
‡Could not be determined from report.

the perioperative period, much of it in the operating room. For this reason anesthesiologists are clearly involved and concerned with the administration of blood and blood products. Indeed, blood transfusion may be the most common non–pain relieving therapeutic maneuver performed by anesthesiologists.

In the United States over 12 million units of blood products are administered annually, up from 8 million units in 1975, and these units have been donated by 8% of the population, which is an increase from the 3% who provided more than 97% of the blood collected in 1975.[4] On occasion the supply-to-demand ratio of blood has been perilously thin despite this increase in the absolute number of units and the percentage of donors. Both the increase in the number of operations and an increase in the complexity of procedures such as liver transplants have increased the demand. More aggressive chemotherapy in oncology has further increased the demand for platelets especially.

To make the available supply go further, two major developments have occurred. First, the shelf life of red blood cells was extended in steps from 21 days in 1979 to the current 42 days. This extension was particularly helpful in avoiding the shortages during and just after the Christmas–New Year holidays. Second, fractionation of whole blood into its several components, in addition to facilitating goal-directed therapy, permits one unit of blood to be used to treat several patients. Fractionation has increased steadily to the point that well over 80% of blood collected in the United States is now routinely fractionated. In cases of trauma, gastrointestinal hemorrhage, and massive surgical bleeding many clinicians prefer to administer whole blood and question whether 80% fractionation will leave enough whole blood for these cases.[5-6] The time required to infuse more viscous red blood cells or to dilute them with crystalloid are disadvantages of component therapy. Additionally, the use of red blood cells in large numbers may require the administration of units of albumin, fresh-frozen plasma (FFP), and platelets, thereby increasing donor exposure, chance of infection, and cost.

Articles discussing the administration of large volumes of homologous blood to patients usually contain words such as "complications"[7] or "problems"[8] in the title, and indeed complications ranging from logistics (such as obtaining an adequate amount of blood or having sufficient large lines through which the blood can be administered) to hypothermia and hemostasis are commonly seen in cases of massive transfusion. However, just one 30 ml unit of red blood cells can be lethal by inducing a hemolytic transfusion reaction.[1] There is a clear dose-response relationship in some complications, such as hypothermia, that is directly proportional to the volume transfused and the rate of transfusion. Similarly, although less than one unit can transmit a fatal disease, the incidence of several infections is directly proportional to the number of units transfused, until a plateau is reached.[9]

I. RECIPIENT ALLOIMMUNIZATION

In 1900, Carl Landsteiner discovered the ABO red blood cell groups, the first step to making homologous transfusion relatively safe. The ABO groups are most important because they are the only blood groups with naturally occurring antibodies. Persons who lack A or B antigens naturally form anti-A and anti-B antibodies, and these antibodies are capable of immediately hemolyzing incompatible red cells.

The A and B antigens have been determined to be short-chain sugar molecules on lipid or protein backbones, with only the terminal sugar differing to determine A or B antigenicity. A and B antigens are also present in many body tissues and certain body fluids and can be found in nature in animals, plants, and bacteria. This is believed to be the stimulus for the formation of anti-A and anti-B antibodies early in life. Incidences differ among different populations and races, but 40% of United States whites possess the A antigen, and only 11% possess the B antigen. Both A and B are present in only 4% of the population. Thus the most frequent blood groups are A and O. Although 45% of American whites are group O, the frequency of this blood group is higher in blacks and American Indians.

In the 90 years since Landsteiner's discovery, over 600 blood group antigens have been discovered.[10] Naturally occurring antibodies do not exist for non-ABO red blood cell antigens, but antibodies form after exposure to foreign red cells either through transfusion or transplacental hemorrhage during pregnancy. Because of the large number of antigens, homologous blood is never perfectly "matched," and autologous transfusion is the only method of red cell transfusion that avoids the possibility of antibody formation.

When homologous transfusion is necessary, compatible blood is identified in the blood bank through multiple steps. In addition to the ABO group, the D antigen from the Rh group is the only other blood group antigen for which the donor's red cells are routinely typed. Antibodies to D antigen are responsible for hemolytic disease of the newborn. After the group and Rh determination, the *antibody screen* is performed to allow one to identify any unnatural antibodies present. For this test, the patient's serum is mixed with red blood cells from two donors predetermined to contain all antigens whose antibodies are known to cause hemolytic reactions. Weak antibodies can be uncovered by the addition of albumin and certain enzymes to the RBC/serum mixture and by incubation at room temperature and 37° C. Similar steps are used when recipient serum is "crossmatched" with donor red cells, and these steps necessitate at least 45 minutes for completion of either an antibody screen or a crossmatch. If agglutination is detected and one or both of the screening cells used during the antibody screen agglutinates with the recipient serum, more serum is then mixed with a panel of 10 selected cells and the same incubation steps are repeated. The pattern of reactions encountered among the antibody panel cells will permit identification of any antibody present. Donor units can then be typed for this antigen, and units negative for the antigen are selected for the cross match.

In addition to the well-known red blood cell alloantibodies, alloimmunization to donor white blood cells, platelets, and serum proteins frequently occurs after homologous blood transfusion.[11] This complication is usually not life threatening, nor does it cause immediate symptoms. Although most antigenic challenges elicit a circulating antibody in 10 to 14 days, red blood cell antibodies may not appear initially for 3 to 4 months. The subsequently administered blood or blood components need to be negative for the specific antigen to which the recipient has become alloimmunized to avoid serious reaction. In addition to blood administration, prior pregnancy may have stimulated red blood cell antibodies, all of which should be detected in the antibody screen before transfusion.

Clinically, platelet antibodies are the most troublesome, and their presence often results in the failure of subsequent platelet transfusions to produce a beneficial effect. Until there is a demonstrated lack of efficacy from random donor platelets suggestive of alloimmunization, random donor platelets are used. Other possible causes for the apparent development of a refractory state to platelet transfusion are continuing platelet consumption with disseminated intravascular coagulation (DIC), nonviable platelets, splenomegaly, fever, and sepsis. Human leukocyte antigen (HLA)–compatible platelets obtained by apheresis is the most feasible method

for treating patients with platelet-reactive antibodies. Unfortunately this technique is ineffective in one third of the cases.[12]

II. HEMOLYTIC TRANSFUSION REACTIONS

Acute hemolysis after transfusion is a life-threatening reaction which will often be regarded as preventable on review. Although some incorrectly refer to red blood cell antibodies as "major or minor," whether acute hemolysis occurs after antigen-antibody reaction is determined by whether this reaction binds complement on the surface of the red cell. Anti-A and anti-B do bind complement, and intravascular hemolysis can be expected when ABO-incompatible red blood cells are transfused. Many antibodies of antigen groups other than ABO also bind complement and cause hemolytic transfusion reactions.

In a review of 54 cases at Mayo Clinic, only 5 of 54 cases were caused by ABO group antibodies.[13] Anti-Kell, anti-Kidd, anti-Duffy, anti-E, anti-c, and anti-D were more common culprits of hemolytic transfusion reactions. This series contrasted with several later reports indicating that ABO incompatibility was responsible for the majority of hemolytic reactions.[14-18] Since the operating room and the intensive care unit were the site of the incompatible transfusion for many of these patients, anesthesiologists should be aware of this severe risk. Proper patient identification procedures should always be strictly adhered to. Patient name and number must be compared on the patient's bracelet, the anesthesia record, and each unit of blood brought into the operating room. The contrast between the types of antibodies reported in the Mayo study and those reported from the FDA data indicates that transfusion procedures at Mayo may already be consistent with the transfusion management system advocated by Sazama.[1] In addition to the emphasis placed on identification procedures in the operating room, blood banks staffed by transfusion nurses are located in each operating suite at Mayo. Non–operating room transfusions are started by nurse transfusionists who specialize in that activity.

Once a red cell is coated with antibody in vivo, extravascular hemolysis will occur as the red cells are phagocytized by macrophages in the reticuloendothelial system. Alternatively, intravascular hemolysis will follow if the antigen-antibody reaction binds complement. The pathophysiology of acute hemolysis has been reviewed by Goldfinger.[19] In most hemolytic reactions, some red cells are probably destroyed by both intravascular and extravascular mechanisms. When complement is bound, a lesion is produced on the red cell membrane and hemolysis follows by one of two mechanisms. The "detergent mechanism" indicates that disorganization of the lipid bilayer may cause an area of the cell wall to become permeable to ions. Alternatively, the "donut hypothesis" is a proposal that the five late-acting components of complement actually form a ring on the cell wall that extends through the membrane, creating a pore through which ions pass until the red cell ruptures.[20]

Renal vascular ischemia and activation of the coagulation system leading to disseminated intravascular coagulation characterize the pathophysiologic process of the hemolytic reaction. Renal vascular ischemia is a more important mechanism of renal failure than is the plugging of renal tubules by hemoglobin casts, which are more likely an effect of the renal injury than its cause. Mortalities between 17% and 53% are reported after hemolytic reactions.[13] Symptoms of the hemolytic reaction are depicted in Table 21-4. Most signs and symptoms are masked by general anesthesia. Fever is actually the most common symptom in awake patients; thus a hemolytic transfusion reaction should be ruled out any time a febrile reaction follows a transfusion. Also, note that hives and skin rash were not observed in patients undergoing hemolytic reactions, a finding that differentiates this serious reaction from more common mild allergic reactions.[13,20]

Therapy for the hemolytic transfusion reaction is aimed at preventing renal failure and DIC. Although mannitol has been the traditional drug of choice, volume loading with crystalloid and use of furosemide (Lasix) to increase renal blood flow and urine output are now recommended. Of course, the transfusion must be stopped as soon as the reaction is suspected. Both that unit and all other units should be rechecked in the blood bank, since a systematic clerical error may have cleared all units crossmatched at the same time. The coagulation system must be monitored for the development of DIC. Platelet concentrates and fresh-frozen plasma may be indicated if DIC develops.

When a hemolytic reaction is suspected, the blood bank must be contacted to assist in establishing the diagnosis. In addition to repeating all clerical checks, antibody screens, and crossmatches, the recipient's cells are checked with anti-human globulin (Coombs' serum) to determine if red cells have been coated with antibodies. Acute hemolysis will also cause a decrease in the level of the recipient's serum haptoglobin, a plasma globulin that binds free plasma hemoglobin.

III. TRANSFUSION-RELATED ACUTE LUNG INJURY

Transfusion-related acute lung injury (TRALI) is a rare but serious reaction in which patients present with noncardiogenic pulmonary edema within 2 to 6 hours after transfusion.[21] The cause is usually leukoagglutinating and lymphocytotoxic antibodies in donor blood products. Intubation and mechanical ventilation are often required. Although Sazama reports 31 deaths from acute respiratory failure secondary to transfusion,[1] patients usually recover completely with supportive therapy. The reaction probably takes place more frequently than rec-

Table 21-4. Hemolytic transfusion reaction symptoms

Acute intravascular hemolysis		Chronic extravascular hemolysis and delayed hemolytic transfusion reaction
Awake patients	Anesthetized patients	
Fever	Fever	Fever
Tachycardia	Tachycardia	Anemia
Hemoglobinuria	Hemoglobinuria	Mild jaundice
Diffuse bleeding	Diffuse bleeding	
Back pain	Hypotension	
Nausea		
Flushing		
Dyspnea		
Apprehension		
Chest pain		
Chills		

ognized and should be suspected any time a patient shows signs of pulmonary edema after a transfusion when there is little clinical suspicion of volume overload.

IV. DISEASE TRANSMISSION

Although viral, bacterial, and parasitic diseases can be transmitted by blood transfusion, viral disease transmission is the major problem. There are two characteristics necessary for a donor to provide a unit of blood that is infected. First, the donor is either an asymptomatic carrier, has a clinically inapparent disease, or is in the prodromal stage of infection. Otherwise, the potential donor would have been rejected from donating blood on the basis of history or physical examination. Second, the disease must be in the early stage where serologic markers of infection have not developed, the so-called window, or the disease is one for which routine screening is not available.

In an editorial addressing the issue of a "zero-risk blood supply" Zuck points out that although totally safe blood may be the only politically acceptable solution it is a futile goal. A corollary of the politically acceptable solution is the risk of legal accountability; that is, someone should be held financially responsible to those injured when transfusion-associated disease ensues.[22] The futility of a zero-risk blood supply is based on the fact that all homologous blood transfusions are genetically incompatible and potentially infectious with the biologic processes of some diseases defying detection of every infected unit.

A. Viral disease

1. Hepatitis. Despite the recent publicity surrounding transfusion-associated AIDS, the most common infection associated with homologous blood transfusion is posttransfusion hepatitis (PTH), which produces long-term as well as short-term morbidity and mortality. Hepatitis A, B, C (the most recent identified), and delta are the identified viruses. Two groups in the mid-1960s contributed significantly to our knowledge of hepatitis. Krugman et al. clearly distinguished two types of hepatitis, infectious and serum, on the basis of incubation period and duration.[23] At the same time Blumberg identified the antigen responsible for serum hepatitis, the so-called Australian antigen, originally found in an Australian aborigine.[24] This is now known to be the unassembled viral coat or surface antigen, HBsAg.

Hepatitis A (HAV), infectious hepatitis, is a rare cause of PTH for three reasons. There is only a very brief 7- to 10-day viremia during the prodromal phase when patients would be acceptable donors. Second, passively transfused anti-HAV antibodies from other transfused units would prevent HAV from infecting a recipient. Finally, there is no carrier state for HAV.

Hepatitis B (HBV) remains a source of PTH with an estimated frequency of 1:200 to 1:300 despite the existence of a serologic test since 1971.[25] Administration of blood in emergency cases without testing or collection of blood during the "window" period before serologic markers develop explain the continued production of PTH by HBV. Of all patients who develop HBV, 90% will have a self-limited course, with the majority being asymptomatic (70% nonicteric), 5% to 10% will go on to a chronic state, and 1% will have a fulminant form of hepatitis with a mortality greater than 50%. Of the 10% who develop a chronic state, half will evidence one of the chronic forms of hepatitis and the remainder become asymptomatic carriers. This last is the group without symptoms or history of hepatitis whose blood donation would transmit HBV were their unit not tested for HBsAg. Approximately 0.1% of volunteer blood donors in the United States are positive for HBsAg, most being chronic carriers rather than in the prodromal state.[9]

In addition to the surface antigen, HBsAg, two other HBV antigens have been identified, the inner protein core (HBc) and the e antigen, HBeAg, which is a free protein in serum. The development of antibody to HBsAg indicates that immunity to HBV has developed and resolution of the acute infection is occurring, whereas failure to develop anti-HBs and persistence of detectable anti-HBc and HBsAg indicate chronic infection.[26]

Hepatitis C (HCV) has only recently been identified, having previously been known by the unwieldy term "non-A, non-B hepatitis" (NANBH), and it is quite likely that some as yet as undetermined portion of NANBH is not attributable to HCV.[27] This virus has a shorter incubation period than HBV at 35 to 70 days and a milder initial course, with 75% being nonicteric, but 50% will develop a chronic state, with 10% progressing to cirrhosis.

Before the development of a specific serologic marker for HCV, exclusion of donors with either of two "surrogate" markers, alanine aminotransferase and anti-HBc, was instituted. These became a standard in the United States in late 1986 without conclusive demonstration of a beneficial effect by the usual prospective randomized studies. It is now impossible in this country to perform the study that would confirm the value of the surrogate markers, which are not used in the United Kingdom. Although the incidence of HCV is not precisely known after establishment of the surrogate markers in the United States, the incidence is estimated to be less than 1:100.[9]

Delta virus (HDV) is a defective RNA virus that infects individuals only previously infected usually with HBV because HDV requires the helper function of a DNA virus. HDV may occur simultaneously with HBV infection or subsequently in someone who develops a chronic carrier state. The average transfusion recipient is not at risk for HDV because few persons are HBV carriers.

The demonstration that blood obtained commercially was associated with a higher incidence of PTH than blood obtained from voluntary donors provided the impetus for an all-volunteer blood system and was the first positive step to decrease the incidence of PTH. Two studies of cardiac surgical patients at NIH who received large volumes of homologous blood have demonstrated that patients who received primarily commercial blood in the early 1960s developed either icteric or nonicteric hepatitis in 50% of the cases whereas 7 years later with exclusive use of volunteer blood that was HAA negative the PTH had dropped to 7.1%[28-29] The use of HBV vaccine, especially in groups such as hemophiliacs, who are at greater risk of PTH, would be an additional way to confer HBV immunity. Fear of developing AIDS from the HBV vaccine is not warranted because the procedure for preparing the vaccine has been shown to inactivate all known infectious agents including HIV.[30]

2. Human immunodeficiency viruses (HIV). Human immunodeficiency viruses (HIV) are RNA retroviruses first reported to be transmitted by transfusion when a 20-month-old child who had received blood products from 19 donors in the first month of life during exchange transfusions to treat hemolytic disease of the newborn developed AIDS.[31] The 1984 Centers for Disease Control report received widespread publicity and created, for want of a better term, hysteria in the minds of many patients whose fear of blood transfusion was totally irrational.[32] Approximately 2% of AIDS cases are attributed to the transfusion of single-donor products and 1% to clotting concentrates in patients with hemophilia. Most of these cases were the result of blood transfusions before the advent of serologic testing in March 1985. To decrease the risk of transfusion-associated AIDS, five steps have been taken:

1. Certain high risk groups have been identi-

fied and are excluded from donating blood, including intravenous drug users, sexually active homosexual or bisexual males, persons with symptoms suggestive of AIDS, and sexual partners of persons with AIDS or at risk for AIDS.

2. Confidential designation by donors of their blood "for lab use only" has been added to the voluntary self-deferment to avoid potential donor embarrassment or peer pressure to donate.

3. Screening all donor units for HIV antibodies.

4. Heat or chemical treatment of blood products manufactured from pooled donor plasma to inactivate HIV and other viruses that might be present.

5. Complete investigation of all cases of transfusion-associated AIDS to identify asymptomatic donors. All recipients of material from the same unit of blood must be followed up. When donors develop AIDS or an AIDS-related condition or are found to be HIV positive at some time after giving blood, recipients of all their prior donations should be investigated.

Despite these five steps, new cases of transfusion-associated AIDS continue to occur. The current incidence of transfusion-associated AIDS is estimated to be between 1:40,000 and 1:1,000,000.[25] Although most such cases were attributed to blood donation during the 6 to 14 week "black window" between infection and HIV antibody development, there have been reports that seropositive asymptomatic homosexual men may lose HIV antibodies without disease progression.[33]

3. Human T-cell leukemia/lymphoma viruses I and II (HTLV-I, HTLV-II). Human T-cell leukemia/lymphoma viruses are also retroviruses. HTLV-I has the capacity to induce neoplastic transformation of infected cells and has been demonstrated to be etiologically associated with adult T-cell leukemia and chronic progressive myelopathy, also called "tropical spastic paraparesis." However, except for a Japanese report that chronic progressive myelopathy can be transmitted with a mean incubation period of 4 years, no cases have clearly been related to blood transfusion.[33] A survey of 40,000 donors in the United States showed a low frequency (0.025%) of antibodies to HTLV-I. Nevertheless with the general concern about transfusion-transmitted retroviruses in January 1989 screening for HTLV-HTVL-I and HTLV HTVL-II was begun.[34]

4. Cytomegalovirus (CMV). Cytomegalovirus is a member of the herpes family, all of which are DNA viruses found intracellularly in leukocytes. Thus there is little risk of transfusion from acellular blood components such as plasma or cryoprecipitate and minimal risk with leukocyte-poor red blood cells. CMV infection is common, with 50% of the donors having demonstrated prior exposure as manifest by antibodies, but only 5% to 12% of seropositive donors may be infectious. Posttransfusion CMV may be primary in previous unexposed persons or reactivation of a latent CMV virus. Normally only a mild febrile illness is associated with viremia and viruria followed by seroconversion 13 to 16 weeks later. The incidence of transfusion-associated CMV has been reported at 7% after a single unit up to a plateau of 21% after 15 units.[35]

In contrast to the mild infection described above, the immunocompromised patient may develop serious, often fatal multisystem disease with pneumonia, hepatitis, and meningoencephalitis. The only certain way to avoid CMV infection in transplant patients is for a CMV-negative patient to receive an organ from a CMV-negative donor and receive only CMV-negative blood.

Low-birth-weight babies (less than 1250 g) whose mothers are seronegative (that is, no transplacental passive immunization) and receive seropositive blood are similarly at great risk. This was first reported by Yeager who subsequently showed that this could be avoided when only CMV-negative blood was transfused.[36]

5. Epstein-Barr virus. Another potential cause of the postperfusion syndrome in patients without detectable CMV antibodies is Epstein-Barr virus (EBV). Over 90% of donors have antibodies to EBV, and blood is not screened for them because most patients are immune to the EBV and are not susceptible to infection. EBV, like CMV, remains in a latent form in host cells and so cannot be transmitted by acellular blood components. For that matter, studies in children indicate that antibodies in donor blood may protect recipients from EBV infection.[37]

B. Bacterial disease

Contaminants generally do not present a problem because both the preservative and the storage temperature of 4° C are bacteriostatic for almost all bacterial genera. For this reason the rare bacterial contaminant seldom produces a clinical picture of sepsis when the blood is administered. Meticulous cleansing of the puncture site and use of a closed bag system will continue to make bacterial contaminants a rarity. The final step in prevention of infusing blood contaminated with bacteria is an inspection of the unit before the administration. Hemolyzed or cloudy units should be returned to the blood bank for examination.

Platelets have been stored at room temperature for 20 years, since their longer survival in vivo was established, but bacteremia after platelet transfusion was not recognized until 1981 when new plastic storage containers were introduced and improved gas exchange and permitted shelf life to be extended from 5 to 7 days.[38] As a result of this bacterial sepsis, shelf life was returned to 5 days.[39]

Yersinia enterocolitica produced seven cases of sepsis with five deaths after RBC administration between April 1987 and May 1989. These occurred in units stored 26 to 40 days before transfusion.[40] This bacteria is unique in that 4° C is not so bacteriostatic as with other genera. There has been a dramatic increase in the frequency of isolation of this organism from both clinical and nonclinical specimens.[41] Whether these cases are just the tip of the iceberg is uncertain, and what steps should be taken are not clear. Although a return to a 21-day shelf life might solve the problem, the impact of that action on the available blood supply would be likely to create more problems than it solves.

Syphilis is no longer common and *Treponema pallidum* is unlikely to survive more than 72 hours in citrated blood stored at 4° C. All donor units are routinely checked, and the serologic tests for syphilis (STS) must be negative as required by federal law, which takes precedence over the AABB (American Association of Blood Banks) standards, which dropped the requirement for serologic testing in 1981. Individuals with syphilis may engage in sexual practices that put them at higher risk for HIV infection, and so serologic testing may further protect the blood supply from transfusion-transmitted hepatitis and AIDS.[33]

C. Parasites

Plasmodium species (causing malaria), *Trypanosoma cruzi* (Chagas's disease), *Leishmania* (leishmaniasis, or kala-azar), *Toxoplasma gondii*, *Babesia microti*, and five species of microfilaria have all been transmitted by blood transfusion. None presents a significant problem in the United States.

V. GRAFT VERSUS HOST DISEASE

Graft versus host disease (GVH) is attributable to donor lymphocytes acting against the host and is a potential major complication in bone marrow transplant patients where the recipient is incapable of responding against allogenic lymphocytes. Viable lymphocytes in a unit of blood can also initiate the same response. Clinical findings are fever, rash, liver function abnormalities, and massive diarrhea in both bone marrow and transfusion-induced GVH; pancytopenia is more common with the latter. Prevention of GVH is readily accomplished by irradiation, and this should be considered in patients who are immunosuppressed, especially if there has been a suggestion of GVH with prior transfusions.

VI. FEBRILE REACTIONS

Approximately 1% of all transfusions are accompanied by a temperature elevation with or without chills. These reactions are usually caused by antibodies to leukocytes or platelets and occur in patients who have been previously sensitized. Leukocyte-poor components will prevent these reactions.[42]

There is no definitive test with which to make the diagnosis of a benign febrile reaction, which may also be the first sign of a hemolytic reaction or the infusion of a grossly contaminated unit. For this reason temperature elevation requires that other more ominous causes be ruled out. When necessary, the fever can usually be effectively treated with antipyretic medication if caused by leukocyte or platelet antibodies.

VII. ALLERGIC REACTIONS

Signs and symptoms of an allergic reaction occur in 1% to 2% of recipients and vary from localized urticaria to rare severe anaphylactic reaction. Although their exact cause is unknown, allergic reactions are probably caused by antibodies against plasma proteins. Fortunately most reactions are mild and respond to antihistamines.

Severe reactions manifest by bronchospasm, dyspnea, and pulmonary edema will require treatment with epinephrine and steroids. These reactions may be caused by IgG or antibodies to IgA in IgA-deficient patients. If IgA antibodies are found in recipients' serum, only extensively washed RBCs and IgA-deficient plasma should subsequently be administered to them.[42]

VIII. HEMODYNAMIC EFFECTS

The administration of blood, especially in large volumes, to the hypovolemic patient will have a beneficial effect on both blood pressure and cardiac output. However, in the patient who is in borderline heart failure the administration of even small volumes of blood may produce frank congestive heart failure and pulmonary edema.

More difficult is the situation where large volumes of blood are being administered rapidly to patients hemorrhaging massively and the hemorrhage is finally controlled. Unless the transfusion is stopped or slowed abruptly the possibility of an overshoot exists in which the hypotensive, hypovolemic patient is at risk for developing the complications related to volume overload. This latter situation is a particular risk in the elderly, patients of small stature, and patients with chronic severe anemia where there is a decreased RBC mass and an increased plasma volume.[3]

Hypotension during the administration of plasma protein fraction (PPF) was initially reported by two groups of anesthesiologists.[43-44] Because PPF was being administered rapidly to treat hypotension secondary to hypovolemia, the persistence of hypotension was interpreted as an indication for more PPF. This set up a viscous cycle associated with significant morbidity and mortality.[45] Subsequently investigation established that increased concentrations of bradykinin were present in PPF, the concentration varying greatly between lots.[46] Bland et al. commented that after the syndrome was identified more cases were quickly recognized, demonstrating once again that when an adverse reaction is defined, its apparent incidence often increases rapidly.[43]

IX. DEPLETION OF PROCOAGULANTS AND PLATELETS

Factors V and VIII, the "labile factors," and platelets are the three hemostatic agents that decay during storage. However factors V and VIII will decrease from 100% of the normal concentration levels to 20% to 50% after 2 weeks' storage, well above the concentration required for hemostasis, whereas few hemostatically viable platelets will remain after 5 days. A dilutional thrombocytopenia is the most common cause of bleeding associated with massive blood transfusion and only after significant volumes of blood have been transfused rapidly.[7-8]

X. IMMUNOSUPPRESSION

That fact that blood transfusion can effect the recipients' immune system was clearly established with the recognition that renal transplant recipients are less likely to reject their donor kidney if they had previously been transfused.[47] This is an example of a "beneficial" side effect of blood transfusion, which had equally potentially adverse effects on other disease states.

Perioperative transfusions have been correlated with early recurrence and poor prognosis in several forms of malignancy as well as increased risk of bacterial infection.[48-49] Patients receiving exchange transfusions as newborns, during cardiac surgery, or with ulcerative colitis have all demonstrated alterations in immune parameters. Most startling may be the observation that these alterations may persist for 20 years.[50] Burrows and Tartter originally suggested that blood transfusion adversely affected survival in colorectal cancer.[51] The logical suggestion that the need for blood may indicate a more advanced cancer has been refuted by other detailed studies that suggested that not only survival of colorectal cancer was adversely affected, but also that of the lung, prostate, kidney, and others. Indeed, only breast cancer studies have failed to indicate an adverse effect on survival rates. This effect is seen more clearly after whole blood transfusion than with RBCs and has been attributed to an as yet unidentified component of stored plasma (or associated cellular damage debris).[50] Currently it is believed that the effect of blood transfusion on natural killer cell function may be intimately involved with tumor progression and metastasis.

XI. METABOLIC COMPLICATIONS
A. Hypothermia

Hypothermia is a risk of administering large volumes of cold blood. Warming each unit of whole blood from 4° to 37° C requires 15 kcal, which is approximately 25% of the recipient's normal resting caloric expenditure.[8] The re-

quirement for one unit will not have a great effect on body temperature. However, in cases of massive transfusion or small recipient size, body temperature can decrease greatly. Theoretically the rapid administration of large volumes of cold blood through a central line could cool the heart selectively. Serious rhythm disturbances with adverse hemodynamic consequences may follow.

To prevent this decrease in temperature in large transfusions one should pass each unit through a blood warmer en route to the patient. Even when heat transfer is impaired by rapid infusion rate, increasing temperature from 4° to 20° to 25° C decreases the impact of the cold blood on body temperature and the recipient's caloric expenditure to maintain normothermia[52] (Fig. 21-1).

B. Citrate toxicity

Citrate toxicity was originally described by Bunker in 1955 when he reported that patients with liver disease were unable to handle the citrate load associated with massive transfusion.[53] That observation remains valid today. The advent of the ionized calcium electrode permitted a better definition of the problem. The ionized calcium concentration will decrease in direct proportion to the rate of administration of blood and return to the pretransfusion level at the same rate in the absence of liver disease. Originally the return was attributed to mobilization of calcium stores from bone and carti-

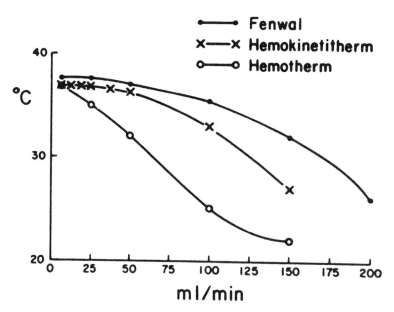

Fig. 21-1. Effect of rate of administration of blood on temperature of the infused blood. At 100 ml/min (1 unit in 5 minutes) the blood will be warmed to a range of 25° to 35° C depending on the blood warmer. This is still better than infusing blood at 4° C. (From Zauder HL: Int Anesth Clin 20:157, 1982.)

lage. Denlinger et al. clearly demonstrated that the ionized calcium was the reciprocal of the citrate concentration, confirming that the metabolism of citrate returned the ionized calcium concentration to that existing before transfusion[54] (Fig. 21-2).

The decrease in ionized calcium will be manifest in the myocardium, not the coagulation mechanism. Continuous monitoring of the ECG during rapid transfusion and looking for prolongation of the QT interval are essential during rapid transfusion, and judicious use of calcium may be indicated, especially in burn or trauma patients or those with liver disease.[52,54]

C. Acidosis

Acidosis theoretically should be a problem in that stored blood is acidotic from the instant of collection and becomes progressively worse, starting with pH 7.16 at the time of collection and decreasing to 6.73 at 35 days.[42] The combined respiratory and metabolic acidosis reflects ongoing glycolysis with lactic acid formation and CO_2 production without an escape mechanism for the latter.

The practice of empirical bicarbonate administration (such as 44.6 mEq per 5 units) to treat this acidosis is no longer recommended. Extensive analysis of patients during the Vietnam

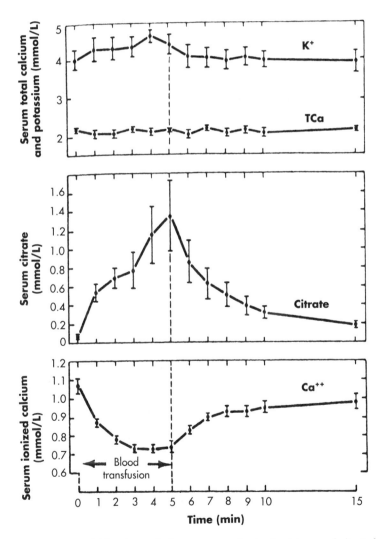

Fig. 21-2. Effect of rapid blood transfusion on serum ionized calcium and citrate levels demonstrating that as the citrate level increases the ionized calcium level decreases. Upon cessation of transfusion in patients with normal liver function the citrate will be metabolized rapidly (*TCa*, total calcium; Ca^{2+}, ionized calcium) and ionized calcium levels will return to base-line levels as the citrate level decreases. (From Denlinger JK et al: Br J Anaesth 48:995, 1976.)

War led to the recommendation that bicarbonate therapy should be based on the actual diagnosis of metabolic acidosis in the patient. In that patient population when blood pressure and perfusion were restored by transfusion the infused acid load was easily handled and any preexisting metabolic acidosis was neutralized. When the hemorrhage could not be controlled, acidemia persisted because of shock, not transfusion.[7-8]

XII. MISCELLANEOUS COMPLICATIONS

A. Microaggregates

Microaggregates form progressively in blood during storage and an industry has grown up to prevent the complications that they may cause ever since Swank originally postulated that they were a source of neurologic problems seen in patients after CPB.[55] The standard blood filter is 180 μm, and the microfilters are 20 to 40 μm. An impressive amount of debris that passes through a standard filter can be trapped in a microfilter,[56] but the clinical importance of this observation is doubtful. Clearly their role in pulmonary toxicity remains unproved speculation.[57]

B. Hyperkalemia

Hyperkalemia has been referred to by Zauder as a "myth" in that the absolute number of milliequivalents of potassium in a unit of whole blood or red blood cells is constant, and any increase in plasma potassium is mirrored by a decrease in the intracellular potassium.[52] Although hyperkalemia can be seen in hypoperfused acidotic patients, that is not a function of the transfusion—that is, as the transfused RBCs regain the ability to maintain the normal intracellular/extracellular potassium ratio, potassium will move back into the cell. In fact, hypokalemia occurs more often than hyperkalemia.

XIII. SUMMARY

The administration of blood is not without risk as this chapter has documented. Nevertheless, more than 12 million units of blood or blood components are administered annually to over 4 million patients in the United States. Their administration is undoubtedly lifesaving in many cases. Their administration may also have lethal consequences as attested to by the list of complications above. Perhaps Sherman stated it best in his editorial, "Blood transfusion is like a marriage: it should not be entered upon lightly, unadvisedly or wantonly, or more often than is absolutely necessary."[58] Conservation in the administration of all blood components is essential.

REFERENCES

1. Sazama K: Report of three hundred fifty-five transfusion-associated deaths: 1976 through 1985, Transfusion 30:583-590, 1990.
2. Sherwood WC: To err is human. . . , Transfusion 30:579-580, 1990.
3. Circular of information for the use of human blood and blood components, Washington, DC, 1987, jointly by American Association of Blood Banks, American Red Cross, and Council of Community Blood Centers.
4. Ellison N and Wurzel HA: The blood shortage: Is autotransfusion an answer? Anesthesiology 43:288-290, 1975.
5. Mollison PL: Summary of reports presented at the Sixteenth Congress of the International Society of Blood Transfusion, Vox Sang 40:289-290, 1982.
6. Ellison N: A commentary on three consensus development conferences on transfusion medicine, Anesth Clin North Am 8:609-625, 1990.
7. Miller RD: Complications of massive blood transfusion, Anesthesiology 39:82-93, 1973.
8. Collins JA: Problems associated with the massive transfusion of stored blood, Surgery 75:274-295, 1974.
9. Rutherford CJ: Transfusion-associated diseases. In Churchill WH and Kurtz SR: Transfusion medicine, Cambridge, Mass, 1988, Blackwell Scientific Publications, pp 107-127.
10. Issitt PD: Applied blood group serology, ed 3, Miami, 1985, Montgomery Scientific Publications.
11. Walker RH, Lin D-T, and Hartrick MB: Alloimmunization following blood transfusion, Arch Pathol Lab Med 113:254-261, 1989.
12. Consensus Development Conference: Platelet transfusion therapy, JAMA 257:1777-1780, 1987.
13. Pineda AA, Brzica SM Jr, and Taswell HF: Hemolytic transfusion reaction: recent experience in a large blood bank, Mayo Clin Proc 53:378-390, 1978.
14. Edinger SE: A closer look at fatal transfusion reactions, Med Lab Observer 17:40-45, 1985.
15. Myhre BA, Bove JR, and Schmidt PJ: Wrong blood—a needless cause of surgical death, Anesth Analg 60:777-778, 1981 (Editorial).
16. Honig CL and Bove JR: Transfusion-associated fatalities: review of Bureau of Biologics report 1976-1978, Transfusion 20:653-661, 1980.
17. Myhre BA: Fatalities from blood transfusion, JAMA 244:1333-1335, 1980.
18. Schmidt PJ: Transfusion mortality with special reference to surgical and intensive care facilities, J Fla Med Assoc 67:151-153, 1980.
19. Goldfinger D: Acute hemolytic transfusion reactions—a fresh look at pathogenesis and considerations regarding therapy, Transfusion 17:85-98, 1977.
20. Faust RJ, Cucchiara RF, and Messick JM Jr: Transfusion medicine and cardiovascular anesthesia. In Tarhan S, editor: Cardiovascular anesthesia and postoperative care, ed 2, St. Louis, 1989, Mosby–Year Book, Inc.
21. Popovsky MA, Abel MD, and Moore SB: Transfusion-related acute lung injury associated with passive transfer of antileukocyte antibodies, Am Rev Respir Dis 128:185-189, 1983.
22. Zuck TF: Greetings—a final look back with comments about a policy of a zero-risk blood supply, Transfusion 27:447-448, 1987.

23. Krugman S, Giles JP, and Hammond J: Infectious hepatitis: evidence for two distinctive clinical, epidemiological, and immunological types of infection, JAMA 200:365-367, 1967.

24. Blumberg BS, Gerstley BJS, Hungerford DA, et al: A serum antigen (Australia antigen) in Down's syndrome, leukemia, and hepatitis, Ann Intern Med 66:924-931, 1967.

25. Consensus Development Conference: Perioperative red blood cell transfusion, JAMA 260:2700-2703, 1988.

26. Berry AJ: Viral hepatitis, Anesth Clin North Am 7:771-794, 1989.

27. Mosley JW, Aach RD, Hollinger FB, et al: Non-A, non-B hepatitis and antibody to hepatitis C virus, JAMA 263:77-78, 1990.

28. Walsh JH, Purcell RH, and Morrow AG: Post-transfusion hepatitis after open heart operations, JAMA 211:261-265, 1965.

29. Alter, Holland PV, Purcell RH, et al: Post-transfusion hepatitis after exclusion of commercial and hepatitis-B antigen donors, Ann Intern Med 77:691-699, 1972.

30. Francis DP, Feorino PM, McDougal S, et al: The safety of hepatitis B vaccine: inactivation of the AIDS virus during routine vaccine manufacture, JAMA 256:869-872, 1987.

31. Ammann AJ, Cowan MJ, Wara DW, et al: Acquired immune deficiency in an infant: possible transmission by means of blood products, Lancet 1:956-958, 1983.

32. Curran JW, Lawrence DN, Jaffe H, et al: Acquired immune deficiency syndrome (AIDS) associated with transfusions, N Engl J Med 310:69-75, 1984.

33. Whitsett CF: Infections acquired through blood transfusion, Anesth Clin North Am 7:897-921, 1989.

34. Inaba S, Sato H, Okochi K, et al: Prevention of transmission of human T-lymphotropic virus I (HTLV-I) through transfusion by donor screening with an antibody to the virus: one year experience, Transfusion 29:7-11, 1989.

35. Prince AM, Szmuness W, Millian SJ, and David D: A serologic study of cytomegalovirus infections associated with blood transfusions, N Engl J Med 284:1125-1131, 1971.

36. Yeager AS, Grumet FC, Hafliegh EB, et al: Prevention of transfusion-acquired cytomegalovirus infections in newborn infants, J Pediatr 98:281-287, 1981.

37. Henle W and Henle G: Epstein-Barr virus and blood transfusions, Prog Clin Biol Res 182:201-209, 1985 (Review).

38. Brain HG, Kickler RS, Charache P, et al: Bacterial sepsis secondary to platelet transfusion: an adverse effect of extended storage at room temperature, Transfusion 26:391-393, 1986.

39. Reduction of the maximum platelet storage period to five days in an approved container, FDA Bull, June 2, 1986.

40. Tipple MA, Bland LA, Murphy JJ, et al: Sepsis associated with transfusion of red cells contaminated with *Yersenia enterocolitica,* Transfusion 26:209-213, 1990.

41. Aber RC: Transfusion-associated *Yersenia enterocolitica,* Transfusion 30:193-195, 1990.

42. Pisciotto PT, editor: Blood transfusion therapy, a physicians handbook, American Association of Blood Banks, ed 3, Arlington, Va, 1989, p 5.

43. Bland JHL, Laver BM, and Lowenstein E: Basodilator effect of commercial 5% plasma protein fractions solutions, JAMA 224:1721-1724, 1973.

44. Harrison GA, Torda TA, and Schiff P: Hypertensive effects of stable plasma protein solution (SPPS): a preliminary communication, Med J Aust 2:1038-1039, 1971.

45. Alving BM, Hujima Y, and Pisano JJ: Hypotension associated with prekallikrein activator (Hageman-factor fragments) in plasma protein fraction, N Engl J Med 299:66-70, 1978.

46. Ellison N, Behar M, MacVaugh III H, and Marshall BE: Bradycardia, plasma protein fraction, and hypotension, Ann Thorac Surg 29:15-19, 1980.

47. Wakeley E, Shelby J, and Corry J: The effect of peripheral blood components on allograft survival, Transplantation 40:113-114, 1985.

48. Schriemer PA, Longnecker DE, and Mintz PD: The possible immunosuppressive effects of perioperative blood transfusion in cancer patients, Anesthesiology 68:422-428, 1988.

49. Warner MA and Faust RJ: Risks of transfusion, Anesth Clin North Am 8:501-517, 1990.

50. Blumberg N and Heal JM: Transfusion and recipient immune function, Arch Pathol Lab Med 113:246-253, 1989.

51. Burrows L and Tartter P: Effect of blood transfusions on colonic malignancy recurrence rate, Lancet 2:662, 1982 (Letter).

52. Zauder HL: Massive transfusion, Int Anesthesiol Clin 20:157-170, 1982.

53. Bunker JP, Stetson JB, Coe RC, et al: Citric acid intoxication, JAMA 157:1361-1363, 1955.

54. Denlinger JK, Nahrwold ML, Gibbs DS, and Lecky JH: Hypocalcemia during rapid blood transfusion in anesthetized man, Br J Anaesth 48:995-1000, 1976.

55. Swank RL: Alteration of blood in storage: measurement of adhesiveness of "aging" platelets and leukocytes and their removal by filtration, N Engl J Med 265:728-731, 1961.

56. Marshall BE, Wurzel HA, Ellison N, et al: Microaggregates formation in stored blood. III. Comparison of Bentley, Fenwall, Pall, Swank Micropore filtration, Circ Shock 2:249-263, 1975.

57. Snyder EL and Bookbinder M: Role of microaggregate blood filtration in clinical medicine, Transfusion 23:460-470, 1983.

58. Sherman LA: The implications of trends in transfusions, Transfusion 28:511-512, 1988.

Chapter 22

Causes and Consequences of Maternal-Fetal Perianesthetic Complications

H.S. Chadwick

Brian K. Ross

Obstetric anesthesia has had a long and slow course in establishing itself as a genuine subspecialty. Although dedicated physicians such as Bonica, Crawford, and Marx have for many years practiced and taught the art and science of obstetric anesthesia, this subspecialty has not attracted interest equal to that of other areas. All too often obstetric anesthesia has been and continues to be provided by nonanesthesiologists.[1] Many obstetric suites make do with older-generation anesthesia machines and monitors no longer considered suitable for nonobstetric anesthesia. Anesthesiology-provided epidural services and dedicated full-time anesthesia coverage is the exception rather than the rule for labor and delivery. When anesthesia service is available, it is often provided by anesthesia personnel with little training or interest in the special problems of the obstetric patient. Although it is unfortunate, we believe it is timely that the current medical liability crises in obstetrics and anesthesiology are forcing the medical community to focus attention on the quality of care provided to obstetric patients.

To improve the quality of care for obstetric patients, we must study and understand the complications and consequences of obstetric anesthesia. In this way we learn from experience and can improve the safety and efficacy of anesthetic care. Such information has been derived from maternal mortality statistics, case reports, and a variety of experimental studies. Recently the American Society of Anesthesiologists' Closed Claims Study has provided a new source of information concerning complications of obstetric anesthesia.[2]

I. MATERNAL MORTALITY

Maternal mortality, defined as the number of maternal deaths per 100,000 (or 10,000) live births, has decreased dramatically in the last 30 years. The maternal mortality in the United States was reported as 83 per 100,000 live births in 1950, but by 1984 it had declined to 7.8 per 100,000.[3] The *Report on Confidential Enquiries into Maternal Mortality in England and Wales* provides one of the most comprehensive and accurate sources of information concerning maternal mortality. Each maternal death is carefully reviewed by an obstetric assessor and since 1973 by an anesthetic assessor (if an anesthetic was given). The cause of death is determined and classified using the ICD-9 (International Classification of Diseases—9th Division) scheme. These reports have been compiled for 3-year periods beginning in 1952. Maternal death is usually defined as the death of a woman while pregnant or within 42 days of termination of pregnancy from any cause related to or aggravated by the pregnancy or its management but not from accidental or incidental causes. This arbitrary time limit has been shown to miss as many as 17% of deaths because of maternal causes.[4] For this reason, recent authors have extended the time period to 90 days[3,5] or even 1 year.[6,7]

The most recent comprehensive data on maternal mortality in the United States are from Kaunitz et al.[7] Data for the years 1974 to 1978 were compiled from various sources, including maternal death certificates identified by the National Center for Health Statistics and state health departments and from state maternal mortality reports. The leading causes of death, excluding those associated with abortive outcomes, were pulmonary embolism of all types, hypertensive disease of pregnancy, obstetric hemorrhage, obstetric infection, cerebrovascular accidents, and anesthetic complications. The data from England and Wales for 1976 to 1978 are similar except that anesthetic complications were responsible for 12.4% of maternal deaths compared to the 4.0% reported by Kaunitz et al. (Table 22-1). Kaunitz et al. speculated that some anesthetic-related deaths may, because of medicolegal concerns,[7] have been attributed to other (unavoidable) causes, such as amniotic fluid embolism. Although anesthesia is by no means the leading cause, it clearly ranks among the main causes of maternal death.

The rapid decline in maternal mortality has been attributable to fewer deaths because of infection, hemorrhage, and preeclampsia. Mortalities related to anesthesia have tended to parallel the overall decline in maternal mortality.[8] Although the percentage of deaths attributable to anesthesia in England and Wales has trended upward since 1952 (Table 22-2),[9] the actual number of deaths from anesthesia reported in the *Report on Confidential Inquiries into Maternal Deaths in England and Wales* has declined since 1952. Thus, given the increase in number of anesthetics administered for cesarean section, labor, and legal abortion, one must conclude that there has been an impressive reduction in the overall risk of anesthetic-related maternal death.[9]

The leading causes of anesthetic deaths have changed over the years. Deaths caused by se-

Table 22-1. Major causes of maternal deaths in the United States and in England and Wales*

| | United States | | England and Wales | | | | | |
| | 1974-78 | | 1976-78 | | 1979-81 | | 1982-84 | |
	No.	%	No.	%	No.	%	No.	%
Embolism								
Thrombotic	271	10.9	43	19.8	23	12.9	25	18.1
Amniotic	189	7.6	11	5.1	18	10.1	14	10.1
Hypertensive disease of pregnancy	421	17.0	29	13.4	36	20.2	25	18.1
Obstetric hemorrhage	331	13.4	24	11.1	14	7.9	9	6.5
Obstetric infection	199	8.0	15	6.9	8	4.5	2	1.4
Anesthesia	98	4.0	27	12.4	22	12.4	18	13.0

*The major causes of maternal deaths in the United States and England are shown. The actual numbers and percent of all maternal deaths are indicated. Data from Kaunitz AM et al: Obstet Gynecol 65:605-612, 1985, and from Turnbull A et al: Report on confidential enquiries into maternal deaths in England and Wales 1982-1984, London, 1989, Her Majesty's Stationary Office. (Some figures in the data from London and Wales differ from previously published data because of reclassification of some deaths in the most recently published report.)

Table 22-2. Maternal deaths caused by anesthesia in England and Wales*

Years	Maternal mortality per 100,000 total births	Number of deaths caused by anesthesia	Percent of all deaths caused by anesthesia
1961-63	26	28	4.0
1964-66	20	50	8.7
1967-69	16	50	10.9
1970-72	13	37	10.4
1973-75	11	31	13.2
1976-78	11	30	13.2
1979-81	11	22	12.2

*Table adapted from Morgan M: Br J Anaesth 59:842-855, 1987.

vere hypotension associated with spinal anesthesia have decreased, and now most deaths are associated with the induction of general anesthesia.[9-11] In recent years, difficult tracheal intubation has superseded inhalation of gastric contents as the leading cause of anesthesia-related maternal mortality.[12,13] This may be attributable to the routine use of tracheal intubation, cricoid pressure, and antacid prophylaxis with general anesthesia in obstetrics. In the report from England and Wales covering the years 1982 to 1984, 10 of 18 deaths directly attributed to anesthesia were related to difficult intubation. Seven deaths were attributed to pulmonary aspiration, and 2 of these were precipitated by difficult intubation.[13] Other less common causes of death include misuse of drugs and difficulty with anesthesia equipment. In the 1982-1984 report, all anesthetic-related deaths were judged to be caused by some form of substandard care. One specifically noted factor was the frequency with which inexperienced anesthesiologists are involved in such cases. Several other risk factors that are often associated with anesthetic fatalities have been identified. In a review of anesthesia-related maternal mortality in Michigan for the years 1972 to 1984, 12 of 15 deaths were associated with the induction of general anesthesia under emergent conditions and an equal number were associated with obesity; in over half the cases hypertensive disease was a risk factor.[3]

II. CLOSED CLAIMS DATA

In 1985 the American Society of Anesthesiologists' Committee on Professional Liability began a study of insurance company files involving closed claims against anesthesiologists (see Chapter 26). Recently the subset of claims involving obstetric anesthesia was analyzed and compared to the set of nonobstetric claims.[2] Although retrospective case review studies such as this can provide useful information, they cannot provide information on the relative frequency of various complications because neither the total number of injuries nor total number of anesthetics administered is known. The most common injury for which a claim was filed was maternal death (22% of all obstetric claims), newborn brain injury (20%), and headache (12%)(Table 22-3). Seventeen of the 38 claims for newborn brain injury were judged to be caused by complications of anesthetic care. The primary anesthetic was a regional technique in 13 of these 17 claims. Included in these were 8 convulsions caused by local anesthetic toxicity and 3 unintentional high blocks. When cases involving a claim only for newborn injury were excluded, the most common injuries were maternal death (27%), headache (15%), and pain during anesthesia (11%). The high proportion of claims for relatively minor injuries such as headache, backache, and pain during anesthesia illustrate that in the obstetric setting even minor side effects and complications may result in litigation. Convulsions, most from local anesthetic toxicity, were much more common in the obstetric claims (10%) compared to the nonobstetric claims (1%) and represent the single most common event leading to an injury in the obstetric claims. As with maternal mortality data, events related to the respiratory system were the most common cause of significant complications, with difficult tracheal intubation, inadequate ventilation, pulmonary aspiration, and esophageal intubation being the most common. Although there were fewer claims involving general anesthesia in the group of obstetric claims, complications associated with general anesthesia resulted in more severe injuries and higher payments than complications involving regional anesthesia. The median payment was significantly greater in the obstetric claims than in the nonobstetric claims.

Table 22-3. Most common injuries in obstetric anesthesia claims

	Nonobstetric claims (n = 1351)		Obstetric claims (n = 190)	Obstetric regional (n = 124)		Obstetric general (n = 62)
Patient/maternal death	39% (524)	*	22% (41)	12% (15)	*	42% (26)
Newborn brain damage	NA		20% (38)	19% (23)		24% (15)
Headache	1% (10)	*	12% (23)	19% (23)	*	0% (0)
Newborn death	<0.5% (1)		9% (17)	7% (8)		10% (6)
Pain during anesthesia	<0.5% (5)	*	8% (16)	13% (16)	*	0% (0)
Patient/maternal nerve damage	16% (209)	*	8% (16)	10% (12)		7% (4)
Patient/maternal brain damage	13% (174)	*	7% (14)	7% (9)		8% (5)
Emotional distress	2% (30)		6% (12)	7% (9)		5% (3)
Back pain	1% (8)		5% (9)	7% (9)	*	0% (0)

From Chadwick HS et al: A comparison of obstetric-and non-obstetric anesthesia malpractice claims, Anesthesiology 74:242-249, 1991.
The most common injuries for which claims were made in obstetric anesthesia are shown in order of decreasing frequency. Percentages are based on the total claims in each group. Some claims had more than one injury and are represented more than once. Cases involving brain damage include only patients who were alive when the claim was closed. Statistical comparisons are made between obstetric and nonobstetric claims and between obstetric regional and obstetric general anesthetics.
*$p \leq 0.01$
NA, Not applicable.

III. MATERNAL COMPLICATIONS

A. Maternal pathophysiology and pharmacology

Pregnancy, in and of itself, is accompanied by many physiologic alterations that increase the risk for maternal complications. In some instances complications may be difficult to ascribe to a specific cause that is, anesthetic related or attributable to inherent risks associated with pregnancy. The anesthesiologist who provides care for obstetric patients must be aware of the physiologic alterations of pregnancy, the medical risks associated with pregnancy and delivery, as well as the risks associated with anesthetic interventions and how these are modified in the pregnant patient.

1. Bleeding. Obstetric hemorrhage ranks as one of the main causes of maternal mortality.[6,7] Conditions associated with an increased risk of bleeding include abruptio placentae, placenta previa, prior cesarean delivery (especially if associated with an anterior placenta), uterine atony, uterine rupture, retained placenta, and coagulation disorders. Although obstetric hemorrhage is not considered an anesthetic complication, when anesthetic care is involved, the anesthesiologist must share responsibility for assessing risk of hemorrhage, ensuring availability of blood and blood substitutes, as well as establishing a mechanism to recruit additional help if needed. Primary responsibility for ensuring adequate venous access and appropriate replacement of fluids and blood components must be assumed by the anesthesiologist. In the presence of coagulopathy, the anesthesiologist must consider the risks associated with regional anesthetic procedures, central venous catheter insertion, and potential for unexpected bleeding with obstetric procedures.

2. Embolism. Pulmonary embolism is the leading cause of maternal mortality, with thromboembolism being most common.[7,13] The hypercoagulability associated with pregnancy and the sluggish venous blood flow in the pelvis and lower extremities predispose the parturient to deep venous thrombosis and thromboembolism.[14] Massive pulmonary embolism of any type results in sudden hypotension and cardiac collapse. Smaller embolic events can present with a variety of nonspecific signs and symptoms including dyspnea, tachypnea, hypoxemia, cough, and rales. Amniotic fluid embolism is considered to be a rare and usually fatal complication of pregnancy;[15] respiratory distress, cyanosis, and cardiovascular collapse may occur rapidly. Unlike with other forms of embolism, disseminated intravascular coagulation is believed to accompany amniotic fluid embolism.[15] If a central venous or pulmonary artery catheter is in place, it may be possible to confirm the diagnosis by recovering fetal squamous cells, fat from vernix caseosa, or lanugo hair. Some authors believe that embolism of fetal or placental tissue may be much more common than previously believed.[16,17] Air embolism, once believed to be a very rare complication in obstetrics, has been detected using precordial Doppler monitoring in 11% to 52% of cesarean deliveries.[18,19] Malinow et al. found that chest pain and dyspnea were closely associated with evidence of air embolism.[19] Because of the nonspecific nature of signs, symptoms, and results of diagnostic tests, it may not always be clear whether a pulmonary or cardiac problem was the result of an embolic event or some other cause. Acute cardiac failure, pulmonary aspiration, and drug reactions may mimic pulmonary embolism. In the event of death, an autopsy may be necessary to confirm the diagnosis.

3. Tocolysis. Modern tocolytic agents such as the beta mimetics (such as terbutaline and ritodrine) and magnesium sulfate allow obstetricians to manage preterm labor or temporarily stop labor for maternal or fetal indications. These drugs can have potent physiologic effects that may complicate anesthetic management. Although it is the $beta_2$ effect that is responsible for inhibition of uterine activity, all commonly used beta-mimetic tocolytic agents have some $beta_1$ activity. Schneider et al. studied 32 women receiving ritodrine as therapy for preterm labor and found cardiac symptoms in 31%, significant dysrhythmias in 10% to 20%, and ECG changes consistent with ischemia in 10% to 20%.[20] Pulmonary edema has also been associated with the use of tocolytics.[21] The pathophysiologic processes involved are not clear, but risk factors include preeclampsia, multiple gestation, preexisting cardiac or pulmonary disease, and signs of infection. Anesthesiologists should look for decreasing hematocrit without bleeding, dyspnea, tachypnea, wheezing, and cough. Particular consideration should be given to appropriate monitoring, careful fluid balance, and choice of anesthetic agents.[22] Halothane should be avoided because of its propensity to sensitize the heart to epinephrine-induced premature ventricular beats.

4. Pregnancy-induced hypertension. Pregnancy-induced hypertension (PIH) affects up to 30% of pregnancies in some populations[23,24] and is the second leading cause of maternal mortality in the United States.[7] Most of these deaths occur in patients with preeclampsia or eclampsia, which affects about 7% of all pregnancies.[25] Preeclampsia is characterized by the triad of hypertension, proteinuria, and generalized edema, usually occurring after the twentieth week of gestation. The proximate cause of death in half of these cases is intracranial hemorrhage or cerebral edema.[26] Despite the prevalence of this disease, little is known about its etiology. The peripartum period is the time of greatest risk for the parturient.

Preeclampsia involves many pathophysiologic alterations that can pose particular problems for the anesthesiologist. Coagulation problems are common and can include decreased platelet count, abnormal platelet function, and prolonged thrombin time.

Thrombocytopenia occurs in 18% of women with preeclampsia[27] and even those without thrombocytopenia may have prolonged bleeding times.[27,28] Preeclampsia is the most common cause of consumptive coagulopathy in the obstetric population though it is usually not severe.[29] The anesthesiologist must pay particular attention to the risks associated with regional anesthetic procedures as well as risks of hematoma associated with placement of central venous and pulmonary artery catheters.

Hypertension, by definition a hallmark of preeclampsia, may be severe and can present problems in anesthetic management. Of particular concern is the potential for an exaggerated hypertensive response to trachial intubation. This could lead to intracranial hemorrhage, the leading cause of mortality in preeclamptic women,[26] transtentorial herniation in the presence of cerebral edema,[30] or pulmonary edema caused by acute left ventricular failure.[31]

Another characteristic of preeclampsia is generalized edema often accompanied by intravascular volume depletion and hemoconcentration. Sympathetic blockade associated with regional anesthesia can quickly lead to hypotension and fetal distress. For this reason, some recommend against the use of epidural anesthesia in patients with preeclampsia or eclampsia.[32] Others, however, have pointed out the advantages of epidural analgesia, particularly in preeclamptic women. These include maternal analgesia without the need for systemic depressant drugs, reduced maternal catecholamine levels,[33] improved placental blood flow,[34] and the ability to facilitate obstetric procedures. Careful attention must be given to restoring adequate intravascular fluid volume before and during onset of epidural block. This process must be undertaken with great care because of the risk of precipitating pulmonary edema[35] or cerebral edema,[36,36] or both. Epidural analgesia can, however, be used safely, even in many severely preeclamptic patients, by careful titration of intravascular volume and epidural local anesthetic.[37] In some patients this may require a central venous or pulmonary artery pressure catheter in addition to the usual monitors.

5. Aorto-caval compression. Aorto-caval compression, although not a complication of anesthetic care, can modify actions of anesthetics to increase the likelihood of adverse outcomes. Supine hypotension syndrome in pregnancy was first described in 1953.[38] Ten percent to 15% of patients at term will develop hypotension, tachycardia (or bradycardia), and sometimes nausea when they are supine. Although only a minority of patients will become hypotensive, up to 90% will have decreased venous return and decreased cardiac output because of compression of the inferior vena cava by the gravid uterus.[39] Most patients are able to compensate for the decrease in cardiac output by increasing systemic vascular resistance. When this compensatory mechanism is attenuated, as with epidural block, the result can be unexpected and profound hypotension. Since uterine perfusion is in large measure pressure dependent, even relatively modest degrees of hypotension may not be well tolerated by the fetus.[40] Even in the absence of hypotension, the increased systemic vascular resistance or direct compression of the aorta by the uterus may result in decreased uterine perfusion and may adversely affect fetal well-being. Maintaining laboring women in the supine position is associated with a progressive decrease in fetal blood pH. We continue to be amazed at how frequently, even in the modern tertiary care center, the effects related to aorto-caval compression are allowed to occur and go unrecognized by trained health care professionals.

B. Complications associated with general anesthesia

The majority of anesthetic deaths in the obstetric population are associated with general anesthesia. The two main causes of these deaths are inhalation of gastric contents and failure to intubate the trachea.

1. Aspiration of gastric contents. Aspiration of gastric contents is the only cause of maternal death that has not declined in the last 20 years,[41] accounting for 6% to 22% of the anesthetic-related deaths in nonpregnant patients and between 28% to 36% of maternal deaths.[42]

Pregnancy increases the threat of aspiration. Gastric emptying is decreased after the thirty-fourth week of pregnancy because of mechanical displacement of both the gastroesophageal junction and pylorus and the combined effects of increased plasma progesterone concentra-

tion[43] and decreased plasma levels of the hormone motilin,[44] which result in slowed gastric motility. Gastric motility is also slowed by the pain of labor, fear, apprehension, and the use of opioids for treating labor pain. Roberts and Shirley found that 25% of women undergoing cesarean section may be at risk for aspiration of acid gastric contents, regardless of the interval between the last meal and the onset of labor.[45]

Antacids increase gastric fluid pH and should reduce the risk of acid-aspiration injury. Gibbs, however, demonstrated that dilute solutions of particulate antacids introduced in the lungs of dogs produce acute pulmonary injury comparable to that produced by instillation of acid.[46] Recent studies using 0.3 molar sodium citrate, a nonparticulate antacid, have demonstrated it to be effective for increasing gastric pH.[47,48] A disadvantage of sodium citrate is its brief duration of effectiveness (2 to 3 hours), necessitating its use shortly before induction of anesthesia.

Blocking gastric histamine (H_2) receptors reduces both gastric volume and acidity without adversely affecting the neonate.[49,50] However, there has been concern that the pharmacokinetic interaction between H_2 antagonists and local anesthetics might lead to inhibition of local anesthetic metabolism resulting in local anesthetic toxicity.[51,52] This concern applies less to ranitidine than to cimetidine, and less to bupivacaine than to lidocaine. Dailey et al. suggest that the cimetidine-lidocaine interaction may not be as clinically important as was first believed.[53] Nonetheless, ranitidine may be the preferred H_2 blocker, since its duration of action exceeds that of cimetidine and it is less likely to interfere with hepatic metabolism.

Emptying the stomach has been suggested to be useful in the prevention of pulmonary aspiration. Brock-Utne et al., however, found that, in addition to being unpleasant, gastric suction by means of a large-bore tube does not guarantee an empty stomach or decrease the number of patients at risk from acid aspiration.[54] Metoclopramide may be a useful adjunct to decrease the risk of aspiration because it increases lower esophageal sphincter tone, speeds gastric emptying, and does not adversely affect the neonate.[55,56] At least 15 minutes is required for metoclopramide to reduce gastric volume.[57]

In summary, an H_2-receptor antihistamine combined with a nonparticulate antacid, such as sodium citrate, seems to be most effective at minimizing the risk of acid aspiration.[58] Remember that no drug or combination of drugs removes completely the risk of acid aspiration.

2. Difficult or failed intubation. Difficulty

with tracheal intubation during anesthetic induction is a life-threatening situation. There is little doubt that the trachea of obstetric patients may be more difficult to intubate than that of their nonobstetric counterparts. The parturient, especially the preeclamptic, may have pharyngeal and laryngeal edema.[59,60] The airway mucosa is hyperemic and prone to bleed. Large breasts may impair proper laryngoscope positioning for visualization of the cords and hamper proper application of cricoid pressure. Improperly applied cricoid pressure can distort or displace laryngeal anatomy or occlude the esophagus inadequately. Additionally, the thorax may be lifted into an unusual position by a hip wedge. Finally, there is a tendency to attempt tracheal intubation before the muscle relaxant has taken full effect.

To minimize the complications of failed intubation, the entire labor and delivery staff should be familiar with a failed tracheal intubation protocol. There are no hard and fast rules as to the techniques and steps one should utilize. New devices that have been found to be useful during difficult intubations and with which anesthesiologists should become familiar are the woven endotracheal tube introducer (Eschmann stylet) and a jet ventilating device that may allow oxygenation or ventilation through a cricothyroid or cricotracheal membrane puncture (Sanders device).[61] The parturient is prone to rapid desaturation because of increased oxygen consumption and reduced oxygen reserve because of a reduced functional residual capacity.[62] Therefore keep in mind that options may be limited because of the foreshortened time interval from apnea to desaturation. Preoxygenation is a standard technique for minimizing hypoxemia during induction. The use of pulse oximetry has led some to believe that 4 vital capacity breaths are as efficacious as 3 minutes of preoxygenation before induction.[63,64] Recent studies looking at denitrogenation as an end point of preoxygenation have shown that 8 to 10 vital capacity breaths or 3 full minutes of normal ventilation with the anesthetic system fully "charged" with oxygen are required for adequate denitrogenation.[58,65] There are few

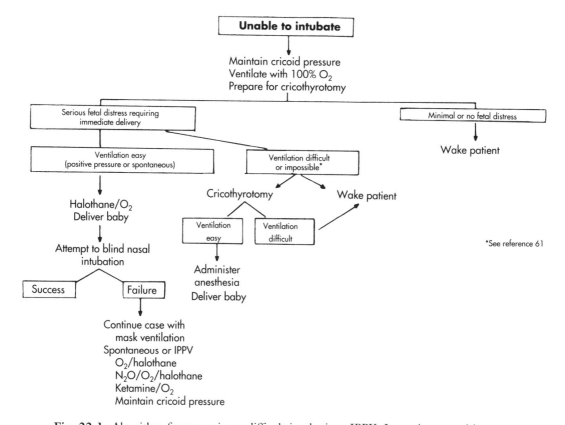

Fig. 22-1. Algorithm for managing a difficult intubation. *IPPV,* Intermittent positive-pressure ventilation. (From Shnider SM and Levinson G: Anesthesia for cesarean section. In Shnider SM and Levinson G: Anesthesia for obstetrics, ed 2, Baltimore, 1987, Williams & Wilkins.)

situations, even in obstetrics, which are of such emergency that even 30 seconds cannot be devoted to thorough denitrogenation before induction of anesthesia. In the event of inability to intubate the trachea, bag-mask ventilation with correctly applied cricoid pressure must be promptly initiated and a decision made whether to continue with the procedure or awaken the patient. Fig. 22-1 is an example of an algorithm used in the event of a failed tracheal intubation in the obstetric patient.

Related to the problem of difficult tracheal intubation is unrecognized esophageal intubation. The signs of esophageal intubation should be obvious, but anesthesiologists continue to be misled. Signs such as bilateral breath sounds, fogging of the endotracheal tube, and absence of sounds over the epigastrium are time-honored indications of proper endotracheal tube placement. However, the continuing presence of carbon dioxide in exhaled gas is the only absolute diagnostic test of correct placement of the endotracheal tube.[66,67] Every obstetric anesthetizing location must be equipped with a device for detecting exhaled carbon dioxide. These detectors can be as sophisticated as mass spectrometry or infrared capnography, or as simple as qualitative CO_2 detectors. Recently, chemical indicators capable of detecting CO_2 in 1 or 2 breaths have become available (Fenem Airway Management Systems, New York, NY).[68] List 22-1 summarizes suggested precautions to be taken to minimize complications from the induction of general anesthesia in the parturient.

3. Awareness during general anesthesia. Maternal awareness is a concern that must be addressed when general anesthesia is employed. The incidence of awareness in the obstetric population can vary from 7% to as high as 25%.[69,70] A major conflict arises when a general anesthetic is provided to the parturient to render her unconscious and at the same time have minimal effects on the uterus and infant. There are three periods during which maternal awareness is likely to occur: during or shortly after tracheal intubation (usually an implication of inadequate dose of induction agent); at the time of delivery (an implication that an insufficient anesthetic agent has been provided); during the insertion of the final skin sutures or staples (insufficient anesthesia in an attempt to provide rapid awakening).

The ideal induction agent has not been found for the obstetric patient. Thiopental in doses of 4 mg/kg has been found to be safe for the mother and reliable at producing amnesia during induction.[71] However, because thiopental readily crosses the placenta, there are concerns

---

List 22-1. Suggested Precautions for the Induction of General Anesthesia in the Parturient

1. Familiarization with a failed intubation protocol for all delivery room personnel
2. Careful evaluation of the patient's airway—if difficult, consider:
   • Awake tracheal intubation
   • Regional anesthesia
3. Routine prophylaxis with a nonparticulate antacid, H_2-blocker, metoclopramide
4. Rapid sequence induction of anesthesia with properly applied cricoid pressure (Sellick's maneuver)
5. Immediate verification of proper endotracheal tube replacement by:
   • Electronic end-tidal CO_2 monitor
   • Fenem CO_2 detector
6. Assessment to rule out right main-stem endobronchial intubation
7. Awake tracheal extubation

---

of neonatal depression. Methohexital provides adequate early amnesia but confers no advantage over thiopental in its neonatal effects.[72] Ketamine in doses of 1 mg/kg has been shown to be an alternative to thiopental in reducing early maternal awareness with little or no neonatal depression.[73] A new induction agent, propofol, has recently been released in the United States. Fetal well-being, as judged by Apgar scores and cord blood gases, was not different from that of infants whose mothers underwent thiopental induction.[74] Propofol, however, should not be used until further studies can be performed to evaluate its efficacy and safety in obstetric patients.

Minimizing drug-induced depression of the neonate can result in a high incidence of maternal awareness. Moir demonstrated that lack of maternal awareness could be ensured with an inspired mixture of 0.5% halothane in 50% oxygen and 50% nitrous oxide without harm to the neonate.[75] Similar results have been noted with equipotent concentrations of other potent inhalation anesthetics.[69] The incidence of awareness varies inversely with the concentration of nitrous oxide and the volatile anesthetic.[70] It is now apparent that a small amount of volatile anesthetic (0.5 MAC) and nitrous oxide (50%) reaching the fetus during the interval between induction of anesthesia and delivery is of little or no consequence to the ultimate well-being of the infant.[76] The maternal stress response, likely to be evoked by awareness, may lead to reduced uteroplacental perfusion and is potentially much more harmful to the infant.[77]

4. Uterine atony. Uterine atony occurs in approximately 2% to 5% of all vaginal deliveries.[78] In a report by Gibbs of 501 consecutive maternal deaths in Texas, postpartum uterine atony was the leading cause of death in the parturient.[79] The risk of uterine atony is increased with high parity, multiple births, polyhydramnios, large infants, retained placenta, and general anesthesia. Local anesthetics have not been associated with uterine atony.

The volatile anesthetics produce a dose-related decrease in uterine contractility and tone thereby increasing the risk of postpartum bleeding.[80] Increased blood loss, however, has not been consistently demonstrated with low-dose halothane (0.1% to 0.8%), enflurane (0.5% to 1.5%), or isoflurane (0.75%).[81,82] The uterine relaxation induced by low-dose volatile anesthetics can be overcome with intravenous oxytocin after delivery.[83] Fear of uterine atony should not preclude the use, at least initially, of volatile anesthetics during general anesthesia for cesarean section. If after delivery there is evidence of uterine atony, the volatile anesthetic can be discontinued, nitrous oxide concentration increased to 70%, and an opioid and benzodiazepine can be added to ensure maternal anesthesia and amnesia.

C. Complications associated with regional anesthesia

1. Global concerns. A national survey by Gibbs and colleagues indicates that most of the anesthetic interventions for obstetric patients in this country involve regional anesthesia.[1] Not surprisingly many complications have been associated with the use of regional anesthesia. Many complications are common to both spinal and epidural techniques, whereas others are usually associated with the particular type of regional anesthetic.

a. Hypotension. The most common causes of maternal death associated with regional anesthesia are mismanagement of hypotension and local anesthetic toxicity. Hypotension is undoubtedly the most common complication seen with spinal or epidural anesthesia in the parturient. One of the major reasons for hypotension is decreased venous return to the heart because of partial occlusion of the inferior vena cava by the gravid uterus.[39,84,85] Hypotension may be worsened by obvious or occult peripartum blood loss. In the face of a regional block, acute intravascular volume changes may be poorly tolerated, since the normal physiologic compensatory mechanisms are blocked by sympathectomy.

Maternal organ systems will tolerate moderate degrees of hypotension. However, since the uterus is essentially a nonautoregulating organ,[86] uterine blood flow will decrease linearly with decreased perfusion pressure. Because of this, the placenta may be inadequately perfused while the parturient remains asymptomatic. It is difficult to predict at what maternal blood pressure fetal asphyxia will develop. It appears that uteroplacental anatomy, base-line maternal blood pressure, and duration of hypoperfusion are all critical. Fetal bradycardias, acidosis, and low Apgar scores have been reported with maternal systolic blood pressures of less than 100 mm Hg for periods of 5 to 15 minutes.[40,87,88] Clinical experience has shown that signs of fetal distress often occur at systolic blood pressures greater than 100 mm Hg in hypertensive patients. On the other hand, fetuses of mothers who normally have systolic blood pressures of less than 100 mm Hg seem to tolerate this without difficulty.

Patients with pregnancy-induced hypertension are at particular risk of becoming hypotensive with regional anesthesia. Reduced intravascular volume, which may be less than 80% of normal pregnant values,[89] predisposes these patients to significant hypotension with the onset of even partial sympathectomy. The risk of fetal distress is further compounded by the fact that these patients often have abnormal placental vasculature and uteroplacental insufficiency. Any intervention that may decrease maternal blood pressure, such as antihypertensive therapy or regional block, must be initiated in a slow, controlled fashion with attention to intravascular volume status.[37] Fetal heart rate monitoring, when available, should be used by the anesthesiologist in conjunction with more routine monitors to gauge the effects of anesthetic intervention.

To prevent potential complications to mother or fetus, it is imperative that the anesthesiologist take all necessary steps to avoid hypotension in the obstetric patient. This includes avoiding aorto-caval compression, adequate fluid preloading, and vasopressor therapy when necessary. Ephedrine has been shown to have the least detrimental effect on uterine perfusion and is considered to be the vasopressor of choice in obstetric patients.[90] As a rule of thumb, a systolic blood pressure of 100 mm Hg should be used as a lower limit in previously normotensive patients. In the hypertensive patient, any sudden decrease in blood pressure of greater than 20% should be treated. A recent clinical study in which low-risk patients were treated in accordance with this usual rule of thumb demonstrated that changes in maternal blood pressure were not correlated with any signs of fetal distress.[91]

b. High segmental blockade. Higher-than-anticipated blocks can be a cause of complications in the obstetric patient. The most common complication associated with high block is hypotension. If hypotension is severe, loss of consciousness will occur resulting in loss of protective airway reflexes. Nausea and vomiting is commonly associated with hypotension and in the presence of depressed airway reflexes may lead to pulmonary aspiration of gastric contents. If neuraxial block extends into the cervical segments, respiratory insufficiency can occur from intercostal and diaphragmatic paralysis.

There is controversy regarding local anesthetic requirement of pregnant patients having epidural or spinal anesthesia.[92] It is generally believed that the epidural and subarachnoid requirements of the parturient are approximately one third those of nonpregnant women.[93-95] In the case of epidural blocks this may be attributable to wider spread of anesthetic solution because of epidural venous engorgement. Similarly, spinal cerebrospinal fluid volume may be reduced resulting in greater spread of anesthetic solution administered into the lumbar subarachnoid space. Recently, several studies have indicated that peripheral neuronal tissue in gravid animals and humans may be more sensitive to the effects of local anesthetics.[96,97] Although there exists some controversy about the local anesthetic requirements for pregnant patients, it is evident from clinical experience that there is great variability in the extent of block achieved with usual doses of local anesthetic in parturients. It behooves the practitioner to be aware of potentially decreased anesthetic requirements and to take a conservative approach.

c. Neurologic injury

(1) NEUROPATHIES IN THE PERIPARTUM PERIOD. Among complications of childbirth, neurologic injury can result from both obstetric and anesthetic causes. Regional anesthesia always carries some risk of neurologic injury; therefore a postpartum neurologic deficit in a patient having a regional anesthetic will inevitably focus suspicion on the anesthetic. The obstetric anesthesiologist must therefore be able to distinguish among symptoms of preexisting disease, symptoms attributable to pregnancy or delivery, and complications related to the anesthetic. Postpartum neurologic complications are much more likely to arise from obstetric or natural causes than from peripartum regional anesthesia. The

incidence of neurologic complications after regional anesthesia is estimated at 1 in 11,000[98] to 1 in 20,000,[99] well below the 1 in 3000 that may be expected in parturients not having an anesthetic.[100]

Any form of neuritis may occur in pregnancy. Refer to several excellent articles reviewing both the common neuropathies of pregnancy and those associated with the administration of anesthesia in the parturient.[100-104] Although most neuropathies have unknown causes, some are attributable to unsuspected trauma, excessive weight gain, fluid retention during pregnancy, the hormonal changes of pregnancy, and underlying medical conditions often aggravated by pregnancy. Peripartum polyneuropathies are usually the result of pregnancy and are seldom seen as a result of anesthetic trespass. The differential diagnosis in patients with diffuse peripheral polyneuropathy is no different from that in the nonpregnant patient and includes metabolic disease, collagen vascular disease, and medications.

Mononeuropathies are the most troubling of the neuropathies for the obstetric anesthesiologist because these can often mimic complications of general or regional anesthesia. Any of the cranial nerves can be affected. The brachial plexus may be compressed between the clavical and first rib from the increased weight of the breasts and abdomen combined with sagging of the shoulder. Sensory loss, pain, and shoulder wasting may ensue. Neuropathy of the ulnar nerve, sometimes in association with median nerve involvement, has been described in the peripartum period. Full recovery usually occurs after delivery. Median neuropathy at the wrist (carpal tunnel syndrome), the most common mononeuropathy in the upper extremity, occurs in at least 7% or more of parturients.[105]

Neuropathy of the lateral femoral cutaneous nerve (meralgia paresthetica, meaning 'paresthetic thigh pain') was first described by Burnhart and Roth in 1895.[105] Mild sensory loss to touch and pinprick with occasional hyperesthesia may develop; because this nerve is purely sensory, no motor impairment is seen. During pregnancy, symptoms usually begin in the last trimester.[106] The lateral femoral cutaneous nerve has a very long course and thus may be stretched by the increased weight and exaggerated lordosis of pregnancy.[107] The exact cause of damage to the nerve is unknown, but injury may occur inside the pelvic wall, as it passes beneath the inguinal ligament, or at the fascia lata. Symptoms may be permanent but most often resolve within 3 months after delivery. The femoral nerve may be injured during vaginal delivery, cesarean section, hysterectomy, or other lower abdominal procedures.[108,109] This nerve is vulnerable to compression from retractors positioned against the greater psoas muscle, from hemorrhage into the iliopsoas muscle, and from trauma as it leaves the abdomen adjacent to the femoral artery. The prognosis is good in most cases; however, on occasion there may be pain and persistent weakness for several months. Neuropathy of the obturator nerve is rare but may be caused by a difficult labor, hematoma, or compression from the fetal head or high forceps. Sciatic neuropathy may occur during pregnancy, particularly during the last trimester as the sacral plexus is compressed by the fetus.[110] Pain is sometimes severe enough to warrant bed rest. Permanent injury is rare, and symptoms clear quickly after delivery. The lateral peroneal nerve may be compressed as it crosses the fibular head by poorly positioned leg supports resulting in foot drop.[102] Alternative theories for this nerve lesion include compression of the lumbosacral trunk, particularly after prolonged labor and mid–forceps delivery in females with platypelloid pelvices. Foot drop, in these circumstances, should be unilateral and on the same side as the infant's brow. Prognosis is good for complete resolution of this injury. Radiculopathies caused by a combination of physical effects of pregnancy (effect of relaxin on joint ligaments) and trauma (changing posture and weight associated with pregnancy) are also relatively common. Radicular symptoms have been observed to appear during pregnancy in 39% of parous females with surgically proved lumbar disk protrusions,[111] most often involving the L5-S1 disk. Symptoms may occur at any time during pregnancy, labor, delivery, or early postpartum period. Motor weakness may be severe.

Bladder dysfunction is seen frequently in the obstetric patient. Although bladder symptoms are common during pregnancy, nervous system lesions causing these symptoms are infrequent. Prolonged pressure on the pelvic nerves by the fetal head in the second stage of labor or during a difficult delivery can lead to partial denervation of the bladder resulting in a hypotonic, distended bladder with frequency, and postvoid residual volume.

Backache is frequently attributed to spinal or epidural anesthesia. Grove reported the incidence of backache after nonepidural vaginal deliveries to be 40% in patients with spontaneous deliveries and 25% in patients with instrumented deliveries.[112] Crawford reported an incidence of 45% in parturients treated with epidural anesthesia, which is only slightly greater than that in parturients not receiving epidural anesthesia, in Grove's study.[113] It appears that the incidence of backache in the parturient is 30% to 40% regardless of whether regional or general anesthesia is used. The cause is probably related to ligamentous strain from pregnancy.

(2) ANESTHETIC-ASSOCIATED NEUROPATHIES. Nerve injury associated with general anesthesia in obstetrics can and does occur (Table 22-3). These injuries are not discussed here because they are covered elsewhere in this text. The complications from regional anesthesia are also not discussed in detail because they are covered in Chapters 3 and 4. However, those symptom complexes associated with obstetric anesthesia are discussed briefly.

Prolonged neural blockade attributable to local anesthetic action must be considered with any of the local anesthetic agents used for spinal or epidural anesthesia. However, prolonged neural blockade (greater than 48 hours) has been reported only after repeated epidural injections of 0.5% bupivacaine for labor.[114-116] Extended blockade in obstetric patients has been attributed to accumulation of highly lipid-soluble agents. The block usually resolves without long-lasting untoward effects.

Trauma to nerve pathways from spinal or epidural needles and catheters is extremely rare.[98,117] If nerve roots are injured, symptoms may occur over the segment or segments involved, and symptoms usually resolve spontaneously. Sensory roots are more often affected than motor roots are. Nerve root injury is more common after spinal than after epidural anesthesia. Trauma to the spinal cord can be avoided if dural puncture or epidural placement is caudal to the conus medullaris (L1-L2). Nerve root trauma is usually heralded by severe lancing pain with needle placement, which, if elicited, should result in immediate withdrawal of the needle. Epidural and intrathecal catheters have been suspected of causing trauma to spinal roots. There is little objective evidence in the literature of trauma caused by an epidural catheter. The use of intrathecal catheters, particularly of the microcatheter design (26 to 32 gauge), has increased significantly in the last year. Intrathecal catheters may be more likely to damage the spinal cord and roots of the cauda equina. In addition to the possibility of direct trauma, a recent report by Rigler et al. detailed four cases of cauda equina syndrome occurring after continuous spinal anesthesia using microcatheters. They postulated that the combination of maldistribution and a relatively high dose of local anesthetic resulted in neurotoxic injury.[117a] In addition, catheter breakage with the microcatheters has been reported. The risk of neurologic injury and loss of catheter tips with the use of subarachnoid catheters should not be dismissed lightly.

The anesthesiologist should have an organized and thorough approach to the patient presenting with neurologic symptoms. Questions that are helpful to ask include: What is the nature of the symptom (sensory, motor, both; unilateral, bilateral); what is the location of the suspected lesion, can it be explained on an anatomic and physiologic basis; are there related medical conditions that might explain the symptoms; are there circumstances surrounding the pregnancy, labor, and delivery that might be the cause of the suspected lesion (that is, protracted labor, difficult or instrument delivery, cesarean section, and use of retractors); and were there any difficulties during the anesthetic that might explain the lesion? A careful physical exam should document sensory and motor deficits as either segmental or peripheral. The results of the history and physical exam will dictate the need for additional consultation and diagnostic tests.

d. Regional anesthesia in patients with coagulopathy. Coagulopathy has been considered an absolute contraindication to regional anesthesia in the obstetric patient.[118] This is especially true for labor analgesia where there may be no clear medical indication for the procedure other than the relief of pain associated with a normal physiologic process. The risk of epidural, subdural, or subarachnoid hematoma with neuraxial block seem obvious, though it is difficult to quantify such risk. Hematomas may occur spontaneously even in the absence of risk factors.[119] Neuraxial hematoma formation has been reported as occurring after lumbar puncture, often in association with anticoagulation therapy.[120] However, no case reports can be found in which a regional anesthetic procedure in an obstetric patient with coagulopathy resulted in neurologic injury as a result of hematoma formation.[121] This may be because regional anesthetics are avoided in such patients or because such cases have not been reported in the literature.

Anesthetic interventions in obstetrics are frequently required on an urgent or emergent basis, often before laboratory results and coagulation studies are available. Retrospective studies have indicated that a significant number of parturients have received epidural anesthetics with platelet counts being considerably below normal.[121,122] This can be a particular problem in preeclamptic patients who, in addition to thrombocytopenia, often have a defect in platelet function, which can prolong bleeding time.[28] None of the studies above have found neurologic injury as a result of neuraxial hematoma even in the obstetric patient at risk. A review of the American Society of Anesthesiologists' closed claims data base containing over 250 closed claims involving obstetric anesthesia for the years 1976 to 1989 found no claims related to neuraxial hematoma formation. Although neuraxial hematoma is a devastating complication requiring immediate surgical decompression, the incidence appears to be exceedingly low. Prudence would dictate avoiding regional procedures in parturients with abnormal coagulation parameters; however, in cases where conduction anesthesia offers particular advantages, the benefits may outweigh the potential risks.[37,121]

e. Regional anesthesia in patients with infection. The potential for spreading infection to the neuraxis has been the main contraindication of regional anesthetic techniques in patients with active infections. Skin infections over the site of needle insertion might allow spread of infection to the epidural space or to the subarachnoid space. Vascular trauma during regional procedures may allow blood-borne organisms to seed infection in the epidural or subarachnoid space, resulting in epidural abscess or meningitis.

Epidural abscesses have usually been the result of osteomyelitis or spontaneous hematogenous spread, and the risks associated with epidural anesthesia seem to be very low.[123] Most cases related to regional anesthesia were reported in the early days of caudal anesthesia for labor.[124] Meningitis after regional anesthesia is also rare, though 3 cases were reported recently in association with epidural anesthesia. One case may have involved the introduction of blood-borne bacteria into the cerebrospinal fluid during unintentional subarachnoid puncture or during subsequent blood patching.[125] The second case involved an uncomplicated epidural anesthetic for labor and delivery with subsequent meningitis caused by a bacterium common in dental carries.[126] In the third case, introduction of bacteria from the skin surface may have been the likely cause of meningitis.[126] In another recent case report, meningitis was described as occurring after obstetric spinal anesthesia for removal of a retained placenta.[127] In that case it was not clear whether the cause was chemical irritation or a partially treated bacterial infection. Although such cases are very rare, the potential for neuraxial infection, introduced either from the skin or from organisms in the blood, must be considered.

The use of regional anesthesia in patients with chorioamnionitis is controversial.[128,129] Since these patients frequently have positive blood cultures, the risk of seeding infection is a possibility. Some anesthesiologists will, however, initiate regional anesthetics in parturients with amnionitis if antibiotic therapy is being given, and they are not grossly septic. This practice has not resulted in reports of epidural abscess or meningitis.

Similar concerns about spreading infection by needle trauma have been raised in pregnant patients with herpes infections. Herpes simplex virus, type 2 (HSV-2) is an increasingly common infection in women of childbearing age. In the greater Seattle area approximately 30% of women of childbearing age are seropositive for HSV-2, and 8% to 10% have symptoms consistent with recurrent outbreaks (Z.A. Brown, personal communication, 1990). Approximately 30% to 50% of women with a history of recurrent HSV-2 infections are delivered by cesarean section.[130] Regional anesthesia seems to be safe in patients with recurrent HSV-2 infections[131,132] perhaps because these recrudescences are not associated with viremia. However, since primary infections are associated with viremia and often severe generalized symptoms such as fever, lymphadenopathy, and headache, it is advisable to avoid regional anesthesia in patients with primary infections.

f. Pain and emotional injury. Examination of obstetric anesthesia closed claims files reveals that 32% of the injuries claimed were for headache, backache, pain during anesthesia, and emotional injury (Table 22-3.)[2] These problems are rarely considered to be significant anesthetic complications, but it is clear that many women are distressed sufficiently to initiate legal action. Most of these cases involved anesthesia for cesarean section, and most of the anesthetics involved were regional techniques. Obstetric patients may be at greater risk for some of these complications (such as post–dural puncture headache) by virtue of age, gender, and the popularity of regional anesthesia in this setting. However, even allowing for a greater risk of such complications, there appear to be a disproportionate number of claims for relatively minor injury in obstetric anesthesia compared to nonobstetric anesthesia. The reasons for this are not clear; however, postpartum emotional liability and depression[133,134] or unrealistic expectations may play a role. Birthing educators should include preparation for unexpected operative delivery, and anesthesiologists should compassionately but accurately describe the procedures and experiences that a woman may encounter during anesthesia for obstetric procedures.

2. Spinal anesthesia. In addition to the general concerns of regional anesthesia in the obstetric patient outlined above, two deserve particular emphasis with relation to spinal anesthesia. These are the risks of hypotension and post–dural puncture headache (PDPH).

a. Hypotension. As discussed previously, hypotension is of particular concern in the obstetric patient because of the necessity to maintain adequate uterine perfusion pressure. Spinal anesthesia can result in sudden and profound hypotension, especially in the hypovolemic patient, because of the rapidity with which sympathetic block develops. Intravascular volume status may be difficult to assess in the presence of occult hemorrhage (such as abruptio placenta) or in the patient with pregnancy-induced hypertension. In such circumstances, the rush to provide an emergently needed anesthetic with a spinal block may result in maternal or fetal death. A review of all maternal deaths in Michigan directly related to anesthesia between 1972 and 1984 found that at least 3 and perhaps all 4 deaths in patients with spinal anesthetics were related to hypotension. Two of these patients had pregnancy-induced hypertension.[3]

b. Post–dural puncture headache. Post–dural puncture headache (PDPH) is a well-known complication of procedures in which the dura mater of the spinal cord is perforated. However, headache is also a frequent symptom in the early postpartum period, even in the absence of anesthesia. The incidence of postpartum headache may be as high as 30% to 40% at the end of the first postpartum week, but in many cases its cause is unknown.[135,136] Pregnancy can modify the course of several headache syndromes, and thus the incidence and severity of headache can be increased during the peripartum period. List 22-2 lists causes of postpartum headache sometimes confused with PDPH.[137] When a headache occurs after spinal or epidural anesthesia, it must be considered a potentially serious complication and must be differentiated from other causes of headache in the postpartum period. Table 22-4 lists those clinical features found to be most useful in differentiating PDPH from other peripartum headaches.[135,138] However, the most distinguishing characteristic of a PDPH is its dependence on the position of the patient. Headache severity is always maximal when the patient is in the upright position and diminishes significantly, if not completely, when the patient is in

---

List 22-2. Differential Diagnosis for Headache in the Parturient

---

Acute migraine
Cluster headache
Tension (psychogenic) headache
Chronic paroxysmal hemicrania
Meningitis
Cortical vein thrombosis
Pseudotumor cerebri
Tumor
Preeclampsia and eclampsia
Subarachnoid hemorrhage

Table 22-4. Clinical features of post–dural puncture and postpartum headache

Post–dural puncture headache	Postpartum headache
Onset: Within first 5 days after dural puncture (90% within 3 days)	*Onset:* Between 3 and 6 days post partum
Duration: Usually 2 or 3 days, seldom longer than 1 week	*Duration:* May last 12 hours
Characteristics: 50% frontal 25% occipital 25% diffuse	*Characteristics:* Primarily bifrontal
Severity dependent on patient position	Patient position unimportant
Throbbing in nature	Continuous in nature
Associated symptoms: Blurred or double vision	*Associated symptoms:* Vision rarely affected
Photophobia	Mild photophobia
Dizziness, tinnitus, decreased hearing	No auditory component
Nausea and vomiting	Mild nausea and vomiting
Unresponsive to minor analgesics	Responds to minor analgesics
	Previous family history common

the horizontal position. The caution of Bonica continues to be applicable today: "A headache should not be attributed to spinal puncture unless it is brought on or aggravated by assuming the erect position and relieved by assuming the horizontal position or flexion and extension of the head."[139]

The problem of PDPH is better avoided than treated. Obstetric anesthesiologists who wish to include spinal anesthesia in their practice should be familiar with the factors that have been implicated in influencing the development of PDPH. These have been reviewed recently and include needle size, increasing incidence with larger diameter of needle; needle bevel orientation, higher incidence with perpendicular insertion to the longitudinal orientation of dural fibers; angle-of-needle approach to the dura, decreased incidence with more acute angle of approach; needle-tip design, lower incidence with pencil-point or conical-point needles; number of dural punctures, higher incidence with increased number of dural punctures; gender, higher incidence in females; age, higher incidence in younger patients; and history of prior PDPH, higher incidence in patients with a previous history of PDPH.[138,140] The obstetric patient is at particular risk of developing PDPH because these patients are young and female, and many will experience a period of bearing down that appears to increase the headache incidence.[141] However, this latter finding has not been observed universally.[142]

PDPH usually occurs 1 to 5 days after dural puncture and characteristically persists for 3 to 5 days. On rare occasions the headache can last for months.[143,144] Because a PDPH is self-limiting and often disappears within 1 week,[138] initial treatment can be conservative. However, remember that the incapacitating nature of this headache significantly impairs mother-infant

bonding and the parturient's ability to care for her newborn. Analgesics (such as acetaminophen, codeine) may provide some relief until the headache resolves. Bed rest is advisable because of the postural nature of the symptoms but does not reduce the incidence of headache.[145,146] Prolonged bed rest may actually be contraindicated in the postpartum period because of the risk of deep venous thrombosis. In an effort to return the cerebrospinal fluid pressure toward normal, fluids (3000 ml/day) by mouth or intravenously and abdominal binders have been recommended.[147] Epidural saline solution, either by bolus injection or continuous infusion has been shown, in some studies, to be effective in controlling the symptoms of PDPH.[141,148,149]

Caffeine has been used in managing PDPH. The cerebral vasoconstrictor activity of caffeine has been credited for the relief of symptoms in 80% of patients.[150] It has been shown to be an effective and inexpensive treatment both in intravenous and oral forms.[151-153] A typical treatment regimen is 500 mg of caffeine sodium benzoate given over 4 hours by intravenous infusion or 300 mg of caffeine given orally. One disadvantage of caffeine is that it may result in only temporary relief of symptoms.

The most effective treatment of PDPH appears to be the closure of the dural rent with the injection of autologous blood into the epidural space, "the epidural blood patch." The discovery of the efficacy of epidural blood patch (EBP) in the treatment of PDPH by DiGiovanni and Dunbar in 1970[154] was a terrific boon to patients and anesthesiologists alike. EBP has been shown to be efficacious in 95% to 100% of patients.[155,156] There has been much discussion regarding the optimum volume of blood to use,[156-158] the level at which the blood patch should be performed,[159] and the optimal timing of the procedure after dural puncture. In one study, EBP within 24 hours had a failure rate of 71% compared to 4% if performed after 24 hours.[158] However, in another study, prophylactic EBP was effective at preventing a significant number of PDPH.[160] Epidural blood patches have been shown to be effective months after dural puncture.[150,161] However, current practice at many institutions is to perform an epidural blood patch 24 to 48 hours after the onset of symptoms. Ten to 15 ml of autologous, nonheparinized blood is injected into the epidural space near the level of the suspected dural rent. Because epidural blood patches are simple, effective, and relatively free of serious complications, there is little reason to delay treatment, particularly when headache is severe. However, the injection of blood into the epidural space is commonly associated with backache and mild signs of meningeal irritation. Potential complications, though very rare, include epidural infection, obliteration of the extradural space, and nerve root compression. Subarachnoid injection of blood can potentially result in adhesive arachnoiditis.

3. Epidural anesthesia

a. Unsatisfactory block. Although rarely considered a true complication of epidural anesthesia in obstetrics, unsatisfactory or inadequate block has been reported to have an incidence of 6% to 15%.[162] Doughty found that catheter manipulation was required in 18.6% of patients before satisfactory analgesia was achieved.[163] The importance of the problem is demonstrated by the ASA Closed Claims Study in which 8% of obstetric anesthesia malpractice claims alleged inadequate anesthesia (Table 22-3). One of the most common causes of inadequate block is catheter malposition. In some cases the malpositioning problem may be attributable to migration of the catheter out of an intervertebral

foramen because of insertion of an excessive length of catheter.[164] Placing the catheter no more than 3 to 4 cm into the epidural space seems to be associated with more reliable blocks.

Recently a new mechanism has been proposed to explain some cases of patchy blocks. Dalens et al., using mixtures of local anesthetic and radiographic contrast solution, found that the technique of using air for the loss of resistance creates air bubbles in the epidural space, which physically displace local anesthetic solutions and may result in patchy blocks or skipped segments.[165]

Studies of epidural anatomy using advanced imaging techniques and epiduroscopy have confirmed the existence of a dorsal median septum (plica mediana dorsalis) in the lumbar epidural space.[166,167] Using contrast epidurography and wide-range gray-scale computerized tomography, Savolaine et al. have demonstrated dorsolateral transverse membranes in addition to the plica mediana dorsalis.[167] These structures subdivide the epidural space and may impede the symmetric spread of local anesthetic solutions. The current trend of using continuous epidural infusions of very-low-concentration local anesthetic solutions (often combined with opioids) may compound the problem of asymmetric blocks. In a study reported by Mogensen et al., half of the patients receiving 0.125% bupivacaine infusions for postoperative analgesia had a primarily unilateral block.[168]

b. Uterine rupture. Some obstetricians have raised the concern that epidural anesthesia may block the pain associated with uterine rupture and delay diagnosis, thereby increasing maternal and fetal morbidity or mortality.[169,170] Because of the growing trend for encouraging a trial of labor in patients with prior cesarean sections,[171] this concern must be considered. As has been pointed out by Chestnut, pain is neither a specific nor a sensitive sign of uterine scar rupture.[172] Among 32 patients with rupture of a previously scarred uterus, Golan et al. reported that 47% were completely asymptomatic and 75% were not associated with unusual pain.[170] Fetal heart rate monitoring may provide the best indication of uterine rupture.[173] Rupture of a previously unscarred uterus is usually a more catastrophic event, which may be associated with continuous abdominal pain. It is unlikely that this type of pain would go unrecognized with typical low-dose epidural analgesia for labor. Nonetheless it is our opinion that epidural analgesia for labor is not advisable in patients at risk for uterine rupture (such as prior uterine instrumentation, grand multiparity, oxytocin stimulation of labor) unless fetal heart rate and intrauterine pressure are monitored continuously.

Concern has also been raised that the process of flexing the torso of a parturient during epidural placement, particularly in the sitting position, may result in abnormal intraabdominal pressures, which could result in uterine rupture.[170,174] The small number of cases in which an association was claimed between the flexed position during epidural placement and uterine rupture seems unconvincing. In those cases, evolving uterine rupture could have been the cause of the pain necessitating epidural analgesia.[172] A recent study of intrauterine pressures in patients having epidural catheters placed, found no increase in maximum intra-amniotic pressure during flexion, in either the sitting or the lateral decubitus positions.[175]

c. Unintentional subdural block. The subdural space is a potential space between the dura and the arachnoid membranes. Several reports have confirmed the unintentional catheterization of this potential space as well as delayed subdural migration of an epidural catheter.[176-179] Typically, the onset of block is similar to epidural anesthesia, and for this reason test doses to rule out subarachnoid block will not allow detection of a subdural injection.[177] The extent of block produced from a given volume of local anesthetic is, however, usually much greater with subdural injection. It is not uncommon to have spread of block to the cervical level with 6 to 10 ml of local anesthetic solution.[177,178] When small volumes of water-soluble contrast media are injected into the subdural space, they rapidly spread over a large number of segments, usually cephalad. Subdural blocks may be patchy or asymmetric.[178] To avoid this complication, one should initiate epidural blocks slowly with incremental doses, taking particular care to notice any signs of unexpected high levels during onset of the block. Subdural blocks should be managed in the same way as high spinal blocks, with support of blood pressure, ventilation, and protection of the airway as necessary. Recently the subdural administration of morphine was reported in the management of a patient with cancer pain.[180] The authors noted a greatly reduced dose requirement compared to that required by the epidural route, suggesting the potential for respiratory depression with unintentional subdural morphine administration.

d. Unintentional subarachnoid block. Unintentional dural puncture during epidural placement is a relatively common complication with a reported frequency of 1.6% to 2.9%;[176] how-ever, the frequency can vary widely depending on the skill and experience of the practitioner. It is usually recognized at the time of occurrence and has a high likelihood of resulting in subsequent PDPH. Unrecognized injection of local anesthetic into the subarachnoid space either through an epidural needle or catheter is a much less common, though potentially fatal, complication. If large volumes of local anesthetic are injected, the result is sudden and massive spinal blockade (total spinal) characterized by severe hypotension, loss of consciousness, and apnea. To avoid catastrophic consequences, one must secure the airway immediately and establish ventilation. Blood return to the heart must be facilitated by a left-lateral, head-down position and rapid intravenous fluid administration. Vasopressors should be used as required to restore adequate perfusion pressure. To decrease high subarachnoid pressure and minimize potential neurotoxic effects from a large volume of subarachnoid local anesthetic, some authors have recommended draining cerebrospinal fluid.[181]

e. Systemic local anesthetic toxicity. Systemic local anesthetic toxicity has been one of the main causes of maternal mortality associated with epidural anesthesia. Central nervous system and cardiovascular toxic reactions have long been recognized as complications of local anesthetic overdose or, more commonly, unintentional intravascular injection. However, before the widespread use of long-acting amide local anesthetics such as bupivacaine, these reactions rarely led to fatal cardiac arrest. In 1979, Albright reported 6 cases of cardiac arrest after bupivacaine or etidocaine injections.[182] Albright speculated that the long-acting amide local anesthetics may be more cardiotoxic and that resuscitation from cardiac arrest induced by these agents may be more difficult. Since then, he has collected at least 44 cases of maternal cardiac arrest, 30 of which have been fatal.[183] Data from the ASA Closed Claims Study indicate that convulsion was the single most common critical event that led to serious complications among the obstetric-related claims.[2] Of 19 convulsions in the group of obstetric claims, 17 were likely attributable to local anesthetic toxic reactions with epidural anesthesia. In 10 of these 17 cases, epinephrine was not used in the test dose, and in the remaining 7 insufficient data was available to know if epinephrine-containing test doses were used or not. Bupivacaine was the local anesthetic used in 15 of the 17 cases. In the remaining 2 cases the anesthetic was not specified. Two of the 19 convulsions appeared to be eclamptic seizures. Eighty-three percent of the convulsions resulted in neurologic injury or death to the mother, newborn, or both.

Many factors influence the toxicity of local anesthetic agents. One important factor is the relative potency of the anesthetic. Numerous studies have indicated that the seizure-producing potential is directly related to anesthetic potency.[184,185] The relationship between anesthetic potency and cardiovascular toxicity is less clear. Liu et al., using cumulative doses of lidocaine or bupivacaine in anesthetized and ventilated dogs, concluded that the cardiotoxicity was similar to the intrinsic potency of the drugs when hypotension and asystole were used as the end point.[186] Since then, other studies using a variety of animal models have demonstrated that bupivacaine has a greater potential for causing dysrhythmias.[187-191] Bupivacaine is different from other local anesthetics (such as lidocaine) in that it can induce cardiac dysrhythmias such as ventricular tachycardia and fibrillation. Other local anesthetics typically produce progressive conduction block with widened QRS complexes and eventual asystole. Research has been directed toward explaining these observations, but the answers are not clear. Clarkson and Hondeghem have proposed that differential binding properties of local anesthetic at the sodium channel may explain the greater dysrhythmogenic potential of bupivacaine.[192] Others have emphasized the role of the central nervous system in explaining the potential for bupivacaine, but not lidocaine, to induce cardiac dysrhythmias.[193,194]

Factors that may lower the cardiotoxic threshold for bupivacaine are hyperkalemia,[195] pregnancy,[190] as well as hypoxia and acidosis.[196] Morishima et al. showed that the pregnant sheep is more sensitive to the cardiotoxic effects of bupivacaine than the nonpregnant sheep is.[190] This sensitivity appears to be attributable to decreased plasma protein binding for bupivacaine in the pregnant animal.[197] When ventilation is supported during experimental infusions of local anesthetics, the margin of safety between central nervous system toxicity and cardiovascular collapse is much wider than when ventilation is not supported. Moore et al. have demonstrated significant acidosis and hypoxia within 30 seconds after the onset of local anesthetic–induced convulsions in humans.[198,199] In the event of a local anesthetic convulsion, it is imperative to rapidly initiate effective ventilation and oxygenation to prevent cardiovascular collapse. Animal studies have shown that it is possible to resuscitate animals after massive bupivacaine infusions[188,200] and

that it is not more difficult to resuscitate after bupivacaine-induced than it is after lidocaine-induced cardiac arrest.[188] It may, however, be much more difficult to resuscitate a pregnant patient than a nonpregnant patient because of partial occlusion of the inferior vena cava by the gravid uterus.[201] For this reason, emergent delivery should be performed if resuscitation efforts are not quickly successful. Cases where resuscitation was not accomplished until after emergent delivery of the infant have been reported.[202]

Since the editorial by Albright,[182] the anesthesia community has become increasingly aware of the potential problems with local anesthetic toxicity in general and bupivacaine cardiotoxicity in particular. In 1983 the Food and Drug Administration issued a warning against the use of bupivacaine 0.75% in obstetrics.[203] Since then, we have become aware of only one or two deaths from bupivacaine toxic reactions (Albright, personal communication, 1990). It goes without saying that local anesthetic systemic toxic reactions are better avoided than treated. To this end, the practice of not injecting more than 5 ml of anesthetic solution at one time and the use of an effective test dose have surely improved the safety of epidural anesthesia in obstetrics.

Aspiration of blood from an epidural needle or catheter is an unreliable sign of intravascular placement. To minimize the chances of unintentional intravascular injection, we advocate the use of a test dose. The test dose in obstetric patients should fulfill a number of criteria: (1) it must contain a marker to identify an intravascular injection of anesthetic; (2) the changes seen with the test injection should be discernible from the cyclic changes seen during active labor; (3) the marker must not be toxic to the mother or fetus; (4) the test dose should be relatively easy to perform. The most commonly used marker for detecting intravascular injection has been epinephrine, since Moore and Batra reported that 15 µg of epinephrine, when injected intravascularly, resulted in a 30 beat per minute increase in heart rate within 20 to 45 seconds.[204] Opponents, however, have suggested that epinephrine, if given intravenously, might have deleterious effects on uterine blood flow thus leading to fetal distress.[205,206] In addition, heart rate changes seen with intravenous epinephrine might be difficult to distinguish from the 20% to 30% changes that may occur with uterine contractions.[207,208] Although these concerns are real, there are few case reports in the obstetric literature linking epinephrine test doses with adverse outcomes, whereas there are reports of large numbers of patients benefiting from the advantages of the epinephrine test dose.[209] Epinephrine test doses should be used with caution, or perhaps not at all, in patients with uteroplacental insufficiency or in those who have a potential for an exaggerated response to intravenous epinephrine (as with pregnancy-induced hypertension).[210] Some patients, such as those being treated with beta-adrenergic receptor blockers, may develop hypertension and bradycardia, not tachycardia in response to epinephrine.[211,212] One can avoid complications by identifying these patients before an epinephrine test dose is administered. Recently, alternatives to the epinephrine test dose have been proposed: a bolus of plain local anesthetic solution,[213,214] isoproterenol,[215] or air.[216] However, significantly more validation of these techniques is necessary before one can recommend replacing the epinephrine test dose. Regardless of the type of test dose one chooses, there is no substitute for close observation of the patient by someone trained to detect adverse signs and symptoms of local anesthetic toxicity.

f. Neurotoxicity. Neurotoxicity from clinically used concentrations of local anesthetics is extremely rare. Drug manufacturers go to great lengths to ensure that their products cause a minimum of local tissue reaction. Nonetheless, it is clear that virtually all local anesthetics in sufficiently high concentration will cause injury to nerve tissue.[217,218] Case reports have linked neurologic injury from spinal anesthesia with various local anesthetics[219] though it has not always been clear if the local anesthetic or a contaminant was the cause. One of the most serious sequelae is adhesive arachnoiditis. This condition involves a gradual proliferation of the arachnoid resulting in scarring and obliteration of the subarachnoid space. The signs and symptoms of the resulting cauda equina syndrome may be progressive over months or years and usually involve weakness and numbness in the lower extremities with bowel, bladder, and sexual dysfunction.

In recent years the local anesthetic most often linked with neurotoxicity has been 2-chloroprocaine. This agent has been very popular in obstetrics because of its rapid onset, short duration of action, and very low systemic toxicity. In most of the reported cases of neurologic injury it appears that the local anesthetic was unintentionally injected subarachnoid[220] though this may not always have been the case.[221] A considerable amount of research has been directed at determining if the cause of neurotoxicity was the drug itself or the antioxodant sodium bisulfite with which the local anesthetic was formulated to minimize oxidation. Some laboratory[222] as well as animal studies[223] have indicated that the sodium bisulfite was the most likely cause of neurotoxicity. Other studies, however, indicate that the drug itself may be more neurotoxic than other commonly used local anesthetics.[224] Presumably because of the concern regarding sodium bisulfite, the manufacturers now use EDTA as the antioxidant in commercially available 2-chloroprocaine. The drug continues to be available to the practitioner, but due care should be exercised in its use. Recent reports have indicated that the epidural use of the newly formulated 2-chloroprocaine may be associated with severe spasmodic back pain.[225,226]

One should use all local anesthetics as directed without exceeding the recommended concentration or total dose. Before injection of significant volumes of local anesthetic a test dose should be given to rule out subarachnoid as well as intravascular placement. In addition, it is advisable to use disposable equipment whenever possible to minimize the risk of introducing contaminants, such as detergents or cleaning solutions, during regional anesthetic procedures.

g. Drug administration errors. Errors in drug or blood product administration are responsible for a small but consistent number of anesthesia-related maternal complications and deaths.[2,13,227] The *Report on Confidential Enquiries into Maternal Deaths in England and Wales* for the last two triennia indicate that approximately 5% of anesthetic-related deaths may be attributable to such errors.[6,13] It is likely that many more errors do not result in obvious complications and go unreported. Contributing to the occurrence of such errors is the emergent nature of many obstetric procedures, as well as lack of attention and judgment because of sleep deprivation. Some drug administration errors have included the injection of thiopental, diazepam, or potassium chloride into the epidural space.[228-230] In most of these cases patients have recovered without permanent sequelae. The popularity of continuous epidural infusions for labor analgesia increase the likelihood of errors involving the infusion apparatus.[230] To minimize the chances of infusing magnesium, oxytocin, or other drugs into the epidural space, epidural infusion devices should be uniquely different from those used to infuse intravenous medications. Connecting tubing should not have injection ports, and epidural catheters should be labeled clearly. All medication errors are avoidable and indefensible; they remind us of the continual need to maintain vigilance and attention to detail.

4. Spinal opioid complications. Spinally injected opioids have been used in the obstetric population since Wolfe and Nichols first described the use of epidurally injected fentanyl in postcesarean patients.[231] Since then the use of spinal opioids in obstetrics has continued to grow. Numerous studies have demonstrated the superiority of epidural compared to intramuscular or intravenous opioid administration for providing postcesarean analgesia.[232-234] The efficacy of epidural opioids, when used alone, for providing labor analgesia has been disappointing.[235,236] Various combinations of low-dose local anesthetic and opioids, however, have proved to be effective for managing labor pain. These combinations appear to act synergistically to provide analgesia[237] but minimizing the undesirable side effects of either agent alone. Chestnut et al. found that a continuous infusion of bupivacaine 0.0625% with fentanyl 0.0002% provided analgesia comparable to that of bupivacaine 0.125% alone but with significantly less motor block.[238] The advantage of this is that patients have more mobility, are easier to care for, and can push effectively. Spinal opioids are, however, associated with several side effects and potential complications. The most common side effects are pruritus, nausea and vomiting, and urinary retention. More serious problems are the potential for oral herpesvirus recrudescence and the most feared complication, respiratory depression.

Pruritus is undoubtedly the most common side effect seen with epidurally injected morphine. The reported incidence in obstetric patients varies from 60% to 90%.[239] Obstetric patients may be more sensitive to both the analgesic effects as well as the side effects of epidural morphine.[240] In one study in which postcesarean patients were given a mean dose of 4.3 mg of epidural morphine the incidence of pruritus was 70%. In 43% the itching was mild and no treatment was required, in 22% treatment was effective, and in 6% symptoms were troubling despite treatment with diphenhydramine, 25 mg IM or naloxone 0.1 mg IV.[241] The incidence of pruritus may be less with other opioids such as fentanyl and meperidine[234,242] and may not be seen at all with agonist-antagonist opioids such as butorphanol.[243]

Nausea and vomiting is common in obstetric patients though most studies indicate a higher incidence in women treated with epidural (or intrathecal) morphine compared to those given narcotic or nonnarcotic analgesics intravenously or intramuscularly. The mechanism of neuraxial opioid-induced nausea and vomiting may involve direct stimulation of the chemoreceptor trigger zone in the medulla. The incidence has been reported as high as 53% in obstetric patients after epidural morphine, but more commonly the reported incidence is in the range of 16% to 25%.[239] Treatment of nausea and vomiting associated with epidural opioids consists in conservative doses of metoclopramide (5 to 10 mg IV), droperidol (0.625 mg IV), or transdermal scopolamine.[244]

The mechanism responsible for urinary retention with spinal opioids is poorly understood but is believed to involve a direct effect of the opioid at the sacral spinal cord. Obstetric patients commonly have voiding difficulty because of genitourinary trauma associated with vaginal or cesarean delivery. Surprisingly, urinary retention has rarely been cited as a clinically significant problem associated with neuraxial opioid analgesia in obstetric patients. One of the reasons for this may be the common practice of catheterizing the bladder of patients during labor and the use of indwelling catheters for 12 to 24 hours after cesarean delivery.

A new complication of epidural morphine in postcesarean patients has become apparent in the past few years. Two retrospective studies suggested that parturients given epidural morphine may be more susceptible to recrudescence of oral herpes infections.[245,246] A recent prospective study compared the incidence of oral herpes outbreaks in postcesarean patients given morphine epidurally or intramuscularly. Fourteen of the 96 women in the epidural group (14.6%) developed herpetic lesions, whereas none in the intramuscular group suffered a recurrence.[247] Postulated mechanisms for this phenomenon include local trauma associated with scratching in response to facial pruritus, or a direct stimulation of virion reactivation in the trigeminal ganglia by morphine. The severity of some of these outbreaks raise the concern for potential transmission of infection to the newborn. If recurrent oral herpetic lesions have been a problem for a woman, it may be advisable to avoid giving neuraxial opioids.

Respiratory depression is potentially the most serious complication of neuraxial opioid administration. Case reports describing respiratory depression appeared soon after spinal opioids were introduced into clinical practice. Large retrospective and prospective studies have estimated the incidence in the general surgical population at between 0.25% and 0.9%.[248,249] Most cases of respiratory depression have occurred within 8 hours of drug administration and are probably attributable to direct depression of brainstem respiratory centers by opioid spread within the cerebrospinal fluid. Low respiratory rates and somnolence have only rarely been reported in obstetric patients. It has been postulated that the parturient may be particularly resistant to ventilatory depression because of the increased respiratory drive that occurs during pregnancy.[250] Depressed CO_2 response slopes, however, have been documented in postcesarean patients after epidural morphine or butorphanol.[243] In a prospective study of 1000 cesarean section patients given morphine, 5 mg, for postoperative pain control, Leicht et al. found four patients with respiratory rates of less than 10 breaths per minute.[251] Two of these patients were given naloxone though only one was documented to have true respiratory depression. These data are the best available in this patient population and indicate that the incidence of respiratory depression may be as high as 0.1% to 0.2%.

It has been suggested that the use of more lipophilic opioids such as fentanyl may be safer than morphine because the drug would be rapidly absorbed in the lumbar spinal cord making it unavailable to cause respiratory depression by cephalad spread in the cerebrospinal fluid.[252] However, in a recent case report, 100 mg of epidural fentanyl, given during cesarean section, resulted in severe respiratory depression.[253] It is clear that the use of neuraxial opioids in all patients must be accompanied with great vigilance. Respiratory rate alone is a poor indicator of ventilatory depression.[254,255] Somnolence may be a more reliable indicator and should be specifically evaluated.[256] The use of neuraxial opioids in obstetrics should be predicated on an organizational structure that assures knowledgeable staff and the ability to provide the necessary monitoring for a as long as indicated.[257]

IV. FETAL COMPLICATIONS

Adverse fetal outcome is one of the most common causes for liability claims involving obstetric anesthesia. Although in half of such claims anesthetic care may have been completely appropriate,[2] the importance of ensuring fetal well-being while providing maternal anesthesia cannot be overemphasized. Protecting the fetus from complications of anesthesia necessitates maintaining adequate uterine perfusion, optimizing fetal oxygenation, and limiting the use of drugs in the mother that may cause newborn depression. The importance of avoiding aortocaval compression and hypotension has been discussed. Supplemental oxygen should be ad-

ministered to laboring women if there is any question of fetal distress, since this has been shown to improve neonatal oxygenation.[258]

All systemic medications commonly employed during labor for anxiolysis and analgesia readily cross the placenta and can cause neonatal depression. Meperidine may produce neonatal depression as a function of both the dose given and the time interval between maternal administration and delivery of the infant, with the second hour after administration being the most worrisome.[259] Morphine in doses of 5 to 10 mg intramuscularly or 2 to 3 mg intravenously has a duration of 4 to 6 hours and in equianalgesic doses produces more respiratory depression than meperidine does.[260] Fentanyl is a highly lipid-soluble, rapid-acting opioid. In doses of 25 to 50 μg intravenously or 50 to 100 μg intramuscularly, fentanyl has a duration of action of 60 to 120 minutes respectively. In one study, fentanyl (1 μg/kg) was administered intravenously just before cesarean delivery and did not produce adverse effects on neonatal Apgar scores, neurobehavioral scores, or blood gas values.[261] Fentanyl might therefore be a reasonable adjunct to labor analgesia or cesarean section anesthesia. Butorphanol (Stadol) and nalbuphine (Nubain) are two synthetic agonist-antagonist opioid analgesics. Both cross the placenta and have depressant effects on the newborn, similar to those seen with meperidine.[262,263] Benzodiazepines are sometimes used for the treatment of maternal anxiety before delivery of the infant. Both diazepam and midazolam have the potential for causing neonatal respiratory depression; however, low doses of diazepam (2.5 to 10 mg) intravenously have been used with minimal neonatal effects.[264] Despite these findings, it is best to avoid central nervous system–depressant drugs in obstetric patients until after delivery of the infant.

A potential hazard of general anesthesia in obstetrics is that of neonatal depression. Large doses of thiopental (8 mg/kg) can result in neonatal depression.[265] However, single doses of 4 mg/kg will not expose the fetal brain to high concentrations of thiopental and not result in significant neonatal depression.[266] Ketamine in doses of 0.2 to 0.5 mg/kg was not found to cause newborn depression[267] and when given in doses of 1 mg/kg IV for induction of general anesthesia resulted in slightly better neurobehavioral scores than when thiopental was used.[268] Etomidate has a rapid onset and short duration of action and has also been used in obstetrics. The maternal-to-fetal base excess differences and clinical status of the newborn were found to be superior to that when thiopental was used.[269] Etomidate carries with it the concern for adrenal suppression. In the neonate this is not a significant problem when etomidate is used as the induction agent for elective cesarean section.[270] Midazolam provides no real benefit over thiopental as an induction agent for elective cesarean section.[271] Midazolam was shown to have no advantage in Apgar scores, time to first cry, and need to provide supplemental oxygen to the newborn. There were no real differences in neurobehavioral scores; however, general body tone, response to changes in body temperature, and arm recoil were somewhat depressed compared to those in neonates whose mothers were given thiopental. Use of propofol, the newest induction agent, for elective cesarean section at a dose of 2.8 mg/kg has been shown to result in lower 1- and 5-minute Apgar scores. The lower scores were attributable to somnolence and hypotonus. Central nervous system depression was evidenced by significantly lower neurobehavior scores.[270] Propofol will require further study before one can recommend its use as an induction agent, particularly in the setting of fetal distress.

The controversy of general versus regional anesthesia for cesarean section continues to draw attention from obstetric anesthesiologists. Since Virginia Apgar reported her conclusions in 1957,[273] it has generally been believed that neonates are more vigorous after cesarean section under regional anesthesia than general anesthesia. Early studies found that neonatal depression (measured by Apgar scores) resulted from the use of potent halogenated agents for cesarean section.[274] Neonatal depression may be related to the duration of anesthesia before delivery as reported by Stenger et al. and Finster et al.[275,276] What is probably of greater importance is the uterine incision–to–delivery interval. Depressed infants in deliveries in which the uterine incision–to–delivery intervals have exceeded 90 to 180 seconds have been reported.[277,278] It is now evident that with prudent use of low-dose halogenated agents, left uterine displacement, supplemental oxygen, and expeditious delivery (particularly short uterine incision–to–delivery intervals), general anesthesia does not result in significant newborn depression.[33,279,280] A recent comparison of the effects of general versus regional anesthesia for elective cesarean section demonstrated no difference in neurobehavioral responses of newborn infants.[281] It is currently unclear whether regional or general anesthesia confers any advantage to the fetus in distress. Well-conducted regional or general anesthetics appear to be equally safe.[282]

Regional anesthesia in obstetrics is not without its potential neonatal or fetal complications. The most frequent complications are attributable to placental hypoperfusion. Epidural anesthesia is preferred over subarachnoid blocks by many anesthesiologists because the block level is more easily controlled, sympathectomy occurs less rapidly, and hypotension is easier to prevent. However, subarachnoid anesthesia exposes the fetus to less anesthetic drug, thus minimizing potential toxic effects. No clear answer exists as to which method of regional anesthesia is superior with respect to the fetus. In addition, the best agent to use for regional anesthesia continues to be debated.[283] Despite potential problems with cardiotoxicity, bupivacaine continues to be used extensively in obstetrics. Its long duration of action and superior sensory-to-motor blocking properties offer particular advantages in obstetric anesthesia.

Some neonatal complications are associated with particular regional anesthetic techniques. Paracervical blocks were at one time popular in obstetrics for providing pain relief during labor. However, depending on the local anesthetic used, dose, and preexisting fetal condition, fetal bradycardia and fetal death have been reported to have an incidence of 2% to 70%.[265,284] Because of this, paracervical blocks are rarely used today. Caudal anesthesia continues to be popular in some anesthetic practices. Placement of the caudal needle must be performed with care, and a rectal examination should be performed to exclude the possibility of accidental puncture of the fetal presenting part. Sinclair et al. have reported fetal local anesthetic toxicity as a consequence of direct fetal injection during caudal anesthesia.[285]

It is clear that the perinate may be influenced by anesthetic effects on placental perfusion, placental transfer of depressant drugs, and anesthetic effects on the course of labor. However, small amounts of systemic medication or properly conducted general or regional anesthesia should have no significant effect on the course of labor or infant well-being.

V. SUMMARY

The care of obstetric patients can be challenging for the anesthesiologist. Often obstetric patients are not well informed and not well prepared for anesthetic interventions. Care is often emergently required with little time for proper assessment and examination of the patient. Maternal physiologic and pathologic conditions may further complicate anesthetic management. Perhaps for these, as well as other reasons, anesthesia-related complications remain one of the leading causes of maternal mortality. It is incumbent upon us to do all we can in an attempt to eliminate adverse consequences of anesthetic care.

REFERENCES

1. Gibbs CP et al: Obstetric anesthesia: a national survey, Anesthesiology 65:298-306, 1986.
2. Chadwick HS et al: A comparison of obstetric- and non-obstetric anesthesia malpractice claims, Anesthesiology 74:242-249, 1991.
3. Endler GC et al: Anesthesia-related maternal mortality in Michigan, 1972 to 1984, Am J Obstet Gynecol 159:187-193, 1988.
4. Rochat RW et al: Changing the definition of maternal mortality: a new look at the postpartum interval, Lancet 1:831, 1981.
5. Lehmann DK et al: The epidemiology and pathology of maternal mortality: Charity Hospital of Louisiana in New Orleans, 1965-1984, Obstet Gynecol 69:833-840, 1987.
6. Turnbull AC et al: Report on confidential enquiries into maternal deaths in England and Wales 1979-1981, London, 1986, Her Majesty's Stationary Office.
7. Kaunitz AM et al: Causes of maternal mortality in the United States, Obstet Gynecol 65:605-612, 1985.
8. Bassell GM and Marx GF: Anesthesia-related maternal mortality. In Shnider SM and Levinson G: Anesthesia for obstetrics, ed 2, Baltimore, 1987, Williams & Wilkins. p 325.
9. Morgan M: Anesthetic contribution to maternal mortality, Br J Anaesth 59:842-855, 1987.
10. Greiss FC and Anderson SH: Elimination of maternal deaths from anesthesia, Obstet Gynecol 29:677-681, 1967.
11. Klein MD and Clahr J: Factors in the decline of maternal mortality, JAMA 168:237-242, 1958.
12. Marx GF and Berman JA: Anesthesia-related maternal mortality, Bull NY Acad Med 61:323-330, 1985.
13. Turnbull A et al: Report on confidential enquiries into maternal deaths in England and Wales 1982-1984, London, 1989, Her Majesty's Stationary Office.
14. Ramanathan S: Thromboembolism. In Ramanathan S: Obstetric anesthesia, Philadelphia, 1988, Lea & Febiger.
15. Morgan M: Amniotic fluid embolism, Anaesthesia 34:20-32, 1979.
16. Plauché WC: Amniotic fluid embolism, Am J Obstet Gynecol 147:982-983, 1983.
17. Ross M, Nowicki K, and Rangarajan NS: Asymptomatic pulmonary embolism during pregnancy, Obstet Gynecol 37:131-133, 1971.
18. Karuparthy VR et al: Incidence of venous air embolism during cesarean section is unchanged by the use of a 5 to 10 degree head-up tilt, Anesth Analg 69:620-623, 1989.
19. Malinow AM et al: Precordial ultrasonic monitoring during cesarean delivery, Anesthesiology 66:816-819, 1987.
20. Schneider EP, Jonas E, and Tejani N: Detection of cardiac events by continuous electrocardiogram monitoring during ritodrine infusion. Obstet Gynecol 71:361-364, 1988.
21. Wheeler AS, Patel KF, and Spain J: Pulmonary edema during beta-2-tocolytic therapy, Anesth Analg 60:695-696, 1981.
22. Dailey PA: Anesthesia for preterm labor. In Shnider

23. Pritchard JA, MacDonald PC, and Gant NF: Hypertensive disorders in pregnancy. In Pritchard JA, MacDonald PC, and Gant NF: Williams obstetrics, ed 17, Norwalk, Conn, 1985, Appleton-Century-Crofts, p 539.
24. Easterling TR, Benedetti TJ, and Schmucker BC: Maternal cardiac output in preeclamptic pregnancies: a longitudinal study, Society of Perinatal Obstetricians, New Orleans, abstracts:4, 1989.
25. Gutsche BB and Cheek TG: Anesthetic considerations in preeclampsia-eclampsia. In Shnider SM and Levinson G: Anesthesia for obstetrics, ed 2, Baltimore, 1987, Williams & Wilkins, p 225.
26. Hibbard LT: Maternal mortality due to acute toxemia, Obstet Gynecol 42:263-270, 1973.
27. Ramanathan J et al: Correlation between bleeding times and platelet counts in women with preeclampsia undergoing cesarean section, Anesthesiology 71:188-191, 1989.
28. Kelton JG, Hunter DJS, and Neame PB: A platelet function defect in preeclampsia, Obstet Gynecol 65:107-109, 1985.
29. Weiner CP: The obstetric patient and disseminated intravascular coagulation, Clin Perinatol 13:705-717, 1986.
30. Donaldson JO: Eclampsia and other causes of peripartum convulsions. In Donaldson JO: Neurology of pregnancy, Philadelphia, 1978, WB Saunders Co.
31. Fox EJ et al: Complications related to the pressor response to endotracheal intubation, Anesthesiology 47:524-525, 1977.
32. Pritchard JA and Pritchard SA: Standardized treatment of 154 consecutive cases of eclampsia, Am J Obstet Gynecol 123:543-552, 1975.
33. Abboud T et al: Sympathoadrenal activity, maternal, fetal, and neonatal responses after epidural anesthesia in the preeclamptic patient, Am J Obstet Gynecol 144:915-918, 1982.
34. Jouppila P et al: Lumbar epidural analgesia to improve intervillous blood flow during labor in severe preeclampsia, Obstet Gynecol 59:158-161, 1982.
35. Benedetti TJ, Kates R, and Williams V: Hemodynamic observations in severe preeclampsia complicated by pulmonary edema, Am J Obstet Gynecol 152:330-334, 1985.
36. Benedetti TJ and Quilligan EJ: Cerebral edema in severe pregnancy-induced hypertension, Am J Obstet Gynecol 137:860-862, 1980.
37. Lechner RB and Chadwick HS: Anesthetic care of the patient with preeclampsia, Anesth Clin North Am 8:95-114, 1990.
38. Howard BK, Goodson JH, and Mengert WF: Supine hypotensive syndrome in late pregnancy, Obstet Gynecol 1:371-377, 1953.
39. Kerr MG, Scott DB, and Samuel E: Studies of the inferior vena cava in late pregnancy, Br Med J 1:532-533, 1964.
40. Zilianti M et al: Fetal heart rate and pH of fetal capillary blood during epidural analgesia in labor, Obstet Gynecol 36:881-886, 1970.
41. Moir D: Anaesthesia and maternal deaths, Scott Med J 24:187-189, 1979.
42. Tomkinson J et al: Report on confidential enquiries into maternal deaths in England and Wales 1976-1978, London, 1982, Her Majesty's Stationary Office.
43. Csapo A: Prosgesterone "block," Am J Anat 98:273-291, 1956.
44. Christofide ND et al: Decreased plasma motilin con-

centrations in pregnancy, Br Med J 285:1453-1454, 1982.

45. Roberts RB and Shirley MA: The obstetrician's role in reducing the risk of aspiration pneumonitis, Am J Obstet Gynecol 124:611-617, 1976.

46. Gibbs CP et al: Antacid pulmonary aspiration in the dog, Anesthesiology 51:380-385, 1979.

47. Gibbs CP and Banner TC: Effectiveness of Bicitra as a preoperative antacid, Anesthesiology 61:97-99, 1984.

48. Dewan DM et al: Sodium citrate pretreatment in elective cesarean section patients, Anesth Analg 64:34-37, 1985.

49. Thompson EM et al: Combined treatment with ranitidine and saline antacids prior to obstetric anaesthesia, Anaesthesia 39:1086-1090, 1984.

50. Gillett GB, Watson JD, and Langford RM: Ranitidine and single-dose antacid therapy as prophylaxis against acid aspiration syndrome in obstetric practice, Anaesthesia 39:638-644, 1984.

51. Freely J et al: Increased toxicity and reduced clearance of lidocaine by cimetidine, Ann Intern Med 96:592-594, 1982.

52. Knapp AB et al: The cimetidine-lidocaine interaction, Ann Intern Med 98:174-177, 1983.

53. Dailey PA et al: Effect of cimetidine and ranitidine on lidocaine concentrations during epidural anesthesia for cesarean section, Anesthesiology 69:1013-1017, 1988.

54. Brock-Utne JG et al: Influence of preoperative gastric aspiration on the volume and pH of gastric contents in obstetric patients undergoing caesarean section, Br J Anaesth 62:397-401, 1989.

55. Brock-Utne JG et al: The effect of metoclopramide on the lower oesophageal sphincter in late pregnancy, Anaesth Intensive Care 6:26-29, 1978.

56. Bylsma-Howell M et al: Placental transport of metoclopramide: assessment of maternal and neonatal effects, Can Anaesth Soc J 30:487-492, 1983.

57. Wyner J and Cohen SE: Gastric volume in early pregnancy: effect of metoclopramide, Anesthesiology 57:209-212, 1982.

58. Carmichael FJ et al: Preoxygenation: a study of denitrogenation, Anesth Analg 68:406-409, 1989.

59. Brock-Utne JG, Downing JW, and Seedat F: Laryngeal oedema associated with preeclamptic toxaemia, Anaesthesia 32:556-558, 1977.

60. MacKenzie AI: Laryngeal oedema complicating obstetric anaesthesia, Anaesthesia 33:271, 1978.

61. Benumof JL and Scheller JJ: The importance of transtracheal jet ventilation in the management of the difficult airway, Anesthesiology 71:769-778, 1989.

62. Archer GW and Marx GF: Arterial oxygen tension during apnoea in parturient women, Br J Anaesth 46:358-360, 1974.

63. Gambee AM, Hertzka RE, and Fisher DM: Preoxygenation techniques: comparison of three minutes and four breaths, Anesth Analg 66:468-470, 1987.

64. Norris MC and Dewan DM: Preoxygenation for cesarean section: a comparison of two techniques, Anesthesiology 62:827-829, 1985.

65. Russell GN et al: Pre-oxygenation and the parturient patient, Anaesthesia 42:346-351, 1987.

66. Birmingham PK, Cheney FW, and Ward RJ: Esophageal intubation: a review of detection techniques, Anesth Analg 65:886-891, 1986.

67. Guggenberger H, Lenz G, and Federle R: Early detection of inadvertent esophageal intubation: pulse oximetry vs. capnography, Acta Anaesthesiol Scand 33:112-115, 1989.

68. Strunin L and Williams T: The FEF end-tidal carbon dioxide detector, Anesthesiology 71:621-622, 1989 (Letter).

69. Juul J, Lie B, and Nielsen SF: Epidural analgesia vs. general anesthesia for cesarean section, Acta Obstet Gynecol Scand 67:203-206, 1988.

70. Crawford JS: Awareness during operative obstetrics under general anaesthesia, Br J Anaesth 43:179-182, 1971.

71. Hodgkinson R et al: Neonatal neurobehavioral tests following cesarean section under general and spinal anesthesia, Am J Obstet Gynecol 132:670-674, 1978.

72. Morgan M, Holdcroft A, and Whitwam JG: Comparison of thiopentone and methohexitone as induction agents for caesarean section, Anaesth Intensive Care 8:431-435, 1980.

73. Schultetus RR et al: Wakefulness during cesarean section after anesthetic induction with ketamine, thiopental, or ketamine and thiopental combined, Anesth Analg 65:723-728, 1986.

74. Moore J et al: A comparison between propofol and thiopentone as induction agents in obstetric anaesthesia, Anaesthesia 44:753-757, 1989.

75. Moir DD: Anaesthesia for caesarean section: an evaluation of a method using low concentrations of halothane and 50 percent oxygen, Br J Anaesth 42:136-142, 1970.

76. Crawford JS, Lewis M, and Davies P: Maternal and neonatal responses related to the volatile agent used to maintain anaesthesia at caesarean section, Br J Anaesth 57:482-487, 1985.

77. Morishima HO, Pedersen H, and Finster M: Influence of maternal psychological stress on the fetus, Am J Obstet Gynecol 131:286-290, 1978.

78. Newton M: Postpartum hemorrhage, Am J Obstet Gynecol 94:711-717, 1966.

79. Gibbs CE and Locke WE: Maternal deaths in Texas, 1969 to 1973, Am J Obstet Gynecol 126:687-692, 1976.

80. Munson ES and Embro WJ: Enflurane, isoflurane, and halothane and isolated human uterine muscle, Anesthesiology 46:11-14, 1977.

81. Stallabrass P: Halothane and blood loss at delivery, Acta Anaesthesiol Scand 25(suppl):376, 1966.

82. Thirion AV et al: Maternal blood loss associated with low dose halothane administration for cesarean section, Anesthesiology 69:A693, 1988.

83. Marx GF et al: Postpartum uterine pressures under halothane or enflurane anesthesia, Obstet Gynecol 51:695-698, 1978.

84. Kerr MG: Cardiovascular dynamics in pregnancy and labour, Br Med Bull 24:19-24, 1968.

85. Bieniarz J et al: Aortocaval compression by the uterus in late human pregnancy, Am J Obstet Gynecol 100:203-217, 1968.

86. Griess Jr FC: Pressure-flow relationship in the gravid uterine vascular bed, Am J Obstet Gynecol 96:41-47, 1966.

87. Hon EH, Reid BL, and Hehre FW: The electronic evaluation of fetal heart rate. II. Changes with maternal hypotension, Am J Obstet Gynecol 79:209-215, 1960.

88. Moya F and Smith B: Spinal anesthesia for cesarean section: clinical and biochemical studies of effects on maternal physiology, JAMA 179:609-614, 1962.

89. Bletka M et al: Volume of whole blood and absolute amount of serum proteins in the early stage of late toxemia of pregnancy, Am J Obstet Gynecol 106:10-13, 1970.

90. Ralston DH, Shnider SM, and deLorimier AA: Effects of equipotent ephedrine, metraminol, mephrentermine and methoxamine on uterine blood flow in

the pregnant ewe, Anesthesiology 40:354-370, 1974.

91. Lechner RB, Droste S, and Chadwick HS: Lumbar epidural analgesia and changes in the fetal heart rate pattern: a blinded study of 139 patients, Anesthesiology 71:A853, 1989.

92. Grundy EM, Zamora AM, and Winnie AP: Comparison of spread of epidural anesthesia in pregnant and nonpregnant women, Anesth Analg 57:544-546, 1978.

93. Shnider SM and Levinson G: Obstetric anesthesia. In Miller RD: Anesthesia, ed 2, New York, 1986, Churchill Livingstone, p 1688.

94. Bromage PR: Epidural analgesia, Philadelphia, 1978, WB Saunders Co, pp 522-525.

95. Cheek TG and Gutsche BB: Maternal physiologic alterations during pregnancy. In Shnider SM and Levinson G: Anesthesia for obstetrics, ed 2, Baltimore, 1987, Williams & Wilkins, p 9.

96. Flanagan HL et al: Effect of pregnancy on bupivacaine-induced conduction blockade in the isolated rabbit vagus nerve, Anesth Analg 66:123-126, 1987.

97. Butterworth JF, Walker FO, and Lysak SZ: Pregnancy increases median nerve susceptibility to lidocaine, Anesthesiology 72:962-965, 1990.

98. Usubiaga JE: Neurological complications following epidural anesthesia, Int Anesthesiol Clin 13:1-153, 1975.

99. Hellmann K: Epidural anaesthesia in obstetrics: a second look at 26,127 cases, Can Anaesth Soc J 12:398-404, 1965.

100. Hill EC: Maternal obstetric paralysis, Am J Obstet Gynecol 83:1452-1460, 1962.

101. Massey EW and Cefalo RC: Neuropathies of pregnancy, Obstet Gynecol Surv 34:489-492, 1979.

102. Massey E: Mononeuropathies in pregnancy, Semin Neurol 8:193-196, 1988.

103. Brown JT and McDougall A: Traumatic maternal birth palsy, J Obstet Gynaecol Br Emp 164:431-435, 1957.

104. Philip BK: Complications of regional anesthesia for obstetrics, Reg Anesth 8:17-30, 1983.

105. Massey EW and Cefalo RC: Managing the carpal tunnel syndrome in pregnancy, Contemp Obstet Gynecol 9:39-42, 1977.

106. Rhodes P: Meralgia paraesthetica in pregnancy, Lancet 2:831, 1957.

107. Pearson MG: Meralgia paraesthetica with reference to its occurrence in pregnancy, J Obstet Gynaecol Br Emp 64:427-430, 1957.

108. Donaldson JO, Wirz D, and Mashman J: Bilateral postpartum femoral neuropathy, Conn Med 49:496-498, 1985.

109. Adelman U, Goldberg GS, and Puckett JD: Postpartum bilateral femoral neuropathy, Obstet Gynecol 42:845-850, 1973.

110. Whittaker WG: Injuries to the sacral plexus in obstetrics, Can Med Assoc J 79:622-627, 1958.

111. O'Connell JEA: Lumbar disc protrusions in pregnancy, J Neurol Neurosurg Psychiatry 23:138-141, 1960.

112. Grove LH: Backache, headache, and bladder dysfunction after delivery, Br J Anaesth 45:1147-1149, 1973.

113. Crawford JS: Lumbar epidural block in labour: a clinical analysis, Br J Anaesth 44:66-74, 1972.

114. Bromage PR: An evaluation of bupivacaine in epidural analgesia for obstetrics, Can Anaesth Soc J 16:46-56, 1969.

115. Cuerden C, Buley R, and Downing JW: Delayed recovery after epidural analgesia for labour, Anaesthesia 32:773-776, 1977.

116. Pathy GV and Rosen M: Prolonged block with recov-

ery after extradural analgesia for labour, Br J Anaesth 47:520-522, 1975.

117. Vandam LD and Dripps RD: A Long-term follow-up of 10,098 spinal anesthetics. II. Incidence and analysis of minor sensory neurological defects, Surgery 38:463-469, 1955.

117a. Rigler ML et al: Cauda equina syndrome after continuous spinal anesthesia, Anesth Analg 72:275-281, 1991.

118. Shnider SM, Levinson G, and Ralston DH: Regional anesthesia for labor and delivery. In Shnider SM and Levinson G: Anesthesia for obstetrics, ed 2, Baltimore, 1987, Williams & Wilkins, p 119.

119. Dawson BH: Paraplegia due to spinal epidural haematoma, J Neurol Neurosurg Psychiatry 26:171-173, 1963.

120. Owens EL, Kasten GW, and Hessel II EA: Spinal subarachnoid hematoma after lumbar puncture and heparinization: a case report, review of the literature, and discussion of anesthetic implications, Anesth Analg 65:1201-1207, 1986.

121. Rasmus KT et al: Unrecognized thrombocytopenia and regional anesthesia in parturients: a retrospective review, Obstet Gynecol 73:943-946, 1989.

122. Rolbin SH et al: Epidural anesthesia in pregnant patients with low platelet counts, Obstet Gynecol 71:918-920, 1988.

123. Baker AS et al: Spinal epidural abscess, N Engl J Med 293:463-468, 1975.

124. Bromage PR: Epidural analgesia, Philadelphia, 1978, WB Saunders Co, pp 682-690.

125. Berga S and Trierweiler MW: Bacterial meningitis following epidural anesthesia for vaginal delivery: a case report, Obstet Gynecol 74:437-439, 1989.

126. Ready LB and Helfer D: Bacterial meningitis in parturients after epidural anesthesia, Anesthesiology 71:988-990, 1989.

127. Roberts SP and Petts HV: Meningitis after obstetric spinal anaesthesia, Anaesthesia 45:371-377, 1990.

128. Bromage PR: Neurologic complications of regional anesthesia for obstetrics. In Shnider SM and Levinson G: Anesthesia for obstetrics, ed 2, Baltimore, 1987, Williams & Wilkins, p 321.

129. Behl S: Epidural analgesia in the presence of fever, Anaesthesia 40:1240-1241, 1985.

130. Brown ZA, Berry S, and Vontver LA: Genital herpes simplex virus infections complicating pregnancy; natural history and peripartum management, J Reprod Med 31:420-425, 1986.

131. Ramanathan S, Sheth R, and Turndorf H: Anesthesia for cesarean section in patients with genital herpes infections: a retrospective study, Anesthesiology 64:807-809, 1986.

132. Crosby ET, Halpern SH, and Rolbin SH: Epidural anaesthesia for caesarean section in patients with active recurrent genital herpes simplex infections: a retrospective review, Can J Anaesth 36:701-704, 1989.

133. Hopkins T, Marcus M, and Campbell S: Post-partum depression: a critical review, Psychol Bull 95:498-515, 1984.

134. Thirkettle JA and Knight RG: The psychological precipitants of transient postpartum depression: a review, Curr Psychol Res Rev 4:143-166, 1985.

135. Stein G et al: Headaches after childbirth, Acta Neurol Scand 69:74-79, 1984.

136. Pitt B: Maternity blues, Br J Psychiatry 122:431-433, 1973.

137. Reik L: Headaches in pregnancy, Semin Neurol 8:187-192, 1988.

138. Gielen M: Post dural puncture headache (PDPH): a review, Reg Anesth 14:101-106, 1989.

139. Bonica JJ: Principles and practice of obstetric analge-

sia and anesthesia, Oxford, Engl, 1967, Blackwell Scientific Publications, pp 721-725.

140. Lybecker H et al: Incidence and prediction of postdural puncture headache, Anesth Analg 70:389-394, 1990.

141. Okell RW and Sprigge JS: Unintentional dural puncture: a survey of recognition and management, Anaesthesia 42:1110-1113, 1987.

142. Ravindran RS et al: Bearing down at the time of delivery and the incidence of spinal headache in parturients, Anesth Analg 60:524-525, 1981.

143. Abouleish E: Epidural blood patch for the treatment of chronic post-lumbar puncture cephalgia, Anesthesiology 49:291-292, 1978.

144. Abouleish E et al: Long-term follow-up of epidural blood patch, Anesth Analg 54:459-463, 1975.

145. Jones RJ: The role of recumbency in the prevention and treatment of postspinal haedache, Anesth Analg 53:788-796, 1974.

146. Carbaat PAT and van Crevel H: Lumbar puncture headache: controlled study on the preventive effect of 24 hours' bed rest, Lancet 2:1133-1135, 1981.

147. Moore DC: Anesthetic techniques for obstetrical anesthesia and analgesia, Springfield, Ill, 1964, Charles C Thomas, Publisher.

148. Baysinger CL et al: The successful treatment of dural puncture headache after failed epidural blood patch, Anesth Analg 65:1242-1244, 1986.

149. Usubiaga JE et al: Effect of saline injections on epidural and subarachnoid space pressures and relation to postspinal anesthesia headache, Anesth Analg 46:293-296, 1967.

150. Jarvis AP, Greenawalt JW, and Fagraeus L: Intravenous caffeine for postdural puncture headache, Anesth Analg 65:316-317, 1986 (Letter).

151. Sechzer PH and Abel L: Post-spinal anesthesia headache treated with caffeine: evaluation with demand method, Curr Ther Res 24: 307-312, 1978.

152. Baumgarten RK: Should caffeine become the first-line treatment for postdural puncture headache? Anesth Analg 66:913-914, 1987.

153. Camann WR et al: Effects of oral caffeine on postdural puncture headache: a double-blind, placebo-controlled trial, Anesth Analg 70:181-184, 1990.

154. DiGiovanni AJ and Dunbar BS: Epidural injections of autologous blood for postlumbar-puncture headache, Anesth Analg 49:268-271, 1970.

155. Brownridge P: The management of headache following accidental dural puncture in obstetric patients, Anaesth Intensive Care 11:4-15, 1983.

156. Ostheimer GW, Palahniuk RJ, and Shnider SM: Epidural blood patch for post-lumbar-puncture headache, Anesthesiology 41:307-308, 1974.

157. Crawford JS: Experiences with epidural blood patch, Anaesthesia 35:513-515, 1980.

158. Loeser EA et al: Time vs. success rate for epidural blood patch, Anesthesiology 49:147-148, 1978.

159. Szeinfeld M et al: Epidural blood patch: evaluation of the volume and spread of blood injected into the epidural space, Anesthesiology 64:820-822, 1986.

160. Cheek TG et al: Prophylactic extradural blood patch is effective: a preliminary communication, Br J Anaesth 61:340-342, 1988.

161. Wilton NCT, Globerson JH, and DeRosayro AM: Epidural blood patch for postdural puncture headache: it's never too late, Anesth Analg 65:895-896, 1986.

162. Brownridge PR, Taylor G, and Ralston DH: Neural blockade for obstetrics and gynecology. In Cousins MJ and Bridenbaugh PO: Neural blockade in clinical anesthesia and management of pain, Philadelphia, 1980, JB Lippincott Co, p 480.

163. Doughty A: Lumbar epidural analgesia—the pursuit of perfection, with special reference to midwife participation, Anaesthesia 30:741-751, 1975.

164. Bromage PR: Epidural analgesia, Philadelphia, 1978, WB Saunders Co, pp 226-228.

165. Dalens B, Bazin J, and Haberer J: Epidural bubbles as a cause of incomplete analgesia during epidural anesthesia, Anesth Analg 66:679-683, 1987.

166. Blomberg R: The dorsomedian connective tissue band in the lumbar epidural space of humans: an anatomical study using epiduroscopy in autopsy cases, Anesth Analg 65:747-752, 1986.

167. Savolaine ER et al: Anatomy of the human lumbar epidural space: new insights using CT-epidurography, Anesthesiology 68:217-220, 1988.

168. Mogensen T et al: No tachyphylaxis during postoperative continuous epidural 0.125% bupivacaine infusion, Reg Anesth 13:117-121, 1988.

169. O'Driscoll K: An obstetrician's view of pain, Br J Anaesth 47:1053-1059, 1975.

170. Golan A, Sandbank O, and Rubin A: Rupture of the pregnant uterus, Obstet Gynecol 56:549-554, 1980.

171. ACOG committee opinion: Guidelines for vaginal delivery after a previous cesarean birth, number 64, Washington, DC, 1988, American College of Obstetricians and Gynecologists.

172. Chestnut DH: Uterine rupture and epidural anesthesia, Obstet Gynecol 66:295, 1985.

173. Elkins T et al: Uterine rupture in Nigeria, J Reprod Med 30:195-199, 1985.

174. Plauché WC, von Almen W, and Muller R: Catastrophic uterine rupture, Obstet Gynecol 64:792-797, 1984.

175. Parker L and Dewan DM: Epidurals and uterine rupture. Does acute anteflexion alter intraamniotic pressure? Society for Obstetrical Anesthesia and Perinatology, Madison, Wisc, abstracts:E-29, 1990.

176. Boys JE and Norman PF: Accidental subdural analgesia:a case report, possible clinical implications and relevance to "massive extradurals" Br J Anaesth 47:1111-1113, 1975.

177. Lee A and Dodd KW: Accidental subdural catheterisation, Anaesthesia 41:847-849, 1986.

178. Manchanda VN et al: Unusual clinical course of accidental subdural local anesthetic injection, Anesth Analg 62:1124-1126, 1983.

179. Hartrick CT et al: Subdural migration of an epidural catheter, Anesth Analg 64:175-178, 1985.

180. Brown G, Atkinson GL, and Standiford SB: Subdural administration of opioids, Anesthesiology 71:611-613, 1989.

181. Shnider SM, Levinson G, and Ralston DH: Regional anesthesia for labor and delivery. In Shnider SM and Levinson G: Anesthesia for obstetrics, ed 2, Baltimore, 1987, Williams & Wilkins, p 115.

182. Albright GA: Cardiac arrest following regional anesthesia with etidocaine or bupivacaine, Anesthesiology 51:285-287, 1979.

183. Albright GA: Local anesthetics. In Albright G, Ferguson IJ, and Joyce IT: Anesthesia in obstetrics, ed 2, Boston, 1986, Butterworth & Co, pp 115-150.

184. deJong RH, Ronfeld RA, and DeRosa RA: Cardiovascular effects of convulsant and supraconvulsant doses of amide local anesthetics, Anesth Analg 61:3-9, 1982.

185. Liu PL et al: Comparative CNS toxicity of lidocaine, etidocaine, bupivacaine, and tetracaine in awake dogs following rapid intravenous administration, Anesth Analg 62:375-379, 1983.

186. Liu P et al: Acute cardiovascular toxicity of intravenous amide local anesthetics in anesthetized ventilated dogs, Anesth Analg 61:317-322, 1982.

187. Rosen MA et al: Bupivacaine-induced cardiotoxicity in hypoxic and acidotic sheep, Anesth Analg 64:1089-1096, 1985.

188. Chadwick HS: Toxicity and resuscitation in lidocaine- or bupivacaine-infused cats, Anesthesiology 63:385-390, 1985.

189. Kotelko DM et al: Bupivacaine-induced cardiac arrhythmias in sheep, Anesthesiology 60:10-18, 1984.

190. Morishima HO et al: Bupivacaine toxicity in pregnant and nonpregnant ewes, Anesthesiology 63:134-139, 1985.

191. Sage DJ et al: The cardiovascular effects of convulsant doses of lidocaine and bupivacaine in the conscious dog, Reg Anaesth 10:175-183, 1985.

192. Clarkson CW and Hondeghem LM: Mechanism for bupivacaine depression of cardiac conduction: fast block of sodium channels during the action potential with slow recovery from block during diastole, Anesthesiology 62:396-405, 1985.

193. Heavner JE: Cardiac dysrhythmias induced by infusion of local anesthetics into the lateral cerebral ventricle of cats, Anesth Analg 65:133-138, 1986.

194. Thomas RD et al: Cardiovascular toxicity of local anesthetics: an alternative hypothesis, Anesth Analg 65:44-450, 1986.

195. Avery T et al: The influence of serum potassium on cerebral and cardiac toxicity of bupivacaine and lidocaine, Anesthesiology 61:133-138, 1984.

196. Sage DJ et al: Influence of lidocaine and bupivacaine on isolated guinea pig atria in the presence of acidosis and hypoxia, Anesth Analg 63:1-7, 1984.

197. Santos AC et al: Does pregnancy alter the systemic toxicity of local anesthetics? Anesthesiology 70:991-995, 1989.

198. Moore DC, Crawford RD, and Scurlock JE: Severe hypoxia and acidosis following local anesthetic-induced convulsions, Anesthesiology 53:259-260, 1980.

199. Moore DC, Thompson GE, and Crawford RD: Long-acting local anesthetic drugs and convulsions with hypoxia and acidosis, Anesthesiology 56:230-232, 1982.

200. Kasten GW and Martin ST: Successful cardiovascular resuscitation after massive intravenous bupivacaine overdosage in anesthetized dogs, Anesth Analg 64:491-497, 1985.

201. Kasten GW and Martin ST: Resuscitation from bupivacaine-induced cardiovascular toxicity during partial inferior vena cava occlusion, Anesth Analg 65:341-344, 1986.

202. DePace NL, Betesh JS, and Kotler MN: 'Postmortem' cesarean section with recovery of both mother and offspring, JAMA 248:971-973, 1982.

203. FDA Drug Bulletin: Adverse reactions with bupivacaine, Rockville, Md, 1983, US Department of Health and Human Services, p 23.

204. Moore DC and Batra MS: The components of an effective test dose prior to epidural block, Anesthesiology 55:693-696, 1981.

205. Hood DD and James DM III: Maternal and fetal effects of epinephrine in gravid ewes, Anesthesiology 64:610-613, 1986.

206. Chestnut DH et al: Effect of intravenous epinephrine on uterine artery blood flow velocity in the pregnant guinea pig, Anesthesiology 65:633-636, 1986.

207. Cartwright PO, McCarroll SM, and Antzaka C: Maternal heart rate changes with a plain epidural test dose, Anesthesiology 65:226-228, 1986.

208. Leighton BL et al: Limitations of epinephrine as a marker of intravascular injection in laboring women, Anesthesiology 66:688-691, 1987.

209. Moore DC et al: Maternal heart rate changes with a plain epidural test dose—validity of results open to question, Anesthesiology 66:854, 1987.

210. Talledo OE, Chesley LC, and Zuspan FP: Renin-angiotensin system in normal and toxemic pregnancies. III. Differential sensitivity to angiotensin II and norepinephrine in toxemia of pregnancy, Am J Obstet Gynecol 100:218-221, 1968.

211. Hom M, Johnson P, and Mulroy M: Blood pressure response to an epinephrine test dose in beta-blocked subjects, Anesthesiology 67:A268, 1987.

212. Popitz-Bergez F, Datta S, and Ostheimer GW: Intravascular epinephrine may not increase heart rate in patients receiving metoprolol, Anesthesiology 68:815-816, 1988.

213. Grice SC et al: Evaluation of 2-chloroprocaine as an effective intravenous test dose for epidural anesthesia, Anesthesiology 67:A627, 1987.

214. Roetman KJ and Eisenach JC: Evaluation of lidocaine as an intravenous test dose for epidural anesthesia, Anesthesiology 69:A669, 1988.

215. Leighton BL and Gross JB: Isoproterenol is an effective marker of intravenous injection in laboring women, Anesthesiology 71:206-209, 1989.

216. Leighton BL and Gross JB: Air: an effective indicator of intravenously located epidural catheters, Anesthesiology 71:848-851, 1989.

217. Meyers RR et al: Neurotoxicity of local anesthetics, Anesthesiology 65:119-120, 1986.

218. Ready LB et al: Neurotoxicity of intrathecal local anesthetics in rabbits, Anesthesiology 63:364-370, 1985.

219. Marx GF: Maternal complications of regional anesthesia, Reg Anaesth 6:104-107, 1981.

220. Reisner LS, Hochman BN, and Plumer MH: Persistent neurologic deficit and adhesive arachnoiditis following intrathecal 2-chloroprocaine injection, Anesth Analg 59:452-454, 1985.

221. Ravindran RS et al: Prolonged neuronal blockade following regional analgesia with 2-chloroprocaine, Anaesth Analg 59:447-451, 1980.

222. Gissen AJ, Datta S, and Lambert D: The chloroprocaine controversy. II. Is chloroprocaine neurotoxic? Reg Anaesth 9:135-145, 1984.

223. Wang BC et al: Chronic neurological deficits and Nesacaine-CE: an effect of the anesthetic, 2-chloroprocaine, or the antioxidant, sodium bisulfite? Anesth Analg 63:445-447, 1984.

224. Meyers RR et al: Neurotoxicity of local anesthetics: altered perineural permeability, edema, and nerve fiber injury, Anesthesiology 64:29-35, 1986.

225. Fibuch EE and Opper SE: Back pain following epidurally administered Nesacaine-MPF, Anesth Analg 69:113-115, 1989.

226. Ackerman III WE: Back pain after epidural Nesacaine-MPF, Anesth Analg 70:224-226, 1990.

227. Chopra V, Bovill JG, and Spierdijk J: Accidents, near accidents and complications during anaesthesia: a retrospective analysis of a 10-year period in a teaching hospital, Anaesthesia 45:3-6, 1990.

228. Tessler MJ et al: Inadvertent epidural administration of potassium chloride: a case report, Can J Anaesth 35:631-633, 1988.

229. Forestner JE and Raj PP: Inadvertent epidural injection of thiopental: a case report, Anesth Analg 54:406-407, 1975.

230. Lin D, Becker K, and Shapiro HM: Neurologic changes following epidural injection of potassium chloride and diazepam: a case report with laboratory correlations, Anesthesiology 65:210-212, 1986.

231. Wolfe MJ and Nicholas ADG: Selective epidural analgesia, Lancet 2:150-151, 1979.

232. Cohen SE and Woods WA: The role of epidural mor-

phine in the postcesarean patient: efficacy and effects on bonding, Anesthesiology 58:500-504, 1983.

233. Rosen MA et al: Epidural morphine for the relief of postoperative pain after cesarean delivery, Anesth Analg 62:666-672, 1983.

234. Brownridge P and Frewin DB: A comparative study of techniques of postoperative analgesia following caesarean section and lower abdominal surgery, Anaesth Intensive Care 13:123-130, 1985.

235. Hughes SC et al: Maternal and neonatal effects of epidural morphine for labor and delivery, Anesth Analg 63:319-324, 1984.

236. Writer WDR, James FM III, and Wheeler AS: Double-blind comparison of morphine and bupivacaine for continuous epidural analgesia in labor, Anesthesiology 54:215-219, 1981.

237. Akerman B, Arweström E, and Post C: Local anesthetics potentiate spinal morphine antinociception, Anesth Analg 67:943-948, 1988.

238. Chestnut DH et al: Continuous infusion epidural analgesia during labor: a randomized, double-blind comparison of 0.0625% bupivacaine/0.0002% fentanyl versus 0.125% bupivacaine, Anesthesiology 68:754-759, 1988.

239. Chadwick HS and Ross BK: Analgesia for post-cesarean delivery pain, Anesth Clin North Am 7:133-153, 1989.

240. Writer WDR et al: Epidural morphine prophylaxis of postoperative pain: report of a double-blind multicentre study, Can Anaesth Soc J 32:330-338, 1985.

241. Chadwick HS and Ready LB: Intrathecal and epidural morphine sulfate for postcesarean analgesia: a clinical comparison, Anesthesiology 68:925-929, 1988.

242. Naulty JS et al: Epidural fentanyl for postcesarean delivery pain management, Anesthesiology 63:694-698, 1985.

243. Abboud TK et al: Epidural butorphanol or morphine for the relief of post-cesarean section pain: ventilatory response to carbon dioxide, Anesth Analg 66:887-893, 1987.

244. Kotelko DM et al: Transdermal scopolamine decreases nausea and vomiting following cesarean section in patients receiving epidural morphine, Anesthesiology 71:675-678, 1989.

245. Gieraerts R et al: Increased incidence of itching and herpes simplex in patients given epidural morphine after cesarean section, Anesth Analg 66:1321-1324, 1987.

246. Crone LAL et al: Recurrent herpes simplex virus labialis and the use of epidural morphine in obstetric patients, Anesth Analg 67:318-323, 1988.

247. Crone LAL et al: Herpes labialis in parturients receiving epidural morphine following cesarean section, Anesthesiology 73:208-213, 1990.

248. Stenseth R, Sellevold O, and Breivik H: Epidural morphine for postoperative pain: experience with 1085 patients, Acta Anaesthesiol Scand 29:148-156, 1985.

249. Gustafsson LL, Schildt B, and Jacobsen K: Adverse effects of extradural and intrathecal opiates: report of a nationwide survey in Sweden, Br J Anaesth 54:479-486, 1982.

250. Korbon GA et al: Intramuscular naloxone reverses the side effects of epidural morphine while preserving analgesia, Reg Anesth 10:16-20, 1985.

251. Leicht CH et al: Epidural morphine for analgesia after cesarean section: a prospective report of 1000 patients, Anesthesiology 65:A366, 1986.

252. Bromage PR: The price of intraspinal narcotic analgesia: basic constraints, Anesth Analg 60:461-463, 1981.

253. Brockway MS et al: Profound respiratory depression after extradural fentanyl, Br J Anaesth 64:243-245, 1990.

254. Ready LB et al: Development of an anesthesiology-based postoperative pain management service, Anesthesiology 68:100-106, 1988.

255. Rawal N and Wattwil M: Respiratory depression after epidural morphine: an experimental and clinical study, Anesth Analg 63:8-14, 1984.

256. Ready LB, Chadwick HS, and Wild LM: Additional comments regarding an anesthesiology-based postoperative pain service, Anesthesiology 69:139-140, 1988.

257. Ready LB and Wild LM: Organization of as acute pain service: training and manpower, Anesth Clin North Am 7:229-239, 1989.

258. Ramanathan S et al: Oxygen transfer from mother to fetus during cesarean section under epidural anesthesia, Anesth Analg 61:576-581, 1982.

259. Shnider SM and Moya F: Effects of meperidine on the newborn infant, Am J Obstet Gynecol 89:1009-1015, 1964.

260. Way WL, Costley EC, and Way EL: Respiratory sensitivity of the newborn infant to meperidine and morphine, Clin Pharmacol Ther 6:454-461, 1965.

261. Eisele JH, Wright R, and Rogge P: Newborn and maternal fentanyl levels at cesarean section, Anesth Analg 61:179-180, 1982.

262. Quilligan EJ, Keegan KA, and Donahue MJ: Double-blind comparison of intravenously injected butorphanol and meperidine in parturients, Int J Gynaecol Obstet 18:363-367, 1980.

263. Miller RR: Evaluation of nalbuphine hydrochloride, Am J Hosp Pharm 37:942-949, 1980.

264. Rolbin SH et al: Diazepam during cesarean section: effects on neonatal Apgar scores, acid-base status, neurobehavioural assessment and maternal and fetal plasma norepinephrine levels, Society of Obstetrical Anesthesia and Perinatology, Seattle, Wash, abstracts:447, 1977.

265. Shnider SM et al: Paracervical-block anesthesia in obstetrics, Am J Obstet Gynecol 107:619-625, 1970.

266. Finster M et al: Plasma thiopental concentrations in the newborn following delivery under thiopental–nitrous oxide anesthesia, Am J Obstet Gynecol 95:621-629, 1966.

267. Akamatsu TJ, Bonica JJ, and Rehmet R: Experiences with the use of ketamine for parturition: I. Primary anesthetic for vaginal delivery, Anesth Analg 53:284-287, 1974.

268. Hodgkinson R et al: Neonatal neurobehavioral tests following vaginal delivery under ketamine, thiopental and extradural anesthesia, Anesth Analg 56:548-553, 1977.

269. Downing JW et al: Etomidate for induction of anaesthesia at caesarean section: comparison with thiopentone, Br J Anaesth 91:135-140, 1979.

270. Reddy BK, Pizer B, and Bull PT: Neonatal serum cortisol suppression by etomidate compared with thiopentone for elective caesarean section, Eur J Anaesthesiol 5:171-176, 1988.

271. Ravlo O et al: A randomized comparison between midazolam and thiopental for elective cesarean section anesthesia. II. Neonates, Anesth Analg 68:234-237, 1989.

272. Celleno D et al: Neurobehavioral effects of propofol on the neonate following elective caesarean section, Br J Anaesth 62:649-654, 1989.

273. Apgar V et al: Comparison of regional and general anesthesia in obstetrics, JAMA 165:2155-2161, 1957.

274. Benson RC et al: Fetal compromise during elective cesarean section, Am J Obstet Gynecol 91:645-656, 1965.

275. Stenger VG, Blechner JN, and Prystowsky H: A study of prolongation of obstetric anesthesia, Am J Obstet Gynecol 103:901-907, 1969.

276. Finster M and Poppers PJ: Safety of thiopental used for induction of general anesthesia in elective cesarean section, Anesthesiology 29:190-191, 1968.

277. Datta S et al: Neonatal effect of prolonged anesthetic induction for cesarean section, Obstet Gynecol 58:331-335, 1981.

278. Crawford JS and Davies P: Status of neonates delivered by elective caesarean section, Br J Anaesth 54:1015-1022, 1982.

279. Warren TM et al: Comparison of the maternal and neonatal effects of halothane, enflurane, and isoflurane for cesarean delivery, Anesth Analg 62:516-520, 1983.

280. Crawford JS, Burton OM, and Davies P: Anaesthesia for section: further refinements of a technique, Br J Anaesth 45:726-731, 1973.

281. Kangas-Saarela T et al: Comparison of the effects of general and epidural anaesthesia for cesarean section on the neurobehavioural responses of newborn infants, Acta Anaesthesiol Scand 33:313-319, 1989.

282. Marx GF, Luykx WM, and Cohen S: Fetal-neonatal status following caesarean section for fetal distress, Br J Anaesth 56:1009-1013, 1984.

283. Kuhnert BR, Kennard MJ, and Linn PL: Neonatal neurobehavior after epidural anesthesia for cesarean section, Anesth Analg 67:64-68, 1988.

284. Rosefsky JB and Petersiel ME: Perinatal deaths associated with mepivacaine paracervical-block anesthesia in labor, N Engl J Med 278:530-533, 1968.

285. Sinclair JC et al: Intoxication of fetus by a local anesthetic, a newly recognized complication of maternal caudal anesthesia, N Engl J Med 273:1173-1177, 1965.

Chapter 23

Anesthesia Complications Occurring Primarily in the Very Young

Frederic A. Berry

The very nature of anesthesia practice is to carefully review any potential or actual bad outcome and determine, when possible, causation. In this way, the art and science of anesthesia can continually improve and grow. Sometimes a situation or condition that was believed to be a result of negligent medical practice turns out to be another of Mother Nature's cruel twists. An example of this is the infant with cerebral palsy. It was and often is still believed that cerebral palsy is primarily caused by birth asphyxia and therefore there must have been negligence on the part of the anesthesiologist and obstetrician.[1,2] Recent studies have documented the lack of significant adverse antenatal events in the vast majority of mothers who delivered infants who later were found to have cerebral palsy.[3,4] Obstetric and anesthetic care in the United States has steadily improved over the years, but the frequency of cerebral palsy has remained steady.[5] A study from Australia would suggest that in about 8% of infants with cerebral palsy an intrapartum hypoxic episode was the *possible* cause.[3]

Unfortunately, the legal profession with the assistance of the medical profession has pursued and won many medicolegal suits for children with cerebral palsy, where there is no evidence of negligence. Undoubtedly the medical profession needs to evaluate objectively potential medical negligence cases and give informed responsible opinion. These opinions should be subject to the same analysis and accountability as any scientific paper presented at a meeting. Unfortunately, at present, there is little accountability in this field. Therefore there are many plaintiffs' experts, among them academic anesthesiologists who travel the country giving outrageous opinions about medical negligence cases to the severe detriment of the medical profession as well as the unfortunate persons involved.

It is hoped that this chapter will provide the anesthesiologist with an understanding of some of the complications that occur in the very young. It is also the goal of this chapter to provide the anesthesiologist with information so that the pitfalls can be avoided wherever possible but also so that they can recognize that there are certain unavoidable complications that will occur regardless of the degree of skill and care and that a bad outcome is not equivalent to negligent care.

I. THE NEWBORN

A newborn is defined as an infant in the first 24 hours of life. This is the period of transition or adaptation where the dependent fetus becomes the relatively independent newborn. The fetus depends on the umbilical circulation for nutrition, oxygenation, and metabolism. At birth, there is adaptation of all the various organ systems, a process that is mainly completed within the first 72 hours but goes on for approximately the first month of life. It is evident that the condition of the infant at birth is related to both the condition of the mother and the maternal fetal circulation. Changes in the maternal fetal circulation that may result in fetal damage may not be evident during the pregnancy and become manifest only in the neonatal period or in the several months thereafter. Meconium staining or aspiration is an example of a condition that may be present at birth but whose cause may have been present for a much longer period of time. Meconium aspiration is discussed in greater detail later. Cerebral palsy is an example of a condition where there may have been long-term asphyxia of the infant, which interferes with cerebral function, resulting in cerebral palsy but the infant may appear normal at birth.

Various catastrophic events may occur at the time of delivery. These catastrophic events may be attributable to the preexisting medical condition of the mother, such as toxemia with seizure activity, or they may be attributable to the process of anesthesia, that is, the inability to intubate or the aspiration of gastric contents. The effect upon the fetus will be directly determined by the length of time of the problem and the ability to resuscitate the mother. In general, if there is an acute problem with the mother, resulting in either hypotension or hypoxia, the fetus is left in utero until the mother can be resuscitated and then the mother can resuscitate the fetus. Reversability depends on the cause of the asphyxia, the length of time it has existed, and the rapidity with which the infant is resuscitated.

A. Anesthetic complications of the mother with a potential acute direct effect on the newborn

Certainly any acute maternal hypoxia or hypotension can reduce the oxygen delivery to the fetus and therefore result in a newborn infant that is depressed from hypoxia. The causes of hypoxia or hypotension include a difficult airway, aspiration, and hypotension from regional anesthesia. At times, the mother may also have received anesthetics, which undergo transplacental passage, and these are discussed later. The major issue for the anesthesiologist is often a mother who needs resuscitation. In situations where the mother needs acute resuscitation, it is always better to delay delivery until the mother is completely resuscitated because the mother can resuscitate the fetus. At times, however, in a situation such as a failed intubation or the regurgitation and aspiration of gastric contents, the situation may not allow a period of delay to deliver the infant, and in that situation the newborn may need resuscitation as well as the mother.

B. Transplacental passages of anesthetic agents resulting in a depressed newborn

As a general rule, all anesthetic agents will cross the placenta. However, there are some exceptions to this rule. Moya et al. demonstrated that in the usual clinical doses succinylcholine did not cross the placenta.[6] A very large (300 mg) intravenous dose of succinylcholine was required before it could be detected in the umbilical vein blood at birth.[7] Even though succinylcholine was detected, there was no apparent effect on the newborn infant.

Succinylcholine is metabolized by plasma cholinesterase. There is a case report where the mother and fetus were homozygous for plasma cholinesterase deficiency and the situation arose in which the newborn was paralyzed by the transplacental passage of a normal dose of succinylcholine.[8] In this situation, an apneic newborn with no muscle tone would represent a real diagnostic as well as therapeutic challenge. The Apgar score would be 2 at best, with no immediate improvement because all the muscles would be paralyzed. It took a period of several hours for the infant to begin to demonstrate muscle activity. This is obviously a very difficult management situation, since the condition of the infant would be compatible with what might be seen with brain death. This would be a rare situation, but it does demonstrate that the placenta is not an absolute barrier to the passage of succinylcholine.

In general, the usual clinical doses of pentothal, that is, 3 to 4 mg/kg does not cause any fetal depression because the fetal liver is active in taking up the thiopental that is in the umbilical venus blood.[9] Prolonged inhalation anesthesia may cause some depression of the newborn, but this should be easily reversed with the normal ventilation of the infant. Lidocaine is also taken up by the fetal liver, and unless there are large overdoses, this should have relatively little effect on the fetus.[10] In this situation one would expect a major effect to be on the mother. At times the mother has received rather generous doses of narcotics, and so these infants are at particular risk, since the narcotics cross the placenta relatively easy and may result in an infant who is depressed at birth and will need narcotic reversal. Finally, A recent study was conducted to determine the effect that fetal acidosis and poor maternal placenta blood flow would have on the transplacental passage of two commonly used drugs in labor: bupivacaine and meperidine.[11] The studies were done in rabbits. The conclusion of the studies was that in the presence of fetal asphyxia there may well be an exacerbation of the adverse effects of the drugs.

C. Maternal fluid therapy with dextrose

The advent of regional anesthesia has resulted in increased amounts of intravenous fluids being administered to the mother. It was recognized early that regional anesthesia with its accompanying sympathectomy often resulted in a decreased blood pressure necessitating the generous administration of a balanced salt solution or vasopressors. This is the reason why it is recommended that before epidural anesthesia, particularly for cesarean section, 1 to 2 liters of balanced salt solution be administered. Dextrose should not be included in this fluid, since it was shown years ago that when a bolus of dextrose and salt solution was administered some of the infants developed an acidosis that was evident shortly after birth. The acidosis was found to be caused by hypoglycemia. The mechanism for the hypoglycemia was that the dextrose would cross the placenta stimulating the fetus's pancreas to release insulin in order to regulate the blood levels of glucose. After birth, the extra supply of dextrose from the mother was discontinued, and the insulin released by the pancreas in some newborn infants resulted in hypoglycemia.

D. Meconium aspiration

Considerable controversy has developed in the last several years about the management of the infant who is delivered from a mother in whom there has been either meconium staining of the amniotic fluid or the frank passage of meconium.[12,13] Intrauterine hypoxia can cause the fetus to pass meconium. If the hypoxia occurs in the immediate time of the delivery, the meconium is often of a thick and tenacious character. This form of meconium mechanically obstructs the airway and needs to be removed by endotracheal suction. Various techniques have been described to accomplish this. On the other hand, meconium staining of the amniotic fluid may be a result of either a short or long period of hypoxia that occurred before the period of delivery. Depending on the length of time that the meconium has been present in the amniotic fluid, there will be varying degrees of meconium staining of the infant's skin and fingernails. At times the reason for the interruption of the maternal placental oxygen flow has been corrected and the meconium-stained infant will have a normal Apgar score at birth. At other times, however, the reason for the longterm occurrence of hypoxia may still be present and the Apgar score may be low at birth. If there is chronic intrauterine hypoxia, the fetus is susceptible to developing increased amounts of muscle in the blood vessels of the lung with the result that the newborn infant may well have a condition known as "persistent pulmonary hypertension"[14] (Fig. 23-1). Therefore the presence of meconium in the amniotic fluid or meconium staining of the infant may be a marker for an episode of intrauterine hypoxia or a chronic state of hypoxia, or it may be an indicator of an acute episode of hypoxia during the delivery period. These infants may have a low Apgar score at birth, need extensive resuscitation, and, depending on the degree of persistent pulmonary hypertension with its rightto-left shunt, varying degrees of respiratory failure. As soon as these infants are identified and it becomes evident that the normal resuscitative and supportive techniques are not successful, these infants may be candidates for ECMO (extracorporeal membrane oxygenation). Even with that, they may have well have a fatal outcome if they have severe pulmonary hyperten-

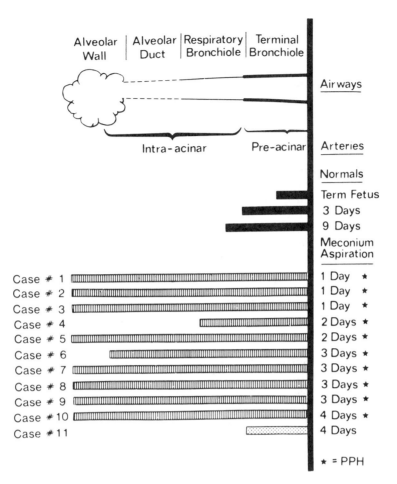

Fig. 23-1. Diagram of muscle extension along pulmonary arterial branches, *shaded bars*. In the normal newborn infant, virtually no intra-acinar artery is muscular. In nine of 10 infants with meconium aspiration with persistent pulmonary hypertension, PPH, muscle extended into the most peripheral arteries; the infant with meconium aspiration without PPH (case 11) had normal intra-acinar arteries. (From Murphy JD, Vawter GF, and Reid LM: J Pediatr 104:758, 1984.)

sion.[14] It must be obvious from this discussion that it is difficult to tell immediately at birth what the various ramifications of meconium staining of the amniotic fluid or the infant are. Infants who have the meconium aspiration syndrome and who require intubation and ventilation when studied later in childhood are often found to have long-term pulmonary sequelae. The problems include airway hyperreactivity, elevated closing volumes, and hyperinflation. The long-term pulmonary sequelae then of the meconium aspiration syndrome is less severe but similar to that found in infants who are premature and those with bronchopulmonary dysplasia.[15]

In the early days of the description of the meconium aspiration syndrome, it was not clear whether the problem was that of airway obstruction or pulmonary hypertension with respiratory failure, or both. Therefore, at that time, it was recommended that all infants be intubated, suctioned, and given supportive care, regardless of the degree of meconium passage or the character of the meconium.[16] In recent years, a change in opinion about the management of meconium aspiration has occurred. There are many infants who have meconium staining who are born with Apgar scores of 7 to 9. In the past, it was recommended that even these infants be intubated and suctioned. However, a recent article has strongly suggested that the risk-to-benefit ratio of this therapeutic technique needs to be reevaluated.[12] In their prospective study of the routine suctioning of meconium-stained infants, regardless of Apgar score, they found a 2% incidence of pulmonary and laryngeal disorders. Although there was no mortality reported, this incidence certainly is a significant morbidity. Esophageal perforation has been reported as a result of the routine suctioning of a meconium baby with an Apgar score of 8.[17] Therefore it is time that we appreciated that meconium staining and the presence of meconium indicates an entire spectrum of disease. In some infants, there is chronic and acute hypoxia with a low Apgar score where the infant needs immediate intubation, suctioning and resuscitation. There are infants who may be obstructed by tenacious meconium that needs to be suctioned from the airway. There are also other infants, though, in whom the presence of meconium is a marker for a hypoxic episode that has long since past. There is no benefit and potential harm in the routine intubation of these infants.

II. THE NEONATE

The neonate is defined as an infant in the first 30 days of life. This is the time during which most of the life-threatening congenital anomalies become evident. These include congenital heart defects, congenital diaphragmatic hernia, tracheoesophageal fistula, and anterior abdominal wall defects. The most frequent cause of mortality in the first 30 days of life is prematurity. The second most frequent cause of mortality and morbidity in the first 30 days of life is congenital defects. Some infants will have the problem of both prematurity and a congenital defect. Another subtle and fortunately infrequent complicating factor in the neonate is the problem of birth asphyxia and a congenital defect. Birth asphyxia may result in heart failure, renal failure, central nervous system instability, or a combination of all three. Fortunately, none of the congenital defects except for gastroschisis require immediate therapy, and so a period of stabilization can be achieved before the necessity for surgery. Because additional congenital anomalies occur more frequently in infants with one congenital anomaly, cardiac evaluation should be undertaken in any infant in whom surgery is contemplated. In congenital anomalies such as a tracheoesophageal fistula, the major risk of death and illness in an infant greater than 2 kg is not from the surgical condition itself, but from congenital heart disease. As a general statement, congenital heart defects are found in approximately 20% of the infants with congenital diaphragmatic hernia, tracheoesophageal fistula, and omphalocele.

At present, there are few lifesaving emergency surgical procedures that need to be performed on newborns. Therefore in most circumstances, if the local surgical team does not believe itself capable of managing the neonate, arrangements can be made for transport to a facility that is capable of their care. The major issue would be stabilization of the infant and then safe, rapid transport to the tertiary facility. In most locations within North America, this is certainly possible.

A. Specific congenital anomalies

1. Hypoplastic left heart syndrome. Fortunately, hypoplastic left heart syndrome is a relatively rare congenital defect occurring in 1 in 6000 live births; however it accounts for 15% of all neonatal deaths from congenital heart disease.[18] It has an extremely high mortality within the first month of life, approaching 95%. In the recent years, there have been palliative and hopefully definitive surgical procedures to repair this defect. The palliative repair is that of the Norwood procedure, and the definitive repair is heart transplant. However, both of these operations have a high mortality and morbidity, and heart transplantation has many problems that have yet to be solved. One of the problems with heart transplantation and immunosuppression is that of accelerated atherosclerosis. Hypoplastic left heart syndrome is one of the classic examples where there is a potential for both additional congenital defects as well as morbidity that is associated with the surgical procedure.

There is a 29% incidence of either a major or minor central nervous system abnormality in infants with hypoplastic left heart syndrome.[19] These abnormalities included agenesis of the corpus callosum, micrencephaly, ocular defects, and an immature cortical mantle. A recent report describes the acquired neuropathologic lesions that have been associated with infants undergoing surgery for hypoplastic left heart syndrome.[20] The study included 40 infants who had detailed postmortem neuropathologic examinations. Of the infants, 55% were free of acquired brain lesions, whereas 45% had a combination of hypoxic ischemic lesions and intracranial hemorrhage. The major associated findings with infants with cerebral necrosis included low diastolic blood pressures during surgery with cardiopulmonary bypass and hypothermic circulatory arrest and hyperglycemia. Although acidosis and hypercapnia were not associated with significant problems, hyperglycemia was. This report suggested that the acquired brain lesions in some of these infants may have resulted from the augmentation by hyperglycemia of the effects of hypoxia on the central nervous system.[21,22]

2. Congenital diaphragmatic hernia (CDH).

The mortality for infants born with congenital diaphragmatic hernia remains approximately 50%, which is not much different from what it was 20 years ago. The reason for this is not the lack of technology that is available but the underlying anatomic defect. For a long time, the basic pathologic condition was believed to be a lung that was compressed by an intestine that herniated through a hole in the diaphragm. The compression of the lung was believed to result in varying degrees of underdevelopment of the lung tissue. It was hoped that if the hernia could be reduced and the lung reexpanded then there should be a positive outcome. Unfortunately, this has not proved to be the case.

There is an alternative hypothesis as to the underlying pathophysiologic condition of CDH. Some believed that the primary defect is underdevelopment of the lung and that the hernia is a secondary or associated defect.[23] In some infants, the underdevelopment of the lung is only minimal and these infants do well after surgery. In other infants, the defect is severe, resulting in a lung bud, not only of the ipsilateral side, but also of the contralateral side, resulting in a fatal outcome. Then there are those infants who are somewhere in between. Their outcome depends on the degree of underdevelopment of the lung as well as the supportive care. Some of these infants will survive, and some will not. A recent study in infants after surgery for CDH demonstrated that the majority had a decrease in compliance and a worsened outcome than might be expected.[24] For that reason, the current thinking among the majority of physicians is that these infants should have a period of intubation and stabilization before surgery. If the infant has a $Paco_2$ greater than 40 and a Pao_2 less than 60 on 100% oxygen with maximum ventilation, which reflects severe pulmonary hypoplasia, then there is almost a 100% mortality.[25]

There are several critical times in the clinical management of these infants. One of these is at the time of expansion of the lung after the reduction of the hernia. At that point, pressurizing the lung to 30 cm of water under direct vision will allow the lung to expand in a gentle way. Any pressures greater than this may result in a contralateral pneumothorax. Any sudden deterioration in oxygenation and vital signs after expansion of the lung is strongly suggestive of a contralateral pneumothorax and the need for a chest tube. Often regardless of the underdevelopment of the lungs, the anes-

thetic can be successfully managed. It is the postoperative recovery in the infant with marginal lung function that is very difficult. The current techniques for supportive care are mainly those of ventilation with paralysis and narcotics for sedation. In cases of respiratory failure, where maximum ventilatory efforts are unsuccessful, the use of ECMO has been suggested.

3. Tracheoesophageal fistula (TEF).

The infant with tracheoesophageal fistula has three potential areas for problems: (1) prematurity and the respiratory distress syndrome (RDS), (2) congenital heart disease (20% incidence), and (3) aspiration pneumonia and dehydration. Some premature infants have the respiratory distress syndrome as well as a TEF. These patients represent an enormous challenge for the management team because the stomach has a much higher compliance than the lungs, with the result that positive-pressure ventilation may be quite ineffective in ventilating the lungs but quite effective in the expansion of the stomach with gas, which predisposes the infant to regurgitation and aspiration. Distension of the stomach with gas also will elevate the diaphragm with the potential of reducing ventilation. For that reason, these infants are often managed with an emergency ligation of the TEF and then a definitive repair later when conditions have improved. The other management technique is the passage of a Fogerty catheter down the trachea and into the fistula and then ventilation of the infant until improvement occurs. Surgical repair follows later.

In the usual infant with TEF, the anesthesiologist is faced with the problem of the placement of the tip of the endotracheal tube below the fistula. Most fistulas originate in the membranous posterior part of the lower trachea and connect into the distal end of the esophagus. Excessive positive-pressure ventilation may fill the stomach with gas, setting up the potential for regurgitation, aspiration, and reduced ventilation. Therefore the placement of the endotracheal tube below the fistula is a useful technique in the management of these infants. It would appear that the easiest technique to achieve this placement would be to pass the endotracheal tube into one mainstem bronchus as is evidenced by chest movement and breath sounds and then slowly withdraw the tube until there are bilateral breath sounds and chest movement. If a gastrostomy tube is in place, the end of the gastrostomy tube should always be open and left at the head of the table beside the anesthesiologist, so that it cannot be obstructed. A patent gastrostomy tube is very useful for decompressing the stomach if gastric distension occurs with ventilation.

4. Anterior abdominal wall defects. Gastroschisis is a developmental problem that is associated with the intrauterine interruption of the blood supply to the anterior abdominal wall, leading to a hernia of the abdominal contents that is not covered by any membrane.[26] The result is a situation where the potential for the complication of fluid loss and infection is great. The incidence of associated congenital anomalies is very low. The other major anterior abdominal wall defect is an omphalocele. An omphalocele is an embryologic defect. The normal division by the diaphram of the thoracoabdominal cavity from a single cavity into a double cavity occurs at approximately 6 to 10 weeks of fetal life.[23] At this point, the intestines will herniate into the umbilical cord while the diaphragm develops. Somewhere between 10 and 14 weeks of fetal life, the intestines return to their final resting place within the abdomen. In the situation of an omphalocele, varying amounts of the intestines remain in their extraabdominal location covered by amnion. The incidence of associated congenital heart defects is approximately 20%. Some anterior abdominal wall defects are simple to close and result in little intra-abdominal tension. Other defects are moderately large, and there is insufficient peritoneum to cover them, and so a skin closure is accomplished. In the most severe form of an anterior abdominal wall defect, there is insufficient peritoneum, skin, and muscle to cover the defect. Therefore the intestinal contents are contained with a Dacron silo, and then the silo is reduced in a stepwise fashion over a period of a week to 10 days. The major problem these infants have is an increased intra-abdominal pressure. This increased intra-abdominal pressure may be transmitted to the blood vessels of the lower extremities, reducing venous return and causing edema of the lower extremities. This increased intra-abdominal pressure may also result in a reduction of blood flow to the abdominal organs. In the case of the kidney, this reduced flow will lead to renal ischemia, the activation of the renin-angiotensin-aldosterone system, resulting in renal failure and hypertension. In addition, the increased intraabdominal pressure may elevate the diaphragm, thereby reducing ventilation. All these factors need to be taken into consideration in the repair and postoperative care of these infants. It has been shown that an intra-abdominal pressure of approximately 20 to 25 cm of water or less is compatible with a successful primary closure of this defect. Pressures greater than this will result in ischemia of the kidneys and abdominal structures resulting in the need for reoperation for the placement of the Dacron silo.[27]

B. Extracorporeal membrane oxygenation (ECMO)

ECMO is a technique of supportive care that has developed over the past 6 to 8 years. Its primary use in infants has been in the respiratory failure that occurs with meconium aspiration syndrome and the respiratory distress syndrome; however it is used in any type of respiratory failure. The object of ECMO is to allow the lung to rest, minimizing alveolar hyperoxia, and barotrauma. The period of ECMO varies from hours to days. The technique involves cannulization of the internal carotid as the vessel that will provide the blood supply for the pump oxygenator and cannulization of the internal jugular vein for the return of oxygenated blood to the infant. The lungs remain inflated with an FiO_2 of 30% at 5 cm of PEEP. As the infant's lungs improve and the PaO_2 improves, the infant is slowly weaned from ECMO. There are several problems associated with ECMO. These include (1) heparinization and the dangers of bleeding and (2) ligation of the internal carotid artery. Many of the infants who have had ECMO have been critically ill at the time that they were placed on ECMO, and so it is difficult to tell in these instances of residual damage or bad outcome if the damage was present before the ECMO was begun. On the other hand, there are certain post-ECMO observations that are being made in these infants, such as the occurrence of focal seizures, changes in the retina, and changes in the pattern of cerebral circulation.[28,29] It will take time for these issues to become sorted out.

C. Pharmacokinetics in the neonate

There are special problems in the neonate of anesthetic drugs that require the liver for metabolism. The two drugs that have attracted the most attention are fentanyl and vecuronium. Two studies in neonates have shown that there is greatly reduced metabolism of fentanyl. The result of reduced metabolism was that some infants required prolonged periods (up to 40 hours) of intubation and ventilation because of the prolonged effects of fentanyl. It is not clear whether this is attributable to alterations of liver blood flow after surgery or the immaturity of the liver, or both.[30,31] (Fig. 23-2). Vecuronium depends on the liver for metabolism. In the neonate there is a reduction in the speed of this metabolism, and so vecuronium in the neo-

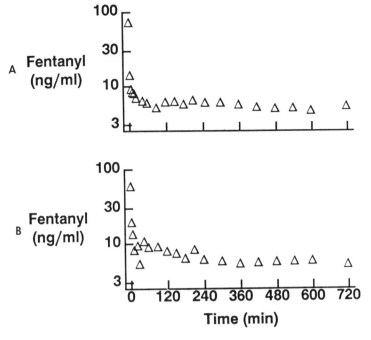

Fig. 23-2. Plasma concentration versus time data are shown for two neonates. **A,** Data for a 1-day-old infant who had repair of an omphalocele and received fentanyl, 52.5 µg/kg, as a 2-minute infusion. **B,** Data for a 3-day-old infant who had repair of hydronephrosis and received fentanyl, 56.5 µg/kg, as a 2-minute infusion. For both patients, after the initial distribution phase there is no further decrease in the plasma concentration during the remaining 10 hours. The data indicate that no clearance may have occurred during this period. (From Gauntlett IS, Fisher DM, Hertzka RE, et al: Anesthesiology 69:683, 1988.)

nate is not a medium-length muscle relaxant, that is, 30 to 45 minutes. Its time course is more like that of curare or pancuronium. Atracurium is the muscle relaxant of choice when a medium-length muscle relaxant is needed in the neonate.

D. Prenatal cocaine exposure and its effects upon the infant

The use of cocaine by Americans has increased in a spectacular fashion over the past decade with an estimated 25 million Americans having used cocaine at some point in their life and approximately 5 million using cocaine on a regular basis.[32] *Pediatric News* (February 1986) reported that in Detroit and its suburbs an estimated 10% of pregnant women use cocaine. Cocaine is an amino alcohol base that is structurally similar to synthetic local anesthetics such as lidocaine. One of the pharmacologic actions of cocaine is that it will prevent the reuptake of neurotransmitters such as epinephrine, norepinephrine, and serotonin at nerve terminals. This leads to increasing levels of the neurotransmitters and an exaggerated responsiveness or su-

persensitivity that can effect the central nervous and cardiovascular systems. There is an increase in motor activity, hyperthermia, and a host of cardiovascular effects, including tachycardia, vasoconstriction, and hypertension. The surprising thing is that fetal cocaine exposure is apparently not associated with a substantially increased risk of teratogenesis.[33]

In some pregnant mothers who use cocaine in the first trimester of pregnancy, abruptio placenta and stillbirth have been reported to occur shortly after either the intranasal or intravenous injection of cocaine later in pregnancy. Also, there is reported to be an increased incidence of spontaneous abortion.[34]

The second period when cocaine abnormalities become obvious is at the time of birth. There is an increased incidence of prematurity, inhibited intrauterine growth, retardation, and various developmental defects. These developmental defects have included cavitary central nervous system lesions, limb-reduction defects, cardiac anomalies, genitourinary anomalies, and intestinal atresia or infarction. The exact cause of this spectrum of developmental problems is not fully understood, but there are several possibilities for the mechanism by which it may occur.[34] The underlying pathogenesis for the mechanism is that of vascular disruption. The vascular disruption may occur either because of hemorrhage, emboli, or vasoconstriction. The mechanism by which hemorrhage could occur is that if there was a rapid increase in systemic and cerebral blood pressure this might lead to a hemorrhage within the various vascular beds of the central nervous system. A recent report describes a stillborn infant with limb deformities who was found to have multiple areas of infarction within the placenta that could have embolized the thrombosed blood to the extremities.[34] Another possible mechanism is that of vasoconstriction secondary to the pharmacologic effects of cocaine. This could lead to uterine, placental, or fetal vasoconstriction. This disruption of the blood supply could lead to altered morphogenesis of the developing structures. Disruption of the superior mesenteric artery early in fetal life may lead to intestinal atresia, and if it occurs later in fetal life, it might result in bowel infarction, which has been described. The stigmas of cocaine use may then be present at birth. The surprising factor is that there is not an increase in eclampsia. Depending on when the mother last used cocaine, the infant might also undergo a neonatal abstinence syndrome.

1. Cardiovascular changes found in newborns of mothers who use cocaine. Fifteen full-term newborn infants whose mothers had a history of cocaine use during pregnancy were recently studied.[35] Table 23-1 reveals the data. The cocaine-exposed infants had a reduced cardiac output and stroke volume and a higher arterial blood pressure in keeping with either a

transplacental passage of catecholamines or of cocaine, which then resulted in an increased level of circulating catecholamines. It is of interest that by day 2 the differences between the cocaine and the control group had completely disappeared. It would appear from these data that if an infant of a cocaine-using mother is born with a congenital anomaly requiring surgery and unless the surgery is of an extremely urgent or emergency nature, that surgery should be postponed until at least the second or third postnatal day to allow the effects of the cocaine to abate.

2. Mortality and cocaine use. There is a higher incidence of intrauterine growth–retarded infants in mothers who have used cocaine and a higher mortality has been reported for intrauterine growth–retarded infants. In addition, a high percentage of the infants born of mothers who have used cocaine have been reported to have a continued delay in the various indexes of motor ability and perceptual performance for several years.[33] Lastly there has been a report that suggests that there is an increased incidence of sudden infant death syndrome (SIDS) in infants who have had an in utero cocaine exposure.[36] SIDS is the leading cause of death between the ages of 1 month and 1 year of life. It is evident that the infant born of the mother who uses cocaine is at increased risk for many, many problems in the fetal as well postnatal period. The delay in development as well as the occurrence of SIDS may be subtle causes of a bad outcome. If one of these infants should have a surgical procedure that is associated with a critical incident and then if there is a bad outcome, that is, developmental delay or sudden infant death, the causative factor for this may be incorrectly alleged

Table 23-1. Cardiac function in cocaine-exposed and control full-term newborn infants on the first and second day of life

	Day 1			Day 2		
	Cocaine-exposed group ($n = 15$)	Control group ($n = 22$)	P value	Cocaine-exposed group ($n = 15$)	Control group ($n = 22$)	P value
Cardiac output (ml/ kg/min)	183 ± 12	235 ± 13	$<.05$	222 ± 10	240 ± 8	NS
Stroke volume (ml/ kg)	1.3 ± 0.1	1.9 ± 0.1	$<.005$	1.6 ± 0.1	1.8 ± 0.1	NS
Heart rate (beats/ min)	142 ± 11	133 ± 20	NS	140 ± 11	134 ± 12	NS
Arterial blood pressure (mm Hg)	60 ± 2	41 ± 2	$<.001$	55 ± 1	56 ± 2	NS

From van de Bor M et al: Pediatrics 85:31, 1990.
Results are given as means $\pm$ SD; P values were obtained from student's test for unpaired observations; *NS,* not significant.

to be an event in the perioperative period, whereas the true cause for the problem may well be the in utero exposure to cocaine. This is yet untraveled ground.

III. THE PREMATURE INFANT

A premature birth is defined in terms of gestational age, that is, conception until birth, and the premature infant is an infant born below 37 weeks of gestational age. Prematurity is one of the leading causes of infant mortality. The reasons for it are multiple and are not discussed here. Medical technology has brought about an increased survival of these very small infants, many of whom have catastrophic short-term and long-term medical problems. Unfortunately, quality of life has not been part of the formula for the management of these infants, and even a superficial exposure to this unfortunate group of infants would reveal that technology has far exceeded humanity. Nonetheless, the anesthesiologist is faced with the anesthetic management of these infants. The discussion of this particular part of the chapter is primarily concerned with the complications that may accompany the management of the premature infant. These include the retinopathy of prematurity, hernia repair, and the ever present and unresolved issue of the management of the premature nursery graduate and the concern of postoperative apnea. This last issue primarily involves whether these patients can be done on an ambulatory basis.

A. Retinopathy of prematurity

In the last 40 or so years, the clinical picture and management of infants with retinopathy of prematurity has undergone major change.[37,38] It was recognized in the early and middle 1950s that the unrestricted use of oxygen, particularly in the small infant, was associated with a very high incidence of retinopathy of prematurity. After this, there were very restricted policies that were followed concerning the use of oxygen in the newborn infant. Certainly at that time, the analysis of blood gases was in its infancy and attempts to correlate arterial oxygen values with retinopathy of prematurity proved to be fruitless. However, one thing became evident with the restrictive management of oxygen administration to newborns. Up until this point, there had been a progressive decrease in the mortality and morbidity of infants. After the restrictive oxygen policies, there was a leveling off and in some countries an increase in the incidence of central nervous system damage that were attributed to the restrictive use of ox-

ygen.[39,40] Over the ensuing years, attempts were made at determining a "safe" level of oxygenation as determined by transcutaneous oxygen values and later by the pulse oximeter. Despite modern technology, there is still no study that can document what level of oxygenation will result in the retinopathy of prematurity. Rather, what has been found is that the more immature the infant, the higher is the incidence of the retinopathy of prematurity regardless of intensive attempts to evaluate and control the administration of oxygen. Therefore it would seem that the retinopathy of prematurity represents a normal state of the retina of some premature infants and does not represent a breach of care. This leaves the anesthesiologist in somewhat of a management quandary. In the 1970s, a case report in the anesthesia literature suggested that the oxygen that was given during the period of anesthesia might be associated with the retinopathy of prematurity and various recommendations were made at that time.[41] There has never been any documentation that the relatively short time of an anesthetic is sufficient for the development of the retinopathy of prematurity. There are differences of opinion as to how the anesthesiologist should attempt to control the Pao_2 of the premature infant. One opinion is that attempts should be made to control oxygenation by monitoring the oxygen saturations and keeping them between approximately 94% to 97%. The other opinion is that the short period of anesthesia is relatively insignificant and that hypoxia is much more of a danger than the retinopathy of prematurity. There would appear to be no consensus on this issue.

B. Prematurity and incidence of inguinal hernia

Hernias that appear in infants under 1 year of age have a natural course different from that of hernias that appear after a year. The incarceration rate of infants under 1 year of age approaches 31%, compared to a 15% to 18% incidence in hernias that appear after 1 year of age.[42] In addition, the incidence of hernias in premature infants is much higher than the incidence of hernias in full-term infants.[43] One of the best studies to document the problems of the premature infant and hernia repair is that of Rescorla and Grosfeld.[42] They reported a series of 100 infants who were operated on by the time they were 2 months of age: 30% of these infants were premature, 42% had a history of the respiratory distress syndrome, and 16% had been ventilated for this condition. A congenital heart defect was found in 19%. Of these infants, 31% had an incarcerated hernia, and 9% were found to have an intestinal obstruction. Two percent of the infants had a gonadal infarction. It becomes evident that the infant who develops a hernia shortly after birth, or during the period in the premature nursery, represents a relatively high-risk situation for the development of an urgent or emergent surgical problem. For that reason, these infants need to be operated on within a reasonable period of time after discovery of the hernia, rather than discharging them home to grow until some arbitrary age, in the hopes that there will be no supervening incarceration or intestinal obstruction.

The anesthesiologist may be presented with two major different clinical scenarios for the management of premature infants: (1) the infant who is still in the premature nursery and who may have varying degrees of heart disease or lung disease who needs an urgent hernia repair or even perhaps an emergency hernia repair or (2) the infant who is scheduled to appear in the ambulatory surgery clinic for "elective" hernia repair. The issues are those of the age at which premature infants can be managed as ambulatory patients and the anesthetic techniques that might have the best outcome in this very vulnerable group of infants. These issues are discussed later in the chapter.

C. Periventricular-intraventricular hemorrhage (PV-IVH)

There is no question but that the premature infant runs a much higher risk of developing PV-IVH. Also, it is believed that newborn infants, regardless of gestational age, who have suffered from acute hypoxia have decreased autoregulation.[44,45] Decreased autoregulation results in a condition in which cerebral blood flow is pressure passive, and any increases in blood pressure will increase cerebral blood flow and the potential for PV-IVH. At any rate, some of the manipulations performed by the anesthesiologists have the potential to induce hypertension, particularly if these manipulations are done in the unanesthetized state. This would include manipulations such as starting of intravenous fluids and awake intubation.

The other potential for increasing blood pressure is the use of anesthetic techniques that have the potential for the development of hypertension such as an opioid-pancuronium combination. Recent studies in a group of premature infants who were observed for PV-IVH have provided some concepts about the natural history and incidence of PV-IVH and some of the factors that might possibly be associated with it.[46] These studies were performed because it has been suggested for a long time in the pediatric literature that increases in blood pressure, which often occur with intensive care procedures, manipulations, and so on, are associated with increases in blood pressure, and the increases in blood pressure were believed to be implicated in the pathogenesis of PV-IVH.[47,48] Other studies have shown that hypoxic episodes that frequently occur in prematures have been associated with cerebral hyperremia.[45] The other factor that may be important in the high incidence of PV-IVH is the fact that the germinal matrix receives a relatively low blood flow under normal physiologic conditions, which may make it more vulnerable to various blood pressure or hypoxic insults. It is also becoming well recognized that not only is the initial insult, that is, hypertension or hypoxia, important, but also varying degrees of injury may occur with reperfusion.

The natural history of PV-IVH was described in a recent study of some 53 infants less than 1500 g.[46] The infants were divided into two groups, those below 1000 g and those over 1000 g. In infants who weighed less than 1000 g, 85% had a PV-IVH, whereas the incidence for infants weighing more than a 1000 g was 14%. Approximately 65% of the infants who developed a PV-IVH did so in the first 24 hours and the rest had developed the PV-IVH by 72 hours. The authors developed what they referred to as a "stability boundary" for blood pressure. When infants' blood pressure went beyond the "stability boundary," the incidence of PV-IVH was significantly higher, that is, 70%. When the blood pressure remained below this stability boundary, the incidence was 13%. Fig. 23-3 also would indicate that smaller prematures have lower blood pressures and that the base-line blood pressure needs to be taken into consideration when determining the "stability boundary." It can be seen from the data that a systolic blood pressure in an infant below 750 g of 100 mm Hg can be associated with PV-IVH, whereas in the larger infant there is no such association. Approximately 75% of the highest peak systolic blood pressures were associated with motor activity of the infant. The motor activity either was spontaneous or had been induced by nursery procedures. Of much more interest is the fact that 25% of the infants had peak systolic pressures associated with no discernible handling or spontaneous activity. It was not known whether noise in the nursery such as would occur from telephones or beepers was responsible for the infants' blood pressure response without any motor response.

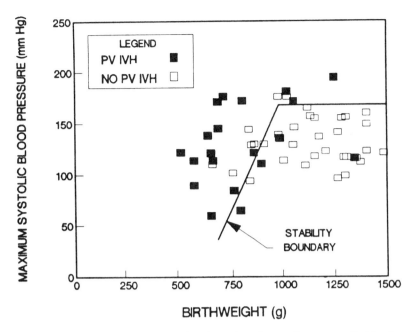

Fig. 23-3. Birth weight–dependent stability boundary for maximum systolic blood pressure. (From Perry EH, Bada HS, Ray JD, et al: Pediatrics 85:727, 1990.)

What is the bottom line for the anesthesiologist? Since it would appear that there is some correlation between these peak systolic pressures and the development of PV-IVH, at least in the first several days of life, it would appear that, when possible, all procedures (that is, intubations) should be done with sedation or anesthesia, unless the infant is so critically ill that to do so would increase the risk compared to the benefits. There is insufficient data to draw any conclusions, but the general belief is that all procedures, whether or not they require sedation or anesthesia, need to be thought of in a risk-benefit fashion. As an example, if an infant is vomiting and has the risk of aspiration during induction and intubation, an awake intubation should be considered, but a rapid sequence induction and intubation may be as safe depending on the circumstances. On the other hand, if there are no compelling reasons for an awake intubation, the infant deserves the same consideration as older patients and should receive the appropriate anesthesia or sedation. Just because a premature infant can be overpowered is not a reason to withhold appropriate anesthetic techniques.[49]

D. The premature nursery graduate

It follows that with the increasing number of premature infants who survive there is an increasing number of premature nursery graduates. They present medical problems in three different areas: (1) chronic lung disease, (2) subglottic stenosis, and (3) apnea.[50]

1. Chronic lung disease. Any infant who has been intubated and ventilated is a candidate for chronic lung disease. The majority of the infants who have this problem are those premature infants who were born with a deficiency of surfactant, resulting in the respiratory distress syndrome. In recent years, there has been an enormous thrust to develop a human surfactant replacement that could be used in these infants of very low birth weight to prevent or treat the respiratory distress syndrome.[51-53] In some trials, all premature infants below a certain weight have been immediately intubated and surfactant has been instilled down the trachea. In others, the treatment was begun after the infant had been intubated and started on ventilatory support for the respiratory distress syndrome. The results of these various studies indicate that there appears to be an immediate improvement in lung function and short-term outcome. Also, the infants that have received surfactant have a decreased incidence of pulmonary interstitial emphysema and pneumothorax compared with control infants who did not receive surfactant.[53] Perhaps most importantly, there would appear to be a major reduction in the occurrence of bronchopulmonary dysplasia in infants who have been treated with surfactant. The future does look promising for the amelioration of the effects of lack of surfactant.

However, there still will be infants who have chronic lung disease. This chronic lung disease will present as a spectrum of clinical problems. In the infant with mild disease, there may be only increased secretions and mild reactive airway disease. At the far end of the spectrum is the child with severe bronchopulmonary dysplasia who is oxygen dependent.[54] There is a significant mortality among this latter group of infants. Then there is a range of infants in between. The important issue for the anesthesiologist is to be able to identify the infant with residual lung disease. The infant with severe chronic lung disease represents no problem of identification. Many of these infants will be on chronic diuretic therapy, and the diuretics should be continued in the perioperative period.[55,56] It is the one with mild respiratory disease and the reactive airway that may present a problem for the anesthesiologist. The red flag for the possibility of residual lung disease is a history that the infant was intubated and ventilated. If the infant is growing normally, is feeding normally, and has had insignificant respiratory infections or symptoms, this infant can be considered normal. However, if the infant has frequent episodes of coughing, recurrent respiratory tract infections, and so on, a high index of suspicion is aroused that this infant is going to present some clinical challenges. Infants with varying degrees of residual airway disease will present with varying degrees of increased airway reactivity, increased secretions, and decreased compliance and in general represent an increased risk of respiratory complications. Infants with moderately severe to severe degrees of residual lung disease need to be managed as inpatients, whereas those patients who have mild residual disease can be managed expectantly as outpatients. These infants benefit from generous doses of anticholinergics to reduce secretions and dilate large airways. Because of the reactive airway disease, they are prone to problems with laryngospasm, bronchospasm, and secretions and are best managed with an endotracheal tube except for the shortest of anesthetic procedures. In addition, they should remain intubated until awake. Infants with mild residual lung disease might slip through the preoperative screening and develop problems with bronchospasm or laryngospasm during induction. In other infants the troubles occur at the end of surgery. Premature extubation of these infants often results in a tumultuous postoperative course, since they will not have normal ventilation and will be unable to effectively remove the inhalation anesthetics from their system. For that reason, any infant who appears to be having any degree of reactive airway disease should be left intubated until awake and able to manage his or her protective reflexes and airway. This period of intubation can be smoothed over by the administration of intravenous anticholinergics as well as 1 to 1.5 mg/kg of lidocaine, which can be repeated.

2. Subglottic stenosis. In 1981, Jones et al. reported on a group of premature infants who had been intubated and ventilated for respiratory problems[57] and 20% of whom subsequently developed subglottic stenosis after discharge. At the time of discharge from the premature nursery, they were believed to be asymptomatic and without airway difficulty. The subglottic stenosis became evident only when the infants acquired a respiratory infection. The increased secretions and edema from the airway infection when added to the previously unrecognized subglottic stenosis caused the infants to have problems with respiratory distress leading to their diagnosis of subglottic stenosis. The anesthesiologist may obtain that history from the parent, or there may be no history of any problems. The first time that the anesthesiologist may become aware that an infant has unrecognized subglottic stenosis is when endotracheal intubation is attempted. If an infant cannot be intubated with the normal-size endotracheal tube and the next-size endotracheal tube cannot be passed or there is no air leak, serious concern for the presence of subglottic stenosis arises. At that point, the anesthesiologist is faced with somewhat of a quandry. If this is emergency surgery that cannot be delayed, an endotracheal tube needs to be used even if it is small and the infant is ventilated for the surgical procedure. Extubation may be possible at the end of surgery with the use of dexamethasone (Decadron) and racemic epinephrine. If the surgery is elective, in this situation postponement until the airway can be evaluated would seem to be the most conservative approach. At times, a pediatric surgeon familiar with airway disease may be immediately available, at which time an evaluation of the airway can be made and then a judgment made as to whether to proceed with the surgery.

3. Apnea. Apnea is a frequent finding in the premature infant and is believed to be caused by an immature respiratory center. The incidence of apneic episodes is inversely correlated with conceptual age. As premature infants approach the conceptual age of 44 to 48 weeks, the incidence of apnea decreases rapidly to almost nil.[58] One of the problems with the various studies is the definition of apnea. Welborn et al. have recently defined the various types of apnea used in their clinical studies.[59,60] Brief apnea is defined as a respiratory pause of less than 15 seconds, not associated with bradycardia, whereas prolonged or potentially life-threatening apnea is defined as a respiratory pause of 15 seconds or longer or less than 15 seconds if accompanied by bradycardia. Bradycardia is defined in this situation as a heart rate of less than 100 beats/min for at least 5 seconds. There has been a concern that the administration of anesthetics and other depressants might increase the incidence of apnea in premature infants. There have been many studies that have been done in premature infants at the various conceptual ages.[58,60,61] It is important to use the term "conceptual age," which is defined as the age from the time of conception until the current age. It is the gestational age plus postnatal age. The majority of studies have demonstrated that in cases of hernia repair and other types of superficial surgery apnea may develop postoperatively in those premature infants who have a postconceptual age (PCA) of less than 44 to 46 weeks.[58,60] Over 44 to 46 PCA, the incidence of apnea was nil. One study has reported that apnea may occur at a later postconceptual age, that is, up to 55 to 60 weeks.[61] However, in this study, the type of surgery was not limited to superficial surgery but rather included such procedures as exploratory laparotomy and a ventriculoperitoneal shunt. Therefore, when studies of postoperative apnea are being evaluated, it is crucial to take into consideration not only the conceptual age, but the health of the infant as well as the type of surgery.

The importance of the issue of apnea is when one considers at what PCA to allow superficial and hernia surgery to be done on an ambulatory basis. There are two current opinions. One is that infants under 50 weeks of PCA should be admitted for all surgery and should be monitored overnight for apnea and bradycardia.[58,60] In some institutions, in addition, these infants are administered caffeine. For infants over 50 weeks of PCA, the infants can be managed as ambulatory patients with no special precautions. The other opinion is that all patients under 60 weeks of PCA need to be admitted and monitored and that these infants can be managed as ambulatory patients only when they are greater than 60 weeks of PCA.[61]

There is also a difference of opinion about whether the choice of anesthesia makes any difference in the outcome. Several studies have suggested that regional anesthesia is the preferred technique in relatively high-risk infants.[62,63] However it has been shown that the administration of sedatives to a infant with regional anesthesia causes an incidence of apnea that is similar to that seen with general anesthesia.[64] In addition, both spinal anesthesia and caudal anesthesia have an incidence of complications that is significant enough so that the choice of technique is not simple.[65,66] The other issue that is somewhat controversial at present concerns the use of caffeine to eliminate the problem of apnea. Welborn and her colleagues have demonstrated quite conclusively that caffeine can greatly alter the incidence of postoperative apnea, and they recommend that 10 mg/kg be given intravenously at the beginning of surgery.[60] This is for infants who are under 48 to 50 weeks of PCA. They still need to be monitored and admitted overnight. It would appear that caffeine in this particular group of infants is safe with a risk-to-benefit ratio that is in favor of the administration of caffeine. Caffeine is a relatively long-lasting drug in these infants, that is, up to a period of several days. The only apparent disadvantage is that the infant may have a higher degree of awareness and may be irritable during this period of time. Caffeine has the distinct advantage over theophylline of being a more potent central nervous system and respiratory stimulant and having fewer side effects.

IV. COMPLICATIONS OF ANESTHETIC TECHNIQUES IN INFANTS

Any discussion of anesthetic techniques in infants must consider the current trend in regional anesthesia, which has been touted by some to be extremely safe and to avoid many of the difficulties associated with postoperative apnea. Certainly the learning curve plays a significant part in the incidence of complications as the anesthesiologist acquires the necessary skills in mastering each anesthetic technique. This is not to suggest that the anesthesiologist should be proficient only in general anesthesia. The requirements of anesthesia practice mandate that the anesthesiologist continue to adapt new techniques and drugs to his or her practice.

A. General anesthesia

Most anesthesiologists are more comfortable using general anesthesia for infants, particularly the high-risk infants. The major complications with general anesthesia in the infant are associated with the establishment and maintenance of the airway as well as the period of extubation and recovery from the anesthetic.[67] Many anesthesiologists do an awake intubation to establish the airway in the small infant. The complications in the premature infant and in the asphyxiated infant have been discussed previously. Other complications associated with awake intubation include trauma to the airway as well as hypoxia. The degree of hypoxia was not fully appreciated until the advent of the pulse oximeter. However, anyone who has performed or watched an awake intubation in the small infant can appreciate the struggle, which is expressed by coughing, breath holding, desaturation, and so on. Insufflation of oxygen, either with the laryngoscope or by whatever technique, may reduce but will not circumvent the problem because it is related to the fact that the infant is breath holding or coughing and not ventilating.

A recent study by Coté sponsored by the Anesthesia Patient Safety Foundation revealed that children less than 2 years of age had a higher incidence of major hypoxic events than older children do.[68] The major finding of this study was the value of the pulse oximeter in both detecting and preventing intraoperative hypoxemic events in infants. The value of the capnograph was also studied. It did not appear to be of value in the detection or prevention of hypoxia but rather was important in evaluating alterations in ventilation that may result in hypercapnia and hypocapnia as well as detecting esophageal intubation before hypoxia occurs.

B. To intubate or not to intubate? Potential complications

The question often arises in the small infant who is going to have a short procedure,that is, under 30 minutes: Does the patient need to be intubated? There is no question but that the very skilled clinician can usually manage even the most difficult airway with a mask, but the flip side of this is that the clinician who does the infrequent infant might not have the skills to maintain a mask airway for a procedure. For that reason, most clinicians would intubate most infants under 6 months for most surgical procedures. The exception to this is an examination under anesthesia that is going to require 5 or 10 minutes or hernia repair with a fast and skilled surgeon. In the older infant, airway management is considerably easier and with the use of the pulse oximeter and capnograph,an ongoing assessment of the success in airway management is much more immediately available. If there is any question about airway management, particularly if documented by the various monitors, endotracheal intubation is the airway management technique of choice.

C. Timing of extubation and postoperative ventilation and avoiding premature extubation

One of the most difficult judgment calls for the anesthesiologist is when to remove the endotra-

cheal tube. If the condition of the infant is marginal, or there is any question about whether the infant will be able to maintain its protective reflexes or ventilation, the endotracheal tube should be left in place and the infant sent to the recovery room or directly to the pediatric or newborn intensive care unit. There has been a changing trend in recent years in where alleged medical malpractice occurs. In the past, the primary location for such claims was from incidents that occurred in the operating room. In the last several years, there has been a major increase in the incidents that are reported to come from the recovery room. Many of the complications of anesthesia in the infant are related to the issue of the timing of extubation.

If the infant is relatively healthy, with appropriate anesthetic planning the infant can be extubated at the end of the procedure in the operating room with protective reflexes intact. The second group of infants is managed with the same type of anesthetic plan, which tailors the anesthetic for extubation at the end of surgery; however if they are not ready for extubation at the end of surgery, they are taken to the recovery room. Then a decision can be made in an unhurried fashion about whether they are appropriate for extubation. If so, they are extubated and observed until the infant is stable and then transferred to the intensive care unit. If after a reasonable period they are still not ready for extubation, they are transferred to the intensive care unit, where the care of the infant is transferred to the medical staff of the intensive care unit. The final group of infants are those in whom it is known that they will need postoperative ventilatory support. The anesthetic in this case is tailored to maintain a degree of sedation and paralysis at the end of the surgery so that the infant may be more safely transported to the intensive care unit where the care of the infant is transferred from the anesthesiologist to the intensive care medical staff. It is usually anticipated that these infants will be extubated in a matter of hours or days.

How does the anesthesiologist then avoid the complication of premature extubation, which can include airway obstruction, hypoxia, pulmonary edema, bradycardia, and delayed awakening because of inability to adequately ventilate? The key is that the infant should be extubated when awake, with protective airway reflexes intact and the neuromuscular system optimal. The signs that the infant is ready is opening of the eyes, crying, coughing, swallowing, and reaching for the endotracheal tube. Even with the most diligent of care, the complication of airway obstruction after extubation cannot be completely avoided, and the clinician must be prepared to reintubate the infant. In some infants, there is always some degree of doubt whether intubation will be successful. These infants should be extubated in the post-anesthesia care unit in an unhurried manner.

D. Complications of regional anesthesia

Regional anesthesia has been highly touted as a very safe technique for infants. However, there are some special factors that make the infant more susceptible to complications in certain areas. One of the most popular and effective regional anesthetic techniques in the infant is caudal epidural anesthesia.[69] However, it should be remembered that the dural sac in the infant may end as low as the S3 level, whereas in the older child and adult the dural sac ends at the S1 level. The technique described for the older child and adult is to penetrate the sacrococcygeal ligament at the sacral hiatus and then advance the needle a short distance in the caudal canal. It is obvious in the small infant that great care must be taken as to how far the needle is advanced.[70] Most clinicians would suggest that after penetrating the sacrococcygeal ligament the needle should be advanced only 1 or 2 mm. Aspiration is then performed to determine the presence of cerebrospinal fluid or blood, and then the drug is administered. Despite extreme care and negative aspiration, total spinal anesthesia has been reported in an infant after a carefully performed caudal epidural block.[71] Another potential complication with caudal anesthesia is the fact that the posterior bony plate of the sacrum is very soft and it is quite easy for the caudal needle to penetrate the bone and terminate in the bone marrow. This can be avoided by both aspiration and by awareness of the most important clinical sign for the correct needle placement for a caudal epidural injection, which is ease of injection of the solution. As with a lumbar epidural, if the solution cannot be easily administered, the needle needs to be relocated.

E. Spinal anesthesia

Spinal anesthesia is another of the regional anesthetic techniques that has become very popular, particularly in the high-risk infant. However, the infant has some differences from the older child and adult that need to be appreciated. One of these is the fact that it takes a very large dose of the spinal anesthetic to accomplish anesthesia, and the second is that, even with the large dose, the duration of the block is shorter than that found in the adult.[70] As an example, the dose of tetracaine in an infant is 0.5 mg/kg.

In a 70 kg adult, this would represent a dose of 35 mg and would last much longer than it does in an infant. This large dose of tetracaine will provide only 60 to 90 minutes of anesthesia for the infant. Therefore one of the "complications" of spinal anesthesia in the infant is the short duration of the block, which may not be appreciated until the infant begins to move and then the various adjuncts need to be added. Usually this requires the administration of intravenous sedation, which in one series of premature infants was reported to result in a similar incidence of apnea as general anesthesia.[64] In some institutions, the intravenous instillation is not begun until after the spinal anesthetic is administered. The reason for this is that the veins of the lower extremities are then more easily cannulated after the regional anesthetic is given and that sympathectomy rarely causes pressure changes in infants.[72] However, the flip side of this is that precious time may be required for starting the intravenous instillation that needs to be subtracted from the surgical time.

Another complication of spinal anesthesia is the occurrence of a high spinal block. The sympathetic nervous system of the infant is not fully developed for several years. Dohi et al. studied the effects of spinal anesthesia on blood pressure and found that for the first several years of life there was little in the way of cardiovascular effects of a spinal anesthetic.[72] This is a double-edged sword. On the one hand, hypotension is relatively infrequent in the infant and child from regional anesthesia. On the other hand, however, is that in the case of a very high regional anesthetic one of the early warning signs is a decrease in blood pressure. This decrease is not found in an infant, and the first sign of total spinal block may be interference with ventilation as was reported by Bailey et al.[65] The first sign of trouble that the infant experienced was desaturation followed by evidence of paralysis of the upper body. This report also demonstrates that there are potential complications of anesthetic management that are associated with the positioning of infants. Some surgeons request a cautery be used. This requires the placement of a ground plate. Some surgeons lift the feet and torso of the infant and place the Bovie pad on the upper back of the infant, thereby flexing the entire body on the neck (Fig. 23-4). This maneuver may cause the spinal anesthetic to migrate cephalad and cause respiratory insufficiency, as in the case reported by Bailey et al. Removal of the pad at the end of surgery can also provide difficulty if the infant has just been extubated and is attempting

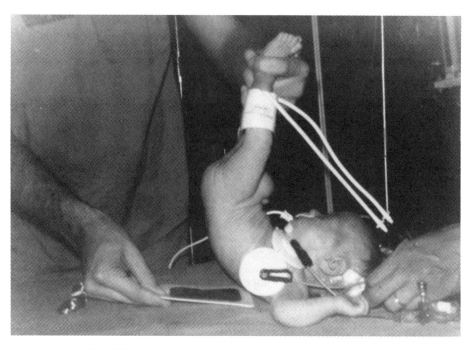

Fig. 23-4. Incorrect technique for placement of Bovie pad.

to regain control of his airway. If the infant is then lifted by the feet and rotated on the neck to remove the pad, this step can interfere with ventilation and precipitate an episode of laryngospasm, which has happened on several occasions to me. Therefore the Bovie pad should be placed either on the upper chest, buttocks, or the leg.

These various complications emphasize the importance of close monitoring with both a stethoscope and a pulse oximeter regardless of whether regional anesthesia or general anesthesia is being used. One must always be cognizant of the fact that Murphy (of Murphy's law) is the constant companion of the anesthesiologist. The next point to remember is that the anesthesiologist must always believe the monitors until the patient and the monitors have been checked.

F. Always believe the monitors!

If there is one theme that the anesthesiologist must remember when dealing with the small infant and child, it is the fact that you must always believe the monitors. If any abnormal values appear on a monitor, the infant requires a check for ventilation and circulation. This should include an analysis of the anesthetic mixtures, the ventilation, feeling the pulse, and so on. Also, if there is any question, the surgeon should be informed. I have reviewed many medical malpractice cases where monitors have

been ignored for several minutes because they were believed to be inaccurate. Then it was discovered after the blood pressure cuff had been moved or the ECG patches replaced or a new oximeter probe attached that the problem was actually the patient. There is no question but that the equipment needs to be checked if the values appear to be wrong, but this is done after there has been a check of the ventilation and circulation of the patient. The caveat for the anesthesiologist is that whenever there are unexpected findings on the monitor first the patient should be checked, the surgeon informed, and then a check made of the monitors.

G. Sudden onset of hypotension or bradycardia as a complication

The complication of the sudden onset of hypotension or bradycardia has undergone an etiologic reevaluation in the past several years because of the pulse oximeter and the capability of monitoring end-tidal gases. Previously, the sudden appearance of either hypotension or bradycardia was attributed to progressive hypoxia that had been missed by the nonvigilant anesthesiologist. There are many plaintiff's experts who travel the country espousing such a view. The pulse oximeter has revealed several things. First of all, complete or nearly complete airway obstruction with progressive hypoxia does not lead to the sudden appearance of bradycardia or hypotension. Severe hypoxia will result in alterations in the heart rate or rhythm as well as the blood pressure before severe bradycardia and hypotension. Put in another way, the sudden onset of bradycardia or hypotension is suggestive of a severe cardiovascular collapse attributable either to a rare but profound vagal response or to an anaphylactic-anaphylactoid reaction. The signs of such a reaction with the percentage of patients involved is found in Table 23-2. The classic triad of anaphylaxis is involvement of the skin, respiratory system, and cardiovascular system. One can rapidly appreciate from the table that all three systems do not need to be present for such a diagnosis to be made.

The classic teaching with the acute onset of bradycardia is that atropine should be administered. If the peripheral circulation remains intact so that venous return is adequate to maintain a reasonable degree of circulation, the intravenous administration of atropine may be effective in treating bradycardia. However, when the bradycardia is severe and the peripheral circulation inadequate, atropine is not the drug of choice, since an increase in heart rate will not be helpful and in all probability, unless cardiac massage is being performed, the atropine will not circulate. Therefore the treatment of the acute onset of hypotension or bradycardia is epinephrine, 5 to 10 μg/kg intravenously. If there is any question about the adequacy of the peripheral circulation, external cardiac massage also needs to be accomplished to maintain or increase the circulation. The remainder of the treatment consists in turning off anesthetics, ventilating with 100% oxygen, expansion of the vascular volume with a balanced salt solution, informing the surgeon, and seeking the cause of the problem. The patient may well need additional doses of epinephrine.

H. Complications of fluid management associated with glucose control

The major perioperative complication in fluid management in the infant is glucose control. The two major potential complications in glucose control are those of hypoglycemia and hyperglycemia.

1. Hypoglycemia. One of the difficulties in the control of glucose in the infant and older child is a definition of what hypoglycemia is. The results of a recent Ciba Foundation discussion meeting was reported by Cornblath et al.[73] The title of the paper certainly characterizes the problem: "Hypoglycemia in Infancy: The Need for a Rational Definition." This paper may help to clear the air about what is hypoglycemia, at least from the standpoint of the infant, but they

Table 23-2. Signs of an anaphylactic-anaphylactoid reaction

Signs	% of patients involved
Tachycardia	94
Circulatory collapse	92
Widespread flush, edema	79
Bronchospasm	39
Cardiac arrest	14
Bradycardia	6
Arrhythmias	4

did not address the issue in the older child. A quotation from this paper brings the problem into focus: "Albert Aynsley-Green returned to the clinical problem of defining neonatal hypoglycemia and illustrated the current dilemma by citing various definitions ranging from 18 to 72 mg/dL glucose from 36 pediatric textbooks and from 178 British pediatricians, the majority of whom used levels of less than 36 mg/dL in full-term infants and less than 20 mg/dL in premature small-for-gestational-age babies as their definition of hypoglycemia." These figures would seem to be very reasonable and worth adopting in our anesthesic practice. Years ago, the issue of hypoglycemia was rarely a problem for the anesthesiologist, since great quantities of glucose were given to all infants. However, as discussed on the next page, hyperglycemia has some potentially serious consequences.

There are several situations where the metabolic status of the baby may be a potential problem for the anesthesiologist. We know that premature infants who are small for gestational age, infants of diabetic mothers, and infants with heart failure all have the potential to become hypoglycemic. As a general rule, it would be useful to know what their blood glucose levels are before and during anesthesia and surgery. It has been well documented, at least in normal older infants and children, that the blood glucose levels remain stable or increase during the period of anesthesia and surgery. In infants who have had problems with their blood glucose, it would be useful to document a blood glucose value during the surgical period. If an infant has had problems with hypoglycemia, a constant infusion of glucose during the perioperative period would avoid the potential problems of hypoglycemia. This is usually given in a constant infusion in a dose of 5 to 7 mg/kg/min. Infants who have been on hyperalimentation should have the infusion continued during the perioperative period.

2. Hyperglycemia: the dangers of glucose and cerebral ischemia. Over the past several years, there has been an enormous interest in the association between the administration of glucose and its effects on worsening the outcome after cerebral ischemia.[21,22] In several of the experimental studies that have been performed, the animals who did not receive glucose but who suffered an ischemic episode appeared to recover normally, whereas those who had received glucose during the period of ischemia and resuscitation had a much worse neurologic outcome.[74,75] This is extremely important for the anesthesiologist because there may occasionally be transient unavoidable episodes of ischemia of the central nervous system secondary to either ventilatory or circulatory problems. It would appear that if intravenous glucose has been administered during this period or in the immediate recovery period the glucose may adversely effect the outcome. The suggested mechanism is that the intravenous glucose, though it may not greatly increase blood glucose, may well increase brain glucose. In the face of ischemia sufficient to trigger anaerobic metabolism, the presence of increased brain glucose will result in a greater production of lactic acid in the central nervous system, which will result in a decrease in the brain pH. Kraig et al. have shown that this will aggravate neuronal injury.[76] In the normal patient, it is prudent to administer glucose-free solutions.

The normal infant does not need to have routine glucose monitoring during surgery, only those infants in whom there is a problem or strong suspicion that there may be hypoglycemia or who received 10% dextrose solutions before surgery. One of the obvious questions about this concern of glucose and brain ischemia is whether there should be tighter control of glucose and whether glucose should be routinely monitored and, if hyperglycemia occurs, treated with insulin. There are no data at present to indicate that a tight control of blood glucose has any clinical application or that there should be routine determination of blood glucose levels during surgery.

V. COMPLICATIONS FROM GENETIC DISORDERS

It is beyond the scope of this chapter to list all the potential complications or the actual complications that have been reported with the various genetic diseases. However, several examples are given to show the complexity of the problems and the enormous challenges that the anesthesiologist must sort out on a daily basis to practice safe anesthesia. One of the problems

with these genetic disorders is that they occur rarely and in some situations may not initially be recognized for what they are. However some syndromes have frequent postoperative complications.[77]

A. Complications of the cervical spine

There are two genetic diseases that have potential complications of the cervical spine. These are Down's syndrome, occurring in approximately 1 in 1000 births, and achondroplastic dwarfism occurring in 2 per 100,000 live births.[78,79] Both of these syndromes are readily recognizable at birth, and both of them have similar potential problems with their cervical spine, that of atlantoaxial instability, which may result in compression of the spinal cord with varying degrees of disability.[80] The problem is that of ligamentous laxity of the transverse ligaments. Normally the connective tissue helps to stabilize the cervical spine; however both of these syndromes have abnormalities of the connective tissue. Approximately 10% to 15% of all children with Down's syndrome will have laxity of the connective tissue, resulting in atlantoaxial instability. Of this number, approximately 10% will become symptomatic sometime in their life. The earliest age that this instability has been reported is 3 years. There are ongoing studies as to the natural history of this problem, but the anesthesiologist needs to be aware of this potential in both of these genetic defects and maintain the head in as neutral a position in the perioperative period as is possible.[81]

B. Complications from genetic neuromuscular disorders

There is a whole host of genetic diseases that result in varying degrees of neuromuscular disorders that in some instances will result in premature death. Duchenne's muscular dystrophy (DMD) is an example of a neuromuscular disorder with a potential for anesthetic complications. Even though the usual onset of the symptoms of DMD is sometime during the second to third year of life, the underlying neuromuscular disease may come to the attention of the anesthesiologist at an earlier age.[82] Alterations within the muscle cell in patients with DMD will result in a flux of K+ when succinylcholine is administered. This flux of potassium may result in varying degrees of hyperkalemia, which apparently, in most patients with DMD, would appear to be of little clinical significance. However, at times, the hyperkalemia has resulted in cardiac arrest or severe circulatory instability.[82,83] Therefore, in any infant in a family with a history of DMD, succinylcholine should be avoided because of this concern for hyperkalemia. In approximately 30% of children with DMD, there is no family history, and so there is no way to avoid this very rare problem. The other problem that is associated with DMD is myocardial involvement. However, this is not a problem in the young infant but becomes a problem as the DMD progresses.

Another problem in the child with DMD is the issue of malignant hyperthermia. Both DMD and malignant hyperthermia are diseases of the control of intracellular calcium. There are various opinions about whether there is an increased incidence of malignant hyperthermia in patients with DMD. There is considerable research at present in both of these conditions, and it is hoped that this issue will be clarified in the near future. One of the reasons for this confusion is that there have been several clinical reports that have confused the issue of hyperkalemia associated with succinylcholine with the hyperkalemia that occurs later in the course of malignant hyperthermia.[83] In malignant hyperthermia the hyperkalemia occurs later on in the syndrome after the injury to the muscle cells and a leaking of potassium into the circulation. In DMD, when hyperkalemia occurs, it occurs within minutes after the administration of succinylcholine. Treatment in this case is directed toward lowering the potassium level, which includes the administration of epinephrine and sodium bicarbonate.[84]

C. Malignant hyperthermia

There has been a great deal of very productive research in the area of masseter spasm, succinylcholine, and malignant hyperthermia in the last several years. Malignant hyperthermia is a genetic disease that results in a state of hypermetabolism. This hypermetabolism is secondary to abnormalities with the intracellular control of calcium resulting in high levels of intracellular calcium. The cellular attempts to maintain normal calcium levels results in a hypermetabolic state that can causes increased oxygen consumption and leads to a respiratory and then a metabolic acidosis as well as muscle rigidity, hyperthermia, and in 50% of the cases, if untreated, death.

VI. COMPLICATIONS OF SUCCINYLCHOLINE
A. Masseter spasm

Recent studies concerning the normal response of the masseter muscle to succinylcholine have caused us to completely reevaluate the issue of "masseter spasm."[85,86] These studies have revealed that the normal response of the masseter muscle to succinylcholine is an increase in tone. As seen in Fig. 23-5, this increase in tone is maximum at the time when the fasciculations

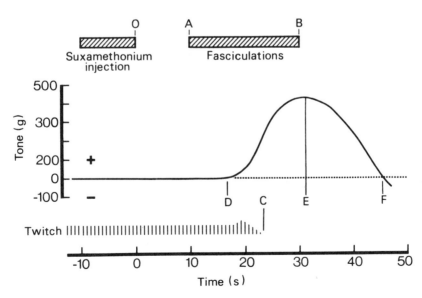

Fig. 23-5. Diagram of study. *A-B,* Period of observed facial muscle fasciculation; *C,* cessation of muscle twitch from ulnar nerve stimulation; *D,* onset of increased muscle tone; *E,* maximum muscle tone; *F,* offset of increased muscle tone. (From Leary NP and Ellis FR: Br J Anaesth 64:488, 1990.)

and the nerve twitch have terminated. Attempts to perform laryngoscopy of the patient at this point occur at a time when the masseter muscle will have its maximum tone. A small but significant number of patients will have sufficient masseter muscle tone (1 in 100), and so it will be difficult to open the mouth.[86] This may well explain some of the previous reports of "masseter spasm." What has also been found in these studies is that low doses of succinylcholine will delay the time of onset of the increase in masseter muscle tone. Therefore, to avoid the complication of "masseter spasm," two techniques are suggested—waiting 20 seconds until fasciculations have stopped and using a larger dose of succinylcholine, that is, 2 mg/kg in infants and children and 1.5 mg/kg in adults.

B. Myalgia

Another of the complications of succinylcholine that is almost completely preventable is that of myalgias. Succinylcholine, particularly in infants and small children, will result in damage to the muscle cell as evidenced by increased levels of creative phosphokinase (CPK) and by myoglobinemia and in some cases myoglobinuria. This is a normal response to succinylcholine. It can be minimized or prevented by the pretreatment with nondepolarizing muscle relaxants (curare or atracurium 0.05 mg/kg). This pretreatment will result in a pronounced reduction in the levels of CPK and so on and a considerable reduction in myalgias. Infants who are not of walking age will be a little bothered by the myalgias, but infants and children of walking age should be pretreated, even though our ability to evaluate this problem in these patients is difficult. For older children and adults the problem of myalgia is so frequent that if the clinician is not going to use pretreatment before succinylcholine that clinician should seriously consider not using succinylcholine except in the most unusual of circumstances because of the complication of myalgia.

C. Malignant hyperthermia (MH)

It is most difficult to determine the youngest age at which MH has occurred in infants. One paper that reported the age to be as young as 7 weeks.[83] In reading the clinical case report, I doubt whether this infant had MH. The imminent development of a genetic test for MH will greatly clear up the issue of the diagnosis in some of these case reports. It has been strongly suggested by recent studies that the increase in masseter muscle tone described on the previous page is not a marker specifically for MH. Two studies address the issue of predicting MH susceptibility by clinical signs.[87,88] One study involved pediatric patients, whereas the other study involved primarily adults. All the patients were suspected of having had a MH episode based on alterations in blood gases, masseter spasm, generalized muscle rigidity, elevated temperature, arrhythmias, myoglobinuria, and elevations of CPK. All the patients were subjected to a muscle biopsy. In the pediatric group, 42% of the patients had a positive muscle biopsy, whereas 62% of the adults had a positive muscle biopsy.[87,88] Attempts to find clinical signs that would aid in the prediction of malignant hyperthermia susceptibility revealed that there was no single finding that was predictable. Table 23-3 gives the results in the study in adults. Generalized rigidity was found in 76% of the children with a positive biopsy but in only 47% of the adults. Masseter spasm was found in approximately an equal incidence between the groups with a negative muscle biopsy (47%) as compared with those with a positive biopsy (34%).

Several papers in the past have strongly suggested that masseter spasm is highly correlated with the development of malignant hyperthermia and point out that 50% of patients with masseter spasm have a positive muscle biopsy.[89,90] The reported incidence of masseter spasm or trismus in one study was 1 in 100 anesthetics when a combination of succinylcholine and halothane was used.[91] However, MH occurs in only approximately 1 in 220,000 general anesthetics.[92] It is evident that this tremendous discrepancy would be suggestive of the need for another explanation for the significance of "masseter spasm." The recent data reported above would strongly indicate that masseter spasm is not a significant indicator of MH but in reality may well be a normal finding. This is relatively new information, and it will take time for this evidence to be fully assimilated in practice. The result is that the clinician is faced with two diametrically opposed positions on what to do in the patient who develops increased masseter muscle tone after succinylcholine. One opinion is that masseter muscle tone is associated with MH and that therefore the case should be immediately stopped, dantrolene administered, and the patient have a muscle biopsy.[93] The other opinion is that masseter muscle tone is not an indicator of MH but is normal with the administration of succinylcholine.[94,95] However, to be on the safe side, these patients need to be carefully monitored with an end-tidal CO_2 and, if there is any ques-

Table 23-3. Incidence of clinical signs in patients found to be malignant-hyperthermia susceptible (MHS) or malignant-hyperthermia negative (MHN) with in vitro testing

Clinical sign	n	MHS incidence n (%)	n	MHN incidence n (%)	p
Masseter spasm	38	13 (34)	23	11 (47)	NS
Generalized rigidity	38	18 (47)	23	1 (5)	0.0001
Tachycardia	38	26 (68)	23	12 (52)	NS
Ventricular arrhythmias	38	15 (39)	23	3 (13)	0.02
Cyanosis	38	23 (60)	23	5 (21)	0.003
Myoglobinuria	17	12 (71)	19	4 (21)	0.003

From Hackl W: Br J Anesth 64:426, 1990.
NS, Not significant.

tion, blood gases. At the same time, the dantrolene should be located and, in the rare instance that malignant hyperthermia is diagnosed, the appropriate treatment regimen instituted.

VII. SUMMARY

The anesthesiologist dealing with infants is walking through a minefield of various potential complications and bad outcomes, some of which are preventable and some, regardless of effort, nonpreventable. Preparation to avoid or identify these complications includes continuing medical education, consultation with colleagues, careful monitoring of the patient, and luck. The one caveat to remember, particularly in infants, is always to believe the monitors.

ACKNOWLEDGMENT

The editorial assistance of Mr. Robert Bland is greatly appreciated.

REFERENCES

1. Stanley FJ: The changing face of cerebral palsy, Dev Med Child Neurol 29:263-265, 1987.
2. Hey E: Fetal hypoxia and subsequent handicap: the problem of establishing a causal link. In Chamberlain GVP, Orr CJB, and Sharp F, editors: Litigation and obstetrics and gynecology, London, 1985, Royal College of Obstetricians and Gynecologists.
3. Blair E and Stanley FJ: Intrapartum asphyxia: a rare cause of cerebral palsy, J Pediatr 112:515-519, 1988.
4. Torfs CP et al: Prenatal and perinatal factors in the etiology of cerebral palsy, J Pediatr 116:615-610, 1990.
5. Freeman JM and Nelson KB: Intrapartum asphyxia and cerebral palsy, Pediatrics 82:240-249, 1988.
6. Moya F and Kvisselgaard N: Placental transmission of succinylcholine, Anesthesiology 22:1-6, 1961.
7. Kvisselgaard N and Moya F: Investigation of placental thresholds to succinylcholine, Anesthesiology 22:7-10, 1961.
8. Baraka A et al: Response of the newborn to succinylcholine injection in homozygotic atypical mothers, Anesthesiology 43:115-116, 1975.
9. Finster M et al: Tissue thiopental concentrations in the fetus and newborn, Anesthesiology 36:155-158, 1972.
10. Finster M et al: The placental transfer of lidocaine and its uptake by fetal tissues, Anesthesiology 36:159-163, 1972.
11. Gaylard DG, Carson RJ, and Reynolds F: Effect of umbilical perfusate pH and controlled maternal hypotension on placental drug transfer in the rabbit, Anesth Analg 71:42-48, 1990.
12. Linder N et al: Need for endotracheal intubation and suction in meconium-stained neonates, J Pediatr 112:613-615, 1988.
13. Wiswell TE, Tuggle JM, and Turner BS: Meconium aspiration syndrome: have we made a difference? Pediatrics 85:715-721, 1990.
14. Murphy JD, Vawter GF, and Reid LM: Pulmonary vascular disease in fetal meconium aspiration, J Pediatr 104:758-762, 1984.
15. Swaminathan S et al: Long-term pulmonary sequelae of meconium aspiration syndrome, J Pediatr 114:356-361, 1989.
16. Ting P and Brady JP: Tracheal suction in meconium aspiration, Am J Obstet Gynecol 122:767-771, 1975.
17. Topis J, Kinas HY, and Kandall SR: Esophageal perforation: a complication of neonatal resuscitation, Anesth Analg 69:532-534, 1989.
18. Morris CD, Outcalt J, and Menashe VD: Hypoplastic left heart syndrome: natural history in a geographically defined population, Pediatrics 85:977-983, 1990.
19. Glauser TA et al: Congenital brain anomalies associated with the hypoplastic left heart syndrome, Pediatrics 85:984-990, 1990.
20. Glauser TA et al: Acquired neuropathologic lesions associated with the hypoplastic left heart syndrome, Pediatrics 85:991-1000, 1990.
21. Nakakimura K et al: Glucose administration before cardiac arrest worsens neurologic outcome in cats, Anesthesiology 72:1005-1011, 1990.
22. Hoffman WE et al: Brain lactate and neurologic outcome following incomplete ischemia in fasted, non-fasted, and glucose-loaded rats, Anesthesiology 72:1045-1050, 1990.
23. Berry FA: Physiology and surgery of the infant. In Berry FA, editor: Anesthetic management of difficult and routine pediatric patients, New York, 1990, Churchill Livingstone.
24. Sakai H et al: Effect of surgical repair on respiratory mechanics in congenital diaphragmatic hernia, J Pediatr 111:432-438, 1987.
25. Bohn D et al: Ventilatory predictors of pulmonary hypoplasia in congenital diaphragmatic hernia, confirmed by morphologic assessment, J Pediatr 111:423-431, 1987.

26. Hoyme HE, Higginbottom MC, and Jones JL: The vascular pathogenesis of gastroschisis: intrauterine interruption of the omphalomesenteric artery, J Pediatr 98:228-231, 1981.

27. Yaster M, Buck JR, Dudgeon DL, et al: Hemodynamic effects of primary closure of omphalocele/gastroschisis in human newborns, Anesthesiology 69:84-88, 1988.

28. Campbell LR et al: Right common carotid artery ligation in extracorporeal membrane oxygenation, J Pediatr 113:110-113, 1988.

29. Patrias et al: Ocular findings in infants treated with extracorporeal membrane oxygenator support, Pediatrics 82:560-564, 1988.

30. Koehntop DE, Rodman JH, Brundage DM, et al: Pharmacokinetics of fentanyl in neonates, Anesth Anal 65:227-232, 1986.

31. Gauntlett MD, Fisher DM, Hertzka RE, et al: Pharmacokinetics of fentanyl in neonatal humans and lambs: effects of age, Anesthesiology 69:683-687, 1988.

32. Abelson HI and Miller JD: A decade of trends in cocaine use in the household population, National Institute on Drug Abuse Research Monogr Ser 61:35-49, Rockville, Md, 1985, National Institutes of Health.

33. Hadeed AJ and Siegel SR: Maternal cocaine use during pregnancy: effect on the newborn infant, Pediatrics 84:205-210, 1989.

34. Hoyme HE et al: Prenatal cocaine exposure and fetal vascular disruption, Pediatrics 85:743-747, 1990.

35. van de Bor, M, Walther FJ, and Ebrahimi M: Decreased cardiac output in infants of mothers who abused cocaine, Pediatrics 85:30-32, 1990.

36. Chasnoff IJ: In-utero cocaine exposure increases risk of SIDS, Pediatr News 21:22-31, 1987.

37. Valentine PH, Jackson JC, Kalina RE, and Woodrum DE: Increased survival of low birth weight infants: impact of the incidence of retinopathy of prematurity, Pediatrics 84:442-445, 1989.

38. Gibson DL et al: Retinopathy of prematurity: a new epidemic? Pediatrics 83:486-492, 1989.

39. Avery ME: Recent increase in mortality from hyaline membrane disease, Pediatrics 57:553-559, 1960.

40. Bolton DPG and Cross KW: Further observations on cost of preventing retrolental fibroplasia, Lancet 1:445-448, 1974.

41. Betts EK, Downes JJ, Schaffer DB, and Johns R: Retrolental fibroplasia and oxygen administration during general anesthesia, Anesthesiology 47:518-520, 1977.

42. Rescorla FJ and Grosfeld JL: Inguinal hernia repair in the perinatal period and early infancy: clinical considerations, J Pediatr Surg 19:832-836, 1984.

43. Peevy KJ, Speed FA, and Hoff CJ: Epidemiology of inguinal hernia in preterm neonates, Pediatrics 77:246-247, 1986.

44. Lou HC, Lassen NA, and Friis-Hansen B: Impaired autoregulation of cerebral blood flow in the distressed newborn infant, J Pediatr 94:118-121, 1979.

45. Milligan DWA: Failure of autoregulation and intraventricular hemorrhage in preterm infants, Lancet 1:896:898, 1980.

46. Perry EH et al: Blood pressure increases, birth weight—dependent stability boundary, and intraventricular hemorrhage, Pediatrics 85:727-732, 1990.

47. Long JG, Philip AGS, and Lucey JF: Excessive handling as a cause of hypoxemia, Pediatrics 65:203-207, 1980.

48. Omar SY, Greisen G, Ibrahim MM, et al: Blood pressure responses to care procedures in ventilated preterm infants, Acta Paediatr Scand 74:920-924, 1985.

49. Berry FA and Gregory GA: Do premature infants require anesthesia for surgery? Anesthesiology 67:291-293, 1987.

50. Leonard CH et al: Effect of medical and social risk factors on outcome of prematurity and very low birth weight, J Pediatr 116:620-626, 1990.

51. Kendig JW et al: Surfactant replacement therapy at birth: final analysis of a clinical trial and comparisons with similar trials, Pediatrics 82:756-762, 1988.

52. Collaborative European Multicenter Study Group: Surfactant replacement therapy for severe neonatal respiratory distress syndrome: an international randomized clinical trial, Pediatrics 82:683-691, 1988.

53. Lang MJ et al: A controlled trial of human surfactant replacement therapy for severe respiratory distress syndrome in very low birth weight infants, J Pediatr 116:295-300, 1990.

54. Tay-Uyboco JS et al: Hypoxic airway construction in infants of very low birth weight weight recovering from moderate to severe bronchopulmonary dysplasia, J Pediatr 115:456-459, 1989.

55. Engelhardt B et al: Effect of spironolactone-hydrochlorothiazide on lung function in infants with chronic bronchopulmonary dysplasia, J Pediatr 114:619-624, 1989.

56. Albersheim SG et al: Randomized, double-blind, controlled trial of long-term diuretic therapy for bronchopulmonary dysplasia, J Pediatr 115:615, 620, 1989.

57. Jones R, Bodnar A, Roan Y, et al: Subglottic stenosis in newborn intensive care unit graduates, Am J Dis Child 135:367-368, 1981.

58. Liu LMP, Cote CJ, Goudsouzian NG, et al: Life-threatening apnea in infants recovering from anesthesia, Anesthesiology 59:506-510, 1983.

59. Welborn LG, Ramirez N, Oh TH, et al: Postanesthetic apnea and periodic breathing in infants, Anesthesiology 65:656-661, 1986.

60. Welborn LG, Hannallah RS, Fink R, et al: High-dose caffeine suppresses postoperative apnea in former preterm infants, Anesthesiology 71:347-349, 1989.

61. Kurth CD, Spitzer AR, Broennle AM, et al: Postoperative apnea in preterm infants, Anesthesiology 66:483-488, 1987.

62. Abajian JC, Mellish PRW, Browne AF, et al: Spinal anesthesia for surgery in the high-risk infant, Anesth Analg 63:359-362, 1984.

63. Harnik EV, Hoy GR, et al: Spinal anesthesia in premature infants recovering from respiratory distress syndrome, Anesthesiology 64:95-99, 1986.

64. Wellborn LG, Rice LJ, et al: Postoperative apnea in former preterm infants: Prospective comparison of spinal and general anesthesia, Anesthesiology 72:838-842, 1990.

65. Bailey A, Valley R, and Bigler R: High spinal anesthesia in an infant, Anesthesiology 70:560, 1989.

66. Watcha MF, Thach BT, and Gunter JB: Postoperative apnea after caudal anesthesia in an ex-premature infant, Anesthesiology 71:613-615, 1989.

67. Berry FA: Physiology and surgery of the infant. In Berry FA: Anesthetic management of difficult and routine pediatric patients, New York, 1990, Churchill Livingstone.

68. Cote CJ: APSF-sponsored research reveals that capnograph supplements oximeter, Anesthesia Patient Safety Foundation Newsletter 5(2):13, Summer 1990.

69. Dalens B and Hasnaoui A: Caudal anesthesia in pediatric surgery: success rate and adverse effects in 750 consecutive patients, Anesth Analg 68:83-89, 1989.

70. Kahana MD: Acute pain management in children: neural blockade and patient controlled analgesia. In Berry FA: Anesthetic management of difficult and routine

pediatric patients, New York, 1990, Churchill Livingstone.

71. Desparmet JF: Total spinal anesthesia after caudal anesthesia in an infant, Anesth Analg 70:665-667, 1990.

72. Dohi S, Naito H, and Takahashi T: Age related changes in blood pressure and duration of motor block in spinal anesthesia, Anesthesiology 50:319-323, 1979.

73. Cornblath M et al: Hypoglycemia in infancy: the need for a rational definition, Pediatrics 85:834-837, 1990.

74. D'Alecy LG, Lundy EF, Barton KJ, and Zelenock GB: Dextrose containing intravenous fluid impairs outcome and increases death after eight minutes of cardiac arrest and resuscitation in dogs, Surgery 100:505-511, 1986.

75. Lanier WL et al: The effects of dextrose infusion and head position on neurologic outcome after complete cerebral ischemia in primates: examination of a model, Anesthesiology 66:39-48, 1987.

76. Kraig RP et al: Hydrogen ions kill brain at concentrations reached in ischemia, J Cereb Blood Flow Metab 7:379-386, 1987.

77. Sherry KM: Post-extubation stridor in Down's syndrome, Br J Anaesth 55:53-55, 1983.

78. Reid CS et al: Cervicomedullary compression in young patients with achondroplasia: value of comprehensive neurologic and respiratory evaluation, J Pediatr 110:522-530, 1987.

79. Pueschel SM and Scola FH: Atlantoaxial instability in individuals with Down syndrome: epidemiologic, radiographic, and clinical studies, Pediatrics 80:555-560, 1987.

80. Msall ME, Reese ME, et al: Symptomatic atlantoaxial instability associated with medical and rehabilitative procedures in children with Down syndrome, Pediatrics 85:447-449, 1990.

81. Davidson RG: Atlantoaxial instability in individuals with Down syndrome: a fresh look at the evidence, Pediatrics 81:857-865, 1988.

82. Delphin E, Jackson D, and Rothstein P: Use of succinylcholine during elective pediatric anesthesia should be reevaluated, Anesth Analg 66:1190-1192, 1987.

83. Wilhoit RD, Brown RE, and Bauman LA: Possible malignant hyperthermia in a 7-week-old infant, Anesth Analg 68:688-891, 1989.

84. Follett DV, Loeb RG, Haskins SC, and Patz JD: Effects of epinephrine and tritodrine in dogs with acute hyperkalemia, Anesth Analg 70:400-406, 1990.

85. Van Der Spek AFL et al: The effects of succinylcholine on mouth opening, Anesthesiology 67:459-465, 1987.

86. Leary NP and Ellis FR: Masseteric muscle spasm as a normal response to suxamethonium, Br J Anaesth 64:488-492, 1990.

87. Larach MG, Rosenbery H, Larach DR, and Broennle AM: Prediction of malignant hyperthermia susceptibility by clinical signs Anesthesiology 66(4):547-550, 1987.

88. Hackl W et al: Prediction of malignant hyperthermia susceptibility: statistical evaluation of clinical signs, Br J Anaesth 64:425-429, 1990.

89. Flewellen EH and Nelson TE: Halothane-succinylcholine induced masseter spasm: indicative of malignant hyperthermia susceptibility? Anesth Analg 63:693-697, 1984.

90. Rosenberg H and Fletcher JE: Masseter muscle rigidity and malignant hyperthermia susceptibility, Anesth Analg 65:161-164, 1986.

91. Schwartz L, Rockoff MA, and Koka BV: Masseter spasm with anesthesia: incidence and implications, Anesthesiology 61:772-775, 1984.

92. Ording H: Incidence of malignant hyperthermia in Denmark, Anesth Analg 64:700-704, 1985.

93. Rosenberg H: Management of patients in whom trismus occurs following succinylcholine, Anesthesiology 68:654-655, 1988 (Reply to letter).

94. Gronert GA: Management of patients in whom trimus occurs following succinylcholine, Anesthesiology 68:653-654, 1988 (Letter).

95. Berry FA and Lynch C III: Succinylcholine and trismus, Anesthesiology 70:161-162, 1989 (Letter).

Chapter 24

Injury to the Anesthetist

Jay B. Brodsky
Mervyn Maze

Physicians are concerned with the prevention and treatment of injury and disease. Therefore it is ironic that the very hospitals in which we work can themselves be hazardous to our health. Each and every workday anesthesiologists are exposed to a wide variety of physical, chemical, biologic, and psychosocial dangers. The nature and extent of these occupational health problems have only recently begun to be appreciated.

I. OCCUPATIONAL EXPOSURE
A. Waste anesthetic gases

Anesthesiologists have come to recognize that some of the drugs we use in our practice may have subtle, long-range effects on our own health and that of our co-workers. One potential environmental health hazard that is almost unique to our specialty is exposure to waste anesthetic gases.

1. Reproductive hazards. How dangerous is exposure to waste anesthetic gases? Most of the studies that have considered this question have focused on the association between waste anesthetic agents, fertility, and pregnancy.

A survey of working conditions in the Soviet Union published in 1967 was the first to report that pregnancies among female anesthetists often ended in spontaneous abortions.[1] The author proposed that this unexpected finding was attributable to some factor or factors in the workplace. Stressful working conditions with long and irregular hours or chronic exposure to trace amounts of anesthetic agents were suggested as the possible causes.

Since publication of this small uncontrolled study, numerous larger epidemiologic surveys have considered the problem of anesthetic practice and pregnancy outcome. Many[2-7] but not all[8] reported an increased risk of spontaneous abortion for women who work in an environment where trace levels of anesthetic gases are present. Although the actual cause of the reproductive complications has not and probably never will be absolutely identified, these studies suggest that chronic exposure to waste gases may be an important factor.

Exposure to *clinical* concentrations of inhalational anesthetics consistently cause toxic effects on experimental animals, possibly because these agents exert physiologic depressant effects on respiratory and cardiovascular function of the mother.[9] When animals are exposed to trace levels of those same gases (that is, levels without physiologic effects), the results have been less dramatic. Only nitrous oxide is consistently teratogenic, even at levels as low as 0.1% (1000 ppm).[9,10] This concentration of nitrous oxide is often present in the ambient air of unscavenging operating rooms. In fact, without gas scavenging, peak concentrations of nitrous oxide can reach levels in excess of 9000 ppm.[11,12]

Among anesthetics, nitrous oxide is unique because it inactivates the vitamin B_{12}–dependent enzyme methionine synthetase.[1,13] Exposure to even low levels of nitrous oxide reduces the production of methionine, which in turn interrupts the conversion of uridine to thymidine. Rapidly dividing tissues are most affected, since methionine synthetase is essential for *normal* DNA production. It is possible that interference with vitamin B_{12} function may account for the high incidence of infertility and undesirable reproductive outcomes in men and women chronically exposed to nitrous oxide.[14]

The epidemiologic studies of occupational exposure to anesthetic gases have been justly criticized because they compared anesthesiologists and nurses exposed to a variety of anesthetic agents with control groups of physicians and nurses working outside the operating room environment.[15,16] Because of controversy regarding the interpretation of these studies, the American Society of Anesthesiologists (ASA) commissioned a group of epidemiologists and biostatisticians to evaluate the health problems attributed to waste anesthetic gases. Their full report was submitted to the ASA in 1982[17] and an abridged version was published in 1985.[18]

The authors reported that the adverse health outcome for spontaneous abortion for pregnant physicians and nurses working in the operating room had a relative risk of 1.3; that is, the risk was increased 30% when compared to the control population. The relative risk for congenital anomalies was only 1.2. These conclusions were reached after 17 articles relevant to the issue were considered, and all but six were rejected. Because of design shortcomings, even the results from these six "best" studies were considered inconclusive, and the true reproductive risk, if any, from anesthetic exposure remains unknown.

One major epidemiologic study that eliminated many of the shortcomings identified in the other studies was unfortunately not included in this report. Unlike anesthesiologists, dental professionals are a unique group to study, since dentists doing essentially the same kind of work may or may not use inhalational anesthetics. What's more, of those that use anesthetics, the majority use only nitrous oxide. Therefore Cohen and his colleagues in the National Dental Study compared nitrous oxide–exposed dental workers with similar controls, that is, dentists and their assistants who worked under the same job stresses, who worked with the same materials, but who were not exposed to any inhalational anesthetics including nitrous oxide.[19]

They found that both paternal (dentists) and maternal (female dental assistants) exposure to nitrous oxide was associated with a significant increase in spontaneous abortions compared to unexposed controls (Fig. 24-1). Women directly exposed to nitrous oxide at work had a doubling in their miscarriage rate. Paternal exposure was not associated with a higher rate of congenital abnormalities; however, rates were higher for assistants directly exposed to nitrous oxide.

Because of experimental evidence that pregnant animals exposed to as little as 1000 ppm nitrous oxide have increased rates of fetal loss, it is easier to explain a toxic reproductive effect for *directly* exposed female dental assistants. How do we explain the increased spontaneous abortion rates for wives of male anesthesiologists and dentists?

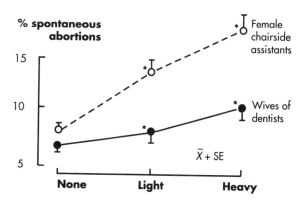

Fig. 24-1. Among female dental chairside assistants and the wives of male dentists who were occupationally exposed to nitrous oxide in the year before conception (* = $p < 0.02$), the incidence of spontaneous abortions per 100 pregnancies increased significantly compared to unexposed controls. Light exposure was 1 to 8 hours of nitrous oxide exposure per week. Heavy exposure was more than 8 hours of exposure per week. (From Brodsky JB: Toxicity of nitrous oxide. In Eger EI II, editor: Nitrous oxide, New York, 1985, Elsevier Science Publishing Co, Inc.)

The sperm or semen of exposed men may be damaged by nitrous oxide. Male rats breathing 20% nitrous oxide develop abnormal sperm and testicular damage within 2 weeks, some as soon as 3 days.[20] Male rats exposed to 10% nitrous oxide for 1 hour had a pronounced reduction in testicular methionine synthetase activity, which required up to 72 hours for that enzyme activity to return to normal.[21]

A study of males anesthesiologists found no differences in sperm morphology or sperm count among anesthesia residents at the start of their training and after 1 year of exposure to anesthetics.[22] However, each of those residents had worked in modern operating rooms with gas scavenging, and so their exposure to waste gases presumably was minimal.

2. Neurologic and other organ toxicity.
Besides its effects on the reproductive system, clinical concentrations of nitrous oxide under experimental conditions are also toxic to the hematologic, immune, and nervous systems in both animals and man.[13] There is indirect evidence that indicates that *occupational exposure* to nitrous oxide may also be a health hazard for man.

For example, a study of 21 dentists habitually exposed to nitrous oxide found that bone marrow function was depressed in 3 of the 21, and 2 of these 3 had abnormal white cells in the periphery.[23] The National Dental Study reported higher rates of liver disease, kidney disease, and neurologic disease among dental professionals using nitrous oxide.[19]

The most striking finding of the National Dental Study was the difference in neurologic complaints between nitrous oxide–exposed people and the unexposed controls.[24] Dentists heavily exposed to nitrous oxide complained of numbness, tingling, and muscle weakness four times as often as unexposed dentists (Fig. 24-2). The combination of halogenated agents and nitrous oxide did not increase the incidence of these problems, an indication that the symptoms were associated with nitrous oxide exposure only!

Layzer described a polyneuropathy characterized by numbness, paresthesia, or clumsiness in the extremities, which he called "*nitrous oxide neuropathy.*"[25,26] With continued exposure to nitrous oxide, the disease progresses to severe weakness, gait disturbances, loss of sphincter control, and impotence. Although many of his patients abused nitrous oxide for recreational purposes, two had been exposed to it only during routine clinical use.

Nitrous oxide neuropathy is identical to the

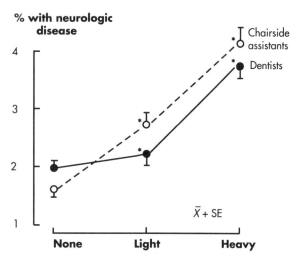

Fig. 24-2. Among both dental chairside assistants and dentists who were exposed to nitrous oxide (* = p <0.02), neurologic complaints were increased significantly compared to unexposed controls. Light exposure was less than 3000 hours of occupational exposure to nitrous oxide per 10-year period. Heavy exposure was more than 3000 hours of occupational exposure to nitrous oxide over a 10-year period. (From Brodsky JB: Toxicity of nitrous oxide. In Eger EI II, editor: Nitrous oxide, New York, 1985, Elsevier Science Publishing Co, Inc.)

neuropathy of pernicious anemia. Monkeys develop neuropathy only if they are fed a vitamin B_{12}–deficient diet for 5 years.[27] However, those same monkeys breathing 15% nitrous oxide develop neuropathy after several weeks.[28] Nitrous oxide, even at chronic low levels, oxidizes B_{12}, reducing methionine synthetase activity.[29] Since low levels of B_{12} result in pernicious anemia, there is a biochemical basis for the neurologic complications of occupational exposure to nitrous oxide. What remains unknown is how much exposure, at what concentration, and what duration of time is needed for nitrous oxide to be neurotoxic to man.

Waste gas exposure can have more subtle effects. In a series of studies Bruce and his colleagues exposed volunteers to 500 ppm nitrous oxide for 4 hours with different trace levels of halothane.[30,31] They reported significant decreases in performance during several audiovisual tasks and short-term memory tests in the exposed groups. Others have been unable to duplicate these findings,[32] and studies of volunteers in unscavenged operating rooms have failed to detect impairment in psychomotor performance even when levels of nitrous oxide exceeded 2000 ppm.[33] There is still no convincing evidence that exposure to subclinical levels of anesthetic agents have any effect. However, the speculation remains that if anesthetics can render a patient completely unconscious at one concentration, lower concentrations of those same agents might impair the thought process of exposed personnel.

3. Anesthetic standards and practices. Up to now, the greatest amount of information on long-term exposure to anesthetic agents in man has come from epidemiologic surveys. However, these surveys cannot prove a cause-and-effect relationship, since they are not controlled scientific experiments. At best they are useful in assessing adverse environmental factors, one of which may be exposure to anesthetic gases. Additionally, problems with inadequate response rates, possible responder bias and inaccurate recall of events,failure to verify medical data, and lack of comparable control groups are serious limitations of the studies of health and reproductive hazards in the operating room.[15,34,35]

Conditions in the operating room have changed since the data in the epidemiologic surveys were collected. Equipment maintenance programs, monitoring for gas leaks, changes in anesthetic practices, and scavenging of waste anesthetic gases are now universally practiced in the United States.[36-38] These efforts have resulted in a tenfold reduction in exposure to waste anesthetic gases when compared to the levels present when the various health surveys were conducted.[36] Thus the potential for health and reproductive problems from waste anesthetic gas exposure has probably been significantly reduced or perhaps even eliminated.

The National Institute of Occupational Safety and Health (NIOSH) recommended as a standard the routine use of scavenging and control measures to keep maximal concentrations of nitrous oxide below 25 ppm and halogenated agents below 5 ppm.[39] These levels were chosen because they were believed to be technically achievable though NIOSH realized that a safe level of exposure to anesthetics could not then (or now) be defined.

The study of dental personnel was the best designed of the epidemiologic surveys.[19] Its findings combined with animal studies demonstrating significant toxic effects of nitrous oxide indicate that long-term exposure to nitrous oxide may have serious health consequences. However, there is still no firm evidence that exposure to trace concentrations of any anesthetic gas is a health hazard to man, but there is no proof that it is not. Until a cause-and-effect relationship is proved or disproved it would seem prudent to minimize unnecessary waste gas exposure in the workplace.

Many questions remain unanswered about the consequences of chronic exposure to waste anesthetic agents. Are the effects in the workplace similar to the experimental findings seen in the laboratory? Is there a real health risk for anesthesiologists and nurses working in an environment where exposure to these gases occurs daily? What are the legal implications? Should the government regulate the levels of exposure to waste anesthetic gases as it regulates other potentially hazardous industrial exposure? Should we even continue to use nitrous oxide?[40] Is it possible to produce an anesthetic that is totally risk free?

The anesthesia community should remain concerned about the potential hazards of waste gas exposure until we know what levels of exposure are safe and how those levels should be determined.

B. Infections

Because of our close contact with patients, many of whom have contagious diseases, anesthesiologists are particularly vulnerable for contracting viral infections.[41,42] Exposure can range from the benign and common (rhinovirus) to the extremely rare and dangerous (Creutzfeldt-Jakob virus). Although exposure to most infectious agents presents no significant threat to the immunocompetent anesthesiologist, two viruses, human immunodeficiency virus (HIV) and hepatitis B virus (HBV), are potentially lethal and are of great concern to us all.

1. Acquired immunodeficiency syndrome (also see Chapter 21). HIV, the retrovirus that causes acquired immunodeficiency syndrome (AIDS), has also been called "human T-cell lymphotropic virus, type III" (HTLV-III) and "lymphadenopathy-associated virus" (LAV).[43,44] As we learn more and more about AIDS we are recognizing how broad the spectrum of diseases caused by HIV is. Most commonly, HIV is associated with problems with the pulmonary, neurologic,and gastrointestinal systems, the skin and mucosal surfaces, lymph nodes, and the retina. However, any organ or system can be involved.

HIV is most often spread through infected blood,vaginal secretions, and semen and is usually transmitted by sexual contact, needle sharing, and transfusion of contaminated blood products and from mother to newborn in the perinatal period. HIV is not transmitted by casual contact.[45] Live HIV has been isolated from blood, semen, urine, saliva, vaginal secretions, bone marrow, lymph nodes, spleen, cerebrospinal fluid, and tears of infected patients.

Patients in high-risk groups include homosexual or bisexual men (67%), heterosexual intravenous drug users (21%), hemophiliacs (1%), and other recipients of blood products (2%) (Fig. 24-3). The remaining members of the high-risk group are sex partners of AIDS patients, Haitians and Africans, and infants of mothers in a high-risk group. The percentage of patients infected with HIV who have no identified risk factor is 3% to 4%. Since it is impossible to identify all patients as HIV seropositive without specific screening tests, it is necessary to treat every patient as potentially infected with HIV or other blood-borne pathogens.[46]

The latent period between exposure and infection to seropositivity in health care workers exposed to HIV is 90 to 180 days.[47] Currently the median time from seropositivity to the clinical diagnosis of AIDS is approximately 43 months, though this figure may change as we learn more about the disease.

Few diseases have created greater anxiety among the health care workers than AIDS. The Centers for Disease Control (CDC) defines a health care worker as a person whose activities involve contact with patients or patients' blood or body fluids. As a group, anesthesiologists are among those health care workers at greatest risk for HIV exposure. What are the risks of contacting AIDS from a patient?

Statistics published in 1987 reported that, of the 32,395 adults then identified to the CDC as having AIDS, 1875 (5.8%) were health care workers.[48] Of those HIV-positive health care workers, 95% belonged to a high-risk (homosexual, intravenous drug abuser) group. For the remaining 5% the means of transmission was initially undetermined, but after careful review of follow-up information, more than half of this group were reclassified when recognized risk factors were identified.

By 1987, among health care workers, only 6 cases out of 2000 documented accidental exposures to HIV resulted in seroconversion.[48] Exposure usually occurred after needle puncture.

The CDC conducted a prospective evaluations of health care workers with documented percutaneous or mucous membrane exposure to body fluids or blood from HIV-infected patients. Seroconversion did not occur in any of 74 workers with nonpercutaneous exposures.[49] In 3 of 351 percutaneous exposures to infected blood, seroconversion did occur. In each in-

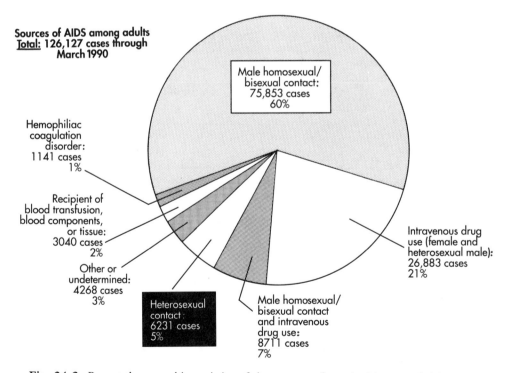

Fig. 24-3. Recent demographic statistics of the sources of acquired immunodeficiency syndrome (AIDS) in the United States. Patients in high-risk groups include homosexual or bisexual men, drug users, hemophiliacs, and other recipients of blood products. The percentage of patients with AIDS who have no identified risk factor is 3%; therefore all patients should be considered potentially infectious.

stance the worker had a small break in the skin, and in one some blood also splattered into the mouth. Two were not wearing gloves!

Although these and other prospective studies have claimed that the risk of occupationally acquired HIV infection is very low,[49-54] documented infection from patients does occur.[48] The growing numbers HIV-positive patients we are treating increases the chances that more health care workers will be exposed and become infected.[55] No one knows the real incidence of HIV infection in the general population, but it seems to be increasing at an alarming rate. For example, more than 4% of patients presenting at an inner-city emergency department, when tested, had unrecognized HIV infection.[56] Because of the long symptom-free period between infection and clinical disease, the risk and incidence of acquired AIDS in the workplace may be higher than now believed.

The incidence of HIV seropositivity among anesthesiologists is unknown. Up to now, there has been no report of any anesthesia personnel becoming infected through his or her work, but the documented cases of AIDS transmission from patients to health care workers underscores the need for strict adherence to the infection-control guidelines issued by the CDC (see the discussion of the prevention of blood-borne infections, p. 579).

If exposure to blood or other fluids does occur, the patient should be approached for consent for HIV testing. If the patient is already known to have AIDS or AIDS-related conditions (ARC), refuses testing, or is tested positive for HIV, the worker should be informed and followed serially for evidence of infection. Testing shortly after the incident will help rule out prior infection.

2. Hepatitis. Although HIV has become a major concern, the risk of similar exposure to hepatitis is often ignored. This cavalier attitude is unfortunate, since hepatitis B virus (HBV) is probably the most serious occupational health danger facing anesthesiologists. Whereas worldwide fewer than 10 health care workers (from non–high risk groups) have contracted AIDS through occupational exposure, more than 20% of anesthesiologists have serologic markers denoting previous exposure to HBV.

The two common human hepatitis viruses hepatitis A virus (HAV) and HBV have been well described, whereas two others, hepatitis C virus (HCV) and hepatitis D virus (HDV, delta virus), have recently been identified.[57,58]

There is minimal risk to the anesthesiologist of parenteral transmission of HAV because of the absence of a chronic carrier state. HAV is spread predominantly by the fecal-oral route, though it can be transmitted from contact with gastrointestinal fluids.[59] If contamination occurs, serum immune globulin should be taken within 2 weeks of exposure.

In many patients with hepatitis, failure to detect HAV, HBV, cytomegalovirus (CMV), or Epstein-Barr virus (EBV) is suggestive of the existence of another pathogen or pathogens. Formerly the diagnosis of non-A, non-B (NANB) hepatitis required negative HAV and HBV serology and the exclusion of a drug history of exposure to hepatotoxic drugs.[60] Recently HCV has been isolated and identified as a major cause of NANB hepatitis.[58] The diagnosis of HCV can now be definitely established serologically. Although no vaccine is currently available for HCV, remission can be induced with alpha-interferon. Precautions against HCV are similar to those for HBV.[61]

HDV depends on HBV for replication, and although no specific vaccine is available, HBV vaccine or hepatitis B immunoglobulin (HBIG) given as a prophylaxis or after exposure can prevent both HBV and HDV infection.

The real risk to the anesthesiologist is from HBV. Approximately 18,000 of the 300,000 people in the United States infected annually with HBV are health care workers.[62] Each year over 10,000 patients with HBV are hospitalized and several hundred die from hepatic failure (Fig 24-4).

Anesthesia personnel are among the highest risk group for HBV, since occupational exposure results primarily from handling blood and blood products.[63-65] The risk of HBV exposure begins during residency training and continues throughout the professional career of the anesthesiologist.[66] Using assays for HBV antigens for evidence of prior or current infection, serologic markers for HBV are present in 20% to 49% of anesthesiologists, an incidence five times greater than the rate for the general public.[64,65,67] Similar high rates of HBV seropositivity have been reported among Canadian[68,69] and European anesthesiologists.[70-72]

About one fourth of individuals positive for HBV antigen develop clinical hepatitis, for the remainder the HBV infection resolves without significant hepatic damage. Fewer than 1% of patients with HBV develop fulminant hepatitis, but this is associated with a 60% mortality.

Unlike HIV where 100% of infected patients become carriers, 6% to 10% of persons infected with HBV become chronic carriers. Carriers not only have the potential to infect others, but also about 25% of the HBV carriers develop

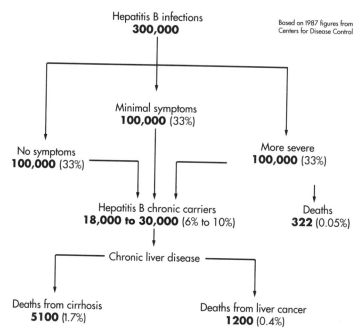

Fig. 24-4. Annual incidence of hepatitis B viral infection. Approximately 18,000 of the 300,000 people in the United States infected annually with hepatitis B virus (HBV) are health care workers. Each year over 10,000 people are hospitalized because of HBV. Several thousand die as a result of acute infection, chronic cirrhosis, or the development of hepatic cancer related to HBV infection.

chronic active hepatitis, which often progresses to cirrhosis. The risk of hepatocellular carcinoma is 200 times greater in HBV carriers than among noncarriers. Over a thousand patients die of HBV-related hepatocellular carcinoma each year in the United States.

As with HIV, certain populations have a high prevalence of HBV. These include all patients with liver disease, patients undergoing hemodialysis or who have had a renal transplant, patients with leukemia, all immunosuppressed patients, intravenous drug abusers, male homosexuals, and immigrants from the Southeast Asia. Although fewer than 10% are carriers, all HBV-positive patients and their secretions must be considered infectious.

It is estimated that 0.1% of the general population are asymptomatic HBV carriers, and between 1% and 1.5% of all hospital patients are seropositive for HBV. Thus an anesthesiologist managing 100 patients per month is likely to encounter an HBV-positive person at least once a month. Unfortunately, since many patients with serum markers for HBV have no clinical history of hepatitis and are not members of any recognized high-risk group, occupational exposure risk is usually greatest from patients not suspected of being carriers.[73] Therefore wear-

ing gloves and taking special precautions only when working with a patient from a high-risk group does not prevent exposure to HBV.

Although contact with blood is probably the most important risk factor, every body secretion from a carrier is potentially dangerous. If any exposure occurs, such as a skin puncture with a dirty needle, hepatitis B immunoglobulin (HBIG) should be immediately administered. If the patient is known to be antigen positive and the exposed health care worker is antigen negative, administration of HBIG within 48 hours of exposure followed by the first dose of HBV vaccine within 7 days is recommended.[74] In groups such as anesthesiologists who are at high risk for repeat exposure, HBV vaccine should be administered simultaneously with HBIG, since this will initiate lasting immunity.

There is a potential risk of catching AIDS from HBIG because it is prepared from plasma, and viral inactivation may not be complete or effective. There have also been reports of HBV and NANB hepatitis transmitted through HBIG.

HBV vaccine is the only effective way to prevent infection. Anesthesiologists are strongly advised to be vaccinated during their residency.

After vaccination, the person should be checked to determine whether he or she became seropositive. A seroconversion rate of 85% to 95% is reported. Revaccination produces adequate antibody titers in only 30% to 50% of those who initially failed to respond to vaccination.

It is estimated that only 30% to 40% of susceptible medical personnel in the United States have been vaccinated. This is surprising, since the vaccine is safe, immunogenic, and effective in preventing HBV infection.

All persons exposed to patients or blood products should be immunized. Anesthesiologists with prior exposure to HBV should be tested first for the presence of antibodies and then vaccinated if necessary. New house staff should receive the vaccine without prior serologic testing. The vaccine is given as a series of three intramuscular injections at 0, 1, and 6 months.[74] Follow-up serologic testing is performed 6 to 8 weeks after the last dose to be sure adequate levels of antibody have developed.

The following recommendations are made for anesthesia personnel who have received HBV vaccine before being stuck with a needle. If antibody levels to HBV were tested within the past year and are known to be positive, nothing has to be done. Anyone who was antibody positive to HBV in the past but who has not been tested in several years should be rechecked for seropositivity. If there is a long delay in obtaining the results, it is advisable to take an HBIG or a booster shot. Anyone previously vaccinated who did not seroconvert should receive HBIG and a full course of the vaccine.

Although it has been recommended that everyone exposed to blood be tested annually for antibody status, adults with normal immune status do not require such frequent routine serologic testing. After vaccination, protection against clinical or viremic HBV lasts more than 5 years.

The side effects of HBV vaccine are minor, the most common problem being soreness in the arm at the site of inoculation. Although it is less painful to receive the vaccination in the buttocks, there may be a suboptimal response for those vaccinated at this site. There are no adverse effects to receiving the vaccine in HBV carriers or immunosuppressed patients.

One reason that many anesthesiologists have resisted being vaccinated has been concern that the vaccine introduced in 1982 might transmit HIV. This vaccine is prepared with plasma, some of which may have been collected from homosexual males. The concern has persisted even though the HIV virus, and all other known human viruses, are killed by the steps involved in the preparation of HBV vaccine. Extensive studies found no evidence that AIDS was transmitted by the plasma-derived vaccine.[75] There have been no reports of AIDS after HBV vaccination in people who did not belong to a high-risk behavior group for HIV. The vaccine is considered safe though several cases of Guillain-Barré syndrome occurred after vaccination.

A second vaccine, prepared with recombinant DNA technology from noninfectious material, was introduced in 1986.[75-77] Because only a portion of the HBV viral genome that codes for the surface coat of HBV is present, no potentially infectious viral DNA (such as HIV) can be produced. No human or animal plasma or other derivatives are used in the preparation of this vaccine. It appears to be almost equivalent in its immunogenicity and protective action to the older, plasma-derived vaccine.[78,79] The new vaccine offers increased safety, immunogenicity, and lower cost with absolutely no risk of HIV exposure.[77]

3. Prevention of blood-borne infections. The CDC has published practice recommendations to prevent the transmission of blood-borne infections in the health care setting.[49,62,80] The American Society of Anesthesiologists Committee on Occupational Health of Operating Room Personnel republished these recommendations.[81] Because HBV is more infectious than the HIV, recommendations to prevent the former also prevent the latter. Anesthesiologists must adhere rigorously to these precautions to minimize their risk of exposure.

The foremost dictum is that all patients must be considered as potentially infected, either with HIV, HBV, or other blood-borne pathogens.

Accidental needlesticks and cuts account for most incidents of percutaneous exposure to blood and so represents the major risk for HBV and HIV infection.[52] Anesthesiologists have a very high incidence of needlesticks in their practice.[65,82] Of the health care workers who became infected with HIV in the workplace, the majority did so after needlestick exposure. Although continued analysis of needlestick injuries and cuts with sharp instruments indicate that the risk of infection is extremely low, all sharp items must be considered potentially infective and handled with care. Needles should *not* be recapped, bent, broken, removed from syringes or manipulated by hand. Recapping needles is the most common cause of inadvertent skin puncture. Contaminated disposable syringes and needles and other sharp items should be placed immediately after use in puncture-resistant containers located in the anesthesia work area.

Barriers should be placed between the potential source of infection and the anesthesiologist. Gloves must always be readily available and should be worn at all times, but especially when in contact with blood, blood products, body fluids or any item soiled with these fluids. Care still must always be exercised with uncapped needles, since gloves will not prevent penetrating injuries. Surprisingly the routine use of gloves alone did not reduce the incidence of HBV infection in new anesthesia residents.[66]

Gloves should be worn when in contact with mucous membranes or nonintact skin of all patients. It is a common practice to double-glove when the diagnosis HIV or HBV is known. Gloves should be changed between patient contacts. Protective new products continue to be introduced, including a surgical glove with a thin layer of polyurethane foam sandwiched between two latex layers. The foam creates a more effective barrier to punctures than latex gloves do and yet transmits tactile pressures more accurately. High cost may restrict the use of such items to only high-risk patients.

Protective eyeware should be worn in situations in which blood or saliva can be spread. Standard surgical masks do not adequately protect against blood-bearing aerosols, which can contaminate the mucous membranes of the eyes, nose, or mouth. Masks and goggles and glasses should be used for procedures that are likely to produce droplets of blood or body fluids. Surgical masks that combine face protection and a plastic eye shield are available. The eye shield is treated with an antifogging agent similar to that used on ski goggles, and the mask contains a fluid repellent so that splattered fluids bead up on the mask surface.

Even though there are no documented cases of either HIV or HBV being transmitted by airborne aerosols to the respiratory tract, prevention of exposure to saliva by using mouthpieces, resuscitation bags, and other ventilation devices during cardiopulmonary resuscitation is currently recommended. Mouth-to-mouth breathing should be avoided, whenever possible.

Gowns or aprons should be worn to protect against splashes of blood or body fluids during procedures. Clothing should be changed as soon as possible if soiled.

Health care workers with exudative skin lesions or dermatitis should refrain from direct patient care until the skin condition resolves. Anesthesiologists with chapped hands, open cuts, or abrasions must protect the involved skin areas. Hands must be washed immediately if they come into contact with blood or other fluids, as well as before and after any patient care procedure. After inadvertent percutaneous or mucous membrane exposure to blood or body fluids the affected area should be thoroughly washed immediately.

A major differences between HIV and HBV exposure is that the latter can be prevented by vaccination. Both the HBV vaccines currently available are safe and effective. All anesthesiologists should be immunized against HBV unless they are serologically positive from previous exposure. There is currently no vaccination for HIV.

Every hospital should develop protocols for handling accidental exposure in the workplace, and all injuries or exposures should be reported. After an exposure (such as a needlestick, contamination of mucosa or conjunctiva, open wound or skin abrasion, or splash) the health care worker should be followed and tested for HIV and HBV. The safety and effectiveness of short-term zidovudine (AZT) administration after accidental percutaneous exposure to HIV-positive blood is unknown. The drug has unpleasant side effects. It is recommended that when the blood serologic status is unknown the likelihood of seroconversion is a function of the local prevalence of HIV infection, and because the benefits of AZT do not clearly outweigh the risk when that prevalence is below a range of 10% to 20%,[83] one probably should not administer AZT.

After administration of general anesthesia to a patient known to be HIV or HBV positive, the anesthesia machine and other nondisposable equipment should be treated. HIV is very weak and does not readily survive outside the body. It is easily killed by many common disinfectants, including household bleach. Techniques that produce high level disinfection (those that are tuberculocidal) should be routinely used for processing equipment that comes into contact with mucous membranes (that is, laryngoscope blades, breathing circuits), since this is effective in eliminating HBV and HIV. Items that enter sterile cavities (needles, endotracheal tubes) require sterilization before use and optimally should be used only once. Equipment in contact with intact skin (that is, blood pressure cuffs) need not be cleaned after use unless they are contaminated with blood or body fluids.

Blood and body fluid spills should be cleaned as soon as possible using soap and water, since HBV is a hardy virus that may remain infectious for at least 1 week in dried blood on an environmental surface.[84] After this, an appropriate disinfectant or germicide can be used. With patients known to be HIV or HBV positive, disposable equipment including soda lime, esophageal stethoscopes, endotracheal tubes, and laryngoscope blades should be used whenever possible and then discarded.

4. Herpes. The herpes simplex virus (HSV) can infect oral mucosa (HSV I and II) or the genital area (HSV II). Oral HSV is quite common in adults, and the fingers of anesthesiologists can be inoculated by direct contact with saliva from infected patients. Because of the frequency of hand washing in the operating room, fingers are frequently traumatized around the nail bed area predisposing the anesthesiologist to herpetic whitlow.[85-87]

The infection begins at the site where the skin integrity has been broken. There is itching and pain, followed by the appearance of a vesicle surrounded by erythema. Generalized symptoms of malaise, fever and lymphadenopathy may also occur. The infection is usually self-limiting, lasting up to 3 weeks. The antiviral drug acyclovir can be used to treat the primary infection.

The infected anesthesiologist represents a risk of cross infection to the patient and therefore should be very cautious with any local cutaneous lesions on his hands. Gloves, now routinely used to protect against HBV and HIV, prevent contamination by HSV as well.[88]

C. Environmental exposure

1. Chemical. Methylmethacrylate, the acrylic cement used to secure surgically implanted prostheses to bone is supplied in two components, a liquid and a powder, which are mixed together before use. Potentially toxic vapors are released during mixing.

Rats exposed to these vapors develop severe liver damage, tracheal mucosal inflammation, and other side effects.[89] Factory workers producing methylmethacrylate have a high incidence of abnormal blood chemistry values (glucose, blood urea nitrogen, albumin, cholesterol, and bilirubin) and respiratory, genitourinary, and cutaneous problems.[90,91] In man, bronchospasm has resulted from inhaling methylmethacrylate vapors.[92-94] There is a case report of a systemic reaction including hypertension, dyspnea, and generalized erythroderma in an operating room nurse exposed to methylmethacrylate.[95] Methylmethacrylate monomers

can affect the nervous, cardiovascular, cutaneous, gastrointestinal, and respiratory systems.[95] Although the Occupational Safety and Health Administration (OSHA) set a maximum 8-hour exposure to methylmethacrylate at 100 ppm, a NIOSH study found evidence of harmful effects at half that level.[96] In fact, the maximum permissible exposure concentration in the United States is 20 times higher than that allowed in the Soviet Union.

Methylmethacrylate should always be mixed so that the fumes are vented outside the operating room. Scavenging devices can reduce the vapor concentration by as much as 75% and should always be used.[97]

2. Radiation. We are all familiar with the potential dangers of long-term exposure to ionizing radiation. Unfortunately, invisibility and absence of an immediate effect of radiation often gives rise to complacency among nonradiologic personnel. Anesthesiologists are frequently exposed to radiation during diagnostic radiologic procedures as well as during surgical procedures. Those examinations performed outside the radiology department are more likely to be hazardous than those performed within, since protection is never as complete as in the specialized department.[98]

Few studies have even attempted to measure the amount of radiation exposure by anesthesiologists. In one study measuring chambers were placed in various locations in the operating and radiology suites during procedures requiring the presence of an anesthesiologist.[99] The measured radiation was only a small fraction of the amount of whole body exposure per week considered permissible. In a second study, 10 anesthesiologists wore radiation dosimeters at work.[100] Their average radiation exposure during the 10-week study period was well below the acceptable limit. But most of the exposure occurred during the first week of the study; thereafter individual and average values all tended to decrease sharply and then level out. The investigators believed that wearing the dosimeter made the anesthesiologist more conscious of the radiation hazard and thus more cautious.

Any radiation that does not pass directly from the source through the patient to the recording material is hazardous because x rays are reflected from surfaces causing a scattering effect.

Anesthesiologists should make a special effort to avoid manipulating patients during examinations. Unless their immediate presence is essential, they should leave the room. If you must stay in a room with the patient, a minimal distance of 3 feet is recommended, with exposure decreasing sharply as distance is increased. Six feet of air provides the protection equivalent to 9 inches of concrete or 2.5 mm of lead.[98] Aprons and other lead-rubber protective devices are not always completely protective, and any cracks in the apron can completely destroy any protection.

Radiation exposure should be kept to the absolute minimum, since the threshold below which radiation is completely harmless probably does not exist.[101]

3. Magnetic fields. Magnetic resonance (MR) studies are becoming an important diagnostic tool. Anesthesiologists are often exposed to magnetic rays during studies involving pediatric or uncooperative patients. Since high-strength MR imaging may require several kilowatts of radiofrequency power, there is a concern about exposure risks to the anesthesiologist who must stay in close physical contact with the patient during the study.

Patient exposure is often limited to a scan time of 20 minutes per study because studies of microwave radiation have shown that such short exposure times limit neuroendocrine responses in laboratory animals.[102] The risk to the anesthesiologist, particularly if his or her presence is frequently required in an active radiology department is unknown.

MR is known to be dangerous in certain circumstances. Individuals with pacemakers or implanted stimulators, ferromagnetic vascular clips, or any other ferromagnetic metal must avoid these strong magnetic fields. Orthopedic prostheses are tolerated.

The noise generated by MR imagers has caused temporary hearing loss.[103] Although studies in animals have suggested that exposure to MR imaging is safe, the effects of exposure of the pregnant health care worker remains unknown.[104]

4. Lasers. Light amplification by stimulated emission of radiation (LASER) technology has mushroomed over the past decade with a variety of different lasers being used in the operating room. The immediate health hazard to the anesthesiologist is eye injury from either direct exposure or from reflected radiation. Burn injuries to the cornea, retina, and optic nerve have been reported. Protective eyeware, designed for the specific wavelength of the laser being used, must be worn.

There is some concern that the vapors and cellular debris (the plume) resulting from the laser may be harmful.[105] Most surgical masks do not trap the small particles released, and the

plume may contain bacteria or intact viral DNA as well.[106-108] Until the actual health risks are known, vaporized debris should be scavenged and care must be taken not to inhale the material.

5. Noise. The government defines hazardous noise as levels that reach 90 adjusted decibels (dBA) for 8 hours per day.[96,109] The time for permissible levels are halved for every increase of 5 dBA, and so 95 dBA exposure is permissible for 4 hours. Twenty years ago the measured noise levels in operating rooms approached 90 dBA.[110] Loud noises have greatly increased with the introduction of numerous electronic monitoring devices since then. Noise from monitors and surgical equipment, particularly when they are alarming, are disruptive. Noise pollution decreases work performance and may reduce vigilance.[111] It is believed that during long, complicated operative procedures normal fatigue levels are increased by the presence of these noises, which actually lessens the competence of the anesthesiologist. At higher levels workers show signs of irritability. Loud sounds stimulate the hormonal stress response and have been associated with elevation in blood pressure.

II. PERSONAL STRESS
A. Physical hazards

Each year there are over 200,000 on-the-job injuries in the United States. At one time or another, every anesthesiologist experiences some physical injury at work.

A partial list of potential physical hazards in the hospital environment include conjunctivitis from the splash of solutions, slippery floors (especially around scrub sinks), airborne contaminants from improperly functioning air-conditioning systems, electric shock from poorly grounded equipment, and punctures and skin lacerations from needlesticks and from breaking glass ampules.[109] Such minor injuries as skin punctures now assume far more importance with the risk of exposure to HIV and HBV.

The 1967 study of working conditions in Russian operating rooms drew attention to health problems besides the reproductive hazards already discussed.[1] The majority of anesthesiologists interviewed for that study experienced headaches, backaches, fatigue, frequent upper respiratory tract infections, and other complaints.

One of these complaints, "anesthesiologist's back" is now recognized as a major occupational disease. In fact, it was described as the "most prevalent noninfectious occupational morbidity" for anesthesia personnel.[112] Over 70% of the anesthesiologists interviewed experienced either back pain or radiculopathy. Although back pain can be attributable to strain from lifting and transferring patients, it most often is a result of poor posture during patient monitoring.

B. Substance abuse

1. Drugs and alcohol

a. Definition. A variety of terms are used in discussing substance abuse and chemical dependency.[113] Drug or substance *abuse* is said to occur when drug or alcohol use interferes with a person's health, economic, and social function. Drug *addiction* is characterized by progressive and compulsive use of drugs despite destructive consequences. These operational definitions indicate a difference in degree between abuse and addiction. The crossover point between these two conditions is not sharp but includes loss of voluntary control of drug use and denial of any problems relating to such use.

Physical *dependence* involves pharmacologic tolerance and a characteristic withdrawal syndrome upon discontinuance of chronic drug use. Unlike addiction, dependency can be produced in anyone given the appropriate drug.

b. Etiology. Addictive disease seems to occur only in susceptible persons. The susceptibility may be hereditary resulting in a neurochemical derangement.[114,115] The amount of drug exposure necessary for addictive disease to develop depends on the specific drug, the circumstances of exposure, and the person's susceptibility. The synthetic opioids used in the practice of anesthesia have an extremely high addictive potential. When exposed to a critical combination of drugs and external conditions, susceptible persons become dependent on chemicals.

c. Clinical manifestations. Often, the first sign is withdrawal from outside interests, since all activities, such as working, sleeping, and socializing, revolve around the use of drugs. As the illness continues, the entire focus of the addict's life is dedicated to the acquisition and use of drugs. Drug use continues compulsively, despite adverse consequences with eventual isolation and deterioration of personal relationships at home and at work. The addict's personality often acquires the traits of fear, guilt, emotional lability, and loss of self-esteem.[116] There may be frequent unexplained illnesses and multiple job changes in an attempt to thwart discovery of their addictive illness.

Addicted anesthesiologists isolate themselves from their peers by working alone, often on long cases, to facilitate their access to drugs. They may frequently volunteer to relieve other anesthesiologists because it gives them an opportunity to divert drugs for their own use.

Although the association seems logical, there are no published reports to demonstrate that impaired physicians are more likely to commit malpractice than nonimpaired physicians. Typically the professional life of the person is the last to be affected by addiction.[117]

At higher doses anesthetic drugs of abuse are potentially lethal. In a recent review of 180 case reports of drug-abusing anesthesia residents, there were 26 instances in which the initial presentation of the problem was death of the resident from overdose.[118] The extreme potency of the opioids used may explain why anesthesiologists become chemically dependent and suffer from premature deaths from overdose and suicide.[119] In a study of drug abuse in anesthesiology residency programs, of 334 confirmed cases of substance abuse where follow-up study was possible in 235 cases, 30 subjects (12.8%) died of drug overdose.[120] Even higher mortalities were reported by others.[121]

d. Prevalence. Chemical dependency and drug addiction has reached epidemic proportions in our society, and the medical profession is certainly not immune.[122-126] In fact, alcohol and drug dependency are more common among physicians than among the general population, and as a group, anesthesiologists are particularly at a high risk of developing this illness.[116,127] The full extent of this problem has not yet been assessed[128] because most of the statistics are based on data from rehabilitation programs.

Although anesthesiologists comprise less than 4% of physicians in the United States, they are overrepresented in treatment groups of chemically dependent physicians, accounting for over 10% of physicians in treatment.[116,129,130] The largest group of physicians (±12%) treated in the Medical Association of Georgia Impaired Physicians Program (MAG-IPP) has been anesthesiologists.[119,131,132] These data may be partly a function of the zeal with which our clinical discipline has addressed the problem to the extent that we are better than other clinical specialties at recognizing addicted colleagues and referring them to appropriate treatment facilities. A recent poll found a substance-abuse prevalence rate of 2% among all anesthesia residents.[118]

e. Epidemiology of the addicted anesthesiologist. Large-scale epidemiologic data are not available to help explain the undue susceptibility of anesthesiologists to this condition though speculation abounds as to possible causative factors. The most prevalent viewpoints, though opposite, are not necessarily mutually exclusive. On the one hand, it has been suggested that physicians with an addictive potential or personality choose this clinical discipline in order to satisfy their needs. Alternatively the specialty of anesthesiology may provide the environment that drives a susceptible individual to addictive disease. The most often-cited environmental factors include excessive job stress and the ready availability of drugs.[133]

The majority of drug-addicted anesthesia have a family history of substance abuse though 85% of anesthesia residents in the MAG-IPP reported that one reason they were attracted to anesthesia was easy drug access.[119] In fact, nearly 8% chose anesthesia as a specialty *after* they had become addicted.

As the stress of the job or their fatigue becomes overwhelming, they may start out experimenting with anesthetic drugs under the guise of "therapeutic optimism."[134,135] In this mindset, the anesthesiologists believe that they can self-administer the anesthetic drugs to desired effect in the same manner in which they dispense to their patients never considering that they may become addicted. Obvious in this progression is the ease of access to highly addictive drugs. Since many of the drugs used in anesthesia practice require only small amounts for their therapeutic effect, diverting nontraceable amounts of these drugs is relatively easy.

Impaired anesthesiologists when compared with other anesthesiologists in practice tend to be younger, with residents and fellows significantly overrepresented. Outside the academic environment it may be easier for addicted anesthesiologists to isolate themselves and avoid detection, since they rarely have their clinical activities evaluated by one's colleagues.

Compared to other physicians, addicted anesthesiologists are more likely to abuse two or more substances. With the easy availability of opioids, exclusive abuse of alcohol alone is rare.[133] Only older anesthesiologists in the MAG-IPP were more likely to abuse alcohol. Parenteral (intravenous or intramuscular) abuse is far more likely than oral use. Not unexpectedly, compared to other specialties, anesthesiologists are more likely to abuse drugs at work.[119]

f. Prevention. The best prevention for chemical dependency begins with education early in the training program. Counseling and information regarding substance abuse and related material should be added to every residency curriculum.

To discourage abuse and to identify anesthesiologists who may be diverting drugs from the workplace, many anesthesia departments have adopted changes in the ways in which they account for the use of these drugs.[136-138] For example, at the start of each work day our pharmacy releases a locked box to each resident containing controlled substances. Any partially used ampules or syringes are returned with the unused drugs at the completion of the work schedule. On a random basis, boxes are selected and returned syringes are examined by refractometry. If the results of the test are not appropriate, all items returned by that person are examined for a period of 2 weeks. The objective is to distinguish between an occasional labeling or measurement error and a consistent pattern. All materials with an unexpected response to refractometry are saved and submitted for gas chromatographic analysis. The confidential reports are reported to the department chairman.

g. Treatment. Understanding the problem and recognizing that a colleague needs help are in the best interests of that person and his patients. There is a critical need for anesthesiologists to be ready at all times to deal with emergencies, whereas prolonged use of addictive substances have effects on cognitive and perceptual functions.[139] Unfortunately, many anesthesiologists remain poorly informed about impairment and addiction and are therefore reluctant or unable to recognize and respond to a colleague afflicted with this disease. As a result, the chemically dependent physician often remains untreated as the disease progresses, often to a fatal outcome.

The American Medical Association has maintained that chemical dependency should be treated as an illness and that the patient (that is, the impaired physician) is entitled to the same legal rights and medical treatment opportunities afforded patients with other illnesses. On the other hand, in order to protect patients and the public, physicians are required to report to the appropriate regulatory body credible evidence of impairment that affects the competence of their colleagues. Thus we all have an obligation to refer colleagues with suspected chemical dependency for diagnosis and treatment.

The first step in the process involves confronting the addicted anesthesiologist. This should not be done on a "one-on-one" basis because of the difficulty one encounters in breaking down the barrier of denial. Rather , information regarding suspected drug abuse or addiction should be collected and corroborated by as many persons as possible and presented in a structured forum known as "intervention." The setting varies depending on the circumstances but should always be performed in an empathic and nonjudgmental manner. Involvement of the family and close associates may help break down the denial and achieve the objective of referring the addicted anesthesiologist to a specialist facility for diagnosis and to initiate treatment.

Treatment is usually based on the recovery model for Alcoholics Anonymous. There is no cure for addiction, but appropriate treatment and follow-up observation can restore the chemically dependent physician to health and a productive life free of drugs. This process of change is called "recovery" and recovery is a life-long process. During treatment patients identify the factors that trigger drug use and develop coping skills. Self-help group interactions are beneficial. Lack of understanding and support by peers seriously compromises the prognosis for long-term recovery.

Successful treatment is a multidisciplinary effort. Detoxification, intensive education, and behavior modification is usually achieved by inpatient treatment early in recovery. Specific blocking drugs (disulfiram [Antabuse] for alcohol; naltrexone [Trexan] for opiates) are often used. Methadone is never used. Naltrexone is particularly valuable for anesthesiologists, and naltrexone therapy is usually a prerequisite for return to work.

h. Reentry. Before 1980, the most common approach to drug addiction in anesthesiology was to redirect the recovering addicted anesthesiologist into another specialty, since returning to the operating room was believed to be analogous to allowing a recovering alcoholic bartender to tend bar.[120] However, several studies have reported that for all physicians, completion of long-term therapy has a favorable outcome. Of the first 334 chemically dependent physicians to complete a 4-month residential and 20-month aftercare at MAG-IPP, 93% were in recovery and practicing medicine 2½ to 10 years after treatment.[140] The overall death rate from addictive disease for these physicians was 1%. Fifty-five of 56 anesthesiologists who completed the MAG-IPP program were in recovery and were practicing medicine. Of those who returned to anesthesia, 90% (36/40) successfully did so whereas the other 4 switched specialties. Of the 9 anesthesiologists who did not complete treatment, 4 died of their addictive disease.[140]

Based on statistics such as these,[130,140,141] the ASA Committee on Occupational Health of Operating Room Personnel concluded in their 1986 publication that "following adequate therapy and follow-up, it appears that the prognosis for long-term recovery and return to (anesthesia) practice . . . should be encouraged and supported."[142]

But a limited number of follow-up studies reveal that chemically dependent anesthesiologists may have a different prognosis from that of other physicians. Results of a survey sent to the 159 anesthesiology training programs in the United States indicate that drug rehabilitation followed by redirection into another specialty may be a more prudent course for the anesthesiology trainee who abuses parenteral drugs.[118] Of 113 residents who reentered anesthesia training, the success rate (completion of anesthesia residency training and maintenance of a drug-free state during clinical practice) among parenteral opioid abusers was only 34% (27/79) compared to a rate of 70% among the nonopioid abuser group (Table 24-1). There were 14 cases of suicide or lethal overdose among trainees who were allowed to reenter anesthesia programs. Death as the initial relapse symptom occurred in 13 of the 79 (16%). Ward et al. found that at a similar time of follow-up study, 70% of anesthesiologists were lost to medicine and at least 10% died of addictive disease.[143] These chilling statistics have caused many to reevaluate the wisdom of allowing former substance abusers to return to anesthesia training.

Still, approximately 75% of residency programs allowed residents with a history of substance abuse to reenter their program. Proponents of this approach argue that anesthesiologists "in recovery" prove to be a useful resource in the identification and referral of other addicted persons to treatment facilities. Also, the possibility of reentry into clinical practice offers a powerful incentive for seeking treatment. The most recent annual report (1990) of the ASA Committee on Occupational Health of Operating Room Personnel states that an exception should be made for early anesthesia trainees (junior residents) who should be steered into another specialty rather than be given an opportunity to reenter an anesthesia training program.

If the impaired physician is allowed to reenter his department, structured plans must be formalized to facilitate a safe and smooth reintegration of the individual back into the department. Everyone must have a clear understanding of what is to be involved in the physician's

Table 24-1. Case reports of substance abuse in anesthesia residents

Substance abused	Case reports	Cases allowed to reenter training Number (%)	Cases excluded (in training)	Success/failure determinations possible	Reentry successes Number (%)	Reentry failures Number (%)	Deaths after reentry Number (%)
Group 1 (parenteral opioids)	132	87 (70)	8	79	27 (34)	52 (66)	13 (16)
Group 2 (other drugs)	38	26 (76)	3	23	16 (70)	7 (30)	1 (4)
Unknown	10	—	10	0	—	—	—

The success rate (completion of anesthesia residency training and maintenance of a drug-free state during clinical practice) was only 34% among parenteral opioid abusers compared to 70% among nonopioid abusers. Death as the presenting relapse symptom occurred in 16 of the 79 opioid abusers.

From Menk EJ et al: JAMA 263:3060, 1990.

ongoing recovery program and a written contract is mandatory. Clear and direct lines of communications must be maintained, and all parties involved (the physician, his colleagues, the hospital and *his patients*) must be safeguarded. Much of the doubts and concerns about the impaired physician can be allayed through staff education.

The hospital-based impaired physicians committee should serve as the liaison between the returning physician and all the groups interested in monitoring his practice. This advocacy group can also fulfill the function of monitoring the recovery of the addicted anesthesiologist.

The recovering physician must participate in a program of random, unannounced, witnessed urine screening tests. Individual or group therapy is also advised, along with periodic contact with the impaired physicians committee and physician advocate.

If the returning physician has been out of practice for any length of time, participation in retraining or refresher courses should be encouraged. Undue stress at work must be avoided with adequate time off and vacation. Finally, it is in everyone's best interest to record and document the physician's clinical performance, the results of the urine screening tests, attendance at therapy sessions, and other positive actions.

Frequent random drug screening is important. A major problem both for identification and follow-up observation of addicted physicians is that most of the commercially available urine and blood screening tests currently used to detect recent drug use do not accurately measure fentanyl, sufentanil, or alfentanil.[144]

Furthermore, unless the person has already been identified as chemically dependent and is in recovery, most physicians will not voluntarily submit to routine urine and blood screening. It is possible that unscheduled, random urine screening of all anesthesiologists, along with tighter control of narcotics, could help control the problem.

2. Inhalation anesthetics. In the past inhalation agents were widely used for "recreational" purposes. Historically, "ether frolics or jags" and "laughing gas parties" existed long before either of these agents were used during surgery. The clinical application of these gases (that is, the start of anesthesiology as a specialty) began when people noticed the absence of reactions to painful injuries while their friends were under the influence of these agents.

Deaths from nitrous oxide, halothane, and ether sniffing are still reported, usually as a result of associated hypoxia.[145] The inhalational anesthetic of choice is "laughing gas" partly because for many years nitrous oxide was believed to be free of any morbidity. We now recognize that recreational abuse of nitrous oxide is not innocuous but can be associated with several health problems including neuropathy.[25]

C. Stress

Stress is defined as any factor that causes bodily or mental tension by placing demands on an individual. Like most physicians, anesthesiologists are exposed to a multitude of physical, psychologic, and emotional demands that affect both our own health *and* our ability to provide medical care to our patients. Anesthesiologists in particular work continuously in situations where a mistake or error in judgment can result in patient death or injury. Often, the only time an anesthesiologist receives publicity is when a patient care disaster occurs. There appears to be a relationship between high levels of drug and alcohol abuse among anesthesiologists and the effects of stress and fatigue.[134]

Some occupational sources of stress are unavoidable, but others can be modified and controlled.

Jackson cites an example of one of the many subtle stresses facing anesthesiologists.[146] Historically the preanesthetic visit on the night before surgery allowed the anesthesiologist to meet and evaluate his patient. Because of economic restraints, the initial evaluation of many high-risk patients now occurs minutes before the induction of anesthesia. Much of the stress we experience each work day comes from the uncertainty, the depersonalization, the inconvenience, and the uncontrollability of our work practices as exemplified by the hurried preanesthetic process.[146]

1. Professional burnout. Besides the obvious hazards and stresses related to direct patient care already discussed, there are other demands from patients, colleagues, and the institution that may not be met and often lead to physical and emotional deterioration. Although most of us cope satisfactorily with work-related stresses, the incidence of substance abuse and suicide among our colleagues testifies to the failure of many others to compensate.

Professional burnout is emotional exhaustion caused by such stress. Symptoms include physical exhaustion, emotional detachment, boredom and cynicism, impatience, irritability, and a feeling of not being appreciated. The last often leads to paranoia, disorientation, psychosomatic complaints, and depression.[147]

Burnout should be suspected if a colleague demonstrates increased absenteeism, decreasing enthusiasm, declining performance, and lack of focus and communication. Unless the burnout sufferer learns to relax (both mentally and physically), begins to exercise to work off stress, or develops new interests or even changes his career, the outcome can be quite serious.

2. Fatigue. Anesthesiologists often work long hours and suffer considerable sleep loss. There are often financial incentives to work longer and harder. There is always pressure from many sources to be more efficient (that is, to provide more service with fewer physicians). Although efficiency may be defined by cost considerations and is greatest with a heavy work load, effectiveness is highest with a moderate work load.[148] When reasonable limits are exceeded, stress and fatigue are inevitable.

Work efficiency decreases with sleep deprivation.[149,150] Studies performed on medical house officers acutely and chronically deprived of sleep demonstrate impairment in efficiency with difficulty in thinking and learning.[151-153] Performance among anesthesiologists was reduced at the end of a long shift when compared to the beginning of the shift when they were refreshed.[154] The reduction in cognitive function associated with fatigue may contribute to potentially dangerous incidents in the operating room.[155] Decreased work satisfaction and reduced self-concept have also been described with heavy work loads.[156] Marital and sexual dysfunction has also been attributable to fatigue from work.[157] Excessive sleep deprivation and prolonged and uninterrupted stressful work not only fatigues the person, but also can cause personality alterations, cognitive and behavioral deterioration, and eventual progression to emotional and physical illness as well as professional burnout.[158]

We have an obligation to modify whatever factors are controllable so as not to jeopardize our own health and that of our patients. Fatigue is one factor that can be controlled.

Several state legislatures have begun to consider the problems of sleep deprivation among physicians. So far their attempts to set standards for maximum hours of work have been arbitrary, often without objective data to support them. However, since inadequate or irregular sleep patterns do increase the risks of errors,[159] voluntary guidelines for anesthesiologists are recommended. Limiting work hours to reasonable levels and the provision of adequate numbers of physicians to alleviate particularly heavy demands is essential.

The following suggestions are guidelines that limit working hours to numbers less than those that have been shown to produce performance deficits.[134]

1. Any anesthesiologist involved with a procedure lasting more than 3 hours should be relieved for short periods every 2 hours.
2. No anesthesiologist should regularly work more than a 16-hour work day without a full 12-hour recovery period.
3. No anesthesiologist should be on call for more than 24 hours without a full 24-hour recovery period.
4. Anesthesiologists must say no to unreasonable work demands.

Other stress factors can also be addressed.[146,160] There must be flexibility and adaptability in covering case loads. Difficult cases, patients with "unattractive" insurance, and work exposure to "difficult" surgeons should be a fairly distributed among the group. An adequate amount of vacation time should be available.

There must be some mechanism for the anesthesiologist who becomes fatigued or physically ill, or who has demanding administrative responsibilities to be covered by his or her colleagues. Cases with suboptimal outcomes should be discussed in a nonthreatening manner.

D. Personal health

All deaths among members of the American Society of Anesthesiologists over the past four decades have been retrospectively and more recently prospectively examined, and the causes compared with the Metropolitan Life Insurance standardized tables for deaths among similar aged men.[161-163]

Deaths rates among anesthesiologists from 1930 to 1946 were similar to those in the period 1947 to 1956 but greater than those from 1957 to 1971, an indication that exposure to the fluorinated anesthestic agents introduced in the mid-1950s may not be an important health hazard influencing the mortality experience of anesthesiologists.[163]

Coronary artery and other vascular diseases accounted for more than half the deaths; however, the rate was below the expected death rate for controls. Likewise, although malignancies were the next highest cause of death, the incidence of cancer was lower than expected. In fact, all categories of death attributable to illness were lower than the control group, often by as much as 30%. Similar reduction in the rate of cancer among anesthesiologists have been reported in Great Britain.[164]

But each of the studies reveal a single shocking finding. The third highest cause of death among anesthesiologists during the past three decades has been *suicide!* Suicide is discussed in the next section.

The overall mortality experience for both American and British anesthesiologists has been shown to compare favorably with that of other physicians.[161-164] However, these retrospective questionnaire surveys are notoriously inaccurate.[15] Therefore a prospective study of consultant anesthetists in England was attempted.[165] It investigated the records in the National Health Service for rates of early retirement among an-

esthesiologists because of permanent ill health and deaths while they were still employed. The control group consisted of consultants in four other hospital specialty groups.

Approximately two thirds of all consultants in the five specialty groups during the period of 1966 to 1983 were included in this study. Retirement because of ill health among male anesthetists was approximately twice that expected when compared to other physicians. The number of early retirements for any reason was also statistically greater than that for other specialties. The numbers of deaths while they were actively employed was also higher. These same categories were also increased for female anesthetists, but the numbers were too small for analysis. Unfortunately, no information on the nature of the health problems or causes of death were made available. The two usual explanations for the apparent excesses in morbidity among anesthesiologists are exposure to waste anesthetic gases and stress and fatigue.

A third possibility is that the results were attributable to selection rather than environmental factors. It is possible that physicians with a predisposition to poor health are attracted to anesthesiology. This is unlikely since ASA studies have demonstrated a *lower* mortality for anesthesiologists compared to that of the general population.[162] The major cause of mortality among male American anesthesiologists under 55 years of age is suicide.

More subtle health hazards have also been suggested.[166,167] For example, studies in the Soviet Union and Great Britain reported increased rates for liver disease, lumbar disk disease, peptic ulcer disease, hypertension, headaches, insomnia, and reproductive problems.[1,167] Presumably occupational stress, chemical abuse as well as exposure to anesthetic gases may all contribute to these generalized, nonspecific health findings.

E. Suicide

Medicine is a demanding and stressful profession, with high rates of alcoholism, drug abuse, and suicide. Suicide among professionals (physicians, dentists, lawyers) occurs more frequently than in the general population. For example, suicide is reported to be two to three times more common and is the leading cause of premature death among all physicians.[168] Presumably because of the pressures of work and fatigue, substance abuse, or declining health, suicide occurs not only more frequently among physicians, but also at an increased rate in their spouses.[169]

Anesthesiologists commit suicide more often

than other specialists, with the possible exception of psychiatrists. Anesthesiologists have a suicide rate of between 44 and 55 per 100,000. This is twice the rate for surgeons and three-to-five times the rate for pediatricians. Suicide accounted for 19 of 211 (9%) of deaths in the prospective ASA study of causes of death among American anesthesiologists.[170] The retrospective surveys of deaths during the 1950s to 1970s found that suicides accounted for more than 6% of all deaths, four times greater than expected from mortality statistics.[161,162] Furthermore, other deaths reported as accidents may in fact have been suicides, an indication that the actual rate may be even greater.

Fourteen of the 19 suicide deaths in the most recent ASA study were among anesthesiologists less than 55 years of age. A high incidence of suicide has also been reported among anesthesia residents while still in training.[171] For anesthesiologists 65 to 75 years of age the suicide rate was 15 times greater than expected!

Involvement in a malpractice suit has been implicated in cases of suicide.[172] A subpopulation of an already high-risk specialty is the anesthesiologist involved in litigation. An anesthesiologist being sued suffers tremendous emotional stress and anxiety. A study of 192 suits over an 11-year period involving 185 of the approximately 400 anesthesiologists in the State of Washington revealed 4 suicides (2.2%), a suicide attempt in one of every 45 anesthesiologists being sued.[173,174]

Litigation is just one contributing cause. Long work hours, demanding patients and peer pressures, overwork and fatigue are believed to be major factors in physician suicide and are frequently offered by chemically addicted physicians as the conscious reason for their use of drugs.[175]

The association of substance abuse and suicide has not been fully examined. Suicide attempts are known to be frequent among physicians with recognized drug-related problems.[176] Chemical dependency on narcotics is believed to be a relatively recent phenomenon. Before the 1970s alcohol was the major drug of dependency. It is interesting that although the suicide rate among anesthesiologists was high during the period 1930 to 1946 it was nearly equal to that of other physicians, particularly during the depression years (1930 to 1940) when the white male death rate for suicide was high.[163] Accidental drug overdose may play a role in the dramatic increase in deaths listed as "suicide" in more recent years.[121]

Whatever the cause or causes, suicide was called the "*only* major health problem" (as a cause of death) among young American anesthesiologists.[162] Anesthesiologists who commit suicide are generally young, working, and not physically ill. Surprisingly, they seem to use the same means as the general population do and almost never use anesthetic drugs to commit suicide.[177]

F. The impaired anesthesiologist

Many of the problems discussed in this chapter lead to a common end point, the *impaired physician*. A physician is considered impaired when he or she is unable to be a healthy family or community member or can safely practice medicine. Impairment can be attributable to advancing age, physical or psychiatric disability, emotional problems, or substance abuse. Substance abuse and chemical dependency are believed to be the leading causes of impairment among anesthesiologists. To compound the situation, these problems usually occur at a time when the person is most productive.

In general the medical profession has policed its own members by disciplining those members compromised by mental or physical illness, chemical dependence, or lack of diligence in keeping current. Physicians are required to report to the appropriate body credible evidence of impairment that affects the competence of their colleagues. We all have an obligation to urge colleagues with physical or mental illnesses or with chemical dependency to seek treatment.

REFERENCES

1. Vasiman AI: Work in operating theaters and its effects on the health of anaesthesiologists, Eksperimental'naia Khirurgiia Anestesiologiia 12:44, 1967.
2. Askrog V and Harvald B: Teratogen effekt af inhalationsanaestetika, Nord Med 83:498-500, 1970 [in Danish].
3. Cohen EN, Bellville JW, and Brown BW Jr: Anesthesia, pregnancy, and miscarriage: a study of operating room nurses and anesthetists, Anesthesiology 35:343-347, 1971.
4. Knill-Jones RP et al: Anaesthetic practice and pregnancy: a controlled survey of women anaesthetists in the United Kingdom, Lancet 1:1326-1328, 1972.
5. Rosenberg P and Kirves A: Miscarriages among operating theatre staff, Acta Anaesthesiol Scand 53(suppl): 37, 1973.
6. Knill-Jones RP, Newman BJ, and Spence AA: Anaesthetic practice and pregnancy: controlled survey of male anaesthetists in the United Kingdom, Lancet 2:807, 1975.
7. American Society of Anesthesiologists: Occupational disease among operating room personnel: a national study. Report of an ad hoc committee on the effect of trace anesthetics on operating room personnel, Anesthesiology 41:321, 1980.
8. Axelsson G and Rylander R: Exposure to anaesthetic gases and spontaneous abortion: response bias in a postal questionnaire study, Int J Epidemiol 11:250-256, 1982.

9. Lane GA et al: Anesthetics as teratogens: nitrous oxide is fetotoxic, xenon is not, Science 210:899-901, 1980.

10. Vieira E et al: Effects of low concentrations of nitrous oxide on rat fetuses, Anesth Analg 59:175-177, 1980.

11. Corbett TH: Retention of anesthetic agents following occupational exposure, Anesth Analg 52:614-618, 1973.

12. Harrington JM: The health of anaesthetists, Anaesthesia 42:131-132, 1987 (editorial).

13. Brodsky JB and Cohen EN: Adverse effects of nitrous oxide, Med Toxicol 1:362-374, 1986.

14. Buckley DN and Brodsky JB: Nitrous oxide and male fertility, Reprod Toxicol 1:93, 1988.

15. Vessey MP: Epidemiological studies of the occupational hazards of anaesthesia: a review, Anaesthesia 33:430-438, 1978.

16. Mazze RI and Lecky JH: The health of operating room personnel, Anesthesiology 62:226-228, 1985.

17. Colton T: Evaluation of the epidemiologic evidence for occupational hazards of anesthetic gases, Park Ridge, Ill, 1982, American Society of Anesthesiologists.

18. Buring JE et al: Health experiences of operating room personnel, Anesthesiology 62:325-330, 1985.

19. Cohen EN et al: Occupational disease in dentistry and chronic exposure to trace anesthetic gases, J Am Dent Assoc 101:21-31, 1980.

20. Kripke BJ et al: Testicular reaction to prolonged exposure to nitrous oxide, Anesthesiology 44:104-113, 1976.

21. Brodsky JB et al: Nitrous oxide inactivates methionine synthetase activity in the rat testis, Anesthesiology 61:66-68, 1984.

22. Wyrobek AJ et al: Sperm studies in anesthesiologists, Anesthesiology 55:527-532, 1981.

23. Sweeney B et al: Toxicity of bone marrow in dentists exposed to nitrous oxide, Br Med J 291:567-569, 1985.

24. Brodsky JB et al: Exposure to nitrous oxide and neurologic disease among dental professionals, Anesth Analg 60:297-301, 1981.

25. Layzer RB: Myeloneuropathy after prolonged exposure to nitrous oxide, Lancet 2:1227-1230, 1978.

26. Layzer RB, Fishman RA, and Schafer JA: Neuropathy following abuse of nitrous oxide, Neurology 28:504-506, 1978.

27. Agamanolis DP et al: Neuropathology of experimental vitamin B_{12} deficiency in monkeys, Neurology 26:905-914, 1976.

28. Scott JM et al: Pathogenesis of subacute combined degeneration: a result of methyl group deficiency, Lancet 2:334-337, 1981.

29. Nunn JF and Sharer N: Inhibition of methionine synthetase by trace concentrations of nitrous oxide, Br J Anaesth 53:1099, 1981.

30. Bruce DL, Bach MJ, and Arbit J: Trace anesthetic effects on perceptual, cognitive and motor skills, Anesthesiology 40:453-458, 1974.

31. Bruce DL and Bach MJ: Effects of trace anaesthetic gases on behavioural performance of volunteers, Br J Anaesth 48:871-876, 1976.

32. Smith G and Shirley AW: A review of the effects of trace concentrations of anaesthetics on performance, Br J Anaesth 50:701-712, 1978.

33. Gambill AF, McCallum RN, and Henrichs TF: Psychomotor performance following exposure to trace concentrations of inhalation anesthetics, Anesth Analg 58:475-482, 1979.

34. Ferstandig LL: Trace concentrations of anesthetic

35. Tannenbaum TN and Goldberg RJ: Exposure to anesthetic gases and reproductive outcome: a review of the epidemiologic literature, J Occup Med 27:659-668, 1985.

36. Whitcher CE, Cohen EN, and Trudell JR: Chronic exposure to anesthetic gases in the operating room, Anesthesiology 35:348-353, 1971.

37. Lecky JH: The mechanical aspects of anesthetic pollution control, Anesth Analg 56:769-774, 1977.

38. Whitcher C and Piziali RL: Monitoring occupational exposure to inhalation anesthetics, Anesth Analg 56:778-785, 1977.

39. National Institute for Occupational Safety and Health (NIOSH): Criteria for a recommended occupational exposure to waste anesthetic gases and vapors, HEW (NIOSH) Pub No 77-140, Washington, DC, 1977, US Government Printing Office.

40. Eger EI: Should we not use nitrous oxide? In Eger EI, (editor): Nitrous oxide, New York, 1985, Elsevier Science Publishing Company, Inc.

41. du Moulin GC and Hedley-Whyte J: Hospital-associated viral infections and the anesthesiologist, Anesthesiology 59:51-65, 1983.

42. Schlech WF III: The risk of infection in anaesthetic practice, Can J Anaesth 35:S846-S851, 1988.

43. Barré-Sinoussi F et al: Isolation of a T-lymphotropic retrovirus from a patient at risk for acquired immune deficiency syndrome (AIDS), Science 220:868-871, 1983.

44. Gallo RC et al: Frequent detection and isolation of cytopathic retroviruses (HTLV-III) from patients with AIDS and at risk for AIDS, Science 224:500-503, 1984.

45. Friedland GH et al: Lack of transmission of HTLV-III/LAV infection to household contacts of patients with AIDS or AIDS-related complex with oral candidiasis, N Eng J Med 314:344-349, 1986.

46. Baker JL et al: Unsuspected human immunodeficiency virus infection in critically ill emergency patients, JAMA 257:2609-2611, 1987.

47. Marcus R: Surveillance of health care workers exposed to blood from patients infected with the human immunodeficiency virus, N Eng J Med 319:1118-1123, 1988.

48. Centers for Disease Control: Update: Human immunodeficiency virus infections in health-care workers exposed to blood of infected patients, MMWR 36:285, 1987.

49. Centers for Disease Control: Recommendations for prevention of HIV transmission in health-care settings, MMWR 36(suppl 2S):3S, 1987 (published in JAMA 258:1293, 1987).

50. Gerderding JL et al: Risk of transmitting the human immunodeficiency virus, cytomegalovirus, and hepatitis B virus to health care workers exposed to patients with AIDS and AIDS-related conditions, J Infect Dis 156:1-8, 1987.

51. McCray E: Occupational risk of acquired immunodeficiency syndrome among health care workers, N Eng J Med 314:1127-1132, 1986.

52. Centers for Disease Control: Update: Acquired immunodeficiency syndrome and human immunodeficiency virus infection among health-care workers, MMWR 37:229, 1988.

53. Weiss SH et al: HTLV-III infection among health care workers: association with needle-stick injuries, JAMA 254:2089-2093, 1985.

54. Henderson DK et al: Risk of nosocomial infection

with human T-cell lymphotropic virus type III/lympa-denopathy-associated virus in a large cohort of intensively exposed health care workers, Ann Intern Med 104:644-647, 1986.

55. Howard RJ: Human immunodeficiency virus testing and the risk to the surgeon of acquiring HIV, Surg Gynecol Obstet 171:22-26, 1990.

56. Kelen GD et al: Unrecognized human immunodeficiency virus infection in emergency department patients, N Eng J Med 318:1645-1650, 1988.

57. Jacobson IM et al: Epidemiology and clinical impact of hepatitis D virus (delta) infection, Hepatology 5:188-191, 1985.

58. Williams AE and Dodd RY: The serology of hepatitis C virus in relation to post-transfusion hepatitis, Ann Clin Lab Sci 20:192-199, 1990.

59. Sherertz RJ, Russel BA, and Reuman PD: Transmission of hepatitis A by transfusion of blood products, Arch Intern Med 144:1579-1580, 1984.

60. Tabor E: The three viruses of non-A, non-B hepatitis, Lancet 1:743-745, 1985.

61. Browne RA and Chernesky MA: Viral hepatitis and the anaesthetist, Can Anaesth Soc J 31:279-286, 1984.

62. Centers for Disease Control: ACIP:Update on hepatitis B prevention, MMWR 36:353, 1987.

63. Denes AE et al: Hepatitis B infections in physicians: results of a nationwide seroepidemiologic survey, JAMA 239:210-212, 1978.

64. Berry AJ et al: The prevalence of hepatitis B viral markers in anesthesia personnel, Anesthesiology 60:6-9, 1984.

65. Berry AJ et al: A multicenter study of the prevalence of hepatitis B viral serologic markers in anesthesia personnel, Anesth Analg 63:738-742, 1984.

66. Berry AJ et al: A multicenter study of the epidemiology of hepatitis B in anesthesia residents, Anesth Analg 64:672-676, 1985.

67. Fyman PN et al: Prevalence of hepatitis B markers in the anesthesia staff in a large inner-city hospital, Anesth Analg 63:433-436, 1984.

68. Malm DN et al: Prevalence of hepatitis B in anaesthesia personnel, Can Anaesth Soc J 33:167-172, 1986.

69. Chernesky MA, Browne RA, and Rondi P: Hepatitis B virus antibody prevalence in anaesthetists, Can Anaesth Soc J 31:239-245, 1984.

70. Siebke JC and Degré M: Prevalence of viral hepatitis in the staff in Norwegian anaesthesiology units, Acta Anaesthesiol Scand 28:549-553, 1984.

71. Carstens J, Macnab GM, and Kew MC: Hepatitis-B virus infection in anaesthetists, Br J Anaesth 49:887-889, 1977.

72. Janzen J et al: Epidemiology of hepatitis B surface antigen (HBsAg) and antibody to HBsAg in hospital personnel, J Infect Dis 137:261-265, 1978.

73. Linnemann CC et al: Screening hospital patients for hepatitis B surface antigen, Am J Clin Pathol 67:257-259, 1977.

74. Centers for Disease Control, Immunization Practices Advisory Committee: Postexposure prophylaxis of hepatitis B, MMWR 33:285, 1984.

75. Francis DP et al: The safety of the hepatitis B vaccine: inactivation of the AIDS virus during routine vaccine manufacture, JAMA 256:869-872, 1986.

76. Scolnick EM et al: Clinical evaluation in healthy adults of a hepatitis B vaccine made by recombinant DNA, JAMA 251:2812-2815, 1984.

77. Brown SE et al: Antibody responses to recombinant and plasma-derived hepatitis B vaccines, Br J Med 292:159-161, 1986.

78. Okada N et al: Comparative immunogenicity of plasma and recombinant hepatitis B virus vaccines in homosexual men, JAMA 260:3635, 1988.

79. Goilav C, Prinsen H, and Piot P: Protective efficacy of a recombinant DNA vaccine against hepatitis B in male homosexuals: results at 36 months, Vaccine 8(suppl):S50-S52, 1990.

80. Centers for Disease Control: Recommendations for preventing transmission of infection with human T-lymphotropic virus type III/lympadenopathy-associated virus in the workplace, MMWR 34:681, 1985.

81. Berry AJ: Practice advisory: prevention of blood-borne infections (hepatitis B and AIDS), Am Soc Anesthesiologists Newsletter, July 1988.

82. Mathieu A: Acquired immune deficiency syndrome, hepatitis and herpes: risks and implications for anesthesia personnel, Semin Anesthesia 6:231, 1987.

83. Sacks HS and Rose DN: Zidovudine prophylaxis for needlestick exposure to human immunodeficiency virus: a decision analysis, J Gen Intern Med 5:132-137, 1990.

84. Bond WW et al: Survival of hepatitis B virus after drying and storage for one week, Lancet 1:550-551, 1981 (letter).

85. Orkin FK: Herpetic whitlow: occupational hazard to the anesthesiologist, Anesthesiology 33:671-673, 1970.

86. Rosato FE, Rosato EF, and Plotkin SA: Herpetic paronychia: an occupational hazard of medical personnel, N Eng J Med 283:804-805, 1970.

87. Juel-Jensen BE: Herpetic whitlows: an occupational risk, Anaesthesia 28:324-327, 1973.

88. DeYoung GG, Harrison AW, and Shapley JM: Herpes simplex cross infection in the operating room, Can Anaesth Soc J 15:394-396, 1968.

89. Chan PC et al: Two-year inhalation carcinogenesis studies of methyl methacrylate in rats and mice: inflammation and degeneration of nasal epithelium, Toxicology 52:237-252, 1988.

90. Cromer J and Kronoveter K: A study of methyl-methacrylate exposure and employee health, DHEW Pub No 77-119 (NIOSH), Washington, DC, 1976, US Government Printing Office.

91. Jędrychowski W: Styrene and methyl methacrylate in the industrial environment as a risk factor of chronic obstructive lung disease, Int Arch Occup Environ Health 51:151-157, 1982.

92. Pickering CAC et al: Occupational asthma due to methyl methacrylate in an orthopaedic theatre sister, Br Med J 292:1362-1363, 1986.

93. Lee CM: Unusual reaction to methyl methacrylate monomer, Anesth Analg 63:371, 1984 (Letter).

94. Schwettmann RS and Casterline CL: Delayed asthmatic response following occupational exposure to enflurane, Anesthesiology 44:166-169, 1976.

95. Scolnick B and Collins J: Systemic reaction to methyl-methacrylate in an operating room nurse, J Occup Med 28:196-198, 1986.

96. National Institute for Occupational Safety and Health (NIOSH): Recommendations for occupational safety and health standards, MMWR 35:33S, 1976.

97. Taylor G: A scavenging device for venting methyl-methacrylate monomer vapor, Anesthesiology 41:612-614, 1974.

98. Barker D: Protection and safety in the x-ray department, Radiography 44:45-49, 1978.

99. Keen RI: The radiation hazard to anaesthetists, Br J Anaesth 32:224-229, 1960.

100. Linde HW and Bruce DL: Occupational exposure of

anesthetists to halothane, nitrous oxide and radiation, Anesthesiology 30:363-368, 1969.

101. Lamberton LF: An examination of the clinical and experimental data relating to the possible hazard to the individual of small doses of radiation, Br J Radiol 31:229, 1958.

102. Kido DK et al: Physiologic changes during high field strength MR imaging, AJR 148:1215-1218, 1987.

103. Brummett RE, Talbot JM, and Charuhas P: Potential hearing loss resulting from MR imaging, Radiology 169:539-540, 1988.

104. Prasad N et al: Safety of 4-T MR imaging: study of effects on developing frog embryos, Radiology 174:251-253, 1990.

105. Nezhat C et al: Smoke from laser surgery: is there a health hazard? Lasers Surg Med 7:376-382, 1987.

106. Baggish MS, Baltoyannis P, and Sze E: Protection of the rat lung from the harmful effects of laser smoke, Lasers Surg Med 8:248-253, 1988.

107. Byrne PO et al: Carbon dioxide laser irradiation of bacterial targets in vitro, J Hosp Infect 9:265-273, 1987.

108. Garden JM et al: Papillomavirus virus in the vapor of carbon dioxide laser–treated verrucae, JAMA 259:1199-1202, 1988.

109. DePaolis MV and Cottrell JE: Miscellaneous hazards: radiation, infectious diseases, chemical and physical hazards, Int Anesthesiol Clin 19:131-148, 1981.

110. Shapiro RA and Berland T: Noise in the operating room, N Engl J Med 287:1236-1238, 1972.

111. Davenport WG: Vigilance and arousal: effects of different types of background stimulation, J Psychol 82:339-346, 1972.

112. Bause GS and Black RG: Anesthesiologist's back: epidemiology of a major occupational disease, Anesth Analg 65:S13, 1986.

113. Rinaldi RC et al: Clarification and standardization of substance abuse terminology, JAMA 259:555-557, 1988.

114. Donovan JM: An etiologic model of alcoholism, Am J Psychiatry 143:1-11, 1986.

115. Cadoret RJ et al: An adoption study of genetic and environmental factors in drug abuse, Arch Gen Psychiatry 43:1131-1136, 1986.

116. Spiegelman WG, Saunders L, and Mazze RI: Addiction and anesthesiology, Anesthesiology 60:335-341, 1984.

117. Talbott GD and Wright C: Chemical dependency in health care professionals, State Art Rev Occup Med 2:581-591, 1987.

118. Menk EJ et al: Success of reentry into anesthesiology training programs by residents with a history of substance abuse, JAMA 263:3060-3062, 1990.

119. Gallegos KV et al: Addiction in anesthesiologists: drug access and patterns of substance abuse, QRB 14:116-122, 1988.

120. Ward CF and Saidman LJ: Controlled substance abuse: a survey of training programs, 1970-1980, Anesthesiology 55:345, 1981.

121. Gravenstein JS, Kory WP, and Marks RG: Drug abuse by anesthesia personnel, Anesth Analg 62:467-472, 1983.

122. Keeve JP: Physicians at risk: some epidemiologic considerations of alcoholism, drug abuse, and suicide, J Occup Med 26:503-508, 1984.

123. American Medical Association Council on Mental Health: The sick physician: impairment by psychiatric disorders, including alcoholism and drug dependence, JAMA 223:684, 1973.

124. Bissell L and Jones RW: The alcoholic physician: a survey, Am J Psychiatry 133:1142-1146, 1976.

125. McAuliffe WE et al: Psychoactive drug use by young and future physicians, J Health Soc Behav 25:34-54, 1984.

126. McAuliffe WE et al: Psychoactive drug use among practicing physicians and medical students, N Engl J Med 315:805-810, 1986.

127. Wallot H and Lambert J: Drug addiction among Quebec physicians, Can Med Assoc J 126:927-930, 1982.

128. Brewster JM: Prevalence of alcohol and other drug problems among physicians, JAMA 255:1913-1920, 1986.

129. Gualtieri AC, Consentino JP, and Becker JS: The California experience with the diversion program for impaired physicians, JAMA 249:226-229, 1983.

130. Herrington RE et al: Treating substance use disorders among physicians, JAMA 247:2253-2257, 1982.

131. Farley WJ and Talbott GD: Anesthesiology and addiction, Anesth Analg 62:465-466, 1983 (Editorial).

132. Talbott GD et al: The Medical Association of Georgia's Impaired Physicians Program: review of the first 1000 physicians: analysis of specialty, JAMA 257:2927-2930, 1987.

133. Goodwin DW, Davis DH, and Robins LN: Drinking amid abundant illicit drugs: the Vietnam case, Arch Gen Psychiatry 32:230-233, 1975.

134. Parker JB: The effects of fatigue on physician performance: an underestimated cause of physician impairment and increased patient risk, Can J Anaesth 34:489-495, 1987.

135. McCue JD: The effects of stress on physicians and their medical practice, N Engl J Med 306:458-463, 1982.

136. Shovick VA, Mattei TJ, and Karnack CM: Audit to verify use of controlled substances in anesthesia, Am J Hosp Pharm 45:1111-1113, 1988.

137. Adler GR et al: Narcotic control in anesthesia training, JAMA 253:3133-3136, 1985.

138. Lecky JH et al: A departmental policy addressing chemical substance abuse, Anesthesiology 65:414-417, 1986.

139. Robinson EL, Fitzgerald JS, and Gallegos KQ: Brain functioning and addiction: what neuropsychologic studies reveal, J Med Assoc Ga 74:74-79, 1985.

140. Talbott GD, Richardson AC Jr, Mashburn JS, and Benson EB: The Medical Association of Georgia's Disabled Doctors Program: a 5-year review, J Med Assoc Ga 70:545-549, 1981.

141. Morse RM et al: Prognosis of physicians treated for alcoholism and drug dependence, JAMA 251:743-746, 1984.

142. American Society of Anesthesiologists: Questions and answers about chemical dependency and physician impairment, Park Ridge, Ill, July 1986, American Society of Anesthesiologists.

143. Ward CF, Ward GC, and Saidman LJ: Drug abuse in anesthesia training programs, a survey: 1970 through 1980, JAMA 250:922-925, 1983.

144. Stiller RL et al: A method to increase recovery of fentanyl from urine, J Toxicol Clin Toxicol 27:101-108, 1989.

145. Chadly A et al: Suicide by nitrous oxide poisoning, Am J Forensic Med Pathol 10:330-331, 1989.

146. Jackson SH: Stress in the life of the anesthesiologist, Bull Calif Soc Anesth 39:2, 1990.

147. Ansell EM: Professional burn-out: recognition and management, J Amer Assoc Nurse Anesthetists 49:135-142, 1981.

148. Binner PR, Potter A, and Halpern J: Workload levels, program costs, and program benefits: an output value analysis, Adm Ment Health 3:156-165, 1976.

149. Friedman RC, Bigger JT, and Kornfeld DS: The intern and sleep loss, N Engl J Med 285:201-203, 1971.
150. Morgan BB Jr, Brown BR, and Alluisi EA: Effects on sustained performance of 48 hours continuous work and sleep loss, Hum Factors 16:406-414, 1974.
151. Goldman LI, McDonough MT, and Rosemond GP: Stresses affecting surgical performance and learning. I. Correlation of heart rate, electrocardiogram, and operation simultaneously recorded on videotapes, J Surg Res 12:83-86, 1972.
152. Friedman RC, Kornfeld DS, and Bigger TJ: Psychological problems associated with sleep deprivation in interns, J Med Educ 48:436-441, 1973.
153. Leighton K and Livingston M: Fatigue in doctors, Lancet 1:1280, 1983 (Letter).
154. Narang V and Laycock JR: Psychomotor testing of on-call anaesthetists, Anaesthesia 41:868-869, 1986.
155. Cooper JB, Newbower RS, and Kitz RJ: An analysis of major errors and equipment failures in anesthesia management: considerations for prevention and detection, Anesthesiology 60:34-42, 1984.
156. Yogev S and Harris S: Women physicians during residency years: workload, work satisfaction and self-concept, Soc Sci Med 17:837-841, 1983.
157. Vaillant GE, Sobowale NC, and McArthur C: Some psychologic vulnerabilities of physicians, N Engl J Med 287:372-375, 1972.
158. Friedmann J et al: Performance and mood during and after gradual sleep reduction, Psychophysiology 14:245, 1977.
159. Mitler MM et al: Catastrophes, sleep, and public policy: consensus report, Sleep 11:100-109, 1988.
160. McCue JD: The effects of stress on physicians and their medical practice, N Eng J Med 306:458-463, 1982.
161. Bruce DL, Eide KA, and Linde HW: Causes of death among anesthesiologists: a 20-year study, Anesthesiology 29:565-569, 1968.
162. Lew EA: Mortality experience among anesthesiologists, 1954-1976, Anesthesiology 51:195-199, 1979.
163. Linde HW, Mesnick PS, and Smith NJ: Causes of death among anesthesiologists: 1930-1946, Anesth Analg 60:1-7, 1981.
164. Doll R and Peto R: Mortality among doctors in different occupations, Br Med J 1:1433-1436, 1977.
165. McNamee R, Keen RI, and Corkill CM: Morbidity and early retirement among anaesthetists and other specialists, Anaesthesia 42:133-140, 1987.
166. Spence AA et al: Occupational hazards for operating room—based physicians: analysis of data from the United States and the United Kingdom, JAMA 238:955-959, 1977.
167. Spence AA and Knill-Jones RP: Is there a health hazard in anaesthetic practice? Br J Anaesth 50:713-719, 1978.
168. Rose KD and Rosow I: Physicians who kill themselves, Arch Gen Psychiatry 29:800-805, 1973.
169. Sakinofsky I: Suicide in doctors and wives of doctors, Can Fam Physician 26:837, 1980.
170. Bruce DL et al: A prospective survey of anesthesiologist mortality, 1967-1971, Anesthesiology 41:71-74, 1974.
171. Helliwel PJ: Suicide amongst anaesthetists-in-training, Anaesthesia 38:1097, 1983.
172. Wohl S: Death by malpractice, JAMA 255:1927, 1986.
173. Solazzi RW and Ward RJ: Analysis of anesthetic mishaps: the spectrum of medical liability cases, Int Anesthesiol Clin 22:43-59, 1984.
174. Birmingham PK and Ward RJ: A high-risk suicide group: the anesthesiologist involved in litigation, Am J Psychiatry 142: 1225-1226, 1985 (Letter).
175. Bressler B: Suicide and drug abuse in the medical community, Suicide Life Threat Behav 6:170, 1967.
176. Crawshaw R et al: An epidemic of suicide among physicians on probation, JAMA 243:1915-1917, 1980.
177. Bruce DL: Central nervous system depression: performance decrements, abnormal behavior, suicide, Int Anesthesiol Clin 19:121-130, 1981.

PART THREE

Medicolegal Considerations

Chapter 25

Assessment of Anesthetic Risk

John Peder Erickson
Michael F. Roizen

Patients have always wanted to know what may happen to them perioperatively. Now they are *demanding* to know. They are not interested in statistics, comorbidities, risk adjustment, or whether a perioperative event is caused by anesthesia, surgery, or their medical conditions. They simply want to know what may happen during and after an operation and how likely it is to happen to them. Because of this demand, the once dormant field of assessing anesthetic risk has taken on a new and broader perspective. By the year 2000, anesthesiologists may be expected to know and to provide information about perioperative risks not only for their own patients, but also for other patients as well. To provide these data, it is necessary to understand the various methods by which risk is currently assessed.

Assessment of anesthetic risk was alluded to as early as 1915.[1] Its present popularity derives from its usefulness in cost-containment, quality assurance, and litigation.[2-4] Payers have tried to cut their costs by sending patients to practitioners with better outcomes (and fewer complications), linking payment to quality of care. The result is that hospitals and physicians try to prove to payers that they provide good care, and payers try to deny access or reduce payment for poor outcomes.[5] Similarly, litigation would not proceed without bad outcomes: The patient tries to prove bad outcome was caused by poor care; the hospital and physician try to prove that bad outcome was inevitable because of the severity of the patient's disease. Even in quality assurance when litigation is not involved, it is necessary to account for the inherently greater risk of bad outcome for patients in poor health. Of two patients undergoing knee arthroscopy, the 65 year old with a 90% stenosis of his left main coronary artery will have a greater risk for perioperative myocardial infarction than a healthy 28 year old will.

There are circumstances unique to anesthesiology that both simplify and make more complex the task of assessing anesthetic risk. Anesthesiologists have generally provided a service with other physicians (surgeons, obstetricians, radiologists) in a limited number of physically similar locations (operating room, recovery room). Thus at times it is difficult to determine whether a specific outcome was caused by anesthetic factors, surgical factors, or both. Recently our practice has expanded to include intensive care units, postoperative pain services, pain clinics, and preoperative consultation clinics. Lastly, anesthetic risk has a different weight relative to surgical risk. The risk of anesthesia is now far less than the risk of almost any operative or nonoperative procedure for which it is administered. It is rare for a patient to refuse anesthesia or for a surgeon to refuse to perform a procedure because of anesthetic risk. Because this is true, anesthetic risk is often thought of as nonexistent.

Relevant literature provides some information needed to assess risk, such as randomized, controlled, prospective studies.[6-9] One typical example is the Coronary Artery Surgery Study, which evaluated perioperative cardiac outcomes after coronary artery bypass surgery.[10] Such studies are useful for determining world records of perioperative results (most good outcomes and fewest bad outcomes) and estimates of specific risks in a small number of circumstances. Because of the large number of variables in clinical medicine, these estimates may or may not be applicable to your patients in seemingly similar circumstances. This issue was demonstrated in a striking fashion in Maine after a series of studies on therapy for benign prostatic hypertrophy. Actual perioperative mortality and rate of reoperation after transurethral resection of the prostate were 3 and 20 times greater, respectively, than expected from review of the urologic literature.[11] Mortality after hernia repair and cholecystectomy varied by more than eightfold from hospital to hospital in the national halothane study.

Assessing anesthetic risk for a specific group of patients requires more than the results of available randomized, clinical trials. It also requires information about outcomes and risk factors for those specific patients. In this chapter we deal with assessment of risk for your patients, regardless of whether you are an individual anesthesiologist, a group of anesthesiologists, or a group of healthcare organizations with sites where anesthesia is administered.

I. HISTORY OF RISK ASSESSMENT IN ANESTHESIA

As early as 1915 Codman pointed out that in order to improve care given to patients, hospitals had to determine their results, analyze them to find strengths and weaknesses, compare them with those of other hospitals, and promote members of the medical staff on the basis of the results they achieved with patients.[1] In 1924 Ward suggested the need to follow results in hospitalized patients.[12]

There were several attempts to identify and in some cases quantify undesirable outcomes related to anesthetic care in the post–World War II years.[13] Unfortunately, measuring outcomes was a field that lay dormant until the late 1960s when Donabedian presented a framework for the measurement of health care.[14]

But these good beginnings were sidetracked. Eventually peer review and professional standards review organizations (PSRO) were set up by Congress in the 1970s and early 1980s to evaluate health care and to ensure that all providers were meeting minimum standards.[15] From the 1950s, the Joint Commission on Accreditation of Hospitals (JCAH) had always stressed evaluation of the structural variables of healthcare, that is, manpower, buildings, and equipment. Such evaluations resulted in an impressive push to get buildings, equipment, and paperwork in order for scheduled inspections but had less impact on the outcome of care. The JCAH changed its name to the JCAHO (Joint Commission on Accreditation of Healthcare Organizations) in the mid-1980s and since then has attempted to use outcome measurements to evaluate the patient care provided by the organizations it certifies.[16] In the late 1980s, the Health Care Financing Administration(HCFA) accelerated the process of measuring outcomes by releasing aggregate morbidity and mortality data about Medicare patients.[17] The Health Care Quality Improvement Act of 1986 mandated creation of a national database for problems of licensure and hospital privileges.[18] By the end of the decade, every physician was aware of the need for assessing risk in medicine; even the lay press carried stories on quality in medicine.[19,20] Risk assessment had become a politically and economically sensitive topic.

II. WHAT IS RISK ASSESSMENT?

Risk is the degree of likelihood that an undesirable event will occur. The field of risk assessment in medicine is broad in scope but as yet insufficiently developed to allow one to assess risk comprehensively. The science of risk assessment crosses many disciplines including medicine, biology, mathematics, politics, economics, law, psychology, sociology, and philosophy. Risk assessment itself encompasses three related but dissimilar activities: risk estimation, risk evaluation, and risk management.

A. Risk estimation

Risk estimation involves quantifying risk. The most effective way to do this is to understand the science behind the risk in question. Unfortunately, the scientific basis for individual risks related to anesthesia in particular and medicine in general is not completely understood; if it were, each risk would probably be eliminated in the first place. The use of randomized, controlled, prospective data to which the scientific method can be applied is the next best alternative. Thus clinical trials are of great value, despite the difficulty of completing them for many medical questions. Clinical outcomes for anesthesiology, however, are difficult to study because of the many variables that affect outcome. Often the available clinical studies are limited by not being controlled for physician, institution, socioeconomic class, or patient comorbidity.

The third best approach is to use data that are retrospective, uncontrolled, and nonrandomized (past experience).[21] These data can be effective as long as their limits are appreciated—predictions cannot be made as reliably as with the results of a controlled, blinded, scientific study. On the other hand, this retrospective, epidemiologic approach is used by various tumor registries, and data from a large segment of the world can be analyzed.

Another example of data gathered in this way is found in the Coronary Artery Surgery Registry compiled by the National Heart, Lung and Blood Institute. Data from more than 24,000 patients having coronary artery bypass surgery between 1974 and 1979 have been recorded. From many pieces of information collected for each patient, estimates of the incidence of various perioperative events can be made. Because the number of patients is so large and the time period so long, most physicians should be able to achieve better results than those reported because many improvements in medical care have been made since 1979 (such as cardioplegia, better care in the intensive care unit). Thus one can assume that if adverse events at the hands of a physician are not equal to or less than those reported, that physician's results may be inferior. Two examples of events reported are perioperative myocardial infarction and congestive heart failure, for which incidence can be determined for different preoperative groups (that is, those patients with uncompensated heart failure, unstable angina, or uncontrolled dysrhythmias).[10] Although not so reliably predictive of future risk, experience is useful for predicting risk in the hands of the group from whom the data were drawn. A nonmedical example of the success of this method for predicting risk is provided by Lloyd's of London. Using accurate records of shipping losses to estimate probabilities of future losses, Lloyd's of London has survived as an insurer for over 300 years. Limitations of a retrospective method are that, unlike the results of a scientific study, data can be interpreted in more than one way; data will usually not be as complete as from randomized, clinical trials; and past data will not be able to help in allowing one to assess new risks.

Other methods of quantifying risk are useful in situations when no or limited data exist, as in nuclear plant meltdowns or the long-term effects of air pollution. In these cases, risk estimation involves extrapolation from current knowledge using mathematical methods to deal with incomplete data. Unfortunately, these non–data based methods are much less accurate for prediction than data-based methods are. Fortunately, in anesthesiology as in most of medicine, the data do exist. We should not confuse failure to collect and examine information with lack of information.

B. Risk evaluation

Risk evaluation involves determining whether a patient's risk category and medical condition reduce or increase reported risk rates for adverse outcomes. This process is more subjective than estimation of risk because risk evaluation is highly dependent on circumstances. Risk adjustment is the part of risk evaluation of most interest to anesthesiologists who want to separate bad outcomes caused by patient disease or factors over which no one has control from those caused by poor care.

C. Risk management (see also Chapter 29)

Preventing undesirable events, decreasing their severity, and minimizing the damage in the event of their occurrence is called "risk management." This aspect of risk assessment is the most important since measuring and evaluating risk are meaningless if nothing is done about the problem.

Despite attempts to base risk assessment upon a scientific foundation, political, social, and economic agendas play major roles. Because of these agendas, risk assessment tends to be undertaken with goals that may not always be objective or scientific.[22-23] Payers want to "prove" care was bad or, more subtly, render a hospital and physicians unable to prove care was "good." Similarly, physicians want to prove to regulators and colleagues that they give good care. These powerful biases must also be considered in the process of risk assessment.[24]

III. ESTIMATING ANESTHETIC RISK

Estimating anesthetic risk requires identifying potential risks, determining the relevant ones (for our purposes, those caused by anesthesia), collecting the necessary data, and calculating the estimates.

A. Identifying risks

Identifying risks is the easiest part of estimating risk. Long lists of good and bad perioperative outcomes can be found in books dealing with anesthetic and surgical complications.[6,7] When informing the patient of potential risk, it is important not to restrict consideration only to risks caused by anesthesia. Relevant outcomes are sometimes referred to as indicators. As of now, all risk is bad; there are no "best" risks or indicators to be guided by in choosing the most desirable anesthesiologist. The absence of serious adverse outcomes is desirable. But is absence of stroke better than absence of death or myocardial infarctions? The JCAHO has spent several years trying and has not succeeded in identifying the key indicators that reflect good or poor care often enough to be scientifically valid.

B. Collecting the data

Collecting the data is the most difficult part of estimating anesthetic risk. The easiest way to collect data is to get it from someone else who already has it. If the cardiology department keeps track of the incidence of congestive heart failure and myocardial infarctions in your hospital, getting this list may be easier than trying to compile your own list of the patients who had congestive heart failure or infarctions. The next easiest way is to find the randomized, clinical trials in the literature that contain the data and draw the appropriate conclusions. The drawbacks of such data have already been discussed: the population may not be the same as your patient population, rendering the conclusions inappropriate for your patients; the experience of the care-givers involved may be different from the experience of those at your institution.

Using billing information is another way to collect information useful for estimating anesthetic risk. Procedure and diagnostic codes (CPT and ICD-9 codes respectively), types of monitors used (arterial catheters, transesophageal echocardiography), and medications delivered (nitroglycerin, epinephrine) are examples of information collected for billing from which conclusions may be drawn about outcomes. But these data, too, have several limitations. Since some CPT* and ICD-9† codes pay more than others, systematic errors in favor of the more highly reimbursed codes may be present. Billing codes can have a moderately high error rate (as much as 10% to 15% for hospital discharge coding) or be unavailable until after the patient is discharged, which may be too late. Even if readily available, billing information may not answer all questions with respect to the risk of anesthesia. This concern was exemplified in a study of carotid endarterectomy, gastrointestinal endoscopy, and coronary angiography; the authors concluded that appropriateness of care could not be predicted from easily available information about patients, physicians, and hospitals.[25] Because bureaucracies that are part of the billing process are comfortable with and well served by coding schemes, physicians will have to deal with this information in order to be reimbursed for their services. It would be an advantage if anesthesiologists could influence the process so that variables relevant to anesthetic risk, perioperative risk, and risk adjustment were included.[26] One study of outcome after coronary artery bypass graft surgery found that adding only three variables to data already collected accounted for 90% of the difference in mortality between institutions, as opposed to 36% of the difference with risk adjustment by Medicare without these three variables.[27]

Another way of obtaining information on risk is to review insurance records, as was done in the American Society of Anesthesiologists Closed Claims Study.[28,29] This method may uncover the cause of risks, but one often does not know the population from which the numbers were drawn (for example, do the participating insurers insure 20% or 80% of the people who give anesthesia in the United States?). The data obtained with this method also are not practical for risk assessment by individual anesthetists for their patients, since the data come from closed malpractice claims and therefore apply to a small, select population. On the

---

*CPT refers to the 5-digit code assigned to procedures performed on patients. The codes are taken from the AMA's *Physician's Current Procedural Terminology,* available in book form and on magnetic tapes from the AMA Order Department, 535 N. Dearborn Street, Chicago, IL 60610.
†ICD-9 refers to the 6- to 8-character codes assigned to diagnoses of disease as approved by the United States Center for Health Statistics. The full initials are ICD-9-CM, that is, *International Classification of Diseases, 9th revision, Clinical Modification.* The codes are available in book form and on disk or tape from Health Care Knowledge Resources, P.O. Box 971, Ann Arbor, MI 48106, and from the American Medical Association. The medical coding division of 3M also has an automated coding package.

other hand, such data are useful for risk management because they allow anesthesiologists to learn from the mistakes of others.

Despite the availability of different sources of data for risk assessment, there are several obstacles that stand in the way of successfully using them. One of the obstacles is, embarrassingly enough, the anesthesiologists themselves. Not unique to our specialty are the unwritten medical mores that good doctors do not inquire about the results of the care other doctors give to patients.[30] The specter of Big Brother and fears of litigation are raised in defense of this behavior. The release of aggregate Medicare data on mortality and morbidity by the Health Care Financing Administration and the demand by third-party payers to see evidence of quality of care is rapidly making this concern moot.[2] By the year 2000, patients may refuse to go to a physician whose results are not available for audit. This channeling of patients to certain physicians applies to anesthesiologists as well.

Another reason this obstacle may soon be removed is that peer review is ineffective if peers are shut off from information about each other's outcomes. Moore provided an apt analogy to describe the current system for the regulation of the quality of open heart surgery:

Imagine a country served by hundreds of small airlines, each of which kept its safety record a tightly held secret. Flight safety was under the total control of the pilots of each airline, and their deliberations and actions, if any, were legally secret in many states. The accepted doctrine was that the pilot is the captain of the ship, and ordinarily is the sole judge of what is safe. About the only way to get rid of an unsafe pilot was through a vote of the pilots of that airline. If a crash occurred, a total news blackout was imposed to maintain public confidence. The airlines varied widely in how thoroughly they investigated crashes, if at all, and the secret inquiries were normally headed by the pilot's closest colleagues.

Large differences in safety records developed among the many airlines. However, the air traveler rarely got access to such information. Even when accident records were occasionally revealed, industry spokesmen insisted that routes, weather, and aircraft were so different that comparisons were meaningless. Other than paying the airfare of all elderly passengers, the federal government had practically no role in airline safety.

Most of us would consider this a bizarre and homicidal way to run an airline industry. However, it accurately describes the much riskier business of hospital care for heart patients.[20]

Other obstacles to data collection are the sheer volume of information and the impossi-

bility of collecting everything that may be needed at some future time. One way to circumvent these obstacles is to periodically get information about perioperative events that are fairly common (nausea, perioperative delays). Some outcomes can be recorded automatically, such as the measurements on monitors in the operating room. Others are as readily detected postoperatively as at the time they occur, such as deaths and cardiac arrests, both brought to the attention of other departments in a hospital anyway. Still other events can be detected by postoperative visits, phone calls, or postcards to be returned by patients.[31]

Whatever collection method is used, the information obtained must be complete. One of the advantages of the ASA Closed Claims Study was that a reviewer made a complete summary of the relevant events in each case.[29] Such a summary allows for future reexamination of the data unhampered by incomplete information. Recording and tracking only indicators will be of limited usefulness because such information is incomplete. It is important, then, not to store an indicator code alone but to include sufficient information so that what happened can be reconstructed later. Keats suggested that the following information should be included for outcome:

1. Identifying information
   - Name
   - Medical record number
   - Date of surgery
2. Date and time of
   - Occurrence of outcome
   - Discovery
   - Therapy
   - Resolution
3. Severity of outcome
4. Temporal nature of the problem (how long it lasted)
5. Conclusion about cause and actions taken[29]

Lastly, there is the issue of computers. The amount of information needed for risk assessment even for individual practitioners makes a computer necessary. Physicians may be able to handle their own information for a time, but larger practices will not be able to do so without computers. Fortunately, computers are becoming easier to use, and more anesthesiologists with computer skills are in practice with each passing year. This is good because a computer that can perform repetitive tasks rapidly and indefinitely without error is useful in risk assessment. Numerous articles concerning billing and demographic database design and operation have been published;[32-34] there have been very few articles on the subject of design and operation of computer systems for the information needs of risk assessment.[35]

IV. EVALUATING ANESTHETIC RISK

A quantitative evaluation of anesthetic risk is a desirable goal. It is, however, a goal impossible to achieve because understanding of and complete information about many perioperative outcomes is not available. Even if this were not true, the evaluation of risk requires that a judgment be made about the significance of any risk. In the past 20 years, this judgment was made by physicians almost exclusively based on scientific data and often without adequate consideration of the preferences of their patients.

Recently the importance of patient preferences in risk evaluation of medical therapy has been given attention long overdue. Investigators in Maine examined the therapy for benign prostatic hypertrophy over a 4-year period. Although not exactly a new discovery, it was observed that patients had a wide range of tolerance for symptoms indicative of prostatic obstruction. In elegant calculations, the investigators showed that the value a patient placed upon additional years of life determined the level of symptoms he would tolerate before agreeing to undergo surgery.[36] For example, a patient who knows he has a 10% chance of impotence or of "dribbling" after transurethral resection of the prostate may prefer watchful waiting and symptoms of obstruction to these two outcomes if the procedure itself does not prolong life expectancy. In such a situation, accurate data about outcomes are critical, since a decision harmful to the patient may be made if risks are understated or benefits overstated.

The Medical Outcomes Study is another investigation that reveals the relationship between patient preferences and outcome. The intent of this observational study of clinicians and patients in Boston, Chicago, and Los Angeles was to determine if variation in outcomes could be explained by variation in the clinician and the system providing care.[37] The investigators also considered outcomes of the chronically ill beyond medical improvement (like reduction in blood pressure) including social functioning, general health perception, and satisfaction with care (for example, the patient's response to questions like the following: Do you feel well? Do you look forward to getting out of bed?). One of the early reports demonstrated significant decrements in measures of the three non-

medical outcomes listed above in patients afflicted with hypertension, diabetes, congestive heart failure, myocardial infarction, angina, arthritis, and chronic lung, gastrointestinal, or back problems.[38] Heart disease and gastrointestinal disorders had the greatest overall impact on outcomes; hypertension, the least. Patients with more than one condition had greater decrements in nonmedical outcomes than those with only one condition. Both of these excellent studies point to the importance of the patient's view in the evaluation of medical risk. We can safely assume this pertains to anesthetic risk as well.

A. Risk adjustment

The most popular aspect of research in evaluating anesthetic risk is risk adjustment. Risk adjustment involves correcting outcome data for the effects of coexisting diseases in patients. Outcomes must be adjusted because sicker patients have worse outcomes than healthy patients.[39] Risk adjustment helps in separating bad outcomes unrelated to anesthesia, such as death in a patient brought to the operating room with a gunshot wound that destroyed the midbrain, from outcomes related to anesthesia, such as death from esophageal intubation in a healthy 19 year old with normal airway anatomy undergoing shoulder arthroscopy.

Unfortunately, risk adjustment can be misused.[40] Intentionally or unintentionally the cause of bad outcomes may be obscured by risk adjustment. The death of a 75-year-old patient during an endotracheal tube change after a procedure for a ruptured abdominal aortic aneurysm can be explained away on the basis of high perioperative risk for that patient. Administrators may sometimes use risk adjustment to exclude from a hospital patients expected to have worse outcomes and longer stays. Faced with data showing high rates of bad outcome, physicians may use risk adjustment as a defense. ("We do sicker patients."). In some cases, the reason for higher rates may be justified, but not in all.

Another potential misuse of risk adjustment lies in the prediction of outcome. Risk indicators are tools to measure outcome and to adjust it for the effects of patient disease, not tools to predict outcome. For example, diagnosis-related groups are used by some hospitals as guidelines for discharging their patients. Since payment is not greater when costs are greater than those allowed for a given diagnosis-related group, some hospitals see the chance to increase profitability by discharging patients when insurance ends, instead of cutting the costs of delivering care. (The latter was the reason for the establishment of diagnosis-related groups.)

Risk adjustment methods proliferate.[13,41-44] They are easy to create but difficult to validate. Their growth has been fueled by the financial rewards and prestige given to those whose plan is officially adopted by organizations like Medicare or the JCAHO. The caveat in the application of such plans is that there is no single best way to adjust outcomes for multiple preexisting medical conditions, even for outcomes related to an isolated circumstance like delivery of anesthesia. On the other hand, adjusters that are applied to a specific situation encompassing a few variables are generally successful. Examples are the Apgar score for neonates and the Glasgow coma scale for assessment of the extent of head injury. Both are measurements taken in specific clinical situations. The Apgar score is determined within 5 minutes after birth, and the Glasgow coma scale is used only for patients with acute head injury. Each also measures the function of only a few physiologic systems—the Apgar score for the heart, lungs, and brain; the Glasgow coma scale for one organ, the injured brain. This narrow scope eliminates the need to determine appropriate weighting of the various measurements used by a given risk adjuster.

Contrast these methods with the popular approach of searching retrospectively for statistically significant associations between outcomes and risk factors. Were numerically significant risk factors the *cause* of a given outcome or merely associated with it? Causal factors can be weighted equally, since, by definition, each potentially caused the outcome. On the other hand, factors merely associated with an outcome will have different weights. Consider the risk factors for perioperative myocardial infarction in coronary artery bypass graft in an emergency operation and in systemic atherosclerosis. The existence of atherosclerosis systemically may mean a patient's coronary arteries are also affected but not necessarily that the patient will suffer an infarction perioperatively. An emergency coronary artery bypass procedure performed on a patient suffering infarction is a risk factor directly linked to perioperative myocardial infarction.

There is no evidence that complex risk adjustment methods are more successful than simple ones. One of the simplest unofficial ways to judge risk for mortality of hospitalized patients is to observe whether they walked into the hospital or were carried in. It has been suggested that the Food and Drug Administration would not have approved any risk-adjustment method if the method first had to meet the standards of efficacy required for approval of drugs and medical devices.[45]

To adjust anesthetic risk in a clinical setting, the most useful factors to consider are age, procedure, diagnosis, and end-organ impairment. It is not so much systemic disease as end-organ damage from disease that affects outcome. The diabetic patient with coronary artery disease is at increased risk for postoperative myocardial infarction because of arterial occlusion, not because of the metabolic derangements of diabetes.[46]

Table 25-1. University of Chicago Hospitals and Clinics' modification of the Aldrete score

Type	Description	Score
Activity	Able to move all four extremities voluntarily or on command	2
	Able to move two extremities voluntarily or on command	1
	Unable to move extremities voluntarily or on command	0
Respiration	Able to breathe deeply and cough freely	2
	Dyspnea or limited breathing	1
	Apneic	0
Circulation	Blood pressure within 20% of preanesthetic level	2
	Blood pressure within 50% of preanesthetic level	1
	Blood pressure more than 50% different from preanesthetic level	0
Consciousness	Fully awake	2
	Arousable on calling	1
	Not responsive	0
Color	Pink	2
	Pale, dusky, blotchy, jaundiced, other	1
	Cyanotic	0

Below we review some methods of risk adjustment.

B. Risk adjustment methods

1. Aldrete score. The Aldrete score is used to categorize the postoperative condition of patients in the recovery room (Table 25-1).[47] This score has limited usefulness for risk adjustment because the same low numbers can represent widely different clinical conditions, and measurement is taken only at a specific time in the perioperative course of events. Given the score, one still must examine the patient's medical record. The Aldrete score is an example of a risk-adjustment method restricted to a limited clinical situation.

2. Apgar score. Although not directly applicable to assessing anesthetic risk, the Apgar score is the granddaddy of risk-adjustment systems. Devised by an anesthesiologist in 1953, it provides an effective and reliable method to assess the overall status of newborns. The Apgar score measures a limited part of the spectrum of medical illness. The lesson to be learned from this evaluation method is that risk should be assessed for patients from homogeneous groups with respect to age, end-organ function, and procedure and include parts of the perianesthetic spectrum rather than all of it (Table 25-2).[48]

3. American Society of Anesthesiologists assessment of physical status. The ASA assessment of physical status has been in existence for more than 50 years.[49,50] Although not developed as a tool for risk adjustment, the score does exactly that for 40% to 60% of all anesthetized patients.[27] It is best at separating the perfectly healthy (ASA physical status 1) and the deathly ill (ASA physical status 5) from the rest of the surgical population. It is also fairly good at separating the less than healthy (ASA physical status 2) from the critically ill (ASA physical status 4). It is less accurate for determining risk for patients of ASA physical status

3 because criteria for evaluation are comprehensive and not limited to specific organ failures. A patient with congestive heart failure and coronary artery disease in ASA physical status 3, for example, might be at greater risk for perioperative myocardial infarction than for respiratory arrest. The opposite might be true for a premature infant with an ASA physical status 3.

The designation E for emergency in the ASA physical status score is even less useful. Patients classified E vary greatly, and perhaps the lack of attention practitioners can give to the other medical problems of emergency patients makes their outcomes appear worse than those of other patients. Categories that would differentiate the following are needed: patients who go straight to the operating room upon arrival at the hospital; patients who have surgery within the hour, 12 hours, or 24 hours; and patients for whom a procedure is delayed one or more days without ill effect. The outcomes of a so-called emergency group that includes both the critically ill and those who have waited as much as a day or two before surgery may appear worse than the outcomes of an otherwise comparable group of patients undergoing elective surgery. This inaccurate pooling may be the basis for support in the literature for effect of emergency status on outcome. Apart from these difficulties with the E category, grouping patients together with respect to their ASA physical status is a simple, moderately sensitive, and moderately specific endeavor.

4. Acute physiology and chronic health evaluation (APACHE II, III, IV). The acute physiology and chronic health evaluation (APACHE) was developed for an intensive care unit setting by a physician in an anesthesia department.[51] It is based on the assumption that the physiologic measurements obtained in the course of a critically ill patient's stay in an ICU yield an accurate assessment of the severity of that patient's illness.

It takes 12 measures: (1) heart rate, (2) mean

Table 25-2. Apgar score

Features evaluated	No points	1 point	2 points
Heart rate	0	<100	>100
Respiration	Apnea	Irregular, shallow or gasping	Vigorous and crying
Color	Pale, blue	Pale or blue extremities	Pink
Muscle tone	Absent	Weak, passive tone	Active movement
Reflex irritability	Absent	Grimace	Active avoidance

blood pressure, (3) respiratory rate, (4) temperature, (5) Glasgow coma scale, (6) hematocrit, (7) white blood cell count, (8) serum potassium, (9) serum sodium, (10) serum creatinine, (11) arterial pH, and (12) arterial Pao_2. Each measure is then assigned a weight that has been empirically determined. The maximum score is 71, with increasing age counting for up to 6 points and chronic illness or emergency presentation up to 5 points. Higher totals denote more severe illness.

Although the APACHE method of assessment may not be entirely applicable in anesthesia, its organ-based approach is probably the most effective way to handle risk adjustment for anesthetized patients because many undesirable perioperative outcomes are determined more by impaired organ function than by disease processes. For assessment of long-term risk, which tends to be related more to the disease process than to an acute physiologic disorder, the organ-based approach is not so effective.

5. Glasgow coma scale. The Glasgow coma scale is a scoring system to rate the severity of injury to the central nervous system[52] (Table 25-3). It is of limited usefulness to anesthesiologists, since almost all of our patients are awake and conscious preoperatively and postoperatively. It too illustrates the success of risk-adjustment methods that are restricted to a part of the clinical spectrum.

6. Goldman cardiac risk scale. The Goldman cardiac risk scale is a popular method for rating the severity of cardiovascular disease.[53,54] It has the advantage of being restricted to evaluation of one part of the clinical spectrum, patients with cardiac disease undergoing noncardiac surgery (Table 25-4). That the Goldman scale has not become the risk adjuster for perioperative cardiac outcomes is testimony to the difficulty of accurate weighting of multiple risk factors with variable degrees of cause-and-effect linkage.

7. HealthQuiz. HealthQuiz* has been under development for more than 3 years. It was initially begun as an attempt to automate the process of selecting laboratory tests and to ensure thorough history taking. Three methods of combining the results from HealthQuiz are be-

Table 25-3. Modified Glasgow coma scale

Sign	Evaluation	Score
Eyes open	Never	1
	To pain	2
	To speech	3
	Spontaneously	4
Best verbal response	None	1
	Garbled	2
	Inappropriate	3
	Confused	4
	Oriented	5
Best motor response	None	1
	Extension	2
	Abnormal flexion	3
	Withdrawal	4
	Localizes pain	5
	Obeys commands	6

Severe head injury is determined by a score of 7 or less persisting for 6 hours or more.

ing considered to assess perioperative risk accurately. HealthQuiz uses algorithms to determine risk, based on patterns of answers to some of the 134 questions asked by the machine. Patients' responses to some questions will be valuable only in conjunction with responses to others though all the questions are necessary for the algorithm. In statistical terms, these questions influence prediction through "high-order interactions," which often go undetected by classic multivariate methods like logistic regression and discriminant analysis.[55] In the last decade, new multivariate techniques, such as recursive partitioning, have been developed specifically to discover such interactions. These methods are also called "classification and regression trees" because they provide the predictive capability of multiple regression by direct construction of a decision tree instead of through a linear model.

In recursive partitioning, a sample is divided into two subsamples on the basis of the answer to a single question. The goal is for each subsample to be as homogeneous and at the same time as different as possible from the other subsample. If the purpose is to predict need for a preoperative chest roentgenogram among patients over 59 years of age, for example, it may be that taking a roentgenogram is indicated 85% of the time for patients with a history of smoking one pack of cigarettes per day or more and only 20% of the time for those without such a history. The indications for chest roent-

---

*Dr. Roizen developed this video preoperative health questionnaire at the University of Chicago to help ameliorate the problem of inefficient preoperative assessments and test selection methods. The university is developing this system, a laptop video device, into a commercial product. If the product is successful, Dr. Roizen will benefit financially because the university distributes a royalty or partial ownership right in such commercialized inventions to its faculty.

genogram from other questions may be less determinate and hence less informative; that is, taking a roentgenogram may be indicated 35% of the time for those younger than 75 years of age and 50% of the time for those older than 75 years. In recursive partitioning, the most informative responses are selected first. In this example, smoking history would be used before age or other variables to split the sample. The group with no smoking history would then be further subdivided on the basis of its responses to other questions. To subdivide the group of nonsmokers (of whom only 20% may require a roentgenogram), one might best question their age. If additional partitioning made prediction of the need for a chest roentgenogram even more determinate, other questions would be used.

The group of smokers could be partitioned in a similar fashion. The most informative questions to separate the 85% of this group who should have a chest roentgenogram from the 15% for whom a chest roentgenogram is un-

necessary may not be the same questions used to split the nonsmokers. The result of an analysis of this sort is a decision tree, often based on a small number of questions that optimally predict the need for a particular diagnostic test. A hypothetical decision tree based on this example is given in Fig. 25-1.

HealthQuiz suffers from procedural limitations, such as the time it takes for patients to complete all responses to questions (well over 5 minutes). Some patients are physically, mentally, or psychologically unable to use the device without assistance. Attempts are under way to validate the ability of HealthQuiz to predict outcome.[56] If the device becomes more and more extensively used—much as pulse oximetry was widely used years before it was demonstrated to improve care—this problem may be rendered moot. The developers of HealthQuiz plan to publish the calculations currently used for risk adjustment when they are validated. Until such publication, the device may seem

Table 25-4. Computation of the Goldman cardiac risk index

Criteria	Points
1. History	
a. Age > 70 yr	5
b. Myocardial infarction in previous 6 months	10
2. Physical examination	
a. S_3 gallop or jugular vein distention	11
b. Important valvular aortic stenosis	3
3. Electrocardiogram	
a. Rhythm other than sinus or premature atrial contractions on last preoperative ECG	7
b. >5 premature ventricular contractions/min documented at any time before operation	7
4. General status	3
Po_2 <60 or Pco_2 >50 mm Hg	
K <3.0 or HCO_3 <20 mEq/L	
BUN >50 or creatinine >3.0 mg/dl, abnormal	
AST (SGOT), signs of chronic liver disease, or patient bedridden from noncardiac causes	
5. Operation	
a. Intraperitoneal, intrathoracic, or aortic operation	3
b. Emergency operation	4
TOTAL POSSIBLE	53

To calculate a patient's score, one sums up the number of points from all factors he or she possesses. Patients are further segregated into class I (0-5 points), with a risk of 1% to 7% of major complications; class II (6-12 points), risk of 7% to 11%; class III (13-25 points), risk of 14% to 38%; and class IV (≥26 points), risk of 30% to 100%.

Abbreviations: Po_2, partial pressure of oxygen; Pco_2, partial pressure of carbon dioxide; *K,* potassium; *HCO_3,* bicarbonate; *BUN,* blood urea nitrogen; *AST (SGOT),* aspartate aminotransferase (formerly called serum glutamic-oxaloacetic transaminase).

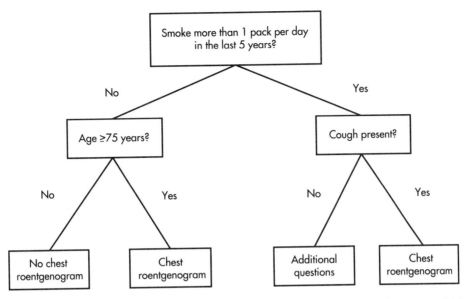

Fig. 25-1. Hypothetical decision tree, an example of how recursive partitioning uses multiple pieces of information to ascertain risk categories, in this case risk of having an abnormal result on the roentgenogram.

Table 25-5. New York Heart Association's (NYHA) and the Canadian Cardiovascular Society's (CCS) classifications of angina

NYHA	CCS
I. Ordinary physical activity, such as walking or climbing stairs, does not cause angina. Angina with strenuous or rapid prolonged exertion at work or recreation or with sexual relations.	I. Ordinary physical activity, such as walking and climbing stairs, does not cause angina. Angina with strenuous or rapid or prolonged exertion at work or recreation.
II. Slight limitation of ordinary activity. Walking or climbing stairs rapidly, walking uphill, walking or stair climbing after meals, or in cold, or in wind, or under emotional stress, or only during a few hours after awakening. Walking more than two blocks on the level or more than one flight of stairs at a normal pace and in normal conditions.	II. Slight limitation of ordinary activity. Walking or climbing stairs rapidly, walking uphill, walking or stair climbing after meals, in cold, in wind, or when under emotional stress or during the few hours after awakening. Walking more than two blocks on the level and climbing more than one flight of ordinary stairs at a normal pace and in normal conditions.
III. Marked limitation of ordinary physical activity. Walking one or two blocks on the level and climbing one flight of stairs in normal conditions and at a normal pace. "Comfortable at rest."	III. Marked limitation of ordinary physical activity. Walking one to two blocks on the level and climbing more than one flight in normal conditions.
IV. Inability to carry on any physical activity without discomfort—anginal syndrome may be present at rest.	IV. Inability to carry on any physical activity without discomfort—anginal syndrome *may be* present at rest.

less inviting to practitioners. HealthQuiz has much to recommend it, but its position in clinical anesthesiology has yet to be determined.

8. Judgment. Judgment is used regularly for risk assessment but, as a general method, is unreproducible and unreliable.

9. New York Heart Association's and the Canadian Cardiovascular Society's classifica-

tions of angina. The classifications of angina provided by the New York Heart Association and by the Canadian Cardiovascular Society appear in Table 25-5.[46] These classifications provide yet another example of the relative success of risk adjusters for limited clinical circumstances.

10. American Society of Anesthesiologists/ Vitez severity scale. The ASA/Vitez severity scale for risk adjustment in anesthesia is the first to take into account the severity as well as the course of adverse outcomes.[57,58] It differentiates events such as death and stroke, which are irreversible or severe, from hypotension and transient hypoxia, which though undesirable are neither severe nor irreversible. It also separates irreversible events from those that take months to resolve or those of a transient nature. The main drawback to this method is the secrecy that has surrounded the evaluation process so far. Effective evaluation is best served by openness. There is no advantage to having only a few individuals aware of potential problems, something not encouraged in the evaluation of risk. When objective criteria are available for the evaluation process, this method may be excellent for adjusting outcomes so that a unified rating system for outcomes can be used to assess performance.

C. Risk adjustment methods of economic import but of limited use to anesthesiologists

1. Diagnosis-related groups. Diagnosis-related groups (DRGs) provide the basis for the Prospective Payment System used by Medicare to determine hospital payments. Although DRGs have been criticized for not classifying patients into homogeneous groups, this deficiency is more a result of inadequacies in the ICD-9-CM coding process than in the DRG plan.[59] DRGs were developed from the best clinical and financial information available at the time. Their use for risk adjustment by anesthetists is limited because they deal with treatment of disease processes rather than end-organ failure. But since DRGs are the basis for hospital reimbursement, we need to be aware of their existence.

2. Disease staging. Clinical Disease Staging (manual version) by SysteMetrics, Inc. has been under development for over 10 years. Disease staging was designed to help hospitals control case mix (severity of illness of patients with a given problem). It identifies a patient's disease from 420 categories and places the patient in one of four stages based on empirically derived criteria rather than on ICD-9 codes: no complications, complications involving one site, complications involving more than one site (poor prognosis), and death.

Facts about millions of patients are entered into databases for nationwide comparisons. Coded Disease Staging (automatic version), developed by Blue Cross of Western Pennsylvania, can be leased in a mainframe or an IBM-compatible PC version. The mainframe version can reportedly stage 10,000 cases in 1 minute. Both versions categorize discharge status, ICD-9 codes, and sex (not age). Disease staging can be done at more than one time after a patient's admission, but since abstracting ICD-9 codes is relatively time consuming, it tends to be done for all patients only upon discharge.

3. MedisGroups. MedisGroups by MediQual, Inc.,[60] is a proprietary measurement of severity of illness based upon a patient's condition at hospital admission. A standardized database of over 500,000 cases is used to generate norms for comparison. Patients are assigned Key Clinical Findings (KCFs) from more than 200 available vital signs and lab tests. Each Key Clinical Finding is given a severity score from 1 to 3. The patient is then placed into one of five severity groups. Because the method of manipulating the data and calculating the severity of a patient's illness is proprietary, MedisGroups has not received widespread evaluation of its scientific merits.

4. Patient management categories. Patient Management Categories (PMC) was developed by the Pittsburgh Research Institute (a nonprofit research wing of Blue Cross of Western Pennsylvania). It is the result of an HCFA grant in 1978 to develop a method of predicting utilization of hospital resources.* Patient Management Categories are used to predict hospitalization requirements on the assumption that categories that determine hospital payment must also predict diagnoses, therapies, and the use of resources. Over 800 patient categories, identified by expert panels including physicians, were associated with relevant ICD-9 and CPT codes, and such associations make it possible to place most patients in the appropriate category by computer. Three products were developed: Patient Management Categories, Relative Cost Weights, and Patient Management Paths. Because this system is used only with inpatients

---

*The final report is in three volumes: I. Descriptions of patient management categories and classification software; II. Cost weighting methodology; III. Physician-specified management strategies based on PMC. The volumes and software are available from the Pittsburgh Research Institute, 301 Fifth Avenue, Suite 1700, Pittsburgh, PA 15222.

and was not intended for the perioperative setting, it is of little use to us.

5. Severity of illness and computerized severity of illness index. The computerized severity of illness scale has been in development at Johns Hopkins for more than 10 years. Its criteria are publicly available and are based upon ICD-9-CM codes, so that existing hospital billing and discharge information can be used.[61,62] This system encompasses the entire spectrum of inpatient illness. The scale determines severity of illness at the time of medical record coding, which usually occurs after discharge. Criteria include signs, symptoms, laboratory values, radiology studies, and physical findings. Treatments are not included. This system can aid hospitals trying to adjust their patient mix in terms of ICD-9 coding, but its value for assessment of anesthetic risk and perioperative outcomes remains to be determined.

6. Quality-adjusted life-years. A successful outcome of medical care is more than just cure of a disease. Also important are the cost of the cure and the kind of life a patient will lead afterwards. Expensive cures may be clinical successes but therapeutic failures if a patient's quality of life is worse after "cure." For several years, economists and decision analysts have tried to incorporate the intangible factors surrounding quality of life into a number that would quantify subjective factors. One result has been the quality-adjusted life-year. The methods used to calculate quality-adjusted life-years are still under development, but the product of the calculation is a number assigned to a therapy that includes both expected outcomes and quality of life. The usefulness of the quality-adjusted life-year is its potential to direct society's health care resources toward treatments that result in the greatest improvement for the most people at the lowest cost. The concept is appealing, but ethical problems arise when clinical decisions for individual patients are based on summaries of community opinions that do not consider patients' preferences. The disadvantages of the widespread application of quality-adjusted life-years have been discussed at length elsewhere;[63] that the method includes criteria in addition to purely medical considerations in its assessment of outcome is an advantage.

V. MANAGING ANESTHETIC RISK

What to do about identified risks is the most difficult and important aspect of risk assessment in anesthesiology. This activity is complicated further by the fact that the impetus for risk management has up to now been almost exclusively financial consideration.[64] Although not necessarily bad, financial motives introduce a bias toward resolving problems with a high cost-benefit potential and away from factors that have a low cost-benefit potential. Enjoyment of life cannot be calculated in dollar value and thus efforts may be directed away from solutions that would increase quality of life.

The simplest way to deal with the risk of anesthesia is not to administer anesthetic. No risk is suffered from an anesthetic that is not given. In other areas of medicine, preventing disease is almost always cheaper, faster, and safer than treating the results of disease. Public health measures aim at prevention of infectious disease or lessening the risk of coronary artery disease by warning of the added risk for smokers or those with untreated hypertension or diets high in cholesterol. Our patients, however, usually do not choose anesthesia; rather they decide to undergo procedures for which anesthesia is necessary.

A variation upon the idea of not administering anesthesia is limiting the types of patients a specific anesthetist may anesthetize. Either because some patients are too sick for a particular anesthesiologist to handle or because an anesthesiologist has had bad results or no experience with the intended techniques, there may be certain patients and anesthesiologists who should not interact. For example, should anesthetist #7 in the Texas heart study,[65] if he or she is unable to improve, be allowed to continue to anesthetize patients with cardiovascular disease? In 1990, this suggestion may seem outlandish. But should payment become linked to outcome, it may suddenly seem fiscally sound and acceptable.

Another method of managing anesthetic risk is to track selected outcomes across the range of all practitioners and institutions, that is, identify the "bad apples" and stop them from practicing anesthesia. This is the JCAHO approach, and it has the advantage of accumulating much data so that statistical analysis can be applied to the problem. Yet because such identification is performed by an external entity, it creates a counterproductive inspector-inspected relationship.[66] If 90% of anesthesiologists' energies are devoted to "looking good" for an inspector, they will not be used for improving care. When anesthesiologists become adept at performing for inspectors, JCAHO will be forced to expend energy on auditing inspections. The result is an endless escalation of effort to catch or avoid being caught, which siphons resources away from patient care. It is a highly optimistic hope that the "new" concentration on indicators garnered from the efforts of external regulation will lead to improvement in care, since this is something that has not happened for the past several decades.

Sanctioning official standards is another approach to risk management.[67-70] It is under the assumption that if correct behavior is identified, mandated, and carried out, good outcomes will result. Unfortunately, human behavior is the most difficult factor to change under any circumstances. It is much more effective to change the system so that potential damage from unwanted behaviors is minimized. Also, if standards follow (rather than precede) changes in practice, they may well codify what already happens instead of leading to positive change. On the other hand, discussions and strong statements about the imposition of standards may have led some hospitals to improve equipment availability, thus allowing a higher quality of care to be delivered. Because of the attention given by the JCAHO and the HCFA to outcomes, more anesthesiologists now take a greater interest in outcomes than they did before.

The most important aspect of risk assessment is getting accurate and complete data. Although less politically and professionally satisfying than deciding what to do with the data, accurate data lead to accurate assessments. Numerous ways to adjust this information for severity of illness exist. Simple adjustment plans can be as effective as complicated ones for certain groups of patients. Currently the cornerstones of adjustment for anesthetic risk are age, procedure, and end-organ impairment. Other factors, both medical and nonmedical, also merit consideration under selected circumstances. Regardless of what method we employ, we must measure how well we take care of patients, we must inform each patient of the risk of having undesirable perianesthetic outcomes, and we must work toward reducing that risk. This is the ultimate clinical utility of risk assessment.

REFERENCES

1. Codman EA: A study in hospital efficiency, Boston, undated (c. 1916), Thomas Todd Co.
2. Roper WL et al: Effectiveness in health care: an initiative to evaluate and improve medical practice, N Engl J Med 319:1197-1222, 1988.
3. Greenfield S: The state of outcome research: are we on target? N Engl J Med 320:1142-1143, 1989.
4. Ellwood PM: Shattuck lecture—outcomes management: a technology of patient experience, N Engl J Med 318:1549-1556, 1988.
5. Grumet GW: Health care rationing through inconvenience: the third party's secret weapon, N Engl J Med 321:607-611, 1989.
6. Ross AF and Tinker JH: Anesthesia risk. In Miller RD, editor: Anesthesia, ed 3, New York, 1990, Churchill Livingstone.
7. Brown DL, editor: Risk and outcome in anesthesia, Philadelphia, 1988, JB Lippincott.
8. Orkin FK and Cooperman LH: Complications in anesthesiology, Philadelphia, 1983, JB Lippincott.
9. Gravenstein N, editor: Manual of complications during anesthesia, Philadelphia, 1991, JB Lippincott.
10. Foster ED et al: Risk of noncardiac operation in patients with defined coronary disease: the Coronary Artery Surgery Study (CASS) registry experience, Ann Thorac Surg 41:42-50, 1986.
11. Fisher ES and Wennberg JE: Administrative data in effectiveness studies: the prostatectomy assessment. In Heithoff KA and Lohr KN, editors: Effectiveness and outcomes in health care, Washington, DC 1990, National Academic Press.
12. Ward GG: The value and need of more attention to end-results and follow-up in hospitals today, Bull Am Coll Surg 8:29, 1924.
13. Blumberg MS: Risk adjusting health care outcomes: a methodologic review, Med Care Rev 43:351-393, 1986.
14. Donabedian A: The definition of quality and approaches to its assessment, Ann Arbor, Mich, 1980, Health Administration Press.
15. Dans PF, Wiener JP, and Otter SE: Peer review organizations: promises and potential pitfalls, N Engl J Med 313:1131-1137, 1985.
16. Agenda for change: update (newsletter), Chicago, 1988, Joint Commission on Accreditation of Healthcare Organizations.
17. Hartz AJ et al: Hospital characteristics and mortality rates, N Engl J Med 321:1720-1725, 1989.
18. Iglehart JK: Health policy report: Congress moves to bolster peer review: the health care quality improvement act of 1986, N Engl J Med 316:960-964, 1987.
19. Ludtke M: Physician, inform thyself, Time, June 26, 1989, p 71.
20. Moore TJ: Heart failure: a critical inquiry into American medicine and the revolution in heart care, New York, 1989, Random House.
21. Couch JB and Nash DB: Severity of illness measures: opportunities for clinicans, Ann Intern Med 109:771-772, 1988.
22. Johnston R: The characteristics of risk assessment research. In Conrad J, editor: Society, technology and risk assessment, New York, 1980, Academic Press.
23. Mazur A: Societal and scientific causes of the historical development of risk assessment. In Conrad J, editor: Society, technology and risk assessment, New York, 1980, Academic Press.
24. Winterfeldt DV: Four theses on the application of risk assessment methods. In Conrad J, editor: Society, technology and risk assessment, New York, 1980, Academic Press.
25. Brook RH et al: Predicting the appropriate use of carotid endarterectomy, upper gastrointestinal endoscopy, and coronary angiography, N Engl J Med 323:1173-1177, 1990.
26. Musen MA: The strained quality of medical data, Methods Inf Med 28:123-125, 1989.
27. Pine M et al: National norms and your surgical mortality rates: how anesthesia records help, Anesthesiology 71:A919, 1989
28. Brunner EA: Analysis of anesthetic mishaps, The National Association of Insurance Commissioners' Closed Claims Study, Int Anesthesiol Clin 22:17-30, 1984.
29. Keats AS: The closed claims study, Anesthesiology 73:199-201, 1990 (Editorial).
30. Beck WC and Meyer KK: Should surgeons know their colleagues wound infection rates? Infect Surg 6:361-400, 1988.

31. Cohen MM and Duncan PG: Postoperative follow-up and quality of care, Semin Anesth 7:270-277, 1988.
32. Chase CR, Merz BA, and Mazuzan JE: Computer assisted patient evaluation (CAPE): a multi-purpose computer system for an anesthesia service, Anesth Analg 62:198-206, 1983.
33. Bashein G and Barna CR: A comprehensive computer system for anesthetic record retrieval, Anesth Analg 64:425-431, 1985.
34. Strauss PL and Turndorf H: A computerized anesthesia database, Anesth Analg 68:340-343, 1989.
35. Erickson JP: Quality assurance and improvement in anesthesiology—is a computer necessary? Regional Refresher Course, Park Ridge, Ill, 1990, American Society of Anesthesiologists.
36. Barry MJ et al: Watchful waiting vs immediate transurethral resection for symptomatic prostatism: the importance of patients' preferences, JAMA 259:3010-3017, 1988.
37. Tarlov AR et al: The medical outcomes study: an application of methods for monitoring the results of medical care, JAMA 262:925-930, 1989.
38. Stewart AL: Functional status and well-being of patients with chronic conditions, results from the Medical Outcomes Study, JAMA 262:907-913, 1989.
39. Knaus WA and Nash DB: Predicting and evaluating patient outcomes, Ann Intern Med 109:521-522, 1988.
40. Perrow C: Normal accidents: living with high-risk technologies, New York, 1984, Basic Books.
41. Laupacis A, Sackett DL, and Roberts RS: An assessment of clinically useful measures of the consequences of treatment, N Engl J Med 318:1728-1733, 1988.
42. Stein REK et al: Severity of illness: concepts and measurements, Lancet 2:1506-1509, 1987.
43. McMahon LF Jr and Billi JE: Measurement of severity of illness and the Medicare prospective payment system: state of the art and future directions, J Gen Intern Med 3:482-490, 1988.
44. Rowe WD: Risk assessment approaches and methods. In Conrad J, editor: Society, technology and risk assessment, New York, 1980, Academic Press.
45. Jencks SF: Issues in the use of large data bases for effectiveness research. In Heithoff KA and Lohr KN, editors: Effectiveness and outcomes in health care, Washington, DC, 1990, National Academic Press
46. Roizen MF: Anesthetic implications of concurrent diseases. In Miller RD, editor: Anesthesia, ed 3, New York, 1990, Churchill Livingstone.
47. Aldrete JA and Kroulik D: A postanesthetic recovery score, Anesth Analg 49:924-933, 1970.
48. Apgar V: A proposal for a new method of evaluation of the newborn infant, Anesth Analg 32:260-267, 1953.
49. Saklad M: Grading of patients for surgical procedures, Anesthesiology 2: 281-284, 1941.
50. New classification of physical status, Anesthesiology 24:111, 1963.
51. Knaus WA: APACHE II: a severity of disease classification system, Crit Care Med 13:818-829, 1985.
52. Shapiro H and Drummond J: Neurosurgical anesthesia and intracranial hypertension: In Miller RD, editor: Anesthesia, ed 3, New York, 1990, Churchill Livingstone.
53. Goldman L: Multifactorial index of cardiac risk in noncardiac surgical procedures, N Engl J Med 297:845-850, 1977.
54. Goldman L: Cardiac risks and complications of noncardiac surgery, Ann Intern Med 98:504-513, 1983.
55. Breiman L et al: Classification and regression trees, Belmont, 1984, Wadsworth.
56. Coalson D et al: Correlation between two physical status measures and the ASA physical status score, Anesthesiology 73:A1253, 1990.
57. Vitez TS: A model for quality assurance in anesthesiology, J Clin Anesth 2:280-287, 1990.
58. American Board of Anesthesiology: Continued demonstration of qualifications for board-certified anesthesiologists, Anesthesiology 73:770-771, 1990.
59. Mullin RL: Diagnosis-related groups and severity: ICD-9-CM, the real problem, JAMA 254:1208-1210, 1985.
60. Iezzoni LI and Moskowitz MA: A clinical assessment of MedisGroups, JAMA 260:3159-3163, 1988.
61. Horn SD and Horn RA: Reliability and validity of the severity of illness index, Med Care 24:159-178, 1986.
62. Horn SD: Measuring severity: how sick is sick? How well is well? reprint, Chicago, 1986, American Hospital Association.
63. LaPuma J and Lawlor EF: Quality-adjusted life-years: ethical implications for physicians and policymakers, JAMA 263:2917-2921, 1990.
64. Couch NP et al: The high cost of low-frequency events, N Engl J Med 304:634-637, 1981.
65. Slogoff S and Keats AS: Does perioperative myocardial ischemia lead to postoperative myocardial infarction? Anesthesiology 62:107-114, 1985.
66. Berwick DM: Continuous improvement as an ideal in health care, N Engl J Med 320:53-56, 1989.
67. Eichorn JH et al: Standards for patient monitoring during anesthesia at Harvard Medical School, JAMA 256:1017-1020, 1986.
68. Eichorn JH: Prevention of intraoperative anesthesia accidents and related severe injury through safety monitoring, Anesthesiology 70:572-577, 1989.
69. Orkin FK: Practice standards: the Midas touch or the emperor's new clothes? Anesthesiology 70:567-571, 1989.
70. Moss E: New Jersey enacts anesthesia standards, Anesthesia Patient Safety Foundation Newsletter 4:13-24, 1989.

Chapter 26

Current Spectrum of Anesthetic Injury

Frederick W. Cheney

The professional liability "crisis of affordability" of the mid-1980s focused attention on the issue of patient injury from anesthesia. To improve patient safety the American Society of Anesthesiologists (ASA) implemented several programs, one of which was the development of a national database of cases of anesthetic injury in the United States. Since 1985 the Committee on Professional Liability has been conducting a study of insurance company closed malpractice claims against anesthesiologists in order to identify major areas of loss because of adverse anesthetic events and the contribution of substandard care to poor anesthetic outcome. This type of in-depth information about contemporary adverse anesthetic outcomes in the United States has not been available previously. The major objective of the closed claims project is the development of strategies to reduce the risk of patient injury.

The ASA Closed Claims Project database is a standardized collection of case summaries of adverse anesthetic outcomes that were retrieved by practicing anesthesiologists from professional liability insurance company closed claims files.[1] As of May 1989, 1,541 claims were collected from 20 insurance organizations throughout the United States. One company processes claims for more than 40 states. The other sources mainly are statewide organizations that include both physician-owned and private companies. Twenty-four anesthesiologists, 14 private practitioners, and 10 academic practitioners participated in the claims review.

To collect data, one or more anesthesiologists visited each insurance company office to review all files for claims against anesthesiologists. Claims for dental injury were excluded. A standardized data collection instrument was completed for claims for which it was believed that there was enough information to reconstruct the sequence of events, nature of the injury, and how the actions of the care providers were linked to the damage that occurred. Typically a closed claim file consists of the hospital record, the anesthesia record, narrative statements of the involved health care personnel, expert and peer reviews, deposition summaries, outcome reports, and the cost of settlement or jury award. The case summaries included detailed information on patient characteristics, date of incident, surgical procedure, personnel involved, anesthetic records, consent, monitors employed, anesthetic techniques and agents, damaging events, clinical clues, complications (outcomes), whether a lawsuit was filed, and the amount of award or settlement. Reviewers wrote a brief summary of each case that summarized the sequence of events and provided additional details. Each reviewer also assessed the overall appropriateness of anesthetic care and its contribution to the adverse outcome. Care was rated by the on-site reviewer as standard (appropriate), substandard (inappropriate), or impossible to judge based upon reasonable and prudent practices at the time of the event. Ninety-two percent of the cases occurred between 1975 and 1985.

It should be recognized that there are major limitations to this sort of analysis. There is no information as to the total number of patients at risk and no information as to the incidence of an injury. There is no geographic balance, and the data obtained depend on which companies agreed to participate in the study. Also, there is a selectivity of claims in that only those in which there is enough information in the file to determine causation and standard of care are entered into the database.

However, a great deal of relevant information can still be gained, and as the data emerged, it became obvious they could be utilized in two major ways. First, broad areas were identified in which changes in practice were suggested by high-incidence occurrence of a single mishap (such as esophageal intubation) and in which the usefulness of preventive measures such as capnography might be inferred. A second way in which the data were utilized was by in-depth study of specific types of injury that occurred without apparent cause. An important example was unexpected cardiac arrest during spinal anesthesia.[2] What follows is a summary of the major findings up to now.

I. ADVERSE OUTCOMES AND INJURY
A. Overview

The database is broken down into two broad categories: (1) complications or adverse anesthetic outcomes, and (2) damaging events. Damaging events were the specific incidents that led to the adverse outcomes. There were fewer damaging events than adverse outcomes because many complications occurred without an apparent damaging event being identified during the perioperative period.

The most frequent adverse outcomes were death (37%), nerve damage (15%), and patient brain damage (12%) (Table 26-1). Claims for low-severity injuries such as emotional damage (3%), no apparent injury (2%), headache (2%), burns (2%), pain during regional anesthesia (1%), and back pain (1%) combined to make up the next largest category or 11% of the adverse outcomes (Table 26-1). Less frequent adverse outcomes were the need for prolonged ventilatory support, airway trauma, eye damage, aspiration, and newborn brain damage. Myocardial infarction represented only slightly more than 1% of the adverse outcomes.

The damaging events or specific critical incidents leading to the adverse outcomes were predominantly respiratory, representing 522, or 34%, of the total claims (Table 26-2). The next most common but by far less frequent damaging events leading to injury were those of the cardiovascular system (6%) (Table 26-2). Most of the claims in the excessive blood loss category (2%) were surgical in nature, and most of

Table 26-1. Adverse outcomes (incidence of 1% or greater) found by the American Society of Anesthesiologists Closed Claims Project

	Number of claims (1541)	Percent of 1541
Death	565	37
Nerve damage	227	15
Brain damage (patient)	188	12
Low-severity injuries	177	11*
Prolonged ventilatory support	87	6
Airway trauma	63	4
Pneumothorax	53	3
Eye damage	46	3
Aspiration	45	3
Pulmonary edema	39	3
Newborn brain damage	38	3
Stroke	33	2
Hepatic dysfunction or failure	31	2
Respiratory distress syndrome	23	1
Myocardial infarction	19	1
Newborn death	18	1
Renal dysfunction or failure	16	1
Localized vascular insufficiency	9	1

*Includes emotional damage (3%), no apparent injury (2%), headache (2%), burns (2%), pain during regional anesthesia (1%), and back pain (1%).

the cases of air embolism (2%) involved sequelae of cardiopulmonary bypass. Finally, the categories of equipment problems (4%), wrong drug or dose (4%), and convulsions (2%) made up the damaging events that led to 10% of the total adverse outcomes in the study.

Adverse outcomes not usually associated with damaging events include nerve damage, headache, pain during regional anesthesia, awareness, myocardial infarction, and hepatic or renal failure.

B. Adverse respiratory events

Difficulties in management of the respiratory system were the most common cause of injury and also the most common cause of severe injury such as death and brain damage. Three mechanisms of injury accounted for approximately three fourths of the adverse respiratory events: inadequate ventilation (196 claims, 38%), esophageal intubation (94 claims, 18%), and difficult tracheal intubation (87 claims, 17%) (Table 26-3). Inadequate ventilation was the most common respiratory mechanism and is a nonspecific incident category in which the patient's lungs were inadequately ventilated or oxygenated but the exact cause was not apparent from the records available. The remaining adverse respiratory events were produced by a variety of low-frequency mechanisms including airway obstruction, bronchospasm, aspiration, premature and inadvertent extubation, inadequate inspired oxygen delivery, and endobron-

chial intubation (Table 26-3). Each of these low-frequency mechanisms represented less than 3% of the overall claims. Respiratory equipment failures (breathing circuit disconnection, misplaced PEEP valves, and so on) represent 1% of the overall claims. Claims for adverse respiratory events generally involved healthy adults undergoing nonemergency surgery with general anesthesia.

Death or permanent brain damage occurred in 85% of the respiratory-related claims. In the group of nonrespiratory claims, these two outcomes accounted for only 30% of cases ($p \leq 0.05$). Death and permanent brain damage occurred in over 90% of the claims for inadequate ventilation and esophageal intubation and 56% of claims for difficult intubation. In the difficult tracheal intubation category many claims were for trauma to the airway.

The reviewers judged that better monitoring would have prevented the adverse outcome in 72% of the claims for adverse respiratory events.[3] This compares to only 11% of the non–respiratory related cases, which were judged preventable by better monitoring. Tinker et al. reported similar data from a review of 1175 cases from the Closed Claims Project.[4] Over 90% of the claims for inadequate ventilation and esophageal intubation were considered preventable with better monitoring, as opposed to 36% of claims for difficult intubation.[3] Monitoring devices that would have prevented the complications were predominantly pulse oximeters and capnographs either singly or in combination.

Claims for esophageal intubation were usually accompanied by detailed descriptions of the events and actions that accompanied this event.[3] Three percent of esophageal intubations

Table 26-2. Damaging events (incidence of 1% or greater) found by the American Society of Anesthesiologists Closed Claims Project

	Number of claims (1541)	Percent of 1541
Respiratory system	522	34
Cardiovascular system	100	6
Inappropriate or inadequate fluid	33	2
Excessive blood loss	29	2
Air embolism	25	2
Electrolyte imbalance	16	1
Wrong blood	11	1
Other	160	10
Equipment problems	67	4
Wrong drug or dose	55	4
Convulsions	38	2

Table 26-3. Distribution of claims for damaging respiratory events

Event	Number of cases	Percent of 522 respiratory claims	Percent of 1541 total claims
Inadequate ventilation	196	38	13
Esophageal intubation	94	18	6
Difficult tracheal intubation	87	17	6
Airway obstruction	34	7	2
Bronchospasm	32	6	2
Aspiration	26	5	2
Premature tracheal extubation	21	4	1
Unintentional tracheal extubation	14	3	1
Inadequate F_IO_2	11	2	1
Endobronchial intubation	7	1	<1
TOTAL	522	100%	34%

From Caplan RA et al: Anesthesiology 72:828-833, 1990.

were detected before 5 minutes, 61% were detected in 5 to 10 minutes, and 36% were detected after 10 minutes. Auscultation of breath sounds was documented in 62 of the 94 claims, or 63%, of claims for esophageal intubation. In about half (48%) of the cases where auscultation was performed, this procedure led to the erroneous conclusion that the endotracheal tube was located in the trachea when it was actually in the esophagus. This diagnostic error was recognized in a variety of ways, including later reexamination with direct laryngoscopy, absence of an endotracheal tube in the trachea at the time of an emergency tracheotomy, resolution of cyanosis after reintubation, and discovery of an esophageal intubation at autopsy.

The major lessons learned from this analysis were that, of the three major mechanisms of adverse respiratory events, esophageal intubation and inadequate ventilation should be preventable by better monitoring. On the other hand, the third major mechanism, difficult tracheal intubation, is less amenable to prevention by better monitoring. To prevent adverse outcomes from difficult tracheal intubation, procedural simulation routines might offer an opportunity for clinicians to obtain a concentrated exposure to a relatively infrequent event. The development of a realistic "Airway Annie" would seem to be a reasonable approach to the problem of realistic procedural simulation routines.

C. Adverse outcomes associated with obstetrical anesthesia

One hundred ninety of the 1541 claims (12%) analyzed were for cases involving obstetric anesthesia[5] (Table 26-4). Among the obstetric claims 127 involved cesarean section and 63 involved vaginal delivery.

It is surprising that the second most common adverse outcome for which a claim was filed was newborn brain damage (38 claims, 20%). Only half of these injuries to the newborn were considered by the reviewers to be anesthesia related. In contrast, in 76% of all obstetric claims and 74% of nonobstetric claims anesthesia was considered as playing a major role in the injury. These data point out a possible high liability risk for obstetric anesthesiologists in that they tend to be sued for adverse newborn outcome regardless of whether the outcome was anesthesia related.

Maternal death accounted for nearly the same number of claims (41 claims, 22%) as newborn brain damage (Table 26-4). The most common damaging events in obstetric claims were inadequate ventilation, difficult tracheal intubation, aspiration, and esophageal intubation (Table 26-5). This is consistent with reports that difficulty with tracheal intubation and pulmonary aspiration are the leading causes of anesthetic-related maternal morbidity and mortality.[6-8] Pulmonary aspiration of gastric contents was cited in 8% of the obstetric claims as compared to only 2% of the nonobstetric claims ($p \leq 0.01$). However, in half the cases aspiration was associated with other problems such as difficult or esophageal intubation. All but two of the obstetric claims involving aspiration occurred in cases in which general anesthesia was utilized.

The high incidence of headache (Table 26-4) among the obstetric claims (12% of total obstetric claims) relative to the nonobstetric

Table 26-4. Most common adverse outcomes among obstetric anesthesia claims found by the American Society of Anesthesiologists Closed Claims Project ($n = 1541$)

	Claims ($n = 190$)	Regional ($n = 124$)		General ($n = 62$)
Maternal Death	22% (41)	12% (15)	*	42% (26)
Newborn brain damage	20% (38)	19% (23)		24% (15)
Headache	12% (23)	19% (23)	*	0% (0)
Newborn death	9% (17)	7% (8)		10% (6)
Pain during anesthesia	8% (16)	13% (16)	*	0% (0)
Nerve damage	8% (16)	10% (12)		7% (4)
Maternal brain damage	7% (14)	7% (9)		8% (5)
Emotional distress	6% (12)	7% (9)		5% (3)
Back pain	5% (9)	7% (9)	*	0% (0)

*$p \leq 0.01$ between proportion of obstetric regional and obstetric general claims for this outcome.

Table 26-5. Most common damaging events among the obstetric claims found by the American Society of Anesthesiologists Closed Claims Project ($n = 1541$)

	Claims ($n = 190$)	Regional ($n = 124$)		General ($n = 62$)
Respiratory system	24% (46)	11% (13)	*	53% (33)
Inadequate ventilation	5% (10)	4% (5)		7% (5)
Difficult tracheal intubation	5% (10)	1% (1)	**	15% (9)
Aspiration	4% (8)	2% (2)		10% (6)
Esophageal intubation	4% (7)	2% (2)		8% (5)
Bronchospasm	3% (5)	1% (1)		7% (4)
Inadequate F_1O_2	2% (4)	1% (1)		5% (3)
Airway obstruction	1% (1)	1% (1)		0% (0)
Premature extubation	1% (1)	0% (0)		2% (1)
Cardiovascular system	3% (6)	3% (4)		2% (1)
Inappropriate fluid therapy	2% (4)	3% (4)		0% (0)
Excessive blood loss	1% (1)	0% (0)		2% (1)
Wrong blood administered	1% (1)	0% (0)		0% (0)
Other				
Convulsion	10% (19)	15% (18)	*	2% (1)
Equipment problems	6% (11)	6% (7)		6% (4)
Wrong drug or dose	4% (8)	2% (2)		10% (6)

*$p \leq 0.01$ and **$p \leq 0.05$ between proportion of obstetric regional and obstetric general anesthesia claims with this event noted.

claims (1% of total nonobstetric claims) was surprising. It is also surprising that relatively minor injuries such as headache, pain during anesthesia, back pain, and emotional injury combined to make up 31% of the total obstetric claims. This compares to an incidence of these injuries of less than 5% in the nonobstetric claims. Claims for pain during cesarean section under regional anesthesia were quite frequent. Of the 77 claims involving cesarean section under regional anesthesia, 19% were for pain during surgery. It is not clear to what extent this reflects true differences in the frequency of such complications in obstetric patients or other factors, such as unrealistic expectations or general dissatisfaction with the care provided.

Regional anesthesia was utilized in approximately two thirds (65%) of the obstetric claims. This is in contrast to the nonobstetric claims in which 76% received general anesthesia and only 20% received regional anesthesia. It is apparent that some damaging events and resultant injuries are much more common with certain anesthetic techniques (Tables 26-4 and 26-5). Claims for maternal death and respiratory system–related adverse outcomes were signifi-

cantly more common in cases involving general anesthesia, whereas claims for headache pain during anesthesia, back pain, and convulsions were significantly more common in cases in which the primary anesthetic technique was regional anesthesia (Tables 26-4 and 26-5). Some complications such as newborn brain damage, newborn death, and maternal nerve damage were not significantly associated with either regional or general anesthesia (Table 26-4). Two claims were brought for lack of anesthesia availability, and in two claims the anesthetic technique was not noted.

The major lesson learned from analysis of obstetric claims is that in some respects the professional liability risk of obstetric anesthesia differs from that of nonobstetric anesthesia. Although adverse newborn outcome was often judged not to be related to anesthetic care, newborn brain damage was a leading cause of claims against obstetric anesthesiologists. As expected, some damaging events, such as aspiration and convulsions, were more common among the obstetric than the nonobstetric claims. However, not expected was that a great percentage of the obstetric claims were for relatively minor injuries such as headache, back pain, and emo-

Table 26-6. Claims for nerve injury

Nerve	Number of claims	Percent of 227
Ulnar	77	34
Brachial plexus	53	23
Lumbosacral nerve root	36	16
Spinal cord	13	6
Sciatic	11	5
Median	9	4
Radial	6	3
Femoral	6	3
Multiple nerves*	5	2
Other nerves*	11	5
TOTAL	227	100%

From Kroll DA et al: Anesthesiology 73:202-207, 1990.
*Includes phrenic, pudendal, perineal, seventh cranial nerve, long thoracic, optic nerves, and unspecified other nerves, each with a frequency of less than 1%.

tional injury. A thorough discussion with patients of the risks of these minor injuries before anesthesia may prevent some of these claims.

D. Nerve injury

Claims for nerve injury were those in which there were clinical, anatomic, or laboratory findings that were consistent with damage to discrete elements of the spinal cord or peripheral nervous system. Nerve injury occurred in 227 patients, or 15%, of the total 1541 claims (Table 26-1). The distribution of claims is shown in Table 26-6. General anesthesia was the primary technique in 61%, and regional anesthesia was the primary technique in 36% of the 227 nerve injury claims. Of the 82 regional anesthetics, the most frequent techniques were subarachnoid block (35%), epidural block (20% lumbar, 6% caudal), and axillary block (20%). No obvious patterns were observed that would indicate an association between nerve injury and surgical procedure. Of the various common surgical positions, only the prone position was associated with claims for nerve damage. The proportion of nerve injury claims associated with the prone position (11%) was twice that of nonnerve injuries (6%, $p \leq 0.01$).

Ulnar neuropathy represented one third of all nerve injuries and was by far the most frequent single nerve injury for which a claim was filed[9] (Table 26-6). Claims for ulnar nerve damage differed from those for other nerves in that they were more often filed by males, the mechanism of injury itself was least often apparent in the claim file, and the injury was more likely to have occurred during general anesthesia than during regional anesthesia. Ulnar nerve injury

occurred despite padding placed over the affected nerves in about 20% of the claims. Symptoms of ulnar nerve injury first occurred 2 days or later after surgery in approximately 20% of the cases.

The medicolegal review process provided very little insight into the mechanism by which ulnar neuropathy occurs after anesthesia. Despite intensive investigation, the mechanism of ulnar nerve injury was observed in the perioperative period in only 6% of the claims. The prone position was the only surgical position in which ulnar nerve injuries were more likely to occur. The only substantive information gained was that 69% of ulnar nerve claims were filed by males as compared to about 40% male incidence for claims for other nerve injuries and for claims not involving nerve damage. These data are in agreement with other studies of perioperative nerve injuries[10,11] and are suggestive of an anatomic predisposition associated with the male body habitus.

The occurrence of ulnar nerve injury in the presence of padding over the affected nerve indicates that some mechanism of injury other than those commonly described in the literature may be operative. This is important not only from the injury-prevention but also from the liability point of view. The unclear mechanism of ulnar nerve injury may be a liability in itself because it leads to the presumption that the anesthesiologist must have done something wrong if the injury occurred in the perioperative period.[9]

Claims for injuries to the brachial plexus and lumbosacral nerve roots were the next most common after claims for ulnar nerve injury (Table 26-6). Spinal cord injuries and isolated median and radial nerve injuries were much less common, as were injuries to femoral and sciatic nerves. The mechanism of injury was noted in about one fourth of the claims for brachial plexus injury and about one third of the claims for lumbosacral nerve root injury. Anesthesic-related causes of brachial plexus injury included the use of shoulder braces and head-down position (three claims), suspension of the patient's arm from a bar (2), other obvious malpositions (4), and regional anesthesia technique (2). All lumbosacral nerve root injuries having identifiable anesthetic cause (36%) were attributed to the administration of regional anesthesia and included technique-related mechanisms such as paresthesia or pain during placement of spinal or epidural needle or pain during injection of a local anesthetic. Of the nerves in the "other" category, the four long thoracic nerve injuries were particularly perplexing as to their cause. In none of these cases was a cause apparent. This is in keeping with a recent paper by Martin,[12] who reported six long thoracic nerve injuries associated with an uneventful anesthetic course.

The major lesson learned from analysis of nerve damage claims is that most anesthetic-related nerve injuries seem to occur without identifiable mechanism. Although the mechanism of nerve injury was noted in a third or less of the cases of brachial plexus injury and lumbosacral nerve root injury, most ulnar nerve injuries occurred without any apparent mechanism.

E. Cardiac arrest during spinal anesthesia

During review of claims in the initial stages of the ASA Closed Claims Project, an unusual number of cardiac arrests in young healthy patients during spinal anesthesia that resulted in death or severe neurologic injury were identified.[1] In order to study this phenomenon in depth the entire claim file was obtained and examined in detail. Fourteen such cases in which all records could be obtained were identified out of the first 900 claims. The patients were relatively young (age 36 ± 15 years) and healthy (8 ASA physical status 1; 6 ASA physical status 2). Nine procedures were elective and five were emergencies. The sites of surgery were pelvic (8 cases), lower abdominal (2 cases), rectal (2 cases), and lower extremity (2 cases). Monitoring included blood pressure cuff in all cases, an electrocardiogram in 13 and a precordial stethoscope in 6 cases. Seven patients were sedated to the point of no spontaneous verbalization, and 5 patients were verbalizing up to the time of arrest. In the sedated patients the doses of opioids and hypnotics were well within customary ranges. Six patients were receiving nasal oxygen before the arrest.

The major conclusions that can be reached from an in-depth analysis of these cases and subsequent reports[13-14] of cardiac arrest during spinal anesthesia are that the phenomenon occurs suddenly and appears to be circulatory in origin. The initial hypothesis of the mechanism of the event was that the patients were relatively oversedated, and such a condition led to hypoventilation with subsequent cardiac arrest from hypoxemia. Since half of the patients were verbalizing at the time of arrest and 40% were receiving nasal oxygen, it seemed unlikely that hypoxemia was the cause of cardiac arrest in all 14 patients.

Subsequently Frerichs et al.[13] reported an episode of sudden asystole in an unsedated patient undergoing arthroscopy under epidural anesthesia who was monitored with a pulse oxime-

ter and who was verbalizing at the time of arrest. Chester[14] reported a similar occurrence in an awake patient in whom spinal anesthesia to T4 was present. The ECG in the latter case showed a normal sinus rhythm with a rate of 80 beats per minute with a sudden cessation of QRS complexes. Both patients were resuscitated without sequelae. It should be pointed out that both reported cases represent the phenomenon with good outcome whereas the closed claims cases represent poor outcomes. The most likely mechanism of the asystole is sudden vagal predominance in the presence of high sympathetic blockade, which blocked the cardioaccelerator fibers.

What factors led to the poor outcomes? First was disbelief of the caregiver that the heart rate could slow so rapidly. In many cases confirmatory diagnostic activity such as attempts to cycle the automatic blood pressure machine preceded pharmacologic treatment of the arrest. By the time atropine or ephedrine were administered intravenously there was no effective cardiac action to circulate the drugs. Sedation often delayed the diagnosis as the signs and symptoms of cerebral ischemia were obscured. Another factor leading to poor outcome was inadequate circulation to the brain and heart engendered by closed chest massage in the presence of the alpha-adrenergic receptor blockade induced by spinal anesthesia. Epinephrine was usually necessary before the return of a spontaneous heart beat.

The lesson learned from these cases is that sudden bradycardia and asystole do occur with high spinal anesthesia. Early treatment of bradycardia with epinephrine should be carried out especially if conventional doses of atropine and ephedrine are not effective. If asystole occurs, a full resuscitation dose of epinephrine should be administered immediately upon recognition of the arrest in order to reverse the alpha blockade and direct perfusion to the heart and brain. Prophylactic treatment of heart rates under 60 with vagolytic agents in patients with a high spinal level may be an effective preventive strategy.

II. IMPACT OF PULSE OXIMETRY ON THE SPECTRUM OF ANESTHETIC INJURY

As of 1 January 1990 use of pulse oximetry became an ASA standard for intraoperative monitoring. This standard was adopted with the expectation that use of the instrument would improve patient safety. Because pulse oximetry first came into clinical use in the middle to late 1980s the ASA Closed Claims database now

Table 26-7. Classification of claims in which the pulse oximeter was used

Damaging event	Number of claims	Number of brain damage or death
Unrelated to use of pulse oximeter	67	8
Probe injury	2	0
Circulatory	10	7
Respiratory	16	15

From Cheney FW: ASA Newsletter 54:10-11, 1990.

Table 26-8. Classification of respiratory-related damaging events in which pulse oximetry was used

Damaging event	Number of claims	Number of brain damage or death
Pulse oximeter mis-used	3	3
Airway obstruction	5	5
False high reading	1	1
Immediate postoperative event after pulse oximeter was disconnected	7	6

From Cheney FW: ASA Newsletter 54:10-11, 1990.[ ]

contains some claims in which a pulse oximeter was in use intraoperatively.[15] Preliminary analysis of approximately 100 claims in which a pulse oximeter was in use during the intraoperative period provides some insight into the nature of the role of pulse oximetry in patient outcome. Table 26-7 shows the overall classification of the damaging events that led to the injuries, the number of cases in each category, and the number of cases in which death or brain damage occurred. Injuries unrelated to the use of the pulse oximeter include nerve damage, burns, awareness, postoperative myocardial infarctions, and purely surgical complications such as uncontrolled hemorrhage. Of the two probe injuries, one was attributable to ischemia and the other was a burn of the finger. Respiratory events include all cases in which the outcome was related to a respiratory system problem. Circulatory events include only those in which cardiac arrest or stroke occurred in the presence of adequate oxygenation determined by the pulse oximeter.

Because pulse oximetry would be expected to play a significant role in the prevention of respiratory-related damaging events, this category was further subclassified (Table 26-8). In the three cases in which the pulse oximeter was misused there were two esophageal intubations and one case in which the anesthesiologist was attempting to adjust the probe while the patient was clearly cyanotic. All three cases resulted in severe injury. Of the five cases of airway obstruction, one was from bronchospasm, one from a mediastinal mass, and three were from upper airway obstruction. In one case the pulse oximeter indicated a high oxyhemoglobin saturation, but the patient was cyanotic when the drapes were removed. Finally, there were seven cases where the pulse oximeter was in use during surgery but the damaging event occurred after its use was discontinued. Three of these cases occurred before or during transport to the patient anesthia care unit (PACU). Four other cases involved respiratory events in the PACU where presumably pulse oximetry would have been helpful in prevention of the incident.

Seven of the 10 circulatory system–related damaging events were sudden cardiac arrests that occurred in the presence of an adequate oxyhemoglobin saturation. In the seven cardiac arrests, pulse oximeter readings indicating high oxyhemoglobin saturation essentially ruled out hypoxemia as the cause of the arrest. Now that the use of the pulse oximeter will rule out the convenient hypothesis of "preexistent hypoxemia" as the cause of unexplained cardiac arrest during anesthesia, attention should become focused on other possible mechanisms such as vagally mediated cardiac events and anaphylaxis.

III. SUMMARY

A review of 1541 anesthesia-related closed malpractice claims, most of which occurred between 1975 and 1985, revealed that the most common adverse outcomes were death (37% of claims), nerve damage (15% of claims), and brain damage (12% of claims). The leading causes of death and brain damage were respiratory in origin. Of the three leading respiratory damaging events, the incidence of adverse outcome from inadequate ventilation and esophageal intubation should be reduced by use of pulse oximetry and end-tidal CO_2 monitoring. Prevention of injury from difficult tracheal intubation requires development of other tactics. A strategy for the prevention of nerve injury was not apparent from this review and more investigation into the pathophysiology of perioperative nerve injury is needed.

REFERENCES

1. Caplan RA, Ward RJ, Posner K, and Cheney, FW: Unexpected cardiac arrest during spinal anesthesia: a closed claims analysis of predisposing factors, Anesthesiology 68:5-11, 1988.
2. Cheney FW, Posner K, Caplan RA, and Ward RJ: Standard of care and anesthesia liability, JAMA 261:1599-1603, 1989.
3. Caplan RA, Posner KL, Ward RJ, and Cheney FW: Adverse respiratory events in anesthesia: a closed claims analysis, Anesthesiology 72:828-833, 1990.
4. Tinker JH, Dull DL, Caplan RA, et al: Role of monitoring devices in prevention of anesthetic mishaps: a closed claims analysis, Anesthesiology 71:541-546, 1989.
5. Chadwick HS, Posner K, Ward RJ, et al: A review of obstetric anesthesia malpractice claims, Anesthesiology 71:A942, 1989.
6. Hughes EC, Cochrane NE, and Czyz PL: Maternal mortality study 1970-1975, NY State J Med 76:2206-2212, 1976.
7. Turnbull AC, Tindall VR, Robson G, et al: Report on confidential enquiries into maternal deaths in England and Wales 1979-1981, London, 1986, Her Majesty's Stationery Office.
8. Turnbull A, Tindall VR, Beard RW, et al: Report on confidential enquiries into maternal deaths in England and Wales 1982-1984, London, 1989, Her Majesty's Stationery Office.
9. Kroll DA, Caplan RA, Posner KL, et al: Nerve injury associated with anesthesia, Anesthesiology 73:202-207, 1990.
10. Cameron MGP and Stewart OJ: Ulnar nerve injury associated with anaesthesia, Can Anaesth Soc J 22:253-264, 1975.
11. Dawson DM and Krarup C: Perioperative nerve lesions, Arch Neurol 46:1355-1360, 1989.
12. Martin JT: Postoperative isolated dysfunction of the long thoracic nerve: a rare entity of uncertain etiology, Anesth Analg 69:614-619, 1989.
13. Frerichs RL, Campbell J, and Bassell GM: Psychogenic cardiac arrest during extensive sympathetic blockade, Anesthesiology 68:943-944, 1988.
14. Chester WL: Spinal anesthesia, complete heart block, and the precordial chest thump: an unusual complication and a unique resuscitation, Anesthesiology 64:600-602, 1988.
15. Cheney FW: The ASA Closed Claims Study after the pulse oximeter, ASA Newsletter 54:10-11, 1990.

Chapter 27

The Cost of Adverse Outcome

Robert A. Caplan

I. WHY STUDY COST?

One of the major challenges in the analysis of health care is *quantification*— the task of finding numbers or values that offer a meaningful representation of a particular process or outcome. Quantitative measures provide a practical means for making comparisons, detecting changes, and evaluating the relationships between risk and benefit.

Cost is an attractive measurement because it readily lends itself to numeric expression. The cost of a particular adverse outcome may be manifest in a variety of quantifiable ways such as extra procedures or medications, extended length of hospital stay, days of rehabilitation, or delayed return to gainful employment. Even the less tangible cost of emotional suffering can be assessed by the use of structured surveys and rating systems.

To varying degrees of completeness and plausibility, many of the costs associated with adverse outcome can be measured in monetary units or "dollars." In simplest terms, these dollars represent the expenses incurred by the need for specific services, or the losses resulting from the inability to work or obtain work-related benefits. An understanding of the dollar cost of adverse outcome can play an important role in risk management. Strategies for minimizing liability can be focused on those classes of injury that are associated with the highest dollar costs. This approach is appealing because it draws attention not only to rare and expensive events, but also to events of relatively low cost that occur frequently enough to produce a significant aggregate impact.

This chapter is an examination of the cost of adverse outcomes from four perspectives. First, the basic economic factors that determine cost are explored. Second, specific factors that contribute to the cost of adverse anesthetic outcomes are examined in detail. Third, the dynamic relationship between the cost of adverse anesthetic outcomes and the cost of professional liability insurance is described. Finally, an overview of psychologic costs is presented.

II. THE COST OF ADVERSE OUTCOME
A. Estimating the Damages of an Adverse Outcome

To provide a general foundation for understanding the dollar cost of adverse anesthetic outcomes, it is helpful to demonstrate the usual method for estimating the damages associated with a particular incident. A hypothetical case of intraoperative death serves as a useful example:

> *Event description. In the late 1980s, a 51-year-old woman in otherwise excellent health was admitted*

621

for elective cholecystectomy. She died during anesthesia because of an unrecognized esophageal intubation. A detailed investigation indicated negligence on the part of the attending anesthesiologist, attributable to drug dependency and impaired vigilance.

Socioeconomic setting. *The patient was employed as a supervisor by a large corporation. She enjoyed her job and planned to work until 65 years of age. The patient was married for 30 years and was responsible for basic management of her household.*

Two types of damages are typically assessed—economic and noneconomic. *Economic damages* include actual expenses or anticipated dollar losses that are associated with the adverse outcome and its consequences. Typical examples of economic damages include hospital bills, fees for rehabilitation, projected costs of long-term care, lost wages, reduced earnings, and inability to have access to previous or anticipated services and benefits. *Noneconomic damages* refer to losses that cannot be directly measured or replaced by dollars but for which dollars will represent partial or symbolic compensation. Typical examples include pain, suffering, disfigurement, loss of companionship, and inability to enjoy previous avocations. In some cases, the symbolic purpose of noneconomic damages is to make an example of the case or serve as a form of punishment.[1]

For the case described here, a simple analysis of economic and noneconomic damages might proceed as follows.

1. Economic damages

a. Lost earnings. The patient's average salary during the 3 previous years of employment was $47,680 per year. Her yearly earnings generally increased at a rate that was equal to or slightly greater than the rate of inflation. Therefore the value of her earnings until 65 years of age can be estimated without discount as:

$$(65 - 51) \text{ years} \times \$47,680/\text{Year} = \mathbf{\$667,520}$$

b. Lost fringe benefits. In the metropolitan area where this patient lived, fringe benefits (such as vacation, medical and dental insurance) usually represented 6% of wages. The estimated present value of these benefits is:

$$(65 - 51) \text{ years} \times \$47,680/\text{Year} \times 0.06 = \mathbf{\$40,051}$$

c. Lost pension benefit. The patient's life expectancy after retirement was estimated at 10 years. Her combined employment pension and Social Security benefit was estimated at $1,750 per month. The face value of this benefit is the product of the monthly benefit and the expected number of months of life after retirement ($210,000). However, these dollars would have been *received in the future.* If the lost

pension benefit is paid as a lump sum *in the present,* a smaller amount will be required because the value of these present dollars, unlike a pension received in the future, is not eroded by inflation. If one assumes an average yearly inflation rate of 4%, this results in a downward adjustment or discount of approximately $107,705. Thus the lost pension benefit in present dollars is calculated as:

$210,000 (face value) − $107,705 (discount) = **$102,295**

d. Loss of homemaking services. The average time spent on household care was estimated at 2 hours per day. The average agency rate for this service in the metropolitan area where the patient lived was $8.50 per hour. The recipient of homemaking services was the patient's husband, whose life expectancy was estimated at 21 years. Assuming, conservatively, that the requirement for homemaking service would remain fairly level over time and that the fee for this service would increase at a rate equivalent to inflation, one can estimate the present value without discount as:

2 hours/day × 365 days/year × 21 years × $8.50/hour = **$130,305**

e. Hospital and physician services. The patient died after 5 days of hospitalization in the intensive care unit. The total charge for hospital and physician services was $11,380. The patient's insurance policy provided for 70% coverage after a deductible of $500. The remaining bill was calculated as:

$$\$(11,380 - 500) \times 0.30 = \mathbf{\$3,264}$$

2. Noneconomic damages. The patient and her husband had a stable marriage and close relationships with their children and grandchildren. Both husband and wife enjoyed excellent health and had planned numerous activities for their retirement years. Although it is impossible to attach a dollar value to these losses, it is quite likely that a jury would respond favorably to a generous request for compensation.

Investigation of this adverse outcome also revealed that members of the hospital staff and administration were aware of the fact that the responsible anesthesiologist had a problem with drug dependency. Preventive action had not been aggressively pursued for a variety of reasons, including a close personal friendship between the chief of anesthesia and the impaired physician. This feature might lead a jury to respond favorably to a generous request for punitive damages.

In the state where this patient lived, a tort-reform law had placed a ceiling on the total

Table 27-1. Estimation of damages associated with an anesthesia-related death

Item	Amount ($)
Economic damages:	
Lost earnings	667,520
Lost fringe benefits	40,051
Lost pension benefits	102,295
Lost homemaking services	130,305
Hospital and physician fees	3,264
SUBTOTAL	943,435
Noneconomic damages:	
Calculated ceiling	242,124
TOTAL	$1,185,559

This estimate of the financial value of damages is based upon a hypothetic case involving a 51-year-old employed woman who died as the result of an unrecognized esophageal intubation in the late 1980s. See text for a detailed description of each component.

amount of noneconomic damages. This ceiling was defined as 43% of the average annual wage for residents of the state, multiplied by the life expectancy of the patient. In this case, the ceiling was calculated as:

$$\$20,110 \times 0.43 \times 28 = \$242,124$$

The total estimate for economic and noneconomic damages in this case was $1,185,559 (Table 27-1). Although this sum may seem astoundingly high, *it could have been substantially greater if the patient had survived.* Suppose this patient sustained hypoxic brain damage and required long-term institutional care or daily assistance from a skilled attendant. Chronic institutional care for a severely brain-damaged patient costs approximately $2,000 per month. Around-the-clock care from a live-in attendant costs about $3,000 per month. (These figures do not include associated medical treatment or special physical therapy.) If the patient's underlying medical status were relatively robust, she might survive for 10 years, thereby increasing the estimated damages by $240,000 to $360,000. These calculations help demonstrate why adverse outcomes that lead to long-term institutional care for a child or young adult often result in total damages exceeding 3 million dollars.

An important purpose of the foregoing discussion is to illustrate the variety of assumptions that enter into the assessment of damages. Many of these are subject to negotiation. For example, if both spouses are employed, is it reasonable to provide *full* future compensation for the wages and benefits that are lost by the de-

ceased? One can argue that death of the injured spouse reduces future living expenses because there is less consumption of food, clothing, shelter, entertainment, and similar services. This line of reasoning can be weakened by specific circumstances. The family may be dependent on two sources of income to meet mortgage payments or pay college tuition fees. Or, it may not be possible for the surviving spouse to single-handedly remain working, rear children, and maintain the household.

Most claims are resolved by an adversarial process in which a defense attorney represents the interests of the physician and the insurance carrier and a plaintiff's attorney represents the injured party. In cases involving large damages, both sides usually hire an economist to calculate lost wages and benefits, discount rates, and consumption factors. The plaintiff's attorney customarily works on a *contingency basis*. If the injured party is successful in obtaining compensation for damages, the plaintiff's attorney usually receives 30% to 50% of the award. Additionally, the injured party must reimburse the plaintiff's attorney for the expenses of pursuing the case. For large awards, the overall reduction can be substantial: an analysis of almost 200 awards exceeding 1 million dollars showed that the injured party ultimately recovered 43% of the original sum.[2] To assure that the injured party receives adequate compensation, the plaintiff's attorney must take a generous approach to estimating damages. Noneconomic damages can play a particularly important role in this regard.

The basic goal of the insurance carrier is to minimize financial loss. When an adverse outcome is the result of negligent care, the insurance carrier usually seeks an out-of-court settlement.* In this situation, a settlement is preferable to a trial because of the expensive nature of a courtroom defense and the likelihood that the jury will award a substantial sum for noneconomic damages. A settlement may be considered preferable to a trial *even if the adverse outcome is not the result of negligence.* This approach may be taken when a case has strong emotional elements that could sway a jury in favor of the plaintiff.

The cost of a courtroom defense is substantial. A variety of basic services contribute to the expense (Table 27-2). The facts of a case are initially established by the process of discovery and deposition. Each deposition results in a

*A discussion of negligence is beyond the scope of this chapter, but the interested reader can find an excellent description in a recent review by Cheney, FW: Anesthesia and the law: the North American experience, Br J Anaesth 59:891-900, 1987.

Table 27-2. Approximate cost of defending a malpractice suit in court

One-week trial	Amount ($)
3 depositions (transcription)	900
3 expert witness fees	3,000
3 simple visual displays	600
1 senior attorney fee	7,500
1 associate attorney fee	5,700
TOTAL	$17,700

Three-week trial	
5 depositions (transcription)	1,500
4 expert witness fees	4,000
1 distant expert witness travel	2,500
3 simple visual displays	600
3 complex visual displays	4,400
1 senior attorney fee	22,500
1 associate attorney fee	17,100
TOTAL	$52,600

Figures are based upon approximate costs for the Northwest region of the United States in the late 1980s. See text for a detailed description of each component.

charge for the court reporter and the cost of transcription and duplication. A relatively simple deposition lasting 2 hours is associated with a fee of several hundred dollars. Three to five witnesses are often deposed before trial. In complicated cases, many more depositions may be required.

Trial testimony by expert witnesses plays a critical role in the courtroom proceedings. Expert witnesses usually charge $1,000 to $2,500 for a courtroom appearance. It is not unusual for the defense to call upon three or four experts. In a complex case, it may be necessary to bring in nationally recognized experts from distant cities. This introduces additional costs for transportation and boarding.

Charts, graphs, and medical illustrations play an important role in the courtroom because jury members may not be able to understand sophisticated medical concepts simply by listening to oral testimony. Visual aids result in charges ranging from $500 for a few simple displays to $5,000 for a complex set of illustrations.

Two defense attorneys are often involved at the time of trial, a senior attorney who takes the leading role in the proceedings and an associate attorney who manages a complex body of legal and administrative issues. Attorneys usually charge an hourly rate in the range of $100 to $200 per hour for a senior attorney and $90

to $125 per hour for an associate attorney. During a trial, both attorneys may work 10 to 12 hours each day.

Overall, the cost of a 1-week trial ranges from $15,000 to $30,000. A complex 3-week trial may incur charges of $40,000 to $60,000. Given these substantial costs, it is easy to understand why insurance carriers (as well as plaintiffs' attorneys) prefer out-of-court settlements when the estimated damages are small. In such cases, the expense of litigation effectively eliminates any economic advantage of a courtroom victory.

B. Cost Data From the ASA Closed Claims Project: Specific Factors

The American Society of Anesthesiologists Closed Claims Project is a structured evaluation of major anesthetic mishaps collected from 23 United States insurance carriers. A basic overview of the project is given in Chapter 26 and detailed descriptions of its methodology have been published recently.[3-5] This chapter is an examination of cost data derived from approximately 1500 cases in the Closed Claims database.

It is important to appreciate the temporal context of the Closed Claims database. Most cases in the database (92%) represent adverse outcomes that occurred in the 10-year period between 1975 and 1985. The interval between an adverse event and closure of a claim typically ranges from 3 to 5 years. Thus the cost data presented in this chapter represent payments made chiefly during the decade of the 1980s.

All cost data are presented in original dollar amounts, without adjustment for inflation. Cost data represent either the amount of out-of-court settlement or the amount of jury award. Transactional costs associated with investigation, analysis, or litigation of a claim are not included. Since these cost data do not necessarily conform to a normal distribution, median values and ranges are used as descriptive statistics.

The limitations of closed claims data have been described in Chapter 26. In brief, data have been obtained only from insurance carriers who have agreed to participate in the Closed Claims Project. Thus the extent to which these data constitute a typical or representative picture of financial liability is uncertain. For the same reason, the validity of comparing closed claims data to information from other sources is difficult to assess.

It is particularly important to recognize that legal factors affecting compensation have been in a state of considerable flux. Tort-reform laws, designed to control the rising costs of liability, were introduced beginning in the 1970s. Many of these laws subsequently underwent challenge, modification, or repeal.[6] Typical features of tort-reform laws include limits on noneconomic damages, regulation of attorney fees, a shorter period for the statute of limitations, and the use of periodic or "structured" payments instead of lump-sum awards. The precise impact of these changes is difficult to define at any one point in time.

1. The three principal features of cost. The first large-scale analysis of the Closed Claims database was reported in 1989.[4] This investigation focused on 1004 cases in which a lawsuit was actually filed, encompassing 85% of the available database. Practicing anesthesiologists reviewed each case and used the concept of "reasonable and prudent practice at the time of the event" as a measure of the standard of care. There was sufficient information to permit a judgment of the standard of care in 869 cases. Overall, 46% of cases exhibited care that met standards, whereas 54% of cases exhibited substandard care. Adverse outcomes were rated using a standardized severity-of-injury scale[7] shown in Table 27-3. Scores of 1 to 5 indicate nondisabling injuries, scores of 6 to 8 indicate disabling injuries, and a score of 9 represents

Table 27-3. Severity of injury scale

Score	Examples
0	**NO OBVIOUS INJURY**
1	**EMOTIONAL INJURY:** awareness, fright, pain during anesthesia
	Temporary injury
2	**Insignificant:** lacerations, contusions, no delay in recovery
3	**Minor:** fall in hospital, delay in recovery
4	**Major:** brain or nerve damage, unable to work
	Permanent injury
5	**Minor:** nondisabling damage to organs
6	**Significant:** loss of one eye or kidney, deafness
7	**Major:** paraplegia, blindness, loss of use of one limb
8	**Grave:** severe brain damage, quadriplegia, lifelong care
9	**Death**

The severity-of-injury scale (SIS) is a standardized rating system for adverse outcomes (from Brunner EA: Int Anesthesiol Clin 22:17-30, 1984). Descriptive categories are shown in bold-faced letters; specific examples are shown in light-faced letters.

death. The median injury score was 7 (a severe, disabling injury). Payments ranged from $0 (295 cases) to $6,000,000 (1 case). A payment of $1,000,000 or greater was found in 39 cases (4%).

Three principal features of cost emerged from this analysis. First, the frequency of payment was linked to standard of care but *not* to severity of injury. Second, the cost of claims was linked to both severity of injury *and* standard of care. Third, adverse events that were judged preventable with better monitoring were associated with far more costly payments than those that were not considered preventable with better monitoring. Each feature is reviewed.

a. Likelihood of payment is a function of standard of care. An important aspect of the cost of adverse outcomes is not just the *magnitude* of damages, but also the *likelihood* that payment will occur. Studies performed in the past two decades indicate that the overall likelihood of payment may be small *if one considers the entire population of adverse outcomes.* The 1974 Medical Insurance Feasibility Study in California estimated that malpractice claims were filed by only 10% of all patients who were injured by negligent medical care.[8] This statistic was recently reaffirmed by the Harvard Medical Practice Study of patients hospitalized in 1984 in the State of New York.[9]

If an injured patient does file a suit, what then is the likelihood that payment will occur? The Closed Claims database offers an opportunity to explore this question specifically for the specialty of anesthesiology. Payment was received in 62% of the lawsuits in the Closed Claims database, whereas no payment was received in 29% of cases. Payment data were missing in 9% of claims.

Severity of injury did *not* exert a significant effect on the frequency of payment (Fig. 27-1). Instead, standard of care was the determining factor. Cases that exhibited substandard care were associated with a higher incidence of payment than cases in which the standard of care was met ($p \leq 0.01$). If care was substandard, payment was received in *at least 80% of cases.* If the standard of care was met, patients received compensation in *approximately 40% of cases.* These data indicate that the current tort-based system results in a pattern of compensation that favors the injured patient. One can readily appreciate, however, that inequities exist for both the injured patient and the physician. Specifically, no compensation was obtained in 10% of the cases in which substandard care was deliv-

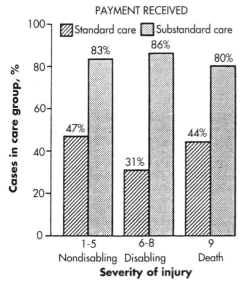

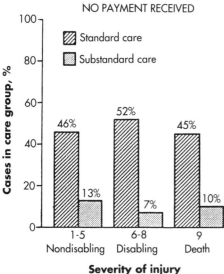

Fig. 27-1. Incidence of payment in malpractice suits from the Closed Claims database. **A,** Lawsuits in which payment was received. **B,** Lawsuits in which no payment was received. Cases exhibiting substandard care were associated with a higher incidence of payment than cases in which the standard of care was met ($p \leq 0.01$). There was no significant relationship between incidence of payment and severity of injury. Cases with missing data and lawsuits without injury are excluded. (From Cheney FW, Posner K, Caplan RA, and Ward RJ: JAMA 261:1599, 1989.)

ered, whereas compensation was provided in 42% of cases where the physician met the appropriate standard.

Litigation under a tort-based system of law is currently the principal tool for resolution of malpractice claims, but it is not the only possible approach. Two other approaches include a

fault-based system and a no-fault system. In a fault-based system, compensation would depend on a finding of substandard care, with this determination presumably being made by peers. In a no-fault system, payment would depend on a demonstration that the injury was caused by medical care, regardless of the relationship of care to the current standard of practice.

How might these alternative compensation systems change the frequency of payment? Since the Closed Claims database contains information on standard of care as judged by peers, the presence and severity of injury, and the incidence of payment, it is possible to generate a comparative view (Table 27-4). The no-fault system produces the highest number of payments (980) because of a projected increase in claims paid in all three categories of injury. Rinaman has cautioned that a no-fault system of compensation could cost approximately 4.5 times more than the current tort-based system,[10] though a recent review by Manuel[11] suggests that the net expenditure would probably be less substantial. The fault-based system results in the lowest number of payments (467) in this analysis. The actual number of payments obtained under the tort-based system occupies an intermediate position (614). The projected reduction in payments under the fault-based system is attributable to substantial decrease in the category of nondisabling injuries and a modest decrease in the category of disabling injuries. Although the tort-based and fault-based systems both show an identical number of pay-

Table 27-4. Number of claims paid under different systems of compensation

Adverse outcome	Compensation system		
	Tort-based	Fault-based	No-fault
Nondisabling injury	201	82	365
Disabling injury	153	125	243
Death	260	260	372
TOTAL	614	467	980

Adapted from an analysis of 1006 lawsuits in the Closed Claims database (from Cheney FW et al: JAMA 261:1599-1603, 1989). Lawsuits with a severity of injury score of 0 have been excluded. Entries in the tort-based column represent the number of cases that *actually* resulted in payment, regardless of care. Entries in the fault-based column represent the number of cases in which payment *would have occurred* because of a determination of substandard care. Entries in the no-fault column represent the number of cases in which payment *would have occurred* because of the presence of an injury.

ments associated with death, the number itself is coincidental—the two groups do not contain precisely the same cases.

At first glance, the fault-based system looks like an attractive alternative, but the result obtained in this analysis may be misleading. Insofar as malpractice claims represent only a small fraction of the total set of adverse outcomes, the availability of an actual fault-based system ultimately might lead to more payments than a tort-based system. This question cannot be answered until there are better estimates of the proportion of injured patients who might access an alternative system of compensation and how the transactional costs would differ from the current tort-based approach. The potential importance of transactional costs merits particular attention. Current evidence indicates that *less than half* of the amount paid in professional liability premiums ultimately reaches patients in the form of financial compensation.[11]

b. Cost is a function of severity of injury and standard of care. The cost of adverse outcomes is linked to severity of injury (Fig. 27-2). Nondisabling injuries are associated with lower median payments, whereas disabling injuries and death are associated with higher median payments. As might be expected from the earlier discussion of the costs of long-term care, the highest median payments are associated with disabling injuries rather than death.

Standard of care produces an important interaction with the relationship between cost and severity of injury. In each of the three main categories of severity of injury, median payments are higher when care is judged substandard as compared to cases in which care meets the appropriate standard. This interaction is most pronounced for disabling injuries, in which the delivery of substandard care is associ-

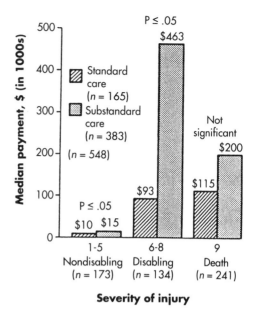

Fig. 27-2. Median payments associated with malpractice suits in the Closed Claims database. Cases with missing data and no payment are excluded. (From Cheney FW, Posner K, Caplan RA, and Ward RJ: JAMA 261:1599, 1989.)

ated with nearly a fivefold increase in median payments ($93,000 for standard care versus $463,000 for substandard care).

Table 27-5 presents a profile of cost for specific complications that occur with a frequency of 3% or greater in the Closed Claims database. Here again, the basic relationship between cost and severity of injury is evident. Examination of the first three lines of this table leads to an important insight: just two complications, death and permanent brain damage, account for almost half the cases. Both of these complications are associated with high severity of injury and,

Table 27-5. Cost profile of common adverse outcomes

Adverse outcome	Number of claims (% of 1541)	Median SIS*	Median payment ($)	Range of payments ($)
Death	565 (37)	9	170,564	750 to 4,000,000
Nerve damage	227 (15)	5	17,500	188 to 2,100,000
Permanent brain damage	179 (12)	7	725,000	10,000 to 6,000,000
Airway trauma	63 (4)	4	10,000	15 to 200,000
Fetal/newborn injury	56 (4)	7	500,000	205,000 to 5,400,000
Pneumothorax	53 (3)	3	6,000	500 to 120,000
Eye injury	46 (3)	6	24,999	45 to 1,000,000
Aspiration	45 (3)	3	40,000	25,000 to 1,100,000
Emotional injury	42 (3)	3	11,750	1,683 to 75,000

Cost of settlement or jury award for adverse outcomes representing 3% or more of 1541 cases in the ASA Closed Claims database (K. Posner, personal communication, 1990).
*SIS, Severity-of-injury score (see Table 27-3).

correspondingly, with high median payments. Although this finding is not outwardly attractive, it does carry an important implication. *If the more common claims are also the most expensive ones, strategies that successfully reduce the incidence of high cost complications, even to a modest degree, are likely to make a significant impact on premium costs.* The applicability of this concept has been emphasized by leading authorities in anesthetic risk management.[12,13]

Adverse outcomes involving the respiratory system account for approximately one third of all cases in the Closed Claims database. An in-depth investigation of 522 adverse respiratory events was recently conducted,[14] and an overview of the major findings has been presented in Chapter 26. Table 27-6 has a comparison of the cost of adverse respiratory outcomes with nonrespiratory complications. Several significant differences are evident. The median cost of adverse respiratory events ($200,000) is over five times greater than the median cost of nonrespiratory events ($35,000). This difference can probably be attributed to the fact that the

Table 27-6. Comparison of cost for adverse outcomes associated with respiratory and nonrespiratory events

	All respiratory events (n = 522)	All nonrespiratory events (n = 1019)
Outcome (% of cases)		
Death	66*	22
Permanent brain damage	19*	8
Other permanent injury	5*	25
Temporary injury	9*	39
No injury	1*	6
Payment ($)		
Range	1,000 to 6,000,000	15 to 5,400,000
Median	200,000*	35,000
Payment frequency (% of claims paid)	72*	51

Based upon an analysis 1541 cases from the ASA Closed Claims database (from Caplan RA et al: Anesthesiology 72:828-833, 1990). Care was judged to be substandard in 76% of the respiratory events and in 30% of the nonrespiratory events.
*P <0.05 compared to nonrespiratory events.

most severe injuries, death and permanent brain damage, constitute 85% of the group of adverse respiratory events as opposed to only 30% of the nonrespiratory events. Another notable finding is the significantly higher *frequency* of payment for adverse respiratory events (72%) as compared to nonrespiratory events (51%). This difference probably reflects the high proportion of ratings of substandard care in the group of respiratory cases (76%) as opposed to the relatively small proportion of substandard ratings in the nonrespiratory cases (30%). Adverse respiratory events represent a particularly urgent target for risk-management efforts because *the cost of these events is driven by three deleterious factors working in unison: frequency of occurrence, substandard care, and severity of injury.*

c. Cost is a function of monitoring and preventability. Can better monitoring lead to a reduction in the cost of adverse outcomes? The ASA Closed Claims database provides an intriguing clue.

As part of the process of data collection, each closed claim was reviewed to determine which, if any, monitoring techniques might have prevented the adverse outcome, even if the monitoring technology was not available at the time of the incident. In making this judgment, the reviewing physicians assumed that the monitor would be properly used and the resultant data would be interpreted and acted upon in an appropriate manner. Significant interrater reliability for this type of judgment has been demonstrated previously.[5]

Tinker and co-workers[15] conducted an analysis of monitoring in 1097 closed claims. This study indicated that better monitoring could have prevented the adverse outcome in 346 of the cases (31.5%). Most of the outcomes considered preventable with better monitoring were associated with respiratory system events (80%). The reviewers determined that a pulse oximeter, a capnometer, or a combination of these two monitors might have prevented the adverse outcome in 322 (93%) of the cases. Perhaps the most striking finding in this analysis was the relationship between preventable outcomes and cost. The median payment for adverse outcomes deemed preventable with better monitoring ($250,000) was *11 times greater* than the median payment for cases that were not considered preventable ($22,500; p <0.01).

Interpretation of these results must proceed cautiously. The reviewers were not asked to consider confounding factors such as equipment malfunction, diversion of attention, misinterpretation and misuse of data, or the impact of false-positive and false-negative results. Thus their judgments must be regarded as a near-maximum (and perhaps unattainable) estimate of the efficacy of better monitoring. Orkin[16] has prepared an excellent overview of confounding factors. Keats[17] has emphasized that the *net* benefit of any new monitor or therapeutic approach cannot be accurately defined until large-scale studies determine whether the innovation is associated with significant side effects or harm. With noninvasive monitors such as the pulse oximeter and capnometer the likelihood of direct physical harm is small, but one cannot arbitrarily exclude the possibility that errors in use or interpretation might be associated with significant damage over a long term.

A related issue is the *cost of prevention*. Would a reduction in adverse outcomes attributable to better monitoring be accompanied by a reduction in insurance premiums *sufficient to offset the expense of the monitors themselves?* An exploratory analysis by Whitcher and colleagues[18] provides an excellent overview of the principal considerations. One must be able to identify the preventable injuries and their cost, define the monitors required for prevention, provide an estimate of the reduction in injury and cost that will occur, and presume that marketplace competition in the insurance industry is high enough to assure that a significant proportion of the savings will pass through to the physician in the form of premium reductions. Using a 50% decrease in preventable injuries as the critical assumption, Whitcher's analysis suggests that oximetry and capnometry could indeed be incorporated in a cost-effective manner.

If one is uncertain about the efficacy of additional monitoring or the magnitude of premium reductions that might occur, it is helpful to consider the *cost per case* of a specific monitor. A useful way to approach this question is to calculate the cost per case that would be required to recover the purchase price and cost of maintenance over a specified period of time.[19] Table 27-7 displays this calculation for a mid-priced pulse oximeter and capnometer in 1990. The key assumptions in this analysis (which can be altered to satisfy specific conditions) are threefold: a 2-year period for recovery of the face value of the purchase price plus maintenance, a yearly maintenance estimate of 10% of the original purchase price, and 1000 uses per year in the anesthetizing location where the monitor is situated. The result is $4.50 per patient for the addition of both a pulse oximeter and capnometer. A 2-year recovery period was chosen in this example as a hedge against rap-

Table 27-7. Estimate of cost per case for a pulse oximeter and capnometer

Description	Oximeter	Capnometer
Purchase price	2,500.00	5,000.00
Two-year maintenance	500.00	1,000.00
TOTAL 2-YEAR COST	$3,000.00	$6,000.00
Patient uses over 2 years	2000	2000
Cost per patient over 2 years	$1.50	$3.00

This analysis is based upon three key assumptions: a 2-year recovery of the face value of the purchase price plus maintenance cost, a yearly maintenance cost equal to 10% of the purchase price, and 1000 patient-uses per year in the location where the device is situated.

idly changing technology (which could make a different device or approach more attractive), uncertain reimbursement factors, and unanticipated breakage or loss. Obviously the estimated cost declines if one can accept a longer period for recovery. The combined cost per case decreases to $2.25 for a 5-year period and $1.82 for a 7-year period. These calculations help the individual practitioner explore attractive but incompletely defined benefits against the likelihood that the extra expense can be absorbed by local economic constraints.

C. The cost of professional liability insurance

The potential for anesthetic care to produce adverse outcomes of high cost creates a distinctive situation: a small number of anesthesia claims can make a disproportionately large contribution to the overall losses incurred by an insurance carrier. The relatively high premium rates paid by anesthesiologists are a direct manifestation of this factor.

What happens if the incidence of high cost outcomes undergoes a change? Since the process of setting future premiums relies strongly upon past experience, the consequences of short-term fluctuations are dampened and the full effects of long-term trends are delayed in their representation. For high cost outcomes, which can have a disproportionate impact on the financial status of an insurance carrier, there may be an added tendency to react swiftly when these events show an apparent increase and, conversely, to adopt a more cautious approach when the incidence appears to decline.

An appreciation of these basic factors can be gained from the general course of anesthesia liability insurance during the past two decades. The National Association of Insurance Commissioners undertook a study of medical claims that had been closed in the interval from 1975 to December 1978. Anesthesia claims represented only 3% of all claims but accounted for 11% of the total payout.[7] This finding succinctly illustrates the potential relationship between a small number of high cost events and overall losses.

During the decade of the 1980s, this distinctive profile seemed to diminish. For the period between 1981 and 1985, St. Paul Fire and Marine Insurance Company (St. Paul, Minnesota)—one of the nation's largest insurers of physicians—reported that anesthetic care produced 4.6% of all claims and accounted for approximately 7% of total losses.[13] By the late 1980s, St. Paul reported that anesthesia care was associated with 3.5% of all claims and only 3.6% of overall losses.[20] On a more focused geographic scale, Zeitlan[21] noted evidence of decreased anesthesia-related mortality in the Commonwealth of Massachusetts, and Eichhorn[22] reported a decrease in major anesthetic morbidity for the nine anesthesia departments affiliated with Harvard Medical School.

How has the insurance industry reacted to these changes? Recent reports indicate a favorable response.[18,20,23,24] The cost of a premium for a given specialty is usually linked to a relative rate factor or equivalent type of modifier. In general terms, a relative rate factor is determined by historical data on the loss per physician for a given specialty. Family practitioners who do not perform surgery often have the lowest relative rate factor, usually a value near 1.0. The base-rate premium is multiplied by relative-rate factors to determine, along with other adjustments, the premium rates for specialties that incur greater risk. This approach distributes the cost of premiums among specialties in approximate proportion to expected losses. St. Paul has lowered the relative rate factor for anesthesiologists from 5.0 to 3.5. The Massachusetts Joint Underwriting Association, the principal professional liability carrier for the Commonwealth of Massachusetts, has decreased the relative rate factor for anesthesiologists from 5.0 to 3.0. Controlled Risk Insurance Company, the insurance carrier for the Affiliated Harvard Hospitals, has also decreased its relative rate factor from 5.0 to 3.0.

Similar changes seem to be making an impact on the overall cost of liability insurance. Nationwide surveys of premium rates for anesthesiologists have been conducted in 1984, 1985, 1988, and 1990.[25-27] These surveys primarily

Table 27-8. Trends in annual premium rates for anesthesiologists

Survey year	Average premium	States represented
1984	$16,165 ± 6,437	40
1985	18,693 ± 7,520	40
1988	32,339 ± 23,647	22
1990	25,637 ± 13,014	38

Figures represent the average price of a 1-year claims-made policy with limits of $1,000,000/$3,000,000 (single claim/total annual claim). Data obtained primarily from physician-owned insurance companies and St. Paul Fire and Marine Insurance Company.[25-27]

reflect data from physician-owned insurance companies and St. Paul. Table 27-8 displays trends in the average cost of a 1-year claims-made policy with limits of $1,000,000/$3,000,000 (single claim/total annual claims). From 1984 to 1988, the average premium doubled in price from $16,165 to $32,339. The average 1990 rate of $25,637 is notable in that it represents a decrease of approximately 20% over the 1988 rate, the first apparent break in the preceding pattern of rising costs. These data must be interpreted cautiously because not every state or carrier is represented.

A detailed display of the 1988 survey of professional liability insurance is shown in Table 27-9. This survey was conducted by the American Society of Anesthesiologists Committee on Professional Liability.[26] Questionnaires were sent to 40 physician-owned companies in the United States, and information was received from 38. Almost all companies (95%) offered claims-made policies. Over half of the companies (58%) offered a claims-made policy with liability limits of $1,000,000/$3,000,000. A notable feature of this data is the wide variation in rates. The average yearly premium for a mature claims-made policy with limits of $1,000,000/$3,000,000 was $105,550 in Florida but only $16,442 in Tennessee. Nearby states often exhibited large differences in rates: compare Missouri ($74,809) and Kentucky ($28,494), or Arizona ($46,102) and Utah ($23,333). The factors contributing to these differences have not been studied in detail.

Some carriers now issue insurance on the condition that the practitioner adhere to specific guidelines. If the practitioner fails to comply, the insurance company may not accept responsibility for damages that occur while the specified guidelines are not in use. Other carriers offer premium discounts of 5% to 20% in exchange for adopting specific guidelines (usu-

Table 27-9. 1988 survey of professional liability insurance

Insurance company (by state)	Annual rate ($)	Type of policy	Limits of liability (event/multiple claim)
Alabama	20,934	MCM	1M/1M
Alaska	67,659	CM	1M/2M
Arizona	46,012	MCM	1M/3M
California Doctor's Co.*	16,803	MCM	1M/3M
California MIEC			
California SCPIE	21,260	MCM	1M/3M
California Norcal*	22,976	CM	1M/3M
Colorado	15,116	MCM	1M/3M
Connecticut	21,448	MCM	1M/2M
District of Columbia	33,561	MCM	1M/4M
Florida Physicians*	27,843	CM	1M/4M
Florida FPIC*	105,550	MCM	1M/3M
Florida Physicians Protect.*	74,628	MCM	1M/3M
Illinois	75,584	MCM	1M/3M
Indiana			
Iowa	27,843	CM	1M/3M
Kentucky	4,762	MCM	100K/300K
Louisiana	29,043	MCM	1M
Maine	28,494	MCM	1M/3M
Maryland*	26,481	MCM	1M/1M
Michigan Physicians*	21,837	MCM	1M/3M
Michigan PICOM*	32,472	MCM	1M/3M
Minnesota	43,473	CM	1M/1M
Mississippi	41,869	MCM	1M/3M
Missouri Medico*	16,836	MCM	1M/3M
Missouri Wedgeworth	17,472	MCM	1M/3M
New Mexico	74,809	MCM	1M/2M
New York*	62,618	CM	1M/2M
North Carolina			
New Mexico	15,446	Occurrence	100K/300K
New York*	27,402	MCM	1M/3M
North Carolina	12,386	MCM	1M/3M
Ohio	40,752	CM	1M/1M
Oklahoma	9,137	Occurrence	1M/1M
Oregon*	27,420	MCM	1M/3M
Pennsylvania*	12,001	MCM	200K/600K
Tennessee	16,442	MCM	1M/3M
Texas	19,151	MCM	1M/3M
Utah	23,333	MCM	1M/3M
Washington	20,575	MCM	1M/3M
Wisconsin	16,756	MCM	400K/1M

A detailed view of the range of insurance products and premium rates provided by physician-owned insurance companies. Data obtained by the American Society of Anesthesiologists Committee on Professional Liability.[26]
CM, Claims made; *MCM,* mature claims made; *K,* $1,000; *M,* $1,000,000.
*Mean value for states in which rates vary by county.

ally the ASA Standards for Basic Intra-Operative Monitoring) or utilizing certain monitors (usually pulse oximetry and capnometry). Premium reductions in the range of $4,000 to $12,000 per policy have been reported.[23]

It is important to recognize that the foregoing changes are fragile. Although there is a strong perception that improved monitoring, especially for hypoxic events, has led to a decrease in highly adverse outcomes, definitive proof is still lacking.[16,17] Other forces contributing to reduced anesthesia losses may include diverse factors such as award limits created by tort reform, marketplace competition among insurers, better legal defense strategies, new anesthetic agents and techniques, improved preoperative management, aggressive postoperative care, and changes in medical training, education, and credentialing. The precise contribution of any one of these factors is difficult to assess. Some generalizations, however, are possible. The role of legal factors such as tort reform must be regarded as unpredictable, because legislation enacted during one year may be modified or repealed at a later time. Marketplace competition may result in some reductions, but this process will be sharply limited by actuarial constraints. *Prevention of adverse outcomes is the single most important factor driving the reduction of premiums.* Continuing efforts to understand the basic causes of adverse outcomes and validate the merits of specific preventive strategies are therefore essential. The basic features of this area of research are just now undergoing formal definition in the field of anesthesiology.[28,29]

D. Psychologic costs

A discussion of the cost of adverse outcomes would not be complete without acknowledging that these events can produce a significant impact upon the physician. During the past decade, Charles and co-workers[30-32] have performed several quantitative studies of the physician's psychologic response to malpractice claims. In the most recent survey of physicians whose malpractice claims progressed to trial, virtually all respondents (97%) acknowledged that the experience was associated with physical or emotional reactions.[32] Symptomatic reactions reported by more than 50% of the physicians included tension, depressed mood, frustration, anger, and insomnia. In addition, two behavioral responses were common: subsequent use of unnecessary tests (67%) and changes in recordkeeping (56%). The use of unnecessary tests is a particularly interesting finding because it demonstrates how adverse outcomes may produce measurable economic effects that extend beyond the strict confines of professional liability insurance. One can also appreciate that symptomatic responses such as mood changes and insomnia might lead to economically significant decrements in work performance.

Ward and Solazzi described a particularly worrisome linkage between adverse outcomes and suicide.[33] As part of an analysis of 192 anesthetic malpractice claims that occurred between 1971 and 1982, three suicides and one suicide attempt were discovered. One anesthesiologist killed himself a few weeks after administration of an apparently routine caudal anesthetic that resulted in paraplegia. Another anesthesiologist committed suicide shortly after his case was dismissed in court. A third suicide occurred several weeks after a favorable award for the plaintiff. An attempted suicide took place while a physician was awaiting trial. Of course, the adverse outcomes and ensuing litigation process may not have been the only factors contributing to these events. A joint study by the American Medical Association and American Psychiatric Association revealed that physicians who ultimately succeed in taking their own lives often have preexisting histories of suicidal intent, drug abuse, and financial difficulties.[34] Perhaps the lesson to be conveyed is that adverse outcomes have the potential for triggering a life-threatening psychologic response.

Some insurance carriers, hospitals, and group practices now take a prospective approach to the psychologic impact of adverse outcomes. Physicians are informed of the availability of relevant reading materials, professional counseling, and "one-to-one" support from fellow colleagues who have previously experienced malpractice proceedings. Not much imagination is required to devise a sound economic rationale for such efforts. The knowledge and expertise of the defendant physician can be vital to the successful defense of a malpractice claim. It is far more likely that an emotionally stable, reassured physician will make a useful contribution to the defense process than one who is depressed, angry, or no longer extant.

III. SUMMARY

Adverse outcomes in anesthetic practice are associated with a wide range of damages. Although not all aspects of damage can be quantified with precision, many can be expressed in terms of dollar cost. This approach provides a workable basis to make comparisons, form aggregate estimates, and focus attention on classes of injury that are associated with the greatest losses.

Analysis of cost data from the Closed Claims Project indicates three principal relationships. Cases involving substandard care are more likely to result in payment than cases in which the physician meets the standard of care. The cost of settlement or jury award is greatest in cases characterized both by substandard care and disabling injury. Finally, adverse outcomes deemed preventable with better monitoring are associated with far higher payments than cases in which monitoring would not have contributed to prevention.

Severe anesthetic injuries are characterized by high economic damages. This feature creates the primary driving force for the high cost of professional liability insurance. Recent reports indicate a probable decline in the incidence of severe anesthetic injuries, along with a parallel but slower reduction in premium rates. These favorable trends can best be preserved by an improved understanding of the basic causes of adverse outcomes and continued efforts to measure the effectiveness of specific preventive strategies.

REFERENCES

1. Peters JD, Fineberg KS, Kroll DA, and Collins V: Anesthesiology and the law, Chapter 1, Ann Arbor, Michigan, 1983, Health Administration Press.
2. Gibbs RF: (Comment), Legal Perspectives on Anesthesia 6(6):1, 1986.
3. Cheney FW: Anesthesia and the law: the North American experience, Br J Anaesth 59:891-900, 1987.
4. Cheney FW, Posner K, Caplan RA, and Ward RJ. Standard of care and anesthesia liability, JAMA 261:1599-1603, 1989.
5. Caplan RA, Posner K, Ward RJ, and Cheney FW: Peer reviewer agreement for major anesthetic mishaps, Quality Review Bulletin 14:363-368, 1988.
6. Walt D and Golin CB, editors: American Medical Association Special Task Force on Professional Liability and Insurance: Profession liability in the '80's, report no 2, Chicago, 1984, American Medical Association.
7. Brunner EA: The National Association of Insurance Commissioners' Closed Claims Study, Int Anesthesiol Clin 22:17-30, 1984.
8. Hiatt HH, Barnes BA, Brennan TA, et al: A study of medical injury and medical malpractice: an overview, N Engl J Med 321:480-484, 1989.
9. Brennan TA, Leape LL, Laird NM, et al: Incidence of adverse events and negligence in hospitalized patients: results of the Harvard Medical Practice study I, N Engl J Med 324:370-376, 1991.
10. Rinaman JC: The tort liability system: overview for the anesthesiologist. In Gravenstein JS and Holzer JF, editors: Safety and cost containment in anesthesia, Boston, 1988, Butterworth & Co.
11. Manuel BM: Professional liability: a no-fault solution, N Engl J Med 322:627-631, 1990.
12. Holzer JF: Current concepts in risk management. Int Anesthesiol Clin 22:91-115, 1984.
13. Wood MD: Monitoring equipment and loss reduction: an insurer's view. In Gravenstein JS and Holzer JF, editors: Safety and cost containment in anesthesia, Boston, 1988, Butterworth & Co.
14. Caplan RA, Posner KL, Ward RJ, and Cheney FW: Adverse respiratory events in anesthesia: a closed claims analysis, Anesthesiology 72:828-833, 1990.
15. Tinker JH, Dull DL, Caplan RA, et al: Role of monitoring in prevention of anesthetic mishaps: a closed claims analysis, Anesthesiology 71:541-546, 1989.
16. Orkin FK: Practice standards: the Midas touch or the emperor's new clothes? Anesthesiology 70:567-571, 1989.
17. Keats AS: Anesthesia mortality in perspective, Anesth Analg 71:113-119, 1990.
18. Whitcher C, Ream AK, Parsons D, et al: Anesthetic mishaps and the cost of monitoring: a proposed standard for monitoring equipment, J Clin Monit 4:5-15, 1988.
19. Duberman SM and Bendixen HH: Concepts of fail-safe in anesthetic practice, Int Anesthesiol Clin 22:149-165, 1984.
20. Pierce EC: Anesthesiologists' malpractice premiums declining, Anesthesia Patient Safety Foundation Newsletter 4:2, March 1989.
21. Zeitlin GL: Possible decrease in mortality associated with anaesthesia: a comparison of two time periods in Massachusetts, USA, Anaesthesia 44:432-433, 1989.
22. Eichhorn JH: Prevention of intraoperative anesthesia accidents and related severe injury through safety monitoring, Anesthesiology 70:572-577, 1989.
23. Holzer JF: Risk manager notes improvement in anesthesia losses, Anesthesia Patient Safety Foundation Newsletter 4:2, March 1989.
24. McGinn PR: Practice standards leading to premium reductions, Am Med News, p 28, Dec 2, 1988.
25. Cheney FW: Cost of malpractice insurance rises 17%, American Society of Anesthesiologists Newsletter 50:5, Feb 1986.
26. Wall RT and Cheney FW: The cost of professional liability insurance for anesthesiologists, American Society of Anesthesiologists Newsletter 52:7, Oct 1988.
27. Stuart M: Postgraduate year (PGY). The cost of medical malpractice insurance, rates across the United States for anesthesiologists, Postgraduate Year 1:8-9, June 1990.
28. Gaba DM, Maxwell M, and DeAnda A: Anesthetic mishaps: breaking the chain of accident evolution, Anesthesiology 66:670-676, 1987.
29. Allnutt MF: Human factors in accidents, Br J Anaesth 59:856-864, 1987.
30. Charles SC, Wilbert JR, and Kennedy EC: Physicians' self-reports of reactions to malpractice litigation, Am J Psychiatry 141:563-565, 1984.
31. Charles SC, Wilbert JR, and Franke KJ. Sued and nonsued physicians' self-reported reactions to malpractice litigation, Am J Psychiatry 142:437-440, 1985.
32. Charles SC, Pyskoty CE, and Nelson A. Physicians on trial: self-reported reactions to malpractice trials, West J Med 148:358-360, 1988.
33. Solazzi RW and Ward RJ: The spectrum of medical liability cases, Int Anesthesiol Clin 22:43-58, 1984.
34. Results and implications of the AMA-APA physician mortality project. Stage II. Council on Scientific Affairs, JAMA 257:2949-2953, 1987.

Chapter 28

Quality Assurance

Terry S. Vitez

Quality assurance has become a familiar term in medicine, primarily because governmental regulations, accreditation agencies, and third-party payers forced the issue upon us. Equating quality assurance with taxation, most of us complied in the most minimal manner possible. However, some took time to actually consider what quality assurance meant. These original few found that our antagonists had actually given us a powerful method to improve our practices. Both by our own impetus and the mandates of outside agencies, quality assurance has become a necessity for every department of every health care institution. In this chapter, I review how the present situation evolved and what quality assurance processes are currently in vogue.

I. ORIGINS OF QUALITY ASSURANCE PROGRAMS

A. Governmental intervention

In an era were most physicians are opposed to, critical of, and fearful of governmental intervention into medicine, it is surprising to learn that medicine has almost always sought outside regulation.[1] Since the eighteenth century, physicians sought to have licensing laws that differentiated between regularly and irregularly trained health care providers. In the late nineteenth and early twentieth century, medical organizations promoted licensing laws and other procedures to restrict the practice of medicine. These laws protected the public and the physi-

cians. The public was protected from charlatans, and the physicians were protected from competition. At the same time that the medical profession promoted licensing laws, it also opposed any rules that interfered with licensed physicians practicing as they wanted.

Outside of state licensing laws, the first substantial laws leading to control of private medicine originated with movements for national health insurance.[2,3] During the Depression, the federal government developed a serious interest in national health insurance. Opposition from the American Medical Association was a key factor in eliminating health insurance from proposals for Social Security. However, as financial difficulties mounted, physicians found their practices suffering and sought to have governmental agencies pay for indigent health care. This medical welfare was envisioned to be only a short-term necessity. Although the AMA leadership encouraged its members to treat the poor without accepting payment from welfare agencies, the economic stress was too great for most doctors.

In the middle to late 1930s, the medical profession had changed its position from strong opposition to reluctant acceptance of certain types of health insurance. A key proviso to this acceptance was that practitioners maintain the right to choose their patients and set their fees. World War II forestalled national health insurance issues until the end of the 1940s. President Truman sponsored a national health plan that was aggressively opposed by the AMA. In 1949, playing upon the fear of communism, the AMA launched a successful $1.5 million dollar campaign against Truman's plan.

The 1950s and 1960s were an era of vast economic growth in the United States. This growth did not apply equally to all classes, and disparities in medical care became more apparent. Care for the aged and the poor became popular causes, leading to the proposal for national health insurance. Originally Congress sought to avoid a confrontation with the AMA by calling for compulsory payment schedules for hospitals only and avoiding the question of physician fees. The AMA opposed the proposal and offered a voluntary plan that, startlingly, included a scheme for physician reimbursement. In 1965, Congress under a stimulus from then President Johnson enacted a plan that combined elements of both congressional and AMA proposals—Medicare. The Medicare Bill contained three parts: Part A created a national insurance for hospital expenses; Part B created a national insurance for physician fees; the last part, Medicaid, increased federal support to states to help pay for medical care for the indigent.

Medicare infused enormous amounts of money into the health care system. Physicians and hospitals flourished because the Medicare reimbursement system paid "costs" and "usual, customary and reasonable" fees. That is, to a certain extent the hospitals and physicians determined the fees. Unfortunately the increase in health care dollars was coupled with a sense that the benefits to the public did not parallel the benefits to the doctors and hospitals. The focus of attention turned from the miracles of modern United States medicine to the abuses and faults of the profession.

B. Professional standards review organizations

The 1970s were characterized by an alarming intrusion of government into medicine. With the enactment of Medicare and Medicaid, the federal government assumed responsibility for one of the most expensive programs in the history of world government. Congress became increasingly alarmed at the escalating costs and abuses. Thus the primary concern of governmental intrusion into the practice of medicine grew from economic concerns. In 1972, Congress passed amendments that created governmental reviews of physician practices.[4,5] The Professional Standards Review Organizations Act was an attempt to oversee health care utilization. The vehicles for this utilization review

were regional organizations directed by physicians. These "professional standards review organizations" (PSROs) were private groups under contract to the government.

The mission of PSROs was to identify unnecessary procedures so that the government would not pay for unwarranted medical services. PSROs were to develop local criteria for evaluating care provided to Medicare and Medicaid patients. Utilization review processes, which included "norms for care" for medical problems (such as normal length of stay for a cholecystectomy) were devised. Utilization review teams identified patients whose care fell outside the norms and reviewed those cases to determine whether care was appropriate. The penalty for falling outside the "norm of care" was denial of Medicare payment.

The AMA proposed that utilization reviews be conducted by physicians. The AMA's proposal was opposed from within and from without. Inside the AMA, some objected to any peer review mandated by the government. Others believed that assessment of adequacy of health care should include representatives of the consumer group. Outside the profession, groups such as Ralph Nader's "Health Research Group" claimed that medical licensing boards and hospital medical review committees were ineffective in eliminating unacceptable care.

Operating as cost-containment units, the PSROs survived for about 10 years. PSRO decisions about appropriateness of care were often made by nurses and clerical personnel on the basis of "paper reviews" or telephone calls. There was little true "peer review." In 1977, the PSROs came under the control of the Health Care Finance Administration (HCFA, the organization that oversees the financing of Medicare). Increasing criticism and complaints about inconsistency in the performance of PSROs led to a plan for their elimination.

C. Peer review organizations (PROs)

The 1980s witnessed attempts by the federal government to finance a publicly popular medical care program that the country could not afford. By 1982, the cost of providing a national health insurance had escalated to the point that it was feared that the Medicare Trust fund would be bankrupted. In response, the Deficit Reduction Act of 1983 created the Diagnosis-Related Groups (DRGs) system. Under this system, hospitals were paid a set amount for providing care to a Medicare patient based upon the patient's diagnosis. It was up to the hospital to provide care for that patient within the limits of the fee set for that diagnosis. After this change in reimbursement, the HCFA again tried to encourage establishment of independent agencies to review the quality of care provided by institutions and individuals receiving Medicare reimbursements. These organizations called peer review organizations (PROs) were given governmental contracts to review care at health care facilities. In fact, the PROs were merely resurrected PSROs.[5]

One of the charges to the PROs was to address quality of care issues: provision of necessary service, reduction of unnecessary procedures, and avoidance of complications and deaths. The PROs responded by dictating how medicine was to be practiced. They made lists of what type of patient should be given what type of care. The HCFA went further, dictating that the PROs review each Medicare case looking for substandard care. PROs were to identify and grade substandard care with a severity score[6]:

Level 1 (25 points) = Mismanagement resulting in significant adverse effects
Level 2 (5 points) = Mismanagement with the potential for significant adverse effects
Level 3 (1 point) = Mismanagement without potential for harm

If any physician or facility received a score of 25 or more in a 3-month period, the PRO was to consider sanctions or report the provider to state licensing organizations and accreditation agencies. This directive bothered both the medical profession and the PROs. The PROs objected to the HCFA about the severity assignments, but the HCFA was unmoved. As it happened, the directives were neither a major threat to physicians nor an effective means of ensuring quality assurance. Only about 100 recommendations for sanctions reached the Office of the Inspector General, and less than half the cases processed were upheld in favor of the PROs.[7]

D. Medicare Program to Assure Quality (MPAQ)

The limitations and problems with the PROs led to reevaluation of how to ensure quality assurance for Medicare. In early 1990, the Institute of Medicine of the National Academy of Sciences published its proposal for the establishment of the Medicare Program to Assure Quality (MPAQ).[7] MPAQ was to be built on the existing PRO structure, with a redirection of the PRO activity away from utilization review and toward quality of care. MPAQ was to be functional by the year 2000. The intervening 10 years would be used for the development of

strategies for collecting data, changing physician decision–making processes, and improving patient outcome. Oversight and advisory committees were attached to MPAQ in a process that described the birth and growth of yet another bureaucratic monstrosity.

II. ACCREDITATION PROCESSES
A. Joint Commission for the Accreditation of Health Care Organizations (JCAHO)

One of the greatest stimuli for the current interest and activity in quality assurance came from the Joint Commission for the Accreditation of Health Care Organizations (JCAHO). The JCAHO affects the daily functions of almost every hospital in the country. The perception of most practitioners is that JCAHO is a bothersome, bureaucratic agency that should be considered an enemy of the private practicing physician. It is surprising how few people know the history and true nature of the JCAHO.

The JCAHO grew out of the American College of Surgery (ACS).[8,9] In the early 1900s, the American College of Surgery became concerned about the level of health care delivered by United States hospitals. In 1912, the college surveyed 692 hospitals that contained 100 or more beds. Eighty-eight percent (88%) failed to meet basic standards of care set by the college. In an effort to improve hospital care, the college expanded its surveying activities. By the 1950s, hospital surveys had become such a large effort that the college sought a coalition with other professional organizations to manage the task. In December 1951, the AMA, the Canadian Medical Association (CMA), the American College of Physicians (ACP), and the American Hospital Association (AHA) agreed to help the ACS create an independent, nonprofit organization known as the "Joint Commission for the Accreditation of Hospitals" (JCAH).

In the 1965, the role of the JCAH was escalated from voluntary to near mandatory when Congress made JCAH accreditation a mechanism for hospitals to be approved for participation in Medicare. In that same era, the JCAH expanded its activities to include a wide range of health care facilities (such as long-care facilities, psychiatric institutions, outpatient centers) and changed from examining for minimal standards to examining for "optimal achievable standards." The power of the JCAH was extended as states incorporated JCAH accreditation into their requirements for licensure. In 1988, the JCAH changed its name to "Joint Commission for the Accreditation of Health

Care Organizations" (JCAHO) to reflect the change in the types of facilities that had developed.

Today, the JCAHO remains an organization directed primarily by physicians, who undertake the inspection and evaluation of health care facilities. The organization is headed by 22 commissioners: 7 from the AMA, 7 from the AHA, 3 from the ACP, 3 from the ACS, 1 from the American Dental Association and 1 private citizen elected annually. The commissioners are advised by professional and technical advisory committees. Committee members are chosen by professional societies on the basis of their expertise in a particular aspect of medical health care. It is through these committees that the ASA gains input into the JCAHO. Anesthesiologists appointed by the ASA president attend meetings with the JCAHO officers and advise the JCAHO as to how a department of anesthesia should be organized, what activities the anesthesia department should be involved in, and what steps an anesthesia department should take to protect the well-being of patients.

In the past few years, the JCAHO has undergone some stressful times, when widely publicized instances of poor medical practices occurred at hospitals that had passed JCAHO inspection. In response the State of New York developed its own state-based review process, and the federal government decided to audit 10% of all JCAHO accreditation.

Using the power of its accreditation program, the JCAHO seeks to enforce the implementation of processes that it believes lead to better care. One of the most prominent processes is quality assurance. Quality assurance was established as a standard for approval as early as 1924, when the ACS prescribed that medical staffs should "review and analyze at regular intervals their clinical experience in the various departments of the hospital."

The process of quality assurance acquired a more directed format in the 1970s when the JCAH began requiring medical audits. Medical audits started with the creation of a set of criteria by which one could indicate proper care of the patent. Several randomly selected patient charts were reviewed in a retrospective fashion. The reviewers marked whether the criteria were present in the patient's record. The concept of audits was that elements of a medical record could be used to identify issues in medical care. Audits were relatively useless because the methodology focused attention on the record, not the care of the patient.

The JCAH made quality assurance a major issue in 1982, when 62% of all contingencies related to a failure to perform adequate quality assurance. In 1984, the JCAHO attempted to establish a hospitalwide quality assurance process with standardization of programs in all departments of a hospital.[9] The device invented to accomplish this goal was "generic" or "occurrence" screening. Under the concept of occurrence screening, a department chose specific areas to investigate in an on-going process. The premise behind occurrence screening was that a department could not possibly review every case but that activity in several important areas would reflect the overall care. Once again this mechanism did not produce quality assurance. Occurrence screening failed because the staff did not know which were the most important areas to investigate, the areas did not necessarily reflect overall care, and the staff still viewed quality assurance as a bothersome bureaucratic process. There was no conviction that JCAHO processes of quality assurance provided insight into medical problems or improved practice. Quality assurance was relegated to clerical personnel by the busy clinician.

Linked to this theme of occurrence screening was the concept of "clinical indicators."[10,12] Clinical indicators were meant to be criteria that facilitated the identification of clinical care problems. The idea was that if certain events occurred or if one event occurred more than a given number of times a problem in patient care might exist. The JCAHO turned to anesthesiology as one of the first specialties for which to develop clinical indicators. A task force was created to identify clinical indicators that would be easily recognized by personnel reviewing a medical record. The detection of an indicator triggered a review of the chart to determine if care had been adequate. The first pilot study to define indicators for anesthesia failed, partly because of the variability of anesthesia and hospital records. Nonetheless, a set of clinical indicators for anesthesia was devised, and departments of anesthesia are required to incorporate clinical indicators into their quality assurance process. In the summer of 1990, the JCAHO began recruiting hospitals to participate in a second attempt to validate these indicators.

Throughout this history, anesthesiologists have held little faith in JCAHO-mandated processes of quality assurance. Despite their disbelief, anesthesia departments found themselves under a great deal of pressure to develop quality assurance programs that adhered to the requirements of the JCAHO. The ASA was surprised when in 1988 a workshop on quality assurance attracted an overflow crowd. Asked how many were attending because of the JCAHO, nearly every hand in the audience was raised.

The criteria used by the JCAHO are published in the *Accreditation Manual for Hospitals*, which is available to hospitals and physicians.[13] The manual stipulates the JCAHO standards for departments of a hospital seeking JCAHO accreditation. The "standards" for Anesthesia services are created with consultation from representatives of various specialties. Although ASA representatives have input, the JCAHO maintains autonomy and does not necessarily heed or implement the ASA suggestions.

The current philosophy of the JCAHO is that hospitals should be able to demonstrate quality improvement. That is, each department should be able to show that a problem of care was identified and resolved with resultant improvement in care. In general, JCAHO requirements are process-oriented requirements that are easily tested by documentation.[14,15] Therefore, gaining JCAHO approval involves recognizing what processes are required by the JCAHO, implementing the processes, and then documenting that the processes are functioning. Documentation is a key to winning the JCAHO game. Departments that are functioning according to JCAHO guidelines but have not adequately documented their organization (with printed and periodically revised rules, regulations, bylaws) and activities (such as regular and acceptable minutes) have difficulty gaining approval.

The JCAHO requirements for an anesthesia department are purposely generic enough to allow for multiple ways to achieve that requirement. Although flexibility is desirable, it brings with it the problem of vagueness. The decision as to whether a department's processes and documentation meet JCAHO standards is made by a JCAHO physician inspector during an extensive on-site examination. The physician inspector may or may not be knowledgeable about the pragmatic problems of providing anesthesia care. The inspector will judge the department according to the JCAHO manual. Thus, where the manual is not specific, the inspector makes a subjective interpretation of the requirements and decides whether the department fulfills this interpretation.

B. Medicare

The government dictates quality of care through its Medicare program. To receive payments for Medicare patients, hospitals must have proof that the facility operates within an acceptable standard. Proof of adequate quality of care was either accreditation by a JCAHO survey or approval by a Medicare survey team. Medicare surveys parallel JCAHO surveys. Both require quality assurance mechanisms to be in place. The HCFA organizes Medicare surveys but calls upon outside agencies, often state health agencies, to perform the surveys. Medicare surveys differ from JCAHO surveys in that Medicare inspections are less peer review and more picayune than JCAHO surveys. In addition, an unsatisfactory Medicare survey may result in a hospital having its Medicare payments suspended, without recourse.

Recently, state and federal governments have questioned the reliability of the JCAHO surveys. The HCFA mandated that JCAHO surveys would have to be validated. To ensure the validity of the JCAHO surveys, the HCFA decreed that 10% of all JCAHO surveys would be followed by a Medicare survey within 90 days. These validation surveys are conducted primarily by nonphysician inspectors reviewing documentation (minutes, rules, regulations, statistics, drug control sheets). In addition to these validation surveys, Medicare occasionally performs unannounced surveys in response to a complaint. Such surveys focus on the area of the complaint and do not address the entire hospital.

III. PROFESSIONAL AND LEGAL OBLIGATIONS

Accrediting agencies notwithstanding, why should we perform quality assurance? A medical staff has an obligation to perform quality assurance and peer review. Where does that obligation come from? It comes from all physicians who have to ensure that they provide the best care possible. Quality assurance is the only manner in which physicians can assure themselves and their patients that care is adequate. Apart from the obligation specific to the patient-physician relationship is the obligation of any profession. By definition, true professions are marked by the characteristic that their members have their abilities and competence judged by their peers. Unquestionably, there is no better judge of good medical care than honest members of the profession. Thus, even if there were no rules and regulations requiring peer review and quality assurance, these functions should be an integral part of any anesthesia department.

In addition to our obligation as a physician and a professional, quality assurance is a legal responsibility. The legal responsibility to perform quality assurance was clearly defined beginning in the 1970s as a result of such cases as

Gonzalez vs *Nork and Mercy Hospital, Johnson* vs *Misericordia,* and *Darling* vs *Charleston Community Memorial Hospital.*[16] In these cases, medical staffs and hospital boards of directors granted privileges to incompetent physicians, without reasonable investigation of the physicians' credentials. Members of the medical staff claimed innocence stating that they were unaware that there was any trouble in the physicians' practice. The court denied that plea stating that the Directors of a department, medical staff, and hospital are liable for malpractice claim if they knew *or should have known* about the malpractice. These cases established the principle of corporate responsibility—that hospitals, medical staff members, and departmental chairpersons have a fiduciary responsibility to the patient to ensure that competent medical care is provided at the health care facility.

At the same time that civil law and national laws demanded peer review, physicians became increasingly more hesitant to perform peer review. Two factors were responsible for this reluctance. The first factor was that there was no well-defined method for judging clinical performance. Without guidelines and criteria for objectively testing competence, physicians felt uncomfortable in making pronouncements that could seriously damage a colleague's career. Secondly, in the face of poorly defined mechanisms for judging competence, medical staffs feared retaliatory civil suits if they acted to restrict or suspend a practitioner's privileges. The result of peer-review proceedings was almost always an unpleasant confrontation. Occasionally, the confrontation grew into a threat of a lawsuit for defamation of character or restraint of trade.

Restraint of trade became a potent deterrent to the peer-review process starting in 1943 when the Justice Department won a conviction against the AMA for attempting to destroy a health cooperative organized in Washington, D.C. In its decision upholding the conviction, the Supreme Court disallowed the AMA contention that antitrust laws did not apply to medicine because it was a profession not a trade.[17] This decision was supported in 1975, when the Supreme Court considered a case charging the Virginia Bar Association with price fixing.[18] In their decision, the Supreme Court judges wrote that antitrust cases could be filed against the "learned professions." In 1976, the Federal Trade Commission (FTC) voted to begin an investigation of medicine. One of the FTC's first targets was the American Society of Anesthesiology. The ASA was forced to accept a 1978 Consent Order involving the relative

value scale.[19] The rationale for investigating the medical field was again economic. The FTC believed that medical care costs could be controlled if more competition could be generated. These developments established a threat to peer review—a peer review action that would affect the income of a practitioner could lead to a federal antitrust suit. Since antitrust awards automatically trebled the amount sought by the plaintiff, the threat of an antitrust suit was rather formidable.

This fear of being sued for performing peer review reached its peak with the famous *Patrick* vs *Burget* case of 1984.[20] In this case, Dr. Patrick's competitors used peer review to try to eliminate his practice. Patrick missed an obvious diagnosis and performed an incorrect operation. Armed with evidence of inadequate care on other occasions, the surgeon's competitors moved to suspend privileges and remove his license. Patrick filed suit claiming restraint of trade.

At the trial, the court allowed certain documents to be entered into evidence, documents that are usually considered privileged information. These hospital documents included accounts and records of meetings concerning the investigation leading to Dr. Patrick's suspension. The court's decision was based on the concept that since the State of Washington did not oversee the peer review process at the hospital the proceedings were not privileged information. With evidence from the hospital proceedings, the court found that Dr. Patrick's competitors had acted outside of a reasonable peer-review process, using the peer-review process for their own benefit. Dr. Patrick was awarded 2 million dollars.

This decision was appealed to the Supreme Court, which supported the original decision. This decision alarmed physicians around the country because it seemed to remove confidentiality and put those participating in peer review at great risk. The response to the Patrick case was unwarranted. There was ample evidence that fair and appropriate peer review had not been performed. Since the case involved unfair peer review, losing confidentiality for appropriate peer-review proceedings was not really a threat. However, for a short period of time, the emotional response to the Patrick case jeopardized the future of effective peer review. As it happened, this perceived threat was eliminated in 1986.

In 1986, the U.S. Congress passed the Health Care Quality Improvement Act of 1986 (HCQIA).[21,22] In the preamble to the law, Congress stated that "medical malpractice and the need to improve quality of medical care have become nationwide problems." Congress was particularly concerned with preventing an incompetent physician from moving from state to state and not honestly revealing his or her previous difficulties in practice. Congress believed that the problems could be solved through effective professional peer review but noted that peer review was discouraged by the threat of civil suit and antitrust laws. Accordingly, Congress mandated peer-review protection for hospitals and physicians participating in fair peer-review processes. The law stipulated that in order to be protected a peer-review process must be conducted fairly and without ulterior motives. The general characteristics of a fair peer-review process are listed:

1. The process must be undertaken in the belief that it will improve quality of care.
2. There must be an adequate effort to obtain the facts.
3. Adequate notice must be given and fair proceedings afforded to the physician involved.

The HCQIA underwent an important test in 1990, when a California neurosurgeon sued a hospital and members of its staff for antitrust.[23] The competence of the neurosurgeon had been questioned by his colleagues. A detailed and lengthy review process resulted in a recommendation that privileges be suspended. The neurosurgeon requested a hearing before the hospital judicial review board. This board found the decision to suspend privileges unreasonable but did note concern about the neurosurgeon's care in a few instances. The neurosurgeon then filed suit against other members of the hospital's neurosurgery department alleging that they had conspired to use the peer review to eliminate their competition. The judge dismissed the case in the pretrial phase, ruling that the peer-review process had met the criteria of the HCQIA. The fact that the peer-review decision was overturned by a higher body was not evidence that the review had been conducted with ulterior motives or in an unfair manner. This ruling was interpreted as a landmark decision guaranteeing protection to physicians who participate in peer review.

Although the first subchapter of the HCQIA was a boon to physicians, the other second subchapter was seen as a peril. In response to the belief that a better mechanism was needed to prevent incompetent physicians from jumping from hospital to hospital, Congress mandated that substantial adverse findings and disciplinary actions be reported to the Department of

Health and Human Services. The Department of Health and Human Services was authorized to establish a "National Practitioner Data Bank for Adverse Information on Physicians and Other Health Care Practitioners." The data bank was designed to contain information about negative actions taken against any physician. The hospital, state medical licensing boards, and other agencies are required to report any reduction, restriction, revocation, denial, or failure to renew privileges to the National Practitioner Data Bank. Malpractice actions are also to be reported. Hospitals and other health care institutions are required to query the data bank about any practitioner when they apply for privileges and about every medical staff member every 2 years. As of the summer of 1990, the data bank was not yet functional.

Individual states have also entered the arena requiring quality assurance processes.[24] The Health Care Quality Improvement Act of 1986 allowed states to choose between complying with federal regulations or establishing their own data bank. Some states opted to create their own data bank. Most others chose to participate in the national data bank. In addition, individual states are creating state laws about standards of care and review processes. New York State Health Commissioner, David Axelrod, took the most aggressive actions relating to ensuring quality of health care by mandating that quality assurance profiles as a basis of relicense.

Although these later developments seem depressing and threatening, there is good evidence that all levels of government would welcome returning control of the assessment of care to the physicians. Speaking to the American Society of Anesthesiologists in 1989, Dr. David Axelrod stated that it is imperative that physicians recapture control of their profession from the government. Noting that only action on the part of the physicians could accomplish this, Axelrod warned that if physicians did not take the responsibility of performing and enforcing peer review, the government would. The alternatives are clearly before the profession and our specialty.

IV. PROCESSES FOR QUALITY ASSURANCE IN ANESTHESIA

How has our specialty responded to these laws, obligations, and demands? Ever since the 1950s anesthesiologists have been attempting to measure the outcome of care. Early studies such as the Beecher-Todd report of 1954[25] examined the incidence of anesthesia-related calamities. In the late 1970s and early 1980s, attempts at a more detailed analysis of adverse events began to appear in the anesthesia literature. The most notable of these were made by Cooper and his colleagues at Massachusetts General Hospital.[27] The MGH group addressed the problems of detecting adverse events and attributing causes. Their data provided a better approximation of the types, the approximate frequency, and the nature of adverse events. This information formed the basis of "standards of practice" that began to be developed for anesthesia.

A. Problem-oriented audit

In the early 1980s there were many publications addressing quality assurance in medicine. Some of these were directed specifically at anesthesiology. These early articles merely reiterated the designs and requirements of accrediting agencies such as the JCAHO. One such article described a quality assurance mechanism for anesthesia called the "problem-oriented audit."[28] This publication was the ASA Peer Review Committee's attempt to help anesthesiology departments implement a quality assurance program that would meet JCAH requirements. The problem-oriented audit involved five steps:

1. Identify problems and concerns
2. Define causes
3. Implement remedial actions
4. Monitor to determine efficacy of remedy
5. Document effectiveness of quality assurance

A basic requirement of the program was that "clinical" performance should be measured by the use of preestablished criteria. The criteria were really acceptable limits for the occurrence of complications. For example, a department would decide on an acceptable rate for the occurrence of accidental dual puncture during the performance of epidural blocks. The rate might be set either by estimate or by published information. If the performance of an individual or a department exceeded the predefined limit, a review would be performed to investigate whether a problem existed. If the frequency of the occurrence was less than the predefined limit, the limit would be decreased until no further improvement could be attained. Theoretically the system would eventually reach the limits of humanly achievable rates for untoward events.

One useful aspect of the "problem-oriented audit" was the philosophy that there were inherent problems in anesthesiology that even the most astute and fastidious practitioner could not eliminate. Another useful aspect was the organizational information about what a quality assurance program should include. At the time, few practitioners knew what quality assurance really meant. The presentation of a generalized process was helpful.

The weaknesses of the problem-oriented audit involved the identification of problems and the determination of cause. The strategy was that since some events were unavoidable and there were so many potential areas to examine, one should start by monitoring areas that anesthesiologists believed were important. Such a strategy was restrictive because it relied on the perceptions of the anesthesiologists of where to look for important problems. Perceptions often looked at easily identifiable problems of low importance. Other more important but less visible or more threatening areas were overlooked. Further, the process was directed at a description of what was happening to the department as a whole. It was not designed to profile the performance of an individual practitioner. Additionally, the process did not address the problem of determining causation and categorizing types of errors.

In 1986, the ASA published a separate monograph entitled *Quality Assurance in the Practice of Anesthesiology*.[29] The monograph provided a convenient resource for history, terminology, and organization. The manual also provided administrative and organizational aids to departments trying to create a quality assurance program for purposes of passing JCAH review. The monograph did not make any progress in resolving the issues facing quality assurance.

In the mid-1980s, more sophisticated programs for quality assurance in anesthesiology appeared. For the first time, some of these programs went beyond basic JCAHO requirements. Common to these programs was the use of computers and databases that allowed quality assurance programs to easily collect and analyze large amounts of information about occurrences. The ability to deal with larger amounts of information led to the ability to make more discriminating analyses.

These types of programs constitute the current quality assurance activities in anesthesia. Several components are the same for each programs. Most programs require a quality assurance form to be completed for each case. Information from these forms is entered into the database. In this manner, "volume indicators" are identified. Volume indicators are merely lists of those types of procedures performed and anesthetics administered most frequently. Volume indicators are used to make "service profiles" and "risk profiles." Theoretically, by knowing the most numerous or most difficult cases, the department should be able to detect the most frequent or the most severe anesthetic-related complications.

To determine what types of events should be investigated, a list of "clinical indicators" is created. Clinical indicators are events that are believed to be markers of instances where patients have suffered harm or been put at risk as a result of anesthetic management. Any cases involving one of these indicators is reported to the quality assurance division of the hospital or the department of anesthesiology. These instances are then investigated with the goal of deciding whether the event was avoidable. Recommendations are made to prevent future occurrences. Finally, subsequent studies are done to determine whether the frequency or severity of complications have decreased. Information about the nature and severity of the case is entered into the computer database. The information includes a code number to identify the anesthesiologist involved. With this information, the computer can generate data about the frequency with which certain complications occur in the department as a whole and to each anesthesiologist. This type of information is used to determine if a problem exists for any practitioner or for the department.

Although these systems offer an advance over the earlier models, most still fall short of effective quality assurance. The shortfall occurs because the systems merely create lists of events. The systems neither search for causes nor set guidelines for evaluating competence. In order for the next step to be taken certain basic problems in quality assurance had to be addressed:

- How can democratic, unbiased peer review be implemented in closely knit, competitive environments?
- What parameters validly reflect quality of care?
- How can adjustments be made for differing types of practice?
- What terms and definitions could be standardized for use across the country?
- Can quality assurance improve anesthesia care?

B. Judging clinical competence ("Vitez model")

Appropriately, these issues were addressed by a model for quality assurance in anesthesiology developed in a private practice setting.[30] Heavily influenced by the pioneering work of Jeffrey Cooper at MGH, the model was developed in Las Vegas, Nevada, between 1984 and 1988. Las Vegas proved an ideal setting to test solutions for the problems facing quality assurance in anesthesiology. Each year, 30,000 to 40,000 anesthetic operations were performed in Las Vegas, at five hospitals. The hospitals ranged in size from as few as 100 to more than 700 beds. Approximately 60 competing anesthesiologists practiced at all five hospitals.

The model was based on three simple concepts:

1. Competence must be decided by knowledgeable, unbiased peers who consider a wide range of evidence.
2. The best indication of competence is outcome.
3. Humans are inherently fallible, and the occurrence of an error, even one of great significance, does not necessarily indicate incompetence.

The model utilizes a semivoluntary system to collect information about anesthesia-related events. A short, general list of clinical indicators focuses attention on clinically significant occurrences, not unrelated happenings or theoretical problems:

1. Cancelation of surgery
2. Respiratory or cardiac arrest
3. Soft-tissue injury to patient
4. New neurologic abnormality (such as coma, seizure, paresis, paralysis)
5. Inability to ventilate the lungs or intubate the trachea
6. Reintubation of the trachea
7. Sustained hypoxia
8. Regurgitation or aspiration
9. Difficulty of patient to breathe
10. Unstable cardiac rhythm, heart rate, or blood pressure
11. New myocardial ischemia or infarction
12. Patient abandonment
13. Death of the patient within 24 hours of surgery
14. Any other event that may be related to anesthesia management

The list is distributed to anesthesia providers and personnel working in anesthetizing locations or in postoperative care units (such as PACU, postpartum, ICU). Any of these events is reported to the anesthesia quality assurance committee (AQAC) of the department of anesthesiology. This committee reviews cases and make recommendations to the department. The quality assurance committee utilizes the hospital's quality assurance department to process the occurrence report and prepare information about the case for review. One important step in this process is the use of copies of the record with names and identifying entries removed. In this manner anonymity is built into the review system. The identity of the practitioner involved in the case is not to be disclosed to the committee or the department. To allow for differences in clinical case mix, institutional setting, and changes in performance over a period of time, codes and information identifying the practitioner, institution, date, type of surgery, ASA physical status are entered into the database by the quality assurance department.

When considering a case, a reviewer classifies the case according to a standard scheme, focusing on what actually happened to the patient. The first step in classifying an occurrence is to decide if there was a clinically significant event that was related to equipment used, a decision made, or action taken by the anesthesiologist. Next, the reviewer decides the seriousness of the event by assigning an outcome score. Outcome scores translate description of an event (nominal data) to a number indicating severity (ordinal data):

0 = No sequelae (such as reintubation of the trachea after esophageal intubation)

1-3 = No harm to patient but escalation of care (such as ventilator required postoperatively because of improper use of relaxant)

4-6 = Reversible damage to integrity of an organ (such as pulmonary edema from fluid overload)

7-9 = Irreversible organ damage (such as myocardial infarction)

10 = Death

This scoring system is important to the process because it transforms narrative and descriptive terms (nominal data) into numeric values (ordinal data), which can be used for more objective comparisons. The third step is for the reviewer to identify and classify any errors committed. Errors are classified by these categories: management area, nature of error, and genesis of error. "Management area" and "nature of error" describe what happened. "Genesis of error" describes why it happened. The categories and their subdivisions are shown here

Management area
Airway, circulatory, neuromuscular blockade, regional

Nature of error
"None"—an unavoidable circumstance
"Mechanical"—failure of device
"Human"—related to formulation or execution of a decision. Human errors are subdivided into three types.
"Judgmental" errors occur when the action taken is the action intended. These are errors of faulty decision processes, such as administration of anesthesia by mask in a "full-stomach" situation.
"Technical" errors occur when the action taken is not the action intended (such as a syringe swap). Such errors involve mistakes in the execution of a decision.
"Vigilance" errors are errors associated with lack of adequate general attention (such as an intravenous infiltration). Judgmental errors are further classified by genesis:

Genesis of judgmental errors
Inadequate knowledge
    Didactic
    Experience
Inadequate data—failure to seek data
Disregard data
    Failure to recognize pattern
    Failure to accept conclusion
Lack of alternative plan

The classification of errors is another key difference between this method and other quality assurance processes. The basic concept that humans are inherently fallible leads to the theory that each practitioner may have a unique pattern of errors that defines his or her clinical performance. Even if different areas of management are involved, the same genesis of error may be repeated in all areas.

Error profiles are created from data collected by the AQAC. After approval of the department, AQAC findings are entered into the practitioners' files in the computer's database. As data accumulate, a picture emerges of the number, type, and frequency of errors made by individuals and the department as a whole. Reviews of the files are made periodically (as whenever a new error is made, at reappointment, annually) or whenever an incident generates concern about the abilities of a practitioner.

Much like athletes use video tapes to study and correct mistakes, error profiles are used to help individuals and the department identify important clinical issues and improve their performance. Without error profiles, it is impossible to know what needs to be repaired. Additionally, once error and outcome profiles are known, limits of acceptability can be set. Competence can be judged from the number, type, and severity of errors made as incompetent practitioners commit errors that are more numerous, less common, or more severe than competent members of the department.

Information from case reviews is used in error analysis. In error analysis, a profile of the practitioner is compared to the profile of the department. A profile contains six comparative elements and three minimal performance levels:

Comparative elements

1. Frequency of anesthesia-related events
2. Average negative-outcome score
3. Number of errors per event
4. Area of clinical management
5. Nature of errors
6. Genesis of errors

Minimal expected performance levels

1. Anesthetizes ASA physical status 1 and 2 patients without outcome score greater than 6
2. Institutes appropriate life-sustaining actions in life-threatening situations
3. Displays insight when involved in significant error

These minimal levels were determined by analysis of quality assessment data collected from four Hospitals in Las Vegas, Nevada. In 4 years, no incident of anesthesia-related organ damage or death occurring in an ASA physical status 1 or 2 patient was been detected. Accordingly, the community adopted "anesthetizing ASA physical status 1 and 2 patients without incurring an outcome score greater than 6" as a minimal level of practice.

In dealing with serious illnesses, not every life-threatening situation was resolvable. However, the most unacceptable outcomes involved evidence that the practitioner had failed to recognize the severity of the problem or react appropriately. Accordingly, a standard was adopted that required evidence that the practitioner institute appropriate life-sustaining actions in life-threatening situations. This minimal level acknowledges that even a competent practitioner may make a fatal error. However, the competent physician recognizes the gravity of the situation and makes appropriate efforts to save the patient.

Finally, "lack of insight" was a common and persuasive factor in decisions to restrict clinical activities. Thus a final standard decrees that when an appropriate peer-review process judges an event to be related to anesthesia, the practitioner involved should pay credence to that judgment.

After establishing comparative and minimal levels, an individual's error profile is compared to the average error profile for the department. This comparison is used to make decisions about clinical performance. As reviews accumulate in the database, it becomes possible to identify which problems occur more frequently and which problems are more onerous for both the department and for the individual provider. It is also possible to identify providers whose performance falls outside the acceptable realm. In order to better understand how to use this mechanism to judge clinical performance and determine competence, consider the following examples.

Examples

CASE 1. An anesthesiologist is applying for reappointment. In order to determine whether the physician should be reappointed, a error

Table 28-1. Comparative quality assurance data (average number per category)

Provider	Number of events per year	Number of errors per event	Average outcome score	Number of minimums violated
1	4	1	4	0
2	2	1	2	0
3	5	4	5	2
Department	2	1	2	0

Table 28-2. Percentage of error by management category

Provider	Airway	Circulation	Relaxants	Ventilation
1	100	0	0	0
2	30	20	30	20
3	40	40	0	20
Department	35	25	25	15

profile is constructed (provider 1 in Tables 28-1 to 28-4). Table 28-1 shows a greater than average frequency of anesthesia-related events and an elevated outcome score for provider 1. No minimal levels are violated, and the practitioner commits a normal number of errors per event. There is a clustering of errors involving airway management (Table 28-2). Table 28-3 shows that provider 1 makes mostly judgmental errors. Table 28-4 illustrates that the practitioner does not collect adequate information about the airway (for example, does not do a physical exam) and fails to recognize the nature of an airway problem. The data support reappointment with counseling, education about recognition and management of airway problems, and periodic reassessment of clinical performance.

CASE 2. The surgery department accuses an anesthesiologist of inadequate clinical performance. Error analysis reveals that the physician has an average error profile (provider 2 in Tables 28-1 to 28-4), is involved in an average number of events, and commits only one error per event. His outcome score is acceptable and no minimal standards are violated. The only significant finding is that the provider has a clustering in "failure to accept conclusions." The data do not support the allegations. In this instance, the system protects the practitioner from unfair criticism.

CASE 3. An individual provider is involved in a serious complication. The question of suspending privileges arises. Error analysis (provider 3 in Tables 28-1 to 28-4) reveals significant deviations from the normal pattern. Table 28-1 shows an increased frequency of events with multiple errors per event. Outcome score is elevated, showing an average of reversible organ damage including an anesthesia-related death. Two minimal standards have been violated. Table 28-2 indicates that the multiple errors include simultaneous mismanagement of airway, circulation, and ventilation accounting for the elevated outcome score. Although Table 28-3 indicates little difference from the norm, Table 28-4 reveals repeated errors involving inadequate didactic knowledge. This clustering represents a significant deviation from normal, not only because it is different, but also because others rarely make this type of error. The practitioner does not collect enough data to help diagnose and treat the problem and is unable to recognize the signs of a serious complication. Lack of knowledge, failure to collect data, and inability to recognize danger constitute a serious combination of deficiencies. Such deficiencies question the advisability of allowing the provider to continue practicing. The data support suspension of privileges.

In addition to judging individual performance, departmental performance can also be improved. In the Las Vegas experience, problems with the use of muscle relaxants became apparent when the computerized database was reviewed. For two consecutive years, complications related to the use of neuromuscular relaxants accounted for 13% to 18% of all complications. In the third year, steps were taken to prevent these complications: purchase of additional nerve stimulators, provision of an educational program, documentation of nerve stimulator results on the anesthetic record, documentation of the patients' ability to breathe before removal of the endotracheal tube. These steps led to a decrease to 3% of problems related to neuromuscular relaxants the next year.

This model of quality assurance relies on computer hardware and software to automate case processing, case analysis, and data analysis. Current software designed especially for the

Table 28-3. Nature of human errors (percentage of errors)

Provider	Judgmental	Technical	Vigilance
1	100	0	0
2	75	20	5
3	75	15	10
Department	75	20	5

Table 28-4. Genesis of judgmental errors (percentage of errors)

Provider	Inadequate didactic knowledge	Failure to seek data	Failure to recognize pattern	Failure to accept conclusion
1	0	75	15	10
2	0	30	10	60
3	30	30	40	0
Department	5	30	30	35

model performs most tasks required by the quality assurance department (Premier Anesthesia, Atlanta, Georgia). The software also acts as an "expert" system guiding physician reviewers through their analysis of the case. Finally, the software contains a database and preset analyses that describe the clinical experience of the department and its members.

Although this model has facilitated quality assurance in anesthesia, many problems still remain. First, detecting events that might be related to anesthesia is one of the most difficult problems facing quality assurance systems. Computerized anesthesia-record devices will enhance detection methods.[31] Computerized anesthesia-record devices consist of computers capable of automatically recording signals from monitors (such as ECG, pressure transducers, gas analyzers) every 15 seconds. In addition, the anesthesiologist enters into the computer information such as events or drugs given. The computer database is then able to produce an accurate anesthesia record and reconstruct any event on a 15-second time scale. Such methodology will allow detection and accurate description of many more perioperative events than is currently possible.

Even with computerized data retrieval, many events will be undetectable except by persons caring for the patient (such as a broken tooth). For this reason, quality assurance systems will probably always rely on the honesty and courage of the physician to report a possible error. Reporting by physicians will improve as they realize that quality assurance systems do not pose a threat to them. On the contrary, quality assurance systems offer the most effective method to improve their clinical expertise.

A second area of difficulty is knowing exactly what happened. Determination of what happened is confounded by the lack of accurate details about events, and the inexperience of peer reviewers. Details of an event are often indistinct because witnesses of any event often have conflicting and inaccurate descriptions of the occurrence. Memory for details fades with time; thus the longer the period of time between the occurrence and the search for information, the greater the loss and distortion of detail. Even when details have been accurately recorded, important parameters may not have been monitored. Computerized data-retrieval systems will provide much more details about clinical events. Still, many aspects of an occurrence will be known only to human witnesses. This means that quality assurance systems must be able to identify and rapidly debrief persons who have knowledge about the event.

A third problem for quality assurance is case analysis. Case analysis is complicated by lack of knowledge about how a case review should be organized. Recently, Robert Caplan has provided a guideline for case review that has useful organizational rules.[32] Caplan's system advises on the chronologic arrangement of events and information. As information is taken from the patient's record and arranged chronologically, the reviewer marks those bits of data that seem important to the event. After looking over the chronology, the reviewer then hypothesizes the mechanism by which the event occurred. The hypothesis is then tested against the facts of the case and the medical literature. Alternative hypotheses are tried to see if they are consistent with the data.

Determining causation is also complicated by lack of information (such as no autopsy) and the presence of mitigating circumstances (concurrent diseases). These factors may obfuscate the assessment of the roles of anesthesia management in the event or injury. The model described above directs that under circumstances of uncertainty, quality assurance decisions favor the practitioner, and the occurrence may be judged as not related to anesthesia care. As experience with formal case review grows, expert systems that will guide reviewers through case analysis will be developed. Expert systems will aid peer review processes, since they will perform more reliably than human reviewers[33] and will provide a uniformity to reviews. Over a period of time a library of peer review cases will aid in rapid analysis of repetitive events.

V. SUMMARY

Although many developments are required to advance peer review and quality assurance to a more sophisticated level, current process do allow for a reasonable assessment of clinical performance. The major obstacle in many settings is the obstinence of the physicians themselves. This obstinence will be overcome by the evidence that quality assurance programs are the only reliable mechanism for improving clinical expertise. Even in the face of this evidence, selfishness, egotism, and paranoia will still cause some practitioners to oppose peer review. As long as the majority of anesthesiologists recognize that quality assurance systems are the key to maintaining the integrity of their profession, those resistant few will harm only themselves.

REFERENCES

1. Starr P: The consolidation of professional authority. In the social transformation of American medicine, New York, 1982, Basic Books.

2. Starr P: The mirage of reform. In The social transformation of American medicine, New York, 1982, Basic Books.

3. Starr P: The liberal years. In The social transformation of American medicine, New York, 1982, Basic Books.

4. Willett DE: PSRO today: a lawyer's assessment, N Engl J Med 212:340-343, 1975.

5. Dane PE, Weiner JP, and Otter SE: Peer review organizations promises and potential pitfalls, N Engl J Med 313:1131-1137, 1985.

6. Hospital Peer Review, pp 133-136, Nov 1988, American Health Consultants, Inc, Atlanta, Ga.

7. Lohr KN and Schroeder SA: A strategy for quality assurance in Medicare, N Engl J Med 322:707-712, 1990.

8. Roberts JS, Coale JG, and Redman RR: A history of the Joint Commission on Accreditation of Hospitals, JAMA 258:936-940, 1987.

9. Oleary DS: The Joint Commission looks to the future, JAMA 258:951-952, 1987.

10. Agenda for change update, vol 2, no 1, 1988, Chicago, 1988, Joint Commission for Accreditation of Health Care Organizations.

11. Agenda for change update, vol 3, no 1, 1989, Chicago, 1988, Joint Commission for Accreditation of Health Care Organizations.

12. Agenda for change update, vol 3, no 2, 1989, Chicago, 1988, Joint Commission for Accreditation of Health Care Organizations.

13. Accreditation manual for hospitals, Chicago, 1990, Joint Commission for Accreditation of Health Care Organizations.

14. Accreditation manual for hospitals, Chicago, 1990, Joint Commission for Accreditation of Health Care Organizations, pp 261-270.

15. Accreditation manual for hospitals, Chicago, 1990, Joint Commission for Accreditation of Health Care Organizations, pp 211-217.

16. Cohen J: Department of Anesthesia quality assurance policy and procedure manual, Gainesville, Fla, 1988, Department of Anesthesiology, University of Florida.

17. Starr P: The triumph of accommodation. In The social transformation of American medicine, New York, 1982, Basic Books.

18. Avellone JC and Moore FD: The Federal Trade Commission enters a new arena: health services, N Engl J Med 299:478-483, 1978.

19. ASA/FTC consent order effective, ASA Newsletter 43, Chicago, 1979, American Society of Anesthesiologists.

20. Rust M: Court decision in *Patrick* to have widespread effect, American Medical News, p 19, Nov 1987, Dearborn, Mich, American Medical Association.

21. Federal Health Care Quality Improvement Act 1986, P.L. 99-660, Title IV, 402, Nov 14, 1986, 100 Stat. 3784, Laws of 99th Congress, 2nd session.

22. National practitioner data bank for adverse information on physicians and other health care practitioners; final regulations, vol 54, Federal Register, 1989, Washington, DC.

23. Meyer H: Immunity law used for first time to dismiss MD peer review suit, American Medical News, p 3, March 23-30, 1990, Dearborn, Mich, American Medical Association.

24. Page L: N.Y.'s Dr. Axelrod: hero or villain? American Medical News, p 3, Aug 1989, Dearborn, Mich, American Medical Association.

25. Beecher HK and Todd DP: Study of deaths associated with anesthesia and surgery based on study of 599,548 anesthesias in ten institutions 1948-1952, inclusive, Ann Surg 140:2-35, 1954.

26. Cooper JB, Newbower RS, Long CD, and McPeek B: Preventable anesthesia mishaps: a study of human factors, Anesthesiology 49:399-406, 1978.

27. Cooper JB, Newbower RS, and Kitz, RJ: An analysis of major errors and equipment failures in anesthesiology: considerations for prevention and detection, Anesthesiology 60:34-42, 1984.

28. Brown EM: Quality assurance in anesthesiology: the problem oriented audit, Anesth Analg 63:611-615, 1984.

29. Duberman S: Quality assurance in the practice of anesthesiology, Chicago, 1986, American Society of Anesthesiology.

30. Vitez TS: A model for quality assurance in anesthesiology. J Clin Anesth 2:280-287, 1990.

31. Cook RI, McDonald JS, and Nunziata E: Differences between handwritten and automatic blood pressure records, Anesthesiology 71:385-390, 1989.

32. Caplan RA: In-depth analysis of anesthetic mishaps: tools and techniques, Int Anesth Clin 27:153-160, 1989.

33. Dawes RM, Faust D, and Meehl PE: Clinical versus actuarial judgement, Science 243:1668-1674, 1989.

Chapter 29

Risk Management

John H. Eichhorn

Risk management (RM) in anesthesia is a comprehensive approach functionally involving all aspects of anesthesia care. RM is intended first to minimize the likelihood of anesthesia-caused or anesthesia-related complications (particularly the large fraction of these complications caused by human error). Second, both because of RM elements already in place before an adverse event and because of actions taken at the time of and after an untoward incident, RM will help minimize the impact of such an event on the patient, the anesthesia provider or providers, and the medical care system.

Some of these elements of RM may at first glance appear to be somewhat defensive in nature, particularly these regarding credentialing, equipment management, informed consent, record keeping, and response to an adverse event. Clearly the overall goal of RM is optimal patient care. Correct and thorough application of the RM principles detailed in this chapter will help minimize complications and thus help optimize patient care. The other side of RM, after the primary efforts to promote the best quality care, is its significant ability to help reduce liability exposure. Unfortunately, it is necessary to be aware of the medicolegal system and the facts of the so-called malpractice crisis of the 1970s and 1980s. Although there are strong suggestions that the medicolegal crunch of astronomically high settlements and awards

with consequent skyrocketing malpractice insurance premiums is lessening in the early 1990s, it has been maintained that this is merely a cycle that will inevitably reverse itself.[1] In either case, it is legitimate to acknowledge that some attitudes and procedures in RM are influenced by the characteristics of the medicolegal system and the insurance industry and also by case precedents that have revealed characteristics that make more difficult the defense of anesthesia practitioners against unwarranted charges of malpractice. In theory it is correct that legal defensive issues (so-called defensive medicine) should not influence health care practices. However, the potentially devastating emotional and financial impact of a malpractice lawsuit on a practitioner—even a suit with no merit at all—is significant enough to justify awareness of and application of proved RM strategies intended to minimize the likelihood of malpractice claims.

Risk management relates to several of the other topics considered in this book. Evaluation of patient risk will reveal cases in which there may be greater than the usual probability of a complication. The insights gained will then lead to possible extra attention to issues of, for example, informed consent, record keeping, and plans for specific action in the event of an untoward incident. Epidemiology of complications reveals in what circumstances or with which patients certain complications may be most expected. Realization of these factors may lead to supplementation or alteration of the anesthetic plan, essentially a classic application of the concept of risk management. An excellent general example of the above is the epidemiologic discovery that unrecognized hypoventilation is the cause of the majority of intraoperative anesthesia-caused catastrophes. This has led over the last several years to the development and implementation of several strategies to minimize this documented risk. Another topic, quality assurance, is often closely related. The quality assurance process uses some of the same problem-solving algorithm. Both programs have the same goal: optimum patient care. The RM program can sometimes be considered an extension or broadening of the quality assurance process into implementation of very practical preventive and remedial measures regarding complications of anesthesia care. Specific discussion of what to do when sued (noting in particular that there is a probability that *all* anesthesia practitioners will be sued eventually, perhaps even multiple times) relates directly to the RM mechanism. Application of the RM principles, especially those involving actions surrounding an adverse event, should make the subsequent response to a malpractice claim significantly easier for the defendant clinician.

Objective documentation and citable sources in the medical literature are less likely available when one is dealing with risk management than when considering, for example, anesthetic complications directly involving physiology and pharmacology, such as whether isoflurane causes myocardial ischemia in patients with severe coronary artery disease through the so-called steal phenomenon. In this chapter, relevant existing references are included, of course. However, by definition, there is also anecdotal reporting, including experiences of multiple various anesthesia practitioners throughout the country. The topics covered here have been identified in some manner as the source of problems or solutions to problems within anesthesia practice. The purpose of this chapter is to explain what issues are involved in each area within anesthesia RM and to offer suggestions based on experience where possible on how best to deal with these issues. Notice that these topics relate directly to the fundamental components of medical care (and many other endeavors) to which all elements can be ultimately reduced: structure, process, and outcome. *Structure* in medical care involves resources, including personnel, facilities, equipment (especially pertinent for anesthesia), and administra-

tion. *Process* involves how things are done, including but not limited to the actual activities of patient care. The result of the interaction of these two is, of course, what happens—*outcome* (such as wellness, length of stay, dysfunction, morbidity, or mortality). Looking at features of clinical practice using this systematic approach helps facilitate the RM process. Concerns about equipment clearly involve structure, whereas policy and procedure and most of the other identified areas of consideration concern process. The larger point is that everything considered here eventually impacts on the outcome of anesthesia care.

I. BACKGROUND

The terminology used in this area has been borrowed by the medical profession from business, industry, and other professions. Medical practitioners usually believe they understand these terms well enough to communicate among themselves, but often this is not true and understanding is inhibited. It is even more difficult when attempting to communicate with others, such as hospital administrators, insurance company personnel, and regulatory and accrediting inspectors. Many medical practitioners still automatically associate "risk management" with reams of apparently irrelevant paper work demanded as fuel by a self-sustaining bureaucracy composed of nonmedical or quasi-medical personnel. Overzealous emphasis early in the development of this still young field on compiling statistics, doing "audits," and filling out forms may have created a legacy of reluctance for involvement by anesthesia practitioners, more used to hands-on activity with rapid feedback. Nonetheless, it is vitally important in the 1990s for all concerned to realize that this type of activity not only is here to stay, but also has the potential, properly utilized, to be enormously beneficial to the practice of anesthesia. Anesthesia providers must learn that this field has advanced significantly. It will continue to do so with the unhesitating, thoughtful involvement of those most interested (anesthesia practitioners themselves) in reduction and eventual elimination of preventable anesthesia complications.

The concept of "risk management" has been traditionally associated with the financial and economic side of business or professional activity. It started with the insurance industry recognizing "risk": certain activities predictably lead to a degree of loss. This risk then became the subject of efforts to (1) plan to pay for the loss and (2) try to reduce the likelihood or magnitude of loss (and consequent cost). Thus there was an attempt to control or "manage" the known risk. Regarding anesthesia, it was clear that data "demonstrate that anesthetic mishaps, although relatively few in number, present considerable risk of loss in the areas of hospital cost, human suffering, and the integrity of the medical profession" and, as a result, providers "have developed formal programs to systematically identify and control risks that may lead to patient injury or financial loss."[2] Financial loss usually means settlements and judgments associated with malpractice claims and suits. The emphasis of medical risk management is correctly on the prevention of any loss-generating untoward incident or outcome. However, a key traditional component also is the effort to limit financial loss once an incident has occurred. A common impression is that the hospital or insurance company risk manager is the person to call as soon as an accident or injury is identified. Although this is true, there needs to be a shift in perception to the fact that prevention is primary and damage control (financial or otherwise), when needed, is a secondary part of the process.

Classic risk management involves four steps: (1) identification of a problem (actual or potential injury or loss), (2) assessment and evaluation of the problem (determining the cause of injury or loss), (3) resolution of the problem (modification or elimination of the cause, by *change*—change of practice, procedures, equipment, or behavior, and enforcement, with sanctions if necessary), and (4) a follow-up check on the resolution (to verify the desired result and to ensure continued effectiveness).

An example of minor injury but no financial loss involves a major medical center with a large volume of facial surgery. Through a combined mechanism of anesthetists' postoperative visits (and reports back to the clinical director of anesthesia), incident reports filed by floor nurses from the postoperative ward and a call from the surgeon doing most of these cases, it was established that a disproportionately large number of corneal abrasions were occurring during one type of operation. Investigative evaluation revealed that all anesthesia practitioners put lubricating ointment in the patient's eyes, which were then taped shut with paper tape. Some anesthetists used gauze pads, and some did not. All the patients receiving corneal abrasions did not have gauze pads over their eyes. The resolution involved the issuance of a guideline, which was distributed in writing, discussed at a department-wide meeting, and put in the procedure manual, stating that gauze pads should be used to cover the eyes of patients having that

procedure. For follow-up evaluation, after several months, the surgeon was asked to confirm the impression that there had not been one identified corneal abrasion associated with the procedure since the new guideline.

A larger scale example: After notification from the malpractice insurer of perceived excessive anesthesia-caused losses, the Risk Management Committee of the Harvard Medical School Department of Anesthesia reviewed the available literature and all the anesthesia-related claims and incidents for the period 1976 to 1986 from the department's malpractice insurer. Considering the substantive identifiable problems discovered, the committee generated a list of subject categories into which problems and incidents were classified. In order of perceived magnitude the list of identified areas associated with problems and incidents included (1) minimal monitoring during anesthesia (far and away the most frequent issue) and in the postanesthetic recovery period, (2) anesthetizing locations outside traditional operating rooms, (3) equipment standards including preanesthetic equipment checkout, (4) equipment maintenance and servicing, (5) record keeping, and (6) preoperative and postoperative visits by anesthesia personnel. This list formed the basis of a program to attempt to devise strategies to improve clinical practice associated with each of the identified areas of attention. Because preventable intraoperative catastrophe accounted, by far, for the greatest cost, mandatory standards for intraoperative monitoring resulted.[3] This effort at the time applied to one institution and seemed likely to be of general interest to most anesthesiologists, but it was first openly publicly offered and evaluated essentially as an example of a new application of the risk management process.[4] Further work along the same lines led to other standards concerning other topics on the original list of identified subject areas associated with problems and incidents.[5] After an appropriate interval, the follow-up component of the classic risk management process led to an evaluation of the potential impact of the original Harvard monitoring standards.[6] Overall, this large-scale example shows the application of risk management techniques that first stress prevention of untoward events and also include but go far beyond the traditional emphasis on financial loss.

In recent years, medical risk management has received significantly increased attention. Among the reasons are (1) the so-called malpractice crisis of the mid-1980s, which heightened awareness of RM among anesthesia practitioners because of intense activity on the part of hospital administrations and malpractice insurance carriers; (2) the major emphasis on containment of the cost of medical care, which has caused thorough critical review of many traditionally accepted practices with particular attention to outcome of care; and (3) great emphasis by both regulators and the public on the quality of medical care and, again, particularly on outcome, which has led to analysis of events at the most basic level in the medical-care delivery system. These three tend to spotlight any adverse outcome of care, both specific instances and trends.

Adverse outcome of anesthesia care spans a spectrum. The most severe untoward results in anesthesia are rivaled in impact only by those in obstetrics. Anesthesia personnel must be constantly aware that anesthesia-related accidents have the potential to cause great harm. Until the late 1980s, anesthesiologists accounted for about 3% of American physicians and correspondingly generated about 3% of the number of malpractice claims filed. These 3% of claims, however, accounted for about 11% of the total indemnity (dollars paid or set aside for future payment) for medical malpractice cases. Serious untoward results in anesthesia tend to have lasting impact (death or permanent injury), which is very unfortunate and very expensive. A comprehensive review of the causes of untoward outcome from anesthesia is beyond the scope of this chapter. This is discussed elsewhere in this book and in several informative reviews and papers.[7-17] Prominent in these discussions is the issue of preventability. Although there is debate about what fraction of adverse incidents might be prevented, it is an inescapable conclusion from study of the literature and from knowledge of current cases that a significant majority of major untoward results (anesthesia accidents) are preventable. There have been many thoughtful discussions of specific clinical strategies and practices for avoiding adverse outcome from anesthesia, including some labeled (probably incorrectly) as dealing with risk management.[18] Discussion of specific monitoring equipment, anesthesia teaching techniques, and case analysis methods is valuable but is only one small component of a comprehensive RM program in anesthesia. Such a program must be intended to cover all relevant aspects of practice. Genuine risk management in anesthesia must emphasize the creation of optimum conditions of structure and process and optimum preparation, awareness, and skill of the anesthesia practitioners. This will help both to prevent complications and to minimize their impact when they occur.

II. ELEMENTS OF RISK MANAGEMENT IN ANESTHESIA
A. The credentialing process and clinical privileges

Most medical practitioners are scrupulously honest. Unfortunately, rare exceptions do occur. There have been examples in which physicians, nurses, or even untrained lay people have forged credentials and lied on applications and in interviews and thus illegally obtained full licensure and privileges. There has been patient injury in a few extraordinary instances. Such cases have received widespread, often sensational, publicity. Probably much less rarely, applicants for professional positions may have stretched the truth somewhat, either by exaggeration of past status and experience or by omitting key details with negative implications (such as investigations, license suspensions, major malpractice judgments, or even criminal prosecutions, including for patient abuse). Because of these persons with their notoriety and because of the general rising expectations by all involved for the quality of care, the health care profession as a whole has significantly tightened up its procedures surrounding credentials. With the radical changes in fundamental patient-doctor relationships in recent years, there seems to be a pervasive public perception that the health care professions are inadequately policed, particularly by their own mechanisms and organizations. Therefore there has been intense public and political pressure on legislatures, regulatory and licensing agencies, and institutional administrators to identify (1) fraudulent, criminal, and deviant health care providers and (2) the incompetent (for whatever reason) or simply poor-quality practitioners who have frequent or severe enough poor results to attract attention. It is in this atmosphere that the risk management implications become very clear. It is reasonable to assume that there will be a lesser likelihood of complications in the practice of those who are appropriately educated, trained, experienced, and competent. Further, unfortunately it has become very important to consider legal doctrines such as vicarious liability and agency. Specific applicability varies from case to case and location to location. However, basically, if an individual, group, or institution hires a practitioner or even simply approves a practitioner (as by securing or granting privileges), the individuals or institutions may be held liable along with that practitioner for the consequences of his or her actions. This, of course, would be especially likely to be true if it were later discovered that there was something questionable in the offending practitioner's past that had not come to light in the credentialing process. Accordingly, for all these reasons, this process must be taken much more seriously than even a few years ago.

To the vast majority of practitioners who are completely honest, this emphasis may seem annoying and unwieldy. Often it is very inconvenient to have to arrange for transfer of certified copies of academic or training records from the distant past. However, the honest majority must recognize that such efforts are fundamentally directed at protecting patients and also the integrity of the profession. It is somewhat analogous to the annoyance caused by the metal detectors and baggage screening at airports, which is tolerated in the interest of the safety of all concerned.

1. Anesthesia department or group. Because of another type of legal case, some examples of which have been highly publicized, medical practitioners may be hesitant to give an honest evaluation (or even any evaluation at all) of persons known to them who are now seeking a professional position elsewhere. Obviously, someone writing a reference for a current or former co-worker should be honest. Adhering to clearly documentable facts is advisable. Stating a fact that is in the public record (such as a malpractice case lost at trial) should not justify an objection from the subject of the reference. Whether omitting such a fact is dishonest on the part of the reference writer is more a gray area. Including positive opinions and enthusiastic recommendation, of course, is no problem. Including facts that may be perceived as negative (such as the lost malpractice case and also personal problems such as a history of treatment for substance abuse) and negative opinions are what some reference writers fear will provoke retaliatory lawsuits (such as for libel, defamation of character, loss of livelihood) from the subject. As a result, many reference writers in these questionable situations confine their written material to very brief and simple facts such as dates employed and position held.

Because there should be no hesitation for a reference writer to include positive opinions, receipt of a reference that includes nothing more than dates worked and position held should be a suggestion that there may be more to the story. Receipt of such a reference about a person applying for a position should always lead to a telephone call to the writer. Such a telephone call may be advisable in all cases, independent of whatever the written reference contains. Frequently, pertinent questions over the telephone can elicit much more candid information than might otherwise be available. In rare instances, there may be dishonesty through omission by the reference giver even at this level. This may involve an applicant who an individual, a department or group, or an institution would like to see leave. The subject may have poor quality practice, but there may also be reluctance by the reference giver or givers to approach licensing or disciplinary authorities (both because of the unpleasantness and also again out of concern about retaliatory legal action). The best way to avoid being victimized by this practice is to telephone an independent observer or source (such as a former employer or associate who no longer has a personal stake in the applicant's success) when any question exists. Because the ultimate goal is optimum patient care, the subjects applying for positions generally should not object to such calls being made. Discovery of a history of unsafe practices or of causing preventable anesthesia morbidity or mortality should cause careful evaluation as to whether the applicant can be appropriately assigned, trained, and supervised to be maximally safe in the proposed new environment.

In all cases without exception, all new personnel of all types in an anesthesia practice environment must be given a thorough orientation and check-out. Policy, procedures, and equipment may be unfamiliar to even the most thoroughly trained, experienced, and safe practitioner. This may occasionally seem tedious, but it is both sound and critically important safety policy. Being in the midst of a crisis situation caused by unfamiliarity with a new setting is not the optimal orientation session.

2. Hospital. There are checklists for the requirements for the granting of medical staff privileges by hospitals.[19,20] Verification of a valid license to practice, medical school graduation, residency training, board certification status, and prior disciplinary action is properly the responsibility of the administration of the hospital, facility, or institution or the medical staff executive department. Usually included, where applicable, are verification of prior hospital privileges and current malpractice insurance (often with minimum prescribed policy liability limits). Even though the state licensing mechanism should theoretically detect any discrepancies, it may be advisable for the institution itself to actually verify these basic credentials. Court decisions in which the hospital was found liable for negligence for failing to discover false statements on the application for privileges of a negligent physician[20] illustrate the key role in patient protection expected of the hospital.

Many states now have reporting requirements that obligate health care facilities to inform the designated state authority (often the medical licensing body) of the occurrence of any of a list of circumstances involving practitioners. Certain major complications and adverse patient outcomes usually are included. Any peer-review action, especially disciplinary findings and suspension, revocation, or modification of clinical privileges, along with knowledge of proved or suspected impairment are always included. Obviously, in states with these laws, it is an integral component of the credentialing process (either granting or renewal of privileges) for the parties involved to check with the state mechanism for any relevant information concerning the applicant.

Potentially even more important is the recent (August 1990) activation of the National Practitioner Data Bank (NPDB). This federal mechanism is one of the responses to all the issues raised above. It particularly is intended to prevent questionable physicians from fleeing a series of adverse events in one state (or many states), concealing their history from another state's licensing authority, and then setting up shop in the new state with the significant potential to continue to generate adverse medical events in a new unsuspecting patient population. The NPDB depends on the reporting of information by all state licensing boards and all medical malpractice insurers. The information collected at the national level would then be available from the NPDB to peer-review components of professional societies, health care facilities of all types, and state licensing boards and to plaintiffs' attorneys in certain limited circumstances involving claims against hospitals. This latter point is related in part to the fact that federal law *requires* hospitals to request information from the NPDB concerning each person appointed to the medical staff or granted clinical privileges. The states and the malpractice insurers report these types of information: (1) indemnity payments made as a result of malpractice claims, (2) adverse privilege actions taken by a health care entity, and (3) licensure actions taken by state authorities. Practitioners themselves have the right to both dispute the accuracy of entries into their NPDB files and to see their own files. In addition to the obvious risk management benefits of hospitals checking this database as part of their credentialing process, it also will be wise for practitioners to verify that their own files are correct so as to prevent any inaccurate negative information being circulated.

Periodic renewal of institutional clinical privileges also involves an obligation to evaluate and verify the competence of the subject practitioner. This process actually may be more important, albeit for different reasons, in the total scheme of health care delivery than the granting of initial privileges. However, renewals all too frequently are essentially automatic, receiving little of the indicated attention or, often, dependent totally on the department chairman's recommendation, which could in some rare circumstances be driven by motives other than optimum patient care. Again, judicious checking of statements on applications for renewal and of any relevant peer review information is required. Groups of physicians or administrators responsible for evaluating hospital staff members and reviewing their privileges are appropriately concerned about retaliatory legal action by a staff member denied renewal. Such evaluating groups must be objective (with total elimination of any hint of political or financial motive) and as close to certain as possible, with documentation, that the staff person whose privileges would be revoked practices below standard and is a danger to patients. Believing this, such groups and individuals within facilities are not only justified in revoking privileges, but also must do so or run the serious risk of being named additional codefendants in any subsequent malpractice action against those in question. Court decisions demonstrate that a hospital can be found liable if the incompetence of a staff member was known or should have been known and was not acted upon.[20] Further, there is an ethical obligation, however difficult to carry out, ultimately to protect the patients' best interests in such situations.

3. State. Specific requirements for medical licensing vary from state to state, but all states focus on the basic credentials of education, postgraduate training, and personal qualifications. For the reasons outlined above, there is now widespread a more thorough verification of claimed credentials. As noted, consequent inconvenience must be accepted as the cost of increased concern about the potential for harm from incompetent or dishonest practitioners.

A relatively recent major involvement of state medical licensing is mandated continuing medical education (CME).[21] Many states specify the number of hours of CME credits that must be obtained, including distribution among categories. Documented CME credits within one's declared specialty may be mandated as well as specific requirements for study of risk-management and patient-safety material. The effectiveness of such programs, especially as they relate to objective indices of patient care outcome, has yet to be thoroughly evaluated.

Currently, the area of state involvement in RM issues receiving the most attention is discipline of incompetent, substance-dependent, and criminal physicians. As noted, many states have reporting requirements specifying that any action taken against a practitioner by a group, department, or health care facility be reported to the state licensing or disciplining authority. In some circumstances, this would include discovery of or treatment for substance dependency. State boards often believe that an independent inquiry by an investigator not from the subject's own workplace can yield the most objective evaluation of fitness to practice. It is very difficult to gauge the effectiveness of such efforts toward the laudable long-term goal of reducing preventable patient morbidity and mortality. However, there have been clear examples in which flagrantly unsafe practitioners have properly had medical licenses revoked. In response to the extant pressures, it is likely that state authorities will continue to increase activity in this area.

4. *Specialty boards and societies.* Of the 23 recognized medical specialty boards, 17 (as of this writing) require some manner of periodic recertification of their diplomates. Many of the recertification programs are relatively recent such as the American College of Surgeons, which conducted its first examination in 1987), and it is likely that it will be some time before a successful attempt is made to assess the impact of such programs on the quality of care delivered or on patient care outcome. As of this writing, the American Board of Anesthesiology (ABA) has announced its intention to start a new program in 1992. This will not be a formal recertification because the original achievement of board certification is considered permanent. Rather the proposal is for a certificate of continuing demonstration of qualifications (CDQ) to be issued by the ABA. Participation will be voluntary and the award of the certificate will culminate a multistep process involving demonstration of valid licensure, freedom from chemical dependence, appropriate clinical case load, competence in the eyes of the department head or supervisor, and current clinical knowledge as demonstrated on a written examination covering both general topics in anesthesia and specialty topics in areas chosen by the applicant from a list of subspecialty interests (such as pediatric, cardiac, obstetric, pain, and intensive care). Whether obtaining this certificate eventually becomes an issue in demonstration of clinical competence during defense against a malpractice action remains to be seen.

Several specialty societies require relevant CME participation.[21] Although the American Society of Anesthesiologists (ASA) offers a large number of extensive CME activities (some directly concerning RM), there is as yet no formal requirement for participation as a condition of membership.

One extremely valuable program available through many state societies of anesthesiology and even, if necessary, involving the ASA is the peer review assessment of an anesthesia group or department. When there are significant RM questions, a group or department may seek (or even be advised to seek) external input and advice from an objective team of volunteer peer reviewers sponsored by the appropriate professional society. In such cases, the suggestions from such a team (offered in a noncritical, nonthreatening manner) can help initiate or enhance RM activities intended to maximize the quality of anesthesia care rendered.

5. *Clinical privileges.* The credentialing process leads ultimately to the granting of initial or renewal clinical privileges to practice in a given setting. The privilege-granting entity or person in a hospital (or facility with anesthesia services) almost always cannot fully evaluate the clinical credentials of an applicant for privileges in anesthesia and must rely on anesthesiologists, usually internal but sometimes outside the institution, for evaluation of clinical competence. How should this evaluation be made? The potential pitfalls of references are mentioned above. However, if an evaluator personally knows a co-worker or supervisor of an applicant, a judicious inquiry should produce valuable information. In the absence of this type of "inside" contact, questions often arise as how best to be certain of an applicant's competence. Most institutions have a mechanism of granting provisional privileges for some trial period during which the clinical practice of the applicant will be observed firsthand before a final decision on granting privileges is made. Before any offer of a position is extended, some institutions now ask an applicant to visit for a day or longer to assume the role essentially of a trainee and render clinical care under the immediate, direct, one-to-one supervision of an evaluating staff member. The wisdom and value of such programs remains to be seen.

A central issue today in the granting of clinical privileges, especially in procedure-oriented specialties, is whether it is reasonable to continue the common practice of approving blanket privileges. These, in effect, authorize the practitioner to attempt any treatment or procedure normally considered in the province of the applicant's medical specialty. Questions surrounding these considerations may have political and economic implications, such as which type of surgeon should be doing carotid endarterectomies or lumbar discectomies. Much more important, however, is whether the practitioner being considered is really qualified to do everything covered by his or her specialty. Specifically, should the granting of privileges to practice anesthesia automatically approve the practitioner to do pediatric cardiac cases, critically ill newborns (such as a 2-day-old baby with a large diaphragmatic hernia), ablative pain therapy (such as an alcohol celiac plexus block under fluoroscopy), or high-risk obstetric cases? These questions raise the issue of procedure-specific or limited privileges. The risk management considerations in this question are strong if practitioners who are not really qualified or experienced enough are allowed, or even expected because of peer or scheduling pressures, to undertake major challenges for which they are not prepared. The likelihood of complications will be increased and the difficulty of defending the practitioner against a malpractice claim in the event of a catastrophe is significantly increased.

There is no clear answer on the question of procedure-specific privileges. Ignoring issues of qualifications has clear negative potential. On the other hand, total adoption of such a system likely would soon result in an anesthesia department or group divided into many small "fiefdoms" with consequent further atrophy of clinical skills outside one's specific area or areas. This is both anti-intellectual and stifling for the individual as well as a disservice to the profession and its future. Each anesthesia department or group will need to address these issues. At the very least, the common practice of every applicant for new or renewal privileges checking off each and every line on the printed list of anesthesia procedures should be reviewed.

B. Peer review organizations

Professional standards review organizations (PSRO) were established in 1972 as utilization-review and quality-assurance overseers of the care of federally subsidized patients (Medicare and Medicaid). Despite their efforts to deal with quality of care, these groups largely were seen by all involved as primarily interested in cost containment. A variety of negative factors led to the PSRO being replaced in 1984 with the peer review organization (PRO).[22] There is a PRO in each state, most being associated with a state medical association. The objectives of a PRO include 14 statements related to hospital admissions (including the shifting of care

to an outpatient basis as much as possible) and five related to quality of care (including the reduction of avoidable deaths and avoidable postoperative or other complications). The PROs comprise full-time support staff and physician reviewers paid as consultants or directors. Ideally, PRO monitoring will discover suboptimal care, and this will lead to specific recommendations for improvement in quality. There is a perception that the quality of care efforts are hampered by the lack of realistic objectives and also that these PRO groups, like others before them, will largely or entirely function to limit the cost of health care services.[22] National physician groups such as the American Medical Association are suspicious enough of the intentions of these groups to establish PRO-monitoring programs.

Aside from the as-yet-unrealized potential for quality improvement efforts, the most likely interaction between the local PRO and an anesthesia provider will surround a request for perioperative admission of a patient whose care is mandated to be outpatient surgery. This frequently will also be a RM issue. If the anesthesiologist believes, for example, that either (1) preoperative admission for treatment to optimize cardiac, pulmonary, diabetic, or other medical status or (2) postoperative admission for monitoring of labile situations such as uncontrolled hypertension will diminish clear anesthetic risk or risks for the patient, then an application to the PRO for approval of admission must be made and vigorously supported. All too often, however, such issues surface a day or two before the scheduled procedure in a preanesthesia screening clinic or even in a preoperative holding area outside the operating room on the day of surgery. This will continue to occur until anesthesiologists educate their constituent surgeon community as to what types of associated medical conditions may disqualify a proposed patient from the outpatient (ambulatory) surgical schedule. If adequate notice is given by the surgeon, as at the time a case is scheduled for the operating room, the patient can be seen far enough in advance by an anesthesiologist to allow appropriate planning.

When the first awareness of a patient with a complex medical problem is 1 or 2 days preoperatively, the anesthesiologist can try to have the procedure postponed, if possible and reasonable, or he or she can undertake the time-consuming task of multiple telephone calls to obtain the surgeon's agreement and PRO approval and make the necessary arrangements. Because neither alternative is particularly attractive, particularly from administrative and reimbursement perspectives, there may be a strong temptation to "let it slide" and try to deal with the patient as an outpatient even though this may be questionable from the RM viewpoint. Because anesthesia-related untoward outcome is generally rare, it is probably likely that there would be no adverse result, yet the patient would be exposed to an avoidable risk. Because of both the workings of probability and the inevitable tendency to let sicker and sicker patients slip by as the lax practitioners repeatedly "get away with it" and are lulled into a false sense of security, sooner or later there will be an unfortunate outcome or some preventable major complication or even death.

The situation is even worse when the first contact with such a patient is immediately preoperative on the day of surgery. There may be intense pressure from the patient, the surgeon, and also even the operating room administrator and staff to proceed with a case for which the anesthesiologist believes the patient is poorly prepared. The arguments made regarding patient inconvenience and anxiety are valid. However, these should not outweigh the best medical interests of the patient. Although this is a point in favor of evaluating all outpatients before the day of surgery, the anesthesiologist facing this situation on the day of operation should state clearly to all concerned the reasons for postponing the surgery, stressing the issue of avoidable risk, and then help with alternative arrangements (including, if necessary, dealing with the PRO).

The other side of risk management considerations is that of liability exposure. Particularly regarding questions of postoperative admission of ambulatory patients whose condition has been unstable in some worrisome manner, it is an extremely poor defense against a malpractice claim to state that the patient was discharged home only later to suffer a complication because the PRO deemed that operative procedure outpatient and not inpatient surgery. As bureaucratically annoying as it may be, it is a prudent RM strategy to admit the patient if there is any legitimate question, thus minimizing the chance for any complication, and later haggle with the PRO or directly with the involved third-party payer. Recalling the great desirability of avoiding malpractice claims, one will understand that such situations constitute a classic application of the old axiom about a gram of prevention being worth a kilo of cure.

C. Policy, procedures, and standards of practice

Developing written policies and procedures often is perceived by medical practitioners as merely more bureaucratic drudgery. This is much less likely to be so for a practitioner who has turned to a detailed, carefully thought-out procedure manual during an actual or impending emergency and found the necessary information to deal with a problem or even prevent an untoward patient care outcome. It is true that the Joint Commission on Accreditation of Healthcare Organizations (JCAHO) requires a policy and procedure manual for anesthesia services within a hospital.[23] This should not, however, be the driving force behind this potentially very useful compendium.

1. Policy and procedure manuals. The first benefit of creating or updating a policy and procedure manual is that it forces those doing it to think about the topics being covered. Multiple examples are possible, but all anesthesiologists are probably aware of at least one instance in which some long-standing routine in a hospital ("That's the way we've always done it") was finally reviewed as a manual was being updated for an impending JCAHO visit. The routine was found not only badly out of date and possibly inappropriate, but also potentially dangerous. After the routine was changed, all involved noted the improvement and stated that the old way was "an accident waiting to happen." Such reviews should occur whenever needed but should be done annually and then particularly thoroughly every 3 years.

The major purpose of having such a written manual in any environment where anesthesia services are provided is to provide an instantly available source of suggestions, guidelines, recommendations, and standards for both the technical skills and the professional conduct of the anesthesia practitioners. There will always be the necessary caveats that specific circumstances differ and the involved practitioners will apply their judgment at any given time along with the outlines provided in the manual.

There are examples of topics that likely would be included in a policy and procedure manual.[24] Combining these with an overview of the intended procedure, the manual logically is divided into two parts: organization and procedural.

Included in the organizational component is the delineation of privileges and responsibilities of and expectations for all involved personnel: that is, the chief or director of anesthesia, the clinical director if different, deputy or division directors, if any, attending staff physicians, resident and fellow physicians, other trainees, certified registered nurse anesthetists, physician assistants, monitoring technicians, equipment engineers or technicians, perfusionists, respiratory therapists, chest therapists, and any others. Immediately associated with this should be a communications section with the verified addresses, telephone and pager numbers, and details of how to reach all personnel associated with the group or department. The intent is to minimize difficulty when help is being sought. Critically important is the delineation of call responsibilities (not a call schedule), a detailed listing of what is expected of a staff member when on one of the various levels of call with regard to presence within the institution at what hours, the telephone availability, pager availability, maximum permissible distance from the institution, and so on. Included also is what is expected from each call person (for example, "second call" covers obstetrics from within the hospital from noon until the next 8 AM unless allowed to take a telephone call from home by the "first call" anesthesiologist staying in the hospital). It is vital to have all such duties spelled out clearly, prospectively, in writing. Unfortunately, this often becomes a key element in the aftermath of an accident in which, it is charged, the appropriate personnel were not available or could not be found. The risk management implications are clear: (1) qualified help should be available through an agreed-upon mechanism, which will help optimize care and reduce complications, and (2) it would be extraordinarily unfortunate after a catastrophe to find members of a department or group pointing fingers at each other trying to shift responsibility and thus blame for the emergency call that was not answered.

Also included in the organizational component of policy and procedure is a clear explanation of the orientation and check-out procedure for new personnel, continuing medical education requirements and opportunities, mechanism of evaluation of all personnel and of communication of this evaluation to them, disaster plans (or reference to a separate disaster manual or protocol), quality assurance activities of the department including membership of any standing committees responsible, and the format for statistical record keeping (number of procedures, types of anesthetics given, types of patients anesthetized, number and type of invasive monitoring, number and type of responses to emergency calls, and so on).

The procedural component of policy and procedure gives specific outlines of proposed courses of action for particular circumstances. Frequently, there are copies of, reference to, or paraphrase of the statements, guidelines, and standards appearing in the back of the *ASA Directory of Members*. Also included are references to or specific protocols for the areas mentioned in the JCAHO standards:[23] preanesthetic evaluation, immediate preinduction reevaluation, safety of the patient during the anesthetic period, release of the patient from any postanesthesia care unit, recording of all pertinent events during anesthesia, recording of postanesthesia visits, guidelines defining the role of anesthesia services in hospital infection control, and guidelines for safe use of general anesthetic agents. In addition, a partial list of other appropriate topics includes:

1. Recommendations for preanesthesia apparatus check-out, as from the United States Food and Drug Administration (FDA)
2. Guidelines for minimal monitoring: infant, child, adult, in the postanesthesia care unit (PACU)
3. Procedure for transport of patients to the operating room, to the PACU, to the intensive care unit (ICU)
4. Policy on ambulatory surgical patients: screening, use of regional anesthesia, discharge home
5. Policy on same-day admissions
6. Policy on recovery room admission and discharge
7. Policy on ICU admission and discharge
8. Policy on physicians responsible for writing orders in the PACU and the ICU
9. Policy on informed consent
10. Policy on the participation of patients in clinical research
11. Guidelines for the support of cadaver organ donors and its termination
12. Guidelines on environmental safety including pollution with trace gases and electrical equipment inspection, maintenance, and hazard prevention
13. Procedure for exchanging personnel during an anesthetic
14. Procedure for the introduction of new equipment, drugs, or clinical practices
15. Procedure for epidural and spinal opioid administration and subsequent patient monitoring (such as type, minimum time)
16. Procedure for initial treatment of cardiac or respiratory arrest
17. Policy on a patient's refusal of blood or blood products including the mechanism to obtain a court order to transfuse
18. Procedure for the management of malignant hyperthermia
19. Procedure for the induction and maintenance of barbiturate coma
20. Procedure for evaluation of suspected pseudocholinesterase deficiency

Individual departments or groups will add to the aforementional suggestions as dictated by their specific needs. A thorough, carefully conceived policy and procedure manual is a valuable RM tool. Many of the components are intended to mandate or encourage practices that will prevent untoward events (such as unfamiliarity with a new anesthesia machine when called "stat." for an emergency case), will help the management of crisis (such as malignant hyperthermia), or will encourage communication in difficult situations (such as refusal of blood). Ideally, each staff member of a group or department would review the manual at least annually and sign off in a log indicating current familiarity with the policies and procedures.

2. Standards of practice. Many elements of policy and procedure could be considered local "standards of practice." Some institutions actively avoid the term "standards" because of the potential medicolegal implications, especially if there is an untoward outcome of practices carried out in a manner other than that contained in the policy and procedure manual. The medicolegal importance of the "standard of care" tends to reinforce the perception that, once promulgated, standards may dictate mandatory practice. Some departments deliberately promote this perception as part of risk management efforts. As detailed above, the Harvard Medical School developed "standards of practice" for minimal intraoperative monitoring for its nine component hospital departments[3] and labeled them standards specifically to emphasize that the practices are perceived as so important as to be mandatory. The same type of thinking was involved when the ASA adopted as national policy "Standards for Basic Intra-operative Monitoring," which includes specifications for the presence of personnel during an anesthetic and for continual evaluation of oxygenation, ventilation, circulation, and temperature.[24] Similarly, several other areas of anesthesia practice are covered by subsequent ASA standards.[24]

The minimal monitoring standards, for example, are "process" standards in that they prescribe actions and are met by carrying out these actions. At various levels (hospital, local, state, national), additional efforts at improving patient care are leading to promulgation of process "standards" or regulations that are mandatory. One of the most detailed examples is the body of regulations issued by the New Jersey State Department of Health in 1989.[25]

Another type of standard is that for "outcome." Hypothetical examples include the statements that "the number of patients experiencing myocardial infarction intraoperatively or within 24 hours of operation should not exceed 0.5% of those anesthetized," or "the number of ambulatory surgical patients experiencing unplanned admission to the hospital for reasons related to the anesthesia should not exceed 1.0% of those outpatients anesthetized." Regulatory and accrediting agencies are moving toward the imposition of such standards. The JCAHO has gone through several versions of a proposed list of outcome indicators for anesthesia care. The overall intention is to encourage the identification of clinical practices that lead to adverse outcome and their replacement with alternatives that will lead to meeting the standards. If realized, this sequence of events should have the additional risk management benefit of reducing preventable morbidity and mortality.

D. Equipment: maintenance and records

Compared to human error, overt equipment failure is relatively very rare as a cause of critical incidents during anesthesia[7] or anesthesia-associated deaths,[26] though anesthesia apparatus problems have been well studied.[27-29] There is a widespread belief that most equipment-related problems in anesthesia (aside from clear human error such as misuse or unfamiliarity) could be prevented by correct maintenance and servicing of the apparatus.

When there is a major equipment failure that, if undetected, would lead to patient harm, the monitoring procedures outlined in the preceding section should detect the development of an untoward situation. If one assumes an appropriate response from the anesthetist (which may even mean completely detaching the patient from the anesthetic-delivery system and ventilator and ventilating with a hand resuscitator bag until a new anesthesia machine can be secured), there should be no adverse patient result. However, there is still occasional damage to a patient from equipment failure. Therefore efforts to minimize these equipment failures must be continued and even increased.

There is an excellent published summary of a complete program for anesthesia equipment maintenance and service.[30] A distinction is made between failure attributable to progressive deterioration of equipment, which should be preventable because it is observable and prompts appropriate action, and catastrophic failure, which often is not practical to try to predict. Emphasis is placed on preventive maintenance for mechanical parts and involves periodic performance checks every 4 to 6 months. Also, there is an annual safety inspection of each anesthetizing location covering 49 points and including the surrounding area and the immediate location as well as the equipment itself. For equipment service, there is a description of a cross-reference system to identify the piece needing service and the mechanism to secure the needed repair.

The general principles of equipment handling are straightforward. Before purchase, it must be verified that a proposed piece of equipment meets all applicable standards, which will usually automatically be true when one is dealing with recognized major manufacturers. Upon arrival, electrical equipment must be checked for absence of hazard (especially leakage current) and compliance with applicable electrical standards. Complex equipment such as anesthesia machines and ventilators should be assembled and checked out by a representative from the manufacturer or manufacturer's agent. There are potential adverse medicolegal implications of relatively untrained personnel certifying a particular piece of equipment as functioning within specification, even if they do it perfectly. It is also very important to involve the representative, if necessary, in preservice and in-service training for those who will use the new equipment. Also, upon arrival, a sheet or section in the master equipment log must be created with the make, model, serial number, and in-house identification for each individual piece of equipment. This not only allows immediate identification of any equipment involved in a future recall or product alert, but also serves as the permanent repository of the record of every problem, problem resolution, maintenance, and servicing occurring until that particular piece is scrapped. This log must be kept up to date at all times. There have been rare but frightening examples of potentially lethal problems with anesthesia machines leading to product-alert notices requiring immediate identification of certain equipment and its service status.

The question of who should maintain and service anesthesia equipment has been widely debated and has significant risk management implications. The point about equipment setup and check-out is above. After that, some groups or departments rely on "factory" service representatives for all attention to equipment, whereas others engage independent service contractors, and still other (usually larger) departments have access to personnel (either engineers or technicians) in their institution, their own department, or a separate bioengineering or medical engineering department within the facility. Needs and resources differ. The single underlying tenet is simple: the person doing preventive maintenance and service must be qualified. Anesthesia practitioners may wonder how they can assess qualification. The best way is to unhesitatingly ask pertinent questions about the education, training, and experience of those involved, including asking for references and speaking to supervisors and managers responsible for those doing the work. Whether an engineering technician who spent a week at a course at a factory can perform the most complex repairs depends on a variety of factors that can be investigated by the practitioners ultimately using the equipment in the care of patients. Failure to be involved in this oversight manner exposes the practitioner to increased liability in the event of an untoward outcome associated with improperly maintained or serviced equipment.

Aside from preventive maintenance and servicing, there must be adequate day-to-day clinical maintenance of equipment. In this era of great emphasis on cost containment, it seems anesthesia technicians are a popular target for budget cutters. It is false economy to reduce these personnel below the number genuinely needed to retrieve, clean, sort, disassemble, sterilize, reassemble, store, and distribute the wherewithal of daily anesthesia practice. Inadequate service in this area truly creates "an accident waiting to happen." An improperly installed canister of carbon dioxide absorbent is only one of multiple possible examples of sources of potential danger from inadequate routine technical support.

When anesthesia equipment becomes obsolete and should be replaced is another problem difficult to solve. Replacement of obsolete anesthesia machines and monitoring equipment is one key element of a risk-modification program.[13] Ten years is cited as an estimated useful life for an anesthesia machine. Certainly, anesthesia machines much more than 10 years of age do not meet the safety standards now in force for new machines (such as vaporizer lockout and fresh gas ratio protection included in gas machine standards in 1979) and do not incorporate the new technology that has advanced very rapidly during the 1980s, much of it being directly referable to the effort to prevent untoward incidents. Further, there is every indication that this technology will continue to advance and appear in the equipment at the same time or even at an accelerated rate in the future. Notice that some anesthesia equipment manufacturers, anxious to minimize their own potential liability, have refused to support (with parts and service) some of the oldest of their pieces (particularly gas machines) still in use. This is a very strong message to practitioners that such equipment must be replaced as soon as possible.

Last, should equipment fail, it must be removed from service and a replacement substituted. Groups or departments are obligated to have sufficient backup equipment to cover any reasonable incidence of failure . The equipment removed from service must be clearly marked with a prominent label (so it is not returned into service by a well-meaning technician or practitioner) containing the date, time, person discovering, and the details of the problem. The responsible personnel must be notified so that they can remove the equipment, make an entry in the log, and initiate the repair. As indicated below in the section on response to an adverse event, a piece of equipment involved or suspected in an anesthesia accident must be immediately sequestered and not touched by anybody, particularly not by any equipment service personnel. If a severe accident occurred, it may be necessary for the equipment in question to be inspected at a specific alter time by a group consisting of qualified representatives of the manufacturer, the service personnel, the plaintiff's attorney, the insurance companies involved, and the practitioner's defense attorney. Also, major equipment problems should be reported to the Medical Device Problem Reporting System of the United States FDA via the Device Experience Network (telephone 1-800-638-6725).[31] This system accepts voluntary reports from users and requires reports from manufacturers when there is knowledge of a medical device being involved in a serious incident. Application of all the principles outlined here should help minimize or even prevent equipment-related adverse outcomes of anesthesia.

E. Informed consent

It is a clear underlying principle that a patient has the right to exercise control over his or her own body and must therefore consent to proposed treatments or procedures.[19] The issue of treatment in the absence of any consent at all (for whatever reason but usually because of gross misunderstandings) involves potential claims by the patient of assault and battery. This is relatively rare and much less likely to involve anesthesia providers than the issue of informed consent would. Informed consent is obtained by a discussion of the potential risks and benefits of a proposed treatment or procedure and any available alternatives and then ascertainment that the patient (or the patient's agent in the cases of a child or an incompetent person) understands and agrees to what is being proposed.

There may still be some residual debate as to whether there needs to be a separate informed consent for the anesthesia for a planned surgical operation or whether consent to the operation implies consent for the anesthesia. In many if not most centers now, anesthesia providers obtain a separate informed consent because there are wholly separate identifiable "material risks" associated with the anesthetic independent of the surgery. It is inadequate to expect the surgeon to fully discuss the anesthetic and, particularly, any special implications for anesthesia of the patient's medical condition. Anesthesia providers do not perform surgery and cannot obtain a genuine informed surgical consent. Likewise, the surgeons are not anesthesiologists and simply do not have the training and experience to discuss the plans and risks of the anesthesia care.

In obtaining informed consent for anesthesia, the question arises as to what risks should be disclosed to the patient during the discussion. There needs to be a balance between giving enough information to allow a reasoned decision and frightening the patient with a long list of potential, extremely rare, severe complications, the latter making a trusting, friendly doctor-patient working relationship very difficult. In times past, the standard was that there should be the disclosure of risks that any reasonable physician would believe appropriate. This doctrine has been significantly altered over time to that involving the "reasonable person" (patient) and now centers on the concept of material risk. A material risk "is one that the physician knows or ought to know would be significant to a reasonable person in the patient's position of deciding whether or not to submit to a particular medical treatment or procedure."[19] The landmark *Harnish* decision[32] stated that *all* risks must be disclosed to the patient in order to obtain informed consent. The equally important subsequent *Precourt* decision[33] added the qualification that there need not be disclosure of every conceivable remotely possible complication whose severity or incidence is "negligible." The decision stressed balancing the patient's right to know with fairness to physicians and avoiding "unrealistic and unnecessary burdens on practitioners."[34]

When the issue of informed consent for anesthesia arises, it unfortunately usually involves questions about the occurrence of rare but devastating complications such as severe neurologic damage or death. Whether the risk of these complications is considered "negligible" in a legal context remains to be determined. Therefore there is no firm guideline as to whether it is wise to tell all patients that general anesthesia might lead to anoxic brain damage or death or that regional anesthesia could cause permanent paralysis. It is possible, however, to state that all anesthesia procedures have some risks, including risks of injury and death, just like riding in a car or crossing the street. Most patients can identify with this analogy and are not threatened by it. Questions as to specific complications prompted by this statement, of course, should be answered. Statistics can be cited to give perspective. Again, patients understand when told that the risk of death or grave injury from an anesthetic for a healthy patient is far less than that from riding in an automobile during the normal course of a year. Any special risks attendant to the patient's medical or surgical condition should be discussed in more detail.

Consent is a state of mind achieved through the establishment of an understanding. It is not an act such as the signing of one's name. Many anesthesia practitioners ask patients to sign a consent form that often has on it a long list of potential complications and any specific additional risks for that particular patient. This is an accepted, reasonable practice. However, both anesthetist and patient must understand that no matter what the form says, it does not release the anesthetist from liability. The form is one way to document that an informed consent discussion took place, but it does not limit the patient's right to later make a claim in the event of an accident. Whether the form is used or a note is written out in the patient's chart (or both), there must be a clear record (created after the discussion) that a discussion took place and that informed consent was obtained. Verbal consent alone is not enough when there is a later question.

In certain life-threatening, emergency circumstances, it may be necessary to administer anesthesia without consent. Case law recognizes this, and the requirements outlined above are necessarily modified. In such an event, it is advisable to write a note in the chart as soon as possible about the necessity to go ahead and also to notify the hospital administrator or counsel, or both, about the situation.

Obtaining genuine informed consent must not be a perfunctory bureaucratic irritation. It is an integral component of the anesthetist-patient relationship. It essentially forces discussion of important issues. Further, the fact today is that it is commonplace for plaintiffs' attorneys to charge lack of informed consent in virtually any case of an unexpected poor patient outcome. Although the charge cannot be avoided,

careful attention to the principles detailed here should be able functionally to eliminate concerns about inadequate informed consent for anesthesia care.

F. Record keeping

It would be difficult to begin to count the number of anesthesia malpractice cases that have been lost, even when there probably was no malpractice, because of inadequate, incomplete, or illegible anesthesia records. The anesthesia chart is the cornerstone of all the information about an anesthetic case for risk management purposes. The old dictum "If you didn't write it down, it didn't happen" is still very much applicable in a medicolegal sense. Even the very best anesthetic care cannot be defended, or even referred to, if there is no clear record that such care took place. "If the record hardly exists, . . . it is tantamount to an outright confession, in the eyes of the law, to careless practice."[35]

Documentation of the preanesthetic evaluation is all too often weak or inadequate in cases of malpractice claims against anesthesiologists. The guiding principles regarding what should be recorded are very simple. The practitioner should document all the information necessary for another anesthesia provider to pick up the chart and quickly obtain a complete enough picture to safely and intelligently conduct the anesthetic. One good way to think of it is for the anesthesiologist doing the evaluation to project him- or herself into the role of picking up the chart and then include everything he or she would want to see. Further, the preoperative evaluation should contain some evidence of the thinking associated with the evaluation. Assigning an ASA Physical Status value is a start. Recording any unusual or dangerous conditions and how these influence plans and risks is mandatory. In all cases, some type of statement about the anesthetic plan (or possible alternatives if the plan is not final) is necessary. Again, it is unfortunate but true that the best possible care may not appear so in the record without some appropriate effort to document what went into that care. Even when thorough notes are written, it is of no help if they cannot be read. All notes must be *dated* and *timed* and made as legible as humanly possible.

A helpful review of the reasoning behind and the elements of the intraoperative anesthesia record[36] cites a study in which 95% of respondent anesthetists believed it important to keep anesthetic records and 74% included medicolegal protection among the reasons given for doing so. Aside from the potential legal uses, an excellent way of approaching the record is to try to do two things: (1) create a legible record of "all pertinent events" (required by JCAHO)[23] and of what went on surrounding the anesthetic and (2) have a compendium of all the salient features (history, allergies, chronic medications, acute medications, positioning, monitoring used, reasons for special monitoring, events, and the patient's responses to these and all factors) in as complete a manner as you would like to see them were you to be the next person, new to the patient, to give anesthesia. Virtually all facilities in which anesthesia is given have a preprinted form that will allow accomplishment of these goals. The only real points about the form are that it should be legible, be as easy as possible to use, encourage completeness, and be reviewed frequently by those using it to see if revision would improve it.

There are now available electronic, computer assisted or driven devices to aid in the maintenance of intraoperative anesthesia records.[37-39] Noninvasive or invasive monitors may be connected to these computers so that vital signs, fractional inspired oxygen (F_IO_2), expired volume and ventilation rate, arterial oxygen saturation (Sao_2), and end-tidal CO_2 ($ETco_2$) are automatically recorded (with no possibility to edit) at preset time intervals. Sensors that would automatically record gas flows and volatile agents and infusions used are being developed. Other drugs and fluids given, blood lost, and events noted can be keyed in by the anesthetist (though alternatives such as light pen or voice could potentially be used).[36,40] The instrument will automatically record the time of the entry, even if its operator states in the entry that an event or action took place at some past time. Studies on the efficacy and desirability of these automated records are being conducted. Proponents state that the technology allows more time to focus on the patient and that a genuinely complete record of vital signs and so on will give a truer picture of events and trends that should aid in evaluation of poor outcome, usually by demonstrating the absence of untoward intraoperative events and also the wide range of normal vital signs that often is "smoothed out" on handwritten records. Others however state that automatic sampling may miss trends by picking up and recording transient major variations and even may record erroneous, grossly incorrect values caused by mechanical or electrical artifact, thus exposing the anesthesiologist later to unjustified charges in the event of a poor outcome. Acceptance and utilization of this technology will depend on the resolution of this typical risk-benefit ratio

question and the ability to both justify and meet the significant capital cost of these instruments.

In the use of any record-keeping method for any anesthetic, a few basics are always true. Medications and vital signs should be recorded contemporaneously and should be entered first when there are many things to record, such as immediately after induction. Descriptive information, important as it is, can wait a moment. During the maintenance phase of the anesthetic, vital signs should be recorded at least every 5 minutes. Numeric values from instruments such as the pulse oximeter, capnograph, spirometer, mass spectrometer, and any other monitoring devices should be recorded at appropriate intervals. It is completely inadequate to note only that these or other devices were used. The generated information must be recorded both for reference (during or after the case) and to prove that the anesthetist was aware of what transpired during the anesthetic usage.

Postoperative documentation is critical in anesthesia risk management. Aside from the fact that it is a JCAHO requirement to see patients in follow-up observation, it is simply good anesthesia care. It also broadens and deepens the relationship with the patient, which is necessarily transient, thus making less likely misunderstanding or misplaced hostility about the outcome of the surgery. Leaving a positive impression can be the key element, for example, in the avoidance of being named a codefendant in a malpractice action against the surgeon. More important, however, is the opportunity to discover any complications or issues with the patient. If one assumes that most of these will be minor, they can be dealt with on the spot, thus eliminating any chance they will grow out of proportion if neglected. It is reasonable to ask the patients what they remember about the operative experience (not directly whether they had recall during general anesthesia), if they were hoarse, if the IV catheter and so on hurt, while also examining the chart and patient for more serious problems. Obviously, the patients' responses should be entered into a postoperative note along with some comment about current status (always including vital signs) and the anesthetist's assessment such as: "No apparent postanesthetic complications. Appears to be doing well."

Should there be an adverse event, with or even without patient injury, a complete account of the facts and, when appropriate, impressions and opinions should go on the chart as soon as possible. One important caution, however, is that the entry thus made must not be influenced by the heat of the moment, by guilt, by the desire to imply blame or innocence on the part of any person, or by the general disorganization that may accompany a significant event. It may be wise for one to seek advice from an objective person, perhaps a co-worker not involved in the case, while recording the account of the event. The one single most important thing in all such cases is to never, ever change the existing record. No matter what is on it, the actual record is better than an altered one. However excellent the anesthetic care may have been, alteration of the record absolutely guarantees the complete inability to defend against any charges, however unjustified they might be. If there is a need to explain, elaborate on, or fill in gaps in the record, it should be done as soon as practical by a dated and timed amendment note in the patient chart. Obviously, the contents of such a note must be carefully thought out. It is potentially advantageous for this note also to be written in the presence of a genuinely objective witness.

Additional benefits in risk management efforts accrue from complete and legible anesthetic records. Certain of the necessary and desirable activities of both RM and quality assurance depend on the ability to retrieve and compile data about the anesthetic practice of both individuals and a group or department.

G. Meaningful morbidity and mortality conferences and continuing education

The JCAHO has a general requirement for all departments in a medical facility that there must be at least monthly meetings at which risk management and quality assurance activities are "documented and reported."[23] Most anesthesia departments, services, and groups have staff meetings or departmental conferences or rounds at least monthly and use those occasions to satisfy the JCAHO meeting requirements. It is likely that some of these meetings might satisfy the letter but not the spirit of the requirement. Having presentations of departmental cases of unusual interest or in which there was a problem and then a thorough group review and discussion of the popular question, "What would you do differently next time?" is a good start. Likewise, staff meetings at which policy, procedure, equipment, and any associated problems are discussed also would help. Inclusion of an open review of departmental statistics including *all* complications, however trivial seeming, brings the effort closer to the intention of the requirement.

Requirements aside, all the suggestions for meetings (whether called "case conference presentations," "morbidity and mortality rounds," or whatever) are intended to encourage a group of anesthetists to combine their thoughts and efforts for the common good—the minimization of untoward outcome in their anesthesia practice. This is an opportunity for application of the classic risk management process, in that future practice should be improved when the participants learn from present experience (failures and successes). The goal of minimizing future complications is obvious. Rapid devolution of a conference into a business meeting or proforma meetings hurried through by a small fraction of the staff benefit no one and waste time. A case presentation needs interactive discussion to genuinely educate.

Formal continuing medical education needs the same thoughtfulness to likewise contribute to the quality of care and the avoidance of complications. Larger groups and departments usually run their own programs, using staff members to speak about areas of their interest and expertise and also bringing in outside speakers to present either reviews of basic material or news of recent developments or ongoing research. By no means should all the presentations deal directly with anesthesia. Not only could this get tedious for even the most committed audience, but also there needs to be updated awareness on the part of anesthesiologists of both the basics and the forefront of many other medical disciplines. Such meetings are excellent opportunities, for example, for surgeons to tell of advancements in their techniques. At the same time there can also be a give-and-take discussion regarding the interrelationship of anesthesia and the surgery in question. Allowing surgeon and anesthetist to see a situation from each other's perspective can do nothing but encourage beneficial cooperation.

Smaller departments or groups need to make deliberate efforts to ensure adequate opportunity for continuing education. This might involve securing access to an accredited continuing medical education (CME) program conducted by a large medical school department and then guaranteeing sufficient time for staff to participate. Also, an additional method involves providing time and in some circumstances financial support for staff to attend local, regional, or national CME programs (either specific workshops, symposia, and "theme" meetings or the CME components of professional society meetings). Most CME requirements for licensing or certification include some acknowledgment of individual reading. Every department, service, or group, regardless of size, needs a library facility of some sort, containing as many current textbooks, manuals, and journals as is practical for the number of people involved.

H. Response to an adverse event (see also Chapter 30)

Despite rigorous application of risk management principles, it is likely that each anesthesiologist at least once in his or her professional life will be involved in a major anesthesia accident. Precisely because such an event is so rare, very few are prepared for it. It is probable that the involved personnel will have no relevant past experience regarding what to do. Although an obvious resource is a colleague who has had some exposure or experience, one may not be available.

The basic outline of an appropriate immediate response to an accident is straightforward and logical. However, unfortunately, the principle personnel involved in a significant untoward event may react with such surprise or shock as to temporarily lose sight of logic. There have been cases of major accidents in an operating room in which the responsible anesthesiologist was so stunned upon realizing what had happened that he or she became nonfunctional or, worse, left the room before help arrived.

At the moment anyone recognizes that a major anesthetic complication has occurred or is occurring, help must be called. A sufficient number of people to deal with the situation must be secured as quickly as possible. For example, in the event an esophageal intubation goes unrecognized long enough during the induction of general anesthesia to cause a cardiac arrest, the immediate need is for enough skilled personnel to conduct the resuscitative efforts, including making the correct diagnosis and replacing the tube into the trachea. Whether the anesthesiologist apparently responsible for the complication should direct the immediate remedial efforts will depend on the person and the situation. In such a circumstance, it would seem wise for a senior or supervising anesthesiologist to quickly evaluate the appropriateness of the behavior and actions of the involved party or parties and decide whether he, she, or they should be asked to step back and allow one of the responding personnel to give remedial care. Even in the heat of the moment, tact must be exercised.

In general, the primary anesthesia provider or providers should concentrate on continuing patient care. The anesthesiologist responsible for supervision of activities in that clinical area, having responded to the call for help, will become the so-called incident supervisor. This person becomes responsible for administrative and investigative activities while the primary anesthesia provider or providers and others (as needed) care for the patient. The supervisor directs the process of immediate prevention of recurrence of the problem, event documentation, and ongoing investigation.

In all circumstances, anesthesia equipment and supplies in use at the time of the untoward event, whether or not believed to be materially involved, should be sequestered under lock and key. Nothing can be altered or discarded. Equipment-support personnel should be enlisted in this effort. There may be reluctance, for example, to take an anesthesia machine out of service. This type of action is mandatory, however, until it is agreed upon by all involved that the equipment is not material to the accident investigation and can be inspected and returned to service or that it is material and plans are made for further investigation. A great many anesthesia malpractice cases have been lost because no one thought in time, for example, to save the endotracheal tube that was plugged with thick secretions thus causing the impaired ventilation.

Immediately after a nonfatal accident, comprehensive evaluation and care of the patient should be carried out quickly and efficiently. Close association and communication with the surgeon at that time and throughout subsequent events should be valuable. Further, do not hesitate to call consultants immediately. Often a cardiologist, neurologist, neurosurgeon, or nephrologist can offer constructive suggestions that might improve the patient's prognosis. It is very unfortunate when such requests are delayed and the consultant is later forced to state that "you might have had a better chance to save the _____ if only you had done _____ immediately after the incident 2 days ago."

As soon as this comprehensive care is underway, it is necessary for the personnel directly involved, often through the supervisor or anesthesia chief, to notify the facility administrator or risk manager. This person may, in turn, choose to notify the facility's malpractice insurance carrier. If different, the anesthetist's malpractice insurer should be called. Depending on the nature of the incident, the risk manager and the insurers may suggest their involvement from the very first contact with the family. If there is an involved surgeon of record, he or she probably will first notify the family, but the anesthetist and others (risk manager, insurance loss control officer or even legal counsel) might appropriately be included at the outset. Full disclosure of facts as they are best known with no confessions, opinions, speculation, or placing of blame is the best presentation throughout all dealing with the family and, when possible, the patient. Any attempt to conceal, withhold, or shade the truth will later only confound an already difficult situation. Obviously, comfort and support should be offered, including, if appropriate, the services of facility personnel such as clergy, social workers, and counselors.

The primary anesthesia provider and any others involved must document relevant information about the incident in the medical record. As noted, never change any existing entries in the record. Write an amendment note if needed with careful explanation of why amendment is necessary, particularly stressing explanations of professional judgments involved. State only facts as they are known. Make no judgments about causes or responsibility and do not use judgmental terms. The same guidelines hold true for the filing of the incident report in the facility, which should be done as soon as is practical. Further, all discussions with the patient or family should be carefully documented in the medical record.

Follow-up investigation after the immediate handling of the incident will involve the primary anesthesia provider or providers but should again be directed by a senior supervisor who may or may not be the same person as the incident supervisor on the scene at the time. The follow-up supervisor verifies the adequacy and coordination of ongoing care of the patient and facilitates communication among all involved, especially with the risk management and quality assurance personnel. Final decisions about the sequestered equipment need to be made. If it is suggested that the equipment was involved in the accident, a plan is outlined on p. 658. Last, it is necessary to verify that adequate postevent documentation is taking place.

Unpleasant as it is to contemplate, it is better to have a plan ahead of time and execute it in the event of an accident. Vigorous immediate intervention after an incident along the lines detailed here may improve the outcome for all concerned.

III. SUMMARY

An anesthesia risk management program should be a comprehensive compendium of efforts related to the topics outlined in this chapter. There will be a necessary significant intertwining of the two themes of quality of patient care and concern for liability exposure. Although many of the elements covered do include medicolegal considerations specifically directed at avoidance or minimization of malpractice claims, the primary goal is optimum patient care. In all circumstances, doing everything possible first to maximize the quality of care should help "manage" or minimize the risks of complications. Minimizing these risks, in turn, minimizes the consequent risk of malpractice claims. It is not at all wrong to have some "defensive" thinking. There is discussion in each section of the chapter concerning issues proved by experience often to be vulnerable points for anesthesia practitioners' defending against malpractice claims, how to anticipate them, and how to best conduct care so as to minimize the risk of exposure to unjustified charges. However, thinking constantly oriented solely toward potential liability issues is unnecessary, inappropriate, and extremely taxing on the practitioner.

Because anesthesia practice is facilitative rather than specifically diagnostic or therapeutic, there is very little tolerance for complications. An expectation has justifiably evolved that no patient should be harmed from anesthesia care. This attitude makes the medicolegal considerations for anesthesiologists probably more acute than for most other medical specialists. Distinguishing between a bad result attributable to the patient's disease and an iatrogenic injury can be difficult. Among the major benefits of an anesthesia risk management strategy are the expectations that the probability of both will be less. As noted, many now believe that there are fewer anesthesia incidents causing complications, though this is debated[1] and likely will continue to be so. However, it is true that some malpractice insurance companies have reduced premiums for all insured practitioners, and even more companies have reduced the risk classification and the resulting premiums specifically for anesthesiologists. Whether risk management efforts of the type outlined here have played a role in this encouraging change can never be proved definitively with "hard-science" statistics. It is the opinion of many insurance company officials and institutional risk managers that such efforts have contributed significantly to the improvement in claims experience. Because insurance actuaries are not by nature charitable people, the reductions in premiums must reflect reductions in insurance payout. Because of the nature of the legal profession today, it is highly unlikely that there are a large number of major complications or injuries that are going unrecognized by the insurance system. These facts add up to an improvement in care, particularly anesthesia care.

It is intuitively reasonable to believe that appropriately educated and trained honest anesthesia practitioners doing work for which they are qualified, under the guidance of sound thoughtful policy and procedure guidelines, using safe equipment, and keeping complete legible records (about patients who understand and consent to their procedures), while pursuing ongoing analysis and improvement of their practice through education and being constantly aware of the appropriate response in the unlikely event of an adverse incident, will give optimal care that minimizes the anesthetic risks to the patient and the medicolegal risks to the anesthesia practitioners themselves.

REFERENCES

1. Keats AS: Anesthesia mortality in perspective, Anesth Analg 71:113-119, 1990.
2. Holzer JF: Analysis of anesthetic mishaps: current concepts in risk management, Int Anesthesiol Clin 22(2):91-116, 1984.
3. Eichhorn JH, Cooper JB, Cullen DJ, et al: Standards for patient monitoring during anesthesia at Harvard Medical School, JAMA 256:1017-1020, 1986.
4. Hornbein TF: The setting of standards of care, JAMA 256:1040-1041, 1986.
5. Eichhorn JH, Cooper JB, Cullen DJ, et al: Anesthesia practice standards at Harvard: a review, J Clin Anesth 1:56-65, 1988.
6. Eichhorn JH: Prevention of intraoperative anesthesia accidents and related severe injury through safety monitoring, Anesthesiology 70:572-577, 1989.
7. Cooper JB, Newbower RS, Long CD, et al: Preventable anesthesia mishaps: a study of human factors, Anesthesiology 49:399-406, 1978.
8. Hamilton WK: Unexpected deaths during anesthesia: wherein lies the cause? Anesthesiology 50:381-383, 1979.
9. Pierce EC Jr: Analysis of anesthetic mishaps: historical perspectives, Int Anesthesiol Clin 2(2):1-16, 1984.
10. Emergency Care Research Institute: Death during general anesthesia, J Health Care Technol 1:155-175, 1985.
11. Keenan RL and Boyan CP: Cardiac arrest due to anesthesia, JAMA 253:2373-2377, 1985.
12. Keenan RL: Anesthesia disasters: incidence, causes, preventability, Semin Anesth 5:175-179, 1986.
13. Pierce EC: Risk modification in anesthesiology. In Chapman-Cliburn G, editor: Risk management and quality assurance: issues and interactions. (A special publication of the Quality Review Bulletin), pp 20-23, Chicago, 1986, Joint Commission on Accreditation of Hospitals.
14. Lunn JN, editor: Epidemiology in anesthesia, London, Baltimore, and Victoria, 1986, Edward Arnold Ltd.
15. Cohen MM, Duncan PG, Pope WDB, et al: A survey of 112,000 anaesthetics at one teaching hospital (1975-83), Can Anaesth Soc J 33:22-31, 1986.
16. Tinker JH, Dull DL, and Caplan RA: Role of monitoring devices in prevention of anesthetic mishaps: a closed claims analysis, Anesthesiology 71:541-546, 1989.
17. Caplan RA, Posner KL, Ward RJ, et al: Adverse respiratory events in anesthesia: a closed claim analysis, Anesthesiology 72:828-833, 1990.
18. Pierce EC, editor: Risk management in anesthesia, Int Anesthesiol Clin, vol 27, no 3, 1989.
19. Peters JD, Fineberg KS, Kroll DA, et al: Anesthesiol-

ogy and the law, Ann Arbor, Mich, 1983, Health Administration Press.
20. Gilbert B: Relating quality assurance to credentials and privileges. In Chapman-Cliburn G, editor: Risk management and quality assurance: issues and interactions. (A special publication of the Quality Review Bulletin), pp 79-83, Chicago, 1986, Joint Commission on Accreditation of Hospitals.
21. Osteen AM and Gannon MI: Continuing medical education, JAMA 256:1601-1604, 1986, and see also Wentz DK, Gannon MI, and Osteen AM: Continuing medical education, JAMA 264:836-840, 1990.
22. Dans PE, Weiner JP, and Otter SE: Peer review organizations: promises and potential pitfalls, N Engl J Med 313:1131-1137, 1985, and see also Peer review organizations (letters), N Engl J Med 314:1121, 1986.
23. Joint Commission on Accreditation of Healthcare Organizations: AMH/90:Accreditation manual for hospitals. Chicago, 1989, JCAHO.
24. American Society of Anesthesiologists: Peer review in anesthesiology, Park Ridge, Ill, 1989, ASA.
25. Moss E: New Jersey enacts anesthesia standards, Anesthesia Patient Safety Foundation Newsletter 4:13, 16-18, 1989.
26. Lunn JN and Mushin WW: Mortality associated with anaesthesia, London, 1982, Nuffield Provincial Hospitals Trust.
27. Rendell-Baker L, editor: Problems with anesthesia and respiratory therapy equipment, Int Anesthesiol Clin, vol 20, no 3, 1982.
28. Spooner RB and Kirby RR: Analysis of anesthetic mishaps. Equipment-related anesthetic incidents, Int Anesthesiol Clin 22(2):133-147, 1984.
29. Cooper JB, Newbower RS, and Kitz RJ: An analysis of major errors and equipment failures in anesthesia management: considerations for prevention and detection, Anesthesiology 60:34-42, 1984.
30. Duberman SM and Wald A: An integrated quality control program for anesthesia equipment. In Chapman-Cliburn G, editor: Risk management and quality assurance: issues and interactions. (A special publication of the Quality Review Bulletin), pp 105-112, Chicago, 1986, Joint Commission on Accreditation of Hospitals.
31. HHS Publ No (FDA) 85-4196, 1985, Food and Drug Administration, Center for Devices and Radiologic Health, Rockville, MD 20857.
32. *Harnish* v. *Children's Hospital Medical Center,* 387 Massachusetts 152 (1982).
33. *Precourt* v. *Frederick,* 395 Massachusetts 689 (1985).
34. Curran WJ: Informed consent in malpractice cases: a turn toward reality, N Engl J Med 314: 429-431, 1986.
35. Lunn JN: The role of the anaesthetic record. In Lunn JN, editor: Epidemiology in anesthesia, pp 136-143, London, 1986, Edward Arnold Ltd.
36. Seed RGFL: Documentation. In Lunn JN, editor: Epidemiology in anesthesia, pp 144-158, London, 1986, Edward Arnold Ltd.
37. Gravenstein JS, Newbower RS, Ream AK, and Smith NT, editors: The automated anesthesia record and alarm systems, Boston, 1987, Butterworth & Co.
38. Whitcher C: Advantages of automated record keeping. In Gravenstein JS and Holzer JF, editors: Safety and cost containment in anesthesia, pp 207-221, Boston, 1988, Butterworth Co.
39. Eichhorn JH: Disadvantages of automated record keeping. In Gravenstein JS and Holzer JF, editors: Safety and cost containment in anesthesia, pp 223-232, Boston, 1988, Butterworth & Co.
40. Bushman JA and Cushman J: The use of computers in anaesthetic records. In Lunn JN, editor: Epidemiology in anesthesia, pp 159-168, London, 1986, Edward Arnold Ltd.

Chapter 30

What To Do If Sued: an Analysis of the Allegation of Malpractice Brought Against an Anesthesia Provider

John H. Tinker
William W. Hesson

I. SITUATIONS WHERE A LAWSUIT MAY RESULT

It is important to understand, at the outset of this chapter, that anyone can sue anyone for anything. This does not always mean that a potential plaintiff can find a lawyer to take his or her case. In discussing the kinds of situations where a lawsuit may result, one can always find exceptions or unusual cases or cases in which the resultant claims seem patently ridiculous, yet a lawsuit was launched anyway. Nonetheless, it is true that there are certain kinds of situations in which a lawsuit should be considered a reasonable possibility by the practitioners involved with the care that was given (or not given).

When you buy a new car, it comes with a warranty. If something goes wrong with that car in 12 months or 12,000 miles or some other time period, you are entitled to return it and get it repaired or replaced free, obviously within the limitations of the fine print of the warranty. Manufacturers of most durable goods know that they cannot compete successfully in today's marketplace without some sort of a "performance bond" or warranty. Today, even housing construction is often warranted. Despite the above, when a patient undergoes a total hip replacement or other surgical operation, no such performance bonding or warranty is given. There are few if any surgeons or hospitals who say to the patient, "If your total hip fails in any way, or gets infected, or is painful, we will fix it free of charge." Physicians reading this likely will rise up in anger and say something like "We can't predict the results of surgery that well" or "There are too many unknowns here with respect to physiology, pharmacology, pathophysiology, etc." Nonetheless, much of today's surgery is rather stereotyped, and the idea of a performance bond whereby, for example, if a patient's total hip became infected, future therapy would be rendered free of charge, is not so far fetched as it may seem. Nonetheless, this idea is still foreign to our health care environment.

This lack of any sort of performance bonding may contribute to the fact that when there are poor results from surgery, the caregivers can expect the following. First, the patient will be angry or disappointed or upset. Second, the patient may be disabled, temporarily or permanently. Caregiver protests to the contrary, it is rare to find the preoperative description of a procedure by a surgeon or an anesthesiologist to a patient to be presented in anything but relatively optimistic terms. We may discuss the complications our patients might suffer, but we almost invariably present the procedures we wish to perform on our patients in relatively favorable terms. We do so, perhaps, partly out of self-deception, stating that we don't want to scare our patients, or they never would agree to the surgery we believe they should have. Whatever the reason, if you could make a tape recording of your own presentation to your next patient about the anesthetic procedure for which you were trying to obtain consent, you would find that it has generally an optimistic tone, not necessarily unrealistic, but definitely optimistic and upbeat. There is nothing inherently wrong with this, but because we do this, we should not be surprised that after a poor result our patients are so angry or disappointed.

This optimistic attitude, if carefully analyzed, probably contributes to our current litigious atmosphere. In other words, after we create expectations of excellence, when something goes awry, it is natural for the patient to assume that something has been done wrong—somebody was negligent, either by omission or commission. Worse, the patient may believe that since the usual and customary results of this procedure are supposedly so good the poor results now evident *must* have been caused by negligence of some sort on somebody's part.

A corollary to the fact that poor results from surgery can be expected to raise litigious interest in the patient or family involved is the problem of *unexpected* results of surgery. For example, a patient who underwent a total hip replacement may now be able to walk fairly well, but there is numbness down one side of his leg. Whether or not he was told about this possibility preoperatively may become a point at issue, but this unexpected result will mar an otherwise beneficial experience and result in similar kinds of disappointment and unhappiness mentioned above. Clearly when we give our very best efforts toward "informed consent" we cannot possibly anticipate all of these surprises, and even if we had mentioned one or more detractive possibilities, there is a remarkable amount of selective forgetting by patients about what they were told.

The unexpected results or complications do not necessarily have to be directly related to the surgery. Many times, patients will have focused their entire emotional and intellectual energies on the disease process itself and will not have considered the possibility that unexpected complications can occur that are not directly related to or located near the actual surgical procedure itself. For example, the patient who suffers an ulnar nerve injury after an arthroscopy can, with some justification, say, "I went into the hospital to have my knee fixed, and now my left hand doesn't work very well and is also numb."

Poor results of surgery, whether they were "expected" (which is rare) or unexpected, whether they were directly related to the surgery itself, and whether they were mentioned in the "informed consent" can lead to litigation. It is a basic tenet of most medical practice, especially procedure-oriented medical practice, that complications *do* occur. It is a basic tenet that it is extremely unlikely, if not impossible, to perform procedures with a zero complication rate. As we get better at doing various kinds of procedures, complication rates do decrease, and, paradoxically, as these procedures become associated with lower complication rates, when such a complication does occur, the patients are *more* likely to assume negligence or else the complication would not have occurred, since it is so rare! The message here is to expect litigation from poor results or complications, whether expected or unexpected, whether the patient was informed or not. The wise practitioner who notes such a complication in one of his or her patients will honestly assess that occurrence for the possibility that indeed something was done wrong, instead of the common tendency to run and hide from the incident (and the patient). A thus-abandoned patient is even more likely to bring suit. Although the latter may simply have been a "judgment call," the practitioner should choose to learn from the incident and perhaps protect the next patient.

Up to this point, we have mentioned only in passing, the issue of informed consent. At one extreme, is it possible for even a board-certified anesthesiologist with many years of experience to give informed consent for himself or herself to have a spinal anesthetic for a particular procedure? If we make the assumption that the procedure is necessary and the disease is causing pain or disability for the anesthesiologist-patient, one could argue that even the physician is unable, because of the pain or disability, to make a particularly wise choice at that time with that level of stress. If that is conceivable, then how can we expect our patients who are not board-certified anesthesiologists to give us informed consent to do anesthesia-related things to them? In truth, the above is *not* legally relevant; our duty is *disclosure*. As every resident today is taught, we do the very best we can during the preoperative visit. We do try to explain the procedure in as much detail as the patient appears willing and able to absorb. We try to explain medical jargon in lay terms. We try to lay out as objectively as possible the fact that complications are possible, which ones are of concern, and, insofar as is known, what the relative risks are. We do inform the patient that death is indeed a possibility, however unlikely. Despite all the above, in many lawsuits one of the allegations against the defendant doctors is lack of informed consent.

Does lack of informed consent, or a hasty, relatively cold or callous-appearing informed-consent taking, actually lead to a lawsuit? Just how important is the "lack of informed consent" claim as a part of a lawsuit? Many have stated that it is very difficult for a plaintiff to win a case based on informed consent. Winning the lawsuit is not the issue. The *process* of obtaining consent, involving compassionate interaction between physician and patient at this critical juncture, is a powerful tool in our risk-management strategy.

In summary, what are the kinds of situations that can result in a lawsuit? When there is a poor result of surgery, the anesthesia caregiver must always consider the possibility that litigation might arise. The same is true when there is a poor result from an anesthesia procedure such as a spinal headache. The indignation with which many newly named defendants greet the claim filed against them on behalf of the plaintiff alleging negligence, which largely appears to be based on the simple fact of a poor result, should be replaced by an understanding of the fact that the patient, though not given a written performance bond preoperatively, probably was given a relatively optimistic explanation of the procedure and its expected results. The surgeon is, in essence, saying "I can help you" to the patient, no matter how many disclaimers follow. So is the anesthesiologist, again irrespective of the number and type of disclaimers. Because

this is true and also because we must continue to "sell," at least to some degree, the treatments for our patients we believe to be appropriate, we are destined to remain caught in the dilemma of having presented something optimistically that then does not turn out so well, coupled with our having not issued any type of specific written performance bond or guarantee to the patient.

II. WHAT EXACTLY IS THE ANESTHETIST BEING SUED FOR?

There are three generic grounds on which a physician can be sued by a patient. Although it is rare, it is possible to sue for *abandonment*. As an example, the responsible supervising physician anesthesiologist leaves the operating room during the administration of anesthesia and does not notify the anesthesia resident (CRNA) or surgical or nursing personnel of his whereabouts. A major crises ensues and contact cannot be made with the physician. In one such case, the physician had, in fact, gone outside the hospital to have breakfast! Although a patient does not have the right to demand medical services of a given physician (that is, a physician cannot usually be compelled to provide medical treatment for a patient), it is a basic tenet of the law that once a physician has entered into a patient-care arrangement with a patient (or patient-care agreement with a third party on behalf of a group of patients) the physician must give the patient reasonable notice when he or she no longer wishes to take care of the patient. The physician who is giving up the patient's care should provide appropriate referrals if possible.

The second major reason for suing a physician involves the allegation of *battery*. Battery is the unauthorized touching of a person and, in the context of medical malpractice, as related to anesthesiology, the allegation usually results when a procedure was performed without an appropriate consent process. If, for example, the procedure performed was radically different from that for which consent was obtained, an allegation of battery might be sustained. A breast biopsy that turns into a mastectomy when consent has been obtained only for the former is a battery. Another example might be a situation where a patient signed an operative consent but was already under the influence of premedicant drugs. To the extent that he or she was not aware of giving consent, the subsequent "touching" may be unauthorized and thus a battery. Yet another example of battery would be a situation where the operative consent was for removal of the gallbladder, but the surgeon went ahead and did an unrelated procedure without permission. An adult Jehovah's Witness patient who refuses blood preoperatively but is transfused anyway could allege battery.

The most common reason for a lawsuit by a patient against medical caregivers is *negligence*. Even if a particular case has elements of abandonment or battery, the lawsuit will most likely be based on grounds of negligence. To prove a case of negligence, the plaintiff needs to convince the jury or judge that (1) the physician had a *duty* to the patient, (2) there was an *act* committed or omitted by the defendant in violation of the duty, (3) the patient was injured, (4) the act *caused* the injury. These are the elements of an action brought against a physician on grounds of negligence. We discuss these in detail below.[2]

III. WHAT TO DO WHEN SUED
A. Early activity by the plaintiff

Long before any lawsuit is actually filed, there is considerable activity on the part of the plaintiff and involved attorneys. A person who believes he or she has been wronged by a medical caregiver or has a case against a caregiver will seek out a plaintiff's attorney. These initial conferences are often quite extensive, and they should be, for the following reasons. Almost always, these cases are taken by plaintiff's attorneys on a contingency-fee basis. Basically, this means that if the plaintiff wins the attorney gets a prearranged percentage of the total settlement or judgment, an amount that often is about one third. If the plaintiff loses, the attorney receives nothing for his or her efforts. A case of negligence against an anesthesiologist almost invariably requires the services of one or more expert witnesses. The attorney must identify these experts, correspond with them, ultimately prepare them for deposition, travel to their location, and depose them. The attorney must also identify and depose witnesses to the events, develop an understanding of the medical facts and medical records, and negotiate with multiple insurance companies for multiple defendants. When one adds all this up, one finds that the time commitment that the attorney must make can be extremely large.

In some ways, the current contingency-fee arrangement by which almost all plaintiff's cases are pursued can be construed as *protection* for the physician. If the patient's injury is inconsequential or minor and therefore the potential for recovery of damages is low, that patient, however angry or litigious, will have considerable difficulty finding a qualified plaintiff's attorney willing to pursue the case on a contingency-fee basis. Therefore one could argue that the contingency fee, so often attacked by tort reformers today, in fact may protect doctors against some potential lawsuits. The contingency fee tends to limit litigation to those cases wherein a major financial settlement or judgment is possible.

During these initial plaintiff-attorney conferences, frank financial discussion therefore occurs. During this time, the patient will sign the appropriate waivers allowing the attorneys to obtain the medical records of the case. Such inquiries are continually received by record rooms in hospitals. Most hospitals or medical centers have risk-management departments. Such an inquiry from a plaintiff's attorney usually triggers a review of that case by the physicians and caregivers involved because it is now known that there is interest. Patients (potential plaintiffs) have the right to see their own medical records and to show those medical records to their attorneys. Caregivers should go to great lengths to make sure that they provide full and complete medical records on such requests because, in the past, there have been cases in which various crucial parts of the medical record were mysteriously lost, misplaced, defaced, or otherwise obfuscated. The plaintiff's side of any such action can always make at least a few points if not an entire case out of such an event, whether inadvertent or not.

On receipt of these medical records, many large plaintiff's law firms employ medically educated individuals to read these medical records and to abstract or interpret them for the attorneys. Often these persons are former nurses, but some law firms employ physicians. The physician author of this chapter (J.H.T.), after considerable experience with these kinds of cases, is still amazed at the facility with which many attorneys can analyze complex medical records to identify the critical issues.

Many plaintiff's attorneys also have networks of contacts, often in the local community or state, with physicians who will read the medical records involved in a particular case and render an opinion to the plaintiff's attorney as to whether the case should be pursued. Often these rather prominent persons are *not* willing to testify on behalf of the plaintiff but are willing to render an opinion to the plaintiff's attorney about the case. These opinions are classified as "work product" and are usually therefore subject to the attorney-client privilege and are not discoverable by the defendant unless and until the reviewer physician agrees to be an expert witness and actually testify in the case.

It is critical to understand the importance of this prefiling period in any lawsuit. The *quality* of the advice being given to the plaintiff's attorneys during this time is variable. If the plaintiff's attorneys are unable to obtain the services of qualified persons in the same subspecialty or specialty of the caregivers the plaintiffs are considering suing, or if the plaintiffs are forced to rely, for their prefiling advice, on physicians who have biased reasons for reviewing the case or who earn large percentages of their incomes from so doing, or whose knowledge base is not up to date or who are not competent for any reason, then the plaintiff's attorneys may receive poor advice as to the advisability of proceeding with a case. Then, after they have filed the lawsuit, gone to the expenses involved, and have sometimes made an assault on the reputations of the defendant caregivers, they sometimes find that they have very little substance in the case. The very best plaintiff's attorneys are successful because they have managed to obtain a network of competent senior physicians who can review their cases and give solid advice as to whether to proceed with the lawsuit. They also have learned to *take* that advice, even when the case looks superficially lucrative. It cannot be overemphasized how important this period of time is.

Eventually, if the plaintiff's attorneys decide to proceed, there will be the actual filing of the lawsuit, which will formally notify the defendants. It is uncommon for the plaintiff to be completely aware at this point exactly who should be sued and who should not. Therefore it is usual that large numbers of caregivers are initially named.

Now intense activity on behalf of the plaintiff begins in earnest. The plaintiff's advisors who rendered opinions about whether there were sufficient grounds to file the lawsuit in the first place will now be either expected to testify themselves or at least expected to help the plaintiff's attorneys find competent persons who will testify against the defendant.

With respect to qualifications of plaintiff's (and defense) experts, many states have addressed this problem in their tort-reform efforts. Tort reform in various states has taken different forms. In some states, for example, physicians testifying against other physicians must be in the active practice of the same specialty of medicine; they cannot be retired and they cannot earn more than a certain percentage of their incomes by testifying. On the other hand, in other states, physicians are still allowed to testify against other physicians even if they have no demonstrable qualifications in the sub-specialty of the defendant. In still other states, retired physicians are still permitted to testify against physicians in active practice. Unfortunately, the problem can be more subtle than that. For example, if the anesthesiologist who is testifying against a defendant anesthesiologist is, himself, board certified, not retired, and in active practice, that may satisfy the requirements of most states. It is still possible, however, that the plaintiff's expert witness could be testifying about obstetric anesthesia when in fact he or she has not done obstetric anesthesia for many years and limits his or her practice to, for example, neurosurgical anesthesia. This nuance goes beyond the tort reform acts currently in existence, though it can certainly be brought to the jury's attention when the time comes to try to impeach (discredit) the person's testimony.

It is important for defendants to understand that the quality and national reputations of the expert witnesses who have agreed to testify against them be carefully assessed by the defendant physicians, their attorneys, and their own expert witnesses. If the expert witnesses lined up to testify against the defendant are themselves nationally known and respectable, this should send a very important message to the defendant and to the defense attorneys.

Early activity by the plaintiff includes the taking of depositions. Each side has the right to find out, in advance and in considerable detail, precisely what the other side is prepared to say in court. Therefore the plaintiff's attorneys will come to the defendant and codefendants and ask them, under oath, to explain their actions in the case. Defendants and codefendants can be expected to be required to answer a long list of questions about their qualifications, their continuing medical educations, and their prior experience in dealing with similar kinds of cases. Defendant physicians can be expected to be asked about other pending or finished malpractice lawsuits, no matter how long ago they occurred or for what kinds of reasons. The defendant physician or caregiver, including the hospital, must have counsel present during this deposition. If a question is asked by the plaintiff's attorney that is considered legally inappropriate, an objection will be raised for the record. Often the defendant will then be instructed by his or her own counsel to go ahead and answer the question if possible. Sometimes, if the question is particularly offensive, or inappropriate, counsel will advise the defendant to refuse to answer the question.

The defendant physician should understand that anything and everything said during the deposition can be utilized in the courtroom, during the trial, before the jury, *as evidence*. The deposition can be introduced as evidence in many ways, up to and including the actual reading of passages from the deposition (or the deposition in its entirety) to the jury and asking the defendant to state from the witness stand whether indeed he or she did say those things that were just read.

During these depositions, plaintiff's and defendant's attorneys may appear relatively casual toward each other, even to the point of laughing and joking or arriving and leaving together. The defendant must not let this relatively informal atmosphere fool him or her into being off guard. "On guard" does not mean that the defendant physician should ever tell less than the whole truth during the deposition or at any other time. What "on guard" means is that answers to questions should be answers to particular questions and should not be expounded upon. A negative attitude by the defendant physician toward the plaintiff or the plaintiff's attorneys will almost invariably be exploited by those attorneys during the depositions and later during court testimony. The defendant physician should therefore provide only the facts, and the deposition phase of the preparation for the trial of the lawsuit can be survived intact. If time is required to review records to provide an accurate response, that time should always be taken.

In addition to the depositions taken from the defendant or defendants, there will be depositions taken of other persons considered *material witnesses*. In cases involving anesthesiology-related activities, these persons are often operating room nurses who are not, themselves, being sued. During these depositions, wide-ranging questions are permitted to be asked by the plaintiff's attorneys of the material witnesses involved. For example, "Was Dr. Jones in the habit of reading while doing anesthesia?" This question may be objected to by Dr. Jones's attorney, but the material witness will almost always be instructed to answer it. If she or he says that Dr. Jones was indeed "often" in the habit of reading during the performance of anesthesia, you can easily see the damage that might be done if this testimony were allowed into evidence at trial. Indeed, it is a *sine qua non* of risk management to be *always* "down to business" in the operating room and the other places where anesthesiologists work.

B. Early activity by the defendant after notification of lawsuit

The actual filing of a lawsuit will usually have come as no surprise to the defendants. The law-suit is almost sure to be based on a poor result from surgery or anesthesia. At the time of the occurrence, it is prudent to notify appropriate insurance carriers and the hospital's risk managers. In any event, when the defendant physician is served with notice of the lawsuit, it is mandatory that the physician or physicians now notify their insurance carriers. Selection of attorneys for defendant physicians is usually done by the insurance carriers and is not often a prerogative of the physician defendant, though it is legitimate for the physician defendant to try to have some say in that selection process. It is also legitimate for any physician who is sued to obtain independent counsel for any reason. Such independent counsel can be obtained either in addition to or instead of the carrier-appointed counsel. In the latter event, dismissal of insurance company–appointed counsel may void coverage from that insurance company and is almost never done. These are sensitive issues, especially if pressure for settlement is coming from other named defendants who are insured by the same carrier.

Next, careful and detailed conferences between attorney and defendant physician or physicians take place. These are critically important to the defendant caregiver or caregivers. During this conference series, the defendant physician will be assessing the attorney but should not forget that the attorney will also be assessing the physician, both as a potential witness and with respect to the veracity or lack thereof of the statements being made by the physician or physicians. An attorney who considers his physician client to be inaccurate or incompetent or to have a poor attitude for being a witness is an attorney who has a problematic case, to say the least. A defendant who is belligerent, defensive, or obviously or apparently covering up some facts, or who has probably altered the records, or who has kept intolerably poor records, will not be highly regarded by counsel. The tendency will be to see if the insurance company can escape this case with as little damage as possible to itself despite the defendant's maintaining no culpability. Attorneys try to be objective, as physicians do in the care of patients, but we are all human in regarding matters subjectively. In sharpest possible contrast, if the defendant physician can establish a trusting solid relationship with the attorney, in these initial conferences, counsel will often respond with remarkable levels of hard work to defend that physician's reputation (not to mention the pocketbooks of all concerned).

Every case, bar none, has weaknesses from the standpoint of the defendant (and the plaintiff). Defendants must understand that plaintiff's attorneys would not have taken this case on a contingency-fee basis unless they strongly believed they could win. Therefore, without exception, there must be weaknesses in the defense. Some weaknesses may appear insurmountable to the defendant physician, and he or she may be reluctant to reveal them to the defense attorneys in these initial conferences. This is wrong thinking for several reasons. First, these weaknesses *will* emerge as time goes by. Second, failure to reveal everything possible initially to the defense attorney, who is not a physician, will damage the attorney-client relationship because later the defendant's own experts will reveal these weaknesses in detail to the defendant's attorneys. The best course for a defendant to take is to discuss in complete candor every aspect of the case with his or her attorney. Some defendants, knowing the weaknesses of the case, have become depressed and have viewed their cases to be hopeless, when in fact competent expert witnesses could testify in favor of reasonable alternative scenarios and convince juries of same. Sometimes defendants who believed initially that no negligence had occurred have been "brow beaten" by plaintiff's expert witnesses into believing that indeed the scenario espoused by said plaintiff's expert witnesses is correct. Competent defense expert witnesses, who often enter the picture later, may need to reconvince the defendant that care was not substandard. Again, these initial conferences between defendant physician or physicians or caregivers and their counsel are critical in establishing the proper foundation for these dynamics.

The next stage is selection of expert witnesses for the defense. Often, defendant physicians will be asked for names of persons who might be considered nationally reputed expert witnesses. These persons will be contacted and themselves may give other recommendations or agree to review the records. It appears that it is easier to retain those who have solid national reputations to testify on behalf of defendants than it is to retain same for the plaintiffs.

How much if any involvement should there be between defendants and defense expert witnesses? Some defendants have developed a "clinging" dependence on the expert witness, bombarding that person with theories, manuscripts, reprints, telephone calls, and the like. If a defendant physician has theories or additional references or statements to make that might be of benefit to the defendant's expert witness, these should be communicated through defense counsel. It is important that a defendant's expert witnesses work mostly with counsel and not with the defendant. It is often considered

optimal if defendant's expert witness has *not* have had prior knowledge of or friendship with the defendant. Lack of a prior relationship lends objectivity. Prior relationships (such as an expert witness testifying for a former trainee) may raise an issue of bias.

The taking of depositions by the defendant's attorneys now begins. These usually include the plaintiff's expert witnesses and material witnesses named by the plaintiffs. The plaintiff himself or herself, if possible, may be deposed, but this is always a delicate matter. In anesthesia-related cases, the plaintiff may be deceased or not competent, and suit has been brought by relatives. Depositions may or may not be taken of any of these persons.

In contrast, depositions of the plaintiff's expert witnesses are usually quite revealing to the defendant's expert witnesses and vice versa. Theories of causation or culpability espoused by plaintiff's expert witnesses will usually need to be countered by defendant's expert witnesses. Knowledge of them allows the work of defense to begin in earnest. Also, qualifications of plaintiff's expert witnesses must be understood in detail because one technique used during cross examination is that of *impeachment,* which means trying to impugn the credibility of that witness.

C. Each side now builds its case, maneuvers, and develops strategy

Now the maneuvering begins (the attorney author of this chapter, W.W.H., prefers to conceptualize this as a process of narrowing the issues). The plaintiff will likely have named a larger number of defendants in the lawsuit than the facts, as they are brought out in the discovery process, will support. Attorneys for various defendants who believe their clients to be either uninvolved or exceedingly peripheral will move to dismiss said clients from the case. The judge may grant such a motion after hearing argument about it, or plaintiff's attorney may agree to drop the individual from the case.

During this time, there may be other reasons for opposing attorneys to confer with each other or make motions. Opposing attorneys have ways of "feeling each other out," that is, finding out how strong each believes its case is relative to that of the opposing side. Physicians believe there is an "art" to our profession. They must concede that right to attorneys. These feelings are important because next comes consideration of possibility of settlement.

Sometimes, especially if the case is complex or plaintiff's counsel believes that there is a real possibility of a major award, the plaintiff may put together a "settlement offer" complete with a written photographically illustrated "brochure" describing terms the plaintiff wishes. Counter offers can be made by counsel for defendants at this time. Often there are several physicians and a hospital or other caregiver or caregivers involved. Some of those involved may all along have been maintaining that they had nothing to do with any aspect of this case and do not want any culpability whatsoever. Other defendants may by this time be angrily demanding vindication before a jury. Other individuals or organizations may also, for various reasons, not want to settle the case. Some of the defendants may opt out by a financial settlement at this time. It is possible that when the trial actually occurs, only a few or even one defendant may remain. The fact that the other original defendants settled, and for how much, is not usually admissible as evidence in the trial of the remaining defendant or defendants. Such "evidence" might be extremely prejudicial because the fact that other defendants have settled might be construed as admission of universal culpability, or the jury, hearing the amount the plaintiff has already received, might say, in effect, "That's enough" and find for the remaining defendant or defendants. Many physicians have trouble with not being allowed to introduce prior settlements in their trials, but calm reflection should convince you that this is proper.

Next comes the difficult problem of setting a trial date and making it stick. Criminal trials have precedence over civil trials, and the judge may need to postpone the case time and again. Various key attorneys will be involved in other trials, which may not be finished exactly as anticipated. Anesthesiologists have considerable difficulty on a day-to-day basis trying to schedule surgery and figure out how to get it done in timely fashion without overlap. They should have an appreciation therefore for the difficulties in scheduling court cases.

Meanwhile, there is consideration by both sides of involving other expert and material witnesses. For example, during the discovery process, various issues regarding handwriting may have come up. In one anesthesiology-related case, there was question raised by plaintiff's expert witness as to whether the defendant anesthesiologist had in fact written at least 1 hour's worth of blood pressures all at the same time. A handwriting expert was consulted and, by microscopic examination of the original ball point pen-written anesthesia record, contended that the blood-pressure tick marks had been written in one continuous application of the pen over at least 1 hour's worth of space. This testimony

was damaging because it spoke against good vigilance. Other nonphysician experts such as chemists or pharmacists may also be called upon for testimony.

During preparation for trial, various visual aids are often constructed. There will be an enlargement view, often 3 feet by 5 feet in dimension, of the anesthesia record. Other pertinent records from the chart are similarly enlarged. One technique used by plaintiff's attorney is to leave the enlargement of the anesthesia record, with its usual less-than-perfect handwriting and legibility, in full view of the jury for many hours during the trial. It is also possible to have graphics done if descriptions of complex anatomy are required. One instance involved a case of truncus arteriosus. You can imagine the difficulty of conveying to a lay jury the anatomy and surgery of truncus arteriosus. To do that, various graphics were obtained including a color cartoon type of panel-by-panel depiction of important surgical stages. That case never went to trial, but you can rest assured that the settlement included the cost of the graphic artist's services!

D. Basic workings of a trial

A lawsuit can be tried before a judge without a jury. However, most cases involving medical malpractice related to anesthesiology are tried before juries. The reason is that most plaintiff's attorneys believe that the injured patient and his or her loss of life, limb, income-earning ability, or whatever, will have a major impact upon a jury.

Defendant physicians not familiar with the trial process often do not understand the critical role of the judge. When the case goes to the jury, the jury has been presented with two sets of "facts," those belonging to plaintiff and those belonging to defendant. The jurors are asked to find for either plaintiff or defendant, whether or not they believe all the "facts" and testimony on that side. So what, then, is the role of the judge? The judge has the critical role in determining the actual permitted *content* of each side. This is done according to the *rules of evidence*. The judge interprets the rules of evidence and decides, preferably in advance, that is, before the jury has heard any statements, what is admissible into evidence and what is not. Since the lawyers are quick to think on their feet and to take advantage of opportunity, things can happen fast during a trial. The judge is responsible at all times for maintaining the equanimity of the situation. If something has "slipped out" that the judge does not believe the jury should include in one or the other set of "facts" or in determining its verdict, the judge must then determine how to prohibit the jury from considering that item. All along, various motions may be submitted for rulings by the judge. These motions can be up to and including a motion by the defense for a directed verdict on grounds that the plaintiffs have presented insufficient evidence to support a decision in his or her favor. After all the evidence has been submitted, the cross examination is finished, the redirect examination is finished, and all the recross examination is finished, the judge charges the jury and interprets the law of the case for the jury. The judge must tell them what they can and cannot do and what their options are in the case.[3]

The jury also determines damages they wish to award, if any, to the plaintiff. This involves their consideration of economic testimony by experts on both sides.

1. What should the caregiver do in preparation for trial? During the attorney-defendant conferences, all pertinent medical facts need to be on the table. The defendant must not be too defensive, must work hard on objectivity, must help the attorney understand the medical record, must interpret the handwriting, and must explain the medical reasons for each act or omission. The defendant caregiver can also help counsel and expert witnesses by providing reprints of pertinent medical literature, especially if recent, including that which might support the plaintiff's position or positions.

Caregivers are not necessarily articulate. Many tend to be relatively nonverbal people who work by thinking about differential diagnoses involved in their minute-to-minute decision making in the operating room and then implementing the decisions, seldom being required to verbalize those decisions to anyone. They are not practiced at having to gain permission or provide verbal or written justification for individual actions. Yet in deposition and at trial, caregivers will be asked to articulate orally the justification for acts or omissions, drugs given and their timing, dosages, and other details about the process of the anesthetic. It makes sense that they now practice, orally, answers to questions they will surely be asked both at deposition and at trial. This is not for any purpose of subterfuge but to allow confidence about verbal answers to such questions. Some attorneys prepare their clients by having, in essence, a mock deposition or mock trial. Others do not do so, believing that some degree of spontaneity would be lost. It is reasonable for a defendant physician or caregiver to practice orally even if this is done alone. Certainly, oral practice of solid succinct answers to questions you will almost surely be asked makes sense.

2. What should the anesthesia caregiver not do? Most important, when one is sued, is to *not* let the lawsuit and the activities associated with it interfere with quality care of any subsequent patients. Anesthesiologists may tend to feel embittered and even a bit paranoid about the fact that they received no accolades for the preceding thousands of patients successfully anesthetized, yet they are being somehow "persecuted" in this case. It is possible to take these attitudes to sufficient extremes so as to have them interfere with quality care of subsequent patients.

It is also important not to get personally or excessively involved with the expert witnesses who are on your side. This does not mean complete avoidance of them, but it means following your attorney's advice to the letter in this regard.

Many defendant physicians also try, to one degree or another, to dictate legal strategy to their attorneys. They may try to dictate the order in which witnesses should be presented, or the kinds of questions that should be asked. It is true that a defendant physician may well be able to help his or her attorney by suggesting certain questions, especially of plaintiff's expert witnesses. Most of the time such activity by the defendant is a hindrance rather than a help.

Most important on the list of "don'ts" is *not to avoid or cover up the weaknesses in your case.* They should be carefully explored early and discussed openly with the attorney, who should in turn discuss them openly with the defendant's expert witnesses, who must develop scenarios that explain or minimize apparent weaknesses. If this cannot be done, either additional expert witness help must be sought or perhaps the case should be settled. Usually, alternative scenarios that fit the facts of the situation and enable a reasonable case to be solidly defended will surface. Sometimes, defendants want to throw up their hands and resort to some form of the "bad things happen" defense. This is *never* sufficient. There must be a scenario alternative to and in sharpest possible contrast to that being presented by plaintiff's expert witness. This scenario must, if possible, absolve the specific defendant from culpability without implicating the other defendants. It is almost never advisable, at least not as a starting point, to have defendants accusing each other, something that the plaintiff's attorneys greatly enjoy.

3. Preparation of the expert witnesses. A potential expert witness has now been contacted by an attorney and asked to review a case. That person's decision whether to take on this case involves the following considerations. After careful review of the medical records, the potential expert witness should ask the following questions. "Would I have managed the case that way? If not, would my way have materially affected the outcome?" It is critical to ask these two questions in tandem. Potential expert witnesses, especially for the plaintiff, may ask only the first of the two questions, and if the case was not handled their preferred way, they agree to provide testimony. The second of the two questions above requires real objectivity. "Would my way, the way I was taught by my mentor, the way I know and love so well, in my honest medical judgment, really have made a major positive difference with respect to the outcome that occurred?" If an expert is asked to be a defendant's witness and the answer is "I'm not really sure that my way would have been better," then this expert may wish to help defend the case even though the anesthetic was not performed in the exact fashion preferred. Next, the potential expert witness for the defense needs to ask: "Is there a scenario that explains the outcome *in my best professional judgment* and is alternative to that being suggested by the plaintiff's expert witness? Is the scenario one in which I can truly believe? Is it supported by the facts in the medical records or sworn testimony?" If these are answered yes, the expert may wish to help.

Many physicians are asked to review plaintiff's cases. Again, the records and testimony must be carefully reviewed. After said study of the medical records, the *same two* questions should be asked. The potential plaintiff's expert witness must be "within a reasonable degree of medical certainty" that the patient would *not* have suffered the negative outcome had the anesthesia been managed another way. The trap here is that, all too often, the potential plaintiff's expert *will* find aspects of the case about which he or she is strongly critical and that emotion may blind the expert to the crucial question of causation, that is, whether another way would have averted the complication. Reading some cases, a qualified anesthesiologist-reviewer might be genuinely outraged. If the two questions above so indicate, that person should agree to testify against the above-mentioned physician. The would-be physician expert witness must also analyze his or her personal biases regarding the case, both medical and financial, before agreeing to testify.

Preparation for testimony must be meticulous. First, the expert witness must know the

facts of the case in considerable detail. Nothing is more embarrassing (and potentially damaging) than getting the facts of the case wrong in the formulation of a particular scenario as to what happened. Next, the expert witness must know or have recently reviewed the relevant medicine and literature. Finally, and most importantly, the expert witness must have carefully developed a scenario that, to his or her best medical judgment, based on experience and training, best explains the facts of the case and the outcome that occurred. The expert witness must *believe* in this scenario and must practice defending it against likely challenges because it will almost certainly be in disagreement with the scenario espoused by the other side.

If the scenario believed in by the defendant's expert witness is one that lays blame on one or more of the other defendants in the case or if other defendants have already chosen to cast aspersions on your defendant, then it may indeed be necessary for the defendant's expert to testify against other defendants. When this happens, as previously mentioned, the plaintiff's side sits back and enjoys. If attorney-attorney conferences have not ironed out these problems in advance, this unfortunate result may occur.

4. Testimony at deposition or trial by defendant physician or caregiver. It is important to understand several differences between deposition and trial. First of all, the deposition is often given in a relatively informal setting and the attorneys for both sides will likely be relatively informal or even friendly together. Sometimes they even come into town on the same airplane, stay at the same hotel, have dinner together, and so forth. At trial, these same attorneys are formal. The difference between the behaviors of these individuals at deposition versus trial can be disconcerting to the uninitiated physician defendant or expert witness. The proper demeanor and attitude of the physician defendant or expert witness should be "all business" at all times both during deposition and trial. No corners should be cut in preparation for the deposition. Everything said by the physician or physician expert witness at deposition can and may well be used at trial. If there are discrepancies in what was said at deposition and what is later believed, these must be discussed in detail with the attorneys involved and strategy agreed upon before trial.

The physician testifying before a jury may be intimidated or arrogant or both. Physicians when intimidated tend to resort to (hide behind?) medical jargon. Perhaps needless to say, this is a gross mistake. Every time you use a term that is *remotely* medical, even terms like

"IV cannula" or "surgical dressing" you must stop and explain by simply defining it to the jury. If you say, "IV cannula," also say, "That's a plastic tube placed in the patient's vein to administer fluids." This is another reason for oral preparation, even if simply done alone by the defendant before testimony. If graphics are to be used during testimony, practice with them is important. Knowing how to use a pointer and when not to use it is not something that is automatic for physicians or other anesthesia caregivers. How to speak to the jury is also not automatic. The defendant needs to *look at the jury* and talk *to* them. You should remember that your testimony is being given *to the jury,* not to the attorneys. Focus on more than one member of the jury and speak directly to them. If you can do this, you also will likely not hide so much behind medical jargon.

The defendant anesthesia caregiver's attorney should, of course, have prepared that person in many ways, including the need to deal with various cross-examination techniques. Anesthesia caregivers deal with milligrams, milliliters, syringes, vapors, and so on. Trial attorneys deal with the spoken word. They are remarkably facile at the nuances and subtleties of our wonderful language. They know that if they can make the defendant somehow emotional or angry or defensive, they can help their case. They may do this with various voice inflections, expressions of incredulity, quizzical looks, arched eyebrows, and other mannerisms that are a part of their professional repertoire. A physician who views himself or herself as somehow superior or above all this usually is rapidly cut down to size. Sticking to the facts and nothing but the facts is the best way to get through one of these experiences. During cross examination of the defendant's testimony, if the plaintiff's attorney uses an insulting or demeaning tone, a tone that suggests that the attorney places no credibility whatsoever in the things the defendant has just said, there is usually nothing defendant's attorney can do about it. For example, during cross examination, the plaintiff's attorney says, "Doctor (you are a medical doctor, I believe; is that not correct?), did you *really* mean to state that you were *certain* that tube went into Mister Jones's trachea?" Even if there is something objectionable about that question, the jury will get the meaning and may be sympathetic, depending in part on whether or not you become belligerent, angry, emotional, or defensive in your answer. Some members of the jury may be eagerly awaiting the defendant doctor's response to such baiting. If you are respectfully honest and none of the attributes mentioned above comes out in your voice, the techniques can backfire badly on the attorney who tries them.

5. Testimony at deposition or trial by expert witness for defendant. As an expert for the defense, you will be expected to explain why you took the case for the defendant. You will explain your scenario to the jury, possibly using visual aids, diagrams, or flip charts. You will then be required to withstand a sometimes lengthy, sometimes peeving, sometimes apparently inordinately ignorant (we say apparently because that is also a technique), and often repetitive cross examination. As with the defendant, various methods can be used to try to intimidate or impeach the defendant's expert witness including demeaning tones, incredulous voice inflections, and simulated (or real) anger by the attorney. If the defendant's expert witness appears arrogant or becomes angry or defensive or emotional, the plaintiff's attorney is likely to pounce (and win). Things are even more difficult for the defendant's expert witness because that person is expected to be a national-level expert in the subject under discussion. Sometimes the plaintiff's attorney may try the so-called "Is this text authoritative?" trap. This trap is set when the attorney for the plaintiff, during cross examination of the defendant's expert witness, holds up one or more volumes of a nationally recognized anesthesia text and asks, "Doctor, is this text authoritative?" Plaintiff's attorney likely knows a passage in that text that counteracts or contradicts something the defendant's expert witness has said. If the defendant's expert witness falls into the trap by saying, "yes, that's an authoritative text," then the plaintiff's attorney will read into the record from that text the passage that tends to refute the expert witness. If, on the other hand, the expert witness keeps his or her wits, a better answer to that question is something like, "Sir, that is a nationally recognized text in anesthesiology; its chapters are written by individual authors and therefore represent their opinions. It is not subjected to the intense level of peer review to which medical journal articles are subjected." Ideally, the expert witness must come to grips with all literature on both sides of the issue and must have carefully examined the case from both points of view, especially that of the other side.

Another trap into which expert witnesses continually fall is the "Are you certain?" trap. In medicine, we generally hedge with respect to being particularly "certain" as to outcome or risk. In the courtroom, one cannot and should not do this. The law respects a person who says, "This is what I believe happened within a reasonable degree of medical certainty." The lawyers for the opposing side may then try to say something like, "Are you really sure?" or "How sure can you be?" or other similar questions attempting to break down your certainty. In medical practice, one can never be totally certain, but in the courtroom the *conviction* with which the expert witness can present his or her scenario as to what happened may be a deciding factor.

Another trap presented to expert witnesses has to do with, "How much is your fee?" The jury knows that the expert witness is being paid for testimony. The jury would expect nothing less. Expert testimony is costly and so are the services of any nationally recognized professional for similar periods of time. The expert witness must not be defensive about forthrightly disclosing his or her entire fee to the jury and must never, ever, take any case on a contingency-fee basis. Forthright answers to the fee questions will *increase*, not decrease the jurors' respect for that witness.

Expert witnesses must understand that they can be held accountable for testimony they have given in other trials, especially if that testimony is related to the subject of the current trial. They will also be held accountable, detail by detail, for the testimony they gave during their own depositions. This is an area that is exceedingly difficult at times, especially if further study of the medical records, something that often happens to a busy expert witness, has revealed weaknesses that were not so evident at the time of deposition. Discussing how to deal with this requires careful preparation between the attorney and the expert witness.

E. What does the plaintiff need to show to make a case of negligence against the anesthesia caregiver?

First, the plaintiff must show that the anesthesia caregiver did have a clear duty and a solid relationship with the patient. You were, for example, the physician on call that night, and you were supervising the residents or nurse anesthetists. The ultimate responsibility for the anesthesia care of all patients in that hospital rested on your shoulders that night. Next, the plaintiff must show that the defendant or defendants did indeed commit or omit the act or several acts related to the case. For example, the surgeons are outside the operating room scrubbing their hands, the scrub nurses are busily working on their instruments, and, while you were anesthetizing the patient, he fell off the operating table. It would be hard to point the "commission or

omission" finger at anyone but you in this unfortunate circumstance.

Next, it must be shown that, as a direct result of the act or acts of omission or commission, the patient did indeed suffer an *injury*, whether permanent or not; that is, the plaintiff must show that the patient's injury was related to or *caused* by the act or acts or nonacts. This is not necessarily easy to do. For example, it might be easily established that the patient fell off the operating table and yet be difficult to establish that the patient's subsequent ulnar nerve paralysis was attributable to the fall off the operating table. Next, the plaintiff must provide evidence that the injury or injuries have monetary value. Things like "loss of consortium" are also said to have monetary value though this escapes the reasoning of many defendant physicians. On the other hand, the patient who is in a vegetative state permanently confined to a care facility and who is estimated to have 20 years of life remaining (by an expert in physical medicine) at a cost of $200,000 per year adjusted for inflation can be reasonably expected to have a patient care–related cost of a certain dollar value over a certain period. This is how the monetary value is calculated. Of course, at each step of the way, plaintiff's experts may be disputed by defendant's experts on the same subjects.

In the usual medical malpractice case, plaintiff must establish that the acts that caused the injury and were done by or omitted by the defendants *were in fact below the then-existing standard of care in the nation for a reasonable and prudent practitioner of anesthesiology.* Occasionally, this can be proved by use of the doctrine of *rēs ipsā loquitur,* which means 'the thing speaks for itself'. There may be the patient who returns in pain 4 months after gallbladder surgery at XYZ Memorial Hospital and during reexploration of the abdomen has had a large lap sponge removed from her abdomen. There, in bold though somewhat faded black letters on the sponge, are the words "property of XYZ Memorial Hospital." To prove that this is below standard of care probably would not require the services of an expert witness because indeed the thing does speak for itself. In most medical malpractice cases, although the doctrine of *res ipsa loquitur* is often employed in one way or another in the initial set of accusations against defendants, it alone seldom suffices to prove that the standard of care was violated. Almost always, one or more qualified expert witnesses for plaintiff are required to testify that certain activities of defendant physicians and other caregivers were below the then-existing national standard of care. The defendant's expert witnesses then must say that the acts or omissions of the defendants were *not* below standard of care, and the jury must decide. This is, of course, the area to which most pretrial attention will be paid and on which the jury's attention should be riveted during the trial. This is the point at which many physicians and medical societies take great issue with some physicians who earn substantial parts of their incomes testifying. Some of these physicians are quick to find fault and quick to state that an act or omission was below the standard of care. This is one reason why societies, such as the American Society of Anesthesiologists, have established their own published standards of care.

1. Establishment of duty and informed consent. With respect to establishment of "duty," the issue of *informed consent* often arises. Sometimes there is sworn testimony by the defendant that verbal consent was given even though the written consent was not specific. For example, the anesthetist testifies that the patient did indeed agree to have a spinal anesthetic even though nothing is written in the chart that so indicates. If so, the credibility of the defendant's testimony will be an issue before the jury. This is one of the many reasons why credible defendant testimony is so crucial. The expert witness can help materially by testifying just how far a "reasonable and prudent" physician should have gone in informing this particular patient about this particular anesthetic. For example, if it was testified by defendant physician that the patient appeared extremely anxious and agitated and defendant physician made a medical judgment that it would unduly disturb the patient to inform her that allergic reaction resulting in death was in fact a possible adverse outcome, the expert witness may be able to gain credibility with the jury by stating that he or she would have done the same thing, if indeed such is true.

2. Establishment of responsibility. If the nurse anesthetist who was supervised by the anesthesiologist did the "act" and the anesthesiologist was not present in the operating room at the time, both persons are likely to be held responsible. But what if the nurse anesthetist was actually employed by the hospital? Under the doctrine of the *borrowed servant*, the hospital will try to be excused from liability by contending that the nurse anesthetist, even though he or she was employed by the hospital, was actually working for the physician anesthesiologist as a "borrowed servant." This same doctrine may be used to try to extricate the hospital from blame for activities by nursing personnel (though it often fails). Perhaps it was the practice to allow the anesthesiologist to take call at home with a nurse anesthetist in the hospital. Does this absolve the anesthesiologist from responsibility? You know the answer. On the other hand, what about the nurse in the recovery room who forgot to give glucose to cover the insulin that was ordered postoperatively even though both the glucose and insulin were ordered in writing? Here, the nurse was acting as a professional nurse, that is, following specific written orders of the physician, but was acting as a professional nurse in the employ of the hospital. In this instance, it is unlikely that the hospital would be absolved because the orders were properly written, the nurse simply failed to obey them, and he or she was *not* the "borrowed servant" of the physician.

3. Establishment of causation of injury by the act. Here, the course of critical events is often crucial. Unfortunately, all too often, the course is poorly documented. There may be two or three different notations about the cardiac arrest, for example, with different time scales on each. Worse, in the middle of the cardiac arrest, there may be a time "gap" where it looks as if nothing was done for 3 or 4 minutes. Another possibility is that blood gases will be noted as having been drawn at a certain time and not having returned until a time much later even though this was not in fact what happened. Record keeping during critical events should be done by *one designated individual*. It is best, in an operating room, to use the wall clock.

It is also difficult sometimes to establish causation of injury if the injury does not become manifest until many days or weeks after the act. For example, the patient who had a surgical operation and then, 3 weeks later, was observed to have developed bilateral ulnar nerve palsy. Is this too long a time after the operation to continue to blame same? What if another patient's blood pressure was "below 40" for a time during the bypass operation but the patient's subsequent brain injury was "focal," not "watershed?" There was considerable aortic valve calcification, and the operation *was* an aortic valve replacement. Which *act* caused the injury? These are the kinds of questions that arise when one is trying to establish that a particular act caused the injury.

4. Establishment of standard of care with respect to the act. What should guide medical experts in decisions as to what was or was not below "standard of care"? It has long been established that *national* anesthesia standards must be used, not local ones. When a defendant testified that it was the "standard of care" in his small town to always use succinylcholine for neuromuscular blockade, this did not suffice as you can imagine. Unfortunately, these cases often do come down to the plaintiff's experts testifying that that care was below standard and the defendant's experts saying it was not. The unfortunate juror is left trying to decide between the credibility of these two expert witnesses. Both came to the courtroom dressed in a conservative suit and tie, and most likely both were well spoken. Both went to medical school. Both had credentials, often certification by the American Board of Anesthesiology. Usually one expert has "more" credentials at least as determined by absolute weight of the curriculum vitae than the other one has. This is why the expert witness for the defendant must have prepared a credible scenario alternative to that presented by the plaintiff that is explained by the facts and is detailed by that expert, possibly with graphics or drawings, for the jury. If either expert can "teach" the jury to understand the pathophysiology and reasoning behind the scenario he or she advocates, that side can carry the day.

F. What are the problems with our current medicolegal system regarding malpractice?

First, these cases may drag on for years. During this time, memories blur and change. Massive expenses are incurred. These cases can consume inordinate amounts of time and energy for everyone involved. Beneath all this there may be an injured patient who needs care. The case is about that injured patient, yet a decision may require years. It *would* be malpractice for physicians to procrastinate or deliberately delay a medical decision! If the patient suffered in the beginning, it is fair to say that often the patient continues to suffer because of the time it takes to get the case adjudicated or settled.

The plaintiff's attorneys usually receive one fourth to one third of any judgment or settlement, that is, the "contingency fee," plus expenses, from the total settlement or judgment. Whether this is bad or good can be debated. It does provide a mechanism whereby patients and families of modest means can obtain redress. In many cases, there are still lump-sum payments to the plaintiff. These payments, after collection of the attorney's contingency fees, go to the patient's families if continuing care is required. Unfortunately, there is not necessarily a mechanism in some cases to assure that the funds directed are actually spent on the patient's care. If the payment is squandered, the

patient may become a ward of the state anyway. This is the subject of many "tort-reform" activities. "Structured settlements" make more sense because they allow for needed care of the injured victim as time goes by. Also, if the estimate of the life span of the injured victim was inaccurate and the total judgment or settlement was therefore excessively high, money held in escrow for the patient's care can be returned to the insurance pool.

With respect to payments to families for "loss of consortium" or "pain and suffering," or both types, several state legislatures have seen fit to put caps on these payments, contending that to do otherwise would unnecessarily further escalate costs. Many plaintiff's attorneys do not see matters quite in that manner. Whether money should be paid for pain, mental anguish, loss of companionship, loss of consortium, and the like is essentially a societal issue.

A most perplexing problem is that of expert witnesses who are not qualified to testify or are no longer in the active practice of the specialty of medicine in which they claim to be experts. Retired physicians are unlikely to be current in their clinical expertise and should not, in most cases, be permitted to testify as expert witnesses. Physicians who earn large percentages of their incomes from testifying are also inherently unlikely to be able to spend a significant amount of time in maintaining clinical expertise. Currently, the system whereby the testimony of these persons in prior similar cases in other jurisdictions is obtained for comparison (or evidence) seems haphazard and inconsistent. Overhaul would require a system of abstracting testimony much like the National Library of Medicine, with extensive computerized cross-referencing, allowing "Medline" type of searches to be performed in each case.

This sets the stage then for what is called *tort reform*. It involves efforts to obtain laws requiring structured settlements, caps on pain and suffering, and demands for valid qualifications of expert witnesses and may also involve various revisions of the contingency-fee mechanism. Other attempts have included pretrial "informal" panels that are supposed to render opinions and discourage further pursuance of unjustified lawsuits. These panels of course simply become minitrials, subjecting both sides to *two* trials. This "reform" is widely viewed as not working. One of the areas in which urgent tort reform is generally agreed upon is in the area of speeding discovery and trial (which can vary from many years to a few months). We now hear of judges who will simply not tolerate requests for continuances or delays and ways of expediting the discovery process may well be the most important tort reform of all. In many jurisdictions progress has been made in requiring that expert witnesses not be retired and have some minimal qualifications before permitting them to testify.[5]

IV. SUMMARY

Anyone can sue anyone for anything, though countersuits and motions to dismiss are always possible. When a physician gets sued, he or she must not panic or become defensive and must especially not allow any recriminations that may occur to affect care of present or future patients. Initial attorney-defendant conferences are critically important. All aspects of the case must be examined carefully, especially the weaknesses. Relationships between the defendant and the defendant's experts must be carefully considered by the attorneys involved. The defendant's experts must construct a scenario about which they can testify with a "reasonable degree of medical certainty." That scenario must be a contrasting alternative that, if possible, does not blame other defendants. It must be supported by the facts of the case as revealed both by the medical record and the sworn testimony. Testimony, both during discovery and trial, must stick to the facts. Oral practice for questions that will be surely asked seems logical. Meticulous preparation for trial including graphics, oral preparation, review of pertinent medical literature and careful consideration of all potential problem areas will allow the case to be presented in the fairest possible fashion. If it becomes obvious during discovery that the case should be settled without trial, every effort should be bent toward doing this in a way that will help the injured patient as fast and as much as possible. Throughout the whole process, though many physicians have become quite cynical, it must be remembered that underneath the inevitable mountain of paper, the oscillation of emotions, the sometimes misleading testimony, and numerous other problems there is a patient. That patient or family *still deserves our attention and care even if they have brought suit against us.* Remembering this is often difficult if the plaintiff's expert witnesses level damaging accusations at the defendants. If we can continue to try to be the good doctors we were trained to be throughout the entire discovery and trial process, despite the latter's inherent negativity, accusations, and innuendos, we can continue competent and compassionate care of our current and future patients.[6]

REFERENCES

These references have been annotated because the medical reader will not likely be familiar with legal texts or citation methodology. They are included for those who wish to pursue these issues from the legal perspective. Notice also that the anecdotes used in this chapter are specifically not referenced. Some did not even become legal cases. All are cases either from the experience of or told to us.

1. Fifty-Six American Law Reports, 2nd series 696, Rochester, NY, 1956, Lawyers Cooperative Pub Co.
   See also updates published yearly entitled "Later Case Service" in this series. These are cases involving allegations of battery.
2. Southwick AF: The law of hospital and health care administration, ed 2, New York, 1988, Health Administration Press, Chapter 3.
3. Pegalis SE and Wachsman HF: American law of medical malpractice, Rochester NY, 1981, Lawyers Cooperative Publishing Co, Chapter 8.
   This contains several cases illustrating the contrasting theories articulated by plaintiff and defendant in anesthesia malpractice cases.
4. Southwick AF, *op cit,* Chapter 10. See also the following cases: *Cobbs* v. *Grant,* 8 Cal. 3rd 229, 104 Cal. Rptr. 505, 502 P. 2nd 1 (1972) and *Canterbury* v. *Spence,* 464 F. 2d 772 (D.C. App. 1972).
   The chapter cited contains a thorough discussion of the doctrine of informed consent. The cases cited are the leading underpinnings of the modern legal theory of informed consent.
5. Havighurst CC: Health care law and policy, New York, 1988, The Foundation Press, Chapter 7.
   This is a recent discussion of various tort-reform initiatives and their fates when analyzed under constitutional or common law scrutiny.
6. Annas GJ, Law SA, Rosenblatt RE, and Wing KR: American health law, Boston, 1990, Little Brown & Co, Chapter 5.
   This is a provocative discussion of the medical malpractice system as a form of quality assurance.

Index